WOMEN'S PRIMARY HEALTH CARE

NOTICE

WOMEN'S PRIMARY HEALTH CARE

Office Practice and Procedures

Editors

VICKI L. SELTZER, M.D.

Chairman, Department of Obstetrics and Gynecology
Long Island Jewish Medical Center
Professor, Gynecology and Obstetrics
Albert Einstein College of Medicine
New Hyde Park, New York

WARREN H. PEARSE, M.D.

The Jacobs Institute for Women's Health
Washington, D.C.

McGraw-Hill, Inc.
Health Professions Division
New York St. Louis San Francisco
Auckland Bogotá Caracas Lisbon London
Madrid Mexico City Milan Montreal New Delhi
San Juan Singapore Sydney Tokyo Toronto

WOMEN'S PRIMARY HEALTH CARE
Office Practice and Procedures

2 3 4 5 6 7 8 9 0 DOCDOC 9 8 7 6 5

ISBN 0-07-056225-3

This book was set in Times Roman by York Graphic Services, Inc.
The editors were Gail Gavert and Steven Melvin;
the production supervisor was Clare Stanley; the cover designer was Karen K. Quigley.
R.R. Donnelley and Sons was printer and binder.
This book is printed on acid-free paper.

Library of Congress Cataloging-in-Publication Data

Women's primary health care / editors, Vicki Seltzer and Warren H. Pearse.
p. cm.
Includes bibliographical references.
ISBN 0-07-056225-3 (alk. paper)
1. Women's health services. 2. Women—Health and hygiene. 3. Women—Diseases. I. Seltzer, Vicki L. II. Pearse, Warren H. [DNLM: 1. Women's Health. 2. Primary Health Care. 3. Genital Diseases, Female. WA 300 W872976 1995]
RA564.85.W687 1995
613′.04244—dc20
DNLM/DLC
for Library of Congress 94-30309

To my wonderful family: Marian and Herbert Seltzer and Richard, Jessica, and Eric Brach

To my father, Harry A. Pearse, M.D.: Obstetrician, poet, and religious historian

Contents

Part IV
Office Gynecologic Procedures 299

Part V
Psychiatric and Psychosocial Issues and Societal Violence 335

Part VI
General Health 381

Contributors

Eric S. Applebaum, M.D.
Fellow, Division of Allergy and Immunology
Departments of Pediatrics and Medicine
Schneider Children's Hospital
Long Island Jewish Medical Center
New Hyde Park, New York [54]

Angeles Badell, M.D.
Chief, Division of Rehabilitation Medicine
Long Island Jewish Medical Center
Professor
Albert Einstein College of Medicine
New Hyde Park, New York [62]

Patricia Bailey, M.D.
Department of Obstetrics and Gynecology
Baystate Medical Center
Springfield, Massachusetts [21]

G. William Bates, M.D.
Department of Obstetrics and Gynecology
Greenville Hospital System
Greenville, South Carolina [2, 17]

Elise Belilos, M.D.
Attending Rheumatologist, Division of Rheumatology, Immunology, and Allergy
Winthrop-University Hospital
Instructor of Medicine
State University of New York
Health Science Center at Stony Brook
Mineola, New York [53]

Fred Benjamin, M.D.
Associate Director, Department of Obstetrics and Gynecology
Queens Hospital Center
Professor of Obstetrics and Gynecology
Albert Einstein College of Medicine
Jamaica, New York [16, 47]

Numbers in brackets refer to chapters written or cowritten by the contributors.

Henny Billett, M.D.
Chief, Division of Hematology
Department of Pathology
Long Island Jewish Medical Center
Associate Professor of Laboratory Medicine
Albert Einstein College of Medicine
New Hyde Park, New York [51]

W. Kenneth Blaylock, M.D.
Chief of the Dermatology Service
McGuire Veterans Administration Medical Center
Richmond, Virginia [56]

Keith L. Blauer, M.D.
Department of Obstetrics and Gynecology
Greenville Hospital System
Greenville, South Carolina [2]

Vincent R. Bonagura, M.D.
Chief, Division of Allergy and Immunology
Departments of Pediatrics and Medicine
Schneider Children's Hospital
Long Island Jewish Medical Center
Professor of Pediatrics, Microbiology and Immunology
Albert Einstein College of Medicine
New Hyde Park, New York [54]

Joanna M. Cain, M.D.
Professor, Department of Obstetrics and Gynecology
University of Washington Medical Center
Seattle, Washington [10, 23]

Steven Carsons, M.D.
Chief, Division of Rheumatology, Immunology and Allergy
Winthrop-University Hospital
Associate Professor of Medicine
State University of New York
Health Science Center at Stony Brook
Mineola, New York [53]

Robert C. Cefalo, M.D., Ph.D.
Professor and Director, Maternal and Fetal Medicine
University of North Carolina School of Medicine
Chapel Hill, North Carolina [4]

David Chelmow, M.D.
Assistant Professor, Department of Obstetrics and Gynecology
Tufts University School of Medicine
Boston, Massachusetts [27, 28]

Frank A. Chervenak, M.D.
Director of Obstetrics and Division of Maternal Fetal Medicine
Department of Obstetrics and Gynecology
The New York Hospital–Cornell Medical Center
Professor of Obstetrics and Gynecology
Cornell Medical School
New York, New York [69]

PonJola Coney, M.D.
Associate Professor and Director, Reproductive Endocrinology and Infertility
Department of Obstetrics and Gynecology
Arizona Health Sciences Center
Tucson, Arizona [4]

Ashley Coopland, M.D., M.P.H.
Department of Obstetrics and Gynecology
Baystate Medical Center
Springfield, Massachusetts [21]

Jeffrey L. Cornella, M.D.
Assistant Professor, Obstetrics and Gynecology
Mayo Graduate School of Medicine
Mayo Clinic Scottsdale
Scottsdale, Arizona [32, 38]

Susan M. Cox, M.D.
Associate Professor, Department of Obstetrics and Gynecology
The University of Texas Southwestern Medical Center
Dallas, Texas [19]

Stephen L. Curry, M.D.
Director, Department of Obstetrics and Gynecology
Hartford Hospital
Professor of Obstetrics and Gynecology
University of Connecticut School of Medicine
Hartford, Connecticut [26]

David R. Dantzker, M.D.
President, Long Island Jewish Medical Center
Professor, Department of Internal Medicine
Albert Einstein College of Medicine
New Hyde Park, New York [43]

Alan DeCherney, M.D.
Louis E. Phaneuf Professor and Chairman
Department of Obstetrics and Gynecology
Tufts University School of Medicine
Boston, Massachusetts [27, 28]

Bruce H. Drukker, M.D.
Chairman, Department of Obstetrics and Gynecology
Michigan State University
East Lansing, Michigan [42]

Leo J. Dunn, M.D.
Professor and Chairman, Obstetrics and Gynecology
Medical College of Virginia
Virginia Commonwealth University
Richmond, Virginia [5]

Roselyn Payne Epps, M.D., M.P.H.
Public Health Applications Research Branch
National Cancer Institutes
Bethesda, Maryland [15]

Arthur L. Frank, M.D., Ph.D.
Associate Director for Medical Education
Topperman Professor of Medicine, Department of Medical Education
The University of Texas Health Center at Tyler
Tyler, Texas [64]

Fredric D. Frigoletto, Jr., M.D.
Chief of Vincent Memorial Obstetrics Division
Massachusetts General Hospital
Charles Montraville Green and Robert Montraville Green
Professor of Obstetrics and Gynecology
Harvard Medical School
Boston, Massachusetts [20]

Stanley A. Gall, M.D.
Professor and Chairman, Department of Obstetrics and Gynecology
University of Louisville School of Medicine
Louisville, Kentucky [11]

Albert B. Gerbie, M.D.
Professor, Obstetrics and Gynecology
Northwestern University Medical School
Northwestern Memorial Hospital
Chicago, Illinois [7]

Thomas Glynn, Ph.D.
Acting Associate Director of Cancer Control Science Program
Division of Cancer Prevention and Control
National Cancer Institute
Bethesda, Maryland [15]

Steven R. Goldstein, M.D.
Associate Professor of Clinical Obstetrics and Gynecology
New York University School of Medicine
New York, New York [34]

Helen Greco, M.D.
Head, Benign Gynecology
Department of Obstetrics and Gynecology
Long Island Jewish Medical Center
Assistant Professor, Obstetrics and Gynecology
Albert Einstein College of Medicine
New Hyde Park, New York [40]

David B. Hale, M.D., Ph.D.
Department of Emergency Medicine
Bowman Gray School of Medicine
Winston-Salem, North Carolina [12, 61]

Ralph W. Hale, M.D.
Executive Director
The American College of Obstetricians and Gynecologists
Washington, D.C. [12, 61]

Joseph A. Hill, M.D.
Associate Professor
Obstetrics, Gynecology, and Reproductive Biology
Harvard Medical School
Department of Obstetrics and Gynecology
Brigham and Women's Hospital
Boston, Massachusetts [20]

Eileen Hilton, M.D.
Department of Medicine
Division of Infectious Disease
Long Island Jewish Medical Center
Associate Professor of Medicine
Albert Einstein College of Medicine
New Hyde Park, New York [50]

Judith Hsia, M.D.
Associate Professor of Medicine
The George Washington University
Washington, D.C. [41]

J. Stephen Hudgins, M.D.
Christiansburg, Virginia [58]

Edward H. Illions, M.D.
Assistant Professor, Obstetrics and Gynecology
University of Florida
Health Science Center Jacksonville
Jacksonville, Florida [29, 37]

Donna D. Johnson, M.D.
Assistant Professor, Division of Perinatal Medicine
University of California San Diego–School of Medicine
San Diego, California [18]

Ronald Kanner, M.D.
Chairman, Department of Neurology
Long Island Jewish Medical Center
Professor of Neurology
Albert Einstein College of Medicine
New Hyde Park, New York [52, 63]

Bruce G. Kay, M.S., R.Ph.
Director, Pharmacy Services
Long Island Jewish Medical Center
Associate Professor, Clinical Pharmacy Practice
St. Johns College of Pharmacy
New Hyde Park, New York [66]

Abbas E. Kitabchi, Ph.D., M.D.
Director, Division of Endocrinology and Metabolism
Department of Medicine
Professor of Medicine and Biochemistry
The University of Tennessee, Memphis
Memphis, Tennessee [48]

Thomas Kwiatkowski, M.D.
Chairman, Department of Emergency Medicine
Long Island Jewish Medical Center
Assistant Professor, Epidemiology and Social Medicine
Albert Einstein College of Medicine
New Hyde Park, New York [65]

Geraldine Lanman, M.D.
Assistant Clinical Professor of Medicine
Albert Einstein College of Medicine
Lake Success, New York [13]

John W. Larsen, M.D.
Acting Chairman, Department of Obstetrics and Gynecology
Professor, Obstetrics and Gynecology
The George Washington University School of Medicine
Washington, D.C. [8]

Anne Y.F. Lin, Pharm. D.
Director, Drug Information Service
Department of Pharmacy
Long Island Jewish Medical Center
Associate Clinical Professor
St. Johns University College of Pharmacy
New Hyde Park, New York [66]

Frederick Neil Lukash, M.D.
Assistant Clinical Professor of Surgery
Albert Einstein College of Medicine
Manhasset, New York [60]

Marc Manley, M.D., M.P.H.
Chief, Public Health Applications Research Branch
National Cancer Institute
Bethesda, Maryland [15]

John H. Mattox, M.D.
Chairman, Department of Obstetrics and Gynecology
Good Samaritan Regional Medical Center
Professor Clinical Obstetrics and Gynecology
University of Arizona
Phoenix, Arizona [22]

Laurence B. McCullough, Ph.D.
Professor of Medicine, Community Medicine, and Medical Ethics
Center for Ethics, Medicine and Public Issues
Baylor College of Medicine
Houston, Texas [69]

Howard Minkoff, M.D.
Professor, Obstetrics and Gynecology
State University of New York Health Science Center at Brooklyn
Brooklyn, New York [49]

Rodrigue Mortel, M.D.
Professor and Chairman, Department of Obstetrics and Gynecology
The Milton S. Hershey Medical Center
Pennsylvania State University
Hershey, Pennsylvania [46]

Susan M. Mou, M.D.
Associate Professor, Department of Obstetrics and Gynecology
University of Missouri at Kansas City School of Medicine
Truman Medical Center
Kansas City, Missouri [25]

Alan S. Multz, M.D.
Director, Medical Intensive Care
Department of Medicine
Long Island Jewish Medical Center
Assistant Professor of Medicine
Albert Einstein College of Medicine
New Hyde Park, New York [43]

Peter A. Mychajliw, D.D.S.
Chief, General Dentistry
Department of Dental Medicine
Long Island Jewish Medical Center
Assistant Professor, Restorative Dentistry
State University of New York at Stony Brook
New Hyde Park, New York [59]

David Myssiorek, M.D.
Section Head, Head and Neck Surgery
Department of Otolaryngology
Long Island Jewish Medical Center
Assistant Professor of Otolaryngology
Albert Einstein College of Medicine
New Hyde Park, New York [57]

Anne B. Namnoum, M.D.
Department of Gynecology and Obstetrics
Division of Reproductive Endocrinology
Johns Hopkins Hospital
Assistant Professor
Johns Hopkins School of Medicine
Baltimore, Maryland [9]

Warren H. Pearse, M.D.
The Jacobs Institute for Women's Health
Washington, D.C.

Richard C. Pees, M.D.
Assistant Professor, Obstetrics and Gynecology
The Milton S. Hershey Medical Center
Pennsylvania State University
Hershey, Pennsylvania [46]

Roy M. Pitkin, M.D.
Professor and Chairman, Department of Obstetrics and Gynecology
University of California Los Angeles–School of Medicine
Los Angeles, California [55]

Thomas M. Price, M.D.
Department of Obstetrics and Gynecology
Greenville Hospital System
Greenville, South Carolina [17]

Kanti R. Rai, M.D.
Chief, Hematology and Oncology
Department of Medicine
Long Island Jewish Medical Center
Professor of Medicine
Albert Einstein College of Medicine
New Hyde Park, New York [51]

William Rennie, M.D.
Department of Emergency Medicine
Long Island Jewish Medical Center
New Hyde Park, New York [65]

Robert Resnik, M.D.
Professor and Chairman, Department of Reproductive Medicine
University of California San Diego–School of Medicine
San Diego, California [18]

John E. Rooney, M.D., Ph.D.
Fellow, Division of Allergy and Immunology
Departments of Pediatrics and Medicine
Schneider Children's Hospital
Long Island Jewish Medical Center
New Hyde Park, New York [54]

Allan Rosenfield, M.D.
Joseph R. DeLamar Professor of Public Health
Professor of Obstetrics and Gynecology
Dean, Columbia School of Public Health
Columbia Presbyterian Medical Center
New York, New York [3]

Leonard J. Rossoff, M.D.
Division of Pulmonary Medicine
Long Island Jewish Medical Center
Assistant Professor of Medicine
Albert Einstein College of Medicine
New Hyde Park, New York [50]

Nanette K. Rumsey, M.D.
Clinical Instructor of Obstetrics and Gynecology
Northwestern University Medical School
Northwestern Memorial Hospital
Chicago, Illinois [7]

Kenneth J. Ryan, M.D.
Department of Gynecology and Reproductive Biology
Brigham and Women's Hospital
Kate Macy Ladd Distinguished Professor of Obstetrics
Harvard Medical School
Boston, Massachusetts [68]

James J. Sciubba, D.M.D., Ph.D.
Chairman, Department of Dental Medicine
Long Island Jewish Medical Center
Professor, Oral Pathology and Biology
State University of New York at Stony Brook
New Hyde Park, New York [59]

Vicki L. Seltzer, M.D.
Chairman, Department of Obstetrics and Gynecology
Long Island Jewish Medical Center
Professor, Gynecology and Obstetrics
Albert Einstein College of Medicine
New Hyde Park, New York [1, 6, 14]

Mark Spitzer, M.D.
Director of Obstetrics and Gynecology
Queens Hospital Center
Associate Professor of Obstetrics and Gynecology
Mount Sinai School of Medicine
Jamaica, New York [24, 35, 36]

John F. Steege, M.D.
Chief, Division of Gynecology
Professor, Department of Obstetrics and Gynecology
University of North Carolina at Chapel Hill
Chapel Hill, North Carolina [30]

Nada L. Stotland, M.D.
Associate Professor, Departments of Psychiatry and Obstetrics and Gynecology
The University of Chicago Hospitals
Chicago, Illinois [39]

Kris Strohbehn, M.D.
Department of Obstetrics and Gynecology
New England Medical Center
Assistant Professor
Tufts University School of Medicine
Boston, Massachusetts [27, 28]

Albert L. Strunk, M.D.
Women's Health Care Specialists, P.A.
Plainfield, New Jersey [67]

Candice A. Tedeschi, O.G.N.P.
Coordinator of DES Screening Center
Long Island Jewish Medical Center
New Hyde Park, New York [24]

Henry A. Thiede, M.D.
Professor and Chairman, Department of Obstetrics and Gynecology
University of Rochester Medical School
Rochester, New York [32, 38]

Robert J. Thompson, M.D.
Professor and Associate Chairman, Department of Obstetrics and Gynecology
University of Florida
Health Science Center Jacksonville
Jacksonville, Florida [29, 37]

Melody Toth, M.S., ATC
Assistant Professor
Senior Women's Trainer
University of Hawaii School of Medicine
Honolulu, Hawaii [61]

R. Edward Varner, M.D.
Associate Professor, Obstetrics and Gynecology
Division Director, Medical and Surgical Gynecology
University of Alabama at Birmingham
Birmingham, Alabama [31]

John D. Wagner, M.D.
Head, Section of Dialysis, Division of Nephrology
Department of Medicine
Long Island Jewish Medical Center
Assistant Professor
Albert Einstein College of Medicine
New Hyde Park, New York [44]

Sandra Welner, M.D.
Department of Obstetrics and Gynecology
Clinical Director of Primary Care
Program for Women with Special Needs
Washington Hospital Center and National Rehabilitation Hospital
Washington, D.C. [62]

Claudia L. Werner, M.D.
Assistant Professor, Department of Obstetrics and Gynecology
The University of Texas Southwestern Medical Center
Dallas, Texas [19]

Renée L. Young, M.D.
Assistant Professor of Medicine
University of Nebraska Medical Center
Department of Internal Medicine
Section of Gastroenterology and Hepatology
Omaha Veteran's Administration Medical Center
Omaha, Nebraska [45]

James P. Youngblood, M.D.
Professor and Chairman, Department of Obstetrics and Gynecology
University of Missouri–Kansas City School of Medicine
Truman Medical Center
Kansas City, Missouri [33]

J. Benjamin Younger, M.D.
Professor and Vice Chairman, Department of Obstetrics and Gynecology
University of Alabama–Birmingham School of Medicine
Birmingham, Alabama [31]

Gerald D. Zahtz, M.D.
Department of Otolaryngology
Long Island Jewish Medical Center
Assistant Professor of Otolaryngology
Albert Einstein College of Medicine
New Hyde Park, New York [57]

Preface

Early in the evolution of the medical profession, the scientific base was so small that a doctor could easily provide the complete range of medical and surgical services to the entire family. During the latter part of the twentieth century, the rapid proliferation of scientific knowledge and technology caused many physicians to narrow their focus and subspecialize. Subspecialization has resulted in the exceptional advances in the quality of care and in the sophisticated and successful therapies that we can offer patients for problems ranging from infertility to coronary artery occlusion.

On the other hand, because of the explosion in knowledge and technology, too many physicians have lost sight of the comprehensive needs of the individual woman by concentrating only on a particular disease process. Clearly, an essential component of medical care is our ability to offer our patients the highest quality care for complex medical problems; however, we will ultimately not be as effective if we are unable to address the overall health needs of women.

Our first goal is to help our patients stay healthy by educating and counseling them about general health strategies and behaviors which promote wellness. Second, we should involve them in programs of early detection. In this way, problems (whether physical, psychiatric, or psychosocial) can be identified at an early stage, when intervention and treatment are most likely to result in cure or optimally address the problem. While it is essential that physicians be able to treat complex disease, this is less effective if we are not also able to promote wellness.

The focus of this book is on the primary and preventive ambulatory health care needs of women. It stresses the role of physicians as educators and promoters of women's wellness. It is as important for the subspecialist as it is for the generalist, since a woman with a narrowly focused problem will often see only one specialist physician over a period of time. Conversely, some women will see many physicians—each for a particular problem that the subspecialist is ideally qualified and most capable of treating—but these women may have no one who is overseeing their total health care needs. Therefore, whether we consider ourselves "generalists" or "subspecialists," we must understand the general health care needs of women and work with them to address their primary and preventive health care needs.

It is clear that no one physician can be all things to all people. For most disease processes, there will come a point at which a given physician believes that the specific problem will be best handled by someone with special expertise. The depth of information in this text extends only to that which would be expected to be handled in a general ambulatory situation.

However, our main emphasis is on the fact that women receive the best health care when their physicians, be they generalist or subspecialist, have a well-rounded approach to health care and understand women's general health care needs.

Part I

Varying Health Care Needs during the Phases of a Woman's Life

The general health care needs of a woman vary during the phases of her life. This section of the book identifies the breadth of important physical and psychosocial issues that physicians can help women to address during their transition through the life phases. The first chapter reviews the most common causes of morbidity and mortality in women of different age groups, as well as age appropriate strategies for screening, laboratory tests, evaluation and counseling, and immunizations. This is followed by chapters that focus on the special needs of the adolescent, the reproductive age woman, the menopausal woman, and the woman who is beyond the menopausal years.

This section of the book is brief, since each of the medical issues identified is reviewed in greater depth elsewhere in the text. It serves to emphasize the broad scope of health care needs that we can and should address with our patients with regard to preventive health and psychosocial issues as well as the most common medical problems in particular age groups of women. By focusing attention on women's general well-being and appropriate preventive interventions at various stages of life, the physician can have the greatest overall impact upon women's health.

1 Screening and Preventive Health Care during the Various Stages of a Woman's Life

Vicki L. Seltzer

One of the main roles of the physician is to help women stay healthy. If disease does occur, it must be diagnosed as early as possible to afford the greatest likelihood of cure or long-term control of the problem, thereby reducing the risk of substantial secondary morbidity. Screening and prevention strategies most important for any given woman will depend on her individual risk factors (genetic, environmental, and behavioral). They will also change as the woman ages and evolves through the phases of her life. This chapter covers a series of preventive and screening strategies that can be used in practice to optimize patients' well-being. The recommendations are based on the report of the American College of Obstetricians and Gynecologists (ACOG) Task Force on Primary and Preventive Health Care.

In the past, emphasis was almost exclusively on the treatment of disease rather than on prevention. However, it has become apparent that physicians can make an enormous impact on their patients' health through preventive strategies. For instance, it is estimated that one-half of premature deaths and one-third of acute disabilities can be prevented by reducing behavioral risk factors and by preventive health care.

While essentially all medical organizations agree that screening and prevention result in a substantial reduction in morbidity and mortality, for many different medical problems debate continues regarding ideal frequency of screening, which studies should be employed, when they should be started, and who should be screened. The recommendations in this chapter follow closely those of the ACOG Task Force on Primary and Preventive Health Care. They attempt to focus on sensible, cost-effective screening and preventive strategies that can be targeted to what is most appropriate to the individual patient's needs. Clearly, our scientific knowledge, screening modalities, available therapies, and preventive capabilities continue to evolve rapidly. As this occurs, recommendations for preventive and screening interventions also will change.

Other organizations have suggested screening strategies that also can be utilized. They may vary somewhat from those of ACOG, which are presented with minor modification in Tables 1-1 to 1-8. Such variations occur because insufficient data are available regarding the benefits of certain interventions as well as the ideal frequency. While it is reasonable to use any one of a variety of strategies, physicians should have some general program for screening and preventive care which they employ regularly in their practices.

Tables 1-1 to 1-8 are intended for periodic screening. It is assumed that the patient is "ongoing" and that the initial history, physical examination, risk assessment, diagnostic testing, and counseling have been done at some time in the past. The tables are also based on the assumption that the woman has no underlying medical problems; if she does, further interventions may be required, and the frequency of certain testing might need to be increased.

TABLE 1-1 Leading Causes of Mortality and Morbidity Ages 13 to 18

Mortality

Motor vehicle accidents
Homicide
Suicide
Leukemia

Morbidity

Nose, throat, and upper respiratory conditions
Viral, bacterial, and parasitic infections
Sexual abuse
Injuries (musculoskeletal and soft tissue)
Acute ear infections
Digestive system conditions
Acute urinary conditions

SOURCE: Adapted with permission from: The Obstetrician-Gynecologist and Primary-Preventive Health Care.

TABLE 1-2 Periodic Health Assessment and Preventive Care Ages 13 to 18

I. Screening
  A. Review problem list and continuity-of-care records
  B. Obtain responses to patient questionnaire
  C. Periodic history: reason for visit; interval medical, surgical, and family history; dietary/nutritional assessment; exercise; tobacco, alcohol, other drugs; abuse/neglect; sexual practices
  D. Periodic physical: height, weight, bp, Tanner staging of secondary sexual characteristics, pelvic examination (yearly when sexually active or by age 18), skin (in individuals with increased sun exposure, family or personal history of skin cancer, or clinical evidence of precursor lesions)
  E. Laboratory tests
    1. Pap test—yearly when sexually active or by age 18
    2. Hemoglobin—testing for women of Caribbean, Latin American, Asian, Mediterranean, or African descent or with a history of excessive menstrual flow
    3. Bacteriuria testing—periodic testing for women with diabetes mellitus
    4. Sexually transmitted disease testing—for women with a history of multiple sexual partners or with a sexual partner with multiple contacts; women who have a partner with an STD; women with a repeated history of STDs; women who attend STD clinics
    5. HIV testing—for women being tested for STDs including all the reasons listed above; for women treated for STDs; past or present history of drug use by injection; current or past history of prostitution; women whose past or present sexual partners are HIV-positive or bisexual or who inject drugs; women born or with long-term residence in an area with a high prevalence of HIV infection; women transfused between 1978 and 1985
    6. Genetic testing/counseling—for women exposed to teratogens; for women contemplating pregnancy who have a partner or family member or who themselves have a history of a genetic disorder or birth defect; for women contemplating pregnancy who are of African-American, Eastern European Jewish, Mediterranean, or Southeast Asian ancestry
    7. Rubella titer—women lacking evidence of immunity; a second measles immunization, preferably as MMR (measles, mumps, rubella) for all women unable to show proof of immunity
    8. Lipid profile—periodic screening for women with an elevated cholesterol level, a history

TABLE 1-2 (Continued)

of a parent or a sibling with a blood cholesterol level of 240 mg/dl or higher; a history of a sibling, parent, or grandparent with documented premature (aged less than 55 years) coronary artery disease; presence of diabetes; smoker

9. Tuberculosis skin test—for women infected with HIV; for close contacts (sharing the same household or other enclosed environments) of persons known or suspected to have Tb; persons with medical risk factors known to increase the risk of disease if infection has occurred; foreign-born persons from countries with high Tb prevalence; medically underserved; low-income populations; alcoholics and IV drug users; residents of long-term care facilities, correctional institutions, mental institutions, nursing homes and facilities, and other long-term residential facilities; health professionals working in high-risk health care facilities

II. Evaluation and Counseling
  A. Sexuality
    1. Development
    2. High-risk behaviors
    3. Contraceptive options
    4. Sexually transmitted diseases
  B. Fitness
    1. Hygiene (including dental)
    2. Dietary/nutritional assessment
    3. Exercise: discussion of program
  C. Psychosocial evaluation: interpersonal/family relationships, sexual identity, personal goal development, behavioral/learning disorders, abuse/neglect
  D. Cardiovascular risk factors: family history, hypertension, hyperlipidemia, obesity/diabetes mellitus
  E. Health/risk behaviors
    1. Injury prevention—safety belts and helmets, recreational hazards, firearms, hearing
    2. Skin exposure to ultraviolet rays
    3. Suicide: depressive symptoms
    4. Tobacco, alcohol, other drugs

III. Immunizations and Supplements
  A. Tetanus-diphtheria booster once between ages 14–16

TABLE 1-2 (Continued)

  B. Measles, mumps, rubella (MMR) for all women unable to show proof of immunity
  C. Fluoride supplement: for persons living in areas with inadequate water fluoridation (less than 0.7 parts/million)
  D. Hepatitis B vaccine: IV drug users; current recipients of blood products; persons in health-related jobs with exposure to blood or blood products; household and sexual contacts of hepatitis B virus carriers; prostitutes; persons with a history of sexual activity with multiple partners in the previous six months. Some experts believe that all adolescents should receive the hepatitis B vaccine.

SOURCE: Adapted with permission from: The Obstetrician-Gynecologist and Primary-Preventive Health Care

TABLE 1-3 Leading Causes of Mortality and Morbidity Ages 19 to 39

Mortality

Motor vehicle accidents
Cardiovascular disease
Homicide
Coronary artery disease
AIDS
Breast cancer
Cerebrovascular disease
Uterine (including cervical) cancer

Morbidity

Nose, throat, and upper respiratory conditions
Injuries (musculoskeletal and soft tissue, including back and upper and lower extremities)
Viral, bacterial, and parasitic infections
Acute urinary conditions

SOURCE: Adapted with permission from: The Obstetrician-Gynecologist and Primary-Preventive Health Care

TABLE 1-4 Periodic Health Assessment and Preventive Care Ages 19 to 39

I. Screening
   A. Review problem list and continuity-of-care records
   B. Obtain responses to patient questionnaire
   C. Periodic history (see Table 1-2, Section I C)
   D. Physical examination
   E. Laboratory tests
      1. Pap test—after three consecutive normal annual tests, physician and patient discretion as to whether this must continue to be annual
      2. Lipids—for low-risk women, cholesterol every five years; more frequent complete lipid profile for: women with an elevated cholesterol level, or with a history of a parent or sibling with a blood cholesterol level of 240 mg/dl or higher; or history of a sibling, parent, or grandparent with documented premature (aged less than 55 years) coronary artery disease; presence of diabetes; smoker
      3. Hemoglobin (see Table 1-2, section I E 2)
      4. Bacteriuria testing: periodic testing for women with diabetes mellitus
      5. Mammography: women aged 35 and older with a family history of premenopausally diagnosed breast cancer in a first-degree relative (see chapter on breast cancer)
      6. Fasting glucose test: every 3 to 5 years for persons with a family history of diabetes mellitus (one first- or two second-degree relatives), who are markedly obese, or who have a personal history of gestational diabetes mellitus
      7. Sexually transmitted disease testing: (see Table 1-2, section I E 4)
      8. HIV testing: (see Table 1-2, section I E 5)
      9. Genetic testing/counseling: for women who are exposed to teratogens or who contemplate pregnancy at age 35 or beyond; patient, partner, or family member with a history of a genetic disorder or birth defect; and persons of African-American, Eastern European Jewish, Mediterranean, or Southeast Asian ancestry
      10. Rubella titer: (see Table 1-2, section I E 7)

TABLE 1-4 (Continued)

      11. Tuberculosis skin test: (see Table 1-2, section I E 9)
      12. Thyroid-stimulating hormone: periodic screening of individuals with a strong family history of thyroid disease and patients with autoimmune diseases (there is some evidence that subclinical hypothyroidism may be related to unfavorable lipid profiles)

II. Evaluation and Counseling
   A. Sexuality
      1. High-risk behaviors
      2. Contraceptive options
      3. Sexually transmitted disease
      4. Sexual functioning
   B. Fitness
      1. Hygiene (including dental)
      2. Dietary/nutritional assessment
      3. Exercise: discuss program
   C. Psychosocial evaluation: interpersonal/family relationships, domestic violence, job satisfaction, lifestyle/stress, sleep disorders
   D. Cardiovascular risk factors: family history, hypertension, hyperlipidemia, obesity/diabetes mellitus, lifestyle
   E. Health/risk behaviors
      1. Injury prevention: safety belts and helmets, occupational hazards, recreational hazards, firearms, hearing
      2. Breast self-examination
      3. Skin exposure to ultraviolet rays
      4. Suicide: depressive symptoms
      5. Tobacco, alcohol, other drugs

III. Immunizations
   A. Tetanus-diphtheria booster every 10 years
   B. Measles, mumps, rubella—for all women unable to show proof of immunity
   C. Hepatitis B vaccine (see Table 1-2, section III D)
   D. Influenza vaccine: residents of chronic care facilities; women with chronic cardiopulmonary disorders; women with metabolic diseases, including diabetes mellitus, hemoglobinopathies, immunosuppression, or renal dysfunction
   E. Pneumococcal vaccine: women with medical conditions that increase the risk of pneumococcal

TABLE 1-4 (Continued)

infections (e.g., chronic cardiac or pulmonary disease, sickle cell disease, nephrotic syndrome, Hodgkin's disease, asplenia, diabetes mellitus, alcoholism, cirrhosis, multiple myeloma, renal disease, or other immunosuppression)

SOURCE: Adapted with permission from: The Obstetrician-Gynecologist and Primary-Preventive Health Care

TABLE 1-5 Leading Causes of Mortality and Morbidity Ages 40 to 64

Mortality

Cardiovascular disease
Coronary artery disease
Breast cancer
Lung cancer
Cerebrovascular disease
Colorectal cancer
Obstructive pulmonary disease
Ovarian cancer

Morbidity

Nose, throat, and upper respiratory conditions
Osteoporosis/arthritis
Hypertension
Orthopedic deformities and impairments (including back and upper and lower extremities)
Heart disease
Hearing and vision impairments

SOURCE: Adapted with permission from: The Obstetrician-Gynecologist and Primary-Preventive Health Care

TABLE 1-6 Periodic Health Assessment and Preventive Care Ages 40 to 64

I. Screening
  A. Review problem list and continuity-of-care records
  B. Obtain responses to patient questionnaire
  C. Periodic history (see Table 1-2, section I C)
  D. Physical examination
  E. Laboratory tests

TABLE 1-6 (Continued)

    1. Mammography: every 1–2 years until age 50; yearly beginning at age 50
    2. Bacteriuria testing: periodic testing for women with diabetes mellitus
    3. Fecal occult blood test: yearly (see chapter on cancer screening)
    4. Sigmoidoscopy (see chapter on cancer screening)
    5. Colonoscopy—for women with a personal history of inflammatory bowel disease or colonic polyps or a family history of familial polyposis coli, colorectal cancer, or cancer family syndrome
    6. Hemoglobin: (see Table 1-2, section I E 2)
    7. Sexually transmitted disease testing (see Table 1-2, section I E 4)
    8. Human immunodeficiency virus testing (see Table 1-2, section I E 5)
    9. Tuberculosis skin testing (see Table 1-2, section I E 9)
    10. Pap test: (see Table 1-4, section I E 1)
    11. Lipids (see Table 1-4, section I E 2)
    12. Fasting glucose test (see Table 1-4, section I E 6)
    13. TSH (see Table 1-4, section I E 12)

II. Evaluation and counseling
  A. Sexuality
    1. High-risk behaviors
    2. Contraceptive options
    3. Sexually transmitted disease
    4. Sexual function
  B. Fitness: hygiene (including dental), dietary/nutritional assessment, exercise (discussion of program)
  C. Psychosocial evaluation: family relationships, domestic violence, job/work satisfaction, retirement planning, life-style/stress, sleep disorders
  D. Cardiovascular risk factors: family history, hypertension, hyperlipidemia, obesity/diabetes mellitus, lifestyle
  E. Health/risk behaviors
    1. Hormone replacement therapy
    2. Injury prevention: seat belts and helmets, occupational hazards, recreational hazards, sports involvement, firearms, hearing

(continued)

TABLE 1-6 (Continued)

3. Breast self-examination
4. Skin exposure to ultraviolet rays
5. Suicide: depressive symptoms
6. Tobacco, alcohol, other drugs

III. Immunizations
   A. Tetanus-diphtheria booster every 10 years
   B. Influenza vaccine to all women annually beginning at age 55 (prior to age 55 it should be given to residents of chronic care facilities; women with chronic cardiopulmonary disorders; and women with metabolic diseases, including diabetes mellitus, hemoglobinopathies, immunosuppression, or renal dysfunction)
   C. Measles, mumps, rubella (MMR): for all women unable to show proof of immunity
   D. Hepatitis B vaccine: (see Table 1-2, section III D)
   E. Pneumococcal vaccine: (see Table 1-4, section III E)

SOURCE: Adapted with permission from: The Obstetrician-Gynecologist and Primary-Preventive Health Care

TABLE 1-7 Leading Causes of Mortality and Morbidity Ages 65 Years and Older

Mortality

Cardiovascular disease
Coronary artery disease
Cerebrovascular disease
Pneumonia/influenza
Obstructive lung disease
Colorectal cancer
Breast cancer
Lung cancer
Accidents

Morbidity

Nose, throat, and upper respiratory conditions
Osteoporosis/arthritis
Hypertension
Urinary incontinence
Heart disease
Injuries (musculoskeletal and soft tissue)
Hearing and vision impairments

SOURCE: Adapted with permission from: The Obstetrician-Gynecologist and Primary-Preventive Health Care

TABLE 1-8 Periodic Health Assessment and Preventive Care Ages 65 and Older

I. Screening
   A. Review problem list and continuity-of-care records
   B. Obtain responses to patient questionnaire
   C. Periodic history: (see Table 1-2, section I C); also ask about polypharmacy
   D. Physical examination
   E. Laboratory tests
      1. Pap: physician and patient discretion after three consecutive normal tests
      2. Urinalysis/dipstick
      3. Mammography annually
      4. Cholesterol every 3 to 5 years; lipid profile for women with an elevated cholesterol level; history of parent or sibling with a blood cholesterol level of 240 mg/dl or higher; history of a sibling, parent, or grandparent with documented premature (aged less than 55 years) coronary artery disease; presence of diabetes mellitus or smoker
      5. TSH: every 3–5 years
      6. Periodic CBC, BUN, creatinine, and fasting glucose
      7. Sexually transmitted disease (see Table 1-2, section I E 4)
      8. HIV testing (see Table 1-2, section I E 5)
      9. Tuberculosis skin test (see Table 1-2, section I E 9)
      10. Fecal occult blood test: (see Table 1-6, section I E 3)
      11. Sigmoidoscopy: (see Table 1-6, section I E 4)
      12. Colonoscopy (see Table 1-6, section I E 5)

II. Evaluation and Counseling
   A. Sexuality
   B. Fitness: hygiene (general and dental), dietary/nutritional assessment, exercise (discussion of program)
   C. Psychosocial evaluation: neglect/abuse, lifestyle/stress, depression/sleep disorders, family relationships, job/work/retirement satisfaction
   D. Cardiovascular risk factors: hypertension, hypercholesterolemia, obesity/diabetes mellitus, sedentary lifestyle
   E. Health/risk behaviors
      1. Hormone replacement therapy

TABLE 1-8 (Continued)

2. Injury prevention: safety belts and helmets, occupational hazards, recreational hazards, hearing, firearms
3. Visual acuity/glaucoma
4. Hearing
5. Breast self-examination
6. Skin exposure to ultraviolet rays
7. Suicide: depressive symptoms
8. Tobacco, alcohol, other drugs

III. Immunizations
   A. Tetanus-diphtheria booster every 10 years
   B. Influenza vaccine (annually)
   C. Pneumococcal vaccine (once)
   D. Hepatitis B vaccine (see Table 1-2, section III D)

SOURCE: Adapted with permission from: The Obstetrician-Gynecologist and Primary-Preventive Health Care

References and Selected Readings

1. American Academy of Family Physicians, Commission on Public Health and Scientific Affairs: *Age Charts for Periodic Health Examinations.* Reprint no. 510. Kansas City, Missouri: AAFP, 1990.
2. American College of Obstetricians and Gynecologists: *The Obstetrician-Gynecologist and Primary-Preventive Health Care.* Washington: 1993.
3. American College of Physicians. *Clinical Efficacy Report.* Philadelphia: 1987.
4. Canadian Task Force on the Periodic Health Examination: The periodic health examination. *Can Med Assoc J* 121:1193–1254, 1979.
5. Hayward RS Steinberg EP, Ford DE, et al.: Preventive care guidelines: 1991. *Ann Intern Med* 114:758–783, 1991.
6. U.S. Department of Health and Human Services, Public Health Service: *Healthy People 2000: National Health Promotion and Disease Prevention Objectives.* Washington: U.S. Government Printing Office, 1991.
7. U.S. Preventive Services Task Force: *Guide to Clinical Preventive Services: An Assessment of the Effectiveness of 169 Interventions.* Baltimore: Williams & Wilkins, 1989.

2 Special Needs of the Adolescent

G. William Bates
Keith L. Blauer

Adolescence often brings turmoil. The adolescent undergoes physical changes, assumes the capacity for reproduction, seeks separation from parents, and searches for self-identity and independence. In addition, adolescents do not want to be labeled as "different" from their peers. The adolescent needs validation and emotional support from adults. Physicians and other health care professionals must recognize the special needs of adolescents and meet these needs in caring, nonthreatening ways. In this chapter, we will identify some of the emotional needs and some of the health-care needs of adolescents, and suggest ways to be open to them as they progress from childhood to adulthood.

There is a broad range of medical needs and social issues which adolescents have in common, but there is also substantial individual variation. Health care and preventive services should be age- and developmentally appropriate and should be sensitive to individual and sociocultural differences.

Adolescents often access the health care system with hidden agendas. In addition to responding to the adolescent's stated reason for seeking care, the physician needs to take the time to identify and address the other issues which are of concern to the adolescent, as well as to provide appropriate preventive and counseling services, as enumerated in this chapter and also in Table 1-2.

Confidentiality is an important issue in providing care for adolescents. Unless the adolescent is assured confidentiality and believes this assurance to be true, she often will not provide a complete history nor receive the full range of needed care. Confidentiality policies should be made clear to the patient, to the adult who has brought her for care if there is one, and to the office staff.

Emotional Concerns of Adolescents

Identity

With the onset of puberty come questions: "Who am I?" "What is my purpose in life?" The adolescent seeks her identity for the first time. Television, video, motion pictures, and print media bombard us with glamorous images of people whose lives are characterized by wealth and leisure. The adolescent must put these fantasies into perspective; the values taught at home, in school, and by religious organizations must be reinforced. Moreover, the adolescent needs strong self-esteem. Self-esteem is developed through success in interpersonal relationships, school, and extracurricular activities. Adolescents with low self-esteem are at much greater risk for early sexual relationships and for exploitation by drug dealers and gangs.

Physicians and other health care professionals have the opportunity to discuss issues of identity and self-esteem with adolescents and to work with them through such youth groups as Scouting programs, athletics, social groups, and religious activities. Physicians often are acknowledged as community leaders, not only by adults, but by adolescents as well. Therefore, physicians have the entrée to become involved in youth activities. In such positions of youth leadership, in addition to traditional medical roles, physicians can reinforce positive identity and high self-esteem among adolescents.

Information

Adolescents need clear, straightforward information about themselves, their changing bodies, their sexual function, and their sexual relationships. Much is said and written about teen-age pregnancy, venereal disease, AIDS, safe sex, sexual exploitation, drugs and alcohol, and tobacco. Few opportunities exist for adolescents to engage in thought and dialogue about these issues. When given the opportunity to serve adolescents as patients, or in other situations where physicians can participate as youth leaders, these critical issues must be raised and discussed. Physicians have credibility that others may not have. We must provide accurate information for adolescents.

Safety

Every person must feel safe in his or her environment. Adolescents need safe homes and schools, safe streets, and safe friends. Some adolescents live in fear of abuse from parents or of abuse of a parent by someone else. Some adolescents fear verbal or physical intimidation in schools. Adolescents can be at risk in their neighborhoods from gangs, on the streets, while riding with a person under the influence of drugs or alcohol, or from friends who can lead them into risky situations.

Health care workers must be aware of the physical and emotional risks to which adolescents are exposed. We must **ask** adolescents about their sense of safety. We ask adult women who may be at risk for spouse abuse. We must have the same awareness of the safety needs of adolescents.

Adolescents may be in jeopardy due to unsafe situations which are apparent to them and about which they are concerned, or because of risk-taking behaviors about which they are unaware or are not concerned. The physician needs to explore both types of situations with the adolescent. Accidents are the leading cause of death in the United States for individuals between ages 13 and 18, followed by homicides.

Self-Reliance

Self-reliance is the road to responsible adulthood. Adolescents want to become self-reliant; often adults do not foster self-reliance for adolescents but create situations that prolong dependency. In our relationships with adolescents, we should ask about their progress in becoming self-reliant, inquire about jobs that adolescents hold, inquire about the extent of self-support adolescents provide (e.g., clothing purchases, paying for part of their automobile insurance, music and miscellaneous entertainment purchases, school books and supplies, and savings for education). We should encourage adolescents to seek jobs that will help them to become self-reliant, and make part-time jobs available to adolescents in the health care fields.

Positive Adult Role Models

Parents are role models for their children. As children move into society through friendships, schools, and other organized activities, they find other positive adult role models in friends' parents and in teachers. As children progress through the stages of puberty to become adolescents and young adults, they seek role models such as coaches, Scout leaders, and camp counselors. As they begin to consider career choices, they seek role models in career fields of interest. Unfortunately, most children and adolescents are also exposed to a wide range of negative role models.

Physicians and other health care professionals can be positive role models at several levels for adolescents. We can become involved as youth leaders and share our own experiences of growing up and seeking identity; we can make ourselves available to adolescents to give career exposure in health care. In our opinion, in addition to their counseling roles while providing health care, physicians should be available to youth as leaders or as career advisers. Several organizations have programs for career exploration for adolescents. Through participation in these, physicians can become involved in organized youth development programs.

Involvement in Society

Adolescents want to be involved in society, even though they may not have reached the age of majority. The word "wait" is anathema to an adolescent. The "age of innocence" about sex, drugs, violence, family relationships, and political affairs has dropped to the pre-teenage years. Adolescents have opinions about common matters of daily life, and they want their opinions valued by adults.

Again, physicians have an opportunity to give adolescents a sense of worth and value along with an involvement in society. When we work with adolescents in our roles as physicians and community leaders, we can affirm their value to society and their place as future leaders of society.

The foregoing issues of the need for identity, information, safety, self-reliance, positive adult role-models, and involvement in society may seem simplistic. However, as primary care physicians, it may not seem obvious to us that we must acknowledge these needs in order to fulfill our responsibilities to adolescents. It is easy to ignore these issues for want of time, or for a seeming lack of relevance to health care. Yet, our recognition of these emotional needs of adolescents may go a long way in helping young people mature into adulthood, ultimately having a substantial positive effect on both their mental and their physical health.

Depression and Suicide

Suicide is the third leading cause of death in the United States among individuals ages 13 to 18. Depression and suicide are discussed extensively in Chap. 39. It is essential that primary care physicians realize the prevalence of depression among adolescents and teenagers. Most individuals who commit suicide access the health care system, often with an unrelated complaint, in the days or weeks before they commit suicide. By making appropriate inquiries, the physician may be able to identify the depressed teenager, and help her to receive needed counseling and treatment.

Medical Needs of Adolescents

Delayed Puberty

Secondary sexual maturation in girls usually begins at approximately 10 years of age; secondary sexual maturation in boys usually begins at approximately 11.5 years. The first outward manifestation of secondary sexual maturation in girls is breast budding. In most young women, this is followed by the appearance of pubic hair about 6 months later. Menarche usually occurs within 18 months of breast budding (about 12 years), and ovulatory cycles usually are established within one year of menarche. This is a predictable sequence of events.

If pubic hair growth is the first event of secondary sexual maturation and precedes breast budding by more than 6 months, it is likely that the affected girl has elevated adrenal androgen production. She should be evaluated for the possibility of late-onset adrenal hyperplasia. If this condition goes unrecognized or untreated, truncated breast development, acne, hirsutism, and irregular reproductive cycles will result.

Girls become concerned if their secondary sexual development does not parallel that of their peers. Young women with either early or delayed breast development often suffer embarrassment. When brought for consultation by a parent, these girls should be able to express their concerns and expectations to the consulting physician. Before reassurance is given, an appropriate history, physical examination, and laboratory studies must be performed.

Girls with delayed puberty must be examined for the presence of breast budding and early sexual hair growth. If there is no breast budding by age 13 (or at latest, 14), gonadotropin levels (FSH and LH) should be obtained to exclude hypothalamic-pituitary dysfunction or ovarian failure. If gonadotropins are in the low range consistent with levels found in a prepubertal child, then olfactory dysfunction, central nervous system tumors, low body weight (including anorexia nervosa), and hyperprolactinemia must be excluded before a diagnosis of constitutional delayed puberty can be established. If gonadotropins are elevated, genetic causes of ovarian failure (Turner syndrome, long-arm deficiency of the X chromosome, Swyer syndrome) must be pursued. In either case, appropriate hormone replacement should be initiated to start secondary sexual development and prevent osteoporosis.

A diagnosis of constitutional delay of puberty is a tentative diagnosis of exclusion. A common mistake in hormone administration to young women with delayed puberty is to begin combination oral contraceptives for hormonal support. The combination of estrogen with progestin administered to a girl who has not achieved secondary sexual development results in truncated breast development because progestins down-regulate estrogen receptors in the breasts. A hormone replacement regimen that will simulate the physiologic pattern of ovarian hormone secretion must be selected for a girl to achieve her normal adult height and to achieve normal breast development. Thus, therapy should begin with low-dose estrogen that can then be slowly and gradually increased until an adequate response is obtained. Progestins should appropriately be added to the regimen after vaginal bleeding begins.

Delayed puberty usually is associated with delayed development of heterosexual relationships. Affected adolescents usually will exclude themselves from activities where group dating and pairing off with members of the opposite sex occur. This problem becomes more pronounced if secondary sexual development is delayed beyond age 15, especially for young women. It is important for the physician to discuss the psychological and social aspects of delayed puberty with affected adolescents. The physician can provide the needed reassurance and counsel that normal heterosexual relationships will develop along with secondary sexual maturation. Moreover, many adolescents with delayed puberty will have concerns about their future fertility. Honest, open answers should be provided if the physician has enough information to give a reasonable prognosis about reproduction.

Acne

Acne is a common problem of adolescents. Nearly all are affected to some degree. The period of maximal acne occurs just at the time of ovulation in young women and at the time of spermatogenesis in young men. Once regular reproductive cycles are established in young women, and spermatogenesis is well established in young men, acne begins to clear spontaneously.

Persistent acne should be investigated. The most common serious cause of persistent acne in young men and young women is late-onset adrenal hyperplasia. Diagnosis should be made early, as late-onset adrenal hyperplasia can be a cause of infertility in both sexes. If the diagnosis can be made during the adolescent years, later problems such as severe facial scarring and abnormal hair growth can be prevented. Ovulatory dysfunction can also be anticipated, and appropriate therapy can be initiated when indicated.

When late-onset adrenal hyperplasia is suspected, dehydroepiandrosterone sulfate (DS) should be obtained as a screening test. If the DS concentration exceeds 2.8 μg/dl, consideration should be given to performing an adrenocorticotropic hormone

(ACTH) stimulation test. If the ACTH stimulation test is abnormal, prednisone 2.5 mg/day usually will be sufficient to control acne and restore normal reproductive function without inducing complete adrenal suppression. Adolescents with acne should not be given empirical courses of Accutane or antibiotics without adequate evaluation.

Body Weight

Weight-consciousness pervades American society. Popular magazines incessantly feature articles on ideal body weight and dietary control. Weight-control programs and physical fitness centers flourish in our society. Having the "right" figure or physique is important to most Americans. This desire for the "right" figure or physique is held by adolescents as well as by adult men and women.

Appropriate diet and exercise in moderation are important for individuals of all ages, and one of the roles of the primary care physician is to ensure that patients are counseled regarding exercise and eating nutritious, low-fat diets. While the adolescent's concerns about nutrition and prevention of obesity are important, fascination with slimness is a major cause of reproductive failure in American society. This fascination with the "waif look" often begins during adolescence, as young teenagers are placed on weight restriction diets by their parents(s), or are told "not to get fat." Lack of appropriate amounts of body fat can lead to delayed puberty, especially in girls, and can lead to secondary amenorrhea.

The extreme forms of dietary control, anorexia nervosa or bulimia, are most common in adolescent girls. Anorexia nervosa and bulimia are serious conditions and can lead to death from cardiomyopathy, electrolyte imbalance, arrhythmia, etc.

When the physician suspects a dietary problem, he/she should counsel the adolescent and (almost always) her parents as well. The parents may be part of the problem by being overly critical of body fat accumulation in an adolescent. Some eating disorders are difficult to overcome. Referral to a psychologist or psychiatrist who is knowledgeable about eating disorders, or to a structured program which addresses eating disorders, may be required to manage these difficult problems—particularly since, as mentioned above, these can be life-threatening illnesses.

Dysmenorrhea

Dysmenorrhea is a common problem for adolescent women who establish ovulatory cycles. Dysmenorrhea develops when the secretory endometrium sloughs because of decreasing ovarian progesterone production. With decreasing progesterone production, the endometrium secretes prostaglandins that may cause uterine contractions, diarrhea, headaches, and vomiting. These symptoms usually can be controlled by prostaglandin synthetase inhibitors or oral contraceptives.

However, uterine cramps that are more severe than the ordinary and that are unrelieved by medical therapy may be the result of endometriosis or congenital uterine deformities. Endometriosis should be suspected in an adolescent woman when the onset of cramps precedes the onset of menstruation, or when cramps last more than three days. Every adolescent woman who is suspected of having endometriosis does not need to undergo diagnostic laparoscopy. However, each can be placed on a trial of combination oral contraceptive tablets to provide relief from pain and to produce suppression of endometriosis. If there is a favorable clinical response to oral contraceptive suppression, endometriosis should be suspected and suppression continued for an extended time. Diagnostic studies such as hysterosalpingography and laparoscopy can be utilized if the physician has a high index of suspicion for anatomical defects of the reproductive tract.

Sexually Transmitted Diseases, Contraception, and Abortion

Sexually transmitted diseases, including HIV infection, hepatitis, chlamydia, and gonorrhea, are an ever-present threat to sexually active adolescents and teenagers. Physicians must discuss responsible sexual behavior, including abstinence, with these young patients.

Adolescents today are often besieged with information about condom use; however, they may get little information about other contraceptives. Physicians have the opportunity and should accept the responsibility to discuss contraception in ways that provide understandable, straightforward information. Adolescents must have the freedom to converse with their physicians alone, without a parent present. The adolescent should be allowed to ask questions and express interest in contraception. Appropriate discussion and establishment of trust will encourage the adolescent to seek effective contraceptives when needed. The adolescent must have the confidence that the physician will not violate confidentiality.

Regardless of the individual physician's attitude about abortion, adolescents should have the opportunity to discuss, in a nonjudgmental fashion, the pros and cons of abortion with the physician. If the physician does not perform abortions, the adolescent can be given the names of reputable physicians who can provide specific abortion information.

Tobacco, Alcohol, Marijuana, and Other Drugs

Adolescents face peer pressure to use tobacco, alcohol, marijuana, and other drugs. They need adult role models who give them the courage to refuse these substances. Many adolescents resort to smoking tobacco in order to withstand peer pressure and to avoid alcohol, marijuana, and other substances. The health dangers of tobacco smoking are often minimized by adolescents. Physicians have the opportunity to educate young people that tobacco is harmful and addicting and that quitting is not easy.

Physicians have a great deal of positive influence on young people in both medical and social settings. We should accept the responsibility of using that influence to help meet the special needs of adolescents and to provide supportive care in nonthreatening ways.

References and Selected Readings

1. Cullins VE, Huggins GR: Adolescent contraception, in Carpenter SE, Rock JA (eds): *Pediatric and Adolescent Gynecology.* New York: Raven Press, 1992, pp 341–352.
2. Council on Scientific Affairs, American Medical Association: Adolescents as victims of family violence. *JAMA* 270:1850–1856, 1993.
3. Frisch RE, Revelle R: Height and weight at menarche and a hypothesis of critical body weights and adolescent events. *Science* 169:397, 1970.
4. "How should we teach our children about sex?" *Time* Vol 141, pp 60–66, May 23, 1993.
5. Marshall WA, Tanner JM: Variations in pattern of pubertal changes in girls. *Arch Dis Child* 44:291, 1969.
6. Steinberg L, Levine A: *You and Your Adolescent. A Parent's Guide for Ages 10–20.* New York: Harper & Row, 1990.

3 Reproductive Health

Allan Rosenfield

Recently, increasing attention has been given to the concept of reproductive health services. These services impact in significant ways on the lives and well-being of women and their families. Reproductive health encompasses a broad range of services for women of reproductive age, including contraception; STD and HIV prevention; testing and treatment of sexually transmitted diseases; prenatal, intrapartum, and postpartum care; and counseling regarding healthy lifestyles and the benefits to health of preventive care. These services are indeed of high priority—yet, the effective provision of comprehensive reproductive health services is an elusive, often neglected target throughout the world, including in the United States.

The provision of family planning services is a critically important part of reproductive health care. For many years, the topic was too controversial to be included in the routine care of women. Margaret Sanger, the founder of what eventually became the Planned Parenthood Federation of America, was imprisoned in the 1920s as a result of her efforts to make contraceptive services available. In a few states it still was illegal to provide contraception as late as the 1960s. The Supreme Court ended this anachronism when it ruled, in Griswold et al. v. Connecticut in 1965, that couples in the privacy of their homes could use contraceptives.[1] Since that time, family planning services have become more readily available throughout the United States. However, although women have better access to contraception, they would benefit by a more active program of counseling and education regarding a variety of issues related to their reproductive health.

Closely related to contraceptive services are education, counseling, and screening aimed at the prevention of sexually transmitted diseases and lower reproductive tract infections. The management of these conditions is a major component of primary reproductive health services. Morbidity secondary to chlamydia or herpes is a significant source of concern to many women. The incidence of STDs has increased significantly, as have ectopic pregnancies. Finally, there is great concern about HIV/AIDS, and many women wish confidential counseling, education, and testing. Primary care physicians need to be knowledgeable about these diseases and to take the initiative in discussing them with their patients.

Teen pregnancy remains a major social problem in the United States, requiring a number of creative initiatives beyond access to services. School-based clinic programs, out-of-school programs, effective sexuality education, and other efforts are of great importance if we are to have an impact on this serious problem.

Without question, the most controversial and difficult topic relates to abortion and the provision of abortion services.[2] Worldwide, the World Health Organization estimates that somewhere between 50,000 and 100,000 maternal deaths each year are the tragic consequences of a botched, usually illegal abortion procedure.[3] Through most of the 19th century, British common law held in the United States, ruling that abortion prior to quickening (between 17 and 20 weeks' gestation) was legal. This changed in the late 1800s, when major efforts were made to make abortion at all stages of pregnancy illegal. By the turn of the century, every state had laws against abortion.

During the first half of the twentieth century,

abortion remained illegal, except for so-called therapeutic abortions, almost all of which were provided to private patients.[4] Efforts aimed at change at the state level began in the late 1960s, and a small number of states legalized abortion by the early 1970s, culminating in 1973 with the landmark Supreme Court decision, Roe v. Wade, which legalized abortion throughout the country, establishing the trimester framework.[5]

While the great majority of physicians in the United States believe that a woman should have the right to terminate a pregnancy, there is an increasing severity in the shortage of abortion providers, with a majority of counties in the United States having no providers.[6] Although the goal clearly is to prevent unintended pregnancy, safe abortion services must be made available.

Prevention of STDs and their early diagnosis and treatment; education of women regarding contraception and the prevention of unintended pregnancy and infectious disease; making available to all women the range of contraceptive and reproductive services; and providing preventive, screening, counseling, and general health care are all major components of providing primary health care for reproductive age women.

References and Selected Readings

1. Griswold v Connecticut 381 US 479 (1965).
2. Rosenfield A: Women's reproductive health. *Am J Obstet Gynecol* 169:128–133, 1993.
3. World Health Organization: *Abortion: A Tabulation of Available Data on the Frequency and Mortality of Unsafe Abortion,* 2d ed. Geneva: WHO, 1994.
4. Hall RE: Therapeutic abortion, sterilization and contraception. *Am J Obstet Gynecol* 91:518–532, 1965.
5. Roe v. Wade 410 US 113 (1973).
6. Henshaw S, Van Vort J: Abortion services in the United States, 1987 and 1988. *Fam Plan Perspect* 22:102–142, 1990.

4 Menopause: Acceptance and Understanding of Its Impact

PonJola Coney
Robert C. Cefalo

Menopause is the second most common and predictable endocrine-metabolic event that occurs in the human female. Puberty is the first. The usual age for the last menstrual period is 50 ± 1.5 years. The classic clinical features of amenorrhea and hot flashes often obviate the necessity for a battery of testing to obtain a diagnosis. The *climacteric* characterizes the period prior to the cessation of menstruation when symptoms and changes in quantity and duration of menstrual flow may appear, reflecting some instability and decline in ovarian function. As life expectancy of the human female increases (it is now 78 years), the impact of menopause on the quality of a woman's life and health assumes greater interest and importance. The physician who is the primary care provider for a woman as she reaches the perimenopausal years and beyond has an extremely important role to play. By making certain that a woman is properly educated about and prepared for the changes which are likely to occur and by making certain that she understands what preventive measures are important and that the physician and the woman are cooperative partners in health care decisions, the primary care physician can make an extremely important positive impact on the woman's physical and emotional well-being.

Body Responses to Estrogen Deficiency

Central Nervous System Responses

The most common affective phenomena seen at the time of the menopause are referable to the central nervous system and include, in order of frequency, hot flashes, fatigue, depression, headache, palpitations, and anxiety. As many as 30 percent of women display some significant degree of stress in response to the menopause. Reports suggest that approximately 16 percent of women are free of noticeable affective symptoms at the menopause.

The hot flash is a sensation of heat that is recurrent and often accompanied by sweating, flushing, anxiety, and chills. The hot flash usually lasts from two to five minutes and may be associated with an increase in body temperature. Hot flashes can begin as soon as estrogen levels begin to decline in the climacteric. Some women endure hot flashes for as long as 10 years, but they can be disruptive to a sense of well-being and to daily function. Hot flashes are the primary reason women seek medical therapy for menopause. They are most prevalent in the first two to three years postmenopause and tend to be more intense and to last longer in women who undergo surgical menopause. Hot flashes do not show a consistent correlation with estrogen or gonadotropin levels. Kronenberg's epidemiologic survey of menopausal women with hot flashes revealed that how long they last is quite variable and that the pattern may change, becoming less frequent and less intense for some women, but continuing into old age for others. In the survey, 50 percent of women who experienced hot flashes said they began before menopause in the presence of regular menstrual cycles; others said they began more than two years after menopause. Hot flashes in this group varied considerably among women, with a frequency of five to 50 per day and lasting from one to five minutes. The women who were surveyed reported other affective discomforts during hot flashes such as irritability, sense of panic, feelings of suffocation, and even occasional suicidal feelings. Some women reported specific triggers of hot flashes, including stressful situations, caffeine, alcohol, confining space, and external heat.

Physical Responses

Estrogen deficiency can have substantial effects on skin. Epidermal and skin-fold thickness diminish, and there are decreases in tensile strength, compressibility, turgor, and total skin collagen after the menopause. Estrogen binding to its receptor is greatest in the uterus, followed by face skin, breast skin, thigh skin, lung cells, and adipose tissue. Estrogen's effect on the vascular system, with its potential to modulate arteriolar and venous tone and alter blood flow, can also influence skin physiology. With estrogen deficiency breast tissue will lose some form and fullness, distribution of body hair changes, and pubic hair becomes sparse. Hirsutism may develop, but is not pathologic. It reflects secretion of androgens primarily, instead of estrogen by the ovary.

In the absence of significant levels of circulating estrogen, the menopausal vaginal epithelium may become thin and dry, which may lead to vaginitis and sexual dysfunction. Lack of lubrication and regression of the upper vagina may lead to dyspareunia. Urethral cellular changes coincide with vaginal changes, and urinary symptoms may appear. Pelvic tissues may lose tone and predispose to prolapse.

Sexual Responses

Sexual response and libido gradually decline with age in both men and women. No obvious relationship between libido decline and menopause has been shown.

Metabolic Responses

Bone loss begins before menopause and may be accelerated after menopause. Postmenopausal osteoporosis affects more than 20 million American women. One-third of women with osteoporosis will suffer vertebral and hip fracture. Prior to fracture, no symptoms are associated with osteoporosis. The key to management is prevention. Lindsay was the first to show the protective effect of estrogen on bone preservation.

More recently, Stevenson randomized 66 early postmenopausal women to either continuous transdermal estrogen (0.05 mg) with norethisterone acetate or oral continuous premarin (0.625 mg) with norgestrel. Thirty women were untreated and served as controls. Bone density was measured by dual photon absorptiometry in the spine and three femoral sites. The untreated group lost 2.4 percent bone from the spine, 3.1 percent from the femoral neck, and 2.1 percent from the trochanteric region. The treated groups did not lose bone at any site, and there were slight gains in bone tissue for both transdermal and oral estrogen users at all sites. Estrogen promotes a decrease in osteoclastic resorption. It is more effective on trabecular bone than cortical bone and will decrease hip and spinal fractures with long-term therapy.

Cardiovascular Heart Disease (CHD)

Cardiovascular heart disease is the chief cause of death in men and women in the western world. Before menopause, CHD mortality is lower in women than in men; after menopause, mortality in women rises to approach that of men. CHD risk is substantially increased in young women after spontaneous and surgically induced menopause. A tremendous amount of experimental evidence—observed, retrospective, and prospective—exists to support the beneficial or protective effects of estrogen against CHD. The exact magnitude of the associated protection is not clear. In 1983, the Lipid Research Clinics Study reported the all-cause mortality in estrogen users to be only half that of nonusers. The one contradictory report was from the Framingham Study, which did not suggest any such cardiovascular benefits; in that study, estrogen use was associated with an increased incidence of stroke and CHD, despite a more favorable cardiovascular risk profile in the estrogen users. It is not difficult to draw the conclusion that estrogen probably protects against heart disease and stroke. Overviews of more than 30 reports, both retrospective and observed, estimate a reduction in CHD risk with the use of hormone replacement therapy.

Prospective cohort studies generally show that estrogen use reduces CHD. The largest cohort study is the Nurses' Health Study, which followed 48,000 menopausal women for 10 years and found the relative risk to be reduced at 0.89 for "ever" used and 0.56 for "current" users of estrogen.

Data suggest that high density lipoprotein (HDL) cholesterol (C) levels might be the biological mechanism by which estrogen confers protection. HDL-C is further subdivided into HDL_2 and HDL_3 subfractions. Sex hormones are known to alter lipid profiles. Estrogen therapy increases the HDL_2-C subfraction. HDL-C is the only hormone-sensitive risk factor marker known, at this time, to predict CHD risk. Within months after menopause, serum concentrations of total cholesterol rise by 6 percent, low density lipoprotein (LDL) cholesterol by 11 percent, and triglycerides by 9 percent, with a gradual fall in HDL cholesterol. Treatment with oral estrogen lowers total serum cholesterol and LDL cholesterol and raises HDL_2. Estrogen typically lowers LDL by 15 to 19 percent and raises HDL by 16 to 18 percent.

Management of Menopause

Behavioral

An exercise program to improve physical fitness will decrease all-cause mortality from a number of disease processes, including coronary heart disease, hypertension, diabetes, colon cancer, and depression. Walking is the best exercise for bone stress and to prevent bone loss. Exercise stimulates HDL_2 production.

Women should also be educated regarding the importance of good nutrition, calcium supplementation, smoking cessation, drinking only in moderation, etc. They should be told that appropriate weight reduction (for the overweight) and moderate exercise will retard bone loss and improve the cardiovascular profile.

Pharmacologic

In addition to behavior modifications—and potentially more important for many women—is the pharmacologic management of menopausal symptoms and effects. The most crucial pharmacologic agent is estrogen. This very important topic is discussed at length later in the text.

General Considerations (What to Tell the Patient)

Education about the menopause is the first and best prescription to give a patient. She should be given comprehensive and accurate information regarding what we know about the menopause, and this information should be provided in a nonpartisan manner. The patient should be armed with accurate information and given full opportunity to make her own decision regarding intervention. She should be cautioned that therapies and recommendations continually change based on ongoing research.

Summary

In summary, menopause is a universal and physiologic event. It can for some women represent a psychological and biological crisis, and counseling and education by health care providers, as well as therapeutic interventions, can have a substantial beneficial effect. Symptoms can become severe, disabling, and intolerable for some, and the decision for medical intervention should be made between the patient and her physician. For those who desire medical therapy, epidemiologic data favor the use of estrogen to protect against accelerated bone mass loss, to reduce the incidence and severity of heart disease, to improve psychological function, and generally to improve the quality of life.

Perhaps as few as 15 to 25 percent of postmenopausal women who have no contraindications to estrogen therapy actually receive estrogen. Approximately 25 percent of women in the United States are at risk for disabling side effects from menopausal osteoporosis. Perhaps the decision to use estrogen for that reason alone should not encompass all candidates; risk assessment at the menopause would enable stratification of individual risk. Approximately 25 percent of women can relate no major affective symptoms coincident with menopause. Some women might wish to rely on genetics, exercise, nutrition, and life-style factors to lower their risks of heart disease and osteoporosis in lieu of estrogen.

Although for many women the benefits of hormone replacement therapy substantially outweigh any potential risk, there is currently no absolute consensus among medical professionals as to what the universal practice should be. For this reason, the patient, her understanding of the benefits and risks, and her participation in the decisions regarding management are instrumental in the approach to menopause. The physician, working with the patient, can contribute greatly to her well-being at this important time in her life.

References and Selected Readings

1. Bilezikian JP, Silverberg SJ: Osteoporosis: A practical approach to the perimenopausal woman. *J Women Health* 1:21–27, 1992.
2. Block E: Quantitative morphological investigations of the follicular system in women. *Acta Anat* 14:108–23, 1952.
3. Bush TL, Cowan LD, Barrett-Connor E, et al: Estrogen use and all cause mortality, preliminary results from the Lipid Research Clinics Program follow-up study. *JAMA* 249:903–906, 1983.
4. Cutler WB, Garcia CR: The menopausal transition and beyond, in *The Medical Management of Menopause and Premenopause,* Philadelphia: JB Lippincott, 1984, p 31.
5. Dupont WD, Page DL: Menopausal estrogen replacement therapy and breast cancer. *Arch Intern Med* 151:67–72, 1991.
6. Feldman BM, Voda A, Gronseth E: The prevalence of hot flash and associated variables among perimenopausal women. *Res Nurs Health* 8:261–268, 1985.
7. Gordon T, Kanel W, Hjortland M, McNamara P: Menopause and coronary heart disease. The Framingham Study. *Ann Intern Med* 89:157–16, 1978.
8. Henderson BE, Ross RK, Lobo RA, et al: Re-evaluating the role of progestogen therapy after the menopause. *Fertil Steril* 49:9S–15S, 1988.
9. Hirvonen E, Malkonen M, Manninen V: Effects of different progestogens on lipoproteins during postmenopausal replacement therapy. *N Engl J Med* 560–563, 1980.
10. Hughes BD, Dallal GE, Krall EA, et al: A controlled trial of the effect of calcium supplementation on bone density in postmenopausal women. *N Engl J Med* 323:878–883, 1990.
11. Kronenberg F: Hot flashes: Epidemiology and physiology, in *Multidisciplinary Perspectives on Menopause,* New York: New York Academy of Science, 1990, vol 592, p 52.
12. Lindsay R, Hart DM, Aitken JM, et al: Long-term prevention of postmenopausal osteoporosis by estrogen: Evidence for an increased bone mass after delayed onset of oestrogen treatment. *Lancet* 1:1038–1041, 1976.
13. *The Medical Letter:* Etidronate for postmenopausal osteoporosis. 32:111, 1990.
14. Meldrum DR: Treatment of hot flushes, in *Menopause Physiology and Pharmacology,* Chicago: Year Book, 1987, p 141.
15. Nachtigall LE, Nachtigall RH, Nachtigall RD, Nachtigall LE: Estrogen replacement therapy. I. A 10-year prospective study in the relationship to osteoporosis. *Obstet Gynecol* 53:277–281, 1979.
16. Nachtigall MJ, Smilen SW, Nachtigall RD, et al: Incidence of breast cancer in a 22-year study of women receiving estrogen-progestin replacement therapy. *Obstet Gynecol* 80:827–830, 1992.
17. Sarrel P, Rousseau M, Mazure C, Glazer W: Ovarian steroids and the capacity to function at home and in the work-

place, in *Multidisciplinary Perspectives on Menopause,* New York: New York Academy of Science, 1990, vol 592.

18. Stampfer MJ, Colditz GA, Willett WC, et al: Postmenopausal estrogen and cardiovascular disease. 10-year follow-up from Nurses Health Study. *N Engl J Med* 325:756–762, 1991.
19. Stampfer MJ, Willett WC, Colditz GA, et al: A prospective study of postmenopausal estrogen therapy and coronary heart disease. *N Engl J Med* 313:1044–1049, 1985.
20. Stevenson JC, Cust MP, Gangar KF, et al: Effects of transdermal versus oral hormone replacement therapy on bone density in spine and proximal femur in postmenopausal women. *Lancet* 336:265–269, 1990.
21. Van Keep PA, Ser DM, Greenblatt, RB, Kopera H: Workshop report in: *Female and Male Climateric: Current Opinion,* Baltimore: University Park Press, 1978.
22. Wahl P, Walden C, Knopp R, Hoover J: Effect of estrogen/progestin potency on lipid/lipoprotein cholesterol. *N Engl J Med* 308:862–867, 1983.

5 Beyond Menopause

Leo J. Dunn

As the patient ages, her needs change and the disorders that may affect her also change. The alterations brought about by aging are gradual, and the age at which such terms as "geriatric medicine" may be properly applied is arbitrary. Whereas much of medicine looks upon individuals age 75 and above as a geriatric population, others consider age 65 as an important landmark—probably because it is a common age for retirement. On the other hand, those who provide care for women often begin their focus on the aging process at menopause, when reproductive life comes to a close. So many physiologic events of importance to continued good health occur at menopause that it is advantageous to use it as a landmark when concerns about the aging process in women should increase.

Young and growing nations usually have a majority of their population in the younger age groups, with a pyramidal rise to a smaller aged population. Older nations that do not have expanding economies tend to reverse this pattern. It is believed that the population dynamics of the United States are now in transition and that the most rapid relative growth is in the older age groups. As a consequence, increasing attention will be paid to health care of the elderly. They are not only growing in numbers; they also are growing in political strength. Importantly, the cost of their care per capita greatly exceeds that of the younger citizen.

The leading causes of morbidity and mortality in women between the ages of 40 and 64 are presented in Table 1-5, and the leading causes of morbidity and mortality in women ages 65 and older are presented in Table 1-7. Physicians clearly must focus substantial attention on these areas with respect to both preventive interventions and care of specific disorders.

The primary care physician provides continuity of care to his or her patient through the menopause and into that phase of life designated as geriatric care. The management of menopause, hormone replacement therapy, and recommendations for health maintenance during this phase of life are covered elsewhere. It is an important responsibility for the physician, who can significantly influence the woman's future health by actions taken at this time.

The disorders that may affect women in their later years include all organ systems and many acute and chronic diseases. They are discussed in several chapters throughout this book. A few specific disorders of substantial importance to women in this age group will be highlighted in this chapter, as well as some general considerations regarding the care of the elderly woman. The physician must realize that in this nation where women significantly outlive men and families are often widely scattered, one is often dealing with an aging individual who lives alone. The potential for isolation and its variety of effects on the individual should be explored at regular health visits.

The Primary Care Task Force of the American College of Obstetricians and Gynecologists has recommended specific items of health care to be addressed at each scheduled primary care visit for women age 65 or above. An adaptation of this information is provided in table form in Chap. 1.

Meeting the Needs of the Elderly

Physicians frequently identify patient needs that require the use of community resources. It is often difficult for individual practitioners to be aware of those resources so that they may incorporate them into their efforts to maintain patients' health and well-being. Some information about existing programs will be discussed below.

Governmental concern regarding the aging population in the United States has been demonstrated in several ways, including the Older Americans Act of 1965. Its purpose was to provide social services to the elderly through a community-based network and to establish the Administration on Aging, a federal agency, as an advocate for the elderly. The six Titles of the Act describe its philosophy and services:

Title I states the policy objectives for services to older persons to include income, health, housing, long-term care, and transportation.

Title II establishes the Administration on Aging and authorizes the Federal Council on Aging to advise the President.

Title III authorizes supportive nutrition and home care service programs, most of which are through home-delivered meals and congregate meals.

Title IV provides federal funding for training, research, and demonstration activities in the field of aging.

Title V awards funds to national organizations and state agencies to create jobs for low-income older workers in a variety of community service activities.

Title VI is a specific program for older Indians and native Hawaiians to provide supportive and nutritional services.

A variety of national programs are available for elderly citizens who qualify. These include:

- Food stamp programs
- Congregate nutrition and home-delivered meals program
- Native American services
- Federal commodity donations
- Social Security
- Supplemental Security Income
- Medicare
- Medicaid
- Federally assisted housing programs
- Employment and training programs for older Americans

Other programs that may be available within a community include adult day-care services, senior centers, transportation services, older American volunteer programs, in-home health aids and personal care services, homemaker and chore services, respite and care-giver support services, and minor home repair services. Information about such services can be obtained by contacting the Agency on Aging.

Table 5-1 provides the telephone numbers for the State Agency on Aging in each state, and was compiled by the National Association of State Units on Aging.

The Nutrition Screening Initiative provides two levels of screening to be applied by a health professional. The Level I Screen uses a nomogram to compute the formula [weight (kg)]/[height (m)]^2 to determine the body mass index (BMI). A BMI <22 or >27, or weight change of plus or minus 10 pounds in six months is indicative of a potential nutrition problem. A series of questions on eating habits, living environment, and functional status are also provided which aid in identifying persons who require nutritional assessment.

The Level II screen also uses the BMI criteria used in Level I but adds anthropometric measurements such as mid-arm muscle circumference and triceps skin-fold. It also requires determination of serum albumin and cholesterol. The questions provided for assessment include drug use, symptoms of

TABLE 5-1 Locating Aging Services and Resources

The following directory lists the telephone numbers for the State Agency on Aging, state or national toll-free numbers, and special hotlines. If no toll-free number is available, contact the State Agency on Aging.

A new service, The Eldercare Locator (1-800-677-1116), is available in all states east of the Mississippi River. It provides callers with the name and telephone number for the source of aging information and referral for each zip code in the country. The service will be available nationwide by the end of 1992.

Alabama
(205) 242-5743
Information & Referral
In State: (800) 243-5463

Alaska
(907) 465-3250

Arizona
(602) 542-4446
Information & Referral
Marlcopa County/
Northern Arizona:
(800) 352-3792
Pima County/
Southern Arizona:
(800) 362-3474

Arkansas
(501) 682-2441
Information & Referral
(501) 682-8150

California
(916) 322-5290

Colorado
(303) 866-5931
Information & Referral
(303) 866-3851

Connecticut
(203) 566-8645
Information & Referral
In State: (800) 443-9946
Out of State: (203) 566-7772

Delaware
(302) 421-6791
Information & Referral
In State: (800) 223-9074

District of Columbia
(202) 724-5622
Information & Referral
(202) 724-5626

Florida
(904) 488-8922
Hot Line MDT—Elder Abuse
In State: (800) 96-ABUSE

Georgia
(404) 894-5333

Guam
(671) 632-4141

Hawaii
(808) 548-2593
Information & Referral
In State: (800) 468-4644

Idaho
(208) 334-3833

Illinois
(217) 785-2870
Information & Referral
In State: (800) 252-9866
Out of State: (800) 252-8600
Hot Line—Nursing Home
In State: (800) 252-8966

Indiana
(317) 232-7020
Information & Referral
In State: (800) 545-7763
Hot Line—Nursing Home
In State: (800) 545-7763
Hot Line—Adult Abuse
In State: (800) 545-7763

Iowa
(515) 281-5187

Kansas
(913) 296-4986
Information & Referral
In State: (800) 432-3535

Kentucky
(502) 564-6930
Information & Referral
In state: (800) 372-2973
Hot Line—LTC Ombudsman
In State: (800) 372-2991

Louisiana
(504) 925-1700

Maine
(207) 626-5335
Hot Line—LTC Ombudsman
In State: (800) 452-1912

Maryland
(301) 225-1100
Information & Referral
In State: (800) 243-3425

Massachusetts
(617) 727-7750
Information & Referral
In State: (800) 882-2003
TDD: (800) 872-0166
Hot Line—Elder Abuse
In State: (800) 922-2275
Alzheimer's Information
In State: (800) 351-2299

Michigan
(517) 373-8230

Minnesota
(612) 296-2770
Information & Referral
In State: (800) 652-9747
Hot Line—LTC Ombudsman
In State: (800) 657-3591

Mississippi
(601) 949-2070
Information & Referral
In State: (800) 222-7622
Hot Line—Personal Care, Nursing Home, Hospital Complaints
In State: (800) 227-7308

Missouri
(314) 751-3082
Information & Referral
In State: (800) 235-5503
Hot Line—Elder Abuse & Neglect
In State: (800) 392-0210

Montana
(406) 444-3111
Information & Referral
In State: (800) 332-2272

Nebraska
(402) 471-2306

Nevada
(702) 486-3545
Information & Referral
In State: (800) 243-3638

New Hampshire
(603) 271-4680
Information & Referral
In State: (800) 852-3345
Hot Line—LTC Ombudsman
In State: (800) 442-5640

New Jersey
(609) 292-4833
Information & Referral
In State: (800) 792-8820

New Mexico
(505) 827-7640
Information & Referral
In State: (800) 432-2080

New York
(518) 474-3585
Information & Referral
In State: (800) 342-9871

North Carolina
(919) 733-3983
Information & Referral
In State: (800) 662-7030

North Dakota
(701) 224-2577
Information & Referral
In State: (800) 472-2622

Ohio
(614) 466-5500
Hot Line—Nursing Home Complaints
In State: (800) 282-1206

Oklahoma
(405) 521-2281
Hot Line—Elder Abuse
In State: (800) 522-3511

Oregon
(503) 378-4728
Information & Referral
In State: (800) 232-3020

Pennsylvania
(717) 783-1550
Hot Line—Alzheimer's
In State: (800) 367-5115
Paid Prescriptions Problems
In State: (800) 225-7223
Hot Line—Fraud & Abuse
In State: (800) 992-2433

Puerto Rico
(809) 721-5710
Information & Referral
(809) 721-4560

Rhode Island
(401) 277-2880
Information & Referral
In State: (800) 322-2880
Hot Line—Alzheimer's
In State: (800) 244-1428

South Carolina
(803) 735-0210
Information & Referral
In State: (800) 868-9095
In Columbia: (800) 735-0210

South Dakota
(605) 773-3656

Tennessee
(615) 741-2056

Texas
(512) 444-2727
Information & Referral
In State: (800) 252-9240

Utah
(801) 538-3910

Vermont
(802) 241-2400
Information & Referral
In State: (800) 642-5119

Virginia
(804) 225-2271
Information & Referral
In State: (800) 552-4464
Hot Line—Nursing Home Complaints
In State: (800) 552-3402

Virgin Islands
(809) 772-4950, Ext. 46

Washington
(206) 493-2500
Information & Referral
In State: (800) 422-3263
Hot Line—Nursing Home Complaints
In State: (800) 562-6028

West Virginia
(304) 348-3317
Information & Referral
In State: (800) 642-3671

Wisconsin
(608) 266-2536
Hot Line—LTC Ombudsman
In State: (800) 242-1060
Hot Line—MEDIGAP Claims
In State: (800) 242-1060

Wyoming
(307) 777-7986
Information & Referral
In State: (800) 442-2766

SOURCE: This listing courtesy of the National Association of State Units on Aging.

oral or dental disease, eating habits, living environment, functional status, and mental and cognitive status. Patients with anthropometric measurements <10th percentile or a skinfold >95th percentile, a serum albumin below 3.5 g/dl, or a cholesterol <160 mg/dl or >240 mg/dl, require further nutritional assessment.

Medications

Physicians who care for the elderly are well aware of the importance of pharmacologic aspects of their care. Older patients are more likely than others to be taking multiple medications, which they often obtain from a variety of sources. Therefore, at each visit it is advisable to ask for a recitation of what medications the patient is now using. A more accurate method is to encourage the patient to bring a list from home, including the correct name and prescribed dose, or to bring in their containers of medicines, which can provide an amazing display of pharmaceuticals.

A common experience is the failure of the patient to take the medication as prescribed. It has been estimated that as many as 50 percent of elderly patients take their medications incorrectly. Written instructions to the patient are often more helpful than the usual directions typed on the container itself.

A general concern in the use of medications by the elderly is a narrowed therapeutic index, as their tolerance decreases and their responses become altered. In addition, the use of many medications increases the risk of drug interactions. Since patients may obtain their medications from different pharmacies, they should be encouraged to take their full medication list with them when they fill any prescription so that the pharmacist may check for potential problems.

Depression

Women are more subject to depression than are men, with a reported ratio of 2:1. Although a common perception is that depression increases in frequency with age, the mean incidence of the disorder is about age 40. It is a condition recognized in adolescence and can occur at any age, including postmenopausal and later years. It is not correct to consider symptoms of depression as an expected event associated with the aging process. Situational changes in anyone's life that involve personal loss—whether economic, social, companionship, health, or loss of a loved one—can give rise to symptoms common to depression. These symptoms are more akin to grief reactions than to true depression. The frequency with which one might face such situations does increase with age, and this may explain the perception of depression as part of the aging process. Although depression is not an uncommon problem in older women, it also may be overdiagnosed. Avoidance of misdiagnosis is important; therefore, a careful interview to expose the life events that may have caused the patient's symptoms is a necessary part of evaluation. The topic of depression is discussed in depth in Chap. 39.

Obviously not every patient with depression will be placed on medication. The importance of counseling and interpersonal interventions, whether or not the woman is placed on medication, cannot be overstated. However, some medications currently considered effective for depression include tricyclic and heterocyclic antidepressants, selective serotonin reuptake inhibitors, and monoamine oxidase inhibitors. The older patient may have conditions that are affected by antidepressants, such as glaucoma, constipation, cardiac arrhythmia, and some neurologic conditions. Patients who have had strokes or dementia such as Alzheimer's disease may have untoward effects from these drugs, such as delirium.

Particularly in the elderly, it is obvious that initiation of pharmacotherapy for depression requires very close follow-up. Since some medications may interfere with cardiac conduction and rhythm, patients receiving these medications require a pretherapy baseline ECG and periodic repeat studies to evaluate the QRS complex. The patient should be informed regarding what to expect from the medication, how soon improvement may be noted, and what risks and side effects are likely. A decision should be made regarding psychiatric consultation. The need for this will depend on the patient's symptoms and the breadth of the primary care physician's experience. Patients with severe symptoms, those who are unresponsive to medication, or those who have recurrences should have in-depth psychiatric evaluation. Any patient who is a significant suicide risk cannot be left alone even for a moment, and requires immediate psychiatric intervention.

Hypertension

In most countries hypertension does not usually make its appearance in later life, but late-onset hypertension is found in the United States. Since cardiovascular diseases are of such importance in the elderly and since hypertension is a major cause of these disorders, all primary care physicians should make an effort to control abnormal elevations of either systolic or diastolic blood pressure. The Joint National Committee on Detection, Evaluation and Treatment of High Blood Pressure, funded by the National Institutes of Health, has provided important guidelines. These are discussed in Chap. 41.

The history taken in evaluation of a patient diagnosed as hypertensive should include both a personal and family history regarding coronary heart disease, cardiovascular disease, stroke, diabetes, dyslipidemia, renal disease, and gout. Specific information should be obtained regarding the duration of the hypertension, previous antihypertensive therapy, weight gain, diet, alcohol use, smoking, and the use of medications that might cause blood pressure elevation.

During the physical examination the physician should document the presence of sustained hypertension in both arms, measure height and weight, perform a funduscopic examination for retinal vascular changes, and examine the neck for carotid bruits, distended veins, or thyroid enlargement. Physical examination should also include examination of the heart for size, rate, rhythm, and sounds, as well as auscultation of the abdomen for bruits and palpation for kidney enlargement or abnormal aortic pulsations. Peripheral pulses should be assessed, a neurologic examination performed, and any edema described.

Routine laboratory tests include urinalysis, complete blood count, a fasting blood glucose, potassium, calcium, creatinine, uric acid, lipid profile, and ECG. Some tests done for specific indication include urinary microscopic and albumin determination, echocardiography, and plasma renin/urinary sodium determination. The management of patients with hypertension is discussed in Chap. 41.

The medical literature offers supportive evidence that when blood pressure is controlled there is a distinct reduction in stroke incidence and a definite but lesser reduction in coronary heart disease. These benefits are seen in older patients whose blood pressure is adequately controlled; they are not limited to younger age groups.

Pelvic Floor Dysfunction—Urinary Incontinence

A major problem for aging women is urinary incontinence. Although this has been the primary focus for investigation and treatment, it is only one manifestation of the broader entity frequency referred to as "pelvic floor dysfunction" (PFD). PFD includes a variety of manifestations of loss of anatomical support and pelvic nerve damage that most commonly are initiated by childbirth and worsened by aging. A spectrum of anatomical changes are well-known manifestations, including cystourethrocele, rectocele, enterocele, and uterine prolapse. Functional loss with urinary incontinence and fecal incontinence are among the most troublesome manifestations. The inability to control urine or feces loss may make the difference between relatively independent living at home versus the need for such institutional care as a nursing home. The economic difference is considerable as well.

The most frequent problem is urinary incontinence, which has been estimated by the Agency for Health Care Policy and Research (AHCPR) of the United States Department of Health and Human Services to affect 15 to 30 percent of noninstitutionalized persons over age 60, and more than 50 percent of 1.5 million nursing home residents. The agency estimates that the costs of caring for these individuals exceeds $10 billion annually. The AHCPR has now published a Clinical Practice Guideline for "Urinary Incontinence in Adults." Although these guidelines will be subject to revision with time, they are the basis for the following information.

Several types of incontinence have been identified:

Urge Incontinence (Fig. 5-1)

Definition: The involuntary loss of urine associated with an abrupt and strong desire to void.

Symptoms: Patients usually complain that they cannot get to the bathroom quickly enough, they leak urine when hearing or touching running water, or they void very frequently day or night and may have bed wetting.

Physical Findings: No specific, characteristic findings.

Laboratory Findings:

- Involuntary detrusor contractions are most common
- Urethral instability with involuntary urethral relaxation
- Detrusor hyperactivity with impaired bladder contractility has also been described.

Stress Incontinence (Fig. 5-2)

Definition: The involuntary loss of urine during coughing, sneezing, laughing, or other physical activities that increase intra-abdominal pressure.

Symptoms: Patients usually complain of urine loss with coughing, sneezing, laughing, rising from a chair, or during exercise.

Physical Findings: Hypermobility or significant displacement of the bladder neck demonstrable by the "Q-tip test." Visible loss of urine with coughing as part of the examination.

Laboratory Findings: No test is absolutely diagnostic. Dynamic urethral profilometry will frequently demonstrate the dominance of intravesical pressure over intraurethral pressure during coughing.

Overflow Incontinence

Definition: Involuntary loss of urine associated with overdistension of the bladder.

Symptoms: Patients usually complain that they lose small amounts of urine day and night, feel that they must void but cannot, void small amounts of urine and still feel full, void frequently at night, spend a long time at voiding and produce only a weak or dribbling stream.

Physical Findings: Usually none except for palpation of a urine-filled bladder. If neuropathy is the cause, neurologic examination may show sensory or motor deficits. If obstruction is the cause, vaginal relaxation or obstructing tumors may be demonstrated.

Laboratory Findings: A cystometrogram would be expected to show an atonic bladder of large capacity. A post-void residual urine volume would be expected to be large. When obstructive pathology is present, a voiding uroflowmetry study should show an obstructive pattern.

Therapy

Not uncommonly, patients will have mixed forms of urinary incontinence (usually urge and stress together), or they may have such complicating conditions as cystitis, respiratory disease, excessive fluid intake, use of diuretics, mental impairment, or emotional problems. A thorough evaluation is necessary before considering a method of therapy.

Algorithms have been proposed by the AHCPR for the management of urge incontinence and stress incontinence as follows:

Treatment methods include behavioral, pharmacologic, and surgical.

Behavior Methods

- Bladder retraining
- Timed voiding
- Prompted voiding
- Pelvic muscle exercises

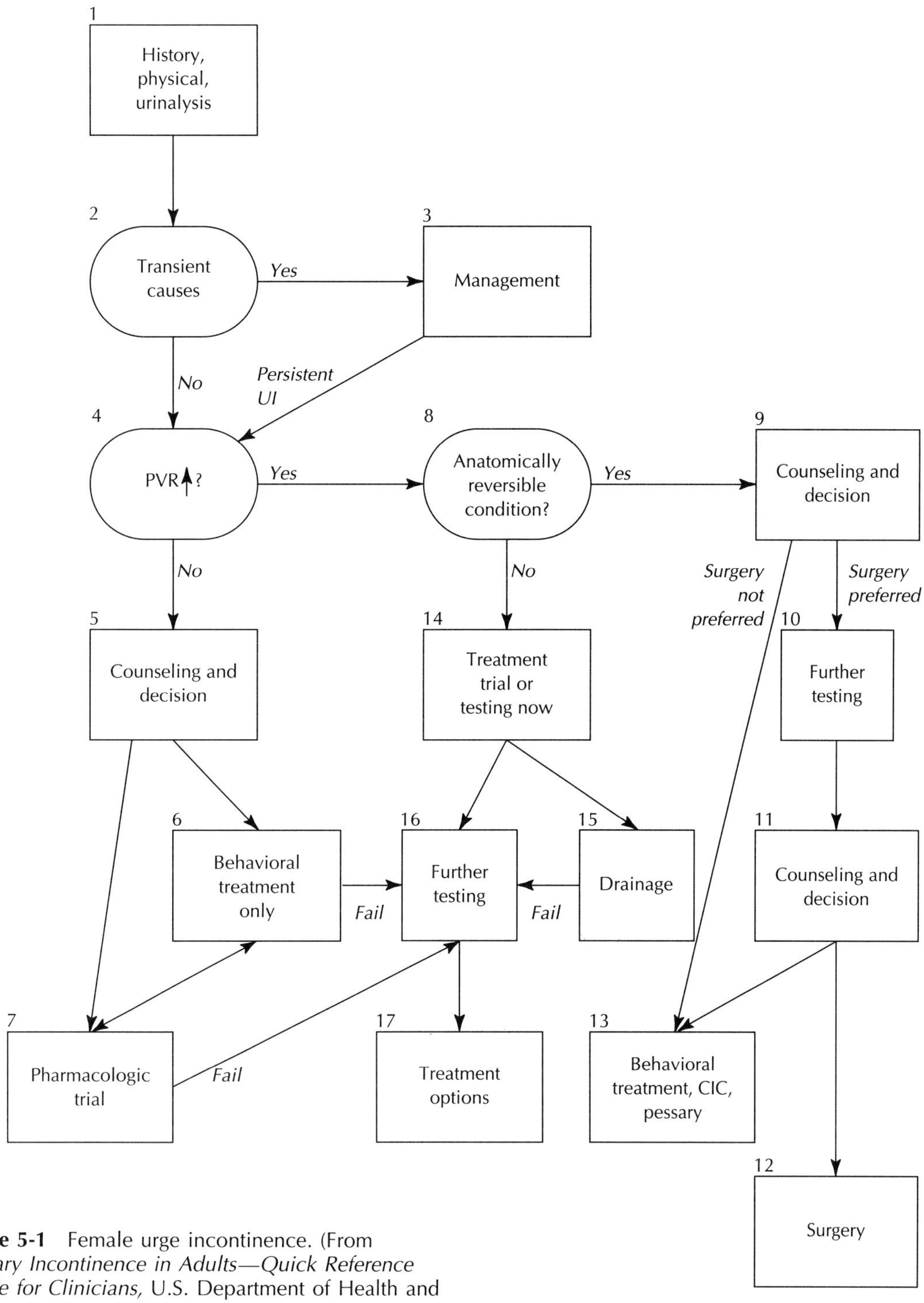

Figure 5-1 Female urge incontinence. (From *Urinary Incontinence in Adults—Quick Reference Guide for Clinicians,* U.S. Department of Health and Human Services, 1992.)

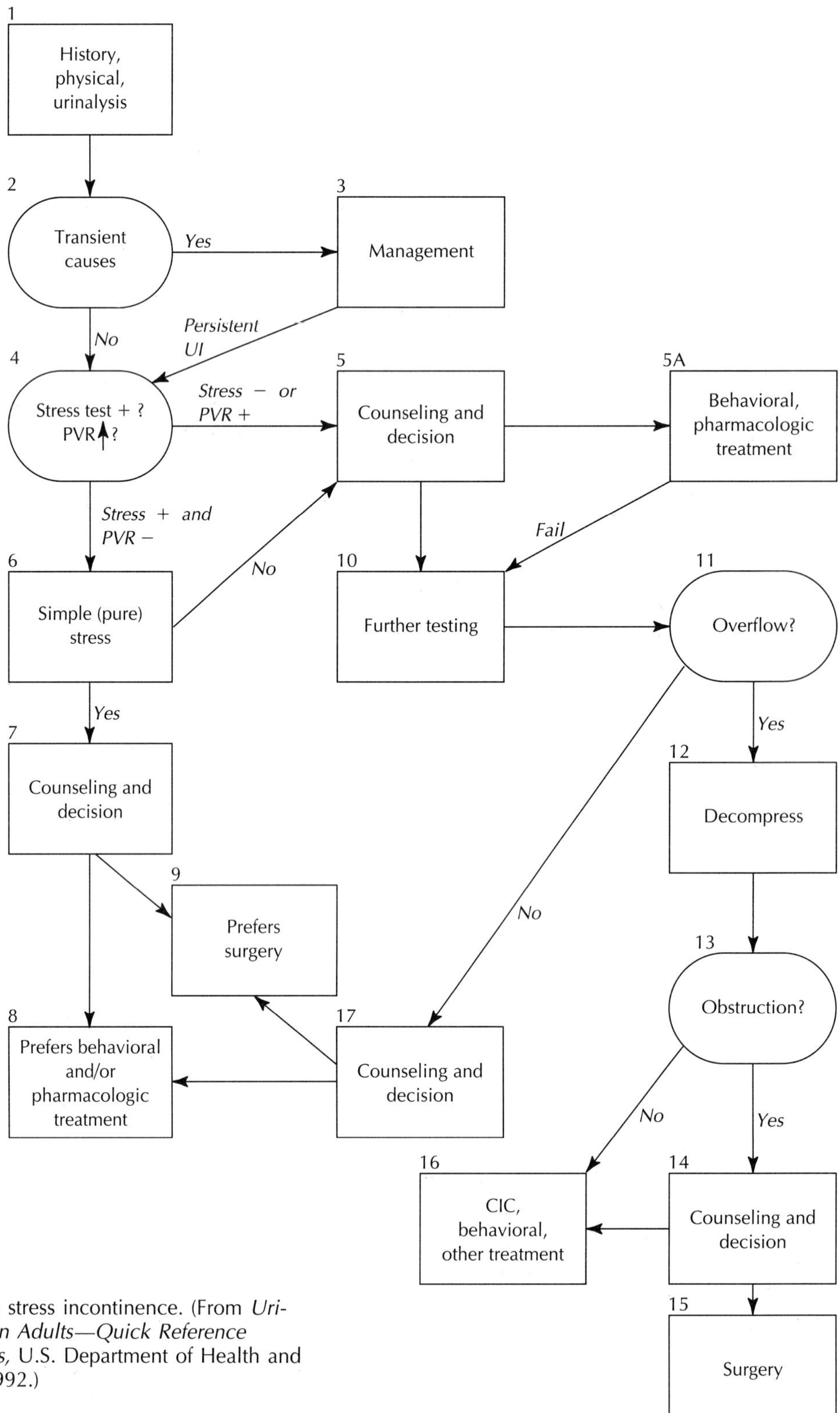

Figure 5-2 Female stress incontinence. (From *Urinary Incontinence in Adults—Quick Reference Guide for Clinicians,* U.S. Department of Health and Human Services, 1992.)

Adjunctive techniques include:

- Biofeedback
- Vaginal cones
- Electrical stimulation

Pharmacologic Therapy

Urge Incontinence: Drugs that have been used include propantheline, oxybutynin, tricyclic antidepressants, and terodiline. These have varying degrees of success and have significant side effects. Physicians prescribing them should be familiar with the risks and benefits before advocating their use.

Stress Incontinence: Drugs that have been used to treat urethral sphincter insufficiency as a cause of stress incontinence are phenylpropanolamine and estrogen. As mentioned above, the risks, benefits, and contraindications should be carefully evaluated by the physician for each patient before using these drugs.

Surgical Therapy

The various procedures devised for treatment of incontinence, their indications, contraindications, complications, risks and benefits are described elsewhere. However, the basic requirements are that the patient has had a work-up sufficiently complete to arrive at an accurate diagnosis and that there has been a trial of nonsurgical therapy of sufficient vigor and duration to assure that surgery is necessary. The operating surgeons should be entirely familiar with the patient's problem and should possess the skills necessary to perform a variety of procedures so that the correct one suited to the patient's specific needs can be performed.

References and Selected Readings

1. The Fifth Report of the Joint National Committee on Detection, Evaluation, and Treatment of High Blood Pressure; National Institutes of Health, 1993.
2. Nutrition Interventions Manual for Professionals Caring for Older Americans. American Academy of Family Physicians, The American Dietetic Association, and National Council on the Aging, Inc., 1992.
3. The Obstetrician-Gynecologist and Primary-Preventive Health Care. ACOG Primary Care Task Force, 1993.
4. Urinary Incontinence in Adults—Quick Reference Guide for Clinicians. Washington: US Department of Health and Human Services, 1992.
5. Hazzard WR (ed): Principles of Geriatric Medicine and Gerontology, 3d ed. New York: McGraw-Hill, 1994.

Part II

Preventive Health Care

6 Prevention

Vicki L. Seltzer

In the distant past, doctors saw only ill patients and they utilized whatever modalities were available to assist them. During the past several years it has become increasingly clear, however, that physicians can do an enormous amount for their patients by utilizing preventive strategies and helping patients to modify high-risk behaviors.

It has been estimated that one-half of premature deaths, one third of acute disabilities, and one-half of chronic disabilities are preventable. The health care team can play a leading role in reducing morbidity and mortality by identifying current or potential high-risk behaviors and emphasizing the importance of healthy life-styles to their patients.

Patient safety is one example of an area in which the health care team can have an important impact. Motor vehicle accidents are the leading cause of death for women between the ages of 13 and 39, and they contribute substantially to morbidity and mortality in all age groups. By simply reminding each patient of the importance of seat belt use for themselves, their passengers, and their families at each visit, and by emphasizing the risks of drinking and driving, the health care team can reduce the likelihood of fatalities. The use of bicycle helmets also should be encouraged.

While auto safety is an important preventive issue for most of the women we see, other safety measures that should be addressed may be more age-specific or season-specific. For instance, during winter, warnings about falls on the ice can be emphasized; in the summer, risks of excess sun exposure and skin cancer should be stressed.

Another important preventive strategy relates to patients' behavior and habits. Cigarette smoking contributes substantially to morbidity and mortality. The health care team should be committed to working with women in individual or group programs for smoking cessation and in counseling adolescents about the risks of smoking before they initiate this habit. Alcohol and drug use are also major contributors to morbidity and mortality. Physicians must be alert to signs of substance use and abuse, must ask direct questions, and must be willing and able to counsel their patients or to refer them when appropriate. Alcohol and drug use are serious and common problems for women in the United States, and physicians can play a role in reducing women's risk.

Exercise and diet are other areas that physicians should discuss with their patients. Proper dietary and exercise habits can substantially reduce the risk of many illnesses and disabilities. Decreasing the number of calories from fat, increasing the fiber content of the diet, maintaining dietary balance and reasonable body weight, and identifying a fitness program that will fit a woman's life-style and in which she will be willing to participate regularly are all important issues for the physician and patient to discuss.

With increasing frequency, sexual behaviors are placing women at risk. In addition to causing lower genital tract infection, sexual practices are placing increasing numbers of women at risk for HIV infection and for hepatitis. Women must be counseled regarding safe sexual practices. The physician must not assume that because a woman is a particular age, of an upper socioeconomic status, or married, that she is not at risk for sexually transmitted disease. Although these discussions are sometimes uncomfortable for the physician and/or the patient, morbidity and mortality can be prevented, and health care providers should be committed to addressing these issues. AIDS is currently the fifth leading cause of death in the United States for women between the ages of 19 and 39. The incidence of sexually transmitted hepatitis is increasing. Despite the difficulty that the physician and/or patient may have, if the physician discusses these issues with true concern for the well-being of the woman, most patients will respond by accepting the importance of the subject and appreciating the physician's concerns.

Prevention of unwanted pregnancy and preconception counseling are other preventive health care areas in which physicians can make major contributions.

Women's psychosocial needs have often been overlooked by the health care team. Here again physicians can have substantial impact in reducing morbidity and mortality. Treatable problems relating to depression, anxiety, and other disorders should be addressed. Women who are subject to domestic violence need to be identified and helped.

Cancer prevention and screening for premalignant and early invasive disease are important responsibilities for women's primary care providers. The mortality from invasive cervical cancer has fallen dramatically in the United States owing to pap smear screening programs. Breast cancer is now diagnosed in earlier, more readily treatable stages due to screening. Many cases of lung cancer are completely preventable with successful smoking cessation programs and behavior modification. The incidence of skin cancer has been rising dramatically. Physicians can help to modify this by patient education. Primary care physicians are in ideal positions to work with patients in screening and prevention programs to reduce cancer mortality.

Unfortunately, infections for which immunizations are available are still a cause of morbidity and even mortality. Clearly, adherence to immunization schedules can greatly reduce this problem, and primary care physicians need to make certain that their patients are being immunized.

For older women, physicians must work with their patients to provide accurate information about the prevention of osteoporosis and heart disease. Education regarding estrogen replacement therapy, exercise, calcium supplementation, and diet is important.

Each of these vital components of women's wellness and preventive health care is discussed in depth in various chapters of this book. It is clear that providing health care to women is not merely an issue of treating illness; at least as important, it is about preventing illness. This requires emphasis on patient education, so that women can play a role in maintaining their own health. Via dialogue and counseling, physicians can have a substantial impact on preventive care.

7 The Importance of a Detailed Personal, Social, and Family History

Albert B. Gerbie
Nanette K. Rumsey

To be successful as providers of primary care for women, clinicians must obtain thorough personal, social, and family histories in addition to performing accurate physical examinations. Effective preventive care, as well as care of specific medical problems, will best be achieved if appropriate emphasis has been placed on a detailed history.

Clinicians' skill, knowledge, and experience are most evident in the taking of a patient's history. In their approach to patient management they should elicit the historical data, perform the physical examination in an organized fashion, and order appropriate laboratory tests. They must then evaluate these data, formulate a logical differential diagnosis of the current illness, and make plans for long-term and preventive care. The history should include all the facts of medical significance up to the time a patient appears; each symptom must be given its own weight. The physician must know when to question more deeply for further details. While the physician will usually aid or guide the patient through the questions, one must avoid the power of suggestion in influencing the patient. Any symptom—trivial, remote, or the one of most concern to the patient—may be the actual key to the problem. Table 7-1 is an outline of the medical history. The focus is broad, with the intent of offering the patient more than the treatment of isolated ailments.

Obtaining such a complete history not only improves care, but also provides an opportunity to address health maintenance and disease prevention, and to initiate and establish a trusting doctor-patient relationship, which is a primary goal of the first and all doctor-patient encounters. Psychosocial issues may contribute enormously to a patient's well-being, and they should be given appropriate emphasis. An in-depth history will also allow the physician to provide appropriate patient education.

In addition, a thorough initial history will insure better outcomes for future problems. Specific examples to illustrate the importance of a thorough medical history are endless. Eliciting a history of past steroid use or an intensive care admission for asthma signals the need for careful pre- and postoperative pulmonary and adrenocortical evaluation. Eliciting a history of excessive bleeding from dental extraction in the patient or her family may uncover a blood dyscrasia (e.g., von Willebrand's disease), thereby avoiding catastrophic perioperative bleeding complications. Taking a thorough immunization history

TABLE 7-1 Medical History

- I. Biographical data
- II. Source of history
- III. Chief complaint and present illness
- IV. Past medical history
  - A. Allergies
  - B. Medications
  - C. Illness/hospitalizations
  - D. Surgery
  - E. Trauma
  - F. Bleeding tendencies
  - G. Transfusion history
  - H. Immunizations
- V. Obstetric and gynecologic history
  - A. Menstrual history
  - B. Sexual history
  - C. Contraception
  - D. Vaginal and pelvic infections
  - E. Pap smear history
  - F. Gynecologic surgery or procedures
  - G. Urologic history
  - H. Breast disease, mammography
  - I. Pregnancies
  - J. DES exposure
- VI. Family history
  - A. Breast, gynecologic, colon, or other cancers
  - B. Genetic diseases, congenital anomalies, twinning, preeclampsia
  - C. Hypertension, diabetes, cardiovascular disease, etc.
  - D. Psychatric and social
- VII. Social history
  - A. Habits—alcohol, tobacco, illicit drugs
  - B. Marital status
  - C. Living arrangements
  - D. Education
  - E. Occupation
  - F. Avocations
  - G. Diet/exercise
  - H. Psychosocial issues
- VIII. Review of systems
  - A. Head and neck
  - B. Cardiovascular/respiratory
  - C. Gastrointestinal
  - D. Genitourinary
  - E. Neurologic
  - F. Psychiatric

identifies the 10 percent of reproductive age women who are still susceptible to rubella, and it identifies those women needing hepatitis B vaccination. No physician should assume that someone else is supervising their patient's general medical status. Every physician should discuss with their patients the issue of who is the individual providing her preventive and screening services in order to make certain that there are neither duplications nor omissions.

Although emphasis must be on the chief complaint, present illness, and past medical history, the family history is exceedingly important. For instance, preventive care can be instituted for entire families if doctors uncover family clusters of colon, breast, and/or gynecologic neoplasms. Taking genetic and ethnic histories will improve the patient's primary care, preconception care, and neonatal outcomes. Unfortunately, the family history is frequently obtained in a routine, cursory fashion. To record the family history simply as "negative" may give an erroneous impression. One should specifically ask about the age, sex, and health of parents, siblings, and other close relatives. Abortions and stillbirths should also be noted. The age and cause of death of deceased relatives should be recorded.

The family history is the leading tool in clinical genetics and can provide important clues regarding the patient's illness. One must remember that the first principle of genetic counseling is to obtain an accurate genetic history, which includes an accurate diagnosis of the disease in question.

Carrier screening usually refers to identification of carriers (heterozygotes) of autosomal or sex-linked recessive disorders. In obstetrics, carrier screening provides prospective parents with reproductive alternatives such as prenatal diagnosis (with options of preparation for care, termination of pregnancy, or treatment of affected fetuses), artificial insemination, or deferral of childbearing. At present it is impossible to screen all individuals for even the most common disorders. Ideally, screening is based on the following criteria: availability of a simple, accurate, inexpensive carrier test; an ethnic, racial, or geographic heritage of increased risk for a specific genetic disorder; and the availability of treatment or reproductive options for the identified carriers. In the near future molecular genetic techniques will increase the reliability and the number of diseases for which carriers may be screened.

In addition to common genetic diseases, the family history should include inquiries about diabetes, heart disease, hypertension, gynecologic cancers, colon cancer, and breast disease. The physician should never lose sight of his or her role in providing preventive care and education to the patient and her entire family.

The psychosocial history is no less important than the medical and family histories. In addition to establishing rapport, taking this history can uncover maladaptive behaviors and identify support systems, both of which are important to patient compliance and outcome—e.g., home bed rest for an obstetric complication might be doomed to failure if family support were unavailable. In taking this personal and social history, it is important to use great tact to avoid embarrassing the patient and to reduce the possibility that the patient may repress or suppress facts.

Specific components of the social history should include tobacco use, alcohol intake, drug use, and any history of sexually transmitted diseases. To inquire about human immunodeficiency virus (HIV), the physician should inquire about the number of sexual partners, contacts with bisexual partners, blood transfusions, intravenous drug use in the patient or her sexual partner, and prostitution. There are characteristic historical and physical findings to suggest substance abuse (Table 7-2). Questionnaires have been devised to assist in screening for alcoholism (Table 7-3).

TABLE 7-2 Characteristics Which May Be Associated with Substance Abuse

Behavioral and Personal	Medical	Obstetric
Noncompliance with appointments	Drug overdose or withdrawal	No or little prenatal care
Difficulty concentrating	Cellulitis, abscesses, or phlebitis	Spontaneous abortion
Poor historian	Septicemia	Preterm delivery
Slurred speech or staggering gait	Bacterial endocarditis	Preterm rupture of the membranes
Bizarre or inappropriate behavior	Sexually transmitted diseases	Birth outside hospital
Psychiatric history	HIV seropositivity	Abruptio placentae
Child abuse or neglect	Tuberculosis	Sudden infant death syndrome
Domestic violence	Hepatitis	Fetal growth retardation
Alcohol or drug abusing partner	Pancreatitis	Fetal distress
Family history of substance abuse	Lymphedema	Intrauterine fetal death
Prostitution	Anemia	Congenital anomalies
Incarceration	Cerebrovascular accident	Fetal alcohol syndrome
Frequent emergency room visits	Myocardial ischemia or infarction	Neonatal abstinence syndrome
Chronic unemployment	Poor dental hygiene	
	Poor nutritional status	

SOURCE: From Verp.[11]

TABLE 7-3 The CAGE Questionnaire Used to Assess the Possibility of a Drinking Problem[a]

1. Have you ever felt you should Cut down on your drinking?
2. Have people Annoyed you by criticizing your drinking?
3. Have you ever felt bad or Guilty about your drinking?
4. Have you ever had a drink first thing in the morning to steady your nerves or get rid of a hangover (Eye opener)?

[a]A yes answer to two or three of the four questions strongly suggests the presence of alcoholism.

SOURCE: From Mayfield et al.[6]

Identifying living arrangements, marital status, and sexual orientation may help to assess stress levels. Occupational histories may reveal environmental hazards or exposures. Educational histories give clues to the amount of patient education needed to insure compliance. Even a patient's postoperative satisfaction and mental health can be predicted if the physician takes a thorough psychosocial history.

In *The Woman Patient: Medical and Psychological Interfaces,* Roeske identified factors that increased a woman's chance of having mental health problems within three months to three years after hysterectomy (Table 7-4). Many of these risk factors would be uncovered only with a very complete, but sensitive, history taking. These risk factors for adverse outcome after hysterectomy underscore the importance of viewing patients in a social context—viewing them not just as patients but as employers, workers, students, sisters, lovers, wives, and daughters. Only with such a broad focus can clinicians provide true primary and preventive care for women.

TABLE 7-4 Risk Factors for Mental Health Difficulties after Hysterectomy

Gender identity (Importance of uterus to a feminine self-concept)
Prior adverse reactions to stress
Personal or family history of depression or other mental illness
Multiple somatic complaints (especially low back pain)
History of multiple surgeries or hospitalizations
Desire for children/more children
Fear that surgery will decrease sexual desire or satisfaction
Partner with a negative view of hysterectomy, marital discord
Age less than 35 years at time of surgery
Lack of vocation or outside interests
Negative cultural or religious views of hysterectomy

SOURCE: From Roeske.[8]

As outlined here, thorough history-taking will provide the foundation needed to offer women high quality preventive and primary care, as well as optimal treatment and counseling.

References and Selected Readings

1. Brooten KE, Chapman S: *Malpractice: A Guide to Avoidance and Treatment.* Orlando: Grune & Stratton, 1987.
2. Dennerstein L, DeSenarclesn M, eds: *The Young Woman: Psychosomatic Aspects of Obstetrics and Gynecology.* Amsterdam: Excerpta Medica, 1983.
3. Droegemueller W, Herbst AL, Mishell DR, Stenchever MA: *Comprehensive Gynecology.* St. Louis: CV Mosby, 1987.
4. Grimes DA: Declining surgical caseload of the obstetrician–gynecologist. *Obstet Gynecol* 67:760, 1986.
5. Judge RD, Zuidema GD, Fitzgerald FT: *Clinical Diagnosis,* 4th ed. Boston: Little, Brown, 1982.
6. Mayfield D, McLeod G, Hall P: The CAGE Questionnaire: Validation of a new alcoholism screening instrument. *Am J Psychiatry* 131:1121, 1974.
7. Pearse WH, Mendenhall RC, Radecki SE, et al: Manpower for obstetrics-gynecology III. Contributions to total female medical care. *Am J Obstet Gynecol* 144:332, 1982.
8. Roeske NCA: Hysterectomy and other gynecological surgeries: A psychological view, in Notman MT, Nadelson CC, eds: *The Woman Patient: Medical and Psychological Interfaces.* New York: Plenum Press, 1978.
9. Scott N, MacGregor SN, Chasnoff IJ: Substance abuse in pregnancy, in Lin C, Verp MS, Sabbagha RE: *The High Risk Fetus.* New York: Springer-Verlag, 1993 p. 570.
10. Simpson JL, Elias S: *Essentials of Prenatal Diagnosis.* New York: Churchill Livingstone, 1993.
11. Verp MS: Genetic counseling and screening, in Lin C, Verp MS, Sabbagha RE: *The High Risk Fetus.* New York: Springer-Verlag, 1993, p. 166.
12. Verp MS: Substance abuse in pregnancy, in Lin C, Verp MS, Sabbagha RE: *The High Risk Fetus.* New York: Springer-Verlag, 1993, p. 570.
13. Wilson JR: Scientific advances, social trends, and the education and practice of obstetrician-gynecologists. *Am J Obstet Gynecol.* 162; 1135, 1990.

8 Preconception Counseling

John W. Larsen

It has been assumed traditionally that the likelihood of a successful pregnancy outcome is greatest when the mother-to-be is healthy and her pregnancy is kept free of hazards. Ideally, good health is the woman's natural state, and pregnancy is easily achieved and maintained with little cause for concern. Unfortunately, 3 to 5 percent of live births are affected by birth defects, and many more pregnancies end prematurely or are compromised in some way by maternal or fetal disorders. Physicians are challenged to improve the outcome of pregnancy for both mother and baby. One substantial contribution that physicians can make to help improve obstetric outcome is through actions taken prior to conception.

It has become popular in recent years to discuss preconception counseling as a specialized, goal-oriented physician encounter designed as a custom tune-up just prior to a very deliberate effort to conceive. This type of visit follows the traditional pattern of history, physical exam, diagnostic testing, and therapy for various conditions. A matrix of maternal disorders, fetal problems, and possible medical actions is contained in Table 8-1.

When Table 8-1 is considered on an item-by-item basis, it is clear that many of the potential problems can be considered and prevented in the course of routine health care many years in advance of a possible pregnancy. The earliest basis for preconception care is early pediatric care. For instance, routine childhood immunization against rubella and hepatitis B will eliminate concern regarding these potential perinatal pathogens in the reproductive years.

Education concerning sexually transmitted diseases, smoking, alcohol, and drugs may come from the family, school, and doctor's office. While cynics may observe that human failing in these areas is abundant, an ounce of prevention can still be more potent than a pound of cure. Consider this in the extreme, but not rare, context of a pregnant teenager who is HIV-positive. Many still have no knowledge of the disease, or think it is somehow limited to homosexual men.

A logical, but underutilized access point for the physician to introduce the topic of preconception care is the young woman's first gynecologic visit. Although that visit may be principally for the purpose of symptom evaluation (e.g., vaginitis or dysmenorrhea) or contraception, there still can be a positive exchange regarding the value of a healthy body for successful reproduction. Depending on the circumstances involved, this communication can be as short as a few words or expanded to include discussion of a pertinent linked topic, such as contraceptive methods that prevent STDs (and thereby preserve tubal function).

Good nutrition is integral to supporting a healthy pregnancy. An appropriate diet can be explained before conception and continued through pregnancy. This is particularly true regarding a therapeutic diet for disorders such as diabetes or phenylketonuria. Women who are overweight may wish to lose excess weight before pregnancy, but should not attept further weight loss after conception. Underweight women should correct dietary deficiencies prior to pregnancy.

TABLE 8-1 Preconception Matrix

Condition	Potential Problem	Action
Infections		
Toxoplasmosis	Acute maternal infection during pregnancy can cause fetal damage.	Check for antibody. • If positive, it is protective • If negative, and the patient is attempting to conceive, counsel her to avoid cat litter and to avoid ingestion of meat that has not been previously frozen or thoroughly cooked.
Rubella	Acute maternal infection during pregnancy can cause fetal damage.	Check for antibody. • If positive, it is protective. • If negative, immunize promptly. Defer pregnancy attempt for six weeks.
Cytomegalovirus (CMV)	Acute infection or chronic infection can cause fetal damage. Risk is much greater when first infection occurs during pregnancy.	Check for antibody. • If positive, check for viral shedding during pregnancy. Follow course of pregnancy with serial ultrasound and consider amniocentesis. • If negative, counsel to avoid direct contact with CMV. Important for health-care and day care contacts to wear latex gloves.
Hepatitis B	Acute or chronic infection during pregnancy can lead to fetal or neonatal infection. Baby may become lifetime HB_sAg carrier.	Check for HB_sAg. • If negative, consider immunization. • If HB_sAg is positive counsel patient about possible in-utero transmission, and prepare to immunize the child at birth.
Syphilis	Acute or chronic infection during pregnancy can cause fetal damage.	Check for antibody • If positive and no prior adequate therapy, give benzathine penicillin G.
Gonorrhea	Can cause cervictitis, salpingitis, infertility, post-partum sepsis, or localized infection. Gonococcal ophthalmia neonatorum can cause blindness in the newborn.	Diagnose by endocervix culture. Treat with ceftriaxone or other appropriate antibiotic for resistant strains.
Chlamydia	Can cause cervicitis, salpingitis, infertility, neonatal conjunctivitis, or neonatal pneumonia.	Diagnose by swab of endocervix for rapid test or culture. Treat with tetracycline (if the woman is not pregnant), erythromycin, or other appropriate antibiotics.
Human immunodeficiency virus (HIV)	Can increase maternal risk for other infections. Transmission to fetus approximately 30%.	Check for antibody. • If positive, counsel regarding ultimate outcome. • Consider contraception rather than pregnancy. • Employ antiviral therapy under protocol.
Genital herpes	Viral shedding at parturition can colonize baby, causing disseminated infection and damage.	Counsel regarding risk and plan C-section if infection active at parturition. Consider acyclovir for suppression at term.
Varicella	Acute maternal infection may cross placenta causing disseminated disease with residual damage in baby. Maternal varicella pneumonia can be fatal.	If no prior history of clinical varicella consider antibody testing and immunization prior to pregnancy. Consider zoster immune globulin for material prophylaxis following significant exposure of susceptible woman who is pregnant or attempting to conceive.

TABLE 8-1 Preconception Matrix (Continued)

Condition	Potential Problem	Action
Infections		
Tuberculosis	Congenital tuberculosis is rare. Maternal disease may become symptomatic during pregnancy. Treatment with isoniazid has potential neurotoxicity for mother and baby.	Skin test if negative history. Chest x-ray followed by completion of chemotherapy, if appropriate, prior to conception.
Maternal diseases		
Diabetes (insulin-dependent)	Poor control increases rate of spontaneous abortion, fetal anomalies, and fetal macrosomia.	Check for acute and chronic complications of diabetes, including measurement of renal function. Counsel regarding risks and need for preconception strict control of diabetes to lower abortion rate, anomaly rate, and during pregnancy to prevent macrosomia. Monitor control by glucose testing and glycosylated hemoglobin.
Hyperthyroidism	Thyroid storm can be fatal. Thyroid suppression therapy can cause fetal goiter. Long-acting thyroid stimulator leads to neonatal thyrotoxicosis.	Stabilize with propylthiouracil and possible surgery before pregnancy. Avoid I^{131} when pregnancy is being considered.
Seizures	Various antiseizure medications can cause fetal anomalies.	Wean off medication if possible. If not, counsel regarding risk and adjust dose to lowest effective range.
Cystic fibrosis	Pregnancy can be fatal if pulmonary function is marginal.	Assess pulmonary function and counsel. Consider contraception rather than pregnancy.
Phenylketonuria	Mental retardation and anomalies in fetus if maternal phenylalanine level is in toxic range.	Low phenylalanine diet before and during pregnancy.
Spina bifida	Fetal risk for NTD; pregnancy may hamper maternal function (varies depending on the extent of preconception deficit).	Begin folic acid 1mg qid 1 month before conception and continue during pregnancy.
Heart disease	Pregnancy can be fatal if preconception cardiac function is marginal. Increased rate of fetal cardiac disease.	Reevaluate cardiac function and counsel. May need contraception.
Renal disease including transplant	Pregnancy can be fatal if marginal renal function preconception. Premature delivery is likely particularly if pregnancy induced hypertension occurs.	Reevaluate renal function including success of prior pregnancy if any. Counsel; may need contraception.
Cystic acne	Maternal treatment with 13-*cis*-retinoic acid during pregnancy can cause multiple severe malformations.	Use effective contraception, and counsel before starting 13-*cis*-retinoic acid.
Smoking	Decreases fertility and may lead to lower birth weight.	Counsel to stop or severely limit. Consider nicotine weaning program preconception.
Narcotics	Addiction of fetus, brain damage, and prematurity. Placental abruption more frequent. Associated risks for STDs and needle-transmitted infections.	Counsel to stop. Consider methadone program if appropriate.

(continued)

TABLE 8-1 Preconception Matrix (Continued)

Condition	Potential Problem	Action
Infections		
Alcohol	Fetal alcohol syndrome associated with steady use throughout pregnancy. Risk increases with increased consumption.	Stop alcohol use.
Caffeine	May be associated with decreased fertility and increased spontaneous abortion rate.	Stop or minimize caffeine consumption.
Family history, ethnicity, or genetic susceptibility		
Neural tube defect (NTD)	NTD in fetus.	Begin folic acid preconception, counsel regarding MSAFP, sonar, and amniocentesis during pregnancy.
Jewish	Tay Sachs disease Gaucher's disease	Screen for carrier status preconception.[a]
Mediterranean	Beta thalassemia in fetus.	Screen for carrier status preconception.[a]
African	Sickle cell disease	Check for carrier status.[a]
Northern European	Cystic fibrosis	Check for carrier status.[a]

[a]Counsel regarding prenatal diagnosis by CVS or amniocentesis if both partners are carriers.

Daily folic acid supplementation may be wise for all women of reproductive age. As little as 0.4 mg of folic acid daily has been shown to significantly decrease the occurrence of neural tube defects (NTDs). Since roughly 50 percent of pregnancies are "planned," daily dosing by a multivitamin tablet containing folic acid would ensure the benefit whether or not a pregnancy is deliberate.

The physician's office setting may also encourage education that promotes preconception counseling through a variety of patient brochures, video educational aides, and physician-extender support staff. A nurse, a physician's assistant, or a genetic counselor can expand on topics that may be particularly pertinent to the individual patient. This type of office visit may be a good opportunity to screen for genetic traits according to ethnicity (Table 8-1), such as sickle trait, thalassemia minor, or carrier status for Tay Sachs disease or cystic fibrosis.

A genetic counselor can be particularly helpful in situations that require study of the family tree for disease or carrier identification or for explaining statistical risks for fetal damage due to disease, genetic factors, or environmental hazards. The genetic counselor's work generally is easier if the patient is not yet pregnant. Even if invasive testing (such as CVS or amniocentesis) is recommended for diagnosis during pregnancy, this advice is given with less decision stress during contemplation of pregnancy, rather than in the first or second trimester of pregnancy.

Beyond urging healthy women to stay that way, the physician has a mission to begin to give preconception advice concomitant with the diagnosis and management of certain medical conditions that will affect a subsequent pregnancy. A representative selection of such conditions is included in Table 8-1. Women with chronic or relapsing infections (such as genital herpes or persistent hepatitis B antigenemia) need to know about the possible changes in their perinatal management. Women who are diagnosed with potentially fatal disorders such as advanced insulin-dependent diabetes, sickle cell disease, cystic fibrosis, severe renal damage, or HIV infection may wish to avoid pregnancy completely.

Physicians giving ongoing medical care to patients with chronic medical disorders such as diabetes, hypertension, renal disease, seizure disorders, hyperthyroidism, autoimmune disorders, and asthma should introduce the issue of pregnancy and make certain that appropriate detailed information is provided to the patient. This may require referral to an obstetric generalist, medical geneticist, or maternal-fetal medicine subspecialist as appropriate to individual circumstances.

When pregnancy is being considered, the physician should review all medications, including nonprescription agents. Certain medical treatments, such as 13-*cis*-retinoic acid for acne, antiseizure medications, antithyroid medications, and chemotherapy for cancer, can be hazardous to the fetus. Women who require such treatment should be advised to use effective contraception while under medical treatment, or in the case of seizure disorders or hyperthyroidism, only to get pregnant when medical control has been optimized, and the risks of therapy have been understood and accepted.

In many urgent or emergent situations it is easy to say that preconception counseling is extraneous to the problem at hand or ''not medically necessary.'' It is very important for primary care physicians to realize that preconception advice can and should be integrated into the broad spectrum of health services for women as a part of overall preventive care.

References and Selected Readings

1. Creasy RK, Resnick R: *Maternal-Fetal Medicine: Principles and Practice,* 3d ed. Philadelphia: WB Saunders Co, 1994.
2. *Immunization during Pregnancy*. Technical Bulletin #160. Washington: American College of Obstetricians and Gynecologists, 1991.
3. Infante-Rivard C, Fernandez A, Gauthier R, et al: Fetal loss associated with caffeine intake before and during pregnancy. *JAMA* 270:2940–2943, 1993.
4. Kitzmiller JL, Gavin LA, Gin GD, et al: Preconception care of diabetes: Glycemic control prevents congenital anomalies. *JAMA* 265:731–736, 1991.
5. Nora JJ, Fraser FC, Bear J, et al: *Medical Genetics,* 4th ed. Philadelphia: Lea & Febiger, 1994.
6. Recommendations for the use of folic acid to reduce the number of cases of spina bifida and other neural tube defects. *MMWR* 41:107, 1992.
7. Sever JL, Larsen JW, Grossman JH: *Handbook of Perinatal Infections,* 2d ed. Boston: Little, Brown, 1989.
8. *Teratology*. Technical Bulletin #84. Washington: American College of Obstetricians and Gynecologists, 1985.
9. *The Obstetrician-Gynecologist and Primary-Preventive Health Care*. Washington: American College of Obstetricians and Gynecologists, 1993.
10. Werler MM, Shapiro S, Mitchell AA: Periconceptional folic acid exposure and risk of occurrent neural tube defects. *JAMA* 269:1257–1261, 1993.

9 Nutrition and Maintenance of Appropriate Weight

Anne B. Namnoum

Diet has always played an important role in health and disease. In the past, nutritional deficiencies were associated with several diseases, such as rickets, scurvy, and beriberi. Undernutrition remains a problem in many parts of the world, but in the United States the abundant food supply has decreased (although certainly not eliminated) the incidence of diseases of nutritional deficiency. Instead, diseases related to dietary excess and imbalance now rank as some of the leading causes of death. Studies have shown that coronary artery disease, stroke, diabetes mellitus, atherosclerosis, and some types of cancer have nutritional risk factors. Obesity has been clearly associated with several diseases, including hypertension, diabetes mellitus, and atherosclerosis. Osteoporosis and diverticular disease may also have nutritional risk factors. Proper nutrition and weight control can thus be viewed as important preventive health measures.

Dietary Recommendations

The U.S. Department of Agriculture, the U.S. Department of Health, and the U.S. Surgeon General have established dietary guidelines for Americans that aim to reverse nutritional patterns that may increase the risk of chronic diseases. Patients should be encouraged to:

1. Eat a variety of foods.
2. Maintain a healthy weight.
3. Choose a diet low in fat, saturated fat, and cholesterol.
4. Eat adequate vegetables, fruits, starch, and fiber.
5. Use sugars only in moderation.
6. Avoid excess sodium.
7. Consume alcohol in moderation if at all.

Clinicians should periodically assess the nutritional patterns of their patients, and provide counseling regarding the recommended intake of calories, fat, cholesterol, complex carbohydrates, fiber, sodium, calcium, and iron. The average individual should have a caloric intake less than or equal to her estimated daily energy expenditure (Table 9-1).

TABLE 9-1 Estimated Daily Energy Expenditure for Women

Category	Age	Median Weight (lb)	Median Height (in)	DEE[a] (kcal)
Nonpregnant	15–18	120	64	2200
	19–24	128	65	2200
	25–50	138	64	2200
	50+	143	63	1900
Pregnant				
1st trimester				2200
2d trimester				2500
3d trimester				2500
Lactating				2700

[a]DEE (Daily Energy Expenditure), estimated based on light-to-moderate activity.

SOURCE: Adapted from National Research Council, Food and Nutrition Board. Recommended Dietary Allowances, 10th edition. Washington, D.C.; National Academy of Sciences, 1989.

Fat and Cholesterol

Total intake of fat should not exceed 30 percent of the daily caloric intake, and saturated fats should be limited to less than 10 percent of calories. Diets high in fat have been linked to increased risks of atherosclerosis and coronary artery disease, some types of cancer, and obesity. One practical way to reduce fat and cholesterol in the diet is to limit the consumption of meat, fish, and poultry to approximately 6 oz/day, choose lean meats, remove skin from poultry, limit the use of butter and oils, and use low-fat dairy products.

Vegetables, Fruits, and Grain Products

Consumption of vegetables, fruits, and grain products should be encouraged. These foods are low in animal fat and cholesterol, and are good sources of numerous vitamins, minerals, and fiber. Certain vegetables and fruits, especially those which are dark green, yellow, and orange, also may be associated with decreased susceptibility to several types of cancers, perhaps owing to their carotenoid or dietary fiber content. Increased intake of dietary fiber improves gastrointestinal motility, and may be helpful in preventing diverticular disease.

Sugar and Salt

While dietary complex carbohydrates are encouraged, refined sugar and sweets are high in calories while providing few nutrients, and thus should be limited. Reduced intake of refined sugars also may decrease the incidence of dental caries.

Salt should be limited to approximately 6 g/day, since doing so is thought by some to possibly decrease the risk of hypertension. The consumption of processed foods that contain high levels of sodium should be avoided, and added salt should be limited when possible. Lemon juice and herbs may be used to flavor foods as an alternative to salt.

Alcoholic Beverages

Excessive alcohol consumption increases the risk of chronic liver disease, hypertension, heart disease, neurologic diseases, nutritional deficiencies, and many other disorders. Alcohol consumption while driving or operating machinery is also associated with accidental injuries and death.

Calcium

Calcium is essential for normal growth, development, and maintenance of bones. More calcium is needed during growth, pregnancy, and lactation than at other times. The Recommended Daily Allowance (RDA) for calcium in different age groups is listed in Table 9-2. Recent evidence has shown that older women may have an increased need for calcium, in

TABLE 9-2 Recommended Daily Allowance (RDA) for Calcium

Category	Age (years)	RDA (mg)
Adolescence	11–18	1200
Adulthood (Nonpregnant)	19+	800
Pregnant	19+	1200
	under 19	1600
Postmenopause[a] (taking estrogen)		800

[a]Postmenopausal women who are not on estrogen replacement require more calcium.

part because of their decreased absorption of the mineral. Calcium intake can be maintained without excessive dietary fat by the use of skim and low-fat dairy products and calcium supplements.

Osteoporosis affects 15 to 20 million Americans, and has direct and indirect costs to Americans of over 7 billion dollars annually. The two most important contributing factors to osteoporosis are postmenopausal estrogen deficiency and a chronically low intake of calcium. The key to the prevention of osteoporosis is to maximize peak bone mass and decrease the rate of bone loss in later years. It is well-documented that estrogen replacement by postmenopausal women is effective in preventing osteoporosis, but an adequate intake of calcium throughout one's lifetime is also important. The National Institutes of Health (NIH) consensus panel on osteoporosis recommended 1500 mg calcium/day for postmenopausal women not on estrogen replacement therapy. In addition, calcium supplements may be indicated for some individuals who are unable to meet their calcium needs through diet.

Vitamins and Minerals

Most healthy individuals who conform to the above dietary guidelines will meet or exceed the RDA for vitamins and minerals, and thus will have no need for supplements. Adequate dietary iron is important to maintain iron stores and prevent iron-deficiency anemia. Menstruating women should include iron-rich foods in their diet, and iron supplements may be indicated during pregnancy owing to increased iron requirements. Vitamin D supplementation may be indicated for those who receive minimal exposure to sunlight or have fat malabsorption.

Diet and Cancer

Some types of cancer have been linked with nutritional risk factors, but conclusive evidence is not yet available. While epidemiologic comparisons of various countries have shown an association between dietary fat consumption and cancer of the breast, colon, and prostate, case-control studies have not shown a causal effect on cancer development. Based on current knowledge, the National Cancer Institute, the National Research Council, and the American Cancer Society have established the following dietary guidelines for cancer prevention:

1. Avoid obesity.
2. Decrease total fat intake to 30 percent or less of total calories.
3. Increase intake of whole-grain foods.
4. Increase intake of dark green, deep yellow, and orange vegetables.
5. Eat salt-cured, smoked, and nitrite-cured foods only in moderation.
6. If alcohol is used, it should be used in moderation.

Nutrition in Pregnancy

Nutrition and healthy eating habits are especially important during pregnancy. Caloric requirements increase during pregnancy, as do requirements for nearly all vitamins and minerals. Iron, folic acid, and vitamin D requirements are doubled, while requirements for other nutrients increase more modestly (Table 9-3). Folic acid and iron are the two nutrients

TABLE 9-3 Recommended Daily Allowances for Nonpregnant and Pregnant Women

Nutrient	Nonpregnant[a]	Pregnant	% change
Folic acid (μg)	180	400	+122
Vitamin D (IU)	200	400	+100
Iron (mg)	15	30	+100
Calcium (mg)	800	1200	+50
Vitamin B_6 (mg)	1.6	2.2	+38
Vitamin B_1 (mg)	1.1	1.5	+36
Vitamin E (mg)	8	10	+25
Zinc (mg)	12	15	+25
Vitamin B_2 (mg)	1.3	1.6	+23
Protein (g)	50	60	+20
Vitamin C (mg)	60	70	+17
Magnesium (mg)	280	320	+14
Energy (kcal)	2200	2500	+14
Nicotinic acid (mg)	15	17	+13
Vitamin B_{12} (mg)	2	2.2	+10
Vitamin A (μg)	800	800	no change
Vitamin K (μg)	65	65	no change

[a]Based on women 25 to 50 years of age.

most likely to be inadequate in a pregnant woman's diet, and are thus important components of prenatal supplements.

Recent data suggest that the periconceptional use of folic acid may decrease the incidence of neural tube defects. Women who are considering pregnancy should be advised to eat a diet high in folic acid (spinach, leafy green vegetables, broccoli, grains) or to consider a multivitamin supplement with 0.4 mg of folate.

Calcium requirements increase 50 percent above nonpregnant levels to 1200 mg/day during pregnancy. Pregnant women should increase their dietary calcium to meet these requirements, or take calcium supplementation when dietary calcium is insufficient.

An individual with a normal weight should gain approximately 25 to 35 lbs during pregnancy; an underweight individual should gain slightly more. The pattern of prenatal weight gain is useful information for the physician when charted according to week of gestation (Fig. 9-1).

Exercise

Regular exercise is an important means of improving health, increasing caloric expenditure, and preventing obesity. Physical activity is known to decrease the risk of coronary artery disease. Weight-bearing exercise also may reduce bone loss in postmenopausal women. Even small increases in activity may have significant health benefits.

Women should be encouraged to exercise on a regular basis when circumstances allow. A reasonable initial goal would be to walk for 30 min at least three times a week. Activity can then be increased gradually, with an ultimate goal of vigorous aerobic exercise three to four times per week. The exercise plan should be tailored to the needs and life-style of the patient.

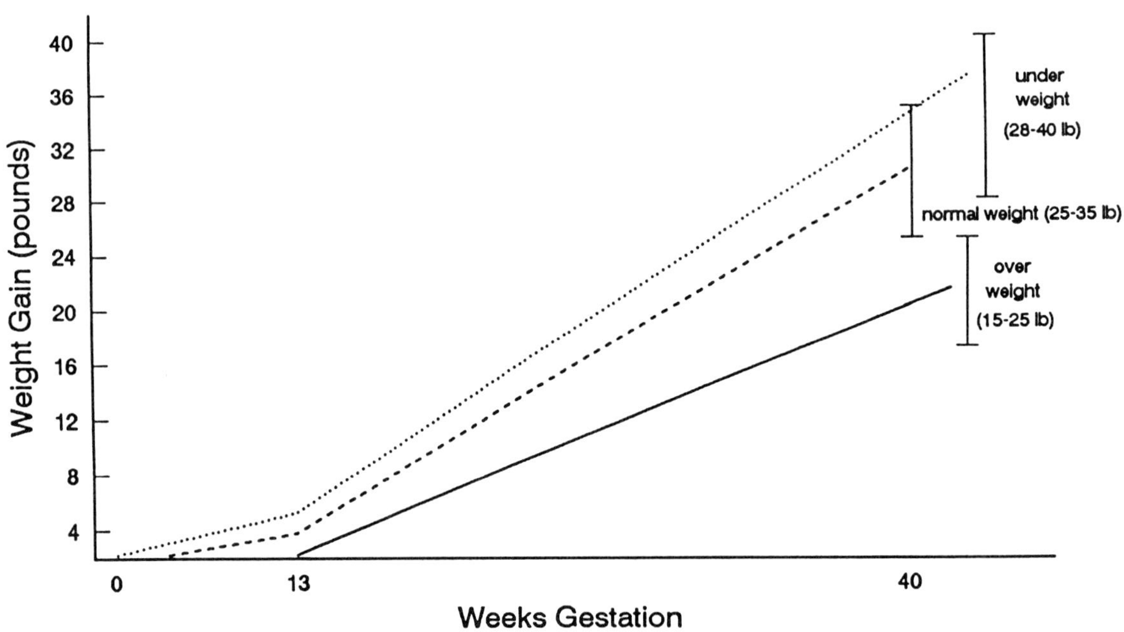

Figure 9-1. Recommended weight gain during pregnancy by maternal pregravid weight status. (Reprinted with permission from Luke B, Keith L: *Principles and Practice of Maternal Nutrition.* Park Ridge, N.J.: Parthenon Publishing Group, 1992, after National Academy of Sciences: *Nutrition during Pregnancy.* Washington, D.C.: National Academy Press, 1990.)

Disorders of Nutrition

Obesity

Obesity has long been considered a health hazard, but recently has been clearly associated with hypertension, diabetes mellitus, atherosclerosis, and several gynecologic disorders. Obesity may also influence the risk of cancer of the colon, breast, and endometrium. Obese individuals have increased morbidity from these and other illnesses, and have reduced life expectancy. Up to 45 percent of Americans are more than 20 percent overweight, and up to 15 percent of Americans are more than 40 percent overweight, making obesity one of the major health risks in our society.

Diagnosis of Obesity Obesity may be defined as the storage of excess calories as fat. Techniques of measuring body fat range from simple and inexpensive to complex and costly. Estimates of body fat may be made with skin-fold measurements, ultrasound of subcutaneous adipose tissue thickness, or densitometry (determined by measuring the water displaced when an individual is submerged in a tank of water). More complex techniques may be used to measure total body fat or percentage body fat, such as total body electrical conductivity, total body potassium, dual photon absorptiometry, electromagnetic scanning, or bioelectrical impedance.

For practical purposes, however, weight tables and/or anthropometric measurements are often used in the clinical setting to define the degree of obesity. The body mass index (BMI) is the body weight (kg) divided by the height (m) squared, and can be obtained from a nomogram (Fig. 9-2). The BMI correlates fairly well with body fat, but an individual with significant muscle mass may have a high BMI without having excess fat.

Accurate measurements of height and weight are the initial steps in the clinical assessment of a patient. The degree of overweight can be expressed as a percentage above the ideal body weight (from a table), or the BMI can be used to assess the severity of the weight problem. As there is a statistically significant increased mortality at 20 percent above ideal body weight, the physician should recommend dietary intervention when a patient approaches this range. A BMI of 27.3 in women similarly warrants intervention.

Body fat distribution should also be assessed, as some types of fat distribution have been associated with greater health risks. Two main patterns of fat distribution have been described. In android obesity, fat is primarily deposited in the central abdominal region. In gynecoid obesity, fat is distributed in the gluteofemoral regions. The patterns can be defined by the ratio between the waist and hip measurements. A waist/hip ratio greater than 0.8 in women may be a predictor of complications of obesity. Android obesity is more strongly associated with insulin resistance, diabetes mellitus, and cardiovascular disease. Gluteofemoral obesity is associated with fewer health risks. Hypertension and hyperinsulinemia may be present, but tend to be less severe. Varicose veins and problems in weight-carrying joints are more common with gynecoid obesity. Deposition of fat in the gluteofemoral region is thought to serve as a storage source for energy during pregnancy and lactation. Adipose cells in the gluteal and femoral regions have lower rates of lipid turnover than do abdominovisceral adipose cells.

Obesity in Pregnancy Obesity may pose special health risks during pregnancy. The incidence of morbid obesity in pregnancy is as high as 10 percent of all pregnancies. Obese women have a higher incidence of antepartum complications such as preeclampsia, hypertension, diabetes, and urinary tract infections (Table 9-4). Severely obese women may also have a higher incidence of cesarean section than non-obese pregnant women, either due to the higher incidence of antepartum complications, or to an increased incidence of cephalopelvic disproportion. Obese women are more likely to have a macrosomic infant, even when they are not diabetic, putting them at risk for shoulder dystocia during a vaginal delivery.

In view of these potential complications, obese patients should be encouraged to lose weight *before* becoming pregnant. When an obese patient is pregnant, she should be carefully monitored for the maternal complications noted above. A glucose screen should be performed between 24 and 28 weeks of gestation, and blood pressure should be observed

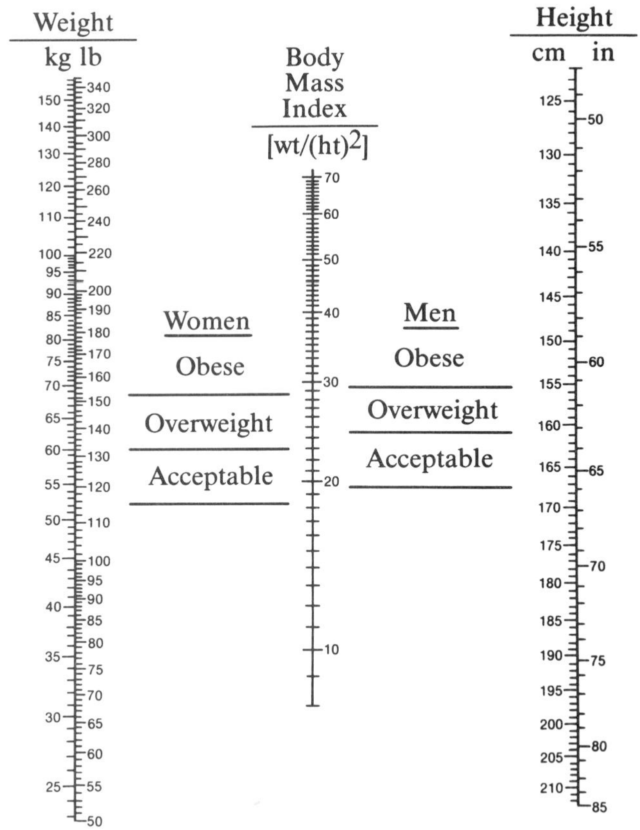

Figure 9-2. A nomogram for determining body mass index (BMI). Place a ruler between the column for height and the column for weight, connecting an individual's measurements. Read the BMI where the straight line crosses the middle line. (Copyright © 1985, *The Medical Journal of Australia;* 142: 52–58. Reprinted with permission.)

closely. Ultrasonography may be necessary to follow fetal growth and watch for macrosomia, and preparations should be made at delivery for the possibility of shoulder dystocia.

Treatment of Obesity In view of the health risks associated with obesity, weight reduction can be viewed as an important preventive health measure. The seemingly simple goal is to reduce caloric intake and/or increase energy expenditure. Unfortunately, the successful treatment of obesity is not easily achieved. Significant weight loss is difficult, and maintenance of weight loss is even more challenging. The resulting situation can be one of frustration for both the patient and the physician.

The objectives of treatment are to promote weight loss, prevent weight gain, reduce the medical complications associated with obesity, and promote psychological well-being. The best form of treatment for the mild to moderately obese person is a combination of diet, behavior modification, and exercise (Table 9-5). The goal should be a realistic target weight, with a 4- to 5-lb weight loss per month. Faster rates of weight loss are unrealistic and can lead to a sense of failure.

Diet An ideal weight-loss diet consists of approximately 1200 kcal per day, is well-balanced, and con-

TABLE 9-4 Complications of Obesity in Pregnancy

A. Maternal Complications
   - Chronic hypertension
   - Preeclampsia
   - Diabetes
   - Urinary tract infections
   - Perioperative/anesthetic risks
   - Wound breakdown

B. Fetal Complications
   - Macrosomia (birth trauma)
   - Shoulder dystocia
   - Hypoglycemia

TABLE 9-5 Treatment for Mild to Moderate Obesity

A. Dietary changes
  1. Choose caloric level (1200–1400 kcal/day for women)
  2. Recommend nutritionally adequate diet:
     Protein—1.5 g/kg ideal body weight
     Carbohydrates—100 g or more
     Fat— < 30% of calories, or <40 g
     Vitamins, minerals—Recommended daily allowances
     Water—1 liter or more
  3. Advise minimizing alcohol, refined sugar, fats

B. Behavioral changes
  1. Instruct patient to keep food diary
  2. Advise how to avoid situations associated with increased food intake
  3. Check in with patients frequently
  4. Recommend support groups

C. Exercise: Encourage regular exercise 3–4 times/week
   Walking
   Swimming
   Exercise bicycle

tains adequate vitamins and minerals. Adequate carbohydrates are necessary to spare protein and avoid ketosis. Sufficient protein is needed to maintain lean body mass and avoid potentially life-threatening side effects such as cardiac arrhythmias. The diet should be low in fat; evidence suggests that a reduction in fat intake, even without a reduction in total calories, may result in weight loss. Fat should be limited to less than 30 percent of the total calories, or approximately 40 g.

Weight loss is faster during the first days of dieting, owing to a loss of glycogen with its associated water loss; a loss of 1 lb of glycogen involves a loss of 3 lb of water. After several days, weight loss is slower, and the dieter may become frustrated if not warned to expect this. Physicians should monitor patients every 3 to 4 weeks in order to assess progress, modify the treatment plan if necessary, and provide support.

Behavior Modification Behavioral changes are an important part of treatment if long-term weight loss is to be achieved and maintained. Food diaries can be used to record times and amounts of food intake, and the situations associated with overeating can then be avoided. Healthier eating habits, decreased snacking, and greater self-control are the objectives. Patients may be advised to prepare smaller portions and to eat more slowly. Techniques to prevent relapse are helpful in maintaining weight loss, such as contacting a support group or engaging in some other preplanned activity when an urge to overeat occurs.

Exercise Exercise alone is not a very effective treatment for obesity because of the amount of exercise required to burn a given number of calories (Table 9-6). The combination of exercise and caloric restriction *is* beneficial, however. Exercise has been shown to decrease insulin levels, blood pressure, and lipid levels, and strenuous exercise causes a temporary decrease in appetite.

Pharmacologic Therapy Pharmacologic agents have been used to increase the effectiveness of weight-loss programs. These drugs can work by decreasing appetite, inhibiting food absorption, or stimulating fat utilization. Most currently available pharmacologic agents are catecholaminergic compounds that have side effects and potential for addiction. Phenylpropanolamine (PPA) is the agent in over-the-counter anorectics. The short-term use of such drugs has been shown to achieve greater weight loss than placebo, but long-term use is not advisable owing to potential problems with addiction and tolerance. In addition, unless long-term dietary and lifestyle modifications are made, the weight lost while utilizing medication will often be regained.

There is growing interest in the use of serotonin agonists such as fenfluramine and dexfenfluramine in the treatment of obesity. These act differently than the amphetamine-like agents, and tend to de-

TABLE 9-6 Approximate Calories Expended in Various Activities

Activity	Calories (per 30 min)
Complete rest	50
Walking	150
Bicycling	200
Swimming	200
Tennis	250
Jogging	350
Running (fast)	450

crease food intake by diminishing meal size and prolonging appetite suppression following a meal. In addition to their anorectic activities, these agents also appear to have a thermogenic effect, and thus may counteract the decrease in basal metabolic rate that occurs with dieting. These drugs have been shown to result in a significantly greater weight loss than placebo, but weight gain occurs when the drug is discontinued. At high doses, serotonin agonists may cause hallucinations or nightmares, but addiction does not seem to be a problem.

As new drugs are proven to be safe and effective in the treatment of obesity, it is possible that long-term pharmacologic therapy may be used, in conjunction with calorie restriction and healthy lifestyle, in the chronic treatment of obesity, just as long-term medical therapy is used in the treatment of hypertension or diabetes mellitus.

Very Low Calorie Diets More drastic modes of therapy may be indicated in cases of severe obesity when traditional diets have failed. ''Very low calorie diets (VLCD)'' or ''supplemental fasts'' are liquid diets that contain 600 to 800 kcal/day and are used for more than one week. Current formulations contain high-grade protein, some carbohydrates, and essential vitamins and minerals. Older versions of these diets used in the 1970s were associated with sudden deaths due to cardiac arrhythmias or myocardial atrophy, believed due to poor quality protein or lack of vitamins and minerals. Very low calorie diets are contraindicated in childhood, pregnancy, lactation, advanced age, and in individuals with serious medical conditions. The diet should only be used under medical supervision, including regular measurements of electrolytes and electrocardiograms. Results of VLCDs show significant weight loss after three to six months (40 to 60 lb), especially when behavioral therapy is included. Much of this weight is regained, however, as shown by long-term follow-up studies.

Jaw wiring has been used with severely obese patients to force adherence to a liquid diet when all other measures have failed. Patients must understand that this is not a cure for obesity, but merely a temporary means of enforcing caloric restriction. The difficult problem of preventing weight regain remains.

Surgical Therapy In selected cases of severe, intractable obesity, surgical treatment may be indicated. Lipectomy, the removal of excess skin and adipose tissue, is not a treatment for obesity, but may be used as a cosmetic adjunct after significant weight loss in order to remove ''sagging'' skin. The most common surgical methods currently used are vertical gastroplasty (gastric stapling) and gastric bypass. Gastric restriction procedures reduce food intake by causing discomfort and/or nausea when the gastric pouch is overdistended. Gastric bypass procedures cause further discomfort when ''dumping''occurs into the small intestine. Some malabsorption may also play a role in weight loss. Weight loss with these methods is significant, averaging 60 percent of excess weight. Perhaps more importantly, associated health risks such as hypertension, diabetes mellitus, and hyperlipidemia are improved in over 90 percent of cases.

The surgical treatment of obesity is not without complications, however. Perioperative complications may occur, as well as such long-term complications as cirrhosis, diarrhea, gallstones, vitamin deficiencies, and arthritis. The most common ''complication'' is weight-loss failure. Gastric restriction procedures can lose effectiveness by gradual enlargement of the gastric pouch. Patients can also acquire the ''maladaptive'' behavior of ingesting calorie-dense foods that negate the effect of the reduced meal size. The risks and benefits of surgical therapy must be weighed, but for morbidly obese patients who have failed all other modes of therapy, surgery may be warranted.

Follow-up Obesity is a chronic and relapsing problem that carries with it significant morbidity and mortality. The etiology is poorly understood, and treatment is often unsuccessful. As with other chronic diseases, such as hypertension or diabetes mellitus, long-term therapy and close follow-up are indicated. Patients should be given every available means of support, and should not be blamed for lack of ''will-power'' when therapy fails. Many patients can benefit from membership in weight-loss support groups such as Weight Watchers, Overeaters' Anonymous, or other local support groups. As research sheds further light on the etiology of obesity, more effective treatment modalities may become available.

Anorexia Nervosa and Bulimia

Anorexia nervosa is an eating disorder characterized by an intense fear of gaining weight, a body weight 15 percent below that expected, a distorted body image, and amenorrhea. Bulimia refers to recurrent episodes of binge eating associated with self-induced vomiting or other forms of purging. Bulimia often begins during a period of dieting, and it has been estimated that 5 percent of obese individuals are bulimic. Any patient who continues to lose weight long after her ideal weight has been attained or who shows evidence of binge eating or purging should be evaluated further, and referred for psychiatric therapy if needed. Other findings that may suggest an eating disorder include:

1. Amenorrhea for several months.
2. Rigid avoidance of certain foods.
3. Compulsive, intensive aerobic exercise.

The complications of anorexia nervosa include metabolic abnormalities, hypothalamic amenorrhea, cardiac arrhythmias, and death. The complications of bulimia include, in addition, gastric dilatation, pancreatitis, enlargement of the parotid glands, and severe dental erosions.

The treatment of anorexia nervosa and bulimia depends on the severity of the problem and the associated psychopathology. Significant medical complications may warrant hospitalization with inpatient therapy. In milder cases, the patient should be followed closely to monitor weight, eating patterns, and attitude. Education plays an important role in overcoming the preoccupation with food and fatness. Antidepressant medications may be helpful in some cases.

Conclusion

Nutrition plays a significant role in heatlh and disease prevention. Clinicians should periodically assess a patient's dietary habits and offer dietary guidelines regarding intake of calories, fat, cholesterol, fiber, salt, sugar, and alcohol. Height and weight should be assessed, and dietary intervention recommended when weight exceeds 20 percent of ideal body weight, or BMI exceeds 27.3. All patients should be encouraged to participate in regular physical exercise appropriate to their needs. Other eating disorders such as anorexia nervosa and bulimia must be recognized and treated.

References and Selected Readings

1. Apfelbaum M, Fricker J, Igoin-Apfelbaum L: Low and very-low calorie diets. *Am J Clin Nutr* 45:1126–1134, 1987.
2. Björntorp P, Brodoff BN: *Obesity*. Philadelphia: JB Lippincott; 2:580, 1992.
3. Bray GA: Obesity: Definition, diagnoses, and disadvantages. *Med J Australia* 142:S2, 1985.
4. Casper RC: The pathophysiology of anorexia nervosa and bulimia nervosa. *Ann Rev Nutr* 6:299, 1986.
5. Department of Health and Human Services: *The Surgeon General's Report on Nutrition and Health*. Washington: U.S. Government Printing Office, 1988.
6. Food and Nutrition Board, Natural Research Council: *Diet and Health; Implications for Reducing Chronic Diseases*. Washington: National Academy Press, 1989.
7. Food and Nutrition Board, Natural Research Council: *Recommended Dietary Allowances*, 10th ed. Washington: National Academy Press, 1989.
8. Gross T, Sokal RJ, King KC: Obesity in pregnancy: Risks and outcome. *Obstet Gynecol*. 56:446–450, 1980.
9. U.S. Preventive Services Task Force: *Guide to Clinical Preventive Services*. Baltimore: William & Wilkins, 1989.
10. Luke B, Keith L: *Principles and Practice of Maternal Nutrition*. Park Ridge, NJ: Parthenon Publishing Group, 1992.
11. Mulinore J et al: Periconceptual use of multivitamins and the occurrence of neural tube defects. *JAMA* 260:3141, 1988.
12. National Academy of Sciences: *Nutrition During Pregnancy*. Washington: National Academy Press, 1990.
13. National Research Council, Committee on Diet, Nutrition, and Cancer: *Diet, Nutrition and Cancer*. Washington: National Academy Press, 1982.
14. Sullivan AC: Drug treatment of obesity: A perspective, in Berry EM, Blondheim SH, Eliahou E, et al (eds): *Recent Advance in Obesity Research,* vol 5. London: John Libbey, 1987, pp 293–299.
15. Van Italie TB. Health implications of overweight and obesity in the United States. *Ann Intern Med*. 103:983–988, 1985.

10 Cancer Epidemiology, Screening, and Prevention

Joanna M. Cain

One of the major roles of the primary care provider is to work with patients to reduce their risk of developing a malignancy and to involve patients in screening programs so that if a malignancy develops it can be identified in an early, more treatable form. Cancer is, in part, a genetic disease propelled by either inherent underlying genetic instability or destabilization due to environmental stimulation or damage at the cellular level. There is no way to prevent, nor even to identify, all exposure to potential carcinogens in the air, the food we eat, or the sun. Furthermore, until better methods are identified for restructuring the genes with which we are born, we cannot avoid risks associated with our own known or spontaneously occurring genetic changes. However, the careful application of the information gleaned from epidemiologic and screening studies can be used to help patients to decrease their risk for malignancy.

Lung Cancer

Epidemiology and Prevention

Lung cancer, the leading cause of cancer death in American women, is the disease associated with the most clear-cut interaction with preventable carcinogens. Both tobacco and asbestos have been implicated in different histologic types of lung cancer.[10–12] As the number of women who smoke has increased, so has the incidence of lung cancer in women. The physician's role in health prevention clearly is counseling and support for smoking cessation.[18] Asbestos-free workplaces and asbestos abatement programs are national initiatives worthy of physician support and patient education. Lung cancer is a disease that, like most cancers, increases in incidence with age.[25] It represents 11 percent of cancers in women.

Screening

Multiple guidelines have been published to evaluate the likelihood that a particular screening test or procedure will be cost-efficient as well as effective.[36] The incidence of the disease should be high in the population, and screening should have a major clinical impact. Screening for a cold virus is not worthwhile because its clinical impact is relatively small, even if the frequency of colds is high. In addition, the preclinical phase does not allow us to intervene to prevent the cold. For a program of cancer screening to be worthwhile, it must identify a premalignant or preclinical phase, so that screening can significantly improve survival. Lung cancer, as an example, is an important clinical problem with subsequent disability and death rates that warrant early intervention. Whether or not there is the capability to identify a significant early malignant or premalignant phase with screening programs that can ultimately improve survival is still an open question.

Screening studies focused on chest radiograms and sputum cytology have failed to show a survival advantage at the present time. These studies included randomization between screening and usual care[14] and between cytology and chest radiographs versus radiographs alone in male smokers over age 45.[22] While the first study showed a tendency toward earlier stage disease in the cancers found in the screened group, in neither that group nor the second was there any difference in mortality. These studies were done in a generally younger population. The highest incidence of lung cancer, however, is in men 65 and older, so these studies do not reflect directly the potential benefits of such screening. Furthermore, the studies excluded women, and the natural history of the disease as well as screening in that population has not been adequately described. While no advisory group recommends screening for lung cancer at this time, it must be acknowledged that the potential benefits or lack of benefits for women or the elderly are unknown.

Recommendation

Encourage patients not to smoke and assist them with smoking cessation. Specific screening for lung cancer is not currently recommended.

Colorectal Cancer

Epidemiology

For women in the United States, colorectal cancer represents the second most common malignancy. This is a cancer that can have a significant inherited tendency. One affected first-degree relative can increase the risk twofold.[37] There are also familial syndromes carrying an increased risk of breast, endometrial, ovarian, and colorectal cancers.[19] Therefore, careful family histories, including both maternal and paternal lines and several generations of family relationships, are important to assess risk and identify patients with a higher potential incidence of colorectal or other malignancies. This higher potential incidence suggests that screening in such populations might be more effective, although definitive studies are not feasible given the relatively small numbers of such patients.

Prevention

There is clear evidence that dietary factors play a role in the development of colon cancers.[34] Recent literature is replete with theories about the presence of toxins, versus transit time, versus stimulation from a high dose of a single food type as the mechanical initiating event for these cancers, and yet the cause remains a mystery. Epidemiologic data give some guidelines in that diets high in fiber and low in fat can considerably decrease the incidence of disease.[28]

Screening

Colon cancer, like lung cancer, is an important clinical problem with subsequent disability and death rates that warrant early intervention. Furthermore, there is a premalignant lesion detectable[13] as an adenoma or neoplastic change. Finally, one potential screening test is relatively cheap and specific for blood in the stool (95 percent), although not specific for colon cancer itself.[33] Fecal occult blood testing (FOT) is only 50 to 78 percent[11,33] sensitive for the diagnosis of colon cancer. Because of its low cost and general patient acceptability (versus invasive procedures), FOT has the best characteristics of screening tests. However, as noted, it tests for blood, not cancer. One major medical organization recommends a six-slide occult blood test annually for patients over 50 years. Others recommend initiating this annual screening at age 40. Others debate this because of the high false positive rate.

Sigmoidoscopy is another potential means of screening, but a major impediment to its utility is poor patient acceptance.[2] Studies of sigmoidoscopy as a screening tool have been compromised by patient failure to comply, and presently may not present strong evidence that this form of screening is cost-effective.[29] Furthermore, the pattern of colon cancer epidemiologically seems to be shifting to a higher incidence in the right colon, an area not accessed by sigmoidoscopy.[6] Flexible sigmoidoscopy may be more comfortable and may confer greater patient acceptability, but the cost per examination still may make its use as a screening tool a problem.[29] Despite its questionable status as a screening test and the problems inherent in poor patient compliance in outcomes of screening studies, it is currently recommended by many that sigmoidoscopy screening begin for the average risk individual at the age of 50, with a repeat one year later. If both tests are normal, repeat every three years. Others debate the routine use of sigmoidoscopy.

Rectal examinations can diagnose the approximately 10 percent of bowel cancers that occur in the distal rectum.[16] They obviously will fail to diagnose the 90 percent of colorectal cancers that are higher. Yet, women commonly have routine screening pelvic examinations on a yearly basis, and the inclusion of a rectal examination for women adds no cost and minimal increased discomfort to the exam.

Serum screening tests hold promise for more specific detection of all cancers, although the presently available serum measure of carcinoembryonic antigen has lacked specificity and has been too costly to promote as a screening tool.[3] The obvious problems as such tests develop will be cost, specificity, and sensitivity, with the potential for overtreatment of patients with false-positive tests.

Recommendation

Rectal examination at the time of pelvic examination for all women. Fecal Occult Screening Tests yearly after 40 years of age. Flexible sigmoidoscopy to begin at age 50, with repeat in one year and then, after two negative examinations, every three years. Patients with a strong genetic predisposition will need to have screening initiated much earlier, and may require screening by colonoscopy.

Breast Cancer

Breast cancer is discussed extensively elsewhere in this text. It is the most common cancer in women in the United States, occurring in approximately 180,000 each year, and resulting in approximately 46,000 mortalities annually.

Screening

In terms of screening, although there is variation among the guidelines espoused by different organizations, one set of guidelines for women who are not deemed to be "high risk" recommends:

1. Monthly breast self-examination.
2. Physician examination every three years until 40 years of age and then annually. (*Note:* Many physicians recommend that, even prior to age 40, breast examination by a health care provider should be performed yearly.)
3. A baseline mammogram between 35 and 40 years of age; every one to two years between 40 and 50 years of age; annual mammography after age 50.

Women who are at high risk for breast cancer, particularly at an early age, may require a more aggressive screening program and an earlier initiation of screening.

Recommendation

Careful evaluation of patient risk factors, including a family history, is important for each patient. Based on such evaluation, screening recommendations for breast cancer may need revision for individual patients. For the typical "normal risk" patient, the screening guidelines discussed above represent one appropriate option.

Skin Cancer

Epidemiology, Prevention, and Screening

The skin is the largest human organ and has the highest exposure to direct carcinogens, particularly sunlight. It is not surprising, then, that squamous cell and basal cell skin cancers are the most common form of cancer. They are not, however, usually associated with major disability or death.

Malignant melanoma of the skin is associated with increased mortality if not diagnosed early. There has been an increase in incidence, thought to be due to increased sun exposure.[27] Physicians should counsel patients regarding sun exposure and the use of sun block. In addition, skin self-examination and information regarding classic signs of melanoma are important health maintenance approaches for these cancers.

Vulvar cancer is a form of skin cancer, and, as such, will be considered in this section. Squamous cell cancer of the vulva has its highest incidence in elderly women, although during the past several years there has been increased incidence in younger women. Educating women regarding the disease, its symptoms, and proper self-evaluation or professional evaluation would be of benefit.

Malignant melanoma of the vulva is a rare disease with a significant mortality if not diagnosed early. The epidemiologic precursors of vulvar melanoma have not yet been elucidated. Removal of vulvar moles, because of the higher relative risk for malignancy, has been proposed by numerous authors. The actual effect of this on decreasing the incidence of vulvar cancer is unknown.[15]

Recommendation

Teaching of skin self-examination, including vulvar skin, should be a routine part of wellness care. All suspicious lesions must be removed and evaluated by a pathologist.

Cervical and Lower Genital Tract Cancer

Epidemiology

Cervical cancer rates have declined steadily in the United States since the 1950s. Even in the last 30 years, the expected number of cases has declined from 20,000 in 1960 to 13,000 in 1991,[35] with a lifetime risk of five per 10,000. The epidemiology of cervical invasive disease, however, retains the same risk factors delineated 30 years ago, at which time it was thought to have an infectious disease component and to be more common in women who had multiple sexual partners, early age of onset of sexual activity, and low socioeconomic status.[5] The search for a sexually transmitted agent involved in this process led to the identification of human papilloma virus (HPV) as integral to the development of such cancers.[17] Other carcinogenic cofactors implicated include smoking and nutritional factors. Furthermore, concurrent human immunodeficiency virus (HIV) infection is associated with a higher incidence of both preinvasive lesions and invasive cervical cancer. Advancing age is a significant risk factor, with the peak incidence between 45 and 60 years of age.[32] There is a twofold higher risk of cervical cancer in African-American, Hispanic-American, and Native American groups. See Table 10-1 for a summary of risk factors.

Prevention

Clearly, changes in sexual practices, encouraging later initiation of sexual intercourse, and limiting partners will decrease risk. Consistent use of male or female condoms may lower risk for transmission of both HPV and HIV.

TABLE 10-1 Risk Factors for Cervical Cancer

Strong:	Age
	Multiple sexual partners
	Early age of initial sexual intercourse
	Human papilloma virus infection
	Human immunodeficiency virus infection
	Low socioeconomic group
	Sexual partners who have multiple sexual partners
Moderate:	Smoking
	Nutritional factors
	Herpes simplex infections (questionable)

Screening

The Papanicolaou smear described by Papanicolaou and Traut in the 1940s[26] remains the classic of screening tests. Although it was never subjected to randomized controlled trials, the test is widely credited for the decline in invasive cervical cancer. The pap smear's success is dependent on important screening characteristics of the disease. For most cervical squamous cancers, there is a clearly defined, preinvasive process. The disease is curable if detected at a premalignant or an early stage. The cost of pap smear screening is low, and its specificity and sensitivity adequate. Repetition of pap smears decreases the false-negative rate.

The interval of screening remains somewhat controversial. Since most cervical dysplasia and invasive cancer is related to onset of sexual activity, screening should begin at that time—even if that is 14 years of age. Because of the large number of young adults who are sexually active by 18 years of age, recommendations have been made to initiate standard screening by age 18.

Once screening has been initiated, the interval between tests is somewhat controversial. Ideally, if a pap smear can identify a preinvasive lesion, the patient can have colposcopy, treatment, and follow-up and never develop cancer. Therefore, in theory, annual pap smears should be able to reduce the incidence of invasive cervical cancer further by identifying almost all cervical lesions when they are preinvasive. For this reason, a substantial percentage of physicians strongly recommend an annual pap test and pelvic examination. The 1993 American College of Obstetricians and Gynecologists Committee Opinion on routine cancer screening indicates that after a woman has had three or more consecutive, satisfactory annual pap smears with normal findings, the pap test may be performed less frequently at the discretion of the physician. It is clear that longer intervals of screening—at five years, for example—result in an increase in invasive cancers developed during the interval, but also in a decrease in the cost of screening. There are many arguments in favor of more frequent screening. These include the problem of false-negative smears, the concern about compliance problems and exceeding the interval, and the question of whether presumed historic patterns of progression are valid in all lesions. A study done by Shy and coworkers[31] showed a marked increase in invasive cancers when the interval of screening extended beyond three years.

Cessation of routine pap smear screening is problematic as well. Ideally, one could assume that by the age of 65, most women have accumulated a significant history of pap smear screening to guide further decision making. Unfortunately, studies of women over age 65 show that 25 to 55 percent have never been screened.[21] Furthermore, of those previously screened, one study found that only 26 percent had been regularly screened. It would be a great error to assume that a woman 65 or older has been screened and to fail to assess or recommend such screening. For women who have been regularly screened and have always had negative pap smears, the benefit of further screening beyond age 65 is questionable.[24] Screening in the older woman must be assessed individually for past history of disease and screening, present exposure changes [new partner(s)], and symptoms.

Finally, the issue of screening intervals for women following hysterectomy needs to be addressed. In this circumstance, a screen for vaginal cancers every three years is suggested by various authors. Of concern are data suggesting that a substantial number of women will still have a cervix or cervical tissue after a ''hysterectomy.''[21] Appropriate screening for these patients can be assessed by careful review of present pelvic examination, review of the pathology for risk factors (e.g., a hysterectomy performed for dysplasia or invasive cancer obviously merits an aggressive screening schedule), and the patient's present risk behaviors. Patients with known infection with HIV, regardless of age, should receive regular pap smear screening.[20]

The issue of concurrent HPV subtype testing with pap screening is one of interest to practitioners and patients. As a screening tool, such tests may be very sensitive and specific for HPV, yet do not detect (nor are intended to detect) CIN or invasive cancer. Therefore, this would not be a screen for the present status of the cervix but, as proposed by some authors, a screen for potential future neoplastic behavior of the cervix. As such, some studies have used HPV testing as a triage for referral for further evaluation or recommendations for screening interval.[30] At present, there are no controlled trials demonstrating the added usefulness or cost-effectiveness of HPV testing for cervical dysplasia or invasive cancer.

Recommendation

All women who are or who have been sexually active or who have reached age 18 should undergo an annual pap test and pelvic examination. After a woman has had three or more consecutive, satisfactory annual examinations with normal findings, the pap test may be performed less frequently at the discretion of her physician. Most physicians recommend continued annual pap smears.

Ovarian Cancer

Epidemiology

Epithelial ovarian cancer is the most common ovarian malignancy, and is highly fatal even if relatively rare. In the United States, the lifetime risk for women is 1.6 percent. However, risk substantially increases in women over 65. Risk factors for the disease include a family history of ovarian cancer, a personal history of breast cancer, older age, and activity of the ovary over time. Both nulliparity and late menopause seem to confer a higher likelihood of developing this malignancy.

Prevention

Prevention would be the first choice for this cancer and, there is evidence that suppression of ovarian function with birth control pills will substantially diminish the risk of this disease.[1] Clearly for any given woman the risks and benefits of oral contraceptives must be assessed, and it is not recommended at present that women use oral contraceptives for the sole purpose of reducing ovarian cancer risk.

Another potential method of prevention for women who are at very high risk of ovarian cancer is removal of the ovaries. The degree of protection conferred by this mechanism for patients with hereditary ovarian cancer syndromes is incomplete. Extraovarian ''ovarian carcinomas'' have been reported in a small number of women who had an oophorectomy because of a hereditary risk. Despite this, recommendations for prophylactic oophorectomy for individuals at clearly documented very high risk for hereditary ovarian cancer are suggested by many groups. For women with one first-degree relative with ovarian cancer, the risk of developing the disease is 5 percent. Prophylactic oophorectomy as an independent operation is not recommended for these women. With two first-degree relatives the risk of developing ovarian cancer is 7 percent. However, 3 percent of women in this latter group have a genetic syndrome which is believed to be associated with an autosomal dominant gene with 80 percent penetrance. If a woman inherits this gene she has an 80 percent risk of developing ovarian cancer. Clearly prophylactic oophorectomy is appropriate for these women.

Screening

Screening for ovarian cancer remains controversial for multiple reasons. First, the incidence in the general population is too low for any but the most specific and low-cost screens to be cost-effective. Second, the presence of a premalignant phase is suggested by some retrospective and pathologic work, but would need to be a prolonged phase to accommodate a reasonable interval between screenings. The concurrent finding of adjacent areas of benign epithelium and transitional epithelium next to malignant epithelium does not insure a premalignant phase in the development of the malignancy. Routine pelvic examination, vaginal and abdominal ultrasound, Doppler studies, and serum marker studies (particularly Ca-125) have been studied, but cost-effective screening for the entire population remains elusive. Ca-125 is not a specific marker for ovarian cancer; in addition, levels may be normal in women who have ovarian cancer. Furthermore, in younger women the value of the Ca-125 can vary throughout the menstrual cycle. Vaginal ultrasound has been widely promoted as a screening tool, but the studies done have failed to deal with the issue of cost versus benefit. They also are structurally difficult because of the failure to assess concurrent control groups or the lack of long-term differences in mortality. In addition, most women who have had surgery because of abnormal findings on screening studies did not have ovarian cancer.

Those most likely to benefit from such screening are the groups at higher risk because of hereditary factors. Even in these women, where every six-month evaluation with pelvic exam, Ca-125, and ultrasound has been proposed, there is no evidence yet of an increase in overall survival for women who are screened. Furthermore, such studies depend solely on historic controls for assessment of efficacy, which will make effective evaluation of these screening methods difficult, if not impossible. Further discussion regarding the use of these diagnostic tools and ovarian cancer can be found in the chapter on malignant and premalignant diseases of the genital tract.

Recommendation

At present, there is no clear benefit for screening for ovarian cancers in any age population. However, the increased incidence of the disease in patients who have a hereditary predisposition suggests that screening these women may be beneficial. Participation in such screening should be understood to be of uncertain, but potential benefit at present. Finally, women who have specific genetic syndromes which place them at extraordinarily high risk for ovarian cancer require very careful evaluation, and the current recommendation for these women is prophylactic bilateral oophorectomy at the completion of childbearing or at least by age 35.

References and Selected Readings

1. ACOG Committee Opinion: Routine Cancer Screening 128:1–5, 1993.
2. American Cancer Society: American Cancer Society report on cancer related health check ups. *Cancer* 30:194–240, 1980.
3. Bates SE: Clinical applications of serum tumor markers. *Ann Int Med* 115:623–628, 1991.
4. Biesecker BB, Boehnke M, Calzone K, et al: Genetic counseling for families with inherited susceptibility to breast and ovarian cancer. *JAMA* 269:1970–1974, 1993.
5. Brinton LA, Fraumeri F: Epidemiology of uterine cervical cancer. *J Chronic Dis* 39:1051–1065, 1986.
6. Cady B, Stone MD, Wayne J: Continuing trends in the prevalance of right-sided lesions among colonrectal carcinoma. *Arch Surg* 128:505–509, 1993.
7. Cecchini S, Palli D, Casini A: Cervical intraepithelial neoplasia III: An estimate of screening error rates and optimal screening interval. *Acta Cytol* 29:329–333, 1985.
8. Collins FS. Medical and ethical consequences of human genome project. *J Clin Ethics* 2:260–267, 1991.
9. Daling JR, Chu J, Weiss NS, et al: The association of condyloma acuminata and squamous carcinoma of the vulva. *Br J Cancer* 50:533–535, 1984.
10. DeVos IH, Lamont DW, Hole DJ, Gillis CR: Asbestos and lung cancer in Glasgow and the west of Scotland. *BMJ* 306:1503–1506, 1993.
11. Diehl AK: Screening for colorectal cancer. *J Fam Pract* 12:625–632, 1981.
12. Eddy DM: Screening for lung cancer. *Ann Int Med* 111:232, 1989.
13. Fleischer DE, Goldberg SB, Browning TH, et al: Detection and surveillance of colorectal cancer. *JAMA* 261:580–585, 1989.
14. Fontana RS, Sanderson DR, Woolner LB, et al.: Lung cancer screening: The Mayo program. *J Occup Med* 28:746–748, 1986.
15. Friedman RJ, Rigel DS, Kopf AW: Early detection of malignant melanoma: The role of physician examination and self examination of the skin. *Cancer* 35:130–134, 1985.
16. Hertz REI, Deddish MR, Day E: Value of periodic examina-

tion in detecting cancer of the rectum and colon. *Postgrad Med* 27:290–294, 1960.
17. Kiviat N, Koutsky L: Specific human papilloma virus types as the causal agents of most cervical intraepithelial neoplasia: Implications for current views and treatment. *J Natl Cancer Inst* 85:934–935, 1993.
18. Kondo AT: The thoracic surgeon's role in smoking cessation and prevention. *Semin Thorac Cardiovasc Surg* 5:184–188, 1993.
19. Lynch H, Kullander S (eds): *Cancer Genetics in Women*. Boca Raton: CRC Press, 1987.
20. Mandelblatt J, Fahs M, Garibaldi K, et al: Association between HIV infection and cervical neoplasia: Implications for clinical care of women at risk for both conditions. *AIDS* 6:173–178, 1992.
21. Mandelblatt J, Gopal I, Wistreich M: Gynecologic care of elderly women. *JAMA* 256:367–370, 1986.
22. Melamed MR, Flehinger BJ, Zaman MB, et al: Screening for early lung cancer: Results of the Memorial Sloan Kettering Study in New York. *Chest* 86:44–47, 1984.
23. Miller AB, Baines CJ, To T, Wall C: Canadian national breast cancer screening study, 1: Breast cancer detection and death rate among women aged 40–49. *Can Med Assoc J* 147:1459–1476, 1992.
24. Muller C, Mandelblatt J, Schechter CB: *Cost and Effectiveness of Cervical Cancer Screening in the Elderly*. Office of Technology Assessment, Paper #4, Washington: U.S. Government Printing Office, 1990.
25. O'Rourke MA, Feussner JR, Feigel P, Laszlo J: Age trends of lung cancer stage at diagnosis: Implications for lung cancer screening in the elderly. *JAMA* 258:921–927, 1987.
26. Papanicolaou GN, Traut HF: Diagnosis of uterine cancer by the vaginal smear. New York: Commonwealth Fund, 1943.
27. Pollack SV. Skin cancer in the elderly. *Clin Geriatr Med* 3:715–718, 1987.
28. Reddy BS, Engle A, Simi B, Goldman M: Effect of dietary fiber on colonic bacterial enzymes and bile acids in relation to colon cancer. *Gastroenterology* 102: 1475–1482, 1992.
29. Rodney WM, Beaber RJ, Johnson R, Quan M: Physician compliance with colorectal cancer screening (1978–1983): The impact of flexible sigmoidoscopy. *J Fam Pract* 20:265–269, 1985.
30. Sheets E, Crum C: Current status and future clinical potential of human papillomavirus infection and epithelia neoplasia. *Curr Opin Obstet Gynecol* 5:63–66, 1993.
31. Shy K, Chu J. Mandelson M, et al: Papanicolaou smear screening interval and risk of cervical cancer. *Obstet Gynecol* 74:838–843, 1989.
32. Silverberg E, Lubera JA: Cancer statistics 1989. *Cancer* 39:3–7, 1989.
33. Simon J: Occult blood screening for colonrectal cancer: A critical review. *Gastroenterology* 88:820–837, 1985.
34. Weisberger JH: Cancer's relevant mechanisms, and prevention of large bowel cancer. *Semin Oncol* 18:316–336, 1991.
35. Wilkinson EJ: Pap smears and screening for cervical neoplasia. *Clin Obstet Gynecol* 33:817–821, 1990.
36. Wilson JMG, Junger G: Principles of early disease detection. *Public Health Pap* 34:27–32, 1968.
37. Winawer SJ, Zauber AG, Stewart E, O'Brien MJ: The natural history of colorectal cancer. *Cancer* 67:1143–1149, 1991.

11 Adult Immunization

Stanley A. Gall

While routine immunization has become an integral part of pediatric practices, the implementation of this concept has not been sufficiently widely incorporated into the health care of adult patients. The result is that adolescents and adults continue to become infected with vaccine-preventable diseases.

Vaccination has proved to be the most effective, cost-efficient means to prevent infectious diseases. The pioneering work of Edward Jenner in the eighteenth century using cowpox to prevent smallpox was the first rational, controlled effort to prevent human disease by vaccination. The first "man-made" vaccine was the attenuated virus vaccine developed by Pasteur in 1885. Inactivated vaccines were introduced in the 1890s.

The technology of cultivating virus in tissue culture, developed in the late 1940s, revolutionized the field of vaccine development. This led to the introduction of an inactivated polio vaccine in 1955 and a live-attenuated oral polio vaccine in 1962. Live attenuated vaccines against measles, mumps, and rubella were introduced in the late 1960s.

The technology of vaccine production improved with vaccines composed of highly purified capsular polysaccharides against three invasive bacterial pathogens, *Streptococcus pneumoniae, Neisseria meningitidis,* and *Haemophilus influenzae* Type b, introduced between 1974 and 1984. In 1986 the first vaccine for human use obtained from recombinant DNA technology was introduced for hepatitis B virus.

Despite impressive accomplishments with immunization programs, infectious diseases continue to kill many people for a number of reasons. First, vaccines for several infectious agents such as *Escherichia coli* and *Plasmodium falciparum* are unavailable. Second, there are numerous logistical problems in the distribution and administration of vaccines.

Third, there is insufficient funding for vaccine research and for vaccine administration. Fourth and probably most important, the general public often fails to understand and comply with recommended vaccine policies. An important public misconception relates to the risk-to-benefit ratio derived from vaccination. Unfortunately, the public perception is that vaccination is essentially free of risks and provides complete protection against disease. Vaccination does have some risks. Rare neurologic sequelae associated with the pertussis vaccine have resulted in a dramatic decrease in pertussis vaccine use and increased litigation.

In most circumstances, the benefits of appropriately indicated vaccination overwhelmingly outweigh the risks. It could reduce the unnecessary occurrence of vaccine-preventable diseases such as polio, diphtheria, tetanus, pertussis, measles, mumps, rubella, influenza, pneumococcal pneumonia, and hepatitis B virus, if health-care providers for adolescents and adults would provide vaccinations as a routine part of their practice. Patients with special life-style behaviors may present additional health problems. International travelers to certain countries may be at increased risk of exposure to vaccine-preventable diseases not present in the United States. In addition, foreign students, immigrants, and refugees either may bring diseases with them or may be exposed to vaccine-preventable diseases in the United States.

General Considerations for Adult Immunization

Organized Physician Programs for Vaccine Delivery

An immunization program is an important part of primary care. The immunization history of all new patients and periodic review of established patients is the starting point. Since the incidence of childhood diseases has been markedly reduced by immunization, a considerable number of adults have missed both immunization and natural infection. Because some diseases, such as measles, are more serious when they occur in the adult, the clinician should insure that patients are protected.

Unfortunately, an accurate immunization history is often difficult to obtain. The patient may have received immunizations from several sources in the past, and patients often do not keep accurate personal histories. However, the most reliable way to determine the patient's immunization history is from information obtained from the patient and her previous physician(s). As a general rule, if there is doubt about previous immunizations, assume that the patient is not immunized.

After obtaining a history, the physician must determine who should be immunized and establish a mechanism for offering necessary vaccines. Experience will indicate that all patients will need immunization except those whose history indicates prior immunization, or those who have a specific contraindication. The actual mechanisms for a successful vaccine program can be simple. The patient can fill out an immunization questionnaire and discuss it with the office nurse, who can indicate which vaccines are needed. Reminder notices can be by postcard or with other correspondence sent out by the office or clinic. Many approaches are successful but they must be initiated and supported with enthusiasm by the physicians involved.

Cost-Effectiveness of Vaccines

There are currently more than 50 types of vaccines in the United States, and some research is available to determine whether these vaccines are worthwhile (i.e., they have positive cost-effectiveness and cost-benefit ratios).

In the analysis of cost-effectiveness and cost-benefit, net medical care costs and net health benefits from the vaccination program are studied. Net medical care costs usually include the cost of the vaccine and its administration, the cost of treating vaccine related complications, and the medical care savings due to prevention of disease. Net health benefits from a vaccination program include reductions in morbidity and mortality from prevention of disease offset by any morbidity and mortality associated with vaccine side effects. Net health benefits may include gains in productivity from reduced absences from work.

Net medical care costs, net health benefits, and net health benefits expressed in dollar terms can all be used to evaluate a vaccination program. If the net benefits exceed costs, or if the ratio of benefits to costs is >1, the vaccination program is considered worthwhile on an efficiency basis. Also, net health-care costs per unit of health benefit can be calculated for different medical programs, with the lowest cost per unit of health improvement being the most cost-effective.

Cost-effectiveness and cost-benefit analysis have demonstrated that immunization programs against measles, pertussis, poliomyelitis, and rubella are clearly cost-effective. Pneumococcal and influenza vaccination programs are reasonably cost-effective, especially in older adults. Studies analyzing hepatitis B screening for health-care workers and other groups at risk have shown a vaccine program to be cost-effective. The cost-benefit analyses of other vaccines used in adult immunizations have not yet been studied.

Vaccine Administration

The package insert that accompanies the vaccine from the manufacturer should be consulted for each specific vaccine. The recommended route of administration should be followed. Adult vaccines usually are administered via the intramuscular (IM), subcutaneous (SC), or intradermal (ID) routes. The injections are usually given in the deltoid muscle in adults. The buttock is not recommended as a vaccine site because of possible injury to the sciatic nerve, and studies with the hepatitis B vaccine have shown its immunogenicity is significantly lower when given in the buttock rather than in the deltoid.

The recommended dose varies with different vaccines. The package insert is specific with regard to dose. There is no advantage to splitting the dose into two injections, and data suggest that the resulting protection could be compromised.

Most of the widely used vaccines are safe and effective when given on the same day. Inactivated vaccines can be given simultaneously at separate sites. Consideration should be given to separate days of administration when using vaccines known to cause pronounced local or systemic side effects (cholera and typhoid vaccines).

The antibody response to simultaneously administered live virus vaccines seems to result in appropriate titers for each without an increase in adverse reactions. Theoretical considerations suggest that live viruses not given on the same day should be given at least 1 month apart to prevent inhibition of the immune response. An inactive and a live virus may be given simultaneously at separate sites as long as the recommendations on the package insert are followed. Data would suggest that vaccination with cholera and yellow fever vaccines, either simultaneously or within 3 weeks of each other, can interfere with the levels of antibody produced by each vaccine. Therefore, these two vaccines should be given at least 3 weeks apart.

The immune globulin and various disease-specific immunoglobulins contain antibodies that can interfere with live attenuated virus vaccines. Passively acquired antibodies to measles, mumps, and rubella can interfere with the active replication of the vaccine virus and limit the antibody response by the patient. It is recommended that at least 6 weeks and preferably 3 months elapse between administration of passive immune globulin and active immunization. The response to oral polio and yellow fever vaccines is not inhibited by immune globulin. Additionally, inhibition of active immunity after an inactivated vaccine is not observed. These two vaccines can be given simultaneously or at any time after immune globulin. If a live vaccine has been administered and immune globulin is indicated, the minimal interval between them is 2 weeks. The patient subsequently must be tested to confirm seroconversion or the need for revaccination.

Contraindications and Misconceptions Concerning Adult Immunizations

Serious reactions such as anaphylaxis are rare. When serious hypersensitivity reactions occur, it is almost always a reaction to a component of the vaccine. These include residual animal proteins, antibiotics, preservatives, or stabilizers. Egg protein is the most common allergic component found in vaccines made from embryonated chicken eggs or chicken embryonal cultures (measles, mumps, influenza, and yellow fever vaccines). Persons who eat eggs may receive these vaccines, but they are contraindicated for patients with a history of anaphylaxis to eggs or egg protein.

Occasionally patients will have an anaphylactic reaction to the MMR (measles, mumps, rubella) vaccine. This is seen in those who have sensitivity to either neomycin or streptomycin, as the two antibiotics are present in the MMR vaccine. Vaccination is contraindicated in those patients. Currently, no licensed vaccine contains any penicillin, so patients allergic to penicillin can be vaccinated. On occasion a patient may experience a severe systemic reaction to cholera, typhoid, or plague vaccines. These reactions are most likely toxic reactions and are true hypersensitivity. Obviously revaccination should be avoided if possible.

Immunization with live virus vaccines should be avoided in individuals who are immunocompromised as the result of disease or medical therapy. Oral polio vaccine is contraindicated if any member of the family is immunocompromised since the usual spread of polio virus is via the fecal-oral route. In the same family the MMR vaccine can be given, because, although recipients can shed vaccine virus, infection is not transmitted to others. The use of oral or topical doses of corticosteroids likely to cause systemic effects contraindicates the use of live virus vaccines.

Most patients who do not receive vaccines do so because of misconceptions concerning adult immunization and *not* because of contraindications to the vaccination.[1] The following list addresses some of the more common misconceptions:

1. Reaction to a previous vaccination consisting of only mild to moderate local tenderness, redness, and/or swelling or fever < 40.5°C is not a contraindication to vaccination.
2. Mild, acute upper respiratory or gastrointestinal illness with fever < 38.0°C is not a contraindication to vaccination.
3. Current antimicrobial therapy or convalescence from a recent illness is not a contraindication to vaccination.
4. Pregnancy in another household contact is not a contraindication to vaccination.
5. Recent exposure to an infectious disease is not a contraindication to vaccination.
6. Breast-feeding is not a contraindication to vaccination.
7. Personal history of ''allergies'' including allergy to penicillin or other antibiotics, but not anaphylactic reactions to neomycin (MMR vaccine) or streptomycin (oral polio vaccine) is not a contraindication to vaccination.
8. Family history of ''allergies,'' adverse reactions to vaccination, or seizures is not a contraindication to vaccination.

Immunization for Healthy Adults*† (Tables 11-1 and 11-2)

Adolescents and Young Adults (15 to 24 years)

Most adolescents and young adults have completed a primary three-dose series of diphtheria and tetanus toxoid by this age. However, if immunization was either incomplete or not done in childhood, the three-dose series should be given. The first two doses should be given at least 4 weeks apart and a third dose 6 to 12 months after the second dose. Those who have completed the entire primary three-dose series should receive a booster dose every 10 years. The combined tetanus and diphtheria toxoids (for adult use) (Td) should be used. Persons whose immunization history is unknown should be considered unvaccinated and should receive the full three-dose primary series of Td.

All persons born after 1956 should have received measles vaccine unless they provide documentation of physician-diagnosed measles or laboratory evidence of immunity. Persons born before 1957 have

*Statements regarding assumptions about vaccinations and history of infection pertain to individuals born in the United States and continuing to reside there. For individuals born and/or living in other countries, the statements may or may not be applicable, depending on the country.

†Physicians should always read the package insert prior to using a vaccine with which they are not totally familiar.

TABLE 11-1 Vaccine Schedules for Adults[a,b]

Vaccine	Primary Schedule and Boosters	Indications	Contraindications and Precautions	Special Considerations
Tetanus-diphtheria toxoid	Two doses IM 4 weeks apart. A third dose 6 to 12 months after second dose. Booster every 10 years.	All adults	1. History of neurologic or immediate hypersensitivity following a previous dose. 2. History of severe local reaction after previous dose. 3. Do not give routine or emergency toxoids for 10 years. 4. Pregnancy not a contraindication.	
Measles vaccine	One dose SC, no routine boosters	1. Adults born before 1957 are immune. 2. For others, if no documented evidence of vaccination, give two doses of vaccine separated by at least one month. 3. Revaccination recommended for students entering college, health care workers, and international travelers.	Pregnancy, immuno-compromised patients, history of anaphylactic reaction following egg ingestion or receipt of neomycin.	1. MMR is vaccine of choice. 2. Live virus vaccine. 3. Persons vaccinated between 1963 and 1967 with a killed measles vaccine should be revaccinated with live measles vaccine.
Mumps vaccine	One dose SC, no booster	1. All adults without documentation of live vaccine or documented disease should be vaccinated. 2. Susceptible travelers. 3. No contraindication to older persons receiving vaccine	Pregnancy, immuno-compromised persons, history of anaphylactic reaction following egg ingestion or receipt of neomycin.	1. MMR is vaccine of choice if recipient is likely to be susceptible to measles and rubella as well as mumps. 2. Live virus vaccine.
Rubella	One dose SC, no booster	1. Adults lacking documentation of live vaccine or laboratory evidence of immunity.	Pregnancy, immuno-compromised persons, history of anaphylactic reaction following receipt of neomycin.	1. A theoretical risk to fetus if vaccinated in first three months of pregnancy is so small as to be negligible.

(continued)

TABLE 11-1 Vaccine Schedules for Adults[a,b] (Continued)

Vaccine	Primary Schedule and Boosters	Indications	Contraindications and Precautions	Special Considerations
		2. Particularly for reproductive age women and persons who work in hospitals, colleges, or on military bases. 3. Susceptible travelers should be immunized.		2. MMR is the choice of vaccine if patient is susceptible to measles and mumps too.
Polio	1. E-IPV is preferred for primary adult vaccination. 2. Two doses SC 4 to 8 weeks apart; third dose 6–12 months after second dose. 3. For adults who have completed primary vaccination and who need a booster; either E-IPV or OPV can be given. 4. For immediate protection either OPV or E-IPV is recommended.	1. Persons traveling outside of U.S. and all health care workers. 2. If an incomplete series of vaccinations was given as a child, the entire series with either OPV or E-IPV should be given.	1. Avoid pregnant women unless immediate protection is needed. If immediate protection is needed, OPV is recommended. 2. OPV should not be given to immunocompromised persons or to individuals with immunocompromised family members. E-IPV is recommended in those situations.	E-IPV = Enhanced-potency inactivated poliovirus vaccine. OPV = Oral poliovirus vaccine (live) E-IPV may not induce a protective immune response in immunocompromised individuals.
Hepatitis B	Two IM doses 4 weeks apart with third dose 5 months after the second. Protection lasts 7 years. Screening with HbsAB should be done before booster given.	1. Adults at increased risk of occupational, environmental, social or family exposure. 2. All health care workers should be vaccinated.	Pregnancy is not a contraindication to vaccination.	1. Recombinant vaccine 2. Prevaccination serologic screening for susceptibility may or may not be cost effective. 3. The vaccine produces neither therapeutic nor adverse effects on HBV-infected persons.

TABLE 11-1 Vaccine Schedules for Adults[a,b] (Continued)

Vaccine	Primary Schedule and Boosters	Indications	Contraindications and Precautions	Special Considerations
Influenza	Annual vaccination with current vaccine. Either whole or split virus vaccine may be used.	1. Adults with high risk conditions, residents of nursing homes or other chronic care facilities. 2. All health care personnel. 3. Healthy person 65 or older.	1. History of anaphylactic hypersensitivity to egg ingestion is a contraindication. 2. No evidence of maternal or fetal risk.	Inactivated whole virus and split virus vaccine.
Rabies	1. Preexposure prophylaxis—two doses IM or ID one week apart, third dose 3 weeks after second. Booster every 2 years if exposure continues. 2. Postexposure prophylaxis—clean wound. If not previously vaccinated: give rabies immune globulin half at bite site; half IM. 5 doses of rabies vaccine IM on each of days 0, 3, 7, 14, 28. 3. Persons who have received postexposure prophylaxis or have a previously documented antibody titer considered adequate: 2 doses rabies vaccine one each on days 0 and 3.	1. Veterinarians, animal handlers, certain laboratory workers and visitors to countries where rabies is a threat. 2. If substantial risk of rabies, preexposure vaccination should be given before pregnancy.	1. History of anaphylaxis to a previous dose of rabies vaccine is a contraindication to further rabies vaccination. 2. Certain steroids and immunosuppressive agents can interfere with the development of active immunity.	1. Human diploid cell vaccine (HDCV) and Rabies vaccine, absorbed (RVA) are the two types of vaccines. 2. Complete preexposure prophylaxis does not eliminate the need for additional therapy with rabies vaccine after a rabies exposure. 3. For postexposure prophylaxis, rabies vaccine should always be administered IM, not ID.

(continued)

TABLE 11-1 Vaccine Schedules for Adults[a,b] (Continued)

Vaccine	Primary Schedule and Boosters	Indications	Contraindications and Precautions	Special Considerations
Yellow fever	One dose SC 10 days to 10 years before travel. Booster every 10 years.	Selected persons traveling or living in area where yellow fever exists.	1. Avoid vaccinating pregnant women unless individual must travel to highly endemic areas. 2. Immunocompromised persons, history of hypersensitivity to egg	1. 17D = Live attenuated. 2. Some countries request a valid international certification of vaccination showing receipt of vaccine.
Cholera	Two 0.5 ml doses SC or IM or two 0.2 ml doses ID 1 week to 1 month apart. Booster doses 0.5 ml IM or 0.2 ml ID every 6 months.	The WHO no longer recommends cholera vaccination for international travels to cholera-endemic areas.	1. No safety data on use in pregnancy. 2. Persons who have had severe local or systemic reactions to a previous dose should not be vaccinated.	1. Inactivated bacterial vaccine. 2. Some countries still require a complete series of vaccination. 3. Cholera and yellow fever vaccines should be administered at least 3 weeks apart.
Mening-ococcus	One dose IM. The need for booster doses is unknown.	Travelers to countries recognized as having epidemic meningococcal disease.	Pregnancy, unless there is substantial risk of infection.	Polysaccharide vaccines (bivalent A and C, tetravalent A, C, and Y, W-135).
Plague	Three IM doses: first dose, second dose 1 month later, third dose 5 months after second dose. Booster doses at 1–2 year intervals if exposure continues.	Selected travelers to countries where exposure to rodents and fleas is likely. Field and laboratory workers working with *Yersinapest-is*.	1. Pregnancy, unless there is a substantial risk of exposure. 2. Persons with known hypersensitivity to vaccine constituents.	1. Inactivated bacterial vaccine. 2. Prophylactic antibiotics may be indicated following definite exposure.
Pneumo-coccal	One IM dose. Revaccination should be considered every 6 years.	1. Adults at increased risk of pneumococcal disease. 2. All adults 65 and older.	Safety in pregnancy not determined and should be used only if risk of infection is high.	1. Inactivated bacterial vaccine. 2. Pneumococcal and influenza vaccines can be given simultaneously at separate sites.

TABLE 11-1 Vaccine Schedules for Adults[a,b] (Continued)

Vaccine	Primary Schedule and Boosters	Indications	Contraindications and Precautions	Special Considerations
Typhoid	Oral vaccine administered in 4 doses every other day. (There is also an inactivated bacterial vaccine which is administered SC in two doses 4 or more weeks apart with a booster dose every 3 years.)	Travelers to areas where there is a recognized risk of typhoid.	Oral vaccine should not be given to immunocompromised individuals.	Live attenuated vaccine.

[a]Always read the package insert prior to using a vaccine, especially if it is used infrequently.

[b]When it is necessary to use a vaccine or toxoid in pregnancy, waiting until the second or third trimester, when possible, is a reasonable precaution that reduces the risk of teratogenicity.

SOURCE: Modified from *Guide for Adult Immunization,* 2d ed. American College of Physicians.[3]

TABLE 11-2 Immunobiologicals[a,b]

Immune Globulins	Schedule	Indications	Major Precautions and Contraindications	Special Considerations
Hepatitis A	1. Preexposure prophylaxis-one IM dose of 0.02 ml/kg for risk of ≤3 months. IM dose 0.06 ml/kg for risk of >3 months. Repeat doses if risk continues.	1. Household and sexual contacts of persons with Hepatitis A. 2. Staff and parents of diapered attendees in day-care center outbreaks.		Immunoglobulin can interfere with the antibody response to administered live virus vaccines.

(*continued*)

TABLE 11-2 Immunobiologicals[a,b] (Continued)

Immune Globulins	Schedule	Indications	Major Precautions and Contraindications	Special Considerations
	2. Postexposure prophylaxis—one IM dose of 0.02 ml/kg given within 2 weeks of exposure.			
Hepatitis B	0.06 ml/kg IM as soon as possible after exposure followed by a second dose 1 month later except when HBV vaccine is given.	1. Following percutaneous or mucous membrane exposure to blood known to be HbsAg positive, sexual exposure or a bite from a person with acute HBV or a chronic carrier. 2. Perinatally for infants born of HBsAg positive mother.		HBV vaccine should be given if person at risk for HBV.
Measles	Postexposure prophylaxis: 0.25 ml/kg IM (maximum 15 ml) given within 6 days of exposure.	Exposed susceptible contacts of measles cases.	IG should not be used to control measles outbreaks.	1. IG given within 6 days of exposure can prevent or modify measles. 2. Recipients of IG should receive live measles vaccine 3 months later.
Tetanus	250 units IM	Part of management of a nonclean, nonminor wound in a person whose history of tetanus vaccination is unknown.		

TABLE 11-2 Immunobiologicals[a,b] (Continued)

Immune Globulins	Schedule	Indications	Major Precautions and Contraindications	Special Considerations
Rabies	20 IU/kg half infiltrate around wound, half IM.	Part of postexposure prophylaxis of persons with rabies exposure who lack history of rabies vaccination.		Rabies immune globulin is usually given with the first dose of vaccine, but it can be given up to 8 days after vaccination.
Varicella	1. Persons ≤50 kg:125 units/10 kg IM. 2. Persons >50 kg:625 units.	1. Immuno-compromised persons likely to have close and prolonged exposure to a contact case. 2. Perinatal prophylaxis and treatment of mothers and prophylaxis of infants born of mothers with varicella.	1. VZIG is not indicated for normal adults exposed to varicella. 2. Not a treatment for herpes zoster.	An acceptable alternative to VZIG is to treat varicella if it occurs with high dose IV acyclovir.

[a]Always read the package insert prior to using a vaccine, especially if it is used infrequently.

[b]When it is necessary to use a vaccine or toxoid in pregnancy, waiting until the second or third trimester, when possible, is a reasonable precaution that reduces the risk of teratogenicity.

SOURCE: Modified from *Guide for Adult Immunization,* 2d ed. American College of Physicians.[3]

been infected with mumps virus and can be considered to be immune. Because of an outbreak of measles in 1989 in school and college settings, a two-dose live virus MMR vaccine has been recommended. It is advisable that young adults attending college or other post-high school institutions should have documentation of having received two doses of live-virus MMR after their first birthday or have evidence of immunity.

Persons vaccinated with killed-measles virus vaccine (1963 to 1967) or with a measles vaccine of unknown type should receive two doses of live measles vaccine given 1 month apart.

Persons are considered immune to rubella only if they have a record of immunization or laboratory evidence of immunity.

Influenza vaccination should be recommended for those who provide essential community service, such as health-care workers including physicians, military personnel, and college students living in dormitories.

Adults (25 to 64 years)

All adults should have completed a primary series of diphtheria and tetanus toxoids. If needed, it should be completed as soon as possible. For those who have completed their primary series, a booster of Td should be administered every ten years.

All adults born in 1957 or later who do not have a medical contraindication should receive one dose of measles vaccine unless they have documented evidence of immunity or documentation of physician-diagnosed disease. Health-care workers and physicians are at a greater risk of exposure to measles and should be offered the vaccine. The clinical diagnosis of rubella is nonspecific, and laboratory documentation of immunity is required. Rubella vaccine should not be administered during pregnancy, but should be given after delivery.

While healthy adults under 65 are not at increased risk for complications of influenza, those who provide community service or who are at increased risk for transmitting the virus to others should be immunized. While pneumococcal vaccination is recommended for adults over 65 years of age, it should be considered for younger patients, based on individual physician judgment.

Hepatitis B immunization should be considered for all health care workers, institutionalized patients, and patients at risk for sexually transmitted diseases. All pregnant patients should be screened for hepatitis B surface antigen. Immunization consists of two IM doses 4 weeks apart and a third dose 5 months after the second dose. Protection lasts 7 years, and booster doses are not recommended during this period.

Adults (65 years or older)

Adults 65 or older are more susceptible to infectious diseases, especially of the lower respiratory tract. This may be caused by a decline in host defense mechanisms primarily affecting cell-mediated immunity.

Adults in this age group should receive influenza vaccine annually. They should receive a single dose of pneumococcal vaccine, with revaccination every six years.

Tetanus and diphtheria boosters should be up-to-date, with revaccination every 10 years. More than half of all cases of tetanus are reported in persons 60 years of age or older. The elderly are capable of mounting a strong antibody response to Td.

Immunization for Special Adult Groups

Pregnant Women

The risks associated with immunization in pregnancy are largely theoretical, and the advantages outweigh the potential risks of adverse reactions. As a general rule, live virus vaccines should not be used during pregnancy unless specifically indicated (e.g., yellow fever vaccine before travel to an endemic area).

Prenatal screening should be done for rubella and hepatitis B. Rubella vaccination should be deferred until postpartum. There is no contraindication to vaccination with hepatitis B vaccine in pregnancy.

Women of childbearing age should be immune to poliomyelitis, measles, mumps, rubella, tetanus, and diphtheria before becoming pregnant. A careful history of illnesses and immunizations may clarify the immune status.

Vaccines that can be used in pregnancy can be used in any trimester. There is no evidence that teratogenicity occurs with vaccines judged safe for pregnancy. It is wise to defer vaccination until the second trimester when the risk of spontaneous abortion is significantly decreased.

Pregnant patients who have not received tetanus and diphtheria vaccine should receive two doses of Td given 4 to 8 weeks apart. This should be followed by a third dose 6 to 12 months later. If the series was not completed earlier, or if it has been 10 or more years since a patient's last dose, a booster should be given.

Vaccination against hepatitis A is not available in the United States, but an excellent vaccine is awaiting approval from the FDA. If the patient is exposed to hepatitis A, she can be screened for the hepatitis A antibody (IgG). If negative, she should receive immune globulin IM within one week of exposure.

Influenza and pneumococcal vaccines are indicated for pregnant women with underlying high-risk conditions, but are not routinely recommended. The vaccines can be given simultaneously at different sites.

MMR vaccine is *not* indicated in pregnancy. Rubella vaccine should be administered postpartum or may be given to nonpregnant women who do not plan to become pregnant within three months.

Pregnant women in the United States should be immune to polio virus; however, immunization during pregnancy is recommended only when the risk of exposure is high. The risk for polio is largely with international travel to endemic areas.

Two vaccines are available to prevent poliomyelitis: oral, live virus vaccine and an inactivated polio vaccine. For an unimmunized pregnant woman at high risk of exposure to poliovirus, a single dose of oral vaccine is recommended if less than 4 weeks are available and immediate protection is needed. If time permits, two doses of inactivated vaccine at 1- to 2-month intervals is recommended. Pregnant women at high risk of exposure, who received polio vaccinations more than 10 years before, should receive a one-time booster of inactivated polio vaccine.

Yellow fever vaccine is an attenuated live virus vaccine but it is not known to be teratogenic. Vaccination is indicated if a pregnant woman must travel to areas where yellow fever is endemic.

As should be done for any patient, before ever vaccinating a pregnant woman, read the package insert carefully for contraindications.

College Students and Other At-Risk Groups

College students are at risk for several vaccine-preventable diseases because of crowding in dormitories, importation of disease from foreign students or after foreign travel, and age-group susceptibility. Several states have laws requiring students to document their immunization status, and some colleges require proof of immunization prior to matriculation. An MMR vaccine (two doses) should be administered to students traveling abroad or entering college unless proof of immunization can be determined.

Td should be given as a booster vaccine if more than 10 years have passed since primary immunization. If the primary three-dose series for tetanus and diphtheria has not been completed, it should be completed.

Hepatitis B vaccination is strongly recommended for groups of college students at increased risk for infection. These include: (a) heterosexually active students with multiple sexual partners or those who have a sexually acquired disease; (b) homosexual or bisexual males; or (c) students with sexual contacts with students from endemic areas. Serologic screening prior to immunization is not cost-effective.

Immunization of Immunocompromised Adults

Patients may be immunocompromised by therapies that cause immune system failure or because they have endogenous diseases that cause immune system failure. In approaching prevention of infection in immunocompromised patients, three principles are important: (1) prevention of infection is better than treatment; (2) the need for preventive efforts is determined by the epidemiology of the exposure to infection; and (3) the likelihood of both acquiring and preventing infection is directly related to the net state of immunosuppression.

Immunosuppressed patients should receive their annual influenza vaccine despite suboptimal antibody response. Pneumococcal vaccine should be given, with revaccination in 6 years. Hemophilus influenza type b conjugate vaccine is of unproven benefit in immunocompromised patients, but should be considered in patients with anatomical or functional asplenia.

Asymptomatic HIV patients should be vaccinated with MMR.

Immunization and Other Measures for International Travel

More than 10 million Americans travel outside of the United States annually; more than half visit areas where tropical diseases are endemic. The physician's advice regarding immunizations is influenced by: (1) the specific itinerary; (2) entry or exit requirements of the countries being visited for yellow fever or cholera vaccination; (3) the type of accommodations; (4) duration of travel; (5) the patient's status regarding routine immunization; and (6) special requirements for people who live within a particular country.

The following immunizations are frequently given: tetanus; diphtheria; polio; hepatitis A; measles; mumps; rubella. Additionally, yellow fever, typhoid, cholera, hepatitis B, meningococcus, rabies, Japanese encephalitis, and plague may be required immunizations based on exposure risk.

Tetanus and Diphtheria

Primary adult immunization of IM injections of tetanus toxoid (in combination with diphtheria at 0, 1, and 6 to 12 months). A booster injection is recommended every 10 years.

Poliomyelitis

Polio is endemic in many areas of the world, and there have been recent major outbreaks in Senegal in 1986 and Taiwan in 1983. Both oral polio vaccine (OPV) and inactivated polio vaccine (IPV) contain the three viral serotypes. Because OPV has been associated with paralytic polio on rare occasion (1 in 2.6 million doses), enhanced potency IPV vaccine is preferred for primary vaccination of the previously unimmunized adult. If the traveler has completed the primary series, a onetime booster of either OPV or IPV is advised. Since IPV does not stimulate immunity for several weeks, previously unimmunized travelers entering an endemic area within 30 days should be given OPV or enhanced potency IPV.

Viral Hepatitis B

Routine immunization against hepatitis B virus is not recommended. However, persons who may be exposed to blood or blood products and persons living in close contact or having sexual contact with infected persons should receive immunization. Hepatitis immunization consists of three IM injections at 0, 1, and 6 months.

Viral Hepatitis A

Active immunization against hepatitis A is not available in the United States. Passive immune globulin IM should be given to persons going to endemic areas. This dose should be effective for 3 to 6 months.

Measles, Mumps, Rubella

MMR vaccine should be given to the international traveler who was born after 1957 who has not previously received two doses and does not have evidence of immunity.

Yellow Fever

Yellow fever vaccination is required for travel in equatorial Africa and parts of South America. Travelers lacking documentation of immunization may be quarantined for 10 days and/or required to receive injection before entry.

Yellow fever vaccine contains attenuated virus and is administered subcutaneously. It is prepared from eggs and is contraindicated in persons with a true egg allergy. It is also contraindicated in immunosuppressed persons and in pregnancy (unless travel to high-risk areas is essential). Protection becomes active 10 days after immunization and continues for 10 years.

Meningococcal Meningitis

Neisseria meningitidis is endemic in parts of sub-Saharan Africa, India, and Southeast Asia. Recently, Saudi Arabia required proof of meningococcal vaccination for all pilgrims traveling to certain parts of the country. The vaccine is a polyvalent polysaccharide vaccine. Antibody development usually takes four weeks, so a person should be immunized at least one month before travel to an endemic area. After immunization, a person is considered protected for 3 years.

Typhoid Fever

Typhoid vaccine is indicated for travelers likely to be exposed to contaminated food and water or those living in rural areas for a prolonged time. In the past this was given by injection. Recently an oral vaccine has become available, but it cannot be given to immunocompromised individuals.

Cholera

Cholera is most prevalent in Asia and Africa. Following natural infection, immunity will last for only 3 to 9 months. Therefore, illness may develop many times. A sterile suspension of phenol-killed *V. cholerae* is used for vaccination. The vaccine only reduces the incidence of clinical disease by about 50 percent for 3 to 6 months.

Japanese Encephalitis

This is a mosquito-borne viral illness endemic to southeast Asia, Japan, Korea, India, and the Philippines. Epidemics occur during the rainy season (June to September). The killed virus vaccine is 75 to 90 percent effective after two injections 1 to 4 weeks apart.

Summary

The concept of immunization and an immunization program should become an important part of a primary care physician's practice. It provides an excellent opportunity to provide primary preventive care. The primary care initiative document published by the American College of Obstetricians and Gynecologists (1993) stresses immunizations as an important function of the primary care physician. Patients and physicians should view immunization against infectious disease as a vital and cost-effective health measure.

References and Selected Readings

1. ACOG Task Force on Primary and Preventive Health Care: *The Obstetrician-Gynecologist and Primary-Preventive Health Care.* 1–22, 1993.
2. Ferenchick GS, Havlichek DH: Primary prevention and international travel. *J Gen Intern Med* 4:247–258, 1989.
3. *Guide for Adult Immunization,* 2d ed. Philadelphia: American College of Physicians. 1990.
4. Handler SC, Francis DP, Maynard JE, et al: Long term immunogenicity and efficacy of Hepatitis B vaccine in homosexual men. *N Engl J Med* 315:209–214, 1986.
5. Hill DR, Pearson RD: Health advice for the international traveler. *Ann Intern Med* 108:839–852, 1988.
6. Immunizations Practice Advisory Committee: Adult immunization. *MMWR* 33 (Supl); 1-68S, 1983.
7. Lancaster D, Elam S, Kaiser AB: Immunogenicity of the intradermal route of Hepatitis B vaccination with the use of recombinant Hepatitis B vaccine. *Am J Infect Control* 17:126–129, 1989.
8. Mulley AG, Silverstein MD, Dienstag JL: Indicators for use of Hepatitis B vaccine, based on cost-effectiveness analysis. *N Engl J Med* 307:644–652, 1982.
9. Nelson KE, Clements ML, Miotti P, et al: The influence of human immunodeficiency virus (HIV) infection on antibody responses to influenza vaccines. *Ann Intern Med* 108:383–388, 1988.
10. Schonberger LB, Bregman DJ, Sullivan-Bolyai JZ, et al: Guillian-Barre syndrome following vaccination in the national influenza immunization program, United States 1976–1977. *Am J Epidemiol* 110:105–123, 1979.
11. Shapiro ED, Berg AT, Austrion R, et al: The protective efficacy of polyvalent pneumococcal polysaccharide vaccine. *N Engl J Med* 325:1453–1460, 1991.
12. Ellis RW: *Vaccines: New Approaches to Immunological Problems.* Boston: Butterworth-Heineman, 1992.
13. Gryz SJ: *Vaccines and Immunotherapy.* Elmsford, NY: Pergamon Press, 1991.
14. Update on adult immunization. *MMWR* 40:1–94, 1991.
15. Willems JS, Sanders CR: Cost-effectiveness and cost-benefit analyses of vaccines. *J Infect Dis* 144:486–492, 1981.

12 Exercise

David B. Hale
Ralph W. Hale

During the last 15 to 20 years, there has been a sudden increase in emphasis on exercise as one of the key aspects of a healthy life-style. When exercise is combined with proper nutrition and preventive health care measures, there can be an increase in the quality as well as the quantity of life. As a result of this emphasis on exercise, women have become more involved in active exercise, extending from general fitness to elite athletic activity. This change in women's life-styles has been accompanied by an increasing need for basic information, and women frequently turn to their physician for this information.

General Fitness

Fitness, or conditioning, is a term used to describe the changes in cardiovascular endurance, muscle strength, coordination, and flexibility that result from an organized, repetitive exercise program. In some instances, it also includes weight control. The major component of fitness will be determined by the type of exercise program selected and the ultimate goal of the program. However, in general, for any program to be successful it must be repetitive and it must be directed. Combining multiple but widely varied activities is unlikely to meet any goal. Since most current programs emphasize aerobic conditioning, the cardiovascular component becomes the key factor.

The source of energy for exercise is dependent on carbohydrates and fats. Glucose is the principal sugar used, and this is either available in the blood or stored in the body as glycogen for later use. Muscle mass is the primary storage area for glycogen, and during exercise enzymatic breakdown occurs that releases the glucose for active cellular metabolism.[11] As exercise continues, there is also a release of lactic acid, which is a by-product of anaerobic metabolism.[16] Resynthesis of lactate to glucose can occur, and lactate measurements are a form of evaluation used by some physiologists and coaches to measure conditioning.[3–5]

Fatty acids stored within the body as fats comprise the largest potential energy stores. They become most important in exercise of longer duration and low to moderate intensity. When intensity increases, the amount of energy obtained from fats decreases.[2] The key factor in this energy cycle is the amount of oxygen available to complete the cycle. Since cellular oxygen is essential for utilization of carbohydrates and fats, any program that increases the presence of cellular oxygen will prolong the ability of the muscle to function. When the amount of oxygen available has been depleted, the energy cycle continues, but becomes anaerobic. Although anaerobic training is utilized in some short, high intensity athletic programs, in the usual aerobic program it signals the end of a meaningful exercise session.

In general, repetitive exercise programs increase the efficiency of the body to utilize these energy sources, and this increases endurance. As training continues, there is an enhanced oxidative capacity as the result of increased mitochondria in the muscle cells and an increase in the capillary support. This results in a reduction in the need for glycogen and an increased reliance on fatty acids.[13] The ultimate outcome is that the longer the exercise program continues, the less efficient it becomes. Thus, for individuals to perceive that they are "in condition," the initial program must be repetitive over long periods as opposed to infrequent long individual sessions. It will take approximately 12 weeks in any program to achieve a significant fitness level.[1]

Cardiovascular Fitness

The goal of most exercise programs will be to obtain a degree of cardiovascular fitness. This will be interpreted as the ability to sustain physical activity over a prolonged period. The level of activity and the length of time will vary with individual goals. Some will seek to become elite athletes, but most will simply wish to improve their general fitness.

The usual format will consist of an aerobic activity performed for 30 min, three or four times a week. In response to this repeated exercise, the body increases its ability to utilize the aerobic energy cycle. The name given to this phenomenon is *aerobic capacity*. The most common method of determining the level of aerobic capacity is to determine the maximum oxygen uptake over a given period of time. The result is called the V_{O_2max} and is measured utilizing a controlled environment such as a laboratory. Aerobic capacity increases in response to sustained repetitive exercise. As aerobic capacity/cardiovascular fitness improves, the V_{O_2max} increases.

A more practical way of measuring this aerobic capacity is to utilize the heart rate change. Since the heart rate increases as oxygen deprivation increases, it provides us with a method to determine the amount of oxygen and resulting glycolysis that is being utilized as a result of exercise.[1] The goal of exercise is to reach and maintain a specific heart rate over a minimum time period. By utilizing this method each exercise session can be monitored to achieve the desired goal. The formula utilized for this determination is: $(220 - \text{age}) \times 60$ percent to 80 percent. The resulting number is the target heart range. For example, a 40-year-old female would have a target heart rate of 108 to 144 beats per minutes $[(220 - 40) = 180 \times 0.6 \text{ or } 0.8]$. See Table 12-1 for other age groups.

Thus, the exercise program can be tailored by the individual to her specific needs. Once the target range is reached, it should be maintained for 20 to 30 min, and this program should be repeated three to four times a week.[8]

It is important to remember that before each exercise program, there should be three to five minutes of gradually increasing activity to reduce the potential for muscle injury. This is referred to as the "warm-up" period. At the completion of exercise, there has been a vasodilation in the muscles and skin, and sudden stopping can result in extensive distal vascular pooling, which could cause a relative central hypovolemia. Thus a period of five to fifteen

TABLE 12-1 Target Heart Rates

	Ranges	
Age	Minimum 60%	Maximum 80%
20	120	160
30	114	152
40	108	144
50	102	136
60	96	128
70	90	120

min at the completion of exercise should be devoted to the gradual reduction of intensity. This is referred to as the "cool-down" period.[18] During this cool-down period, hot baths, hot showers, or any other activity that could contribute to peripheral vascular pooling should be avoided.

There are three key aspects of any exercise program designed to obtain cardiovascular fitness: specificity, progression, and overload.[12] Specificity refers to designing a program that will result in attainment of the goals. For example, if the goal is cardiovascular fitness, the exercise should be aerobic and not increased muscle strength. If the goal is to run a marathon, then training for a short jog is insufficient. Progression refers to starting at a low level of intensity and over time increasing to a higher level of intensity. There is no ideal time length for this to occur, and it varies greatly from individual to individual. A method of measuring progression is again to use the target heart rate. As conditioning, i.e., cardiovascular fitness, occurs, it will require an increased intensity of activity to reach the target rate. The concept of overload refers to the necessity of increasing the demand on the body over and above that which is usual. Since the cardiovascular system is not stable, it will respond by increasing or decreasing activity over a period of time in response to the demands placed upon it. Thus for any exercise program to succeed, it must exceed the current level of performance and stress the system. The target heart rate remains an excellent measurement tool to evaluate the level of stress attained.

Coordination, balance, and flexibility may occur as the result of an exercise program. As muscles work in a group in a repetitive program, they become more efficient as a group. This helps the individual perform activities with less difficulty. Although this is rarely an initial goal of exercise, it is an important benefit.

One final word of caution is that any level of conditioning is reversible, and often this occurs faster than developing the conditioning.[4,15] Therefore, it is necessary to maintain a long-term commitment to exercise if conditioning is to remain.

Injury Prevention

All exercise programs can be harmful if they are improperly performed. Therefore, any of the following signs should signal the need for an abrupt halt until adequate reevaluation has taken place[1]:

- Sudden pain, especially sharp and specific
- Excessive fatigue, acute or chronic
- Respiratory problems
- Nausea and/or vomiting
- Dizziness or light-headedness
- Chronic muscle or joint pain
- Any heart rate irregularity or pain
- Frequent severe headaches
- Recurrent epistaxis

Weight Control

Exercise also can be helpful in maintaining as well as reducing weight. Weight reduction programs that are combined with exercise are more effective than any dieting program by itself.[17]

When utilizing exercise as part of a weight control program, it must be remembered that weight loss is a slow process. Depending on the intensity of exercise, it is necessary to expend approximately 3500 calories for each pound of fat lost. Thus the time span for significant weight reduction can be very lengthy. In addition, as fat is lost, muscle is produced. Per unit volume, muscle is approximately twice the weight of fat. Thus in the initial phases of exercise, weight may increase slightly before a significant decrease occurs. A helpful guide during this period of time is the fit of clothes. If fat is lost, they should become looser, even while weight is stable.

It should be remembered that any exercise program that is part of weight control is based on maintaining a stable or reduced caloric intake. If additional calories are consumed because of the exercise, minimal or no weight reduction will occur.

As a word of caution, strenuous dieting in association with exercise is to be avoided. The resulting energy loss will increase the exhaustion felt with exercise, and usually will lead to cessation of the exercise program.

Muscle Strength

For a muscle to strengthen, it is essential that it work repetitively against a fixed resistance. The result is that the fibers will then hypertrophy. It is this hypertrophy that causes an increased work capacity or strength. For muscle strength to occur, a program for the specific muscle group must be developed. Strength training programs designed for one muscle group will not affect other unstressed groups. The classic example is the tennis player with one large strong arm used to hold the racquet, while the other arm has less muscle mass and is much weaker.

Depending on the program, some cardiovascular effects also may occur. However, if the main goal is cardiovascular fitness, aerobic exercise should be performed; if the goal is strength, a specific strength program is necessary.

An ancillary use of muscle strength is for "toning." This is accomplished by developing specific muscle groups to improve one's appearance. Body builders use this form of weight training.

Effects on Menstruation and Reproduction

The most common effect of exercise on the female reproductive system is to initiate changes in the menstrual cycle. This was first reported in long-distance runners and occurred as oligomenorrhea. Menstrual changes may vary from a sudden cessation of menses to a gradual reduction over an extended period. The exact mechanism is unknown, but probably relates to changes in the hypothalamic-pituitary axis.[14]

It is known that both oligomenorrhea and amenorrhea are related to the amount of exercise. The amount and intensity can vary from individual to individual, but it appears that a minimum exercise expenditure equivalent to running 20 miles per week is needed.[7] On the other hand, some women can exercise far more extensively without any noticeable changes. If changes occur, a reduction in activity usually will result in a return of normal menses within two to three months.

Other areas of concern are the impact on menarche, dysmenorrhea, infertility, and the breast. These areas are all currently being investigated for potential effects. Thus far, there are no consistent findings, and the reader is referred to specific references on these topics for greater details.[1,6] Unfortunately, anecdotal experiences are quoted far more commonly than scientific studies. It appears that the menarche may be delayed if intense exercise is started several years prior to menarche. However, no adverse effects have been noted due to this delay. Dysmenorrhea may or may not be increased. It is theoretically possible that release of prostaglandins during exercise could increase dysmenorrhea. On the other hand, many women report a relief from dysmenorrhea once they began an active exercise program.

The effect of exercise on fertility is still very controversial. Obviously, a woman who becomes amenorrheic usually will be infertile. However, it is unknown whether this amenorrhea will subsequently have an impact on fertility. Some very preliminary evidence suggests that those who would have infertility problems anyway may be more susceptible, but this has not been proven.[7]

It is rare for any exercise program to cause significant injury to the breast. Minor abrasions can occur if an ill-fitting support is used, but no long-term effects have been documented.

Bone Density

Bone density has been shown to increase in women who are involved in an active exercise program.[9] Pressure on the bone results in increased calcium deposition due to increased osteoblastic activity. Thus, a moderate exercise program can be helpful as an adjunct to supplemental estrogen therapy in postmenopausal women. It can also be a primary therapy in menopausal women who do not take estrogens.

Exercises designed to help prevent osteoporosis involve use of large muscles attached to the long bones. It is necessary that stress be placed on the bond to ensure that adequate bone strength is maintained; this facilitates conservation or replacement of calcium. Fortunately, most aerobic exercise programs involve use of enough large muscle mass to accomplish this stress and to help reduce the incidence of osteoporosis. Since osteoporosis probably begins its development when a woman is in her 40s and 50s, it should be emphasized that exercise at this age is an important step in preventing later problems. However, in women over 60, light-to-moderate aerobic exercise apparently can still have a positive effect in improving bone density. When combined with hormonal replacement therapy and adequate calcium intake, bone density will improve.[10]

Summary

Exercise should be a regular part of an individual's daily activities. Whether it is a two- to three-mile vigorous walk or a high-intensity, elite athletic program, it will have long-term benefits on the life-style and health of the individual. Humans throughout history have never been a sedentary species. Activity has always been central to living. However, modern appliances and conveniences have reduced the need for exercise, and thus we must now make an effort to help our patients maintain fitness.

References and Selected Readings

1. ACOG Technical Bulletin #173: *Women and Exercise.* October 1992.
2. Ahlbory G, Felig P, Hagenfeldt L, et al: Substrate turnover during prolonged exercise in man: Splanchnic and leg metabolism of glucose, free fatty acids and amino acids. *J Clin Invest* 53:1080–1090, 1974.
3. Cheetham ME, Boobis LH, Brooks S, Williams C: Human muscle metabolism during sprint running. *J Appl Physiol* 61:54–60, 1986.
4. Coyle EF, Hemmert MK, Coggan AR: Effects of detraining on cardiovascular responses to exercise: Role of blood volume. *J Appl Physiol* 60:95–99, 1986.
5. Gollnick PD: Energy metabolism and prolonged exercise, in Lamb DR et al. (eds): *Perspectives in Exercise Science and Sports Medicine.* Indianapolis: Benchmark Press, 1988, pp 14–15.
6. Hale RW (ed): *Caring for the Exercising Woman.* New York: Elsevier, 1991.
7. Hale RW, Kosasa T, Kruger J, Pepper S: A marathon: The immediate effect of female runners luteinizing hormone, follicle stimulating hormone, prolactin, testosterone and cortisol levels. *Am J Obstet Gynecol* 146:550–556, 1983.
8. Hartley LH: General principles of exercise prescription, in Strauss RH (ed): *Sports Medicine.* Philadelphia: WB Saunders, 1984 pp 45–56.
9. McCulloch RG, Bailey DA, Houston CS, Dogg BL: Effects of physical activity, dietary calcium intake and selected life-style factors on bone density in young women. *Can Med Assoc J* 142:221–227, 1990.
10. National Institutes of Health Consensus Conference: Osteoporosis. *JAMA* 252:799–802, 1984.
11. Newsholme EA: The regulation of intracellular fuel supply during sustained exercise. *Ann NY Acad Sci* 301:81–91, 1977.
12. Prins J, Hale RW: Exercise programs and the prescription of exercise, in Hale RW (ed): *Caring for the Exercising Woman.* New York: Elsevier, 1991, pp 42–50.
13. Prins J. Basic exercise physiology, in Hale, R (ed): *Caring for the Exercising Woman.* New York: Elsevier, 1991, pp 9–11.
14. Russell JB, Mitchell D, Musey PI, Collins DC: The relationship of exercise and anovulatory cycles in female athletes: Hormonal and physical characteristics. *Obstet Gynecol* 63:452–456, 1984.
15. Salten B, Blomquist G, Mitchell JH, et al: Response to exercise after bed rest and after training. *Circu Suppl* 7, 1968.
16. Sherman MS, Lamb DR: Nutrition and prolonged exercise, in Lamb DR, Murray R (eds): *Perspectives in Exercise and Sports Medicine,* vol 1. *Prolonged Exercise.* Indianapolis: Benchmark Press, 1988 pp 213–217.
17. Tremblay A, Despres JP, et al: Effect of intensity of physical activity on body fatness and fat distribution. *Am J Clin Nutr* 51:153–157, 1990.
18. Wilmore JH. *The Wilmore Fitness Program: A Personalized Guide to Total Fitness and Health.* New York: Simon & Schuster, 1981, pp 75–123.

13 Safety and Accident Prevention

Geraldine Lanman

Accidents are significant causes of mortality—and certainly of morbidity—in the United States. In fact, after cardiovascular diseases and malignancies, they are the leading cause of death in the United States, regardless of age. They cause more deaths than infectious diseases, pulmonary diseases, diabetes, and liver or kidney problems. In women the importance of accidents as a cause of death varies by age; from ages 13 through 39, accidents are the leading cause of death. Although accidents are by no means uncommon in middle-aged women, the frequency of accidents as a cause of death diminishes with age until 55, when it starts to climb again, doubling every five years until age 85, when it triples in number. Motor vehicle accidents constitute the majority of the accidents; the remainder are assaults, burns, toxic ingestion, and electrical, household, and sports injuries.

In caring for our patients, we as physicians can be far more to them than "medical people." We can help our patients by anticipating problems and risks, and then educating and advising them about our concerns without causing needless alarm. While there are many ways of identifying risks and still more of advising people of them, I believe the direct face-to-face method to be the most effective. Brochures and other educational aids are best used to augment and enhance rather than substitute for counseling.

Leaving the advice for the "wrap-up" session at the end of a visit sometimes leaves the patient overwhelmed and confused. In addition, the patient may feel that what you are telling her is something you identified during the course of the physical examination and that you are withholding information from her. The best time to identify issues and initiate advice about safety is during the initial conversation, while the history is being obtained. This can then be reinforced at the wrap-up consultation after the physical examination. At subsequent visits, since the patient's condition may change, recurrent issues of safety and accident prevention can be reinforced and new ones introduced.

The following suggestions can be utilized to integrate safety issues into the history. When obtaining the surgical history, make sure to inquire about injuries. Previous injuries will provide an idea of the person's risk, particularly as pertains to driving. This is an important time to emphasize seat-belt use. Also ask about other types of accidents. In older women, make certain to ask about falls. Discuss potential household injuries that represent a significant hazard, particularly in women. Advise about caustic agents, bathtub falls (particularly in the elderly), loose rugs, furniture or clutter obstructing frequently traveled paths (e.g., between the bed and the bathroom, particularly at night), stairs, kitchen utensils, stoves, and sports and recreation equipment. Are there joint instability or limb weakness problems that might predispose to falls? In the winter, warn about injuries on the ice. During the other seasons, yard and garden equipment may cause injuries.

Discuss the details of the woman's occupation to understand its risks, and to advise about any special precautions to be borne in mind. For example, hepatitis and HIV should be discussed with health-care workers, tetanus shots with construction workers, and TB exposure with school teachers. Carefully explore substance abuse issues in relation to occupation and the jeopardy coworkers and others are placed in by those who abuse a substance while working.

Ask about eyeglass frames. Are they shatterproof? Do dentures fit? Oversize dentures are a major choking hazard in the elderly.

With allergies, ask specifically about bee stings. Caution the person with this allergy to keep an EpiPen in her purse, desk, and house. With medications, be sure to ask about over-the-counter drugs, so that any possible adverse drug interactions can be discussed.

Look into the possibility that the smoker may smoke in bed, and caution about the risk of fire. Alcohol and drug use should be discussed, with particular emphasis on driving or involvement in other dangerous activities while not completely mentally alert. A substantial proportion of motor vehicle accidents are the result of persons driving under the influence of alcohol or drugs.

Safety is an important issue. It is more likely that many of our patients will suffer injury or death from preventable accidents than from many of the other medical issues we physicians diligently address. As physicians entrusted by patients with their care, we have an obligation to evaluate potential safety risks for each patient and to offer safety advice.

14 Complications of Alcohol and Drug Use

Vicki L. Seltzer

The majority of adults in the United States drink alcohol socially, and it is estimated that 3 to 5 percent of women have problems related to alcohol use. The use of illicit drugs is also common among women in the United States. The National Institute on Drug Abuse reported that more than half of U.S. teenagers try an illicit drug before they complete high school. The numbers of drug-related emergency room visits and mortalities continue to be substantial. Alcoholism and illicit drug use are problems for women of all age groups and social, cultural, and economic backgrounds, and it is essential that the physician not dismiss these as potential problems without making appropriate inquiries. In addition, even if a woman does not drink excessively nor use illegal drugs, she may be at risk because of drug use by her partner or friends. For instance, she may be involved in an automobile accident because the driver was intoxicated or she may be infected with hepatitis or HIV by having intercourse with a partner who uses intravenous drugs. Physicians need to address these issues with their patients.

Alcoholics have a life span that is, on average, shortened by 15 years. For users of illegal drugs, depending on the drug(s) used, the data may be considerably worse.

Alcohol

The leading causes of death for alcoholics are cardiovascular disease, cancer, accidents, and suicide. Alcoholics have 10 times the cancer risk of the general population (with substantial increases in cancer of the head and neck, esophagus, stomach, pancreas, liver, and possibly breast). Alcoholics are also at risk for Wernicke's and Korsakoff's syndromes, cerebrovascular accidents, esophagitis and gastritis, gastrointestinal bleeding, malnutrition, pancreatitis, cirrhosis, cardiomyopathy, arrhythmias, and psychosocial and psychiatric problems. Excessive drinking will also impair judgment acutely, often leading the patient to take inappropriate risks (e.g., driving unsafely, unprotected intercourse).

The physician has several important roles to play with regard to alcohol-related morbidity and mortality. These include:

1. Primary prevention of inappropriate or excessive alcohol use
2. Identification of women with problems related to alcoholism
3. Prevention of complications of alcohol use
4. Treatment of patients who are withdrawing
5. Assisting abusers of alcohol to stop drinking

The primary physician should not underestimate the role he or she can play in affecting the behavior of many patients. Merely by discussing alcohol and drug use as part of the initial and ongoing history, physicians give the message to their patients that this is an important issue that can impact substantially on their well-being. The risks of all the aforementioned medical problems that may occur secondary to alcohol use—and also the risk of automobile fatalities—should be emphasized.

Several different screening tests can be used by physicians to identify the patient who is an alcoholic [e.g., the CAGE questionnaire discussed in Chap. 7 or the MAST (Michigan Alcohol Screening Test)]. Rather than asking a patient, "Do you drink?", it is probably more useful to ask "How many drinks do you have in a week (day)?" Depending on the answer to the first questions, subsequent inquiries should be directed at helping the physician to determine whether alcohol might be affecting the woman's personal safety, interpersonal relationships, employment, and health. The particular strategy that the primary physician chooses is not as important as the need to determine which patient is at risk (medical, social, or occupational) from excessive alcohol use. In addition to information obtained by the history, abnormal physical findings and laboratory tests may provide clues to excessive alcohol use. Patients who have disorders associated with alcohol use such as cancer of the head and neck, pancreatitis, cirrhosis, or who have laboratory abnormalities such as elevated LFTs may be using excessive alcohol.

Once the physician has determined that a patient is abusing alcohol, the woman must be evaluated for the common medical problems associated with alcoholism and the alcohol problem discussed with her (and possibly her family, depending on the circumstances) in a straightforward fashion. The role of the primary care physician will depend in part on the extent of the problem and the expertise of the physician. At minimum, the primary care doctor should continue to follow the patient and provide support and encouragement. Depending on the circumstances, the woman may require an inpatient or outpatient treatment program, counseling, and rehabilitation. Alcoholics Anonymous (AA) is an important and widely available resource, and the family may derive substantial benefit from involvement with Alanon (a group for families of alcoholics).

Illicit Drugs

A wide range of illicit drugs are currently in common use. Illicit drug users commonly use more than one drug, depending on availability, and many abuse both drugs and alcohol. In addition, health care providers should keep in mind that the drugs they prescribe also may be abused.

The physician's role regarding drug abuse is similar to his/her role regarding alcohol abuse:

1. Primary prevention
2. Identification of users
3. Prevention of complications of drug use
4. Treatment of drug-related problems
5. Helping the woman to discontinue use

Since many of these issues were presented earlier in this chapter, this discussion will focus on specific issues related to a few of the more commonly used drugs.

Although many different terminologies are utilized, it is worthwhile to consider one classification from the psychiatry literature that distinguishes substance abuse and substance dependence—either of which obviously needs to be identified and addressed. An individual is considered a substance *abuser* if she has a pattern of substance use that causes significant distress or life impairment. At least one of the following circumstances will occur related to substance use during a year to fulfill this definition: continued use despite social and interpersonal problems, a legal problem, a physical hazard, or failure to fulfill a major role or obligation. Substance *dependence* is defined as causing distress and life impairment with any three from among the following list occurring within one year: tolerance, withdrawal, increasing and prolonged use, inability to control use, continued use despite known adverse physical or psychological sequelae, expenditure of substantial amounts of time around substance use, and loss or reduction of significant life activities due to substance use.

In addition to the medical and social problems related to substance use, there often are many serious associated psychiatric disorders. It is sometimes difficult to identify which problems were present initially and perhaps led to an increased potential for substance use, and which occurred as a sequela of substance use. For instance, depression and anxiety often precede illegal drug use, but are common problems secondary to drug use as well.

Cocaine

One controlled substance commonly used illegally in the United States is cocaine; its use has increased dramatically in the past decade. It is usually snorted, but also may be smoked or administered intravenously (sometimes combined with heroin). Tens of thousands of emergency room visits each year are associated with cocaine abuse, and there has been an alarming increase in mortality.

Cocaine use may be associated with hypertension, respiratory depression, hyperpyrexia, arrhythmias, seizures, or psychiatric problems. It may cause hyperprolactinemia, menstrual irregularities, and infertility. Cocaine use has been associated with an increased risk of adverse pregnancy outcome, including fetal anomalies, placental abruption, and fetal demise.

Cocaine overdose is an emergency that requires intensive medical care and may result in mortality from the potential complications mentioned above.

Heroin

Intravenous heroin use remains a common problem in the United States. There is a substantial mortality rate among heroin users secondary to infectious diseases such as AIDS, hepatitis, SBE, and drug-resistant tuberculosis; accidents, suicide, and homicide; and a variety of other problems related to drug use. Other problems seen in heroin users include CNS damage, respiratory depression, constipation, anorexia, complications related to adulterants used to "cut" the heroin, and a broad range of psychiatric and psychosocial problems.

Heroin users may overdose and appear in the emergency room with shallow respirations, bradycardia, and hypothermia. They are treated with support of vital signs and naloxone. Heroin overdose may lead to cardiorespiratory arrest and death.

Primary care physicians may also see patients during varying stages of heroin withdrawal, which usually commences approximately 9 to 15 h after the last dose and peaks at 1.5 to 3 days after the last dose. Patients who are withdrawing will exhibit sweating, increased respiratory rate and blood pressure, insomnia, yawning, nausea and diarrhea, rhinorrhea and lacrimation, body pain, and drug craving.

The primary care physician can play a major role in primary prevention, identification of drug users, preventing or treating the complications of drug use, helping patients to understand their situation and enter treatment programs, and providing counseling and support. However, managing these problems usually requires an experienced team effort, and referral will commonly be needed for detoxification, treatment, and rehabilitation.

In addition to everything that the physician can contribute to his or her patient's health pertaining to drug use as discussed above, there is one additional responsibility. The health of women who do not use intravenous drugs is jeopardized when their sexual partners are intravenous drug users. Their partners' drug use may or may not be known to them, and their partners' HIV and hepatitis status also may or may not be known to them. Physicians must make certain that their patients are aware of and understand this potential jeopardy.

Summary

Although only alcohol, cocaine, and heroin use have been discussed here, the physician also needs to be alert to the abuse of other drugs, such as amphetamines, Valium, Demerol, and LSD. Some of these drugs may even be prescribed by a physician but used by the patient either inappropriately or excessively.

Abuse of alcohol and drugs are common problems for both men and women of all social strata, and this may result in a high rate of morbidity and mortality. While they will not be successful with all their patients, primary care physicians are in an ideal position to reduce the incidence of these problems, to prevent drug and alcohol abuse, to identify women who are substance abusers, to prevent or treat complications of substance abuse, and to assist patients in becoming involved in treatment programs.

15 Smoking Cessation

Marc Manley
Roselyn Payne Epps
Thomas Glynn

Cigarettes are the leading cause of preventable death in the United States today. Cigarettes kill more than 400,000 people each year, which is more than alcohol, illegal drugs, car crashes, homicides, suicides, and AIDS combined. For women and men, smoking is a known cause of cancer of the lung, larynx, oral cavity, and esophagus; it also causes coronary heart disease, atherosclerotic peripheral vascular disease, and chronic obstructive pulmonary disease. It is associated with intrauterine growth retardation and low birth weight. Smoking also contributes to infertility, peptic ulcer disease, and skin wrinkling. Smokeless tobacco use causes oral cancer and other oral lesions. Environmental tobacco smoke, a known human carcinogen, causes lung cancer in nonsmoking adults and respiratory illness in children.

An epidemic of lung cancer is now occurring among women. Lung cancer has surpassed breast cancer as the most common type of fatal cancer in women. The number of lung cancer deaths is rising rapidly for women, while remaining constant for men. Women who smoke face a risk of lung cancer 12 times the risk of nonsmoking women. Among women 79 percent of lung cancer deaths are attributable to smoking.

In 1991, 46.3 million Americans, or 25.7 percent of the adult population smoked cigarettes: 28.1 percent of men and 23.5 percent of women. The highest levels of smoking were among people aged 25 to 44. Smoking rates are decreasing for men and women, but a smaller proportion of women than men are quitting.

This chapter provides physicians and other health care providers the information necessary to institute effective smoking cessation techniques for their patients. The interventions described are simple and brief, taking as little as 3 min. They are based on large clinical trials supported by the National Cancer Institute (NCI) that clearly indicate that physicians and other health care professionals can significantly reduce the prevalence of smoking if they provide smoking cessation interventions.

Clinical Interventions

The NCI recommendations for clinical interventions consist of four activities, each beginning with the letter "A":

- *Ask* all patients about smoking
- *Advise* smokers to stop

- *Assist* their efforts with self-help materials, a quit-date, and possibly nicotine gum or the transdermal patch
- *Arrange* follow-up

This intervention plan (often referred to as the "4 *As*") describes a general approach to smoking that can be used in almost any outpatient encounter, whether 30 s or 30 min are available to the clinician. Each element of the intervention is described below.

1. Ask about smoking at every opportunity.

A nurse or other staff member should routinely ask patients "Do you smoke?" or "Are you still smoking?" at each visit, usually while measuring vital signs. Once it is known that a person smokes (or has previously smoked), an identifier should be placed prominently on the patient's chart to remind the physician and staff to discuss smoking at each visit.

2. Advise all smokers to stop.

A clear statement of advice (e.g., "As your physician, I must advise you to stop smoking now") is essential. Many patients do not recall receiving this advice from their physician; therefore, the statement must be easy to understand and memorable. Personalization of the message by referring to the patient's clinical condition, social roles, personal interests, or family history may add to the effectiveness of the advice. Motivations to stop smoking vary greatly from patient to patient. A list of reasons different people might give for stopping is provided in Table 15-1.

3. Assist the patient in stopping

A patient's level of interest in stopping smoking usually is evident in discussions with the physician. If it is not, ask the patient if she wants to stop. For those patients who don't, nagging rarely helps. Physicians must accept the patient's decision, make sure it is an informed decision, and attempt to maintain the patient's trust and confidence so that smoking can be discussed at future visits.

For those patients who express a sincere desire to stop smoking, the physician should help them set a specific date. There is evidence that patients who set a "quit-date" are more likely to make a serious attempt to stop. This date should be soon (generally

TABLE 15-1 Good Reasons To Stop Smoking

For teenagers
Bad breath
Stained teeth
Cost
Lack of independence—controlled by cigarettes
Sore throat
Cough
Dyspnea (might affect sports)
Frequent respiratory infections
For pregnant women
Increased rate of spontaneous abortion and fetal death
Increased risk of low birth weight
For parents
Increased coughing and respiratory infections among children of smokers
Poor role model for children
For new smokers
Easier to stop now
For asymptomatic adults
Twice the risk of heart disease
Six times the risk of emphysema
Cost of cigarettes
Cost of sick time
Bad breath
Less convenient and socially unacceptable
Wrinkles
For symptomatic adults
Upper respiratory infection
Sore throat
Gum disease
Dyspnea
Cough
Angina
Claudication
For any smoker
Money saved by stopping
Feel better
Improved ability to exercise
More likely to enjoy retirement, grandchildren, etc.

SOURCE: Adapted from Glynn T, Manley M: *How to Help Your Patients Stop Smoking: A National Cancer Institute Manual for Physicians.* Bethesda, MD: National Institutes of Health, 1989.

within four weeks), but not immediate, giving the patient the necessary time to prepare.

Once a patient has selected a specific date, information must be provided so that she can prepare. For patients who can read, this is easily accomplished by providing a self-help brochure. Effective brochures provide necessary information about smoking cessation (e.g., symptoms and time course of withdrawal, tips about stopping, good reasons for stopping, answers to common questions). Effective brochures are available from several professional and voluntary organizations, including the American Cancer Society, the American Lung Association, and the National Cancer Institute.

Physicians should consider prescribing nicotine replacement therapy, especially for highly addicted patients. These are smokers who consume more than one pack of cigarettes per day, smoke their first cigarette within 30 min of waking, or have experienced strong withdrawal symptoms during previous quit attempts. In clinical trials, nicotine gum and the nicotine transdermal patch have generally been effective in more addicted smokers, and only when combined with advice and information from a physician or other health professional.

The use of prescribed nicotine during pregnancy is controversial and considered by many to be contraindicated. Blood nicotine levels are generally lower among patch and gum users than among smokers, and the harmful compounds contained in tobacco smoke are avoided, but clinicians must weigh the potential disadvantages of prescribing nicotine during pregnancy with the potential advantage of helping a patient avoid cigarettes during that time.

The transdermal nicotine patch delivers nicotine through the skin. It is relatively easy for patients to use, placing minimal demands on their need for compliance, and often provides a higher level of nicotine replacement than nicotine gum. Several studies suggest that the patch reduces craving for cigarettes, a principal cause of smoking relapse. Randomized, controlled trials of nicotine patches have demonstrated long-term successful smoking cessation rates ranging from 22 to 42 percent amoung active patch users, compared with 5 to 28 percent among placebo patch users. All trials published to date have used nicotine patches in combination with behavioral interventions.

Patients should be provided with an information sheet on the patch and instructed in its proper use. If the patient does not stop smoking, treatment with the patch should be terminated. All brands recommend that the patch be applied once every 24 h, usually in the morning, to a nonhairy, clean, dry skin site on the upper torso or arm. Skin sites should be changed daily, and the same site not reused for at least one week. All brands of patch recommend a higher initial dose of nicotine (21 to 22 mg for the 24-h patches, 15 mg for the 16-h patch) for the first few weeks of treatment. Patients can then be given a lower-dose patch for subsequent weeks. Most brands have a third and lowest dose patch for the final weaning period. A total of six to eight weeks of treatment is recommended. Patients weighing less than 100 lb and patients with cardiovascular disease may begin treatment with a lower dose patch.

The most common side effect of the nicotine patch is mild, transient itching or burning after application. Erythema, sometimes accompanied by edema, may also occur at the patch site. The nicotine patch is contraindicated for patients who have hypersensitivity or an allergy to nicotine, have serious arrhythmias or severe or worsening angina, or who have had a recent myocardial infarction.

An alternative form of nicotine replacement is nicotine polacrilex gum. It should not be used like chewing gum but instead chewed intermittently and then held in contact with the oral mucosa, where the nicotine is absorbed. Patients need careful instruction in the use of this unusual drug delivery system or they will derive no benefit from it. The office staff can review gum use with the patient. When the gum is used appropriately, withdrawal symptoms are reduced.

4. Arrange follow-up visits.

When patients know their progress will be reviewed, their chances of successfully stopping improve. This monitoring may include a letter or telephone call from the office staff just before the quit-date, reinforcing the decision to stop. Most relapses occur in the first weeks after cessation, and a person who comes to the office after being a nonsmoker for one to two weeks has a much improved chance of remaining abstinent. For this reason, it is critical that patients be contacted during their first two weeks of abstinence to reinforce their decision to stop. Follow-up visits consist of an assessment of the patient's progress, discussion of any problems encountered or anticipated, and discussion of nicotine gum or patch use, if prescribed.

It is important to set up a second follow-up visit with the physician or staff member in one to two months. Studies show that the quit-rate improves as the number of follow-up visits increases.

Office Organization

Some simple changes in office procedures will significantly increase the physician's effectiveness in treating patients who smoke. The goal is to ensure that all patients who smoke are routinely identified, monitored, and appropriately treated. Office organizational procedures include selecting an office coordinator, making the office tobacco-free, systematically identifying and monitoring smokers, and involving staff members with the intervention and follow-up.

To act as a coordinated team, all members of the office staff must know their roles. The team approach is facilitated by naming a smoking cessation coordinator, usually a nurse, who will incorporate the intervention into the day-to-day activities of the practice with the help of the other staff members, maintain the staff members' commitment to the program, and ensure that the system is operating smoothly.

The team approach emphasizes staff identification of all patients who smoke. When patients are identified as smokers, their charts should be marked in a prominent manner. The typical identifier is a brightly colored permanent sticker or stamp, but this can be a removable sticker that is put on the chart at each visit. The regular use of these chart reminders has been shown to increase cessation rates significantly in office practices.

Staff members also should attach a progress card or flow sheet to the chart, thereby providing an easy way for the entire team to keep informed about the patient's current smoking status and allowing for brief cessation advice to become a routine part of every office visit for this patient. It is important that all staff members understand and implement this kind of charting system.

A staff member often will schedule the follow-up visits, make the contact just prior to the "quit-date," and also may be the person who conducts some or all follow-up visits. Staff members also can review with patients their self-help materials and instructions for use of nicotine polacrilex gum or transdermal patches, if prescribed.

Steps for making an office tobacco-free include posting no-smoking signs, removing ashtrays, displaying tobacco cessation information prominently, and eliminating tobacco advertising from the office, either by subscribing to magazines that do not carry this advertising or by crossing out tobacco advertisements with bright markers.

Special Issues in Tobacco Control

Weight Gain

The issue of weight gain is important to many patients who try to stop smoking. Some patients cite weight gain as the reason for relapse after previous attempts to stop. The average amount of weight gained after cessation is approximately 5 lb. Some patients gain no weight after cessation, but a small proportion of people gain large amounts.

Advice to a patient concerned about preventing weight gain can include two approaches. First, high-calorie foods should be avoided. Carrot and cinnamon sticks are time-honored, low-calorie foods that patients should have available whenever the urge to eat occurs. Attention to caloric intake may be recommended to patients to avoid weight gain. Second, recommend to weight-conscious smokers that they exercise more, even if this exercise is nothing more than walking. This tactic may help prevent weight gain and provide the patient with an activity usually incompatible with smoking, thus supporting smoke-free behavior.

Lack of Social Support for Stopping

Social factors are frequently given as a reason for relapse, particularly when the patient is confronted by situations and friends who provide strong cues or prompts for smoking. During the time of a brief office visit, major changes in the social skills and support of a patient cannot be expected. However, all patients should be encouraged to tell their family, friends, and coworkers of their decision to stop smoking. Patients with little support for stopping can be referred to group cessation programs, if they are willing to attend. Referral to a counselor or other health professional also may be useful.

It is often difficult for a smoking patient to stop if her spouse also smokes and is unwilling to stop. The unwilling spouse should be encouraged to join in the quit attempt. If this is not successful, the smoking spouse should at least be encouraged to smoke only outside the home.

Preventing Tobacco Use among Youth

This is another group that can benefit from the advice and assistance of physicians. Because most smokers become addicted during childhood and adolescence, advice from physicians during these periods is critical. It is challenging but essential to provide these young people with anticipatory guidance appropriate for their age and developmental stage. Some physicians have used cigarette advertisements to initiate discussions with adolescents, showing them the deceptive nature of the ads. When rapport with a young person is established, a physician can provide reasons for avoiding tobacco use that are relevant to an adolescent and that also can help the patient practice refusal skills. Adolescents who already are regular smokers should be advised and assisted like an adult. However, adolescents are often much more concerned with the immediate effects of smoking, such as odors and poor athletic performance, and are not influenced by the risks of cancer and other diseases that may not appear for many years.

Finally, children of any age should be protected from exposure to environmental tobacco smoke. Parents who smoke should be advised to stop and to keep their children in smoke-free environments, both at home and at day-care and other settings.

Summary

Enormous potential public health impact can be derived from clinical interventions with smoking patients. Even with very modest expectations of cessation rates, 100,000 clinicians using effective intervention can produce more than 3 million new ex-smokers each year. This, in conjunction with other tobacco control efforts in communities, will result in a marked reduction in the morbidity and mortality caused by smoking, one of the most important public health issues of our time.

References and Selected Readings

1. Cohen SJ, Stookey GK, Katz BP, et al: Encouraging primary care physicians to help smokers quit. A randomized, controlled trial. *Ann Intern Med* 110(8):648–652, 1989.
2. Cummings SR, Coates TJ, Richard RJ, et al: Training physicians in counseling about smoking cessation. A randomized trial of the Quit for Life program. *Ann Intern Med* 110(8):640–647, 1989.
3. Epps RP, Manley MW: A physician's guide to preventing tobacco use during childhood and adolescence. *Pediatrics* 88(1):140–144, 1991.
4. Fiore MC, Jorenby DE, Baker TB, Kenford SL: Tobacco dependence and the nicotine patch. Clinical guidelines for effective use. *JAMA* 268(19): 2687–2694, 1992.
5. Glynn T, Manley M: *How to Help Your Patients Stop Smoking: A National Cancer Institute Manual for Physicians.* NIH Publication No. 89-3064. Bethesda, MD: National Institutes of Health, 1989.
6. Hollis JF, Lichtenstein E, Mount K, et al: Nurse-assisted smoking counseling in medical settings: Minimizing demands on physicians. *Prev Med* 20(4): 497–507, 1991.
7. Kenford SL, Fiore MC, Jorenby DE, et al: Predicting smoking cessation: Who will quit with and without the nicotine patch. *JAMA* 278(8):589–594, 1993.
8. Manley M, Epps RP, Glynn T: The clinician's role in promoting smoking cessation among clinic patients. *Med Clin North Am* 76(2): 477–494, 1992.
9. U.S. Department of Health and Human Services: *The Health Consequences of Smoking: Nicotine Addiction. A Report of the Surgeon General.* DHHS Publication No. (CDC) 88-8406. U.S. Government Printing Office, 1988.

10. U.S. Department of Health and Human Services: *The Health Consequences of Smoking: 25 Years of Progress. A Report of the Surgeon General.* DHHS Publication No. (CDC) 89-8411. U.S. Government Printing Office, 1989.

11. U.S. Department of Health and Human Services: *The Health Consequences of Smoking Cessation. A Report of the Surgeon General.* DHHS Publication No. (CDC) 90-8416. U.S. Government Printing Office, 1990.

Part III

Reproductive Health and Disorders of the Reproductive System

16 Anatomy, Physiology, Growth, and Development

Fred Benjamin

The ability of the health-care provider to dispense proper primary care for women presupposes a basic knowledge of female anatomy, the normal growth and development of the reproductive organs, and the physiology of menstruation.

Anatomy

The female reproductive organs consist of the reproductive tract (the vulva, vagina, cervix, uterus, fallopian tubes, and ovaries) and the breasts. However, since the urinary and gastrointestinal tracts develop in close embryological relationship with the genital organs, and since they remain in close contact with the reproductive structures and share many pathological and clinical presentations with each other, knowledge of the anatomy of all of these interrelated organs is also necessary.

Vulva

The vulva is the composite name for the female external genitalia (Fig. 16-1). It includes the mons pubis or veneris, the labia majora and minora, the clitoris, the entrance to the vagina, the hymen, the vestibule, the urethra, and the perineum.

The *mons* is a fatty pad covered by hair-bearing skin; it lies over the upper part of the symphysis pubis. Extending backward from the mons are the *labia majora,* which are folds of skin overlying fat pads on either side of the vaginal orifice that merge posteriorly in the midline; laterally they are covered with hair, but their medial surfaces are smooth. Between the labia majora and vaginal orifice are two delicate flaps of skin called the *labia minora,* which

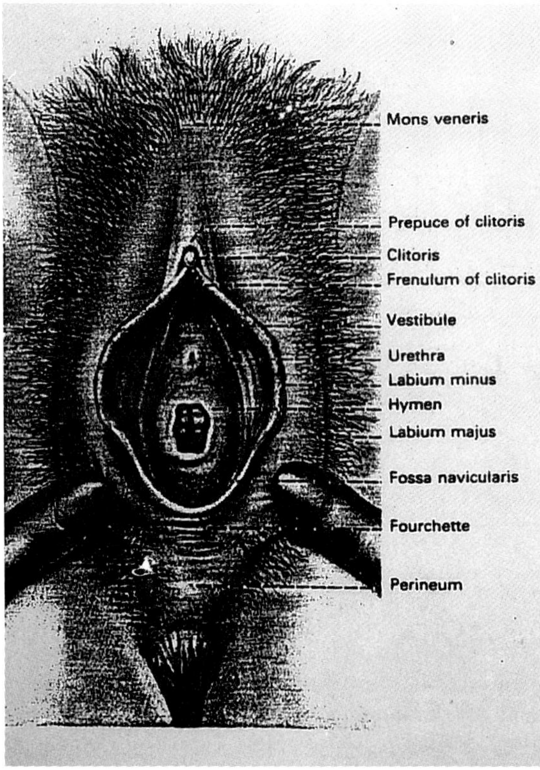

Figure 16-1. External organs of reproduction of women. In nulliparous women, the vaginal orifice is not so readily visible because of the close apposition of the labia minora. (From *Jeffcoate's Principles of Gynecology,* 5th ed, p 16, 1987. Ed: Victor R. Tindale. With permission of publishers, Butterworth-Heinemann, Oxford, England.)

vary in size considerably so that they may be hidden by the labia majora or may project beyond them. Anteriorly they split at the clitoris to supply it with a prepuce superiorly and a frenulum inferiorly. Posteriorly, they form a fold of skin called the *fourchette.* The depression between the fourchette and the hymen is the *fossa navicularis.* The *hymen* is a thin membrane covering the entrance to the vagina. It has one or more apertures to allow the outflow of menstrual blood. Unless the hymen is particularly elastic it is nearly always torn by coitus, but being relatively avascular, bleeding is usually slight. During childbirth it is torn more extensively so that only small remnants or tags remain, called carunculae myrtiformes. The *vestibule* is the space between the labia minora and extends from the clitoris anteriorly to the fourchette posteriorly; the vaginal and urethral openings are seen in it. The *clitoris,* the homologue of the penis, is a small organ lying in front of the symphysis pubis, almost hidden by the anterior portions of the labia majora. It consists of a glans, prepuce, body, and two crura that attach it to the pubic bones. The clitoris consists of erectile tissue, richly supplied with nerves that make it the most erotically sensitive area of the vulva. The *vestibular bulbs* are two elongated collections of erectile tissue passing from the root of the clitoris to either side of the vaginal orifice; they are analogous to the corpus spongiosum or bulb of the penis.

Bartholin's glands (also known as "the greater vestibular glands") are the analogs of Cowper's glands in the male. They are located on the posterolateral aspects of the vaginal orifice at 4- and 8-o'clock. Each gland is about the size of a pea, and has a duct, about 1 cm in length that runs downward and inward to open into the groove between the hymen and the labia minora. The gland is racemose and produces a colorless mucoid secretion, mainly in response to sexual stimulation. *Skene's glands,* or the paraurethral glands, correspond to the prostate gland in the male. They are branched tubular glands that lie next to the distal urethra. They have a duct that runs for 1 cm parallel to the long axis of the urethra, eventually opening into the distal urethra. The perineum is the tissue between the vaginal orifice anteriorly and the anus posteriorly. It consists of nonhairy skin and subcutaneous tissue. Its length anteroposteriorly, which ranges from 2 to 5 cm or more, is directly related to the resistance it offers and the injury it sustains during the delivery of a child.

Vagina

The vagina is an elastic fibromuscular tube that extends upward and backward from the vulva to the uterus (Figs. 16-2 and 16-3). Normally the walls of the vagina are in apposition and flattened anteroposteriorly so that on cross section it has an H-shaped

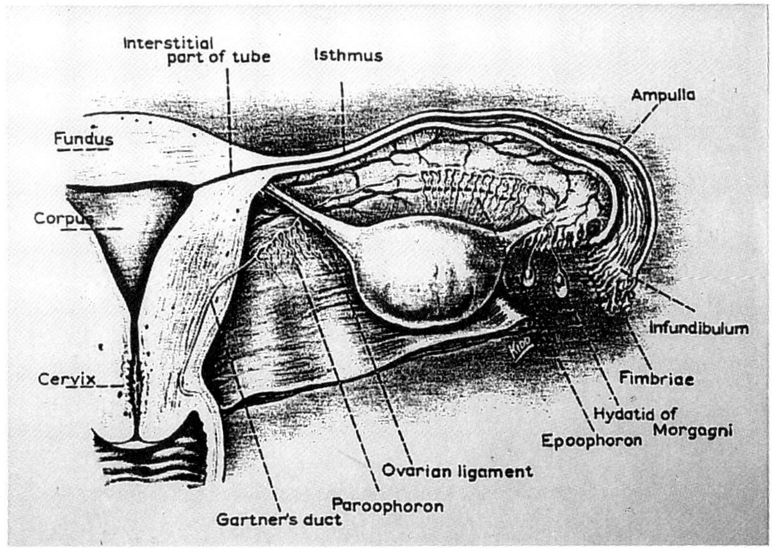

Figure 16-2. The uterus and broad ligament from behind. (From *Jeffcoate's Principles of Gynecology,* 5th ed, p 26, 1987. Ed: Victor R. Tindale. With permission of publishers, Butterworth-Heinemann, Oxford, England.)

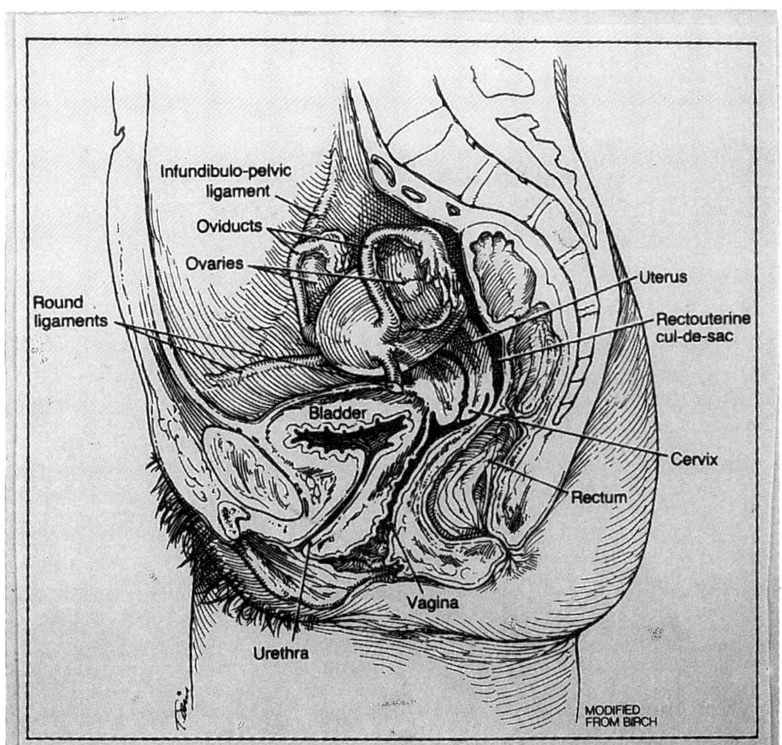

Figure 16-3. Sagittal section of pelvis of an adult woman that is illustrative of relations of the pelvic viscera. (From *Williams Obstetrics,* 17th ed, p 11, 1988. Eds: JA Pritchard, PC MacDonald and NF Gant. With permission.)

appearance. The vagina has a blind upper end except for the external os of the cervix. The cervix protrudes down below the vault, forming four areas: the posterior fornix, which is capacious; the anterior fornix, which is shallow; and two lateral fornices. The result is that the anterior vaginal wall is about 8 cm long, the posterior wall 10 cm, and the diameter is 3.5 cm. However, the length and width vary considerably in different women; functionally, its elasticity and the tone and contractions of the surrounding muscles enable the vagina to accommodate readily to coitus. Folds of epithelium running circumferentially, called *rugae,* contribute to the ability of the vagina to distend.

The vagina is lined by stratified squamous epithelium, which also covers the vaginal portion of the cervix up to the external os. The superficial zones of the epithelium contain glycogen, which is acted upon by a normal inhabitant of the vagina, *Doderlein's bacillus* (or the lactobacillus) to produce lactic acid, resulting in an acid pH of the vagina, about 4.5. This acidity is of major clinical importance, accounting for the excellent resistance of the vagina to infection with common bacteria.

The upper third of the vagina is supported by the cardinal ligaments and parametria, the middle third by the levator ani muscles and lower portion of the cardinal ligaments, and the lower third by the urogenital and pelvic diaphragms. When a woman is standing, the axis of the vagina is close to horizontal. The tissues surrounding the vagina and the vaginal wall itself are extremely vascular. The blood supply is mainly from the vaginal artery, but branches of the uterine artery and internal pudendal artery also contribute, as do small branches from the middle and inferior rectal arteries.

The vagina undergoes considerable anatomical and physiological change from the neonatal period through puberty, the reproductive years, and menopause. The vagina of the newborn child has a well-developed, glycogen-rich epithelium with an acidic pH, due to estrogen from the mother that has crossed the placenta. With the drop in estrogen, the epithelium becomes atrophic after about two weeks, and the pH of the vagina remains at an alkaline level, about pH 7, until puberty, when it reverts to its estrogenized state. The pH becomes even more acidic during pregnancy. After menopause, some thinning of the tissue occurs, the vaginal wall becomes smooth, glycogen and Doderlein's bacilli wane, and the pH rises.

The anatomical relations of the vagina are important in connection with clinical examination, injuries, childbirth, and surgery (Figs. 16-2 and 16-3). Anteriorly, the lower portion of the vagina is related to the ureter and the upper portion to the bladder. Posteriorly, the upper end of the vagina is in contact with the peritoneal cul-de-sac of Douglas, the middle portion is related to the ampulla of the rectum, and the lower third to the perineal body. Laterally, the upper third of the vagina is related to the lower portion of the cardinal ligaments, which are inserted into the lateral fornices. Below the fornices are the levator ani muscles and the tissues of the paracolpos; lower down is the ischiorectal fossa. At the vaginal introitus, on either side, are the sphincter vaginae or bulbocavernosus muscles, the vestibular bulbs, the Bartholin's glands and their ducts, and the triangular ligaments with their muscles.

Uterus

The uterus is a thick-walled hollow muscular organ shaped like a pear. The tapering end is the cervix, which projects into the vagina. The nulliparous uterus is about 8 to 9 cm long, 6 cm wide, and about 4 cm thick. The length of the cavity on sounding is, therefore, about 6 cm. The organ weighs 40 to 50 g. The multiparous uterus weighs about 70 to 80 g.

When seen from the front, the cavity is triangular in shape. The uterus is made up of a body (or corpus) and a cervix. The narrowed area between the cervix and the body is called the isthmus. The part of the body above the insertion of the fallopian tubes is called the fundus; the area where the tube is inserted is termed the *cornu* of the uterus.

The uterus has three layers. The outer serosal layer consists of the visceral peritoneum; the middle layer is the muscular layer *(myometrium)*; the inner layer is the *endometrium,* which, depending on the phase of the menstrual cycle, varies from 1 to 6 mm in thickness. The endometrium is divided into three layers: the superficial stratum compactum; the intermediate stratum spongiosum; and the innermost layer, the stratum basalis, which lies on and often penetrates somewhat into the myometrium. Only the superficial and intermediate layers respond to the hormonal changes of the menstrual cycle and are shed with menstruation. They are therefore referred to as the "functional zone" of the endometrium.

The blood supply of the uterus is furnished by the uterine arteries, derived from the hypogastric arteries, and by the ovarian arteries, which come off the aorta directly.

Fallopian Tubes or Oviducts

The fallopian tubes (oviducts), extend from the cornua of the uterus outward, in the free upper edge end of the broad ligament, toward the ovaries (Fig. 16-2). The lumen of each tube opens into the uterine cavity at its proximal end and into the peritoneal cavity at its distal end. This is the only communication between the peritoneal cavity and the outside, which explains the susceptibility of women to pelvic peritonitis arising from an ascending infection.

The fallopian tubes are between 10 and 14 cm long, and each is divided into four anatomical sections: 1. the interstitial or intramural segment is the part that transverses the uterine wall and is about 2 cm long; 2. the isthmus begins as the tube leaves the uterus; it is straight and narrow (1 to 2 mm in its inside diameter), 4 cm long and has the most highly developed muscular wall; 3. the ampulla is the widest portion of the tube (6 mm in its inside diameter) and is 6 cm long (fertilization normally takes place in the ampulla, and 80 percent of ectopic tubal pregnancies occur in this area); 4. the infundibulum is the most distal, trumpet-shaped end of the tube; it bears the opening into the peritoneal cavity, the "abdominal ostium." About 20 to 25 finger-like projections protrude from the fimbriated end of the tube and surround the abdominal ostium; one of the longest of these is attached to the ovary and is called the *fimbria ovarica.*

The mucosa of the tubes have numerous folds or plicae, which are most prominent in the ampullary portion. The mucous membrane has three different types of cells: columnar ciliated cells, columnar secretory cells, and narrow peg cells situated between the ciliated and secretory cells.

Ovaries

The two ovaries are mainly solid structures, light gray in color. During the reproductive years they measure approximately 3.5 × 2.5 × 1.5 cm, and each weighs about 5 g. After the menopause the ovaries become smaller and firmer, and clinically are nonpalpable. The ovaries are attached to the back of the broad ligament by the *mesovarium,* and are attached to the cornu of the uterus by the ovarian ligament; the part of the ovary attached to the mesovarium is called the *hilum,* and all nerves and vessels enter and leave at this area. In the hilum are groups of "hilus cells," analogous to the interstitial Leydig cells of the testis.

The ovary is divided into an outer zone, called the cortex, and an inner zone, the medulla. Follicles are located mainly in the cortex, the medulla being composed largely of connective tissue and blood vessels. The ovary is the only intraabdominal organ not covered by peritoneum. In early life it is covered by a single layer of cuboidal cells derived from the coelomic-epithelium, the primitive peritoneum. This layer is often called the "germinal epithelium"; however it does not give rise to germ cells, and preferably should be labeled the "surface epithelium" of the ovary.

Physiology of Menstruation

Menstruation is a phenomenon unique to the human species and the higher apes. Its purpose is the periodic preparation for fertilization and pregnancy. The physiology of menstruation consists of the integration of four interdependent activities: 1. the hypothalamus, which secretes the gonadotropin releasing hormone (GnRH); 2. the anterior pituitary gland, which in response to the stimulus of GnRH secretes follicle stimulating hormone (FSH) and luteinizing hormone (LH); 3. these two hormones then act on the ovaries to cause the development of the follicles, ovulation, and the secretion of the two major ovarian hormones, estrogen and progesterone; 4. estrogen and progesterone cause growth and development of the endometrium in preparation for embedding of the fertilized ovum. Each of these four aspects of the menstrual cycle will be considered in turn.

The Hypothalamic Cycle

The hypothalamus secretes hormones that have been identified as small polypeptides. These substances pass through the pituitary portal system to the anterior pituitary to stimulate it to synthesize and secrete its hormones. The hypothalamic hormone responsible for FSH and LH secretion is GnRH, a decapeptide containing 10 amino acids. GnRH is not secreted at a constant steady rate but in a pulsatile fashion, one pulse occurring every one to three hours. Many of the menstrual disorders, such as amenorrhea and dysfunctional uterine bleeding, are basically due to aberrations in the pulsatility of GnRH.

The Anterior Pituitary Cycle

In response to GnRH, the anterior pituitary synthesizes and secretes FSH and LH. FSH causes growth and development of the Graafian follicle, and in concert with LH results in estrogen production. LH, through its surge at midcycle, causes ovulation and the subsequent development of the corpus luteum (Fig. 16-4).

The Ovarian Cycle

The ovary is endowed with a peak of about 6 million ova at 20 weeks of gestation, but this number is reduced to about one million at birth and about 300,000 at puberty. The store of germ cells continues to be depleted by atresia until the process finally is completed about 40 years later at menopause.

Ovulation does not take place until full maturation of the hypothalamic pituitary axis after puberty. Beginning at that time, with each menstrual cycle a large number of follicles begin to develop. With few exceptions, only one of these undergoes full development. This total development consists of three phases: the follicular phase, ovulation, and the formation of the corpus luteum.

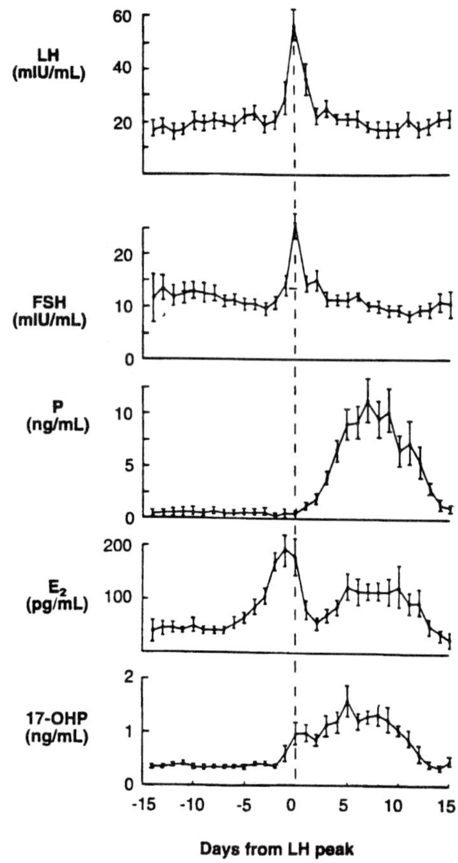

Figure 16-4. Mean values of LH, FSH, progesterone (P), estradiol (E_2) and 17-hydroxyprogesterone (17 OHP) in daily serum samples of 9 women during ovulatory menstrual cycles. Data from different cycles combined with the use of the day of the mid-cycle LH peak as the reference day (Day 0). The vertical bars represent one standard error of the mean. (From IH Thorneycroft, DR Mishell Jr, SC Stone, et al: *Am J Obstet Gynecol* III:947, 1975. With permission.)

The follicular phase begins with the primordial follicle, which is an oocyte arrested in the diplotene stage of the first meiotic division, surrounded by a single layer of granulosa cells. This development then proceeds through ovulation and the formation of the corpus luteum. The ovarian follicles undergo significant development throughout life, beginning even in the fetus during intrauterine life, and then continuing throughout life until menopause. However, the vast majority of these developing follicles become blighted at various stages of their development through the process called *atresia.* Atresia means that a follicle grows and enlarges but fails to ovulate; instead, it degenerates and becomes replaced by fibrous tissue. The follicles that do ovulate rupture; the ovum is extruded and is picked up by the fimbriated end of the tube and transported to the uterus. The ruptured follicle develops into a corpus luteum, which secretes progesterone as well as estrogen. If pregnancy occurs, the corpus luteum persists and there is no menstruation until after delivery. If pregnancy does not occur, the corpus luteum degenerates after its life span of about 14 days, and menstruation ensues.

The Endometrial Cycle

At the beginning of the menstrual cycle, the endometrium is only about 1 mm thick—much of it, except for the basal layer, having been shed with the menstrual flow. The developing follicle now produces estrogens, which cause the endometrium to grow; the glands lengthen, but do not become convoluted nor secrete. These endometrial changes prior to ovulation are called the *proliferative* or *follicular* or *preovulatory* phase of the cycle. Following ovulation and the formation of the corpus luteum, the endometrium, under the influence of progesterone, exhibits coiled and tortuous glands that secrete a clear fluid; this phase of the cycle is therefore called the *luteal* or *secretory* phase. When the corpus luteum degenerates and the estrogen and progesterone wane, the endometrial vessels go into spasm, probably as a result of the release of prostaglandins. This results in necrosis of the endometrium and the shedding of the superficial and intermediate layers of the endometrium (the strata compactum and spongiosum, respectively) causing the menstrual flow. The basal layer remains behind to grow and to develop and form the new endometrium for the next cycle. At its peak the endometrium has grown to a thickness of about 6 mm.

The mean duration of the menstrual flow is 4 ± 2 days, and the mean length of the cycle is 28 ± 7 days. The mean blood loss with each menstrual period is 35 ml; if the mean blood loss is regularly more than 80 ml, iron deficiency anemia will develop.[2]

Primary Amenorrhea

Definition

The mean age for the appearance of the first menstrual period (the *menarche*) is 12.8 years. Girls who do not have their first period by 16 or 17 require evaluation.

Clinical Approach

A useful clinical approach to the patient with primary amenorrhea is to carry out a general physical examination, when it will be found that all of the patients fall into one of three clinical categories: 1. those with absent secondary sex characteristics—i.e., no breast development and (usually) no pubic nor axillary hair; 2. patients with well-developed breasts and pubic and axillary hair; 3. those with evidence of androgenization—i.e., hirsutism and possibly an enlarged clitoris. By using this simple classification, the differential diagnosis becomes logical and easy, because each of these three groups of cases has its own specific causes.

Causes of Primary Amenorrhea (Table 16-1)

Patients with Absent Secondary Sex Characteristics Failure of breast development is due to absence of ovarian estrogen production. In the overwhelming majority of cases, this results from failure of gonadal development and formation of streak ovaries—i.e., *Gonadal Dysgenesis.* Occasionally however, the ovaries are normal and their failure is secondary to hypothalamic or pituitary disease, with resulting absent stimulation of the ovaries. The differential diagnosis between these two types of ovarian failure is readily made by an FSH assay; in pri-

TABLE 16-1 Clinical Presentations and Causes of Primary Amenorrhea

Absent Secondary Sex Characteristics	Well-Developed Secondary Sex Characteristic	Virilization
Primary ovarian failure (gonadal dysgenesis)[a]	Congenital utero-vaginal anomaly[a]	Congenital adrenal hyperplasia (CAH)[a]
Secondary ovarian failure Pituitary failure Hypothalamic failure (Kallmann's syndrome)	Stein-Leventhal syndrome/polycystic ovarian disease (PCOD)	True hermaphrodite
	Testicular feminization syndrome; androgen insensitivity syndrome	Male pseudohermaphrodite, developmental type
	Hyposensitive ovary syndrome/ "Savage" syndrome	Incomplete testicular feminization (AIS)
	Many of the causes of secondary amenorrhea occurring at or before puberty Hypothalamic; psychogenic Nutritional Systemic disease Medical endocrine disease	Stein-Leventhal syndrome/polycystic ovarian disease (PCOD) Rare virilizing tumors before or at puberty Ovarian Adrenal

[a]Most common cause (all others are rare causes of primary amenorrhea).

mary ovarian failure the FSH is high (above 40 mIU/ml), whereas in secondary ovarian failure it is low or absent.

Primary Amenorrhea with Well-Developed Secondary Sex Characteristics In these cases the ovaries function normally, with good estrogen production. The amenorrhea usually is due to a developmental defect in the mullerian ducts, resulting in absence or obstruction of the vagina or uterus. Occasionally, however, an apparent female with primary amenorrhea and well-developed breasts actually has androgen insensitivity syndrome (also called ''testicular feminization syndrome''). This condition can be suspected clinically by the absence of pubic and axillary hair, and the diagnosis can be established by the finding of an XY karyotype. Other rare causes of primary amenorrhea with well-developed breasts include nutritional amenorrhea, systemic disease, and hyperprolactinemia (although these conditions usually cause secondary rather than primary amenorrhea).

Primary Amenorrhea with Androgenization Practically all patients with primary amenorrhea, hirsutism, and an enlarged clitoris have congenital adrenal hyperplasia. Very rare and unusual causes of primary amenorrhea with androgenization are polycystic ovarian disease (this more often presents with secondary amenorrhea), various types of pseudohermaphroditism, and masculinizing ovarian or adrenal tumors.

Diagnosis

When a girl of 16 or 17 has not started menstruating, diagnosis of the cause of the condition can be made with little difficulty by determining which of the three clinical categories the patient fits. Most of those with absent breast development will have primary ovarian failure due to gonadal dysgenesis. If the secondary sex characteristics are normal, most will have a congenital anomaly of mullerian duct development. Those with hirsutism will in most cases have congenital adrenal hyperplasia. Only in the rare cases where these three diagnoses have been ruled out should a workup be done to determine which of the other rarer conditions (mentioned above in the discussion of the causes of primary amenorrhea) is present.

Treatment

The mainstay of the treatment of primary and secondary ovarian failure is estrogen replacement therapy (with the addition of a progestational agent to prevent the development of endometrial hyperplasia or carcinoma). The treatment of mullerian duct anomalies is reviewed later in this chapter. Congenital adrenal hyperplasia is managed by corticosteroid therapy with excellent clinical results.

Normal and Abnormal Sexual Development

Because the interpretation of congenital anomalies of the reproductive tract requires an understanding of the developmental processes involved, this basic embryology will be reviewed briefly. This is done merely to highlight aspects of the embryology essential to an understanding of the various clinical abnormalities.

Normal Sexual Development and Sexual Differentiation

Basically, the sex of an individual depends on the chromosomes which that individual possesses. This is determined at conception according to whether the ovum, which is always X-bearing, is fertilized by an X-bearing sperm, to form an XX or female chromosomal pattern, or by a Y-bearing sperm, to form an XY or male chromosomal pattern. However, although the sex is determined from the very moment of conception, for the first two months of embryonic life there is no real difference between the male and female embryonic form, all the genital structures being the same and having the potential of developing into male or female body form.

Thus, the primitive genital ridge from which the gonad develops appears at about the fourth week of embryonic life; but it is only at the seventh week in the male, and the ninth week in the female, that this genital ridge begins to differentiate into a testis or an ovary. Until then the ridge is the same in both sexes and consists of a peripheral cortex and a central medulla. In the male, the medulla predominates and the cortex atrophies—and this becomes a testis; in the female, the opposite occurs, the cortex predominating and the medulla atrophying—and this becomes an ovary. What makes the undifferentiated gonad develop into a testis or an ovary? A single gene situated on the *short* arm of the Y chromosome with a 1A1 DNA sequence is the essential factor necessary for the development of the testis. It is called the sex-related Y gene (SR-Y gene) or the testis determining factor gene (TDF gene). Without the presence of this gene the testis will not develop, and the gonad will develop into an ovary. It was previously thought that the H-Y gene and its antigen, the H-Y antigen, was the TDF. We now know that it is involved in spermatogenesis and not in testis determination; it is, in fact, situated on the *long* arm of the Y chromosome.

The undifferentiated gonad contains three distinct specialized tissues: primordial germ cells that will become either oogonia or spermatogonia, specialized epithelium that will become either granulosa cells or Sertoli cells; and specialized mesenchyme or stromal cells that will become either theca cells or Leydig cells. Although germ cells do not induce gonadal development and simply take the form of the gonad in which they find themselves becoming either oogonia or spermatogonia, should they fail to arrive, the gonads do not develop and form mere fibrous streaks. This results in the clinical disorder gonadal dysgenesis or Turner's syndrome and its varieties.

As is true of the gonads, the extragonadal genital structures are at first the same in both the male and female embryos. The internal structures are the mullerian (paramesonephric) ducts and the wolffian (mesonephric) ducts. In the male at about the 12th week, the wolffian duct predominates and the mullerian duct atrophies; the wolffian duct develops into the epididymis, vas deferens, and seminal vesicles. At about the same time in the female, the wolffian duct atrophies and the mullerian duct develops into the fallopian tubes, uterus, and upper part of the vagina.

Likewise, the external genital structures in both sexes originally are the same; by looking at a fetus before the 10th week—for example, after a spontaneous abortion—it cannot be determined whether it is male or female. These external structures, which appear at about the fourth week, are the genital tubercle, the genital or labioscrotal folds, and the urogenital membrane. At about the 12th week, the genital tubercle develops into the penis in the male and clitoris in the female; the labioscrotal folds develop into the scrotum in the male and the labia majora in the female; and the urogenital membrane forms the penile portion of the urethra in the male and the labia minora in the female.

The differentiation of the external and internal genital organs along male lines is entirely dependent on two substances produced by the fetal testicle, namely, testosterone produced by the Leydig cells and the mullerian inhibiting factor (MIF) secreted by the Sertoli cells. Testosterone causes the genital tubercle to develop into the penis and the labioscrotal folds into the scrotum. It causes the urogenital sinus to furnish the penile portion of the urethra and the prostate and also causes the wolffian duct to develop into the epididymis, vas deferens, and seminal vesicles. The MIF causes atrophy of the mullerian duct. On the other hand, in the absence of testes and the consequent lack of testosterone and MIF, the mullerian duct develops into the uterus, tubes, and upper part of the vagina.

Abnormal Sexual Development and Reproductive Tract Congenital Anomalies

A knowledge of the embryology as described above permits a ready understanding of the clinical states resulting from abnormalities in sexual development:

Chromosomal Defects Two of the clinical conditions the physician may encounter that are due to sex chromosomal defects are: gonadal dysgenesis (Turner's syndrome) and Klinefelter's syndrome.

Gonadal dysgenesis (Turner's syndrome) can occur in a male or female. In the male, if there is a defect in the short area of the Y chromosome there is absence of the testis determining factor (TDF) and failure of testicular development, the testes presenting as mere streaks. Since there is no testosterone and no mullerian inhibiting factor, these patients present as females, with a vulva, vagina, uterus, and streak gonads; they are indistinguishable phenotypically from the usual female gonadal dysgenesis.

In the female, any abnormality in the second X chromosome (whether it is absent altogether, i.e., XO, or present but abnormal) results in total failure of development of the ovaries, and they become fibrous streaks.

Both these male and female Turner's syndromes present with female genitalia, but with primary amenorrhea and absent secondary sex characteristics. Both are treated with replacement estrogens; however, if the karyotype is male, i.e., if there is a Y chromosome, it is essential to remove the streak gonads because there is a high incidence of malignancy.

Klinefelter's syndrome affects males with an extra X chromosome, i.e., XXY. They present as phenotypic males. However, having an extra X chromosome, they tend to have some feminine characteristics. There is a whole spectrum of clinical presentations, ranging from an apparently normal male who is only diagnosed in the course of an infertility work-up, to a male who is tall and eunuchoidal with somewhat enlarged breasts and small testes. They are all infertile, having either azoospermia or marked oligospermia.

Gonadal Defects The most striking gonadal defect is the well-known but very rare situation where both ovarian and testicular tissue are present—the true hermaphrodite. With the presence of both ovarian and testicular tissue a wide range of clinical presentations has been encountered. In the majority of cases there is a large phallus, so most of these patients are reared as boys. However, when puberty arrives there is much confusion because breasts almost always develop. Diagnosis is made by karyotyping and by evaluating the external and internal genitalia. Eventually, laparoscopy or laparotomy and biopsy of the gonads usually are required to make a definitive diagnosis.

Extragonadal Defects This category includes all congenital defects where the chromosomes and gonads are normal but the extragonadal structures, i.e., the external genitalia and/or the internal genitalia (derived from the mullerian and wolffian ducts) resemble those of the opposite sex. These patients are called pseudohermaphrodites.

Male pseudohermaphrodites are males (with an XY chromosomal makeup and testes), but there are varying degrees of incomplete masculinization of the external and/or internal genitalia. The clinical presentation can range from a simple hypospadias, to a small penis, bifid scrotum (i.e., failure of fusion of the labioscrotal folds), to undescended testes, to almost complete feminization, as seen in the ''testicular feminization syndrome'' or ''androgen insensitivity syndrome.'' In this syndrome, the male pseudohermaphrodite looks like a normal female, with breast development but no pubic nor axillary hair. Since this patient is XY, there will be no menstruation. If a patient presents with any or all of these features, the differential diagnosis is from a female pseudohermaphrodite or a true hermaphrodite, and the main key to the diagnosis is the karyotype: an XY pattern will show that the patient is a male pseudohermaphrodite.

Female pseudohermaphrodites are females with an XX karyotype and ovaries, but there is some degree of masculinization of the external genitalia. The usual way this is shown is by enlargement of the clitoris, but in advanced cases there may also be a single urogenital sinus.

The vast majority of these cases are due to congenital adrenal hyperplasia (CAH), but on rare occasion the condition is due to exogenous masculinizing hormone taken by the mother during pregnancy, or when an ovarian or adrenal tumor during pregnancy produces androgens.

Evaluations, Diagnosis and Treatment of the Intersexual State (Hermaphroditism) When a patient (usually a newborn child) presents with ambiguous genitalia, the main method of evaluating the patient and making a diagnosis is by carrying out a karyotype and by performing appropriate hormone assays. The karyotype will indicate whether the patient is a male or female pseudohermaphrodite, or the very rare true hermaphrodite. The dehydroepiandrosterone sulfate (DHEA-S) and 17-hydroxyprogesterone (17-OHP) will enable a diagnosis of CAH to be made. In some cases the diagnosis cannot be made by these tests alone, and a laparotomy and inspection of the internal genitalia and biopsy of the gonads may be necessary.

Treatment of the young child depends on what the anticipated pubertal changes will be (male or female), and whether the patient will be able to function best as a male or female. Obviously the size of the phallus is an important determining factor. It is much easier by plastic surgery to create a suitable vagina than a penis. If the phallus is inadequate, the child should be feminized and a vaginoplasty should be done. In that case one must make sure that the patient will not have a male puberty. If there is any testicular tissue, it must be removed; if it is a situation of CAH, this must be properly treated with cortisone so that the child does not masculinize at puberty.

If the patient is an older child or is an adult, the most important factor is whether the individual is psychosexually oriented in a masculine or feminine way. It is essential that the patient be treated appropriately so that the individual can live a life dictated by the psychosexual orientation. This may require both surgery and hormonal manipulation. If this is not done it is inevitable that major psychological problems will result.

Mullerian Duct Anomalies A large number of different congenital anomalies result from developmental defects in the mullerian ducts. In practically all of these cases, however, the ovaries are normal; therefore, these patients have well-developed secondary sex characteristics. Another important clinical fact is that, owing to the close embryological relationship between the mullerian and wolffian ducts, anomalies of the kidneys and ureters must be sought, because they are present in about 25 to 30 percent of the cases.

A simple classification of all the mullerian duct anomalies has been proposed by Jones[4]: 1. agenesis; 2. problems of vertical fusion—(a) obstructive and (b) nonobstructive; 3. problems of lateral fusion—(a) obstructive and (b) nonobstructive.

1. *Agenesis of the Mullerian Ducts.* Part or all of the vagina may be absent, and often the uterus also is absent; this disorder is sometimes called the Rokitanski-Kuster-Hauser syndrome.

2. *Problems of Vertical Fusion.* The most common clinical presentation is a transverse vaginal septum. If complete, it will cause obstruction to the outflow of menstrual blood after puberty, and surgical excision is required. If incomplete, surgery may be required later because of dyspareunia.

3. *Problems of Lateral Fusion.* Varying degrees of failure of lateral fusion of the mullerian ducts may occur. The extreme form is total lack of fusion, resulting in a double vagina and uterus (uterus didelphis). In some cases there is full development of one side and rudimentary development of the other. If there is no obstruction of menstrual outflow, there are usually no overt symptoms. Should obstruction be present, menstrual outflow is impaired and surgical management is usually mandatory.

The condition that may be encountered in the office setting is hematocolpos resulting from obstruction at or near the outlet of the vagina. This could be due to a problem of vertical fusion of the lower ends of the mullerian ducts, to an imperforate hymen, or to failure of canalization of the area where the mullerian ducts join the sinovaginal bulb. The patient presents with one of three symptoms: primary amenorrhea; cyclic or continuous pelvic pain; or difficulty in urinating culminating in acute retention of urine. The condition must be suspected in any young girl who complains of any of these symptoms soon after puberty.

References and Selected Readings

1. Crowley WF Jr, Filicori M, Spratt DI, et al: The physiology of gonadotropin releasing hormone (GnRH) secretion in men and women. *Recent Prog Horm Res* 41:501, 1988.
2. Hallberg L, Hillson L: Determination of menstrual blood loss. *Scand J Clin Lab Invest* 16:244, 1964.
3. Hallberg L, Hogdahl AM, Nilsson L, Rybo L: Menstrual blood loss—a population study variation at different ages and attempts to define normality. *Acta Obstet Gynecol Scand* 45:320, 1966.
4. Jones HW Jr: Anomalies of the Mullerian ducts, in Rosenwacks Z, Benjamin F, Stone ML (eds): *Gynecology: Principles and Practice.* New York: Macmillan, 1987.
5. Knobil E: The neuroendocrine control of the menstrual cycle. *Recent Prog Horm Res* 36:53, 1980.

17 Pediatric Gynecology

G. William Bates
Thomas M. Price

Gynecological disorders in prepubertal girls are uncommon. Most disorders result from perineal trauma, foreign bodies placed in the vagina by the child, or inflammatory conditions of the vulva or vagina. Neoplastic and endocrine-metabolic disorders are rare. Developmental abnormalities, precocious puberty, delayed puberty, incomplete puberty, and disorders of menstruation are covered elsewhere in this book. This chapter will present an approach to the pediatric gynecological patient and discuss the common disorders encountered in children and the treatment of these problems.

Examination of the Child with Gynecological Problems

Children (boys and girls) are put in diapers at birth and continue to have clothing on their perineum for the remainder of their lives. Thus, exposure of the perineum during childhood, except while bathing or using the bathroom, is an unusual event. This basic fact must be kept in mind when the physician is required to examine the perineum and genitalia of a prepubertal child or young adolescent. Children are embarrassed when asked to reveal the perineum to a stranger and feel uncomfortable when the external genitalia are touched.

Examination of a child must begin with conversation between the child, her parent(s), and the physician. The physician should include the child in the conversation if the child has passed infancy and is able to talk and participate. It is common, but less than ideal, for the conversation to take place between the parent(s) and physician with the child being the object of the conversation. Children should be included in the conversation from the outset of the medical visit if the child has reached an age to be a participant. The authors find that age to be around 18 months.

The physician should be at eye level with the child. If the child is standing, the physician will be in a squatting position facing the child. If the child is seated on an examination table, the physician will be sitting on a chair facing the child. This initial courtesy diminishes the dominance of the physician over the child and makes the child an immediate participant in the medical encounter.

Children should be examined with the parent(s) present unless the situation is emergent and the parent is unavailable. A nurse or other attendant is not a substitute for a parent, regardless of how reassuring that person may be to the child.

We believe it is best to meet the child when she is fully clothed. Preparation for the examination can come later. When the child is undressed for the examination, the physician should ask her to touch the spot of discomfort or area of interest. If the child touches her own perineum before the physician touches her, she will be more relaxed and will have less tendency to withdraw or adduct the thighs when the physician touches the perineum. Moreover, this helps to make the child feel that her privacy has not been invaded.

The pelvic examination of a child should begin with visual inspection of the mons pubis, the vulva, the anus, and the intertriginous areas of the thighs. Look for bruises, excoriation, inflammation, edema, or distortions of normal anatomical structures. After visual inspection, the labia majora should be separated to reveal the labia minora, clitoris, urethral meatus, and vaginal introitus. The perineal body and its anatomical relationship to the posterior perineum and anus should be observed. (Elongation of the perineal body is a sign of antenatal androgen excess.) If abnormalities are noted, we make a photographic record (with parental consent) of the lesion(s). This is especially helpful if perineal reconstructive surgery is required in the future as in girls with genital ambiguity, vaginal agenesis, or perineal trauma.

Examination of the vagina and cervix of a child need not be a traumatic procedure. A mother is often concerned that her daughter's hymen will be ruptured during vaginal examination. This issue should be raised by the examining physician and reassurance given that injury of the hymen can usually be avoided.

A nasal speculum or small test tube can be used to visualize the vagina and cervix. We prefer a small test tube. Test the structural integrity of the test tube to ensure that it will not break. Remove the rubber stopper from the test tube and moisten the test tube with water. It will slide easily into the vagina. By shining a flashlight into the test tube, the cervix can be visualized. Although a nasal speculum is more like a vaginal speculum than a test tube, opening and closing the speculum produces more sensation for the child than insertion of the test tube. Even in older preadolescent and adolescent girls, a test tube can be used to visualize the vagina and cervix.

We try to avoid a digital examination of the rectum or vagina in an unanesthetized girl. These examinations may traumatize the child and usually produce little information for the physician.

If there is perineal trauma, we recommend that examination be conducted under anesthesia so that the possibility of a broad ligament hematoma or perivaginal hematoma can be better evaluated. Vaginal ultrasound may aid the evaluation. If there is a history of sexual abuse with blunt penetration to the perineum or a history of impact trauma such as that produced by a water skiing or bicycle injury, there may be substantial risk of occult hemorrhage.

The approach to the perineal and genital examination in a child requires concern for the feelings of the child and forethought about the future psychological impact such an examination could have if conducted in a thoughtless manner.

Perineal and Vaginal Infections

Perineal and vaginal infections are the most common gynecological problems in prepubertal girls. Vulvovaginitis occurs with the greatest frequency. Because the genital tract of a girl is different from that of a reproductive age woman, the young girl has greater susceptibility to vulvovaginitis. The labia majora lack fat and the vaginal mucosa is thin and friable.

Labial Agglutination

Of the disorders we encounter, labial agglutination is most common in girls under 3 years of age. These children complain of vulvar itching and may have excoriation of the perineum due to scratching. On physical examination the labia majora are agglutinated in the midline, usually posterior to the urethral meatus. When the agglutinated labia are separated, the surfaces may be raw and ooze blood or serum. On occasion, the labial surfaces may not separate.

Labial agglutination occurs in children who live in hot, humid climates. We see this condition most frequently during the summer months. *Candida albicans* vulvitis may be a cause or consequence of labial agglutination.

Therapy should be directed at relieving perineal pruritis and facilitating healing of the raw skin surfaces of the inner aspects of the labia majora. We recommend that topical terconazole cream be applied twice daily to the vulva to alleviate itching and prevent scratching. After the pruritus is relieved (usually 4 to 5 days), topical conjugated estrogen cream should be applied to the vulva and vaginal introitus. Within 10 to 14 days, the labial adhesions will separate and the vulvar skin will be healed.

We further recommend that girls with labial agglutination keep the perineum uncovered as much as possible during the treatment period and during hot, humid days. This helps prevent recurrence.

Surgical separation of the labial adhesions is a last resort. Surgery should not be considered unless the labial agglutination extends anterior toward the clitoris and obstructs urine flow on micturition. The child should be observed during voiding by a parent or the physician. If the urinary stream is impeded, surgical lysis of labial adhesions is indicated. We have observed incomplete emptying of the urinary bladder utilizing transabdominal ultrasound examination in a child with labial agglutination.

When surgical lysis of labial adhesions is performed, the child should be pretreated with topical antifungal cream and topical estrogen cream to facilitate healing. Another surgical technique to facilitate vulvar healing is the application of a small Goretex membrane on each raw vulvar surface. Also, we have found that daily packing of the introitus will facilitate healing. Good surgical outcome may be compromised by persistent agglutination. Subsequent attempts at surgical correction are unlikely to solve the problem.

Nonspecific Vulvovaginitis

Older girls who participate in athletic programs such as ballet, gymnastics, or swimming are at greater risk for vulvovaginitis because of the persistent moist environment of the perineum. They should be educated about the need to keep the perineum dry once the vulvovaginitis has resolved; this will prevent further episodes. Older girls are not likely to develop labial agglutination.

Vaginal Foreign Bodies

Girls may explore their vaginal introitus, and may insert foreign bodies into the vagina. The foreign body will go undiscovered until the child develops a malodorous vaginal discharge or vaginal bleeding, which is usually detected by the parent. On examination, the vaginal introitus may be erythematous, and a foul yellow exudate will ooze from the vaginal opening. Unless the foreign body has worked its way to the introitus and can be grasped easily, we recommend that the object be extracted under light anesthesia. Several foreign bodies may have been inserted in the vagina, and thus careful exploration is warranted. A flexible hysteroscope is useful in vaginal inspection. Obtaining cultures from the vagina at the time of exploration is also a good precaution to exclude sexually transmitted diseases as a cause of vaginal exudate.

Sexually Transmitted Diseases

Sexual molestation should be suspected in any girl with a sexually transmitted disease. Sexually transmitted diseases can be acquired from the mother at birth, but this is unlikely after the first few weeks of life. Any vaginal discharge or lesion of the vulva should raise the suspicions of the clinician that the child is a victim of sexual molestation. Ulcerated or umbilicated lesions of the vulva, warty lesions of the vulva, and exudate from the vagina demand culture for viral, bacterial, and spirochete infections. Treatment is based on the results of culture.

The vulva and vagina should be inspected for signs of penetration by a blunt object, finger, or phallus. If rape is suspected, the chain of evidence established by the local or state court must be followed to identify the perpetrator. If a girl is withdrawn or uncommunicative, she should be encouraged to describe any sexual attack on her. She may better express herself through pictures and dolls than through words. When sexual molestation is suspected, a person qualified to properly obtain a history should be consulted.

Perineal and Vaginal Trauma

Perineal and/or vaginal trauma results from sexual assault, straddle injuries, and impact injuries to the perineum. A medical history can usually be obtained that identifies the cause of the injury. As discussed earlier, perineal trauma requires a careful examination of the vulva, vagina, cervix, and peritoneal cavity. Any of these injuries can cause avulsion of the uterus from its attachments, perforation of the rectum or sigmoid colon, or occult laceration of the vagina. In our opinion, the pelvic examination of a child who has sustained a traumatic injury must be performed in the operating room under anesthesia. If there is shock or evidence of anemia, there should be no delay in examination. Moreover, blood products should be available along with adequate surgical assistance.

In cases of suspected intraperitoneal hemorrhage or broad ligament hematoma, a diagnostic laparoscopy is warranted to rule out bleeding. Surgical treatment should be as conservative as the clinical situation allows.

Vaginal Agenesis and Imperforate Hymen

Abnormalities of the introitus may be discovered by a parent or grandparent while bathing the child. In our opinion, although it is important that these conditions be explained thoroughly to the parents at the time, surgical correction should be deferred at least until the girl has entered puberty. If an imperforate hymen is suspected, hymeneal incision should be timed to coincide with menstruation or be performed soon after the onset of menstruation. Delay may result in hematometra with regurgitation of menstrual effluent into the peritoneal cavity.

If vaginal agenesis is confirmed, we believe *any* corrective efforts (pressure dilatation of the rudimentary vagina or vaginoplasty) should be postponed until the girl has reached an age of 15 to 16 years, unless she has a functioning endometrium. The young woman with vaginal agenesis must have achieved emotional maturity and an understanding of sexual intercourse before these corrective attempts will be successful.

Parents, upon learning of a congenital anomaly of the reproductive tract, may insist that surgical correction be carried out before puberty. The education of parents and reassurance of appropriate psychosexual development for the girl are the responsibilities of the physician caring for the child.

Gynecological Tumors

Gynecological tumors are rare in girls. The most common tumor is sarcoma botryoides of the vagina. Children with this tumor present with vaginal bleeding or bloody discharge. A soft friable polypoid mass may protrude from the vagina. Chemotherapy is the preferred initial therapy followed by surgical excision. Despite therapy, the prognosis is poor.

Endodermal sinus tumors of the vagina are even rarer, and have a similar clinical presentation. Histologic identification is required to differentiate the two. This tumor occurs in girls under 3 years of age, and the prognosis is poor.

Germ cell tumors are the most common ovarian neoplasms found in girls and young adolescents. Complaints of urinary frequency, rectal pressure, abdominal fullness, increase in girth, lethargy, and change in appetite are clues that suggest ovarian neoplasms. Dysgerminomas have a good prognosis with surgical treatment. If the dysgerminoma is unilateral, conservation of the contralateral ovary preserves reproductive function. Endodermal sinus tumors of the ovary are usually confined to one ovary, and are treated with conservative surgery and chemotherapy. These are usually much more aggressive tumors than the dysgerminoma.

Lymphomas and leukemias may present with gynecological symptoms. Uterine bleeding in a prepubertal girl may be a sign of a hematologic neoplasm; pelvic pressure or tenesmus may be a sign of a pelvic lymphoma.

References and Selected Readings

1. Bates GW, Wiser WL: A technique for uterine conservation in adolescent women with vaginal agenesis and a functional uterus. *Obstet Gynecol* 66:290, 1985.
2. Carpenter SE, Rock JA (eds): *Pediatric and Adolescent Gynecology*. New York: Raven, 1992.
3. Carson SA: Gynecologic examination of the adolescent, in Carpenter SE, Rock JA (eds): *Pediatric and Adolescent Gynecology*, New York: Raven, 1992, pp 67–76.
4. Cowell CA (ed): Pediatric and adolescent gynecology, in *The Pediatric Clinics of North America*, vol. 28, Philadelphia: Saunders, 1981.
5. Fleischer AC, Shawker TH: The role of sonography in pediatric gynecology. *Clin Obstet Gynecol* 30:735, 1987.
6. McCann J, Simon WR, Voris J: Genital findings in prepubertal girls selected for non-abuse: A descriptive study. *Pediatrics* 86:428, 1990.
7. Millstein SG, Adler NE, Irwin CE, Jr: Sources of anxiety about pelvic examination among adolescent females. *J Adolesc Health Care* 5:105, 1984.
8. Wilson MD: Vaginal discharge and vaginal bleeding in childhood, in Carpenter SE, Rock JA (eds): *Pediatric and Adolescent Gynecology*. New York: Raven, 1992, pp 139–51.
9. Wiser WL, Bates GW: Management of vaginal agenesis: A report of 92 cases. *Surg Gynecol Obstet* 159:108, 1984.

18 Planning for Pregnancy

Donna D. Johnson
Robert Resnik

MATERNAL STATUS
Advanced Maternal Age • Medical Disorders
REPRODUCTIVE HISTORY
GENETICS
Genetic Counseling • Prenatal Diagnostic Tests • Screening Tests
GENERAL HEALTH HABITS
Medications • Nutrition • Sexually Transmitted Diseases • Illicit Drug Use • Smoking • Alcohol • Exercise • Vaccinations • Environment

An uncomplicated pregnancy and the birth of a healthy child are the primary goals of every expectant couple. However, many prospective parents do not realize that preparation prior to conception optimizes their chances for a normal pregnancy. Often the only contact the couple has with the medical community is through the woman's annual checkup. If a woman is contemplating a pregnancy, the primary care provider should identify any historical or physical factors that may affect the offspring of the couple. The physician can then encourage the patient to alter any behaviors that may affect the pregnancy or the fetus. In addition, a woman with underlying medical problems should maximize her physical well-being prior to conception.

The best method of identifying any risk factors associated with an adverse pregnancy outcome is by performing a thorough history, physical examination, and *general health assessment.* The medical history should include any medical illness, current medication, vaccinations, and dietary habits. The obstetrical history should contain details of previous preterm deliveries, pregnancy complications, repetitive first trimester losses, second trimester losses, and intrauterine fetal demises. The gynecological history should identify any risk factors for sexually transmitted diseases, including human immunodeficiency virus (HIV). Besides medical problems, the family history should incorporate questions to identify any genetic disorder or congenital malformation in either the paternal or maternal family. In addition, ethnicity of the potential parents should be noted. The social history should include questions regarding tobacco, alcohol, or illicit drug use. A history of exposure to potentially toxic agents and infectious diseases in the workplace and home should also be obtained.

Maternal Status

Preconception counseling begins with an overall assessment of general health status. As part of this evaluation, attention is directed to a complete review of systems in order to determine the presence of any issues that may influence reproductive outcome. Although it is beyond the scope of this chapter to discuss all of the potential medical problems that may influence pregnancy, a few will be mentioned briefly to provide examples of the type of information women require in order to make informed choices prior to conception.

Advanced Maternal Age

It is clear that many women, for professional and personal reasons, are delaying their childbearing until later in their reproductive years. Recent studies strongly suggest that healthy, nonsmoking women over the age of 35 years may ultimately anticipate a good pregnancy outcome, assuming the fetus does not have a genetic disorder.[2] However, women need to be made aware of a few issues that they may confront by delaying their childbearing. First, it is well known that fecundity decreases with advancing maternal age. Further, the risk of chromosomal disorders increases with advancing maternal age: At age 35 the risk of trisomy 21 is approximately 1/260, and at age 40 this risk increases to 1/75. When one considers all chromosomal abnormalities, including trisomy 21, the risk is approximately doubled. Balancing this negative counseling is the fact that other types of congenital malformations, including neural tube defects, do not increase in frequency with advancing maternal age as long as they are not associated with chromosomal defects. Once beyond the first trimester, and with genetic studies indicating a normal fetus, outcomes in this group of women are largely favorable.

Medical Disorders

Diabetes Mellitus Probably more than any other disorder, the experience of women with diabetes mellitus illustrates the benefits of preconceptional counseling. Meticulous metabolic control during pregnancy combined with tests of fetal well-being and fetal lung maturity drastically reduced perinatal mortality among infants of diabetic women (IDM) from 1970 to the present. However, the high frequency of congenital malformations among IDM remained an uncontrolled problem until it was demonstrated that good metabolic control and normalization of blood glucose prior to and during the critical periods of embryogenesis could reduce the risk to that found in the general population.[5] This crucial observation serves to emphasize the singular importance of preconceptional counseling.

Congenital Heart Disease Another example of the role of preconceptional counseling is found in those cardiac disorders in which pregnancy carries a significant risk of maternal mortality. For example, women with Eisenmenger's syndrome, which is associated with pulmonary hypertension and an uncorrected right-to-left shunt, are subject to a maternal mortality risk of 30 to 50 percent. Those with Marfan's syndrome should undergo echocardiographic examination prior to pregnancy inasmuch as their risk of aortic dissection is much higher if the diameter of the aortic root exceeds 40 mm. Those women with artificial heart valves should understand the risk of the various types of anticoagulation prior to conception. These are but three examples of the importance of providing women with adequate and precise information prior to conceiving, rather than placing them in the position of having to make difficult choices after they have become pregnant.

Chronic Renal Disease It has long been known that women with chronic, underlying renal disease have an increased risk of delivering preterm, frequently growth-restricted, infants and of developing superimposed preeclampsia. However, it is also important for women with chronic renal disease anticipating a pregnancy to have their renal function thoroughly evaluated prior to conception inasmuch as various derangements of renal function are correlated with increasingly poor fetal outcome. For example, among patients without hypertension and a serum creatinine of 1.4 mg/dl or less, pregnancy outcome is quite favorable and further deterioration of renal function is unusual. However, in the presence of hypertension or a serum creatinine of 1.5 mg/dl or higher the prognosis for a healthy pregnancy outcome is more guarded. There is a small risk of deterioration of renal function as well as a significant perinatal morbidity, largely due to preterm delivery. Clearly, women who have undergone renal transplantation also need to be counseled regarding the effects of various immunosuppressive drugs on fetal outcome. They also need to understand the criteria most commonly associated with a favorable pregnancy result.

Similar counseling is required for virtually all medical disorders inasmuch as the disease entities themselves or the medication utilized to treat the disorder may have a significant impact on the patient or her fetus.

Reproductive History

The nonpregnant state provides the physician an excellent opportunity to evaluate causes of previous poor pregnancy outcomes. First, the cause for recurrent first trimester losses may be evaluated after two or three spontaneous abortions, depending on maternal age and degree of anxiety. Cytogenetic studies of couples with a history of repetitive spontaneous abortions reveal that there is approximately a 5 percent risk of karyotypic abnormalities. Although this problem is not correctable, genetic screening tests in successive pregnancies may be offered. Next, müllerian anomalies as well as submucosal fibroids have been implicated as a cause of recurrent spontaneous abortions, and they can best be detected by a hysterosalpingogram or hysteroscopy. Advanced techniques in operative hysteroscopy may provide patients with the opportunity to have some of these malformations readily corrected. In addition, luteal phase defects can be excluded with serum progesterone levels or an endometrial biopsy. Finally, several autoimmune factors such as lupus anticoagulant and anticardiolipin antibody have been implicated as a cause of repetitive spontaneous abortions. Although treatment remains controversial, physicians can be alerted to the potential problems associated with these antibodies, such as preeclampsia, stillbirth, and intrauterine growth restriction.

Although second trimester losses may be due to a structurally or karyotypically abnormal fetus, most are associated with maternal causes such as preterm labor, an incompetent cervix, a placental abnormality, uterine anomalies, drug abuse, or infection. Physicians should obtain an accurate history as well as review previous medical records to clarify etiology. Clarification of the diagnosis of an incompetent cervix versus preterm labor is important. Although the classic history of an incompetent cervix (painless dilatation and delivery) is rarely obtained, other historical facts, such as DES exposure, previous obstetrical laceration, or cone biopsy may make a diagnosis of cervical incompetence more likely. Efforts to define cervical incompetence clinically with hysterosalpingograms, Hegar dilators, and Foley catheters have been proposed but are not widely accepted. Ultrasonographic evaluation of the cervix and lower uterine segment during pregnancy may provide additional information. Anticipating the problem of an incompetent cervix can result in timely diagnosis and intervention and a successful pregnancy outcome.

Some third trimester complications in a previous pregnancy may warrant further workup when a patient is planning another pregnancy. For example, a woman who had early onset severe preeclampsia may have persistent hypertension or renal disease. A woman who had a previous pregnancy complicated by insulin-requiring gestational diabetes may now have overt diabetes. Each evaluation must be individualized and based on the patient's prior history.

Genetics

Genetic Counseling

The most valuable tool for identifying couples at risk for transmitting an inherited disorder to their fetus is a thorough history. To simplify the recorded history, physicians may construct a pedigree that includes first-degree relatives (parents, siblings, and offspring), second-degree relatives (grandparents, uncles, aunts, nephews, and nieces), and third-degree relatives (first cousins). Questions should identify family members with congenital anomalies, mental retardation, learning disabilities, blindness, deafness, chronic medical illnesses such as anemia and skin disorders, and genetic disorders such as cystic fibrosis, myotonic dystrophy, and Huntington's chorea. As described below, a careful review of the reproductive history as well as possible drug or toxin exposure is important.

Because some gene mutations are concentrated in specific ethnic populations, ethnic origin should be documented. Ashkenazi Jews and French Canadians are frequently carriers of Tay-Sachs disease. The carrier frequency is 1/27 and 1/30 to 1/50 for the respective populations.

Similarly, hemoglobinopathies are more frequent in specific groups. Approximately one in ten African-Americans is positive for sickle cell trait. Alpha thalassemia is most frequently encountered in Southeastern Asians. Beta thalassemia is encountered in many ethnic groups; however, Italians and

Greeks have the highest carrier frequency. As prenatal diagnostic techniques are now available, appropriate screening tests should be offered.

Parental ages should be documented. In addition to decreased fertility as well as an increased rate of spontaneous abortions and underlying medical illnesses, a woman of advanced maternal age is at risk for problems related to autosomal trisomies and sex chromosome aberrations. Although many women are aware of their increased risk for a child with Down's syndrome, they do not realize their risk for problems related to other chromosomal abnormalities secondary to nondisjunction. Any woman who will be 35 years or older at the time of delivery should be offered genetic counseling and prenatal diagnosis. With the exception of aneuploidy, paternal age over 55 years is not associated with any chromosomal abnormality. However, fathers in their fifth decade of life are at increased risk for offspring with new autosomal dominant mutations such as Marfan's syndrome and neurofibromatosis. Currently, no prenatal diagnostic tests are available to detect these mutations.

Couples who are first cousins have one eighth of their genes in common. Consequently, they are at higher risk for having a child who is homozygous for a deleterious autosomal recessive gene. Although prenatal diagnosis is not beneficial for these couples, counseling should be provided. Genetic counseling may be very emotional and often difficult for patients to comprehend. Counselors should use simple terms, visual aids, and written information to reinforce concepts. Most importantly, the information should be relayed in an objective manner.[10]

Prenatal Diagnostic Tests

Amniocentesis performed at 15 to 18 weeks of gestation is the most commonly used prenatal genetic diagnostic test. The advantage of this procedure is its safety. Although the exact fetal loss rate is debated, the overall risk of abortion appears to be less than 1 percent. The disadvantage of this test is that a woman is often into the mid-second trimester before the results are available. If a couple chooses to terminate their pregnancy based on the information obtained, the procedure may be technically difficult or physically uncomfortable for the patient.

As an alternative to a traditional amniocentesis, an early amniocentesis may be performed at 11 to 14 weeks gestation. An early amniocentesis is performed in the same manner except a smaller aliquot of amniotic fluid (1 ml/week of gestation) is removed. Because the chorion and amnion often do not fuse until after the 14th week of gestation, the procedure is technically more difficult and is associated with a greater percentage of unsuccessful procedures. The associated fetal loss rate has not been clearly established.

Another method, chorionic villus sampling (CVS), may be performed as early as 9 weeks of gestation. Placental chorionic villi tissue is obtained either transabdominally or transvaginally with ultrasound guidance. Although the results are available by the end of the first trimester, this procedure is associated with one- to threefold higher fetal loss rate than traditional amniocentesis. Recently, several studies have raised the possibility of limb reduction defects in the offspring after CVS. Although other studies have failed to confirm such a risk, couples may be more reluctant to utilize this diagnostic procedure. The information obtained from CVS and amniocentesis is the same except that amniotic alpha fetoprotein analysis cannot be performed on CVS samples.

Percutaneous umbilical blood sampling (PUBS) provides the quickest results. Chromosomal studies are available within 72 h. However, this technique is difficult prior to 20 weeks of gestation. The fetal loss rate is dependent on the experience of the physician and the indication for the procedure.[11]

Screening Tests

Trisomy 21 (Down's syndrome) occurs in approximately 1 out of 800 livebirths. Although the risk of giving birth to a child with trisomy 21 increases with maternal age greater than 35 years, most affected infants are born to women who are younger. Low maternal serum alpha fetoprotein (MSAFP) can detect approximately 20 percent of fetuses with trisomy 21. Recently, high maternal serum human chorionic gonadotropin and low conjugated estriol have also been associated with trisomy 21. Initial studies suggest that a combination of age and these three maternal serum biochemical markers may detect 60 to 70 percent of affected pregnancies without greatly increasing the number of invasive tests. If these results are confirmed, routine screening for trisomy 21 in all pregnancies may be available in the near future.[6]

General Health Habits

Medications

Many prescribed and over-the-counter drugs are known to be teratogenic. Medications known to be potentially teratogenic include angiotensin converting enzyme (ACE) inhibitors, antiepileptics, antimetabolites, coumadin, isotretinoin, and lithium. When taking any medication, a woman contemplating a pregnancy and her physician should assess the potential risk to a fetus and the importance of the medication to the patient's well-being. If the medication is needed for only a short duration, such as isotretinoin, the patient may delay childbearing until after the treatment is completed. Although medical illnesses, such as epilepsy, may require a woman to take teratogenic drugs throughout her lifetime, these patients should be informed of such risks prior to conception. In other medical conditions, patients may be able to change from medications associated with malformations to safer alternatives. For example, a patient with chronic hypertension may be changed from an ACE inhibitor to another effective antihypertensive medication. Medications, such as large doses of vitamin A, which are not essential to maternal well-being should be discontinued. Prior to taking any medication a woman should consult her physician regarding the potential effects on a fetus. Prior to advising the patient, the physician should be aware of the teratogenic potential of the medication. Although the drugs mentioned above are not all-inclusive, they are pharmacological agents that have received extensive study.[3]

Nutrition

Inadequate nutrition is often a confounding variable in adverse pregnancy outcomes. Yet, scientific data in humans are frequently lacking regarding the role that specific nutrients play in normal pregnancy. In addition to encouraging all women to eat a well-balanced diet prior to pregnancy, the physician should also make some specific dietary recommendations. Recent studies have indicated that dietary supplementation with 0.4 mg of folic acid reduces the incidence of neural tube defects (NTD) by 50 percent. If a patient has had a previously affected infant with a NTD, she should take 4 mg of folic acid each day. Folic acid supplementation should be instituted several months prior to conception and continued through the first trimester.[4]

The physician may also calculate a woman's body mass index (BMI) by dividing her weight in kilograms by the square of her height in meters.[2] Women with a BMI less than 19.8 kg/m^2 are underweight. Women with low pregnancy weight are at a significant risk for having low birthweight infants and should have extensive nutritional counseling to ensure an adequate caloric intake. On the other hand, women with a BMI greater than 29 kg/m^2 are considered obese. Maternal obesity is associated with an increased incidence of diabetes, hypertension, and fetal macrosomia. In summary, patients should be encouraged to modify their weight appropriately prior to conception to optimize their pregnancy outcome.[7]

Sexually Transmitted Diseases

In the past few decades, there has been a striking increase in the occurrence of sexually transmitted diseases in the United States. A resurgence of old infections, such as *Neisseria gonorrhoeae* has been noted in addition to the recognition of new diseases such as acquired immunodeficiency syndrome (AIDS). Patients who are at high risk for sexually transmitted diseases should be screened prior to pregnancy.

Chlamydial and gonococcal infections often coexist in the same patient, and both are associated with similar perinatal complications. Both infections can cause neonatal conjunctivitis, and chlamydial infections may also cause neonatal pneumonia. *N. gonorrhoeae* can be successfully treated with a single 250-mg dose of ceftriaxone intramuscularly. Chlamydial infections may be treated with tetracyclines prior to pregnancy and erythromycin during pregnancy. Although still requiring extensive investigation, other sexually transmitted diseases have been associated with prematurity. Bacterial vaginosis and *Trichomonas vaginalis* have received more attention in recent years. The drug of choice for both infections is metronidazole. Patients may be treated prior to or during pregnancy.

Other sexually transmitted diseases can be directly detrimental to the fetus. Syphilis is resurging as a public health problem, and congenital syphilis is at its highest rate since 1970. High-risk patients should be screened with a nonspecific serological test such as the rapid plasma reagin (RPR) prior to pregnancy. Positive results should be confirmed by specific antitreponemal tests [fluorescent treponemal antibody − absorption (FTA − ABS) test]. Primary, secondary, and latent syphilis of less than 1 year's duration may be treated with a single dose of 2.4 million units of benzathine penicillin G. Syphilis of more than 1 year's duration can be treated with the same medication, but it should be administered weekly for three successive weeks. Neurosyphilis requires longer treatment. Follow-up quantitative serology at 3, 6, and 12 months should be performed. A fourfold drop (two dilutions) in titer is indicative of successful treatment.

No treatment can eradicate herpes simplex virus, human papilloma virus, or HIV, and these sexually transmitted diseases may adversely affect pregnancy outcomes. The patient should be cautioned about the effects of perinatal transmission. As AIDS becomes an increasing health concern, women at risk for HIV infection deserve special consideration. Prior to conception all women should be offered HIV screening tests.

Illicit Drug Use

As many as 10 to 15 percent of pregnant women may use illicit drugs. Because women often do not volunteer information regarding substance abuse, the physician should ask directed questions about the type, frequency, and quantity of substances abused. Questions should not be posed in a judgmental or confrontational manner. If a patient admits to using illicit drugs, random urine toxicology screens with the patient's permission may be useful in assessing the type and frequency of use. Drug users rarely abuse a single substance. Once a problem with drug addiction is identified, the physician should explore other aspects of the patient's health associated with substance abuse. In addition, the safety of the social environment to which a newborn child will be taken should be evaluated. Ideally, substance abuse should be identified prior to pregnancy, and women should be referred to a drug rehabilitation program before conception. Continued substance abuse during pregnancy has been associated with placental abruption, growth retardation, congenital anomalies, central nervous system (CNS) damage, and drug withdrawal in the neonate. The physician should be familiar with the potential pregnancy complications and adverse fetal effects of each drug.[8]

Smoking

Twenty-six percent of reproductive age women smoke. Besides affecting general health and reproductive capabilities, cigarette smoking adversely affects pregnancy. In pregnancy, an increased incidence of placenta previa, abruptio placenta, premature rupture of the membranes, and low birth weight infants have each been associated with tobacco use. Although over 2500 chemicals are present in tobacco smoke, carbon monoxide and nicotine appear to be the major components that cause health problems. Smoking cessation programs that use adjunctive therapy with transdermal nicotine patches have reported success rates of 50 percent. Although the use of transdermal nicotine patches is controversial in pregnancy, replacing cigarette usage with the patch will reduce fetal exposure to carbon monoxide and other toxins. The physician and the patient must weigh the potential harm of the transdermal patches to the fetus against the risk of continued cigarette use during pregnancy. If a patient cannot stop smoking prior to pregnancy, she should be encouraged to decrease the amount she smokes to less than twenty cigarettes per day.

Alcohol

Because alcohol consumption is popular and legal in our society, many women do not realize the substantial risk that alcohol consumption may confer to the fetus. Fetal alcohol syndrome (FAS) may result from heavy drinking during pregnancy; it consists of growth deficiency, developmental delay, and structural abnormalities. Although children born to mothers who consume even moderate amounts of alcohol during their pregnancy may not have the complete syndrome, many may exhibit some features. Excluding genetic causes, alcohol consumption during pregnancy is the major identifiable cause of mental retardation in the United States. Because the amount of alcohol consumption that is safe in pregnancy has not been established, women who are contemplating pregnancy should be encouraged to abstain from alcohol.

Exercise

As general awareness of cardiovascular benefits of exercise increases, more women will engage in fitness programs. In addition, exercise can assist women in controlling weight as well as improving flexibility and coordination. Although extremely vigorous exercise programs may cause menstrual irregularities, women who are attempting to become pregnant can engage in moderate activity without increasing the likelihood of menstrual disorders. After conception, the patient may need to modify her exercise program. Maternal heart rate with exercise should not exceed 140 beats per minute. Exercises performed in the supine position, those that require strenuous activity for greater than 15 min, and those that employ the Valsalva maneuver should be avoided. Deep flexion or extension should not be performed. Because of the possible association of neural tube defects and hyperthermia, core body temperature should not exceed 38°C. Basic principles of fitness programs, such as avoiding unlevel surfaces and avoiding dehydration, should also be followed. In general, the physician and patient can compose an individual exercise program based on clinical understanding of the physiological adaptations in pregnancy and common sense.[1]

Vaccinations

All women of reproductive age should be immune to measles, mumps, rubella, tetanus, diphtheria, and poliomyelitis by virtue of natural infection or vaccination. However, during recent years, an increasing number of postpubertal females in the United States are seronegative for rubella. Since rubella infection during pregnancy may be devastating to the fetus, the rubella status of women should be documented prior to pregnancy. Susceptible women should be vaccinated. The patient should avoid pregnancy for a minimum of 3 months after her inoculation. In general, live attenuated viral vaccines should be avoided during pregnancy and immediately prior to conception.

Hepatitis B infection during pregnancy can also be detrimental to the mother as well as the fetus. Women who are at high risk for hepatitis B should be vaccinated. High-risk groups include intravenous drug users, health care workers who may be exposed to body fluids, household contacts of chronic hepatitis B carriers, and recipients of clotting factors. Although this vaccination is considered safe during pregnancy, ideally patients should be immune prior to pregnancy. In general, vaccines derived from toxoids or inactivated organisms may be used in pregnancy if needed.

Environment

As more women seek employment outside of the home, physicians providing conception counseling should be aware of the potential exposure to teratogens and infectious agents in the workplace. Doctors should direct questions to the patient regarding her occupation, hobbies, and environment. Although most occupations do not pose a risk to the pregnant women or fetus, some hazards do exist. For example, gardeners and veterinarians who come in contact with cat feces are at higher risk for toxoplasmosis infections. Child care providers and elementary school teachers are at greater risk for varicella, cytomegalovirus, and parvovirus exposure. If a patient is at higher risk for an infectious disease that may affect her pregnancy outcome, her immunity status may be determined prior to conception. Practical advice may be given to a nonimmune female to decrease her susceptibility, and she should be told to report any exposure or symptoms immediately. Women employed in the biomedical industry are often exposed to radiation, organic solvents, and heavy metals.

The intent of this discussion is not to outline every possible risk but to increase physician awareness. Ideally, all hazardous materials should be avoided in pregnancy. However, we do not live in a risk-free environment. Consequently, efforts should be made to minimize exposure to agents that may contribute to adverse pregnancy outcomes. In addition to the references provided, other resources include teratogen registries, occupational health experts, and several governmental agencies.

References and Selected Readings

1. Artal R: Exercise and pregnancy. *Clin Sports Med* 11:363, 1992.
2. Berkowitz GS, Skovron ML, Lapinski RH, et al: Delayed childbearing and the outcome of pregnancy. *N Engl J Med* 322:659–664, 1990.
3. Briggs GC, Freeman RK, Yaffe SJ: *Drugs in Pregnancy and Lactation: A Reference Guide to the Fetal and Neonatal Risks*. Baltimore: Williams and Wilkins, 1993.
4. Centers for Disease Control: Recommendations for use of folic acid to reduce number of spina bifida cases and other neural tube defects. *JAMA* 259:1233, 1993.
5. Fuhrmann K, Reiher H, Semmler K, et al: Prevention of congenital malformations in infants of insulin-dependent diabetic mothers. *Diabetes Care* 6:219, 1983.
6. Garber AP, Hixon HE. Prenatal genetic counseling. *Clin Perinatol* 17:749, 1990.
7. King JC, Weininger J: Nutrition during pregnancy. *Semin Perinatol* 13:162, 1989.
8. Little BB, Gilstrap LC, Cunningham FG: Social and illicit substance abuse during pregnancy, in Cunningham FG, MacDonald PC, Gant HF (eds): *Williams Obstetrics,* 18th ed. (supplement 7). Norwalk, CT: Appleton & Lange, 1990.
9. Pastorek JG (ed): Sexually transmitted diseases. *Obstet Gynecol Clin North Am* 16(3), 1989.
10. Scioscia AL, Resnik R: Preconception counseling: *Curr Probl Obstet Gynecol Fertil* 14:42, 1991.
11. Williamson RA (guest ed): Prenatal diagnosis. *Clin Obstet Gynecol* 31(2), 1988.

19 Diagnosis of Pregnancy

Claudia L. Werner
Susan M. Cox

The health care worker caring for women who are in their reproductive years must constantly ask the question, "Could she be pregnant?" A diagnosis of pregnancy is important before ordering diagnostic tests that employ radiolabeled compounds or involve radiographic imaging [i.e., x-ray, computerized tomography (CT), and magnetic resonance imaging (MRI)] and before initiating therapies with potential to harm the unborn child. Furthermore, early pregnancy diagnosis allows the timely initiation of prenatal care, which will have a favorable impact on the outcome of both mother and child.

The diagnosis of pregnancy is usually based on a delay or cessation of menses and the presence of a positive pregnancy test. Unfortunately, many women do not keep careful track of their menstrual periods and may be unaware that they have missed one or more periods. Also, spotting in early pregnancy may be misinterpreted as a period. Therefore, it is incumbent on the physician caring for a reproductive age woman to elicit the most accurate information possible about the date of the last menstrual period, whether any periods have been missed, whether the woman has been sexually active, what contraceptive method she has used and whether she uses it regularly, and for the physician to obtain a pregnancy test if indicated.

This chapter will review the symptoms and signs of pregnancy and the diagnostic tests currently available. Common symptoms of pregnancy include "morning sickness," frequent urination, fatigue, and the perception of fetal movement. These are *symptoms* as opposed to clinical *signs*. The signs of pregnancy (Table 19-1) are categorized as "presumptive," "probable," or "positive."

In women who have regular, predictable, cyclic menstruation, the abrupt cessation of menses is highly suggestive of pregnancy. This is especially true if there is associated fatigue, morning sickness, and/or breast tenderness. The physical exam may reveal softening and enlargement of the pregnant uterus, bluish discoloration of the vagina and cervix (Chadwick's sign), and softening of the cervix and lower uterine segment (Hegar's sign).

TABLE 19-1 **Signs of Pregnancy**

PRESUMPTIVE
Cessation of menses
Chadwick's sign
Skin changes
Breast changes
PROBABLE
Enlarged abdomen
Fetal outline on physical examination
Positive pregnancy test
Anatomic changes in cervix
Ballotment
Braxton-Hicks contractions
Changes in uterine shape/size
POSITIVE
Identifiable fetal heart tones
Examiner-detected fetal movement
X-ray or ultrasound detecting fetus

The probable signs of pregnancy include an enlarged abdomen and uterus, palpable Braxton-Hicks contractions, ballotment of the fetus, and a positive pregnancy test. None of these is a positive sign of pregnancy since all can be mimicked by a variety of other conditions; for example, the uterus may be enlarged by leiomyomata, and the pregnancy test may be positive secondary to various ovarian tumors (i.e., embryonal carcinoma, choriocarcinoma, or immature teratoma).

The positive, or definitive, signs of pregnancy include identification of fetal heart tones, examiner-detected fetal movements, or recognition of the fetus via ultrasound or incidental x-ray. Fetal heart motion is audible by Doppler at 10 to 12 weeks gestation and by auscultation with a fetoscope at 18 to 20 weeks. Generally, fetal movements can be palpated by 20 weeks gestation. Using ultrasound techniques, both transvaginal and transabdominal, a gestational sac can be visualized by 6 weeks and fetal cardiac activity by 8 weeks. (*Note:* Gestational age is generally measured in weeks from the first day of the last normal menstrual period.)

Pregnancy Tests

The basis for all current pregnancy tests is the presence of human chorionic gonadotropin (hCG), which can be detected in maternal serum 8 to 9 days after fertilization or in the maternal urine somewhat later. Levels of hCG peak approximately 65 days after conception and fall gradually in the second and third trimesters. A variety of techniques are available for the detection of this glycoprotein hormone, including agglutination inhibition tests, radioimmunoassays, and ELISA (enzyme-linked immunosorbent assays). All have in common the use of mono- or polyclonal antibodies directed against hCG in urine or serum samples.

Agglutination inhibition, utilized by the older and less sensitive urine slide tests, makes use of anti-hCG, which is added to the urine sample. This is followed by the addition of erythrocytes or latex particles coated with hCG. In the presence of pregnancy, no agglutination occurs because all the antibody has been complexed with the hCG in the patient's urine and is unavailable. Agglutination, which is seen as clumping of particles within the sample, occurs if hCG is absent (i.e., the patient is not pregnant). Sensitivity varies from 250 to 3000 mIU/ml of hCG. Most tests are positive 1 week after missed menses.

ELISA tests determine the quantity of hCG present by binding the sample hCG to monoclonal antibodies attached to a solid phase. A second enzyme-linked antibody is used to "sandwich" the hCG. A dye color change will occur when substrate for the enzyme is added to samples that contain hCG. Based on the amount of dye released, hCG can be quantitated. This technique is sensitive to levels of hCG in the 25 to 50 mIU/ml range and is usually performed in less than 1 h.

Radioimmunoassays are the most commonly used tests to quantitate accurately serum levels of hCG. By targeting the beta subunit of the hCG glycoprotein, cross-reactivity with LH (luteinizing hormone) is avoided, allowing very sensitive and specific measurements. The assay is based on the competitive displacement of a radiolabeled ligand, $[^{125}I]$hCG, from antibody directed against the β subunit of hCG. The amount of unbound ligand is proportional to the amount of hCG present in the patient's serum. Unbound radioactivity is quantitated and standard curves are used to calculate results. Serum levels as low as 2 to 4 mIU/ml can be detected. Quantitative β-hCG can therefore be positive several days before menstruation is delayed. This assay is commonly used to rule out early pregnancy prior to invasive or radiographic procedures. It is also used to aid in the diagnosis of abnormal gestations by watching the rate at which the serum hCG is rising and by correlating the level of hCG with sonographic findings.

Newer urine and serum pregnancy test kits now available to clinicians combine immunochromatography with the principles basic to ELISA tests. They consist of convenient plastic test devices across which urine or serum samples are allowed to diffuse. Antibody reaction with hCG results in a color change and/or appearance of a symbol in the "window." Results are available in less than 10 min. These kits can detect levels of hCG in urine as low as 25 to 50 mIU/ml. Therefore, they can become positive any time from 1 week postconception to the time of expected menses. They are sensitive enough for urine testing to detect some abnormal gestations, including a significant proportion of ectopic pregnancies.

Numerous home pregnancy test kits are now available and have become quite popular. Older versions utilize hemagglutination inhibition while newer ones utilize immunochromatography as described above. There have been reports of false positive and, much more commonly, false negative home test results. In some cases, the cause of these may be failure to follow package directions correctly or a misinterpretation of results. It is often prudent, therefore, for the clinician to confirm reported home test results. Additionally, clinicians should make patients aware that home pregnancy tests detect hCG but do not guarantee that a normal gestation is present or that it is intrauterine. A careful history and physical examination are always indicated as soon as possible after a positive pregnancy test.

Summary

The diagnosis of pregnancy is generally based on the patient's history, physical exam, and one of a variety of sensitive pregnancy tests. Additionally, ultrasound imaging can be used to help distinguish between normal and abnormal gestation. The possibility of pregnancy should be considered whenever the health care provider cares for a woman of reproductive age, even if she does not initially report a missed period. By always considering the possibility of pregnancy, clinicians will avoid unintentional exposure of the fetus to potentially harmful agents and procedures. Additionally, a diagnosis of pregnancy allows the initiation of prenatal care and the timing and modification of necessary therapeutic interventions in ways that maximize the benefits and minimize the risks to both the woman and her unborn child.

References and Selected Readings

1. Buster JE, Carson SA: Placental endocrinology and diagnosis of pregnancy, in Gabbe SG, Niebyl JR, Simpson JL (eds): *Obstetrics: Normal and Problem Pregnancies,* 2d ed. New York: Churchill Livingstone, 1991:83.
2. Pregnancy: Overview and diagnosis; ovarian function and ovulation, in Cunningham FG, MacDonald PC, Leveno KJ, Gant HF, Gilstrap LC, III (eds): *Williams Obstetrics,* 19th ed. Norwalk, CT: Appleton & Lange, 1993:21–31.

20 Diagnosis and Management of Spontaneous and Recurrent Abortion

Fredric D. Frigoletto, Jr.
Joseph A. Hill

Spontaneous abortion is one of the most common reasons for women of reproductive age to seek medical attention. Of the more than 5 million clinically recognizable pregnancies established each year in the United States, 85 percent or less result in a viable infant. The majority of spontaneous abortions result from fetal chromosomal abnormalities and occur in the first trimester of pregnancy. A significantly smaller number are the result of a maternal condition such as a uterine abnormality, endocrine deficiency, immunologic factor, genital tract infection, or environmental factors such as smoking or alcohol exposure.

Women of reproductive age who experience vaginal bleeding other than at the time of expected menses should be considered to have a pregnancy-related problem until proven otherwise. First-trimester vaginal bleeding occurs in 30 to 40 percent of pregnancies, and one half of these end in abortion. Generally, those that proceed to abortion are preceded by heavier bleeding and cramping. Although vaginal bleeding other than menses is commonly a consequence of pregnancy, other conditions should be considered.

Differential Diagnosis of Vaginal Bleeding in Early Pregnancy

The possible causes of vaginal bleeding in early pregnancy can be divided into those etiologic factors that are solely pregnancy-related and those that are pregnancy-associated (i.e., not caused by pregnancy but which can occur during pregnancy) as listed in Table 20-1.

A quantitative pregnancy test (using bhCG) should be performed on all women of reproductive age with abnormal vaginal bleeding. This test determines whether women are having bleeding during pregnancy, but it does not distinguish whether this bleeding is a direct result of the pregnancy. A thor-

TABLE 20-1 **Etiologies of Vaginal Bleeding in Early Pregnancy**

Pregnancy Related	Pregnancy Associated
Implantation bleeding	Vulvitis
Abortion	Vaginitis
Ectopic pregnancy	Cervicitis
Molar pregnancy	Carcinoma of vagina, cervix
	Foreign body
	Polyp
	Thrombocytopenia
	von Willebrand's disease
	Anticoagulant therapy
	Disseminated intravascular coagulation

ough history will often enable the clinician to arrive at the proper diagnosis. Determining the date of the last menstrual period is important, as implantation bleeding occurs around cycle day 21 while ectopic pregnancies usually do not become symptomatic until 6 to 8 weeks gestation. Bleeding tends to become heavy in cases of spontaneous abortion while ectopic pregnancies more likely present with spotting.[13] Passage of tissue suggests spontaneous abortion; however, passage of decidual tissue may occur in ectopic pregnancies, mimicking spontaneous abortion. Crampy lower abdominal pain in a woman who is pregnant with vaginal bleeding suggests an inevitable abortion.

In ectopic gestations the pain may be described as cramping but more commonly will be sharp and constant, often associated with peritoneal signs resulting from the accumulation of blood in the abdomen and pelvis. Hemorrhage may also result in referred shoulder pain. Often the diagnosis of an ectopic pregnancy is very difficult in early pregnancy (before 5 weeks gestation), because it is difficult to determine whether an intrauterine pregnancy exists by ultrasound assessment before 5 weeks gestation or when the bhCG level is less than 2000 mIU/ml. In cases of a ruptured corpus luteum cyst during pregnancy, spotting associated with pain may mimic an ectopic pregnancy. Furthermore, free fluid in the posterior cul-de-sac may be seen on ultrasound after the release of the cyst fluid, which in appearance is ultrasonically indistinguishable from blood seen in the cul-de-sac after a ruptured or unruptured but bleeding ectopic pregnancy. In such cases a culdocentesis may be helpful, although sophisticated ultrasound techniques with quantitative serum bhCG determinations have largely replaced it as a diagnostic modality.[7,10] Serial quantitative β-hCG titers can be helpful in these cases to determine whether an abnormal pregnancy exists. If the β-hCG titer does not rise by 66 to 100 percent after 48 h, then an abnormal pregnancy (ectopic or potential abortion) may be present.[8] A quantitative bhCG titer > 2000 mIU/ml warrants an ultrasound examination to look for an intrauterine pregnancy. If no intrauterine pregnancy is seen, an ectopic gestation is strongly suggested. Abnormally high bhCG titers associated with vaginal bleeding may be the result of a molar pregnancy, although multiple gestation is also a possibility. Possible risk factors for ectopic pregnancy include the following: prior ectopic pregnancy, a history of pelvic inflammatory disease, pelvic adhesions, prior ruptured appendix, prior tubal surgery, contraceptive failures with intrauterine devices (IUDs) or oral contraceptives, prior tubal ligation, diethylstilbestrol (DES) exposure, and a history of recurrent abortion. One method of assessment to rule out ectopic pregnancy is demonstrated in Fig. 20-1.

Spontaneous Abortion

In approximately 70 percent of human conceptions fetal viability is not achieved, with an estimated 50 percent lost prior to the first missed menses.[12] The actual rate of pregnancy loss after implantation may be as high as 31 percent.[14] *Spontaneous abortion* is defined as the loss of a clinically recognized (blood test or ultrasound) pregnancy prior to 20 weeks gestation, and occurs in 10 to 15 percent of all clinically established pregnancies. Approximately 60 percent of pregnancy losses before eight weeks gestation are chromosomally abnormal, with trisomies being the most common abnormality. However, the most common single abnormality is monosomy X (45,X).[2]

Spontaneous abortions are subdivided into threatened abortion, inevitable abortion, incomplete abor-

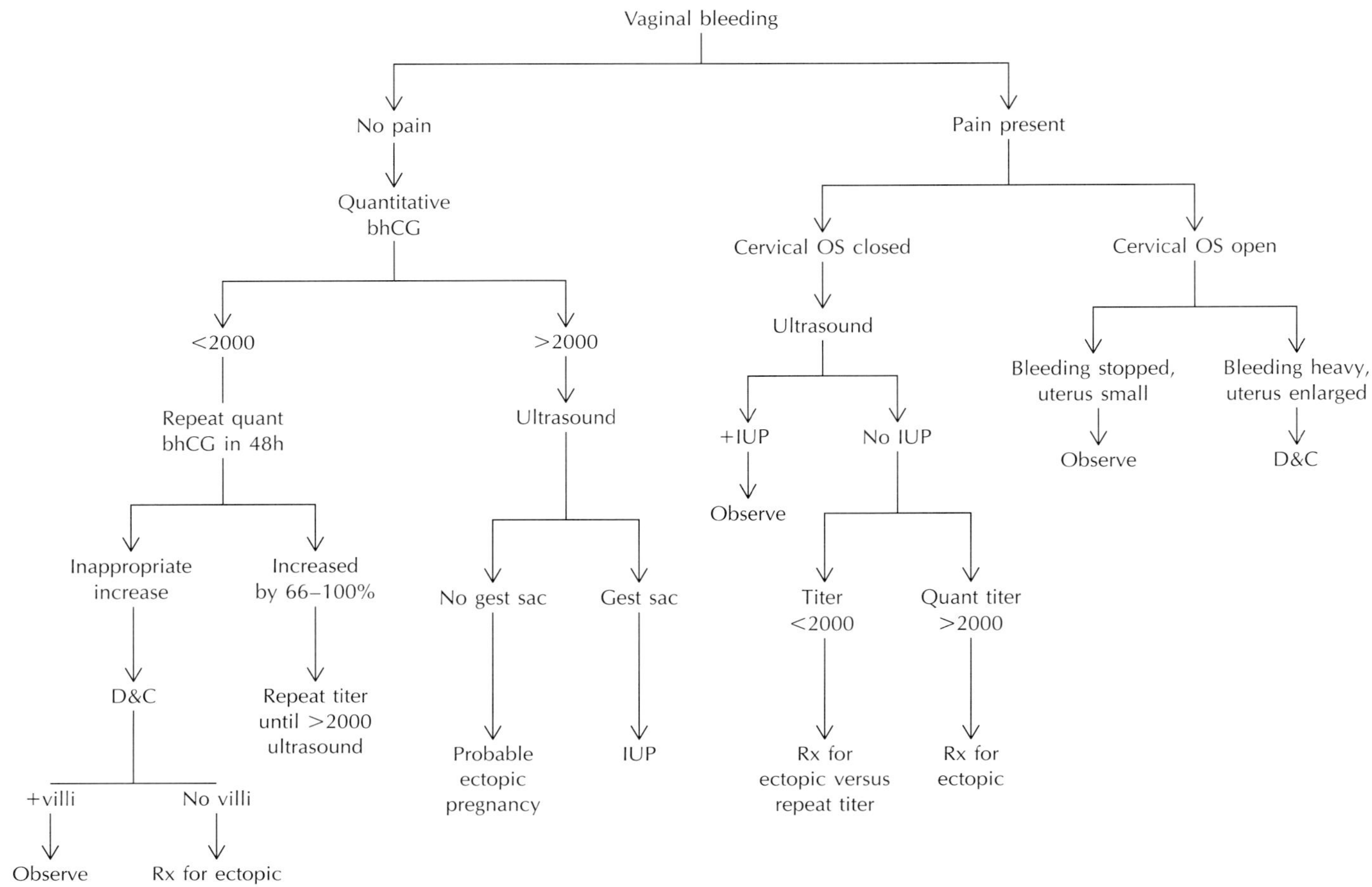

Figure 20-1 An algorithm for ruling out ectopic pregnancy. IUP, intrauterine pregnancy.

tion, complete abortion, missed abortion, and recurrent abortion. Threatened abortion refers to viable clinical pregnancies accompanied by vaginal bleeding. Inevitable abortion occurs during pregnancy in the presence of a dilated internal cervical os or in cases with ruptured membranes. An incomplete abortion occurs when some, but not all, fetal placental tissue has passed through the internal cervical os; while a complete abortion is when all fetal placental tissue has been spontaneously passed through the internal cervical os. A missed abortion is a pregnancy in which the fetus is no longer viable in the absence of vaginal bleeding. Symptoms of pregnancy (nausea, breast tenderness) may or may not be present at the time of a pregnancy loss. Pelvic examination and ultrasound assessment will usually lead to the proper diagnosis.

Recurrent Abortion

Recurrent abortion has been traditionally defined as the occurrence of three or more clinically recognized pregnancy losses prior to 20 weeks gestation, and it occurs in approximately 1 in 300 pregnancies.[1] A clinical investigation of pregnancy loss, however, should be initiated after two spontaneous abortions, especially when the woman is older than 35 years, the couple has had difficulty conceiving, or the couple is anxious to investigate potential causes. It is important to understand the calculated risks for recurrent abortion based on epidemiologic surveys, especially when reviewing the literature on potential success rates with various therapies. These surveys indicate that after one spontaneous abortion the recurrence risk is 24 percent; after two, 30 percent; after three, 35 percent; and approximately 40 percent after four consecutive clinical losses.[1,12]

Etiology

Parental chromosomal abnormalities remain the only uncontested cause of recurrent abortion and occur in approximately 5 percent of couples seeking evaluation. Other associations with recurrent pregnancy loss have been made, including müllerian or anatomic anomalies (10 percent), endocrinologic abnormalities (17 percent), infections (5 percent), and autoimmunity (3 percent). The potential cause in the majority of cases, however, remains unexplained (60 percent) even after a thorough conventional evaluation (Table 20-2).[5,6]

The most common inborn parental chromosomal abnormality contributing to recurrent abortion is balanced translocation. Pericentric chromosomal inversion and sex chromosome mosaicism have also been associated with recurrent abortion. Other genetic causes of abortion include multifactorial inheritance of autosomal recessive genes and x-linked disorders.

Anatomical causes can be divided into both congenital and acquired lesions. Congenital anomalies include incomplete müllerian fusion or septum resorption defects, diethylstilbestrol (DES) exposure, and uterine artery anomalies. Women with a septate uterus may have a 62 percent risk for spontaneous abortion. Second-trimester losses are most commonly seen; however, first-trimester abortions may be caused if the embryo implants on the intrauterine septum, since the endometrium overlying the septum is poorly developed and blood supply to this area is often limited. When abnormal placentation occurs, the pregnancy may end in an abortion. DES-exposure in utero can lead to uterine developmental anomalies, most commonly hypoplasia, which may be associated with both first- and second-trimester abortions. DES-exposed women may also have a predisposition to develop an incompetent cervix and

TABLE 20-2 Investigative Measures Potentially Useful in the Evaluation of Recurrent Spontaneous Abortion

1. Parental peripheral blood karyotypes
2. Hysterosalpingogram
3. Luteal phase endometrial biopsy
4. Thyroid function studies (TSH, T4)
5. Anticardiolipin and antiphosphatidyl serine antibodies
6. Lupus anticoagulant
7. Antisperm antibodies[a]
8. Cervical cultures for mycoplasma and ureaplasma[a]

[a]Not evaluated until late in the workup.

premature labor. Isolated cases of uterine artery anomalies have been reportedly associated with recurrent abortion, most likely due to compromised blood flow to the implanting blastocyst and developing placenta. Acquired anatomical lesions potentially predisposing to recurrent abortion include uterine synechiae (adhesions), submucous or intramural leiomyomata (fibroids), and endometriosis. These associations with abortion are tenuous, but theoretical mechanisms that may be involved include interference with blood supply, as in the case of adhesions and fibroids, and immunological phenomena that may be involved in cases of endometriosis.[3]

Endocrinologic abnormalities associated with recurrent abortion include luteal phase insufficiency, thyroid disorders, and diabetes mellitus. The early maintenance of pregnancy is dependent on progesterone production by the corpus luteum until the placenta takes over progesterone production between 7 to 9 weeks of gestation. Spontaneous abortion could ensue if (1) the corpus luteum fails to produce sufficient quantities of progesterone, (2) progesterone delivery to the uterus is compromised, or (3) progesterone utilization within endometrial-decidual tissue is disordered. Thyroid disorders, most commonly hypothyroidism, have also been associated with recurrent abortion, most likely due to ovulation disorders leading to corpus luteum insufficiency. The mechanism of abortion in women with diabetes mellitus is unclear but may be due to compromised blood flow to the developing conceptus, especially in cases of advanced disease.

Maternal infections have been tenuously associated with recurrent abortion. The most commonly reported association between infection and pregnancy loss has been cervical colonization with mycoplasma and ureaplasma. Causal mechanisms are poorly described, but one theoretical possibility may involve immunologic activation.

Other poorly established associations include environmental factors such as heavy metal toxicity; carbon tetrachloride and trichloroethylene benzene; drugs such as folic acid antagonists, nicotine, ethanol and inhalation anesthetic agents; ionizing radiation; and chronic medical illnesses such as cardiac and renal diseases or any other disorder that compromises uterine blood supply. Thrombocytosis (platelet counts greater than 1 million) has also been associated with recurrent abortion, presumably due to clotting and occlusion of the placental vasculature. It is important to reassure patients that exposure to video display terminals (VDTs) and microwave ovens does *not* cause abortion.

Immunologic phenomena involving allogeneic immunity and autoimmunity have also been associated with reproductive failure.[4]

Evaluation

Diagnostic evaluation of couples experiencing recurrent abortion should begin with a general history that includes medical, surgical, genetic, and psychological factors. A description and sequence of all prior pregnancies is important, as is whether histologic and karyotypic assessment of prior abortions were performed. The practitioner should also ask about chronic illnesses, uterine instrumentation, infection, DES-exposure, as well as exposure to drugs, radiation, and possible environmental pollutants.

A general physical examination of the woman should include an investigation for signs of metabolic illness. On pelvic examination, the examiner should search for signs of infection, DES-exposure, or previous cervical laceration, and on bimanual examination, for irregularity of the size, shape, and contour of the uterus.

Laboratory measurements potentially useful (Table 20-2) include the following: (1) a peripheral blood karyotype of both partners; (2) hysterosalpingogram followed by hysteroscopy and laparoscopy, if indicated; (3) a luteal phase endometrial biopsy, ideally 10 days following the luteinizing hormone (LH) surge after cycle day 24 of an idealized 28-day cycle (If the biopsy is out of phase by more than 2 days according to established criteria, then repeat assessment in a subsequent cycle is required before making the diagnosis of luteal phase insufficiency. In cases of an abnormal biopsy a serum prolactin and androgen profile should also be determined.); (4) thyroid function tests (TSH, free T4); (5) anticardiolipin and antiphosphatidyl serine antibodies; (6) lupus anticoagulant (a PTT or Russell Viper Venom Time); and, as a last resort, (7) antisperm antibodies in the woman's peripheral serum and cervical mucus and (8) a cervical culture for mycoplasma and ureaplasma.

Therapy

Therapy should include appropriate measures for the specifically identified problem. For individuals with recurrent abortion of unknown etiology, expectant management consisting of synchronized ovulation and sperm deposition may be helpful, as dyssynchronized fertilization has been hypothesized to contribute to early pregnancy loss due to chromosomal abnormalities. Early diagnosis and close monitoring during the first trimester may also be psychologically therapeutic. Serial human chorionic gonadotropin (hCG) determinations for the beta subunit (bhCG) should be performed. Once the bhCG attains 1000 to 5000 mIU/ml at 5 to 6 weeks gestation, an intrauterine pregnancy should be confirmed by ultrasound, recognizing that women with recurrent spontaneous abortion have a 2 to 4 percent risk of ectopic gestation.

Rarely, immunotherapy may be considered, but this is experimental and in the authors' opinion should only be utilized under a strict scientific protocol at no cost to study patients. Immunosuppressive therapies have been proposed for recurrent abortion believed due to maternal immune hyperresponsiveness. Most remain untested in randomized, double-blind, placebo-controlled trials and therefore cannot be recommended. Some evidence, however, does exist indicating that aspirin (80 mg/day) and heparin (10,000 units bid) may be efficacious in preventing abortion and other poor obstetrical outcomes associated with maternal antiphospholipid antibody production.[11]

The prognosis for a subsequent live birth (Table 20-3) in couples with a history of recurrent abortion is not necessarily dismal. Most chromosomally abnormal pregnancies abort prior to achieving fetal cardiac activity. Recent evidence suggests that once fetal cardiac activity has been ultrasonically detected between 5 and 6 weeks gestation, the risk of subsequent loss is approximately 23 percent. While this is significantly higher than the 4 percent incidence in the general population, knowledge that a 77 percent chance of fetal viability exists once fetal cardiac activity has been detected can be tremendously reassuring to the couple who has experienced multiple miscarriages, and it helps to set a more realistic prognosis for pregnancy success.

TABLE 20-3 Prognosis for Live Birth

Etiology	Percent Success
Genetic (chromosomal)	30–60
Anatomic	60–70
Endocrinologic	90
Unknown (other)	30–90

Summary

In conclusion, the diagnosis of early pregnancy disorders depends on an accurate assessment of the patient's history, physical examination, and appropriate laboratory tests. Understanding the potential pathophysiologic mechanisms involved in each diagnosis as outlined in this chapter will enable women's health care providers to manage effectively the most commonly encountered disorders that cause early pregnancy wastage.

References and Selected Readings

1. Alberman E: The epidemiology of repeated abortion, in Sharp F (ed): *Early Pregnancy Loss: Mechanisms and Treatment.* New York: Springer-Verlag, 1988, pp 9–17.
2. Boue J, Boue A, Lasar P: Retrospective and prospective epidemiologic studies of 1,500 karyotyped spontaneous abortions. *Teratology* 11:11–26, 1975.
3. Hill JA: Immunological factors in endometriosis and endometriosis-associated reproductive failure. *Infert Reprod Med Clin North Am* 3:583–96, 1992.
4. Hill JA: Sporadic and recurrent spontaneous abortion. *Curr Prob Obstet Gynecol Fertil* 17:113–164, 1994.
5. Hill JA, Polgar K, Harlow BL, Anderson DJ: Evidence of embryo and trophoblast toxic cellular immune response(s) in women with recurrent spontaneous abortion. *Am J Obstet Gynecol* 166: 1044–52, 1992.
6. Hill JA, Ravnikar V: Recurrent abortion, in KJ Ryan,

RS Berkowitz, RL Barbieri (eds): *Gynecology: Principles and Practice,* 5th ed., St. Louis, MO: 1990, pp 406–30.

7. Kadar N, DeVore G, Romero R: Discriminatory hCG zone: Its use in the sonographic evaluation for ectopic pregnancy. *Obstet Gynecol* 58:156, 1981.
8. Kadar N, Freedman M, Zackar M: Further observation on the doubling time of human chorionic gonadotropin in early asymptomatic pregnancy. *Fertil Steril* 34:783, 1980.
9. Laufer MR, Ecker JL, Hill JA: Pregnancy outcome following ultrasound documented fetal cardiac activity in women with a history of multiple spontaneous abortions (submitted).
10. Nyberg DA, Filly RA, Mahoney BS, et al: Early gestation: Correlation of hCG levels and sonographic identification. *AJF* 144:951, 1985.
11. Triplett DA: Obstetrical implications of antiphospholipid antibodies. *Clin Obstet Gynecol* 6:507–18, 1992.
12. Warburton D, Fraser FC: Spontaneous abortion rate in man: Data from reproductive histories collected in a medical genetics unit. *Am J Hum Genet* 16:1, 1963.
13. Weckstein LN: Clinical diagnosis of ectopic pregnancy. *Clin Obstet Gynecol* 30:236–44, 1987.
14. Wilcox AJ, Weinberg CR, O'Connor JF, et al: Incidence of early loss of pregnancy. *N Eng J Med* 319:189–94, 1988.

21 Contraception and Abortion

Ashley Coopland
Patricia Bailey

Prevention of pregnancy and limitation of family size have been sought by individuals and society throughout recorded history; however, it is only in recent years that effective contraception has become available. In the western world, hormonal contraception has become the principal means of preventing pregnancy.

Hormonal Contraception

It had been recognized for years that estrogen would prevent ovulation; however, irregular and unpredictable bleeding, as well as other problems, precluded the use of unopposed estrogen as a contraceptive. With the development of a synthetic orally active progestin in the 1950s, oral contraception became a reality.

Over the past 20 years, we have witnessed rapid developments in the composition of oral contraceptives, most notably a decline in the estrogen content, from 100 μg to as low as 20 μg in some current preparations. We have also become thoroughly familiar with their potential side effects, the more serious of which were encountered earlier when higher doses of synthetic estrogens were being used. The extensive study by Vessey and Doll in the United Kingdom in the late 1960s found an alarming increase in cases of cerebrovascular accidents, deep vein thrombosis, and myocardial infarction. While a history of, or predisposition to, these conditions still constitutes a contraindication to oral contraceptive therapy, it is now realized that the currently used low-dosage agents pose little threat in the absence of other risk factors—most notably smoking and hypertension. Although serious complications associated with oral contraception use are uncommon, it is important for the physician to be familiar with the potential risks and to discuss them with the patient prior to initiation of use. A thorough list of potential associated problems can be found in the *Physician's Desk Reference* (PDR).

By far the most commonly used agents today are the "combination" pills, which contain a low dose

(20 to 35 μg) of one of two synthetic estrogens, ethinyl estradiol or mestranol, and a low dose of any one of a number of orally active progestins. These pills are most often prescribed on a "Sunday start" regimen. The usual pack contains 28 pills, the last 7 of which are inert and serve to keep the patient in the habit of taking a pill every day.

Problems are relatively uncommon, and most patients can use the birth control pill for several years if desired. Although with the older, higher-dose pills it was usual to stop prescribing for patients over age 35, most experts now agree that there is little risk at age 40 or even 45 years old in the absence of other cardiovascular risk factors and provided the woman does not smoke. Nevertheless, patients frequently call their physicians with regard to a number of minor but troublesome complaints. Some examples follow:

"Doctor, I forget how you said to take them." For a Sunday start, tell the patient to begin on the first Sunday after the onset of her period and to take one pill per day for 28 days; after this time, she should start the next pack. Even if she does not have a period, she should start the next pack anyway as long as she has not missed any pills. If she has missed a pill, she should make certain to contact her physician.

"Doctor, some of my friends have told me the pill causes cancer." Actually, the pill reduces the risk of two types of cancer (ovarian and endometrial). Whether the pill may increase breast cancer risk in a very small subset of women is being evaluated, but many health care providers do not feel that there is any convincing evidence of this at present.

"Doctor, I missed taking my pill yesterday." The chances of pregnancy may increase very slightly, but the patient should be told to take the forgotten pill at once and the next one at the usual time. If she misses two pills consecutively, she should be advised to double up on the active pills for the balance of the cycle and use a backup method of birth control.

"Doctor, my period has come nearly 2 weeks early." Depending on the patient's reliability, on whether she has been taking the pill properly, and whether this is the first occurrence, she may require an examination to rule out ectopic or intrauterine pregnancy or any other significant cause of bleeding. If there is no serious problem and the complaint is actually only spotting, the patient can frequently be told to ignore it in the expectation that it will cease to be troublesome in subsequent cycles. If the bleeding is heavier and significant problems have been ruled out, then the patient is probably experiencing "breakthrough" bleeding. She should be advised to double up on the dosage until the end of the cycle. The bleeding should cease and a normal period should follow. If the problem becomes recurrent, the patient should probably be switched to a pill with a higher hormonal content.

Other fairly common problems that women using oral contraceptives may complain of include headache, mastalgia, nausea, weight gain, and depression. These frequently abate after a few cycles, but if not and if a change in pill composition does not improve the situation, then it may be necessary to discontinue treatment and switch to an alternate method of contraception.

The beneficial side effects of oral contraceptives include reduction in the amount of menstrual flow, diminished incidence of anemia, reduced incidence of ovarian cysts, and significantly less dysmenorrhea in most patients. While the theoretical contraceptive efficacy of the combination pill is close to 100 percent, the user outcome is somewhat lower.

In addition to hormonal contraception employing both estrogen and a progestin, there are progestin-only agents. The mechanism of action of pure progestin agents relies partially on their inhibition of ovulation, but, in addition, their effect on cervical mucus is also important as they render it viscid and impenetrable to sperm. As they are free of synthetic estrogen, estrogen-related side effects do not occur. However, progestin side effects—including depression, spotting, irregular bleeding, and amenorrhea—can be troublesome. Progestin agents can be taken orally or administered intramuscularly. One of the newer agents is implanted under the skin of the upper arm.

Several pharmaceutical companies market the continuous, low-dose progestin agent in an oral form, the "mini pill." This typically consists of

0.35 mg of the synthetic progestin norethindrone or 0.2 mg of another synthetic progestin, D-norgestrel. The pill is taken 365 days a year and has a theoretical effectiveness only slightly less than that of the combination pill. However, the side effects mentioned above limit its usefulness, and it is usually prescribed for patients in whom synthetic estrogens are contraindicated. Many practitioners find it particularly useful in postpartum patients who are breast-feeding. One injectable agent has already been approved the Food and Drug Administration (FDA) for contraceptive use. DepoProvera, previously used for a variety of indications (including the treatment of endometrial hyperplasia), can now be used for patients who want relatively prolonged contraception without having to remember to take a pill every day. The recommended dose is 150 mg IM every 3 months. Before initiating treatment with long-lasting progestins, as indeed with most contraceptive methods, it is essential to ensure that the patient is not pregnant. For this reason, the initial dose is frequently administered during a regular menstrual period.

Norplant, another innovation in contraceptive technology, involves the insertion of several capsules containing a synthetic progestin beneath the skin of the upper arm. Progestin is slowly released and the contraceptive effect lasts for up to 5 years. Although the initial cost is relatively high, the manufacturers point out that there is little difference from that of the cost of 5 years of oral contraceptives. Studies are beginning to show that as many as 25 percent of patients request early removal, either because of side effects or because they have decided to have another baby earlier than initially planned. For properly selected patients, this is a good method of contraception, but probably not cost-effective if used indiscriminately.

Barrier Methods of Contraception

Barrier methods of contraception are relatively inexpensive and safe; however, they are not without drawbacks. For barrier methods to be effective, sexual activity must be anticipated or interrupted, and the methods must be used consistently and correctly with each episode of coitus. In addition, there is a substantially higher accidental pregnancy rate with barrier methods than with oral contraceptives (OCs) or intrauterine devices (IUDs).

Diaphragm

The diaphragm is a shallow rubber dome with a firm, flexible rim. Diaphragms come in sizes between 55 and 105 mm. The arcing spring-type diaphragm is recommended for most nulliparous patients because of the ease of insertion. The diaphragm is always used in conjunction with a spermicidal jelly, which should be spread around the entire rim as well as the inside of the dome. It must be left in place for at least 6 h after intercourse. If the woman has intercourse again within the 6-h period, she should add another application of spermicide into the vagina but must be careful not to move the diaphragm while doing so.

Successful diaphragm contraception requires a high level of patient motivation. The diaphragm is usually not the best method of contraception for the younger adolescent who is not yet comfortable with her body.

A diaphragm must be fitted by a health care provider who is willing to invest substantial time and patience. An initial counseling session includes a thorough review of the available methods of contraception and their risks and benefits. The counseling session also involves a discussion regarding the frequency and geographic location of the patient's sexual activity. (For example, if activity occurs ''sometimes at his place, sometimes at my place,'' it might be wise to prescribe two diaphragms for the patient, one to keep at her home and one to leave at her partner's.)

When the practitioner is confident that the patient understands the instructions and that the diaphragm is appropriate for the patient's lifestyle, the device is fitted. Once fitted, the patient is encouraged to palpate the properly placed diaphragm, i.e., feel the cervix behind the contraceptive device. She should then remove the diaphragm and reinsert it under the direct supervision of the practitioner who again checks the fitting. The necessary instructions are reviewed during the fitting process and the patient sent home with a copy of written instructions.

Contraceptive Sponge

The Today sponge was approved by the FDA in 1983. This contraceptive is a dome-shaped device composed of polyurethane foam impregnated with nonoxynol-9. It provides protection from unwanted pregnancy in three ways:

1. The spermicidal activity of nonoxynol-9 (spermicide dose of 1 g).
2. Mechanical protection by absorption of semen.
3. Mechanical blockage by covering the cervical os.

The sponge must be moistened with clean tap water and squeezed at least once before insertion. This procedure helps to release the spermicide and improves protection. The sponge may be inserted just prior to coitus or several hours before.

The advantage of the sponge for the adolescent is that it is available over the counter and does not require fitting by a health practitioner. Because it can be placed well in advance of sexual activity, it offers the advantage of increased spontaneity as well as protection for multiple sex acts with a single insertion.

The risk of toxic shock syndrome (TSS) has been estimated at 10 in 100,000 users; therefore, patients selecting the sponge should not use it during menses and must use alternate contraception at that time. Furthermore, all users should be educated about the warning signs of early TSS. Other disadvantages include sponge tearing, allergic reactions, and vaginal dryness caused by the tendency of the sponge to absorb vaginal fluid during intercourse. This device may be limited for an adolescent patient whose sexual activity does not take place near a source of clean tap water.

Vaginal Spermicidal Inserts

Vaginal spermicidal inserts include jellies, creams, suppositories, and films. The most widely used spermicidal agents in these products are nonoxynol-9 and octoxynol-9. As with the contraceptive sponges, the principal advantage for the patient is that they are available over the counter at a reasonable price. It should also be noted that the suppositories are small enough to fit discreetly into a purse, and the film can easily be carried in a wallet or in one's pocket. Elimination of clumsy applicators should make films and suppositories even more attractive to adolescents.

When vaginal spermicidal inserts are discussed with a patient, specific brand names should be mentioned. The principal foam products on the market are Emko, Ortho-Gynol, and Delfen. The commonly available suppositories include Encare Oval, Semicid, and vaginal contraceptive film (VCF). It is helpful to have samples of these products, especially those that require an applicator so that proper placement can be demonstrated. The patient should be encouraged to read the package insert and to discuss any questions she might have about the product.

Patient instructions for the use of spermicides are the following:

1. Insert the contraceptive foam, suppository, or film high into the vagina so that it will cover the cervix. Use the foam 30 min or less prior to (*not* after) intercourse.
2. Do not douche for at least 6 h after intercourse.
3. Keep an extra condom with the contraceptive foam since use of the combination lessens the risk of failure.

Cervical Cap

The cervical cap is a small dome-shaped contraceptive made of pliable latex that is used in conjunction with a spermicide as a contraceptive. The cap is designed to fit snugly across the cervix and is held in place by suction. It was approved for use by the FDA in 1988; however, it has not achieved great popularity in the United States. There are several disadvantages to this method of birth control, especially for adolescents. Of note is that the clinical trials have primarily involved adult women. The device must be fitted by a trained health care practitioner and insertion may be difficult. In a comparative study with diaphragm users, cap users were more likely to report dislodgement during use at least once (40 vs. 14 percent) and vaginal odor (17 vs. 9 percent). Advantages of this method include the fact that the cap may be left in place for 24 to 48 h, permitting more spontaneity in sexual relations. The cap is also smaller and more durable and uses less spermicide than the diaphragm.

Because of concern about a possible adverse effect of the cap on cervical tissue, the cap should be used only by women with a normal pap smear, and it is recommended that users have another pap smear 3 months after starting to use this method. The use of the cervical cap in adolescent patients is not well studied. The cap, like the diaphragm, may be an appropriate method of contraception for an older, highly motivated adolescent. In contrast, younger adolescents in the United States are unlikely to be good candidates for this method of birth control.

Condoms

In addition to being an effective method of barrier contraception, latex condoms are quite effective in reducing the risk of transmission of sexually transmitted diseases, including human immunodeficiency virus (HIV). In addition to the traditional male condom, a female condom has recently been developed.

Intrauterine Devices (IUDs)

The Progestasert System has been marketed by the Alza Corporation, Palo Alto, California since 1976. It is a T-shaped unit that contains a reservoir of 38 mg of progesterone. Two monofilament nylon retrieval threads are fastened to the base of the T stem. The Progestasert releases progesterone at a rate of approximately 65 μg per day. It must be replaced after 1 year, which is a disadvantage. Advantages include its reduction of average menstrual blood loss and its improvement of primary dysmenorrhea, both presumably effects of topical progesterone on the endometrium.

The second IUD available in the United States is the Paragard 380 (the copper T 380A), which was introduced by GynoPharm, Inc., New Jersey, in 1988. Since its introduction, a half-million of these IUDs have been inserted, and the demand appears to be increasing. The body of the Paragard is wound with approximately 176 mg of copper and carries approximately 66.5 mg of copper on each of its transverse arms, creating an exposed surface area of copper of 380 ± 23 mm^2. The Paragard should be replaced after 8 years.

While the exact mechanism of action of IUDs remains unclear, recent evidence indicates that they exert their effects beyond the uterus. IUDs may prevent sperm from fertilizing ova in several ways, including foreign body response in the myometrium and biochemical changes in endometrial enzymes and prostaglandins that may interfere with sperm transportation in the genital tract and may actually damage sperm and ova. Sivin has concluded that IUDs "act as contraceptives and are not abortifacients."

Both types of IUDs appear to be very effective forms of birth control. Pregnancy rates of 0.1 to 1.3 pregnancies per 100 woman years have been reported for the Paragard, while rates of 1.5 to 4.9 pregnancies per 100 woman years have been reported for the Progestasert.

In the 1960s and 1970s studies suggesting a cause-and-effect relationship between IUDs and pelvic inflammatory disease (PID) began to appear. Because of the increasing expense of litigation, all IUDs except Progestasert were removed from the market in the early 1980s.

A reassessment of the IUD-PID connection reveals that these previous studies had many methodological flaws. There is increasing evidence from randomized, prospective, carefully performed studies that the IUD in itself does not cause PID. The newer findings of these studies are the following:

1. It is the woman's lifestyle, especially her sexual behavior [e.g., number of partners and exposure to sexually transmitted diseases (STDs)] that is responsible for the additional PID risk.
2. Insertion and removal procedures increase PID risk.
3. Copper and hormone-releasing IUDs are associated with the lowest PID risk in IUD users.

Currently, IUDs are recommended for patients who have had at least one child and are in a stable, mutually monogamous relationship.

Natural Family Planning

Some religious groups object to any artificial contraception. For many members of these groups, "natural" family planning is employed. Natural family planning uses the "safe period" calculation, or estimation of the status of cervical mucus. It is variably dependable and requires a good deal of instruction, considerable sophistication, and self-control.

Using the calendar method, the woman determines her fertile period and then abstains from intercourse during this time. Since for many women the interval between menstrual periods has variability, the woman must make her calculations based on a year's worth of prior experience. After determining the length of her shortest and longest cycles during the previous year, the woman calculates her fertile period as follows: The earliest day on which she is likely to be fertile is calculated by subtracting 18 days from the length of her shortest cycle the previous year. The latest day in the month on which she is likely to be fertile is determined by subtracting 11 days from the length of her longest cycle during the previous year. The entire time span between these two days represents the woman's most fertile period during the month.

An example of this calculation is as follows: During the prior year, the woman's shortest intermenstrual interval was 28 days, and her longest intermenstrual interval was 33 days. Her probable first fertile day would be $28 - 18 =$ day 10; her probable last day would be $33 - 11 =$ day 22. Therefore, on days 10 through 22 of each menstrual month (day 1 being the day on which the menstrual period starts), she should not have intercourse.

Other methods of natural family planning employ the calendar method in concert with either the evaluation of cervical mucus (which usually becomes clear and can be stretched into a thin strand around the time of ovulation), the use of commercially available kits which measure hormonal changes, and basal body temperature charts. Natural family planning is associated with a much higher pregnancy rate than any of the other methods of contraception.

Sterilization

For the woman who has completed her childbearing, permanent sterilization may be an attractive option. In mature, mutually monogamous couples, sterilization may be performed on either partner.

Tubal Ligation

Ligation, or blocking of the Fallopian tubes, can be accomplished by a variety of procedures with ease and safety, although the operation is more difficult and carries more risk than ligation of the vas deferens in the male. A regional or general anesthetic is almost invariably used, and the risks of hemorrhage and infection are greater than with a vas ligation. Numerous techniques and approaches have been described, but the most common today are either ligation at the time of cesarean section or laparoscopy or minilaparotomy with tubal occlusion being achieved by ligation, cauterization, or the application of synthetic occlusive devices. Patients must be informed of a failure rate of 4 to 10 per 1000 as well as the fact that there is a 50 percent chance that if there is a subsequent pregnancy it will be in the fallopian tube. It is mandatory to ensure insofar as it is possible that the patient truly desires sterilization and is aware of the fact that it is intended to be permanent. This is particularly true since more and more young women are electing to obtain sterilization.

Vas Deferens Ligation (Vasectomy)

Bilateral ligation of the vas deferens is performed easily and safely under local anesthesia. Recovery is rapid, and there are few postoperative complications. Sexual function is not compromised and the quantity of ejaculate is virtually undiminished, as prostatic secretion, the main component of seminal fluid, is unchanged. On rare occasions sexual dysfunction may result; this can usually be resolved by counseling but emphasizes the need for careful patient selection. The patient must be informed that there is a small failure rate and must be advised to use another method of contraception for about 6 weeks, at which time a seminal fluid sample should show a complete absence of spermatozoa.

Elective Termination of Pregnancy

Woman have sought and obtained abortions for many centuries. In some times and places, abortion has been illegal and was performed in clandestine settings, usually by individuals totally ignorant of anatomy, let alone sterile technique. Abortion became legal in the United States, as a result of the Supreme Court decision on *Roe v. Wade.* Almost overnight, deaths from complications of abortion in the United States were massively diminished.

Abortion can be performed most safely and easily in the first trimester. The procedure most often employed at this time is suction curettage under local anesthesia. The patient may experience slight bleeding and mild to moderate pain for a few hours and is usually able to return to regular activities the following day.

From about 13 weeks to 15 or 16 weeks, the operation becomes considerably more demanding, largely because of the need to dilate the cervical os to a greater diameter. This procedure is termed *dilatation and evacuation* (D&E) and requires more specialized training and experience. In the later weeks, the operation often requires general anesthesia. Physicians vary—usually related to their training and experience—with regard to how late in pregnancy they will perform a D&E, but 18 weeks is usually the upper limit.

From there up to 23 or 24 weeks (the upper limit in the majority of states), the method of choice is amnioinfusion. Amnioinfusion usually employs a mixture of saline and prostaglandin $F_2\alpha$, known as Prostasaline, injected into the amniotic sac. Sometimes oxytocin augmentation is required, and only rarely is D&C or hysterotomy (making an incision in the uterus) required. The last method of abortion is hysterotomy, but it is highly undesirable and only rarely employed.

Complications of abortion are relatively uncommon but on occasion can be serious. They include such problems as uterine perforation, retained products of conception with bleeding, infection, and damage to bladder or bowel. It is also important to realize that a suction curettage performed early in pregnancy is relatively simple and inexpensive, but as pregnancy progresses, the other more complex, slightly more risky, and more costly methods become necessary.

Another method of preventing embryonic development and subsequent birth is RU-486. This is an antiprogesterone agent which, in essence, produces a very early miscarriage. It has been widely used in several European countries but has not yet been approved by the FDA for abortion use. There is great interest in this compound as it has the potential to cut down substantially on the need for an operative procedure for termination of pregnancy.

Summary

Prevention of unwanted pregnancy is a major public health responsibility, with individual and societal ramifications. As with virtually all health problems, effective contraception depends on health education. Even with excellent education and a high level of patient motivation, all contraceptives have a predictable failure rate.

References and Selected Readings

1. Bailey P, Sanfilippo JS: in Shoupe E, Haseltine F (eds): *Contraception.* New York: Springer-Verlag
2. Chi I-cheng: What we have learned from recent IUD studies: A researcher's perspective. *Contraception* 48, August, 1993.
3. Chi I-cheng, Garr, Gasston, Rivera, Roberto: The intrauterine device in the present and future. Curr Opin *Obstet Gynecol* 5:9–832, 1993.
4. Brenner PF, Mishel DR: Contraception, in Glass RH (ed): *Office Gynecology,* 3d ed. Baltimore: Williams and Wilkins, 1988, 53–85.
5. Emans SJH, Goldstein DP: *Pediatric and Adolescent Gynecology.* Boston: Little, Brown, 1990, 451–503.

6. Greydanus DE, Lonchamp D: Contraception in the Adolescent. *Adolescent Medicine* 74:000, 1990.
7. Grimes D: Safety and Efficiency of the IUD, in Shoupe E, Haseltine F (eds): *Contraception.* New York: Springer-Verlag, 1993.
8. Hatcher R, et al: *Contraceptive Technology.* Irvington, 1993.
9. Heaton CJ, Smith MA: The Diaphragm. *J Am Family Practice,*
10. Kulig JW: Adolescent contraception: New hormonal methods. *Pediat Clin North Am* 36:717–730, 1989.
11. Mishell DR: Contraception. *New Engl J Med* 320:177–787, 1989.
12. Reinprayoon D: Intrauterine Contraception. *Curr Opin Obstet Gynecol* 527–530, 1992.
13. Rivera R., Chi I, Farr G: The intrauterine device in the present and future. *Curr Opin Obstet Gynecol* 5:829–832, 1993.
14. Sivin I: IUDs are contraceptives, not abortifacients: A Comment on research and belief. *Study Fam Plan* 20:355–359, 1989.

22 Disorders of Menstruation

John H. Mattox

PRECOCIOUS PUBERTY
PRIMARY AMENORRHEA
SECONDARY AMENORRHEA
OLIGOMENORRHEA
PREMENSTRUAL SYNDROME
DYSMENORRHEA
ABNORMAL UTERINE BLEEDING
Presentation and Management • Most Common Etiologies of Bleeding in the Various Age Groups

Menstrual disorders are a common problem. They are sometimes associated with serious underlying pathology. It is important, as a part of a woman's routine health evaluation, to inquire about her menstrual cycles.

Precocious Puberty

The appearance of sexual development before 8 years of age characterizes precocious puberty (PP). Seventy to 80 percent of cases will be due to an early "awakening" of the hypothalamic-pituitary-ovarian axis, idiopathic PP. The clinical presentation of precocious puberty in the female is almost always isosexual. The onset of secondary sexual characteristics is predominantly estrogen-dependent. Heterosexual precocity resulting in virilization of the female is unusual and will not be discussed in this chapter since it is discussed elsewhere in this text.

Any secondary sex characteristics appearing before the age of 8 years warrant a clinical evaluation that involves trying to exclude serious disease such as neoplasms of the brain, adrenal, or ovary, or some disorder of the thyroid. While the complete onset of puberty is the most dramatic, there are partial presentations that also generate significant parental concern. Premature thelarche, unilateral or bilateral breast enlargement, is usually an isolated event and is mainly self-limiting. It is not unusual to see breast changes related to maternal estrogen production in the newborn for up to 4 to 6 months following delivery.

Until recently, the cause of breast development in early childhood (premature thelarche) was unknown and was thought to be due to temporary increased sensitivity of estrogen receptors in breast tissue because no increase in circulating estrogen could be detected in most of these cases. However, more sensitive assays have demonstrated a subtle, but real, increase in estradiol, and ultrasound has shown an increase in ovarian size with small follicle cysts. The GnRH pulse pattern is not quiescent in these girls as it is normally in the prepubertal period, but is not as active as it is in girls with true precocious puberty. The resultant increased estrogen production is very slight. It is enough to cause some isolated breast development; however, it is not sufficient to cause any other features of puberty.

Premature pubarche, the onset of pubic hair, or premature adrenarche, onset of axillary hair, can also occur as isolated events but may also hail the beginning of abnormal androgen secretion. Some investigation of all of these partial forms is warranted. This should begin with a focused history, a physical examination looking for other signs of secondary sexual maturation, and a bone age determination; if the bone age is advanced, this should lead the cliñician to believe there is a more serious underlying disease.

The most common type of isosexual precocious puberty is constitutional (idiopathic) and is found in 70 to 80 percent of cases. Early activation of the hypothalamic-pituitary-ovarian unit is responsible and denotes premature secretion of GnRH. Besides the obvious phenotypical manifestations there are major psychosocial issues associated with this problem. The parents are often very distressed, and the child may experience problems relating to peers. The behavioral precocity needs to be addressed and may be the more poignant reason for instituting therapy. While in the beginning of constitutional sexual precocity anovulation is more common, ovulatory cycles can be established, and therefore these children are at potential risk for pregnancy. If ovulation can be documented with a well-timed serum progesterone test, no other studies are likely to be necessary; ovulation does not occur during any pathologic or disease states associated with precocious puberty. A thorough history, which includes information about the mother's pregnancy, developmental milestones, family history regarding the onset of puberty, and the possibility that the child may be ingesting sex steroid hormones, is critical. The physical assessment should include documentation of the stage of pubertal development using a system developed by Tanner, grading the breast and pubic hair progression.

TABLE 22-1 A Basic Evaluation for Isosexual Sexual Precocity

Possible Site of Problem	Test(s)
CNS Lesions	MRI, EEG
Thyroid	TSH, ultrasensitive
Adrenal	DHEAS
Ovary	FSH, E_2

NOTE: Bone age assessment using x-rays of the wrist will help in assessing severity.

TABLE 22-2 Important Clinical Issues Regarding Precocious Puberty

- The onset of secondary sex characteristics, usually isosexual, before eight years of age requires evaluation.
- Premature thelarche and premature pubarche are most often isolated and self-limiting problems; some evaluation is required and follow-up is essential to exclude more serious pathology.
- The etiology in the majority of females with PP is an earlier onset of hypothalamic-pituitary-ovarian function.
- The location of possible pathology resulting in PP includes the brain, adrenal, thyroid, and ovary.

As the diagnosis of idiopathic or constitutional precocious puberty is a diagnosis of exclusion, some testing is desirable and can be seen in Table 22-1. It should be recognized that some of the cases are associated with serious CNS problems, hypothyroidism, or neoplasms of the adrenal or ovary; therefore, the therapy is guided by the etiology. If all other etiologies have been excluded and it is determined that the problem is idiopathic, GnRH analog therapy is used for the curtailment of physical and behavioral symptoms. The drug can be administered by injection or nasal spray.

Important clinical issues regarding precocious puberty are reviewed in Table 22-2. Because most clinicians have limited experience with this problem, the optimum management usually requires either close consultation with, or referral to, a qualified endocrinologist. Depending on the consultant's training and clinical experience, this could be a medical, reproductive, or pediatric endocrinologist.

Primary Amenorrhea

The female pubertal sequence usually follows a predictable, chronological pattern initiated by the onset of a growth spurt and breast changes. The absence of breast budding by age 14 and no menses by age 16, primary amenorrhea (PA), constitute reasons for concern. Although this chapter will distinguish between the clinical evaluation and management of primary amenorrhea, secondary amenorrhea, and oligomenorrhea, the clinical reality is that this separation is arbitrary and that there is often overlap in the approach.

Primary amenorrhea may be due to delayed physiological menarche. Other possible reasons include a genetic cause impacting ovarian or gonadal function, a congenital anomaly involving the vagina and/or uterus, and a central problem influencing hypothalamic function and GnRH pulsatile secretion. A clinical evaluation should be directed to different compartments: (1) the uterovaginal tract, (2) ovary, (3) pituitary, (4) CNS-hypothalamus, and (5) other systemic problems.

An average healthy female in the United States usually has menarche by the age of 12½ years; it is not unusual, however, for menarche to be delayed until 15 or 16 years of age. A major consideration influencing the onset of menses is the female having reached a certain body mass with a proportional amount of fat-to-lean body tissue. Any disease state, a psychosocial problem, physical stress (particularly that which results in a sudden increase or decrease in weight) can result in the delay of menstrual function.

Congenital abnormalities associated with primary amenorrhea can be as minor as an imperforate hymen or as major as the complete absence of the müllerian structures; patients with the latter frequently have renal anomalies and skeletal defects along with the underlying vaginal agenesis. The diagnosis of anatomic defects is readily evident on performing a careful physical examination. A lack of sensitivity of androgen receptors, more commonly known as *testicular feminization syndrome,* should also be included in this category. Patients with androgen insensitivity will have some secondary sex characteristics and a 46,XY karyotype. Any female patient with a Y-bearing gonad should have it removed because of the increased risk of neoplasia.

Gonadal causes comprise a substantial number of the cases in this category. Turner syndrome, 45,X, is the most common of the primary gonadal causes. Numerous anomalies have been associated with this problem, and there is individual variation. The major medical problems for these individuals are a high incidence of heart disease, particularly coarctation of the aorta, and renal anomalies. Occasionally some learning disorders are found in such individuals. The FSH will be elevated (> 40mIU/ml). Along with the characteristic 45,X karyotype, 46,XX and a 46,XY (Swyer's syndrome) have also been described. The key physical finding will be the absence of secondary sex characteristics, and the serum FSH will always be elevated, defining the need for karyotypic analysis.

Pituitary causes of primary amenorrhea are uncommon, although isolated gonadotropin deficiencies have been reported. Any patient with a diagnosis of amenorrhea should have a serum prolactin, the elevation of which would require the investigator to exclude a tumor. Whenever a pituitary cause of amenorrhea is considered, careful evaluation dictates that hypothyroidism or hypoadrenalism be excluded.

Central nervous system (CNS) causes of primary amenorrhea should focus on either a primary or a secondary process inhibiting the pulsatile secretion of GnRH. The patient with Kallmann's syndrome, GnRH deficiency associated with lack of the ability to smell (anosmia), presents with the absence of secondary sex characteristics and a low FSH level. A simplified table of the most-common clinical problems in patients who present with primary amenorrhea is presented in Table 22-3.

When considering therapy, disorders of the outflow tract may require surgical correction to either allow for the exit of menstrual flow, as in the case of imperforate hymen, or the creation of a new vagina for sexual function when vaginal agenesis is present. Prior to the latter procedure a trial of vaginal dilators should be considered. Those females with a Y-bearing gonad require gonadectomy, as approximately one third will develop gonadal neoplasia. Individuals with other genetic problems present a fascinating clinical picture, and there is a strong temptation to perform a laparoscopy. However, this almost never adds any additional information that can be used in the patient's clinical management.

TABLE 22-3 Common Diagnoses in Patients with Primary Amenorrhea

Diagnosis	Secondary Sex Characteristics	Serum FSH	Karyotype
Delayed menarche	Yes	Normal	46,XX
Gonadal dysgenesis	No	Elevated	45,X (Turner's syndrome) 46,XX; 46,XY (Swyer's syndrome)
Uterovaginal anomaly	Yes[a]	Normal	46,XX; 46,XY (testicular feminization)
GnRH deficiency (Kallmann's syndrome)	No	Low	46,XX

[a]Partial in cases of androgen insensitivity, in which case patients have breast development.

For those individuals who will not have functioning ovaries, hormone replacement therapy, usually conjugated equine estrogens, 1.25 mg daily, with medroxyprogesterone acetate, 5 mg, calendar days 1 through 13, are sufficient to ensure body function and tissue integrity.

It is not difficult to understand why there are many psychosocial issues that need to be addressed when managing these complicated endocrinopathies; on occasion extensive counseling will be required. Important clinical issues regarding primary amenorrhea are reviewed in Table 22-4. Optimum management by the primary care provider can often be enhanced with liberal dialogue and interaction with a reproductive endocrinologist.

Secondary Amenorrhea

After a previously menstruating individual misses three consecutive periods (if she is oligomenorrheic) or 6 months pass without a period, she has met the definition of secondary amenorrhea. When pregnancy has been excluded, clinical evaluation should be directed to different compartments: (1) CNS-hypothalamus, (2) pituitary, (3) ovary, and (4) the uterovaginal tract. Other systemic problems should be considered in the differential diagnosis, and will need to be ruled out if no other etiology is identified. The most common problem resulting in secondary amenorrhea is hypothalamic dysfunction and includes CNS tumors, weight change–related disorders, severe psychologic stress, and exercise-induced problems. Pituitary causes include neoplasms, the most common being a tumor that either directly or indirectly results in hyperprolactinemia. Premature ovarian failure, the cessation of periods before age 40, is another important cause and is characterized by an elevated serum FSH of > 40 mIU/ml. Intrauterine scarring can be sufficiently extensive to result in amenorrhea. Characteristically, these patients have either had a D&C following a pregnancy episode or have had severe endometritis.

While secondary hypothalamic amenorrhea can be associated with CNS lesions such as craniopharyngioma, glioma, other tumors, head trauma, and external irradiation, the overwhelming majority of

TABLE 22-4 Important Clinical Issues Regarding Primary Amenorrhea

- The absence of breast budding by age 14 or lack of menses by age 16 requires evaluation.
- Delayed menarche is the most common explanation for primary amenorrhea and is self-limiting.
- A careful history (including family history) and a physical examination, documenting the state of development of the secondary sex characteristics and pelvic structures, will usually suggest the diagnosis.
- Gonadal (usually ovarian) failure is the most common pathologic etiology.
- An elevated FSH (> 40 mIU/ml) requires that a karyotype be performed.
- A normal FSH requires that an MRI be obtained.
- Two principles of therapy for women with no ovarian function are most important: (1) providing hormone replacement and (2) addressing future fertility potential (adoption or oocyte donation).
- The most common hormone replacement regimen is conjugated estrogen, 1.25 mg, daily, and medroxyprogesterone acetate, 5 mg, calendar days 1–13.
- Y-bearing gonads should be removed.

patients with this problem have a neurobiochemical disorder affecting GnRH secretion. The diagnosis of hypothalamic amenorrhea is usually suggested by the history and reinforced after the evaluation of the pituitary, ovary, and endometrium have revealed no significant abnormalities. Amenorrhea associated with dramatic or sudden significant changes in weight (plus or minus 15 percent from ideal body weight) are often associated with hypothalamic amenorrhea. Anorexia nervosa is the most extreme form of weight loss associated with amenorrhea, and the patient needs to be referred to an appropriate counseling and support environment. At the other end of the spectrum is pseudocyesis, a strong desire for pregnancy, with mild to moderate weight gain. Pregnancy is excluded by a negative pregnancy test, and pseudocyesis is often self-limiting. Hypothalamic amenorrhea associated with significant forms of exercise such as long-distance running usually is accompanied by loss of body weight. However, there is also a stress component if these individuals are participating in organized competition. In addition, there is a decrease in the percent of body fat below 22 percent, which seems necessary to maintain normal menses.

Any woman who has a disorder of ovulation including amenorrhea should have at least one serum prolactin test. In addition, a serum ultrasensitive TSH level should be part of the evaluation. With any persistent prolactin elevation when pregnancy, hypothyroidism, the use of medication known to elevate prolactin levels, and chest wall trauma have been excluded, the patient should be evaluated for a prolactin-secreting tumor. While there are clinically useful ways of utilizing a TRH stimulation study to help fine-tune the evaluation, the basic assessment is a radiologic study, usually magnetic resonance imaging (MRI).

The diagnosis of premature ovarian failure requires ordering a serum FSH level, which should be greater than 40 mIU/ml in ovarian failure. If ovarian failure is suspected, it must be remembered that disorders of other endocrine systems such as the adrenal, thyroid, parathyroid, and islet cells should be assessed. An SMA 20 or the equivalent along with an ACTH-stimulation test measuring the changes in cortisol will usually point toward any associated disease.

Karyotypic analysis is important to order in women who are under 30 years of age, as XY mosaicism can be present and necessitate gonadectomy. Any patient who has the appearance of hirsutism or androgen excess should have a serum testosterone and DHEAS test.

A very common cause of secondary (and occasionally primary) amenorrhea is polycystic ovarian syndrome (PCO). This is a hyperestrogenic and hyperandrogenic syndrome associated with anovulation. The basic pathogenesis of the disorder is an increase in LH, which stimulates the theca interna of the follicle to produce increased amounts of androstenedione. Androstenedione, being an androgen, is responsible for the androgenic features of the disease; since androstenedione is the major precursor of estrogen, PCO is also a hyperestrogenic disorder. The three cardinal symptoms of PCO are menstrual disorders [amenorrhea, oligomenorrhea, or dysfunctional uterine bleeding (DUB)], which are present in about 80 percent of the cases; hirsutism, which occurs in 70 percent; and infertility, which is the presenting symptom in 75 percent of patients with PCO. The diagnosis is made by the clinical features and by the presence of an elevated serum LH (or reverse FSH/LH ratio). After exclusion of pregnancy, the amenorrhea, oligomenorrhea, and/or DUB are usually treated by endometrial sampling and then either medroxyprogesterone, monthly, or the combination birth control pill. Women who wish to become pregnant may be treated with clomiphene.

Another cause of amenorrhea and/or oligomenorrhea is congenital adrenal hyperplasia (CAH). The "acquired" or "adult onset" form of this disease closely resembles PCO in its clinical presentation. Although it is a common autosomal genetic disorder, clinically it is a far less frequent cause of oligomenorrhea than PCO. The basic defect in CAH is an enzymatic failure in the production of cortisol. The resultant increase in ACTH stimulates the adrenal to produce increased amounts of androgens, causing hirsutism and oligomenorrhea. The diagnosis is made by the family history, clinical presentation, and laboratory findings, including elevated DHEAS, androstenedione, and 17-OHP. The obvious, logical, and specific treatment is oral cortisone administration. This replaces the cortisol that is lacking, suppresses the ACTH of the anterior pituitary, and prevents the excess secretion of androgens by the adrenal cortex. In this way both the oligomenorrhea and the hirsutism are ameliorated.

The most probable diagnoses and the basic evaluation of these problems can be seen in Table 22-5.

The more precise the diagnosis, the more accurate is the plan of therapy. For some women with hypothalamic amenorrhea, all that may be needed to correct the amenorrhea is adequate nutrition, stress reduction, and/or moderation in exercise. If any of the above conditions is coexistent with an extreme form of behavior, consultation with a psychiatrist is important.

Usually individuals with either primary or secondary amenorrhera have estrogen deficiency and therefore require hormone replacement. In young acyclic patients, particularly if androgen excess is present, hormone replacement is most likely provided by a birth control pill, and one with minimal androgen activity should be utilized. Alternatively, a commonly prescribed hormone replacement regimen in patients with amenorrhea is conjugated estrogens 0.625 to 1.25 mg or equivalent, daily, with medroxyprogesterone acetate, 5 mg, on calendar days 1 to 13. This program will provide the needed hormone to prevent osteoporosis and sufficient hormone to keep the other tissues and the vascular system intact. Clomiphene citrate is indicated in women who have some evidence of ovarian function and who desire pregnancy. The initial dose is 50 mg per day from cycle day 5 to 9. In acyclic individuals, after endometrial hyperplasia has been ruled out, progesterone-induced withdrawal bleeding is required before therapy can begin. In women who weigh more than 175 lb, 100 mg as the starting dose should be considered.

TABLE 22-5 Most Probable Diagnoses in Patients with Secondary Amenorrhea

Diagnosis	Study
Pregnancy	HCG determination
Hypothalamic dysfunction	History; other studies negative
Pituitary tumor	Prolactin; MRI
Premature ovarian failure	FSH > 40 mIU/ml
Intrauterine scarring	Hysterogram or hysteroscopy
Polycystic ovarian syndrome	LH, LH: FSH ratio, androstenedione
Adult onset CAH	DHEAS; androstenedione, 17-OHP

Bromocriptine (Parlodel), a dopamine agonist, has been effective in treating prolactin-secreting adenomas. As the majority of patients will have a microadenoma, they should be quite responsive to this medication. Starting with a small dose, 1.25 mg PO at bedtime with a snack, and increasing the dose until euprolactinemia is achieved is the simplest way to effect therapy. There is still significant debate about whether every patient with a microadenoma should be treated with medication or whether they can just be observed.

Intrauterine scarring is strongly suggested by history, and in most patients the history includes a prior pregnancy episode followed by severe endometritis or a postpregnancy hemorrhage that requires curettage. Pelvic irradiation in large doses directed to the uterus can result in obliteration of the endometrical cavity. In addition to the significant history, the diagnosis could be made and often the problem treated as well by performing a hysteroscopy; the hysterosalpingogram can also be of utility. Hormone therapy may be indicated to stimulate uterine lining growth.

Table 22-6 reviews important clinical issues in patients with secondary amenorrhea. If there are any atypical clinical presentations, inconsistent laboratory findings, or the patient fails to respond promptly to therapy, consultation with a reproductive endocrinologist should be considered.

Oligomenorrhea

Most of what has been discussed in the section on secondary amenorrhea applies to the differential diagnosis, evaluation, and treatment of oligomenorrhea as well. The symptom of oligomenorrhea, infrequent uterine bleeding at unpredictable times, is

TABLE 22-6 Important Clinical Issues in Patients with Secondary Amenorrhea

- After pregnancy has been excluded, hypothalamic causes of secondary amenorrhea are identified over 50 percent of the time.
- Hypothalamic-related amenorrhea is most strongly suggested by the history of rapid weight changes, excessive exercise, or serious psychological stress. Laboratory and radiologic studies are usually negative; an FSH is normal.
- Any patient with a disorder of ovulation should have a serum prolactin.
- About one third of patients with amenorrhea and hyperprolactinemia will have a tumor; hypothyroidism and prolactin-elevating medications should be excluded.
- A serum FSH > 40 mIU/ml strongly suggests ovarian failure; the diagnosis should not be made based upon one test; hypothyroidism, hypoadrenalism, and associated autoimmune disorders should be excluded.
- Patients with oligoamenorrhea and hirsutism should be screened with a serum testosterone and DHEAS.
- Women with premature ovarian failure should have a karyotype (if < 30 years old).
- Uterine bleeding following a progesterone challenge does not exclude ovarian failure.
- Intrauterine scarring (synechiae) is usually preceded by a history of uterine curettage associated with a pregnancy episode or severe infection.
- If a patient is not responding to ovulation induction, she may have ovarian failure or a nonprolactin-secreting pituitary tumor.
- Hormone replacement therapy, conjugated equine estrogen 0.625 to 1.25 mg daily (women < 50 years old may need the higher dose), with medroxyprogesterone acetate, 5 mg calendar days 1 through 13 (if the uterus is present), is one of the most widely used regimens in these situations.
- With hypothalamic amenorrheic patients desiring pregnancy, starting clomiphene, 50 mg daily (a higher dose if the patient weighs more than 80 kg), for 5 days is the initial ovulation inducing therapy.
- Neither clomiphene nor menotropin therapy has been successful in inducing ovulation in patients with premature ovarian failure.

arbitrarily characterized as occurring at intervals of greater than 45 days; it signifies an underlying disorder of ovulation and therefore represents a malfunction of the hypothalamic-pituitary-ovarian axis. A small percentage of women will never have normal menses following menarche because the axis does not completely mature. Oligomenorrhea can represent an intrinsic axis disorder such as premature ovarian failure or an extrinsic problem interfering with normal axis function such as hypothyroidism. The more common problems can be detected by utilizing the tests listed in Table 22-7.

Other systemic or metabolic problems (e.g., severe hepatic or renal disease) can be associated with oligomenorrhea; however, the clinical management is usually focused on the primary disease and the menstrual disorder becomes a secondary issue.

Hypomenorrhea, lighter than expected flow, either in amount or in duration (less than 4 days), is more likely to represent an underlying uterine cavity disorder but can be associated with oligo-ovulation. The same tests, also including a hysterogram, would adequately evaluate this symptom.

The evaluation and management of the above disorders are similar to those for amenorrhea.

TABLE 22-7 Tests Commonly Utilized to Identify Potential Problems in Patients with Oligomenorrhea

Test	Significance
hCG	Any oligomenorrheic patient can have an occasional ovulatory cycle. Pregnancy should be excluded prior to any evaluation.
FSH	If it is elevated, ovarian failure may be present; the FSH level is usually normal with other intrinsic or extrinsic axis disorders.
Prolactin (PRL)	Any patient with a disorder of ovulation should have a PRL. When elevated, the etilogy should be identified.
TSH	The current "sensitive" test can screen for hypo- and hyperthyroidism. While being a less likely cause of axis dysfunction, thyroid disease should be considered.
Testosterone, DHEAS, and 17-OHP	These tests are only necessary if the patient has symptoms of androgen excess or is very obese.
LH/FSH ratio	LH is elevated; LH/FSH ratio is inverted in women with PCO usually 3:1.

Premenstrual Syndrome (PMS)

Most women having ovulatory cycles experience alterations in their body's sensation and sometimes their mood prior to the onset of menses. This symptom aggregate is termed *molimina.* If the number and severity of the symptoms increase to the point where they interfere with daily existence, this is considered *premenstrual syndrome* (PMS). The general approach of the primary care provider is to make the patient who has premenstrual symptoms more comfortable and functional. Predominant somatic symptomatology can include the feeling of bloatedness, breast pain, headache, pelvic pain, and alterations in bowel function. The major psychological symptoms can include mood alterations such as irritability, aggressive tendencies, anxiety, depression, extreme lethargy, sleep disorders, crying spells, diminished libido, and loss of concentration. Feeling bloated seems to be the most common somatic complaint while depression is the most common psychological complaint.

There is no single currently understood biochemical etiology to explain satisfactorily the entire symptom complex associated with PMS. Part of the difficulty relates to this multifaceted disease and the investigational limitations in dealing with disorders of brain function and neurotransmitter metabolism. Numerous hypotheses have been tested and include progesterone deficiency, progesterone allergy, hypoglycemia, vitamin B_6 deficiency, inappropriate aldosterone secretion, inappropriate prostaglandin activity, endorphin dysfunction, and disorders of monoamineoxidase or dopamine metabolism. It also becomes readily apparent to the health care provider who has taken care of a number of PMS patients that there can be a serious anxiety or depressive disorder which includes the premenstruum or is intensified around the time of ovulation or in the luteal phase.

Following the initial history and physical, including the pelvic examination, the most practical approach is to have the patient record her symptomatology on a daily basis, identifying both somatic and psychological complaints and quantitating the severity, usually on a scale of 1 to 4, with 4 being the most intense. Concurrently, she should document basal body temperature measurements, which will also serve to localize the major symptomatology to the luteal phase. Concurrent medical problems should be considered and laboratory tests that address those possible problems obtained.

The patient requires constant support and affirmation that improvement will occur, but it is important to identify which symptoms are most bothersome. It is also critical for the patient to understand that there is no single medicine that will take away all the symptoms but that the approach is to try to alleviate the most bothersome ones. The health care provider, on the other hand, must strongly avoid a multiple pharmacologic approach, as this avenue often creates more problems that it solves.

Following clinical evaluation and after concluding that PMS is the most likely diagnosis, different therapies can be considered. This is an opportune time to motivate the patient towards a more healthy diet and to include a moderate amount of exercise. A multiple feeding, high-protein diet and the elimination of caffeine and alcohol have been very effective for certain patients. Vitamin B_6 (pyridoxine) 50 mg daily, has also had a salutary effect on this condition. In Table 22-8 some other medical therapies are

TABLE 22-8 Possible Medications for PMS Symptoms

Symptoms	Oral Drugs[a]
Bloating or fluid retention	Spironolactone, 50 mg q AM
General, multiple symptoms	Low-dose estrogen birth control pill
Sleep disorder	Dalmane 15–30 mg hs
Anxiety, mood swings, crying	Xanax, 0.25–0.5 mg tid
Depression	Prozac, 20 mg qd
Breast tenderness	Danazol, 200 mg qd
Symptoms	**Injectable Drugs**
Severe PMS (not responsive to oral therapy)	GnRH analog with or without add back therapy

[a]Usually required during luteal phase only, except for birth control pills and Prozac. Some contraceptive measures should be used to avoid taking the medication during pregnancy. The pharmacology of these medications should be reviewed before usage.

listed. If depression or other substantial psychiatric problems are a component of the woman's problems, these must be addressed. Formal psychiatric consultation is sometimes needed.

Important clinical issues about PMS are reviewed in Table 22-9.

Dysmenorrhea

Dysmenorrhea, lower abdominal cramping pain with menses and usually with a constellation of other symptoms, is classified as primary or secondary and can be incapacitating. The major tenet when considering this diagnosis is the accurate identification or, more specifically, the exclusion of pelvic disease.

Primary dysmenorrhea (PD) usually appears shortly after the menarche and is associated with ovulatory cycles. Characteristically, it is not caused by or associated with demonstrable pelvic pathology such as adhesions, infection, or endometriosis. The pain is crampy in nature and may sometimes radiate to the back or thighs. Other symptoms such as nausea, emesis, headache, fatigue, and diaphoresis have been associated with dysmenorrhea. The severity may be correlated with the amount and duration of menstrual flow.

While the exact etiology of the pain is unknown, the role of endogenous prostaglandins seems to be important. Women with clinically significant dysmenorrhea have elevated prostaglandin levels in menstrual fluid, increased uterine tone, and increased frequency of uterine contractions, believed secondary to prostaglandins. Once severe cyclic pain is anticipated, there may be an associated fear and anxiety, which, as in other forms of pain, has been shown to intensify the perception of pain.

TABLE 22-9 Premenstrual Syndrome (PMS)

- Premenstrual symptoms may be incapacitating for a small number of women.
- A thorough clinical evaluation should occur prior to making the diagnosis of PMS.
- A daily diary kept by the patient recording her symptoms is the cornerstone of diagnosis and management.
- General health improvement measures addressing exercise, diet, and reduction of alcohol and caffeine will produce improvement in most patients.
- Medications are prescribed to relieve the most bothersome symptom(s).
- Formal psychiatric consultation may be necessary for certain patients.

The diagnosis can usually be made upon taking a detailed history about the character of the pain associated with menstruation and the lack of abnormal physical findings during the pelvic examination. If there is any concern about a possible pelvic finding or a limited exam because of obesity, a pelvic ultrasound should be obtained. At the present time there does not appear to be any significant value to ordering a screening battery of laboratory tests. A hemoglobin or a serum ferritin might prove beneficial if excessive menstrual flow is associated with dysmenorrhea; other tests should be obtained as clinically warranted.

As this problem is often seen in younger women who may have not had prior interaction with a health care professional, it is particularly important to approach the patient with sensitivity and a sympathetic demeanor. Sufficient time should be allowed in the office to avoid giving the patient the impression that she is being rushed through the visit. This visit may also present an opportunity to discuss the need for maintaining physical activity, correcting dietary deficiencies, and considering some relaxation therapy. The initial medical therapy in women who do not desire any contraception is a prostaglandin synthetase inhibitor (PGSI). Over-the-counter ibuprofen with a usual dose of 400 mg 3 times per day will provide adequate relief for many patients. Higher doses of more potent agents may be utilized if over-the-counter medication is not effective. It is important for the patient to understand that the medication is being taken not only for the relief of discomfort but also for reduction of the production of prostaglandins, and therefore it needs to be taken continuously through the entire episode for optimum relief. Low-estrogen-containing birth control pills (BCP) are effective therapy for primary dysmenorrhea in approximately 90 percent of patients. If the patient does not respond to the BCP or PGSI, it is appropriate to consider a diagnostic laparoscopy, as the presence of pelvic pathology (i.e., advanced endometriosis) has been identified in a teenage population who have not been responsive to medical therapy.

The primary care provider must consider secondary dysmenorrhea (SD) as a symptom, requiring an attempt to identify some pelvic pathology. Women presenting with SD are usually over 20 years of age and have experienced a significant period of time during which the pain associated with menstruation was manageable. Historically, the patient will relate that the pain has gradually progressed over some time and is becoming more incapacitating and less likely to be relieved with over-the-counter analgesics. There is frequently a concomitant change in the pattern of menstrual flow, either in the duration or the amount.

While the list of possible pelvic diseases causing secondary dysmenorrhea can be seen in Table 22-10, the most likely possibilities are endometriosis, adenomyosis, and chronic pelvic infection. The same detailed inquiry into the nature of the pain will usually point to one of the diagnoses. There are often significant pelvic findings at the time of the bimanual examination, (e.g., uterine enlargement or a fixed retroflexed uterus). Characteristically, mild analgesic therapy and oral contraceptive steroids have not been effective in relieving the discomfort. The assessment of the endometrial cavity, either with hysterosalpingogram or hysteroscopy, and of the pelvic structures, utilizing a diagnostic laparoscopy, should be incorporated into the clinical evaluation. The rational approach to therapy depends on a specific diagnosis and using whatever medical or surgical therapies are necessary to make the patient more comfortable; on rare occasions a hysterectomy may be indicated. The most vexing problem for the clinician is the patient with chronic pelvic pain that is accentuated at the time of menses. It is thought that this condition might be due to pelvic nerve hypersensitivity or a form of pelvic somatization. If after a complete workup pelvic disease has been excluded, it may be necessary for the patient to be referred to an individual or clinic specializing in the management of chronic pain. Important clinical issues about dysmenorrhea are reviewed in Table 22-11.

TABLE 22-10 Possible Causes of Secondary Dysmenorrhea

Endometriosis
Adenomyosis
Chronic upper genital tract infection
Adhesions
Cervical stenosis
Accentuated by stress, fatigue, or pelvic somatization

TABLE 22-11 Dysmenorrhea

- Primary dysmennorrhea (PD) usually presents shortly after menarche in the absence of any abnormal pelvic findings and is customarily improved with PGSI or BCP.
- A sudden acute episode of PD can be alleviated by a paracervical block injecting 2 ml of 0.25% marcaine at 12, 4, and 8 o'clock.
- Any patient with PD who does not adequately respond to medical therapy should be considered a potential candidate for diagnostic laparoscopy.
- Patients with secondary dysmenorrhea usually have some accompanying pelvic pathology; the most common problems are endometriosis, adenomyosis, and pelvic inflammatory disease (PID) with concomitant pelvic adhesions.
- Dysmenorrhea may be intensified by stress, fatigue, and pelvic somatization.

Abnormal Uterine Bleeding

Abnormal uterine bleeding (AUB) is a frequent complaint of patients and a major reason for gynecological procedures to be performed. Making an accurate diagnosis and ruling out serious etiologies is important. Table 22-12 reviews the differential diagnosis of abnormal uterine bleeding and Table 22-13 reviews the possible causes of anovulation in reproductive age women. It is also important when a woman complains of vaginal bleeding to rule out the possibility that the origin is actually from another site (e.g., bowel, urinary tract, vulva).

Benign organic causes of abnormal bleeding such as endocervical polyps are usually not difficult to diagnose and manage. Gynecologic malignancy (particularly of the uterus and cervix) often presents with abnormal uterine bleeding. The major clinical dilemmas are created by nonorganic, hormonally

TABLE 22-12 Differential Diagnosis of Abnormal Uterine Bleeding

PELVIC PATHOLOGY (ORGANIC)
- Endocervical or endometrial polyps
- Leiomyoma
- Malignancy of the cervix, endometrium, or myometrium
- Premalignant lesions of the cervix (dysplasia) or endometrium (hyperplasia)
- Chronic endometritis
- Adenomyosis
- Endometriosis
- Pelvic inflammatory disease (PID)
- Functional ovarian tumors
- Neoplastic ovarian tumors

HORMONE-RELATED (NONORGANIC)
- Endogenous
  - Anovulatory cycles
  - Ovulatory cycles
- Exogenous
  - Hormone replacement therapy
  - Birth control pill therapy

SYSTEMIC PROBLEMS
- Disorders of coagulation
- Severe liver disease or renal disease
- Thyroid disease

DISORDERS OF PREGNANCY
- Ectopic pregnancy
- Threatened abortion, incomplete abortion, complete abortion, missed abortion
- Gestational trophoblastic disease

related causes of bleeding, 80 percent of which are associated with anovulatory cycles. Pregnancy-related disorders are common causes of abnormal uterine bleeding. Hormone replacement and birth control pill therapy as well as certain systemic disease—for example, disorders of blood coagulation, severe liver disease, and thyroid dysfunction—can also result in AUB.

While the same general approach as outlined in Table 22-14 can be used in any patient regardless of age, it will become apparent that stronger emphasis is placed on specific tests, as the risk of certain diseases varies in different age groups. The exclusion of a premalignant or malignant endometrial lesion is the major reason to sample the endometrium. In anovulatory cycles, the management of AUB focuses on:

- Controlling an acute bleeding episode
- Ruling out the presence of a malignancy
- Preventing unpredictable bleeding
- Treatment to prevent the occurrence of endometrial hyperplasia or endometrial cancer

TABLE 22-13 Possible Etiologies of Anovulation in Reproductive Age Women

PERIPHERAL ETIOLOGIES
- Liver and renal disease
- Neoplasms, producing androgen, estrogen, or chorionic gonadotropin
- Obesity

CENTRAL ETIOLOGIES
- Hypothalamic: malnutrition, anorexia, substantial weight loss, exercise—associated, systemic disease, psychogenic factors
- Kallmann's syndrome (GnRH deficiency)
- Hypothalamic-pituitary damage
- Hyperprolactenemia-galactorrhea—e.g., due to medications, pituitary tumors, hypothyroidism, associated with empty sella syndrome.

OTHER ENDOCRINE ETIOLOGIES
- Congenital adrenal hyperplasia (CAH)
- Thyroid disorders
- Polycystic ovarian syndrome
- Cushing's syndrome
- Acromegaly

TABLE 22-14 Evaluation of Abnormal Uterine Bleeding

BASIC ASSESSMENT
- Problem-oriented history
- General physical and pelvic exam
- Pap smear
- CBC
- hCG
- Endometrial biopsy (if patient is not pregnant)

AS INDICATED
- Transvaginal ultrasound with endometrial thickness measured
- Prolactin
- TSH, ultrasensitive
- Platelet count, PTT, bleeding time
- AST, ALT
- Hysterogram or hysteroscopy
- D&C, laparoscopy
- Other studies as warranted

Presentation and Management

In a woman who is ovulating, normal menstrual periods occur approximately 14 days following ovulation. Women who are ovulating and experiencing regular menstrual periods may have menorrhagia (duration of flow longer than 7 days) or hypermenorrhea (excessive bleeding with normal duration). An estimated blood loss of more than 80 ml during a period is considered excessive uterine flow. *Metrorrhagia* is variably defined as abnormal bleeding between periods (intermenstrual bleeding) or irregular, usually excessive, bleeding with no definable cycle.

When conditions of pregnancy are excluded, a simplistic separation of the causes of abnormal uterine bleeding are those associated with pelvic pathology and those that are a result of the hormonal effect on the endometrium. There are a small number of patients who have systemic disease, such as a disorder of coagulation or severe liver disease, in whom the uterine bleeding problem is secondary. In these instances although the bleeding may be a problem, it is usually not the major issue.

Dysfunctional uterine bleeding (DUB) is abnormal endometrial shedding caused by an endocrine dysfunction. Seventy to 80 percent of DUB is associated with anovulation, and this is more likely to be seen when the hypothalamic-pituitary-ovarian axis begins to mature during adolescence, as well as in women from 40 to 50 years of age. About 20 percent of abnormal uterine bleeding occurs in the peripubertal period, 30 percent during the prime reproductive years, and 50 percent during peri- and postmenopause.

There is a group of conditions associated with ovulatory cycles that are usually not clinically dramatic and are self-limiting. A persistent corpus luteum, a short luteal phase, an irregular shedding of the endometrium have all been associated with unpredictable endometrial bleeding; uterine lining asynchrony is more likely to require hormone therapy to correct.

A constitutional illness producing DUB is uncommon; a factor VIII deficiency, leukemia, and other problems of coagulation are some clinical examples in which interference with blood clotting is manifested by abnormal uterine bleeding.

Most Common Etiologies of Bleeding in the Various Age Groups

Although almost all of the etiologies listed in Tables 22-12 and 22-13 are possible in all age groups, certain problems are more likely to be seen depending on the patient's age, and they will be discussed in the following sections.

Adolescence As the hypothalamic-pituitary-ovarian axis begins to function, there is a period of time required for it to mature completely, which averages approximately 2 years. During this transition, menstrual cycles are frequently anovulatory. If cycles do not normalize within 5 years of menarche it is unlikely that they will through the remainder of menstrual life; this occurs in less than 10 percent of women.

The history should include specific items that address the onset of pubertal changes. It is important to determine whether the adolescent has become sexually active. Depending on the history and, depending on the severity of bleeding, in an adolescent who has definitely not yet become sexually active a rectoabdominal examination or abdominal ultrasound may be all that is necessary. Pap smears are not usually obtained until sexual activity is initiated, and an endometrial biopsy is almost never necessary. With *severe, acute episodes* of DUB, screening for a clotting disorder and an examination (possibly under anesthesia) to exclude malignancy are warranted. With an acute episode of bleeding in a nonpregnant adolescent, a progestin-dominant birth control pill such as LoOvral administered every 8 hours will usually control the bleeding over 3 to 4 days; the pill should be continued in the usual dosage for three to six cycles. In milder cases, medroxyprogesterone acetate (Provera), 5 mg to 10 mg, calendar days 1 through 13 for 3 to 6 months, should achieve normal bleeding. Because of the self-limiting nature of the problem it is unusual to require hormonal treatment for a longer period of time. If contraception is needed, birth control pills will serve the dual role of providing contraception and correcting the problem.

Organic causes are unusual in this age group. However, the presence of endometriosis has been documented in teenagers. In this situation pelvic pain, not abnormal bleeding, tends to be the presenting complaint.

Reproductive Age It is not unusual for a normal menstruating female to have one or even two anovulatory cycles per year, and they may be associated with abnormal bleeding. If cycles are usually regular and pregnancy and other obvious considerations have been ruled out, a brief evaluation and pelvic examination will assure both the physician and the patient that nothing serious is wrong and that the problem need only be monitored. It is not necessary to do a full-scale workup after a single episode for a woman in this age group. However, if the situation becomes repetitive, it must be promptly investigated. There are also women who under normal circumstances have either very heavy flow during their menses, resulting in anemia, or who have menstrual periods lasting 7 to 8 days, placing them at risk for iron deficiency. It has been well documented that the use of prostaglandin synthetase inhibitors during the time of menses will reduce the flow; oral iron therapy is also recommended.

Patients in this age group who have a history of menometrorrhagia of more than two cycles duration require a basic assessment as outlined in Table 22-14. If the pelvic examination is limited for any reason, a pelvic ultrasound using an endovaginal probe is a preferred method of accessing pelvic structures. The assessment of the myometrium and endometrial thickness can help to exclude intramural myomas and make the diagnosis of endometrial hyperplasia or cancer less likely if the total endometrial thickness is under 5 mm. As the risk of malignancy is low in women under age 30, selective endometrial biopsy is preferable and depends on the presence of other risk factors. A pregnancy episode should always be considered when abnormal bleeding occurs in this age group, and a quantitative hCG test is mandatory.

Hypothyroidism can be seen in this group, and an ultrasensitive TSH should be performed; coagulation studies are less likely to be productive.

An endometrial sampling can be performed in the office using a paracervical block with 2 ml of 1% Lidocaine at twelve, four, and eight o'clock to reduce patient discomfort. The Pipelle disposable suction cannula will help determine uterine depth as well as provide an adequate sampling approximately 97 percent of the time. As endometrial polyps or submucous myomas will not be diagnosed with this technique, some patients with chronic or recurring DUB may require a hysterogram or hysteroscopic evaluation of the endometrial cavity to make a precise diagnosis.

In the absence of pelvic pathology, pregnancy, or serious endocrine or systemic problems, the most convenient therapy for the patient is to use the low-dose monophasic birth control pill. The hormones will override the "inappropriate messages" being sent to the endometrium and will induce normal menstrual bleeding. Clearly for each woman the risks and benefits of the birth control pill should be assessed. However, it should be noted that the birth control pill has many noncontraceptive benefits, including a reduction in the risk of developing ovarian and endometrial cancer and pelvic inflammatory disease (Table 22-15). An alternate hormonal therapy is medroxyprogesterone acetate (Provera), 5 mg to 10 mg, calendar days 1 through 13. This will help prevent endometrial hyperplasia, although the patient must be counseled that some form of contraception will be necessary as she can rely neither on her past history of anovulatory cycles nor on the current medication as adequate protection against unwanted pregnancy.

The clinician will readily intuit that organic causes of uterine bleeding are more common in this age group than in the adolescent. The likelihood of serious pathology being present increases as women become older, although this does occur in younger

TABLE 22-15 Noncontraceptive Advantages of Birth Control Pills

Birth control pills reduce prevalence of
Iron deficiency anemia
Ovarian cancer
Endometrial cancer
Irregular bleeding
Pelvic inflammatory disease
Ectopic pregnancy
Premenstrual syndrome
Dysmenorrhea
Breast fibroadenomas

women as well. Adnexal masses, usually ovarian lesions, may require diagnostic surgery, depending on the size and character of the mass. Ovarian unilocular cysts less than 5 cm in diameter are usually functional and will disappear with observation. An ovarian mass that is multilocular or persistent after 8 weeks requires further investigation.

If the workup makes malignancy quite unlikely, diagnostic laparoscopy with cyst resection will answer most questions. As more and more experience is gained with this technique, larger ovarian lesions are being managed in this fashion. The only way to properly diagnose and stage endometriosis is with a diagnostic laparascopy; as fertility potential may be part of the clinical evaluation, chromotubation may be appropriate.

Adenomyosis usually occurs in parous females in their late thirties and forties. In addition to abnormal uterine bleeding, the uterus is often slightly enlarged and globular, and it may be tender. Not every woman with adenomyosis is symptomatic, and, therefore, her clinical presentation should interfere with her lifestyle before surgical intervention is considered. Hormone therapy can be considered on a trial basis but is usually ineffective; the patient's age and her desire to maintain fertility will determine if hysterectomy is the best course.

Endometriosis and ovarian cysts also may result in abnormal vaginal bleeding in women in this age group, and they may require laparoscopy for diagnosis. Following a thorough evaluation when no serious pathology is present and premalignant and malignant lesions have been ruled out, endometrial ablation can often reduce menstrual flow and be a satisfactory alternative for women who are substantially affected by the bleeding but adverse to hysterectomy.

Perimenopause As ovarian function wanes and the cyclic production of estrogen and progesterone varies, the incidence of abnormal uterine bleeding increases. While the more common problem is ovarian insufficiency, the incidence of organic lesions is also increased. Disorders of coagulation are rare at this time in life, and the possibility of pregnancy is lessened. The algorithm suggested in Table 22-14 will provide a satisfactory way to approach these patients and, as a general statement, every woman with AUB should have an evaluation of the endometrial cavity and a pelvic ultrasound. If any endometrial abnormality exists, a diagnostic D&C and hysteroscopy should be considered. If an adnexal abnormality is suggested on sonography, laparoscopy should be considered.

Because hormone-related problems are the most common, some type of management to promote regular uterine bleeding should be considered. Once premalignant and malignant problems and pregnancy have been ruled out, consideration can be given to the use of a low-dose birth control pill; not only will this provide appropriate support for the endometrium, vascular system, and bones, but it may help to reduce the risk of ovarian and endometrial cancer. Current practice dictates that prescribing a birth control pill up until age 50 if there are no contraindications is acceptable; smoking is the most serious contraindication necessitating that birth control pills not be prescribed after the age of 34. Whether or not a women should be required to forego birth control pills exactly at age 50 if there are no risk factors and she is tolerating the medication satisfactorily is a point for debate but most doctors would recommend that this patient be given hormone replacement therapy rather than the birth control pill. As part of the routine health maintenance there should be monitoring of the serum cholesterol, fasting blood sugar, TSH, blood pressure, etc. Although continuous estrogen therapy with cyclic progestin therapy is probably the most efficacious for the patient at this point, there will be withdrawal bleeding, and the patient needs to be counseled and reassured.

Postmenopause Women with postmenopausal bleeding should be considered to have pelvic cancer unless proven otherwise. Approximately 20 percent of women with postmenopausal bleeding who are not receiving hormone replacement therapy do, in fact, have a premalignant lesion or cancer. In addition, it is important to remember that serious pelvic disease and hormone replacement therapy can exist concomitantly, and, therefore, all patients should undergo an evaluation if unpredictable bleeding occurs. The clinician should make the assumption that organic pelvic pathology exists until all possibilities have been excluded. Therefore, the liberal use of endometrial sampling, pelvic ultrasound, and even diagnostic laparoscopy should be considered in patients who have unexplained abnormal uterine bleeding in this age group. With women on long-term hormone therapy the assessment of the endometrium with ultrasound becomes even more valuable; incorporating this adjunct can help to reduce the number of times an endometrial sampling will be required. However, endometrial measurements should never be used as a substitute for a biopsy. Hormone replacement therapy in this group can be modified to continuous therapy, and the most popular regimen currently is 0.625 mg of conjugated or esterified estrogen and medroxyprogesterone, 2.5 mg daily. Endometrial thickness will be less with this treatment, and the regular withdrawal bleeding episodes will be avoided in most of the patients after adjusting to the medication, which may take up to 1 year.

References and Selected Readings

1. Bayer SR, DeCherney AH: Clinical manifestations and treatment of dysfunctional uterine bleeding. *JAMA* 269:1823, 1993.
2. Brenner PF: Precocious puberty in the female, in Mishell DR, Davajan V, Lobo R (eds): *Infertility, Contraception and Reproductive Endocrinology,* 3d ed. Oradell, NJ: Medical Economics, 1990, pp 336–355.
3. Breyer P, Haider A, Pescovitz OH: Gonadotropin-releasing hormone agonist in the treatment of girls with central precocious puberty. *Clin Obstet Gynecol* 36:764, 1993.
4. Caufriez, A: Menstrual disorders in adolescence: Pathophysiology and treatment. *Horm Res* 36:156, 1991.
5. Christensen, L: Effects of eating behavior on mood: A review of the literature. *Int J Eat Disord* 14:171, 1993.
6. Classen EA, Cowell CL: Acute adolescent menorrhagia. *Am J Obstet Gynecol* 87:603, 1981.
7. Freeman E, Rickels K, Sandheimer SJ, Polansky M: Ineffectiveness of progesterone suppository treatment for premenstrual syndrome. *JAMA* 264:349, 1990.
8. Frische RE, MacArthur JW: Menstrual cycles: Fatness as a determinant of minimum weight for height necessary for the maintenance or onset. *Science* 185:945, 1974.
9. Ingram JM: The bicycle stool in the treatment of vaginal agenesis: A preliminary report. *Am J Obstet Gynecol* 1981; 140:867.
10. Kaplan SL, Grumbach MM: Clinical Review 14: Pathophysiology in treatment of sexual precocity. *J Clin Endocrinol Metab* 71:785, 1990.
11. Kauppila, A: The changing concepts of medical treatment of endometriosis. *Acta Obstet Gynecol Scand* 72:324, 1993.
12. Mahnmood TA, Templeton A: Prevalence and genesis of endometriosis. *Hum Reprod* 6:544, 1991.
13. Mattox JH: Amenorrhea, in Wilson JR, Carrington ER (eds.) *Obstetrics and Gynecology,* 9th ed. St. Louis, MO.: Mosby-Yearbook, 1991, pp 94–110.
14. Mortola JF: Applications of gonadotropin-release hormone analogues in the treatment of premenstrual syndrome. *Clin Obstet Gynecol* 36:753, 1993.
15. Muse K: The premenstrual syndrome. *Curr Opin Obstet Gynecol* 3:865, 1991.
16. Rebar RW, Cedars MI: Hypergonadotropic forms of amenorrhea. *Endocrinol Metab Clin North Am* 21:173, 1992.
17. Reindollar RH, Novak M, Tho SPT, McDonough PG: Adult onset amenorrhea: A study of 262 patients. *Am J Obstet Gynecol* 155:531, 1986.
18. Smith RP: The dynamics of nonsteroidal anti-inflammatory therapy for primary dysmenorrhea. *Obstet Gynecol* 70:785, 1987.
19. Stenchever, MA: Dysmenorrhea and premenstrual syndrome, in Herbst, AL, et al (eds): *Comprehensive Gynecology.* St. Louis, MO.: Mosby-Yearbook, 1992.
20. Tanner JM: *Growth in Adolescents,* 2d ed. Oxford, England: Blackwell Scientific, 1962.
21. Vale RF: Endometrial ablation for dysfunctional uterine bleeding: Role of GnRH agonists. *Int J Gynaecol Obstet* 41:3, 1993.
22. Wilmore JH: Eating and weight disorders in the female athlete. *Int J Sport Nutrit* 1:107, 1991.

23 Premalignant and Malignant Gynecologic Lesions

Joanna M. Cain

This chapter is structured by anatomic site and will provide the following for each site:

1. Introduction to common premalignant and malignant gynecologic pathology
2. Standard techniques of evaluation for diagnosis
3. Decision-making flow charts (Figs. 23-1 to 23-4)
4. Information about management of premalignant and malignant gynecologic lesions

Vulva

The skin of the vulva must sustain integrity in the face of multiple insults from body moisture, urine, fecal material, trauma, and infections with local or introduced pathogens. Considering the biologic challenge it faces, it is surprising that vulvar abnormalities are not the most common abnormalities in women. Vulvar cancer only comprises 5 percent of all gynecologic malignancies. In considering premalignant and malignant changes in vulvar tissue it is valuable to remember the axiom for all gynecologic tissues that can be visually inspected: *If it looks abnormal, it should be biopsied.* This is the only way that the clinician can avoid misdiagnosing a premalignant problem or a vulvar cancer.

Vulvar Squamous Changes

The normal color of the vulvar skin is uniform over the labia majora but may vary over the labia minus. There is an obvious change from the pink, unpigmented vaginal mucous membrane to the labia minus at the introitus. The vulvar skin becomes thicker, more stratified, more pigmented, and more keratinized the farther it is from the introital area. Normal vulva should be symmetric in their distribution of pigment changes, underlying fat, and thickness of skin. Changes in pigmentation, thickness, or symmetry should be sought at every examination. Lentiginous changes in the vulva are normal and fairly common.

The most common premalignant change in vulvar skin is vulvar intraepithelial neoplasia (VIN). The physical appearance of VIN can vary from mild whitening of the epithelium with no change in texture to lesions with a tan to brown appearance and lesions that mimic condylomata. It is for this reason that any change of appearance warrants further evaluation and usually biopsy.

VIN has been associated with the human papilloma virus (HPV).[6,17] VIN is most commonly associated with women in the 20- to 30-year age range, while invasive squamous cancers are more commonly seen in older women.[17,34] Verrucous cancer, one of the rarer subtypes of squamous cancers that occurs more frequently in older women, has a gross appearance very similar to that of condylomata acuminata.[24] The fact that these cancers may appear either mimicking condylomata or occurring in concert with apparent HPV infection argues for a high index of suspicion and biopsy rather than presumption of diagnosis and treatment of HPV.

Colposcopy of the vulva can reveal some of the features of neoplasia seen in lesions on the mucous membranes. Obviously, these features are more likely to be present the closer the lesion is to the introital area, since keratinization may obscure the underlying vascular structures. Changes suggestive of VIN are white epithelium, mosaicism and punctation, and irregular surface structure.[19]

Invasive squamous cancers generally share the characteristic of being more friable and more frequently associated with loss of skin integrity or ulceration. As noted, the verrucous subtype does not share these characteristics, as it mimics condylomata. In addition, most invasive cancers will be unilateral, thus destroying the symmetry described earlier. Invasive cancers are associated with thickening and irregularity of the epithelium. Colposcopically, these lesions can display the hallmarks of invasion such as atypical, aberrant blood vessels and marked irregularity of the topography of the lesion. Colposcopic evaluation is rarely required, however, since these lesions stand out as different even in vulva with squamous hypertrophy or other vulvar conditions.

Pigmented Lesions and Nevi

Lentiginous changes are present on the vulva as a normal finding. It is important to note that such changes occur in the basal layer and as such should not disturb in any way the texture of the skin in the area. Nevi also are present on the vulva as a normal finding. However, for the proportionate area of skin represented by vulvar tissue (2 percent), a disproportionate number of malignant melanomas (3 to 5 percent) occur in this area.[25] This has led some authors to suggest removal of all nevi, although the actual benefit in terms of prevention of melanoma is unknown. Certainly, the number of admittedly uncomfortable biopsies with benign findings would be likely to be excessive.

Given these caveats, it is important to document the presence of any presumed nevi on the vulvar skin and to chart the appearance of these areas over time. Any adverse change in appearance warrants removal of the area. In addition, the changes associated with malignant melanoma in other areas of the skin should always be evaluated. These include asymmetry within the lesion/nevus itself; an irregular border; marked color change, including different shades in the same lesion; a diameter greater than 6 mm or size changes; and any evidence of an inflammatory response with weeping, bleeding, or itching. Finally, as distinct from lentigo, the skin is elevated in the area of melanoma.

Paget's Disease

Another change in the vulvar skin of importance is the erythematous and often raised and rough surface associated with Paget's disease.[4,15] This can be unilateral or bilateral but again presents with a departure from previous evaluation and certainly from normal skin appearance. It often appears pink and white and is sometimes said to have a "cake frosting" appearance. This lesion can be difficult to differentiate from chronic skin irritation due to multiple etiologies, such as urinary incontinence.

Vulvar Biopsy

The next step in evaluating all these abnormalities is vulvar biopsy or wide local excision of the area. The decision regarding whether one biopsy, multiple biopsies, or wide local excision is appropriate depends on the area involved, the number of lesions, and the type of potential premalignant or malignant condition that the appearance portends. For a large lesion or multiple affected areas, it must be borne in mind that a single biopsy with a benign or a premalignant diagnosis does not preclude invasive cancer elsewhere on the vulva. As a general rule, a single lesion up to 1 cm can be easily excised in the office setting. Multiple lesions require multiple biopsies. In addition, lesions that are suspicious for melanoma are best served by an initial wide excision that is deep enough to allow for pathologic measurement of depth of invasion. If the lesion suspicious for melanoma is too large for adequate local excision, the biopsy technique must be adequately deep to permit proper measurement of depth of invasion.

Two techniques are appropriate in this area and are summarized below:

PUNCH BIOPSY

Equipment

- Local antiseptic solution
- Local anesthetic and 30-gauge needle
- Topical anesthetic if lesion is on mucosal area
- Keyes punch (disposable); 6-, 8-, or 10-mm, depending on size and depth of lesion
- Iris scissors
- Fine surgical forceps
- Silver nitrate sticks
- Gauze sponges

Note: Have available Monsel's solution, needle holder, 3-0 suture

Procedure After adequate preparation of the area, infiltrate the skin with local anesthetic (if on mucosal area, pretreat area with topical anesthetic). Place the punch over the area and press firmly while twirling the punch between thumb and forefinger. Remove the punch and grasp the specimen below the skin level with forceps. Cut the base cleanly with the iris scissors. Put the specimen in fixative. Cauterize the base or suture as clinically indicated.

Precautions for the Patient The area is at risk for infection and bleeding. Some spotting and bleeding can be expected for 24 h. Ice packs may be applied to control swelling and for comfort for the first 24 h as necessary. Wound care should include one to two sitz baths per day for 2 days and longer if the area is not closed. The area should not be rubbed or wiped but patted dry or dried with a hand-held hair dryer on a low temperature. Any evidence of increasing pain, erythema, fever, or increased bleeding should be reported promptly.

WIDE LOCAL EXCISION

Equipment

- Local antiseptic solution
- Local anesthetic and 30-gauge needle
- Topical anesthetic if lesion is on mucosal area
- No. 15 scalpel (disposable)

- Iris scissors
- Fine surgical forceps
- Needle holder (fine)
- Hemostat
- Suture, 2-0, 3-0, or 4-0 subcuticular (cutting needle)
- Gauze sponges
- Sterile perineal pad

Note: Optional: purple sterile surgical pen, surgical assistant (extremely helpful)

Procedure After adequate preparation of the area, infiltrate the area with local anesthetic (use topical pretreatment if on mucosal area). Outline the area to be resected prior to preparation or at this time, if necessary. Excise the perimeter from inferior to superior. Grasping one edge, dissect the area to be removed from the underlying subcutaneous tissue with the scalpel at a depth appropriate for the lesion type. Put the specimen in fixative, with a suture at 12 o'clock if orientation is important. Grasp areas of major bleeding with the hemostat and tie. Close the incision in layers with 2-0 for the deep subcutaneous layer and 3-0 or 4-0 for the skin closure, using either a subcuticular or an interrupted closure.

Precautions for the Patient These are the same as for the punch biopsy, with the following exceptions: Ice should be applied to the perineum for 24 h. (A damp sterile perineal pad cooled in the freezer makes a good ice pad to use at home.) After 24 h, sitz baths twice a day for 1 week are recommended. Any evidence of increasing pain, erythema, fever, or increased bleeding should be reported promptly.

Management of Vulvar Intraepithelial Neoplasia (VIN) and Invasive Carcinoma [Fig. 23-1]

The underlying phenomenon of VIN is the assumed connection between the propensity to form VIN and infection with HPV. The fact that the virus appears to infect the field—including the perineum, potentially the distal anal squamous area, the vagina, and the cervix at the time of the initial exposure—underlies the clinical pattern of behavior of these lesions. Despite adequate treatment with local excision, laser ablation, or topical solutions such as 5-fluorouracil, these lesions have a 30 to 50 percent chance of recurrence. Since women with VIN and invasive vulvar cancers are at higher risk for cervical and vaginal lesions as well, they must also have an evaluation of the cervix and vagina, usually by colposcopy. Certain patient behaviors or conditions seem to be related to the development of such neoplasias, including smoking and the use of immunosuppressive drugs or immunosuppression associated with infection with human immunodeficiency virus (HIV). Greater age does increase the likelihood of finding invasive disease, so excision is the best choice for therapy.[9,10] No matter how young or old the patient, under no circumstances should a lesion be presumed to be VIN and treated with ablative therapy without adequate biopsies and careful histologic evaluation to rule out the presence of microinvasive or invasive cancer.

Patient Counsel The obvious preventive counsel for patients without the disease is to avoid infection with HPV and HIV a priori. For patients with VIN, smoking cessation and avoidance of infection with the virus are important topics to cover. In addition, patient vulvar self-examination and report of any new lesions is important in follow-up. Appropriate follow-up includes inspection and colposcopy every 3 months for the first year, every 6 months for the next, and then yearly if no other lesions appear. Continued support for smoking cessation and avoidance of sexually transmitted diseases is appropriate.

Invasive squamous cancers and verrucous cancers are appropriately treated by surgical excision. The extent of surgical excision may vary by the lesion size, location, histologic appearance—including depth of invasion and the presence or absence of involvement of regional inguinal lymph nodes—and local structures. As an example, some early invasion (less than 1 mm with no other prognostic risk factors) may be treated by wide radical excision whereas a 1-cm lesion with a spray pattern located in the midline may require full radical vulvectomy and bilateral groin lymph node dissection. Large lesions

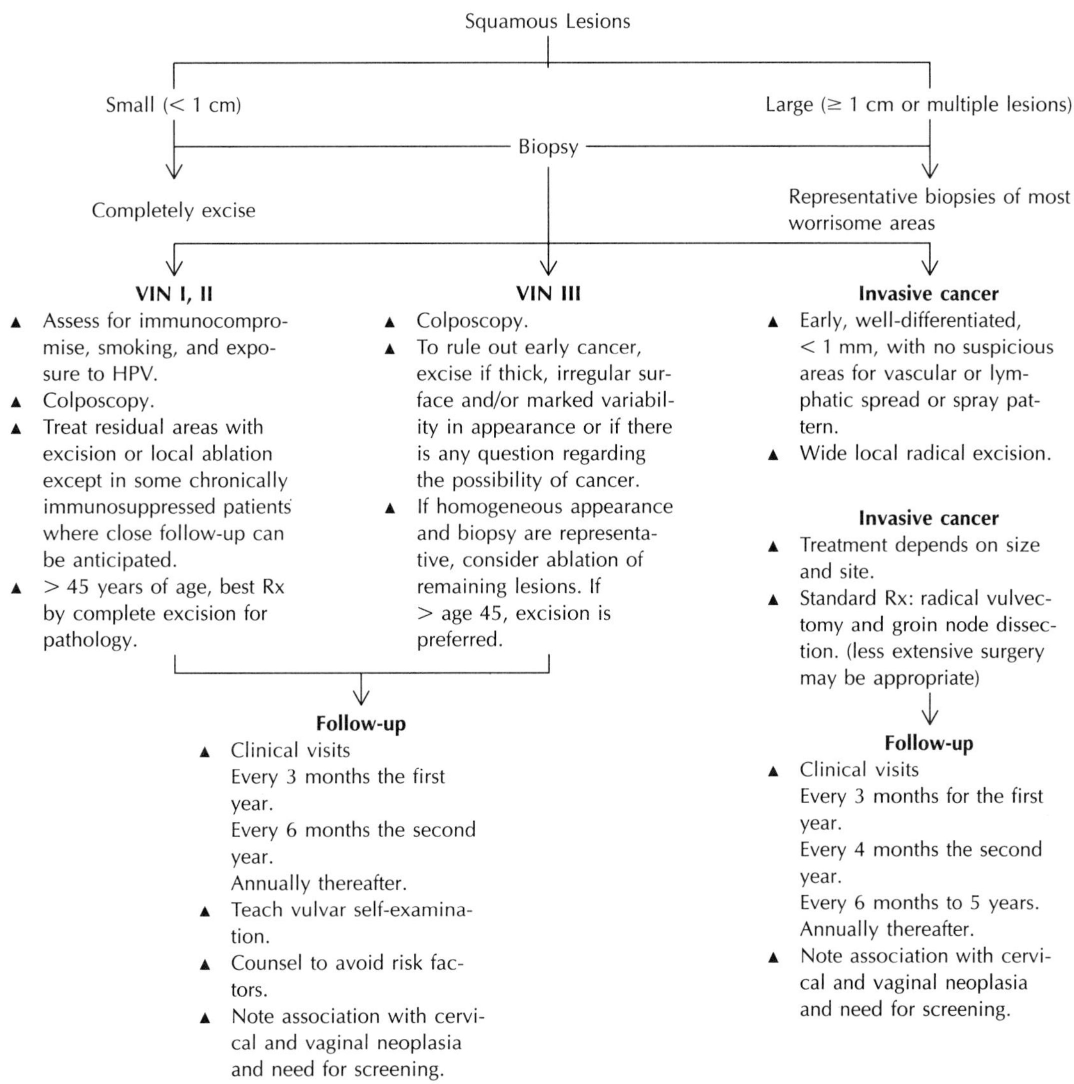

Figure 23-1 Decision flow chart for vulvar cancer.

that compromise surrounding structures such as the pubic arch or the urethra-rectum may be better treated with chemoradiation and potential subsequent excision. Choices of therapy come under the expertise of the gynecologic oncologist and require such consultation.

Overall, squamous cancers of the vulva are found at earlier stages and associated with excellent long-term cure rates (Table 23-1). Follow-up for patients includes an evaluation every 3 months for the first year, then follow-up depending on the prognostic factors of the original lesion. These patients are also at risk for the development of VIN or neoplasia elsewhere in the genital tract or the anorectal area, and clinical evaluation of these areas is required during follow-up.

TABLE 23-1 **Common Invasive Disease and Treatment**

Type of Cancer	Most Common Type	Most Common Stage	5-Year Survival	Common Treatment[a]	Common Side Effects of Treatment
Vulvar	Squamous	I	90%	Radical vulvectomy and bilateral groin node dissection (less extensive surgery may be appropriate for many lesions)	Wound breakdown, leg lymphedema
Vaginal	Squamous	Rare	Variable	Radiation or radical surgery	
Cervical	Squamous	I	75 to 90%	Radical hysterectomy with lymph node dissection	Ureteral fistula (1.6%), bowel and bladder dysfunction
				Radiation therapy	Ureteral fistula (1.6%), long-term bowel, rectal, and bladder dysfunction, including fistula
Endometrial	Adenocarcinoma	I	75 to 90%	Staging laparotomy with total abdominal hysterectomy, bilateral salpingo-oophorectomy, and node sampling	
				May require adjuvant radiation therapy	Radiation may result in bladder and bowel changes
Ovarian	Epithelial carcinoma	III	30%	Staging laparotomy with tumor debulking, TAH-BSO, omentectomy, multiple biopsies possible bowel resection	
				Chemotherapy given after initial exploration	Chemotherapy side effects depend on which agents are used

[a]As noted in text, treatment depends on histopathology and clinical risk factors.

Management of Malignant Melanoma

As opposed to the squamous cancers, malignant melanomas derive their prognosis from depth of invasion and are rarely found in favorable depth.[14,25] The standard therapy remains either vulvectomy or wide local radical dissection, both with regional node dissection. Other forms of therapy such as radiation, chemotherapy, and immunotherapy remain of little benefit for most of the these patients. Again, selection of therapy is the expertise of the gynecologic oncologist, and these patients require such consultation.

Vagina

Normal Vaginal Examination

The normal vagina should have a pale pink appearance demonstrating a good subdermal blood supply throughout. The texture of the walls should be smooth with circular rugae. The underlying tissue should be symmetrical and should not contain cystic or firm structures. The suburethral area should be rubbery, consistent throughout its length and not firm. On inspection it is important to note that either the traditional Graves or the Pedersen metal speculum will obscure the vaginal mucosa underneath, and adequate inspection requires either the use of a clear plastic speculum or careful inspection of the anterior and posterior walls on withdrawal of the speculum. It is also important to note that Pap smears can identify vaginal neoplasia. If the Pap smear is abnormal but there is no cervical pathology, the vagina requires careful inspection, including colposcopy to rule it out as the site of the abnormality.

Vaginal Squamous Changes

The same changes that are seen in the medial vulva when neoplastic lesions are present are seen in the vagina. Because the vagina is not keratinized, colposcopy can identify lesions that are clinically inapparent. Application of 1% acetic acid to the area of colposcopic view and sequential inspection with colposcopy from cephalad to caudad offers a method that should prevent skipping a clinically inapparent lesion. Of practical assistance, given the softness of the vaginal walls and their tendency to collapse into the field of view, a condom (with both ends open) or finger of a large surgical glove applied over the speculum before insertion can assist in the lateral retraction of tissue. Again, the classic changes of whitening of the epithelium or pigment change as well as vascular changes (from punctation to atypical or abnormal vessels) identify the areas for biopsy. Invasive squamous cancers may be friable, may be ulcerated, and have a consistency that is different from the surrounding mucosa. Such lesions should be biopsied regardless of the colposcopic appearance or Pap smear results. Again, remember the axiom: *If it looks abnormal it should be biopsied.*

Cystic areas can be seen in the wall of the vagina. These may be associated with epithelialized islands of adenosis in patients with a history of diethylstilbestrol (DES) exposure or may be remnant cysts. The hallmarks of colposcopic vascular changes associated with DES exposure[35] or with neopolasia must be sought before conservative management is proposed. In addition, for DES patients a drawn map of lesions is of great assistance to the patient and the physician in the long-term management of such lesions. While clear cell adenocarcinoma of the vagina is less common contemporarily, the clinical appearance is of importance. One of the differences between adenocarcinomas and squamous carcinomas in the vaginal mucosa is the fact that these lesions often may not be palpably different from the surrounding tissue and therefore are more likely to be missed at early stages. In addition, adenocarcinomas may have a papillary and cystic appearance as well as the ulcerative and friable nature associated with squamous cancers. Again, the importance of careful inspection of the entire vagina, including the anterior and posterior surfaces, cannot be overstated.

Vaginal Biopsy

Vaginal biopsy presents particular difficulties because of the soft and mobile nature of vaginal tissue. Wide local excision requires significant surgical assistance and rarely is an option for the clinic setting.

Equipment

- Local antiseptic solution
- Local and topical anesthetic solution
- Skin hook
- Allis clamp, long
- Kevorkian or Schubert biopsy forceps
- No. 15 blade scalpel
- Long forceps or Crile clamp
- Long Metzenbaum scissors
- Long hemostat
- Long needle holder
- Gauze sponges
- Sponge stick
- Chromic or Dexon suture material, 2-0 or 3-0 atraumatic
- Silver nitrate and Monsel's solution

The appropriate mixture of equipment depends on the area of the vagina involved and the accessibility of the lesion. The above list is provided because all of these instruments have been found to be of assistance at one time or another, depending on the extent of the lesion.

Procedure In general, lesions near the introitus can be managed much as described in the section on vulvar biopsies. Lesions near the cervix can be managed as described under cervix (see text following). It is the lesions in the deep vaginal fornices and sidewalls which are difficult to grasp that present a greater clinical challenge. Such lesions can be managed with topical application of anesthetic (and infiltration as needed) and grasping with an Allis or skin hook to tent the area so as to enable the use of a biopsy forceps, scalpel, or Metzenbaum scissors. Adequate exposure of the area is important, and readjustment of the speculum or addition of the sidewall support as described previously can be very helpful. There is a tendency, however, to overdistend the vagina in the region, which leads to an inability to tent the vaginal wall. This can be solved by merely releasing the pressure slightly on the speculum.

Precautions for the Patient This area is at risk for infection and bleeding. Spotting and bleeding can be expected for 24 h. No vaginal intercourse, tampons, or douching should be permitted for at least 24 h for small biopsies, and longer depending on the size of the biopsy. Any increasing pain, bleeding, or fever should be promptly reported.

Management

The most common neoplastic lesions in the vagina are vaginal intraepithelial neoplasia (VAIN) and invasive squamous cancer.[2] VAIN can be treated with a multiplicity of options, including wide local excision, laser ablations, and topical measures such as 5-fluorouracil. Of these, the only option that will adequately evaluate the lesion for the presence of early invasive disease is the wide local excision. For this reason, if the biopsy suggests a carcinoma in situ or there is any clinical or pathologic question of invasion, the local excision is usually the best option.

Invasive vaginal cancer is rare, and the appropriate management is predicated on the depth of invasion, the location of the lesion, and the cell type. The majority of vaginal cancers are treated primarily with radiation, although radical surgery is appropriate in some patients with limited lesions. Such choices come under the expertise of gynecologic oncologists and require such consultation.

Patient Counsel While vaginal cancer and intraepithelial neoplasia have not received the study that vulvar and cervical lesions have, the avoidance of infection with HPV and HIV is appropriate in prevention. For patients with such lesions, particularly intraepithelial neoplasia, support for smoking cessation as well as prevention of infection with other sexually transmitted pathogens may be of value.

Cervix

Cervical neoplastic changes are far more common than either vaginal or vulvar changes. For this reason, any woman's primary care physician should be aware of the issues involved in the management of premalignant and malignant lesions of the cervix. The hallmark symptom of invasive cervical cancer, postcoital bleeding, is important to note because lesions may not be clinically apparent, and this symptom should warrant further investigation even if the Pap smear is read as negative. It is important to note that the false-negative rate of one Pap smear may be as high as 10 to 30 percent[10] and cannot be taken as proof that no malignancy exists. In the face of this classic symptom of malignancy, further evaluation is warranted.

Normal Cervix

The normal cervix has a uniform pale pink appearance with a smooth surface. Occasional nabothian cysts can be seen with mucoid material covered by a smooth surface epithelium. These can vary in size but should not be friable or irregular in appearance. The endocervix generally appears velvety red. Previous trauma to the cervix from biopsy or cervical lacerations should present a white appearance with a distribution consistent with the trauma, most often linear. The substance of the cervix is moderately firm and consistent throughout. The shape of the cervix should be symmetrical except in those circumstances in which significant cervical trauma or previous surgery can be documented.

Cervical Abnormalities

Because of early detection of many neoplastic changes of the cervix by Pap smear, these changes may be apparent only colposcopically. Therefore, any patient with a Pap smear consistent with CIN or invasive cancer (unless a tissue diagnosis of invasive cancer has already been obtained)—and often patients with a smear interpreted as atypical squamous cells of undetermined significance—must undergo colposcopic evaluation. The colposcopic hallmarks of a neoplastically active epithelium are described in Chap. 35. The adequacy of view of the most biologically active zone, the *transformation zone,* must be carefully assessed and documented. A careful map should be drawn for further evaluation and management. Areas of abnormality should be biopsied for diagnosis. It is essential that the transformation zone is able to be visualized totally since almost all cervical cancers begin in this region. If the whole transformation zone cannot be visualized colposcopically, the physician cannot be certain that invasive cancer is not present.

Any gross lesion of the cervix requires biopsy, preferably at the time of first notation. Some patients may prefer rescheduling, but a Pap smear obtained at the time of notation of such a lesion is not adequate either to make a diagnosis of the etiology of the lesion or to plan therapy. A negative Pap smear does not alter the mandatory requirement for biopsy of any abnormal lesion noted clinically.

Of importance in the evaluation of the cervix are lesions that occur in the endocervical area. These may present with no gross external abnormality and merely a thickening of the cervical diameter. The ability of Pap smears to detect such lesions is diminished because of their site in the substance of the endocervix. Because of these difficulties, the diagnosis of endocervical lesions can be clinically challenging. The endocervical curettage is often the only way to diagnose such cancers, and, even so, may miss the lesion. A high index of suspicion is therefore appropriate.

Cervical Biopsy

This discussion will confine itself to routine biopsy of the cervix. Loop excision is discussed in the chapter on colposcopy (Chap. 35).

Equipment

- Antiseptic solution
- Topical anesthetic solution
- Shubert, Kevorkian, Tischler biopsy forceps
- Kevorkian curette
- Silver nitrate sticks, Monsel's solution

Note: Optional: tenaculum, paracervical block material (see endometrial biopsy, Chap. 36).

Procedure After identification of the area either visually or colposcopically, topical anesthetic can be applied to the area. In patients with previous traumatic experiences with cervical biopsy, consideration of a paracervical block may be appropriate. In general, simple cervical biopsy is well tolerated. The area for biopsy is located and biopsy forceps chosen based on the site. For some lesions at the transformation zone, the need to grasp the endocervical area may suggest a Kevorkian biopsy forceps as the best choice. If there is difficulty due to excess cervical mobility, use of the tenaculum can be quite helpful. As with all biopsies, the area of highest clinical suspicion should be biopsied first, particularly if discomfort or unusual bleeding occurs. This will assure that the most important area is evaluated. An endocervical curettage is performed with the Kevorkian curette.

Precautions for the Patient There may be spotting and bleeding for 24 h following the procedure. No douching, use of tampons, or intercourse are permitted for 24 h. If fever, increased bleeding, or pelvic pain occurs, this should be reported promptly.

Management [Fig. 23-2]

Management of preinvasive cervical disease is discussed in the Chap. 35.

For patients with CIN III and negative endocervical evaluation who have completed desired childbearing or are perimenopausal, a hysterectomy may be the most appropriate choice, since it produces a

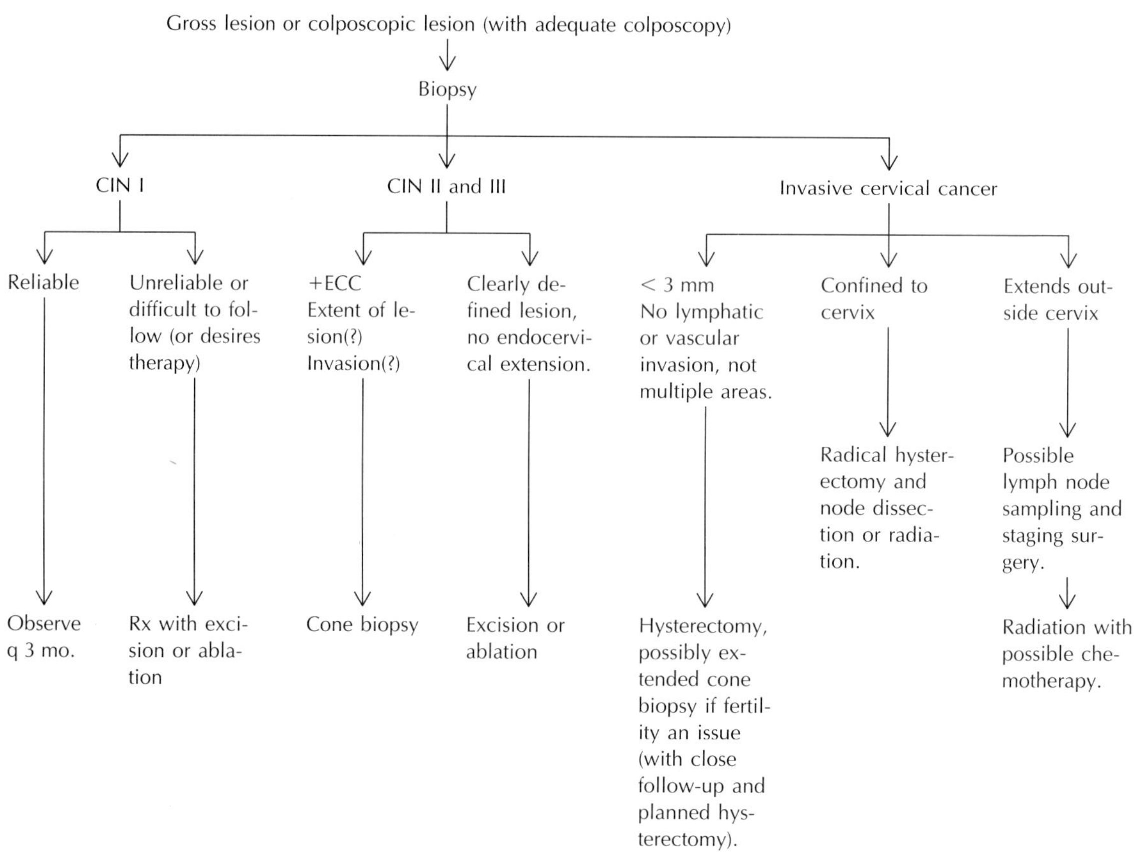

Figure 23-2 Decision flow chart for cervical cancer.

slightly lower chance of recurrence. For these patients as well, the importance of careful compliance with a proposed screening and evaluation management plan cannot be overstated. In particular, even with a hysterectomy, these patients are at risk for vaginal neoplasis and require Pap follow-up of the vaginal apex.

Squamous carcinoma of the cervix generally presents as a stage I lesion.[18] Despite the fact that the new FIGO staging defines subgroups based on a depth of invasion of 5 mm or a width of invasive disease of 7 mm, these are generally not the criteria used to define microinvasive disease for purposes of planning therapy. In the United States, the generally accepted criteria are those proposed by the Society of Gynecologic Oncologists (SGO), which recognizes microinvasion as lesions with less than 3 mm of depth of invasion from the basement membrane and with no vascular or lymphatic invasion or confluent tongues. The reason for this caution is related to the possibility of lymph node involvement at the FIGO microinvasion stage, generally held to be 1 to 5 percent, depending on risk factors.[1] In fact, even using the SGO definition, lymph node involvement may, on rare occasion, occur.

For those patients meeting the criteria set by the SGO for microinvasion, the most common recommendation is hysterectomy, although cone biopsy can be considered in very specific circumstances in young women wishing to preserve childbearing capacity for the immediate future. In general, a hysterectomy would then be recommended when childbearing was completed, although some European-based studies suggest that cone biopsy alone may be adequate. The rate of recurrence of cancer in the cervix is slightly higher in the group managed conservatively than in groups managed by hysterectomy, although generally the risk is less than 5 percent.[26]

For patients with invasion beyond this limit (i.e., not microinvasion but still restricted to the cervix), two options for therapy of equivalent efficacy as measured by 5-year survival rates are available. One option is radical hysterectomy and lymph node dissection, and the other is primary radiation therapy. Removal of the ovaries is not necessary for therapy unless they are diseased. Both options have potential complications, with surgical side effects being the risk of ureteral fistula (1.6 percent) and potential long-term bladder and bowel dysfunction (rarely requiring therapy). These side effects occur because radical hysterectomy entails the removal of the parametrial tissue in the broad ligaments and the uterosacral ligaments, and this removal disrupts the normal nerve supply to the bladder and the rectum; the surgery also requires the complete dissection of the ureter to remove the surrounding parametrium and a wide margin of upper vaginal mucosa. Radiation side effects tend to be long-term (beyond the initial mild nausea and diarrhea) and include the risk of ureteral fistula (1.6 percent), permanent and progressive bowel and bladder injury (occasionally requiring surgical management), and vaginal atrophy and stenosis. Because of the time differential in side effects, surgery is generally recommended for women who are good surgical candidates and particuarly if they are young and/or sexually active.

All other stages of cervical cancer and some subtypes of stage I cervical cancer are treated primarily with radiation therapy. The barrel-shaped stage I cervical cancer often is treated primarily with radiation therapy with a subsequent hysterectomy planned, depending on the lesion and the response.[32]

For patients who present with massive pelvic disease (stage III or IVA), radiation therapy may be augmented with chemotherapy to increase the response rate. Patients with these advanced stages of disease may present with ureteral obstruction and, if so, are best served by nephrostomy to restore renal function during therapy, with the potential for conversion to internal stents if further therapy is required. This can allow these patients an appropriate trial of chemoradiation therapy to control their disease and prolong a disease-free interval. This is different from the choice that might be made in a patient with secondary ureteral obstruction with massive recurrence of disease after adequate primary therapy has failed. In that circumstance, if no other therapy offers reasonable benefit, relief of the renal failure may not be in the patient's best interest. In that setting the patient's own goals with a terminal illness and her comfort (which is potentially augmented by the renal failure) are the primary objectives.

Adenocarcinoma of the cervix is treated in the same fashion as squamous carcinoma of the cervix, although there is some evidence in the literature that the response to therapy may not be as good as with the squamous counterparts.[3] Particular cell types of high metastatic potential include glassy cell cancers and small cell cancers (particularly those with markings for neuroendocrine or oat cell subtypes). These cancers, with their high propensity for early local and distant spread, may be treated by different combinations of all the modalities. At present, therapy has been individualized for such patients, and no one pattern of therapy seems to offer an advantage over another. It is important to note that even microinvasive tumors of these high-risk histologic types behave in atypical fashions, and conservative therapy for them is not appropriate.

Follow-Up

For invasive cancers, follow-up should include examinations and Pap smears every 3 months for at least 1 to 2 years. Following that, the interval for follow-up is dependent on the cell type and stage, with shorter intervals both initially and long-term, depending on the pattern of potential metastases.

Uterus

Endometrial cancers tend to be diagnosed in early stages because of their identifying symptom, uterine bleeding. The majority of these malignancies occur in postmenopausal age groups, but they can occur in women in their thirties or younger. Predisposing factors include large adipose tissue layers (presumed to increase endogenous estrogen), unopposed exogenous estrogen, and, in very rare instances, a genetic component. Patients with previous breast cancer may have a slightly higher rate of endometrial cancers, particularly if receiving adjuvant tamoxifen.

The hallmark of these cancers is postmenopausal or irregular bleeding. Uterine size or shape may not be altered in the presence of malignancy; therefore, the absence of such change on physical examination does not rule out a premalignant or malignant condition.

The presence of rapid growth in an area of presumed myoma, particularly in a postmenopausal woman, may be characteristic of the rare uterine malignancy sarcoma, although this occurs in less than 1 percent of myomas. It is the pattern of rapid growth that is of concern rather than the presence of myomas. Slow growth over many years would not be a significant concern.

Suspected involvement of the cervix in the patient with endometrial cancer will often dictate a different surgical or radiation and surgery choice of management. Because of this, careful description of the cervical appearance, including its shape and size, is important.

Screening with Pap smears is ineffective for this malignancy, as 50 percent or more are not detected with Pap smears. The finding of endometrial cells on a Pap smear of a woman who is postmenopausal or not near a normal menstrual flow may be a warning of underlying pathology and should warrant further investigation. A negative Pap smear, logically, does not rule out this malignancy.[41]

When abnormal bleeding occurs, an office evaluation of the endometrium and endocervix is warranted. Office biopsies with various instruments have been reported to have sensitivities and specificities that range from 80 to 98 percent.[11,27,38] The addition of hysteroscopy may be warranted in some circumstances to identify polypoid lesions or anatomic abnormalities such as submucous myomas that might be the cause of the abnormal bleeding. It is neither warranted nor required in all cases of abnormal uterine bleeding. The procedure for office endometrial evaluation is discussed in Chap. 36.

Management [Fig. 23-3]

If the pathology of an office endometrial biopsy shows hyperplasia, most physicians feel that a formal D&C must be performed to rule out the presence of a synchronous endometrial cancer. Evidence suggests that the use of progestins in patients who only have simple hyperplasia will decrease the inci-

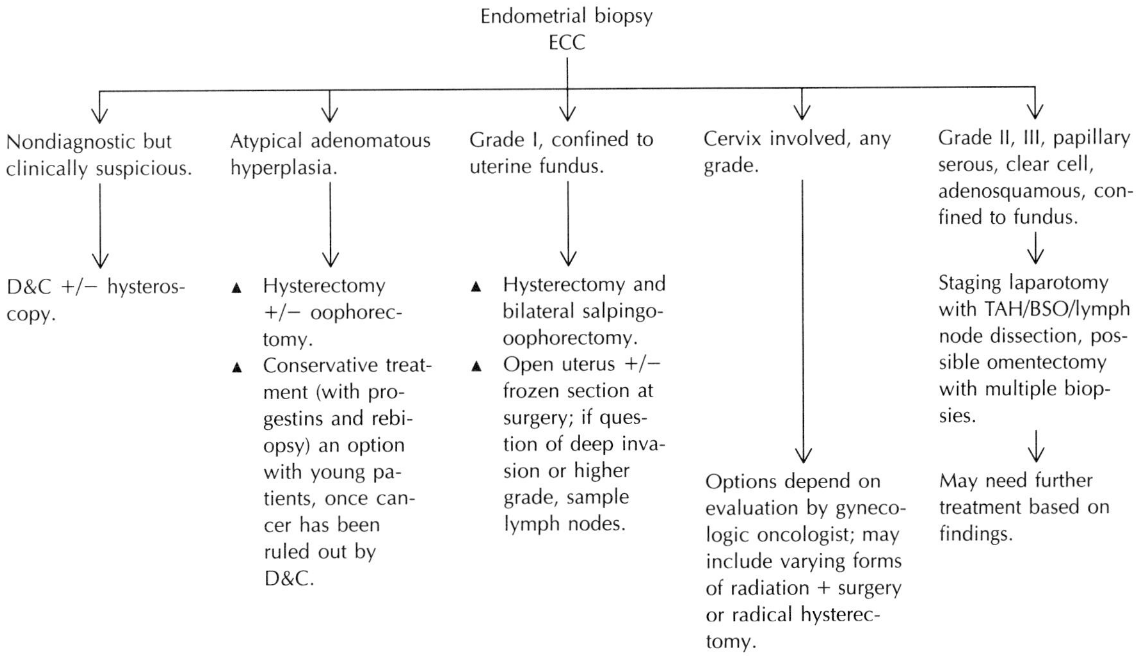

Figure 23-3 Decision flow chart for endometrial cancer.

dence of subsequent endometrial cancers; therefore, its use may be considered in such women.

Atypical endometrial hyperplasia may represent a premalignant lesion. In a perimenopausal woman, the association with concurrent or subsequent endometrial cancer is high enough to warrant removal of the uterus.[28,29] In younger women who desire preservation of the uterus, a conservative approach with higher-dose progestins and follow-up biopsies may be considered if the patient is likely to be compliant with close follow-up.

Adenocarcinoma of the endometrium is generally well differentiated—most often stage I—and highly curable. It is important to recognize the differences among subtypes, however, as their behaviors vary widely from the usual and should be treated differently. Of most importance is the recognition that papillary serous endometrial cancer invades earlier and has a high propensity to spread as though it were a primary ovarian cancer. This cancer requires an approach analogous to ovarian cancer, which is discussed later in the chapter. In addition, clear cell and adenosquamous cancers also have a higher likelihood of spread.

The standard treatment for endometrial cancers is removal of the uterus, cervix, tubes, and ovaries (because of a greater propensity to spread to this region). Lymph node sampling and full lymphadenectomy are based on the grade, the depth of invasion at surgery, and the histologic type. Full staging biopsies are reserved for cell types such as papillary serous or for histologic or surgical findings that place the patient at risk for spread of disease. The surgeon should be able to provide all of these options at the time of surgery as well as to differentiate between the various prognostic factors associated with the cell type and the surgical findings.[16]

Uterine sarcomas, as noted above, may present as rapid growth of a uterine ''fibroid'' in a postmenopausal woman. However, more frequently they present with vaginal bleeding, and an endometrial biopsy returns copious, fleshy, often gray, material. These cancers vary prognostically according to histologic type, mitotic activity, and extent of disease, although they generally confer a much poorer outcome than endometrial adenocarcinoma.[30,48] Their primary management is surgically tailored to the presentation and the histologic type.

Ovaries

Ovarian cancers are the most fatal of all the gynecologic malignancies.[38] Whether or not they have a premalignant phase and, if so, how long a phase that might be is a matter of great interest as the existence of such a phase might allow for the development of a screening system for the disease. Although there has been much interest in serum cancer-related antigens (particularly Ca-125) and ultrasound in screening for these cancers, there is presently no evidence to support the cost and/or efficacy of any screening method.[23,39] The management of both benign and malignant ovarian neoplasms begins with the diagnosis of a pelvic mass.

Normal Ovaries

Normal ovaries in premenopausal and menopausal women differ in shape and consistency. The premenopausal, ovulatory woman usually has ovaries that are palpable, somewhat almond-shaped, with a length of 3 to 5 cm and width of 2 to 3 cm. The normal ovary produces cystic structures on a cyclic basis, some of which can persist through a cycle. These tend to be mobile, nontender, and less than 5 cm in diameter. The postmenopausal ovary undergoes progressive atrophy. Thus the ovary 1 year after menopause will be different from 20 years after menopause. The idea of a nonpalpable ovary being the hallmark of the menopausal ovary merely refers to the small size (1 to 1.5 cm diameter of the senescent ovary). The postmenopausal ovary can be occasionally felt in extremely thin women, and the ovary may be slightly larger if menopause has been fairly recent. (Adherence to the criteria of surgery for every palpable postmenopausal ovary is therefore not warranted.)

Ovarian Masses

The problem of management of ovarian masses is complicated by the fact that biopsy of the ovary is generally discouraged and direct access for evaluation is required. Management must then depend on the likelihood of malignancy for certain presentations at different ages as well as the likelihood of complications from suspected benign ovarian masses. Furthermore, ovarian masses must be differentiated from the multiple surrounding structures that can present as pelvic masses but require entirely different management plans. Clinical examination and evaluation form the major means of providing the plan and differ according to age groups. The differential diagnosis and triage of masses in the premenarchal female will not be included in this discussion, except for the comment that pelvic masses in this young group of patients invariably represent a condition that warrants further investigation.

Ovarian Masses in Premenopausal Women Premenopausal cycling women may have cystic areas of the ovary on a routine basis. As noted above, the persistence of a cyst of greater than 5 cm requires further evaluation. The concurrent nonovarian conditions that need to be differentiated from these include hydrosalpinx, hydatid cysts, and pedunculated fibroids.[8] As with most medical investigations, the history and physical examination can provide most of the major clues as to the cause of the mass. For example, an ovarian mass in a woman who has a history of multiple episodes of sexually transmitted diseases may suggest a tuboovarian abscess or hydrosalpinx, whereas an ovarian mass in a patient with increasing dyspareunia and dysmenorrhea may suggest the presence of an endometrioma. In these examples, it is also important to note that the patient's wishes for present or future fertility may play a substantial role in the therapy chosen. Of course, if there is a significant likelihood of malignancy, surgery is mandatory.

As noted in Fig. 23-4, in the premenopausal population ultrasound, particularly vaginal ultrasound, may be an appropriate next step in narrowing the differential diagnosis. The use of ultrasound in the premenopausal patient is more likely to result in information that will allow for the conservative management of these patients, thus justifying the added cost of such procedures. In particular, the findings that corroborate hydrosalpinx with a normal ovary or a simple cyst suggestive of a physiologic cyst may allow a choice for close observation. The addition of serum tests for cancer antigens such as Ca-125 can be problematic at this point in evaluation because of the increased unreliability in premenopausal, cycling women and because of the potential for Ca-125 elevation in the presence of other conditions, particularly endometriosis, but also infections. For that reason, unless the clinical differential diagnosis at this point in the evaluation includes malignancy, Ca-125 may not be of value.

The clinical characteristics of a malignant process of the ovary in this population are important. In particular, persistence and growth of an ovarian mass through a normal menstrual cycle are potentially worrisome. Additionally, the finding of internal septations, excrescences, and large bilateral cysts on ultrasound are correlated with a higher likelihood of malignancy. For these lesions the inclusion of Ca-125 in the evaluation may be of some benefit with the caveat that malignancy, particularly mucinous and low-malignant-potential epithelial cancers, can have normal Ca-125s in 50 percent of patients or more. If the lesions have clinical criteria suggestive of possible malignancy, despite a normal Ca-125, further evaluation with surgery is warranted.

Rapid growth of an ovary, often with pain and the ultrasound finding of primarily solid consistency, is suggestive of a germ cell malignancy. Germ cell malignancies occur more commonly in younger patients and are usually confined to one ovary. Examples of germ cell tumors are the dysgerminoma (which is not usually an aggressive malignancy), the immature teratoma, endodermal sinus tumor, and embryonal cancers (which are extremely aggressive malignancies). The benign cystic teratoma (dermoid) is a very common benign germ cell tumor. Germ cell malignancies may also have an elevated Ca-125, but the tumor markers more commonly associated with germ cell tumors are α-fetoprotein, β-hCG, and, potentially, LDH. This clinical pattern requires more rapid intervention.

Gonadal stromal tumors are rare ovarian neoplasms that are often hormonally active. The granulosa cell tumor is associated with increased estrogen production and therefore may cause abnormal vaginal bleeding, endometrial hyperplasia, or endometrial cancer. Although uncommon, granulosa cell tumors are seen in postmenopausal women as frequently as in premenopausal women. The arrhenoblastoma often produces androgen and is associated with masculinization.

Ovarian Masses in Postmenopausal Women The differential diagnosis of ovarian masses in postmenopausal women is substantially different than it is with women in their twenties, thirties, and forties because of the absence of physiologic cysts in the older age group and the fact that the incidence of epithelial ovarian malignancy in ovarian masses steadily rises as age progresses. For these reasons, a significant ovarian mass generally warrants surgical exploration in postmenopausal women. Ultrasound or CT scan may be of assistance but is not usually considered completely diagnostic. The possibility of other malignancies such as pancreatic cancer, gastric or bowel cancer, metastatic breast cancer, inflammatory conditions such as Crohn's disease, or chronic diverticulitis should be elicited from the history and physical examination. A history of previous conditions such as pelvic inflammatory disease (PID) with persistance of a known or suspected hydrosalpinx should also be sought. In such circumstances, the utility of a CT scan or ultrasound might be increased. The finding of a large mass with associated ascites or cul-de-sac nodularity is highly suggestive of ovarian malignancy. Ca-125 is warranted, as are other tumor markers for colon or breast cancer, if any of these cancers is suspected in these patients. As noted previously, the finding of a normal Ca-125 does not change the management when the possibility of malignancy is suspected.

Biopsy

Not appropriate for ovarian lesions.

Management [Fig. 23-4]

The surgical management of an ovarian mass depends on the patient's age, the suspected diagnosis, and the associated radiographic, ultrasound, or serum findings if warranted.

Premenopausal masses, particularly those suspected to be benign and requiring confirmatory histology, may be appropriate for laparoscopic management. Drainage of what grossly appears to be a "physiologic" cyst, however, presents particular difficulties. The major problem is that a benign gross appearance does not disprove the presence of malignancy. In addition, the laparoscopic drainage or rupture of malignant "cysts" may be correlated with an increased likelihood of more advanced disease,[31,33] particularly if there is a delay between the drainage or cyst removal with rupture and definitive surgery. For this reason, the choice of evaluating a patient with a persistent ovarian mass needs to be made judiciously with corresponding counsel to the patient that appropriate surgical treatment and staging should be done concurrently if a malignancy is found. If there is sufficient presurgical suspicion of cancer or intraoperative laparoscopic suspicion, a biopsy or drainage should not be attempted; it does not serve to further a diagnosis and potentially increases the likelihood of spread of the disease. The diagnoses of endometriosis, pedunculated fibroid, or hydrosalpinx and associated PID may or may not require a corresponding laparoscopically directed biopsy.

The definitive therapy for ovarian malignancy is a full staging laparotomy.[7,21] The utility of laparoscopic staging is fundamentally compromised by the inability to assess adequately all areas of the abdomen, including the mesenteric folds, as well as the inability to adequately debulk tumor that is present. Both accurate initial staging and aggressive surgical debulking of epithelial ovarian malignancies have prognostic and therapeutic correlates with the patient's survival. These should never be compromised

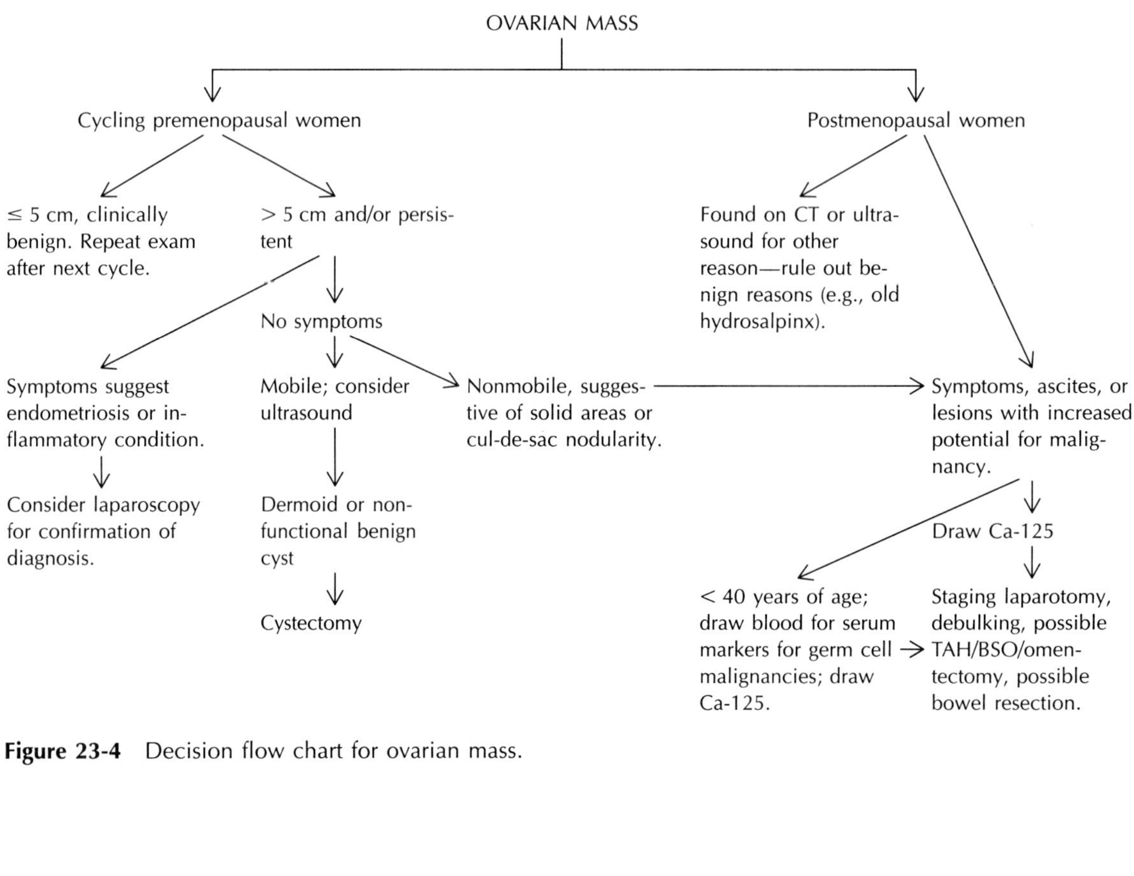

Figure 23-4 Decision flow chart for ovarian mass.

by the use of technology that has not been proven adequate for the circumstances. A full open laparotomy through a vertical or muscle-cutting incision is required for these malignancies. For all but the malignancies restricted to one ovary and of low grade, a hysterectomy and bilateral salpingo-oophorectomy are standard parts of the staging laparotomy. Dependent on the findings at the time of surgery, the ultimate therapy may differ.

The majority of these cancers present with widespread peritoneal disease and with higher grades of tumor. The standard therapy following adequate staging and debulking is chemotherapy. A number of regimens and cytotoxic drugs may be employed, including those restricted to the protocol setting. At present, active agents for ovarian epithelial carcinoma include cisplatin, carboplatin, cyclophosphomide (Cytoxan), ifosfamide, paclitaxel (Taxol),[13] hexamethamelamine, melphalan, and other agents with slightly lower response rates. Standard first-line therapy includes one of the platinum compounds, and with this regimen in the Netherlands registry an improvement in overall survival for ovarian malignancies can be documented. Currently most physicians in the United States believe that platinum plus paclitaxel is the most effective combination of agents for ovarian cancer, and that this combination should be used as first line therapy following primary surgery for advanced epithelial ovarian cancer. Optimal therapy for epithelial ovarian cancer focuses on accuracy and adequacy of initial surgical management and then on aggressive chemotherapy. The Ca-125 serum levels find their best use in the setting of evaluating responses to ongoing therapy.

Germ cell malignancies, as noted, have a presentation that differs from the epithelial malignancies. Their proper surgical and chemotherapeutic management differ as well. In general, these malignancies present as stage I disease, that is, confined to the ovary. Since this disease is more common in young women, the issue of preserving childbearing ability is relevant. In this disease the likelihood of spread to the uterus or other ovary is smaller, and if those organs are grossly normal, they can be retained at the time of staging laparotomy. Following primary surgery, women who have stage I dysgerminomas do not require additional therapy. However, without further treatment (chemotherapy) most germ cell malignancies (endodermal sinus tumor, embryonal tumor, primary ovarian choriocarcinoma, immature teratoma) are usually fatal. Appropriate surgical staging and treatment planning is critical to survival for patients with these malignancies. Present aggressive chemotherapy regimens have altered response rates from less than a 10 percent 5-year survival to greater than 90 percent 5-year survivals for many germ cell tumors.

The issue of quality of life is a frequent problem in patients with progressive malignancy and may be one in which primary care physicians can play an important role assisting their patients. There are multiple issues with which it is important to become familiar, including a durable power of attorney and the "living will" or advance directive documents as well as ethical concerns surrounding the concept of quality of life and treatment planning.[9]

Fallopian Tubes

These are very rare tumors. They are usually not diagnosed preoperatively, but rather the diagnosis is made either at the time of surgery or by the pathologist. The staging that is utilized is the ovarian cancer staging, and both surgery and subsequent chemotherapy follow the guidelines used for ovarian malignancy.

Gestational Trophoblastic Disease (GTD)

This set of diseases is unique to pregnancy as it requires some combination of maternal ovum and paternal sperm to initiate the changes. These diseases include varieties of hydatidiform mole, invasive mole, and choriocarcinoma. Gestational trophoblastic disease (GTD) was the first such malignancy reported to have been cured by chemotherapy. With appropriate management virtually all of these malignancies can be cured, and this makes it important to recognize the classic symptoms and initiate standard evaluation and management. The types most likely to be encountered by primary care physicians are complete mole and partial mole. Complete moles have no identifiable fetal components and are characterized by trophoblastic overgrowth. The usual karyotype is a 46,XX, where both components are paternally derived. This is in contrast to the rarer partial mole where the trophoblastic changes are similar but fetal tissues or fetal development is present. This karyotype is usually triploid, with two components being paternally derived.

Molar Pregnancy

Presenting Signs and Symptoms The majority of patients with molar pregnancy present with two features. The first is a delay in menses related to the pregnancy and the second is the presence of vaginal bleeding. Bleeding occurs in about 97 percent of patients with the most common type of GTD, complete molar pregnancy. In complete mole, the classic presentation also includes a uterine size larger than dates (although present only in about half of patients); early preeclampsia (in about a quarter) that is usually associated with high hCG levels; hyperemesis gravidarum (in about a quarter of patients)—also associated with high serum hCG levels; and the rarer ($<$ 7 percent) hyperthyroidism. In addition, patients may present initially or after evacuation of a mole with transportation of molar tissue to the pulmonary vasculature with tachypnea and tachycardia. Finally, patients may have concurrent ovarian enlargement (theca lutein cysts) of greater than 6 cm correlated with high serum hCG levels.

Evaluation Initial evaluation of a suspected molar pregnancy should include a careful physical examination with particular attention to neurologic function, pulmonary status, size of liver, size of the uterus, and the presence or absence of ovarian enlargement. Occasionaly the classic small grapelike clusters can be seen in the cervical os or in the vagina. Additionally implants of a similar appearance might be seen in the cervical stroma or vagina. If GTD is suspected, biopsy of these lesions is not performed because of the associated risk of severe hemorrhage from these ectopic sites of abnormal trophoblast.

Initial evaluation requires the measurement of a serum β-hCG and performance of a pelvic ultrasound. The hCG will be elevated out of proportion for the gestational age, and the ultrasound will show a classic ''Swiss cheese'' appearance consistent with a molar pregnancy. In partial moles, the placental site will usually show classic changes despite the presence of a fetus. Evaluation for hepatic, cerebral, and pulmonary metastases varies, depending on risk factors identified by the patient's history and the findings of physical examination, laboratory values, and ultrasound. Consultation with a gynecologic oncologist is appropriate after the diagnosis is made.

Management These tumors are usually treated initially by suction and, occasionally, sharp evacuation after careful evaluation for the significant medical complications that can occur with possible attendant hyperthyroidism, preeclampsia, and anemia. The potential for transportation of trophoblastic tissue with pulmonary embolization also exists at the time of evacuation. In general, patients with recognized molar gestations should have their evacuation done at a center that has experience in such uterine evacuations. Alternatives of management can include hysterectomy in patients who do not desire preservation of fertility. Patients who have metastatic disease must receive chemotherapy in addition to having evacuation of the mole or hysterectomy.

Follow-up Follow-up after initial evacuation (or hysterectomy) for a molar pregnancy should be serial β-hCG measurements on a weekly basis until normal for 3 weeks, then monthly until normal for 6 months, then bimonthly for the remainder of the year. Because of the concern about detecting recurrence, prevention of pregnancy during this follow-up time is advisable. The use of oral contraceptives, diaphragm, or an IUD after normalization of hCG levels are all options for patients. If the hCG fails to decline with either a plateau of values or an increase in level, the patient should be referred for evaluation and probable chemotherapy.

Choriocarcinoma

Malignant trophoblastic disease is preceded by hydatidiform mole in 50 percent of cases, by an antecedent normal pregnancy in 25 percent of cases, and by an abortion or ectopic pregnancy in the other 25 percent of cases. In a woman who has a history of a previous hydatidiform mole, it is usually not difficult to make the diagnosis when malignant trophoblastic disease occurs because the physician's index of suspicion is high. However, if the pregnancy event that preceded malignant trophoblastic disease was an abortion, a seemingly normal pregnancy, or an ectopic pregnancy, there is often a delay in making the diagnosis. In a few instances the antecedent pregnancy was many years before.

To make a timely diagnosis the physician needs to have an index of suspicion in any woman with a previous pregnancy who has abnormal bleeding. For instance, hemoptysis in a young woman who has had a previous pregnancy may be from trophoblastic disease metastatic to the lungs. A woman who has bleeding a few weeks, many months, or even years following a pregnancy could have gestational trophoblastic neoplasia in her uterus. Metastatic gestational neoplasia can also be found in the brain, liver, gastrointestinal (GI) or genitourinary (GU) systems. If a patient is not pregnant, a positive beta subunit will be very important in assisting to make the diagnosis. Since gestational trophoblastic neoplasia is most often curable, it is important for the primary care physician to appropriately consider this when formulating a differential diagnosis.

References and Selected Readings

1. Alvarez RD, Soong SJ, Kinney WK, et al: Identification of prognostic factors and risk groups in patients found to have nodal metastases at the time of radical hysterectomy for early stage squamous cell carcinoma of the cervix. *Gynecol Oncol* 35:130, 1989.
2. Ball HG, Berman ML: Management of primary vaginal carcinoma. *Gynecol Oncol* 14:154–163, 1982.
3. Berek JS, Hacker NF, Fu YS, et al: Adenocarcinoma of the uterine cervix: Histologic variables associated with lymph node metastases and spread. *Obstet Gynecol* 65:46–49, 1985.
4. Bergen S, DiSaia PJ, Liao SY, Berman ML: Conservative management of extramammary Paget's disease of the vulva. *Gynecol Oncol* 33:151–156, 1989.
5. Berget A, Lenstrup C: Cervical intraepithelial neoplasia examination, treatment, and follow-up. *Obstet Gynecol Surv* 40:545–551, 1985.
6. Boden E, Rylander E, Evander M: Papilloma virus infection of the vulva. *Acta Obstet Gynecol Scand* 68:179–184, 1989.
7. Bushsbaum HJ, Lifshitz S: Staging and surgical evaluation of ovarian cancer. *Semin Oncol* 1:227–230, 1984.
8. Cain JM: Pelvic mass: Detection, diagnosis and management, Stenchever M (ed): *Office Gynecology*. St. Louis: Mosby-Year Book, 430–440, 1991.
9. Cain JM, Stacy L, Jusenius K, Figge D: The quality of dying: Financial, psychological, and ethical dilemmas. *Obstet Gynecol* 76:149–152, 1990.
10. Cecchini S, Palli D, Casini A: Cervical intraepithelial neoplasia III: An estimate of screening error rates and optimal screening interval. *Acta Cytol* 29:329–333, 1985.
11. Chambers JT, Chambers SK: Endometrial sampling: When? Where? Why? With what? *Clin Obstet Gynecol* 35:28–39, 1992.
12. Chafe W, Richards A, Morgan L, Wilkinson E: Unrecognized invasive carcinoma in vulvar intraepithelial neoplasia. *Gynecol Oncol* 31:154, 1988.
13. Advanced Ovarian Trials Group: Chemotherapy in advanced ovarian cancer: An overview of randomized clinical trials. *Br Med J* 303:884–893, 1991.
14. Chung AF, Woodruff JW, Lewis JL: Malignant melanoma of the vulva: A report of 44 cases. *Obstet Gynecol* 45:638, 1975.
15. Creasman WT, Gallagher HS, Rutledge F: Paget's disease of the vulva. *Gynecol Oncol* 3:133–148, 1975.
16. Creasman WT, Morrow CP, Bundy BN, et al: Surgical pathologic spread patterns of endometrial cancer. *Cancer* 60:2035, 1987.
17. Daling JR, Chu J, Weiss NS, et al: The association of condylomata acuminata and squamous carcinoma of the vulva. *Br J Cancer* 50:533–535, 1984.
18. Delgado G, Bundy BN, Zaino R, et al: Prospective surgical-pathology study of disease free survival with stage IB cervical cancer: A Gynecologic Oncology Group study. *Gynecol Oncol* 38:352–357, 1990.
19. Giuntoli RL, Atkinson BF, Ernst CS, et al: *Atkinson's Correlative Atlas of Colposcopy, Cytology and Histopathology*. Philadelphia: JB Lippincott, 1987.
20. Hendrickson M, Ross J, Eifel P, et al: Uterine papillary serous carcinoma: A highly malignant form of endometrial adenocarcinoma. *Am J Surg Pathol* 6:93, 1982.
21. Hoskins WJ, Bundy BN, Thigpen JT, Omura GA: The influence of cytoreductive surgery on recurrence-free interval and survival in small volume stage III epithelial ovarian

cancer: A Gynecologic Oncology Group study. *Gynecol Oncol* 47:159–166, 1992.

22. Hsiu JG, Given FT, Kemp GM: Tumor implantation after diagnostic laparoscopic biopsy of serous ovarian tumors of low malignant potential. *Obstet Gynecol* 68:902–903, 1986.
23. Jacobs IJ, Oram DH, Bast RC: Strategies for improving the specificity of screening for ovarian cancer with tumor associated antigens Ca-125, Ca-15-3, and TAG 72.3. *Obstet Gynecol* 80:396–399, 1992.
24. Japaze H, Dinh TV, Woodruff JD: Verrucous carcinoma of the vulva: Study of 24 cases. *Obstet Gynecol* 60:462–466, 1982.
25. Karlen JR, Piver S, Barlow JJ: Melanoma of the vulva. *Obstet Gynecol* 45:181–184, 1975.
26. Kolstad P: Follow-up study of 32 patients with stage Ia1 and 411 patients with Stage IA2 squamous cell carcinoma of the cervix. *Gynecol Oncol* 33:265–267, 1989.
27. Koss LG, Schreiber K, Oberlander SG, et al: Detection of endometrial carcinoma and hyperplasia in asymptomatic women. *Obstet Gynecol* 64:1–11, 1984.
28. Kurman RJ, Kaminski PF, Norris HJ: Behavior of endometrial hyperplasia: A long-term study of "untreated" hyperplasias in 170 patients. *Cancer* 56:403, 1985.
29. Kurman RJ, Norris HJ: Evaluation of criteria for distinguishing atypical endometrial hyperplasia from well-differentiated carcinoma. *Cancer* 49:2547, 1982.
30. Leibsohn S, Mishell DR, d'Ablaing G, Schlaerth JB: Leiomyosarcomas in a series of hysterectomies performed for presumed uterine leiomyomata. *Am J Obstet Gynecol* 162:968, 1990.
31. Maiman M, Seltzer V, Boyce J: Laparoscopic excision of ovarian neoplasms subsequently found to be malignant. *Obstet Gynecol* 77:563–566, 1991.
32. Maruyama Y, Van Nagall JR, Yoneda J, et al: Dose response and failure pattern for bulky and barrel shaped IB cervical carcinoma treated by combined photon irradiation and extrafascial hysterectomy. *Cancer* 63:70–76, 1989.
33. Menczer J, Voliovitch Y, Modan B, et al: Some epidemiologic aspects of carcinoma of the vulva in Israel. *Am J Obstet Gynecol* 143:893–896, 1982.
34. Report of the Committee on Terminology of the International Society for the Study of Vulvar Disease. New nomenclature for vulvar disease. *J Reprod Med* 35:483–484, 1990.
35. Robboy SJ, Szyfelbein WM, Goeliner JR: Dysplasia and cytologic findings in 4,589 young women enrolled in the diethylstilbestrol-adenosis (DESAD) project. *Am J Obstet Gynecol* 140:579–586, 1981.
36. Sheets E, Crum CP: Current status and future clinical potential of human papilloma virus infection and epithelial neoplasia. *Curr Opin Obstet Gynecol* 5:63–66, 1993.
37. Silverberg E, Boring C, Squires T: Cancer statistics. *Cancer* 40–49, 1990.
38. Vuopala S: Diagnostic accuracy and clinical applicability of cytological and histological methods for investigating endometrial carcinoma. *Acta Obstet Gynecol Scand* (suppl) 56:1–72, 1977.
39. Willson JR: Ultrasonography in the diagnosis of gynecologic disorders. *Am J Obstet Gynecol* 164:1064–1067, 1991.
40. Yoonessi M, Hart WR: Endometrial stromal sarcomas. *Cancer* 40:898, 1977.
41. Zucker PK, Kasdon EJ, Feldstein ML: The validity of pap smear parameters as predictors of endometrial pathology in menopausal women. *Cancer* 56:2256–2263, 1985.

24 Nonmalignant DES-Related Changes

Mark Spitzer
Candice A. Tedeschi

Diethylstilbestrol (DES), a nonsteroidal estrogen, was used from 1941 through 1971 to prevent miscarriage. DES was marketed by many companies under more than 70 different names. The peak years of its use were the late 1940s and early 1950s, after which its popularity declined. In some parts of the United States, DES continued to be prescribed widely through November 1971. The drug was banned from use during pregnancy after its use was associated with clear cell adenocarcinoma of the vagina and cervix. While this form of cancer is rare (risk between 1.4:1000 to 1.4:10,000 women exposed to DES in utero), the benign changes associated with DES are common. DES-associated changes are most common if the mother took DES during the first 18 weeks of pregnancy, which is the period of fetal life during which the genital tract is being formed.

Pertinent Questions to Ask during History Taking

By asking a patient certain questions, the physician can identify women who may have had in utero DES exposure. Such questions include the following:

1. Did your mother take medication during her pregnancy with you?
2. Did your mother have a history of miscarriages or threatened miscarriages?
3. Has any other health care provider told you about any vaginal or cervical changes seen or felt during prior examinations?

Knowledge of DES-associated problems together with a complete obstetrical and gynecological history should raise the practitioner's level of suspicion regarding DES exposure. Today, with the declining number of unidentified DES-exposed women, these questions are frequently asked only after DES-associated problems have been identified.

Epithelial Changes

Adenosis is the presence of normal glandular epithelium on the vaginal wall. Studies differ in their estimation of the number of DES-exposed women with adenosis, with estimates ranging from 35 to 90 percent. Each woman differs in the amount of adenosis she may have. The most common vaginal walls affected are the anterior and posterior. Adenosis may extend from the fornices and along the entire length of the vagina. This is important because the vaginal walls are frequently covered by the blades of the vaginal speculum; therefore, these changes may be missed. Adenosis will regress spontaneously through the process of squamous metaplasia. Often, by the time a woman reaches her thirties, her adenosis has resolved, but the rate of regression varies.

Structural Changes of the Upper and Lower Genital Tract

Eighteen to 33 percent of DES-exposed women have a variety of structural changes of the cervix and vagina. The most common of these are vaginal and cervical ridges, pseudopolypoid formation, cervical hood or cockscomb cervix, absent pars vaginalis, and apical narrowing of the vagina. The endocervical canal may be about a third smaller. As many as 53 percent of DES-exposed women have abnormal hysterosalpingograms. The most common abnormalities are a T-shaped uterus; a hypoplastic uterus; constriction of the upper, middle, or cornual uterine regions; and irregular uterine margins. Any of the structural changes may be associated with a higher risk of fertility problems or difficulties maintaining a pregnancy.

Pregnancy-Associated Problems

The issue of infertility has not been resolved. Some studies show an increase in the rate of infertility in DES-exposed women; others do not. If one evaluates several of the largest pregnancy outcome studies, it seems that once pregnancy has been achieved, DES-exposed women may be at greater risk for pregnancy problems. These problems include ectopic pregnancy, spontaneous abortion, and premature delivery. The following information represents some of the literature which has been written in support of the concept that DES-exposed women have less successful pregnancy outcomes:

1. The risk of ectopic pregnancy is 8.6 times greater in the DES-exposed population. If the DES-exposed woman also has structural changes of the cervix, vagina, and/or uterus, the risk rises to 13.5 times greater than for unexposed women. Ectopic pregnancies are most commonly located in the isthmic portion of the fallopian tube. The increased incidence of ectopic pregnancy seems to be independent of any history of pelvic infection.
2. Almost 23 percent of DES-exposed women will have at least one spontaneous abortion. The risk of spontaneous abortion may be as high as 1.8 times that in the unexposed population, but if structural changes are present, the risk may be 2.6 times higher.
3. Premature delivery occurs in 13 percent of the exposed population. DES-exposed women may be at greater risk for premature cervical effacement during pregnancy, particularly in the second trimester.

Other Problems Which May Be Associated with DES Exposure

In addition to having an increased risk of invasive clear cell adenocarcinoma of the vagina and cervix, DES daughters may have an increased risk of intraepithelial squamous neoplasia of the cervix and vagina as well. However, colposcopy to identify areas of dysplasia may be very difficult because of the marked colposcopic changes due to metaplasia which are frequently found in DES-exposed women. White epithelium, punctation, and mosaic patterns are all very common on the cervix and vagina of DES-exposed women; dysplastic changes may be admixed with the metaplasia. Colposcopy in DES-exposed women should be done by an experienced colposcopist and preferably by the same one each time so that findings different from the patient's normal metaplastic changes can be recognized.

Despite the potential increased risk for dysplasia, caution is advised when deciding on a mode of treatment. Any mode of surgical treatment (e.g., conization, cautery, or cryosurgery) may be associated with cervical stenosis in a substantial percentage of DES-exposed women. Treatment with laser vaporization may be less associated with stenosis, but the risk is still present. Treatment of a cervical ectropion for mucorrhea should be discouraged.

The DES-exposed population is aging. At this time, it is unknown what additional or increased risk this aging group of women may have.

Health Care Guidelines

The following guidelines have been suggested in the care of DES-exposed women:

1. Annual pelvic examinations including a careful 360° palpation of the vagina, feeling for any induration and nodularity; a cervical Pap smear; and a four-quadrant vaginal Pap smear.
2. Annual colposcopy to monitor the DES-associated changes. This is particularly important if the woman has a history of an abnormal Pap smear. If it is not possible to perform a colposcopy, use half-strength Lugol's iodine solution to stain the vaginal walls. Nonstaining areas of the vagina may indicate adenosis or dysplasia.
3. Routine biopsies are not necessary. They should be reserved for specific indications such as abnormal Pap smears or visualized lesions. If abnormalities are found and the primary care physician does not have expertise with this problem, the primary care physician may need to consult with, or refer the woman to, a physician experienced with treating DES-exposed women.
4. If a DES-exposed woman thinks she may be pregnant, it is important to order a pregnancy test as early as possible. A pelvic ultrasound should be done at 6 to 7 weeks gestation to rule out an ectopic pregnancy.
5. Because of the potential risk of premature cervical effacement, a careful palpation of the cervix should be done every 1 to 2 weeks during pregnancy to monitor the length of the cervix. If effacement occurs, bed rest is recommended. Routine cerclage is not recommended unless there is a history of proven cervical incompetence.

Summary

Nonmalignant changes in DES-exposed women are much more common than malignant ones. Adenosis and structural changes of the cervix and vagina are common findings; however, clinical problems such as an increased risk of ectopic pregnancy, premature deliveries, and premature effacement of the cervix may be of greater concern. DES-exposed women are at risk for cervical and vaginal dysplasia. Careful adherence to certain health care guidelines will help ensure optimal care for these women.

References and Selected Readings

1. ACOG Committee Opinion: Diethylstilbestrol, 1993, 131:1.
2. Barnes AB, Colton T, Gundersen J, et al: Fertility and outcome of pregnancy in women exposed in utero to diethylstilbestrol. *N Engl J Med* 301:609–613, 1980.
3. Cousin L, Karp W, Lacey C, Lucas WE: Reproductive outcome of women exposed to diethylstilbestrol in utero. *Obstet Gynecol* 56:70–76, 1980.
4. Haney AF, Hammond MG, Soules MR, Creasman, WT: Diethylstilbestrol-induced upper genital tract abnormalities. *Fertil Steril* 31:142–146, 1979.
5. Herbst AL, Hubby MM, Azizi F, Makii MM: Reproductive and gynecological/surgical experience in diethylstilbestrol-exposed daughter. *J Obstet Gynecol* 141:1019–1028, 1981.
6. Kaufman RH, Adam E: Genital tract anomalies associated with in utero exposure to diethylstilbestrol. *Isr J Med Sci* 14:353–362, 1978.
7. Kaufman RH, Adam E, Noller KL, et al: Upper genital tract changes and infertility in diethylstilbestrol-exposed women. *Am J Obstet Gynecol* 154:1312–1318, 1986.
8. Mangan CE, Borow J, Burtnett-Rubin MM, et al: Pregnancy outcome in 98 women exposed to diethylstilbestrol in utero, their mothers, and unexposed siblings. *Obstet Gynecol* 59:315–319, 1982.
9. Noller KL, Blair PB, O'Brien PC, Melton LJ, et al: Increased occurrence of autoimmune disease among women exposed in utero to diethylstilbestrol. *Fertil Steril* 49:1080–1082, 1988.
10. Noller KL, O'Brien PC, Colton T, et al: Medical and surgical disease associated with in utero exposure to diethylstilbestrol, in Noller KL (ed): *Clinical Practice of Gynecology*. New York: Elsevier, 1990, pp 1–7.
11. Schmidt G, Fowler WC, Jr: Cervical stenosis following minor gynecological procedures on DES-exposed women. *Obstet Gynecol* 56:333–335.

25 Gynecologic Infections

Susan M. Mou

SITES OF GYNECOLOGIC INFECTIONS
Vaginitis • Mucopurulent Cervicitis • Pelvic Inflammatory Disease (PID) • Bartholin's Duct Cysts/Abscesses • Necrotizing Fasciitis

COMMON SEXUALLY TRANSMITTED ORGANISMS
N. Gonorrhoeae • Chlamydia • Syphilis • Mycoplasma • Human Papilloma Virus • Herpes • Chancroid • Lymphogranuloma Venereum (LGV) • Donovanosis • Molluscum Contagiosum • Pediculosis Pubis • Scabies

COMMON SYSTEMIC DISEASES THAT MAY BE TRANSMITTED VIA THE VAGINAL ROUTE
HIV • Hepatitis B • Toxic Shock Syndrome

Many diseases are transmitted to women by infection via the vaginal route. The site of the ultimate infection may be any one of a variety of organs, or multiple sites may become infected. The patient may present with an infection of the vulva (vulvitis, Bartholin's abscess), vagina (vaginitis), cervix (cervicitis), or uterus (endometritis). An organism may then ascend further (with or without prior clinical symptoms in any of the aforementioned areas) to involve one or both fallopian tubes (salpingitis) or tubes and ovaries (salpingo-oophoritis). It is rare for the ovaries to be infected (oophoritis) without accompanying tubal infection. In addition to being foci of local disease, the lower genital tract is a route of entry for organisms that cause life-threatening systemic disease (e.g., HIV and hepatitis B).

Sites of Gynecologic Infections

Vaginitis

Vaginitis is a common problem for which women seek medical care. Before discussing the usual forms of vaginitis, it is important to understand the normal flora of the vagina. Postpubertally the vagina contains multiple organisms, with a concentration of less than 1×10^7 organisms per gram of vaginal secretion. Lactobacilli are the predominant organisms. The ratio of anaerobes to aerobes is 2:1 to 5:1. Group B beta streptococci can be cultured from the vagina in 20 to 30 percent of women. There are three primary vaginal infections for which women seek care: bacterial vaginosis, candidiasis, and trichomoniasis.

Bacterial Vaginosis Bacterial vaginosis is a disruption of the normal vaginal flora, with an overgrowth of anaerobes. Some women will be symptomatic, complaining of increased vaginal discharge and a foul-smelling fishy odor (especially after intercourse, when alkaline semen mixes with the vaginal discharge). Other women will be asymptomatic, but on physical examination, bacterial vaginosis will be evident. The majority of women who have bacterial vaginosis are sexually active and between the ages of 15 and 44. The lactobacilli that are predominant in a healthy vagina are replaced by anaerobes, with the ratio of anaerobes to aerobes increasing to 100:1. The vaginal pH is elevated. The number of organisms per gram of vaginal fluid increases to 1×10^{11}.

The diagnosis of bacterial vaginosis can be made clinically with three of four of Amstel's criteria present. These are (1) vaginal fluid collected from the side walls of the vagina with a pH greater than 4.5; (2) a thin, homogeneous discharge that looks like skim milk and may roll out of the vagina onto the perineum; (3) a positive amine (Whiff) test (performed by adding 10% KOH to vaginal secretions on a glass slide); (4) clue cells present on a wet preparation of vaginal secretions. The clue cells are epithelial cells coated with bacteria.

Gram stain criteria also have been described for bacterial vaginosis and consist of an absence of lactobacilli with many anaerobic morphotypes present. It is not necessary to culture for Gardnerella since up to 40 percent of healthy women may have Gardnerella as normal flora. Similarly, culture for anaerobes is not necessary since anaerobes can be normal vaginal flora. It is the overgrowth that is associated with bacterial vaginosis.

There are multiple treatment regimens for bacterial vaginosis. Metronidazole, one 2-g oral dose, is effective about 85 percent of the time. An alternate oral regimen of 500 mg metronidazole twice daily for seven days also is similarly effective. Oral clindamycin can be used in a dose of 300 mg twice daily for seven days. Alternatively, topical regimens with fewer potential side effects also are effective. A 2% clindamycin vaginal cream can be used nightly for seven nights. Alternatively, metronidazole gel, 0.75%, applied intravaginally twice daily for five days is effective.

Neither vaginal medications designed to lower vaginal pH nor douching cure bacterial vaginosis. Treatment of sexual partners is advised only when patients have recurrent bacterial vaginosis.

While bacterial vaginosis was once considered a benign, nuisance condition, there is now evidence that it may be associated with postabortal infections, posthysterectomy infections, postpartum endometritis, preterm labor, delivery of low birth-weight infants, and chorioamnionitis.[6]

Candidiasis Vulvovaginal infections caused by Candida species are very common in women. *Candida albicans* is responsible for the infection in 80 to 90 percent of patients; the remaining 10 to 20 percent are due to *C. glabrata, C. tropicalis,* and other species. The role of asymptomatic colonization and infection of other sites (such as the oral cavity and gastrointestinal tract) in subsequent symptomatic vaginal infections are not fully understood at this time. It is known that patients who have depressed cell-mediated immunity, those with high blood glucose levels, and those who have recently received antimicrobials, are at increased risk for vulvovaginal candidiasis.

Patients usually complain of vulvar and sometimes vaginal pruritus, burning, dysuria, and dyspareunia. Some patients note a vaginal discharge. Physical examination reveals vaginal and/or vulvar edema and erythema, signifying a vulvitis. A discharge will be nonodorous to sweet-smelling, possibly thick and white. The vaginal pH is usually less than 4.5.

Microscopic examination of a wet mount of vaginal secretions at 100 × magnification will show branching hyphae and spores. Leukocytes usually are absent and lactobacilli are present. Visualization of the hyphae and spores may be aided by addition of 10% KOH. *C. glabrata* will be seen with spores present without branching pseudohyphae. Yeast culture can be done on Sabouraud's media, but is clinically indicated only when, on the basis of signs and symptoms, Candida is suspected but no confirmation can be made on potassium hydroxide preparation.

Local therapy is usually employed, including imidazole compounds such as clotrimazole, miconazole, and butoconazole. Nystatin also is useful. Triazoles including terconazole may also be used. In patients who do not respond to local therapy, oral fluconazole may be effective. There is no need to treat sexual partners unless a male partner has balanitis.

In patients with recurrent candidiasis, 1% aqueous solution of gentian violet to the vagina and vulva twice weekly for 2 weeks is effective. Oral treatment with ketoconazole, 200 to 400 mg daily for 7 to 14 days, with monitoring of liver function tests as an alternative regimen for recurrent candidiasis.

Trichomoniasis Trichomoniasis is the third of the most common etiologic agents of vaginitis. *Trichomonas vaginalis,* a flagellated protozoan, causes this communicable infection. The asymptomatic carrier rate in women is about 10 percent. Symptomatic patients may complain of dysuria, vaginal discharge, and/or pruritus.

The diagnosis of trichomoniasis can be made at the time of pelvic examination. A thin, yellow-green, sometimes foul-smelling discharge usually is present. The vaginal pH is elevated to between 5 and 7. Vulvar irritation is often present. Motile trichomonads can be seen on saline suspension of vaginal discharge. The wet mount is 50 to 60 percent sensitive, while cultures are usually more than 89 percent sensitive.[5]

Cultures can be done with Trichicult's or Diamond's culture media. Recently, InPouchTV[3], a culture system that can be used at the bedside and then examined under the microscope daily without broth culture, has been marketed and may be helpful in diagnosis.

Treatment consists of oral metronidazole, 2 g once, or metronidazole 500 mg two times per day for 7 days. Partners should be referred for treatment at the same time. Follow-up is necessary only for women who do not become asymptomatic after treatment.

Other causes of abnormal vaginal discharge as well as cervicitis and upper tract disease will be covered in the next section.

Mucopurulent Cervicitis

Mucopurulent cervicitis is a clinical entity characterized by a yellow endocervical exudate, visible either in the endocervical canal or on an endocervical plug specimen, and by polymorphonuclear leukocytes in the endocervical exudate. Mucopurulent cervicitis is found in reproductive age women. It should not be diagnosed during the bleeding phase of the menstrual cycle. Mucopurulent cervicitis may be caused by *Chlamydia trachomatis, Neisseria gonorrhoeae,* herpes simplex virus, or other vaginal organisms. The first two organisms cause 50 to 70 percent of mucopurulent cervicitis.

Clinically, women may be asymptomatic, or they may complain of dyspareunia, postcoital spotting, or abnormal discharge. Patients may have tenderness on palpation of the cervix during a pelvic exam. Criteria for diagnosis include: yellow or green mucopurulent endocervical secretion(s) when viewed on a white cotton-tipped swab (positive swab test); cervicitis as determined by a friable cervix and/or erythema or edema in the cervical ectropion; and ten or more polymorphonuclear leukocytes per microscopic oil immersion field on a Gram stain smear of endocervical secretions. Cultures or a DNA probe for *Neisseria gonorrhoeae* and *Chlamydia trachomatis* should be performed at the same time. Herpes simplex virus infection usually can be diagnosed clinically. It also can be detected about 50 percent of the time on Papanicolaou smears or by viral culture.

Treatment of mucopurulent cervicitis ideally should be based on the results of tests for *C. trachomatis* and *N. gonorrhoeae.* However, if the likelihood of infection with either organism is high or if the patient is unlikely to follow through once culture results are available, treatment should be initiated empirically. Treatment for *C. trachomatis* and *N. gonorrhoeae* should also be prescribed empirically for patients with mucopurulent cervicitis in populations with a high prevalence of these infections. If prevalence of both infections is low, and if compliance is high, test results may be awaited. If the prevalence of *N. gonorrhoeae* is low but the likelihood of Chlamydia is high, treatment for Chlamydia only may be prescribed. Follow-up should be specific for the organisms cultured or otherwise detected. Sex partners of patients treated presumptively should receive the same treatment as the woman with mucopurulent cervicitis.

Pelvic Inflammatory Disease (PID)

Pelvic inflammatory disease encompasses a spectrum of disease, including endometritis, salpingitis, oophoritis, tuboovarian abscess, and pelvic peritonitis. The two most common organisms that cause PID are *N. gonorrhoeae* and *C. trachomatis.* However, many other vaginal microorganisms such as *E. coli* and other gram-negative enteric organisms, Bacteroides species, anaerobic cocci, Provetella species, *Haemophilus influenzae, Streptococcus agalactiae, Gardnerella vaginalis,* and possibly *Mycoplasma hominis* and *Ureaplasma urealyticum* are potential etiologic agents for PID.

The severity of PID varies greatly, ranging from asymptomatic to life-threatening diffuse peritonitis and florid sepsis. A high index of suspicion on the part of the physician is necessary. Risk factors for PID include young age, multiple sexual partners, attendance at an STD clinic, recent insertion of an intrauterine device, vaginal douching, cigarette smoking, and recent gonorrhea or chlamydial infection.[11] Barrier methods of contraception and, to a lesser extent, oral contraceptives reduce the risk of PID.

The most common presenting symptom is lower abdominal pain, which usually is bilateral. Gonococcal and chlamydial PID usually present during the first half of the menstrual cycle. Abnormal bleeding, abnormal vaginal discharge, fever, nausea, vomiting, breakthrough bleeding on oral contraceptives, new onset dysmenorrhea, and dyspareunia also may be present. Some questions to ask the patient include: (1) Have you noticed a change in your vaginal discharge? (2) Do you have spotting after intercourse? (Note: This may also be suggestive of cervical cancer or cervical intraepithelial neoplasia.) (3) Have you noticed a sudden onset of pain with sexual intercourse?[7]

Diagnosis The diagnosis is usually made by employing clinical criteria. Laparoscopy is the gold standard for diagnosis, but may not be necessary or indicated, may not be available universally, and may miss early endometritis. Clinical criteria have a positive predictive value of 65 to 90 percent as compared to laparoscopy.[1] Empirical treatment of PID is recommended by the Centers for Disease Control and Prevention when there is lower abdominal tenderness, adnexal tenderness and cervical motion tenderness, and no other detectable cause such as ectopic pregnancy, appendicitis, bowel disease, endometriosis, ovarian torsion, bleeding into a corpus luteum, or functional pain. Additional routine criteria are: oral temperature >38.3°C; abnormal cervical/vaginal discharge; elevated erythrocyte sedimentation rate or C-reactive protein; documented *N. gonorrhoeae* or *C. trachomatis* infection.

Cultures should be obtained from the endocervix and rectum for *N. gonorrhoeae,* and from the endocervix for *C. trachomatis*. In acutely ill patients, aerobic and anaerobic blood cultures may be obtained, but are frequently negative even in the presence of infection.

Treatment Appropriate treatment (Table 25-1) varies, depending on the clinical presentation and the severity of illness. Many experts believe that all patients with PID should be hospitalized. Certainly most adolescents with PID should be hospitalized,

TABLE 25-1 Antibiotic Therapy in PID

Outpatient	
Regimen A	Cefoxitin, 2 g IM *plus* 1 g probenecid orally concurrently *or:* ceftriaxone, 250 mg IM *or:* other parenteral third-generation cephalosporin (e.g., ceftizoxime or cefotaxime) *plus* doxycycline, 100 mg orally 2 times per day for 14 days
Regimen B	Ofloxacin, 400 mg orally 2 times per day for 14 days *plus* either: clindamycin, 450 mg orally 4 times per day for 14 days *or* metronidazole, 500 mg orally 2 times per day for 14 days[1]
Inpatient[a]	
Regimen A	Cefoxitin, 2 g IV every 6 h *or* cefotetan, 2 g IV every 12 h *plus* doxycycline, 100 mg IV or orally every 12 h
Regimen B	Clindamycin, 900 mg IV every 8 h *plus* gentamicin, loading dose IV or IM (2 mg/kg body weight) followed by a maintenance dose (1.5 mg/kg) every 8 h,[1] with peak and trough levels to check for appropriateness of dose

[a]Either inpatient regimen should continue until the patient is afebrile and nontender for 48 h; then oral doxycycline or oral clindamycin is continued until 14 full days of therapy are completed.

owing to the likelihood of poor compliance and the sequelae of PID. Mild PID is treated by some on an outpatient basis if clinical follow-up within 72 h of antibiotic therapy initiation can be assured. Hospitalization may be required when the diagnosis is uncertain, pelvic abscess is suspected, the patient is pregnant, the patient has HIV infection, severe illness or nausea and vomiting preclude outpatient therapy, the patient is unable to follow or tolerate an outpatient regimen, or when the patient has failed to respond to outpatient therapy.[1] In those who fail to respond to outpatient antibiotics, the diagnosis should be reassessed.

Patients with tuboovarian abscesses need anaerobic coverage and hospitalization and may need laparoscopic follow-up if they do not respond clinically. A ruptured tuboovarian abscess (TOA) is a surgical emergency and may be fatal if not promptly treated.

Treatment of Sexual Partners Sexual partners should be referred for evaluation and empirical treatment of *C. trachomatis* and *N. gonorrhoeae* and screening for other STDs. Treatment of the infected patient and her partner ideally should be simultaneous.

Seven to ten days after therapy, repeat cultures should be obtained. Some recommend rescreening for *N. gonorrhoeae* and *C. trachomatis* four to six weeks after therapy is completed.

Tubal scarring and damage from PID can result in long-term sequelae of chronic pelvic pain, recurrent disease, ectopic pregnancy, and infertility. Westrom et al.[15] found that 8 percent of women had tubal occlusion and infertility after a single episode of PID, 19.5 percent after two episodes, and 40 percent after three or more episodes of PID. Previous serologic evidence of Chlamydia infection is associated with increased infertility and increased ectopic pregnancies.[11]

Pyometra Pyometra is the accumulation of purulent material in the endometrial cavity. It usually occurs as the result of interference with the normal drainage of the uterus. Most often, this obstruction is due to malignant disease, such as cervical or endometrial cancer. However, other causes have been identified, including polyps, leiomyomata, scarring after cervical surgery such as conization, radiation, cervicitis, congenital anomalies, and puerperal infection.

The diagnosis may be difficult. It is essential to consider pyometra in the differential diagnosis of a tender midline pelvic mass, since therapy is different from that for salpingo-oophoritis. Classically, women with pyometra present with vaginal discharge of bleeding, fever, and abdominal pain. Physical examination usually will reveal an enlarged uterus, and the presence of endometrial cavity fluid can be confirmed by ultrasound.

A thorough pelvic examination, of course, is necessary if pyometra is suspected. Dilatation of the cervix and gentle curettage of the cervix and uterine cavity with histologic examination as well as aerobic and anaerobic culturing are important in evaluating the patient. In patients with malignancy, treatment of the malignancy by hysterectomy will also remove the pyometra. In patients with such benign conditions as leiomyomata or polyps causing obstruction of the endocervical canal and resultant pyometra, removal of the uterus or the obstructing lesion will resolve the condition. However, in many situations this may not be necessary or desirable.

Many women with pyometra will prefer to preserve the uterus if possible (e.g., young women with pyometra following surgery for cervical dysplasia). Cervical dilatation, prolonged drainage of the uterus with a catheter, and broad-spectrum antibiotics covering the usual genital tract flora may resolve the problem. Sometimes the myometrial infection cannot be eradicated, and hysterectomy may be necessary even in young women.

Left untreated, pyometra may result in spontaneous perforation and resulting sepsis. Broad-spectrum antibiotics with good anaerobic coverage, surgical exploration, and hysterectomy are necessary with ruptured pyometra. Without aggressive therapy, ruptured pyometra is fatal. Even with surgical exploration and antibiotics, death may occur.

Bartholin's Duct Cysts/Abscesses

An acute abscess of the Bartholin's gland and duct may occur as the result of infection; from trauma, such as an improperly placed mediolateral episiotomy; or after a posterior colporrhaphy where sutures can ligate or injure the duct. Infectious agents causing the abscess include *N. gonorrhoeae, C. trachomatis,* and facultative and obligate anaerobes that are normal vaginal/perineal flora. In women over 40, a cancer of the Bartholin's duct or gland must be considered in the differential diagnosis.

Bartholin's duct cysts may follow acute abscess formation or may be found incidentally during routine pelvic examination. Patients with symptomatic cysts present with pain on walking, sitting, or with intercourse.

Diagnosis Examination of the vulva will reveal a tender, cystic-feeling mass in the area of the Bartholin's duct and gland. It must be differentiated from a hydrocele, from the Skene's glands which are more anterior, and from such solid tumors as fibromas, fibromyomas, lipomas, and hidradenomas.

Treatment An acute abscess must be incised and drained. Marsupialization is sometimes difficult with the acute abscess. Local anesthetic should be sufficient for incision and drainage; however, some patients will require brief general anesthesia. Cultures for aerobes, anaerobes, *N. gonorrhoea,* and *C. trachomatis* should be obtained at the time of incision and drainage. Just as with marsupialization, the incision should be made inside the vaginal mucosa but outside the hymenal ring. Systemic broad-spectrum antibiotics that cover *N. gonorrhoeae, C. trachomatis,* and normal vaginal flora may be administered after cultures are obtained; when culture results are available, the antibiotics may be adjusted to provide the best cover for infecting organism(s). Sitz baths postoperatively are helpful.

A Bartholin's abscess/cyst also may be treated with insertion of a Word catheter for three to four weeks or by marsupialization of the cyst. Both of these procedures usually are performed under local anesthesia in an outpatient setting, but may occasionally need therapy in an operating room. These procedures avoid excising the gland and thus preserve its secretory function.

A Word catheter is inserted through a small incision inside the vaginal mucosa, outside the hymenal ring near the usual duct opening. The bulb is inflated with 2 to 3 ml normal saline. The catheter is removed three to four weeks later, after epithelialization of the incision has occurred.

Marsupialization is performed by making a wedge-shaped vertical incision in the vaginal mucosa, draining the cyst and breaking up any loculations with a Kelly clamp, and everting the cyst wall edges to the vaginal mucosa with number 2-0 delayed absorbable interrupted sutures. Sitz baths are helpful postoperatively. No wick or packing is necessary. Cysts may recur in 10 to 15 percent of patients.

Excision of a Bartholin's duct cyst should be reserved for recurrent cysts that are refractory to other therapies and that are symptomatic. This procedure should be done in the operating room.[9]

Necrotizing Fasciitis

Necrotizing fasciitis is a relatively uncommon but life-threatening soft tissue infection that may progress rapidly. The risk of necrotizing fasciitis increases in patients over 50 years of age, and those with histories of arteriosclerosis, diabetes, obesity, smoking, previous radiation therapy, and operative trauma. Hypertension, renal failure, immunosuppression, and vascular disease are also thought to be risk factors for necrotizing fasciitis.[13]

Diagnosis Patients with necrotizing fasciitis often appear acutely ill with severe systemic toxicity. However, occasionally there is surprisingly little evidence of generalized toxicity. Fever is usually present. There may be erythema, edema, and tenderness of the overlying or adjacent skin. Thick pus is usually not present in the wound; however, there is a thin, ''dishwater'' appearance to wound drainage. Examination of the wound may show necrotic edematous-appearing tissue. The fascia may appear gray. When blunt dissection with a finger or probe is performed, the fascia feels soft, and the adjacent subcutaneous tissue does not bleed.

Laboratory data may show an increased leukocytosis, anemia from hemolysis, or hemoconcentration due to third spacing of intravascular fluid into the wound, and/or hypocalcemia. Radiographic studies may show soft tissue gas. Culture of debrided tissue usually will show a polymicrobial infection. Histology of debrided tissue will show leukocyte infiltration, thrombosis of microvasculature, and focal necrosis of the fascia.

Treatment *Immediate* surgical debridement in an operating room is necessary. The necrotic tissue has to be excised back to margins that bleed easily. Delay in surgical debridement increases the mortality rate to almost 100 percent. Polymicrobial etiology is common, with both aerobes and anaerobes being present in wound cultures; thus, broad-spectrum antibiotics are indicated until culture results are available. Patients who succumb to necrotizing fasciitis usually die in septic shock.

Common Sexually Transmitted Organisms

Patients who have one STD are at high risk for simultaneous or subsequent infection with others, and should be screened appropriately.

N. Gonorrhoeae

Gonococcal infections may be symptomatic or asymptomatic; both can cause infertility and increase the risk of ectopic pregnancy. Screening of high-risk women has been the mainstay of *N. gonorrhoeae* control in the United States. *N. gonorrhoeae* is found most commonly in 15- to 29-year-olds. The primary site in women is usually the endocervix, although the urethra, Bartholin's, Skene's, and periurethral glands may be involved. In women with endocervical infection, a large number also have coexistent rectal infection. Pharyngeal infection also should be considered in evaluation. Symptoms of gonococcal infection that may prompt a visit to a healthcare provider and that should be elucidated in the history include vaginal discharge, dysuria, pelvic pain, dyspareunia, menorrhagia, and intermenstrual bleeding.

Diagnosis Mucopurulent discharge may or may not be present on pelvic examination. After cleansing the cervix to remove exudate, culture should be obtained from the endocervix by inserting a swab 1 to 2 cm into the internal os and rotating it for 5 to 10 s. Alternatively, DNA probes can be used for diagnosis, with one swab needed for both *N. gonorrhoeae* and *C. trachomatis* probes. If prompt transport and prompt incubation of the culture are not possible, DNA probes may be a good alternative method of diagnosis. However, since DNA probes are usually ''batched'' by labs, the turn-around time for results may be up to one week.

Treatment Uncomplicated *N. gonorrhoeae* may be treated with antibiotics. The cost of the antibiotic, side effects, resistance, anatomical site of infection, and possible concurrent infection with *C. trachomatis* or syphilis must all be considered when choosing an appropriate antibiotic. The 1993 CDC–STD guidelines propose ceftriaxone (125 mg IM), cefixime (400 mg PO), ciprofloxacin (500 mg PO), or ofloxacin (400 mg PO) to treat gonococcal infections, *plus* a regimen effective against *C. trachomatis,* such as doxycycline, 100 mg bid for seven days.[1] In pregnancy, quinolones and tetracyclines are contraindicated, and erythromycin may be substituted for tetracycline. Pharyngeal infection is effectively treated over 90 percent of the time with the ceftriaxone or ciprofloxacin regimens. Incubating syphilis can be treated with ceftriaxone or the seven-day course of doxycycline or erythromycin used to treat *C. trachomatis.*

Alternative regimens include spectinomycin for patients allergic to cephalosporins and quinolones. This regimen does not treat incubating syphilis nor pharyngeal gonorrhea. Ceftizoxime, cefotaxime, cefotetan, and cefoxitin are also active against *N. gonorrhoeae*. Other antimicrobials are effective, and the above guidelines are not an exhaustive list of antibiotics used to treat gonorrhea.

Screening for HIV should be offered at the time of diagnosis of gonorrhea. Screening for syphilis and other STDs should be performed when *N. gonorrhoeae* is diagnosed. Patients who do not receive a β-lactam or tetracycline derivative should have the serologic test for syphilis repeated in one month.

Sexual partners within the last 30 days need to be referred for evaluation and treatment if patients are symptomatic. In asymptomatic patients, sexual contacts within the last 60 days should be examined and treated. If the last sexual intercourse took place before these time periods, then the most recent sex partner needs evaluation and treatment.

Disseminated gonococcal infection requires hospitalization, and has been alluded to previously in the section on PID.

Chlamydia

Chlamydial genital infection is common among adolescent and young adult women. Screening of asymptomatic sexually active teenagers and women 20 to 24 is recommended. Other women at risk obviously should be screened as well. Those who do not use barrier contraception or who have new or multiple partners should be screened at the time of routine periodic examinations.

It is generally believed that treatment of asymptomatic cervical infection will reduce the likelihood of upper genital tract disease and such sequelae as infertility and ectopic pregnancy, although few studies have been performed to confirm this. Treatment prevents transmission to partners and may prevent vertical transmission at birth.

Diagnosis Women may be asymptomatic or may have mucopurulent cervicitis with symptoms of vaginal discharge, postcoital bleeding, and/or dyspareunia. Upper genital tract infection may go unrecognized or may produce subtle symptoms of infection, such as abnormal bleeding, dyspareunia, vaginal discharge, low-grade fever, or mild abdominal pain. Endocervical culture, DNA probe, fluorescent antibody tests, or immunoassay tests may be performed for diagnosis. When culturing the endocervix, endocervical cells need to be obtained because Chlamydia is an obligate intracellular organism. The endocervix should first be sampled for the Papanicolaou smear (exfoliative cytology) unless this has recently been performed; then with a cotton-tipped swab for *N. gonorrhoeae;* and lastly for Chlamydia testing with a Dacron-tipped, plastic shaft swab. If only Chlamydia testing is performed, the endocervix should be cleansed with a swab initially, and then a second sample obtained. A sterile cytobrush may facilitate procurement of endocervical cells. In patient populations with a high prevalence of Chlamydia infections, the rapid tests for Chlamydia will be sufficiently sensitive and specific. However, in patient populations with a low prevalence of Chlamydia, there may be a high number of false-positive results. Thus, in children, in alleged assault evaluations, and in women older than 25 to 30, culture should be employed for diagnosis whenever possible.

Treatment: Uncomplicated Chlamydia cervicitis may be treated with doxycycline, 100 mg orally twice daily for 7 days, or azithromycin, 1 g orally (single dose).[1] Cost and compliance should determine which regimen is employed. Alternative regimens include ofloxacin, 300 mg twice daily for 7 days; erythromycin base, 500 mg four times daily for 7 days; erythromycin ethyl succinate, 800 mg orally four times daily for 7 days; or sulfisoxazole, 500 mg orally four times daily for 10 days (lower efficacy).[1] Additionally, amoxicillin, 500 mg orally three times daily for 7 to 10 days, may be used if erythromycin is not tolerated in pregnant women.[2] If 500 mg of erythromycin base is not tolerated four times daily for 7 days, alternative erythromycin regimens during pregnancy include erythromycin base, 250 mg orally four times a day for 14 days; erythromycin ethylsuccinate, 800 mg orally four times a day for 7 days; or erythromycin ethylsuccinate, 400 mg orally four times a day for 14 days.

Syphilis

Presentation, Diagnosis, and Treatment of Early Syphilis Syphilis, caused by *Treponema pallidum,* is a sexually transmitted disease that can manifest a myriad of signs and symptoms, ranging from asymptomatic to neurologic impairment in neurosyphilis or visceral gummas in tertiary syphilis. Syphilis also can be transmitted vertically, causing congenital syphilis and stillbirth. *T. pallidum* gains systemic access through minute abrasions in skin or mucosal surfaces and begins to replicate locally, then extending to systemic disease.

Dark-field microscopy of a moist primary chancre or regional lymph node aspiration can be used for the diagnosis. The chancre is a painless, firm ulcer with raised edges, and often is asymptomatic. The chancre heals spontaneously in three to eight weeks.

Serologic testing with rapid plasma reagin (RPR) or the Venereal Disease Research Laboratory (VDRL) test usually is positive (80 to 90 percent). Confirmatory testing with microhemagglutination assay for antibodies to *T. pallidum* (MHA-TP) or fluorescent treponemal antibody-absorption (FTA-ABS) is necessary after the nonspecific antibody tests.

About six weeks after primary syphilis, almost all untreated patients will progress to secondary syphilis. Multiple symmetrical skin lesions may develop, as well as any of the following: lymphadenopathy, hepatitis, nephrosis, alopecia, condyloma latum. Serologic testing is positive. The untreated secondary syphilis lesions resolve after three to 12 weeks. Following secondary syphilis, there is syphilis of less than one year's duration, termed "early-latent."

All of the above types of syphilis can be treated with benzathine penicillin G, 2.4 million units IM in a single dose. Penicillin allergic nonpregnant patients may be treated with doxycycline, 100 mg orally two times a day for 2 weeks, or tetracycline, 500 mg orally four times a day for 2 weeks, or, with a higher failure rate, erythromycin, 500 mg orally four times a day for 2 weeks. A single dose of ceftriaxone is not effective for treating syphilis, but a regimen producing eight to ten days of treponemicidal blood levels may be used.[1]

Follow-Up of Patients with Early Syphilis The serologic test titers should be repeated and a clinical exam performed at 3 and 6 months post-treatment. Titers should decline fourfold by 3 months with primary and secondary syphilis, and by 6 months with early latent syphilis. Patients with continuing signs or symptoms of persistent infection or reinfection, or with a fourfold increase in serologic titer should have their HIV status checked and a lumbar puncture performed to examine the cerebrospinal fluid (CSF) for signs of infection. Retreatment should be with benzathine penicillin G, 2.4 million units IM for three weekly injections, unless neurosyphilis is present. Just like any patient being treated for syphilis, pregnant patients may develop a Jarisch-Herxheimer reaction after penicillin, with fever, headaches, myalgia, and flushing, but this should not be a reason to delay therapy. Patients should be instructed to watch for decreased fetal activity and preterm labor. Penicillin-allergic pregnant patients should be hospitalized for desensitization to penicillin, then treated with penicillin. Follow-up of pregnant patients should consist of HIV testing and monthly serologic titers until antibody titers decrease appropriately.[1]

Late Latent Syphilis or Latent Syphilis of Unknown Duration Late latent syphilis or latent syphilis of unknown duration includes patients who have had syphilis for more than one year on the basis of documented seroconversion or who have latent syphilis of unknown duration. These patients are usually asymptomatic. They need to be evaluated for evidence of tertiary disease. A CSF examination is necessary for patients with any of the following criteria:

- Neurologic or ophthalmic signs or symptoms
- Other evidence of active syphilis (e.g., aortitis, gumma, iritis)
- Treatment failure
- HIV test positive
- Serum nontreponemal titer $\geq$1:32, unless the duration of infection is known to be $<$ 1 year
- Nonpenicillin therapy planned, unless the duration of infection is known to be $<$ 1 year[1]

Treatment consists of:

- Benzathine penicillin G, 7.2 million units total, administered in three doses of 2.4 million units IM each, at one-week intervals.
- For penicillin-allergic patients (after neurosyphilis is excluded): doxycycline, 100 mg twice daily for 2 weeks if $<$ 1 year *or* for 4 weeks if duration of infection is unknown or $>$ 1 year, *or* tetracycline, 500 mg four times a day for 2 weeks if duration of infection is $<$ 1 year *or* for 4 weeks otherwise.

Penicillin-allergic pregnant patients need to be hospitalized and desensitized.[1]

Follow-up: Quantitative nontreponemal serologic testing should be repeated at 6 months and 12 months. If titers increase, if a titer $\geq$ 1:32 does not decline fourfold (two dilutions) within 12 to 24 months, or if the patient develops signs or symptoms of syphilis, the patient needs to be evaluated for neurosyphilis and re-treated as necessary.

Tertiary (Late) Syphilis Tertiary (late) syphilis develops only after a latency of many years, and occurs in only 20 to 30 percent of untreated patients. Tertiary syphilis encompasses patients with gumma and cardiovascular syphilis. A CSF examination is necessary at the time of diagnosis. Consultation with an expert should be sought.

Recommended treatment is benzathine penicillin G, 7.2 million units IM total, given in three doses of 2.4 million units at 1-week intervals.[1] Penicillin-allergic patients should receive doxycycline or tetracycline as in late-latent syphilis. Penicillin-allergic pregnant patients need to be desensitized.

Neurosyphilis Ophthalmic or auditory symptoms or cranial nerve palsies can occur at any stage of syphilis and warrant a CSF examination. Syphilitic eye disease, such as uveitis, neuroretinitis, or optic neuritis is frequently associated with neurosyphilis. Patients with syphilis and eye disease should be treated as if they have neurosyphilis.

The recommended treatment regimen by the Centers for Disease Control is 12 to 24 million units aqueous crystalline penicillin G daily, administered as 2 to 4 million units IV every 4 h, for 10 to 14 days, *or,* in a compliant patient, 2.4 million units procaine penicillin IM daily, plus probenecid, 500 mg orally four times per day, both for 10 to 14 days. In addition, some physicians recommend benzathine penicillin, 2.4 million units IM, after completion of the above regimen, to have therapy last as long as the therapy for late latent syphilis. Penicillin-allergic patients need to be desensitized and treated as above.

If CSF pleocytosis was present initially, follow-up CSF should be examined every 6 months until there is a normal cell count. If the cell count has not decreased by 6 months, or if there is an abnormal cell count at 2 years, retreatment needs to be considered.

HIV and Syphilis All patients with syphilis should be screened for HIV infection as well as for other STDs. Syphilis in HIV-infected patients requires special care owing to reported treatment failures, occurrence of neurosyphilis, and bizarre nontreponemal titers. The reader is referred to the *1993 Centers for Disease Control—Sexually Transmitted Disease Guidelines* for specifics.

Partner Evaluation Sexual partners of all patients with syphilis (any stage) should be evaluated serologically and clinically. Sexual transmission only occurs with mucocutaneous lesions. The Centers for Disease Control recommend the following:

- Persons who are exposed to a patient with primary, secondary, or latent (duration < 1 year) syphilis within the preceding 90 days might be infected even if seronegative, and therefore should be treated presumptively.
- Persons who are sexually exposed to a patient with primary, secondary, or latent (duration $<$ 1 year) syphilis $>$ 90 days before examination should be treated presumptively if serologic test results are not available immediately and the opportunity for follow-up is uncertain.
- For purposes of partner notification and presumptive treatment of exposed partners, patients who have syphilis of unknown duration and who have high nontreponemal serologic test titers ($\geq$ 1:32) may be considered to be infected with early syphilis.
- Former and current sex partners of patients with late syphilis should be evaluated clinically and serologically for syphilis.[1]

The time periods before treatment used for identifying at-risk partners are 3 months plus duration of symptoms for primary syphilis, 6 months plus duration of symptoms for secondary syphilis, and 1 year for early latent syphilis.

Mycoplasma

These are organisms that have no cell wall but can grow in cell-free media. The presence of *Mycoplasma genitalium* is of uncertain clinical significance. *M. hominis* is present in about 50 percent of public clinic patients and 20 percent of private obstetric patients. *U. urealyticum* is present in 80 percent of women in public clinics and 50 percent of private patients.[10] Both of the latter species are present more often in women with bacterial vaginosis.

Along with other organisms, both have been found in patients with intraamniotic infection, pelvic inflammatory disease, and postpartum endometritis. Ureaplasma have been associated with low birth weight infants, infertility and habitual abortion.

Cultures for these organisms currently have no place in routine clinical practice. However, if cultures are needed, the vaginal mucosa rather than the endocervical canal should be cultured. Genital Mycoplasma can be cultured from specimens transported by an anaerobic transport device within 2 to 3 h of obtaining the specimen. Special mycoplasma transport broth contains antibiotics and cannot be used for any other cultures. Rapid delivery to the laboratory is important.[8]

Since Mycoplasma usually are associated with other organisms, broad-spectrum antibiotics will usually be employed to treat associated pathogens. *U. urealyticum* is treated with tetracyclines or erythromycins. *M. hominis* is susceptible to clindamycin. *M. hominis* is not susceptible to erythromycins, and some isolates are resistant to tetracycline. Upper genital tract infections should be treated with an antibiotic that is effective against these organisms.

Human Papilloma Virus

Human papilloma virus causes a broad spectrum of disease, ranging from subclinical infection in 70 percent of infected patients to overt genital warts in 30 percent of patients. HPV prevalence is greatest between ages 15 and 35. As with trichomoniasis and bacterial vaginosis, HPV is associated with other sexually transmitted diseases. Human papilloma virus can be detected by cytology, histology, and DNA probes. HPV is associated with squamous genital tract malignancies. HPV usually occurs multicentrically in the cervix, vagina, vulva, and perianal regions.

Some condylomas will be seen grossly on physical examination; others will be visible with colposcopy. Cytology, histology, HPV antigen detection, and HPV DNA molecular hybridization also may be used for detecting HPV.

Treatment of HPV is difficult, with recurrences and failure to treat all involved areas common. The goal should be to rule out significant neoplasia, to eradicate exophytic warts, and to decrease symptoms. The goal is not to remove all HPV completely, since this usually cannot be achieved.

In patients with external symptomatic disease, once colposcopic evaluation (of the vulva, vagina, and cervix) and biopsy (of the lesion and of other areas as needed) have been performed to rule out the presence of a malignancy or a premalignant lesion, trichloroacetic acid, 80 to 90 percent, may be applied to warts. Patients are retreated every week for up to 6 weeks. An alternative regimen that can be used at home is purified podophyllin resin, podofilox (Condylox) 0.5 percent, which may be applied to obvious lesions twice daily for 3 days, followed by no treatment for 4 days. This cycle may be repeated up to four times. Podophyllin, 10 to 25% in compound tincture of benzoin, can also be used externally. It must be washed off in 1 to 4 h, and can be repeated weekly up to six times. As with podofilox, ≤ 0.5 ml of solution can be used in daily treatment, and $< 10\ \text{cm}^2$ of tissue per day can be treated. TCA can be used in pregnancy, but podofilox and podophyllin are *contraindicated* in pregnancy.

5-Fluorouracil, 5%, can be used for vulvar and vaginal lesions; however, it may cause severe ulceration of normal tissue. Treatment with cryotherapy, laser, and LEEP procedures also may be helpful.

Cervical warts must be examined for coexistent dysplasia or carcinoma before treatment. Cervical warts can be treated with cryotherapy, LEEP, or TCA. Because of the role of HPV as a cocarcinogen for lower genital tract squamous carcinoma, all women with HPV should be followed regularly with Papanicolaou smears and usually colposcopy.

Herpes

Herpes simplex is the most common cause of genital ulcers. After an incubation period of three to five days, 2- to 4-mm vesicles appear, and subsequently become painful ulcerations. Genital herpes may be caused by two serotypes, HSV-1 and HSV-2. HSV-2 is most common in genital disease.

Diagnosis of acute genital herpes is made by recognizing clinical lesions and culturing unroofed vesicles or ulcers. Cytology with a Papanicolaou smear or a Tzanck smear has lower sensitivity.

Treatment for primary herpes in immunocompetent patients is acyclovir, 200 mg orally, five times daily for 7 to 10 days. Systemically ill patients with herpes should be treated with intravenous acyclovir, 5 to 10 mg/kg body weight, every 8 h for 5 to 7 days or until clinical resolution occurs. Treatment for recurrent herpes in immunocompetent patients may be acyclovir, 200 mg orally five times a day for 5 days, or acyclovir, 400 mg orally three times a day for 5 days, or acyclovir, 800 mg orally two times a day for 5 days. Daily suppressive therapy in patients with six or more recurrences per year may also be used. Safety and efficacy have been shown with therapy for as long as 5 years, but after 1 year a trial without acyclovir should be allowed to assess the patient's recurrence rate. Daily suppressive therapy dosing is acyclovir, 400 mg orally twice daily; the CDC's alternative regimen is acyclovir, 200 mg orally three to five times a day. The lowest dose that provides relief should be used.

HIV-infected women and other immunosuppressed women who have an acute herpes infection may need an increased acyclovir dosage of 400 mg three to five times daily until clinical resolution occurs, and intravenous therapy should also be considered.

Resistant herpes strains may respond to foscarnet, 40 mg/kg body weight injected every 8 h until clinical resolution.[1]

HIV and other STDs may be transmitted more easily when open ulcers are present; thus, patients with herpes should be counseled and appropriate screening performed.

Chancroid

Chancroid has an incubation period of 1 to 14 days. A small papule or pustule erodes into an ulcer, which usually is deep, painful, and indurated. The ulcerated area is softer than that present in syphilis or granuloma inguinale. Painful adenopathy is present in 30 to 60 percent of patients. Diagnosis of chancroid is usually clinical, with one or more painful genital ulcers present, no *Treponema pallidum* and no HSV clinical symptoms nor positive tests. Tender inguinal adenopathy with a painful ulcer is suggestive, and suppurative inguinal adenopathy is almost pathognomonic of chancroid. Laboratory confirmation is difficult, but can be made by culture of *Haemophilus ducreyi,* using direct inoculation of ulcer exudate onto selective blood agar media with vancomycin and then incubation at 33°C with 5 percent CO_2. Cytologic examination of the ulcer base exudate with a Giemsa or Gram stain will show gram-negative rods, but this is not very sensitive nor specific. Biopsy of the ulcer base shows three zones: one of neutrophils, red blood cells, and fibrin; one of blood vessel formation and endothelial cell proliferation; and one deeper level with plasma cell and lymphocyte infiltrate.

Treatment regimens include azithromycin, 1 g orally in one dose; ceftriaxone, 250 mg IM; or erythromycin base, 500 mg orally four times a day for 7 days. Alternative regimens are oral amoxicillin, 500 mg, plus oral clavulanic acid, 125 mg three times daily for 7 days; or ciprofloxacin, 500 mg orally, twice daily for 3 days. Patients with chancroid should be screened for HIV, syphilis, and other STDs.

Lymphogranuloma Venereum (LGV)

Lymphogranuloma venereum, caused by *Chlamydia trachomatis,* serotypes L1, L2, or L3, is endemic in tropical areas. There are three stages of this disease. The incubation period for the first stage is 5 to 7 days. A pustule or papule forms and rapidly ulcerates. In women, this is commonly on the vaginal wall, vulva, posterior fourchette, or posterior lip of the cervix. Fifty percent are asymptomatic and heal spontaneously. Stage II presents with a tender, firm, lymph node collection (bubo). Proctitis may be found with anal involvement. Infrequently, systemic symptoms of fever, headache, and meningismus occur. These lesions resolve in 2 to 3 months. Stage III results from fibrosis of lymphatic tissue with elephantiasis, rectal strictures, and perineal fistulas. Diagnosis is by a serologic complement fixation test or microimmunofluorescence test. Alternatively, tissue culture of an aspirate from an enlarged lymph node can be used for diagnosis. Histologic identification of chlamydia elementary or inclusion bodies in secretions or infected tissue also may be used. The differential diagnosis includes other sexually transmitted ulcerative diseases, Hodgkin's disease, non-Hodgkin's lymphoma, cat scratch fever, and bacterial lymphadenitis. Treatment is with doxycycline, 100 mg orally twice daily for 21 days. The CDC recommends alternative regimens of erythromycin, 500 mg orally four times per day for 21 days, or sulfisoxazole, 500 mg orally four times per day for 21 days. Pregnant and lactating women should be treated with erythromycin.[1] As in all sexually transmitted diseases, when one is present the woman is at risk of infection with multiple other STDs. She should be tested for these, and also counseled.

Donovanosis

Granuloma inguinale (donovanosis) is caused by *Calymmatobacterium granulomatis,* and is endemic in tropical regions. The incubation time is 8 to 80 days. Single or multiple genital ulcers occur; these are painless, irregular, and hard, with a rolled border and a clean base. Labial lesions are most common, but cervical and vaginal lesions may occur. Lymph nodes are not enlarged, but a "pseudo bubo," which is a deep granuloma, may mimic a fluctuant node. If left untreated, sequelae include lymphatic obstruction and elephantiasis. Diagnosis is by histologic evidence of short, pleomorphic rods in ulcer border biopsies. Giemsa, Wright's, Dieterle, or Warthin-Starry staining will enhance diagnosis by identification of intercytoplasmic inclusion bodies (Donovan bodies) within histiocytes. Pap smears may reveal Donovan bodies in women who have cervical lesions. For treatment, tetracycline, 500 mg orally four times daily for 10 to 14 days, is the drug of choice. Trimethoprim/sulfamethoxazole, two tablets twice daily for 14 days is an alternative regimen.

Molluscum Contagiosum

Molluscum contagiosum is caused by an unclassified pox virus. It is seen most often in children. However, it is also a sexually transmitted disease in adults, occurring in adults on the lower abdomen, thighs, genitalia, or buttocks. The incubation period is 1 week to 6 months; if untreated in immunocompetent hosts, the infection remits spontaneously in about 6 months to 3 years. Diagnosis is by clinical recognition of dimpled papules. Confirmation is by biopsy or staining a smear of the caseous material from the dimple, in which inclusion bodies of virions can be seen. Treatment is by mechanical removal of the lesions with liquid nitrogen, direct curettage, or trichloroacetic acid.

Pediculosis Pubis

Phthirius pubis, the crab louse, is usually spread through sexual contact. Patients with this problem commonly complain of itching. Small hemorrhages in the skin from lice bites may be visible. Patients may see the lice moving. Microscopic examination of nits or adult lice is diagnostic. Treatment is with lindane 1% shampoo, used for four minutes and then washed off; permethrin 1% cream rinse, used for 10 min, then rinsed off; or pyrethrins with piperonyl butoxide for 10 min and then rinsed off. Lindane should not be used in pregnant or lactating women or in children under age 2. Machine washing and drying (hot cycles) or dry cleaning of bedclothes and clothing is recommended. Eyelash involvement should be treated with occlusive ophthalmic ointment to eyelids twice daily for 10 days. Patients should be reevaluated in one week.

Scabies

Scabies is caused by *Sarcoptes scabiei,* var. hominis, and is transmitted both by sexual contact and by contact with infected bedding, clothes, or other fomites. Patients complain of intense itching, usually worse at night. Linear burrows 5 to 10 mm long and tiny brown and white specks at the ends (the mites) are pathognomonic. A scraping of the burrow examined microscopically can confirm the diagnosis. Treatment is with 5% permethrin cream applied from the neck down and washed off after 8 to 14 h, or 1% lindane 1 oz of lotion or 30 g of cream applied from the neck down and washed off after 8 h. Lindane should not be used in pregnant or lactating women, in children less than 2 years old, after a bath, or in individuals with extensive dermatitis, as it may cause seizures. An alternate therapy is 10% crotamiton applied from the neck down for two nights and washed off 24 h after the second application. Bedding and clothes should be machine-washed and dried (hot cycles) or dry cleaned. Pruritus may persist for several weeks, even with adequate therapy.

Common Systemic Diseases that May Be Transmitted via the Vaginal Route

HIV

Human immunodeficiency virus (HIV), the virus that causes AIDS as a late manifestation, is another sexually transmitted virus. HIV testing should be offered to all women at risk, including but not limited to women with other STDs, women whose partners are bisexual or drug users, women who are drug users, women with multiple sexual partners, and women whose partners have multiple sexual partners. HIV infection is discussed extensively in Chapt. 49.

Hepatitis B

Hepatitis B is sexually transmitted. One-third to two-thirds of the 200,000 to 300,000 new cases that have occurred annually in the United States in the past 10 years have been due to sexual transmission.[1] Hepatitis B virus (HBV) infection can result in death due to fulminant disease, jaundice, chronic HBV, and long-term sequelae, including cirrhosis of the liver and hepatocellular carcinoma.

The use of HBV vaccine should be advised for women at risk of acquiring HBV. This includes, but is not limited to, health-care workers, persons with multiple sex partners, sex partners of HBV carriers, sex partners of injecting drug users, injecting drug users, and women whose partners have multiple partners. The ACIP recommends HBV vaccination for persons who have had more than one sex partner in the last 6 months, men and women with another STD diagnosis, and sexually active homosexual and bisexual men. Older patients ($\geq$ age 25) may have a higher incidence of past infection as measured by anti-HBC; those immune due to vaccination will have a positive anti-HBsAg. Depending on the patient population, the physician will need to determine whether serologic screening for past infection/immunization is cost-effective before vaccination.

Vaccination DOSAGE: 1 ml of HBV vaccine IM in the *deltoid* at 0, 1, and 6 months. Depending on vaccine manufacturer, the dose for adolescents (11 to 19 years) is either 0.5 or 1 ml. Universal vaccination is recommended for newborns.

Exposure to HBV through Sexual Contact Patients sexually exposed to HBV should receive 0.06 ml/kg of HBIG IM once within 14 days of last exposure, plus the first (0) dose of HBV vaccine, followed by the 1- and 6-month vaccine doses. Pregnancy is not a contraindication to HBV or HBIG. As patients age, there may be less of an antibody response to HBV vaccine. Repeat dosing is recommended if seroconversion does not occur after the first vaccine series.

Sequelae In young adults who survive HBV, 6 to 10 percent become carriers, and over 25 percent of these patients will develop chronic active hepatitis with cirrhosis. An HBV carrier's risk of liver cancer is 12 to 300 times higher than that of non-HBV carrier adults.

Toxic Shock Syndrome

Toxic shock syndrome (TSS) is caused by infection or colonization with bacteriophage-specific strains of *Staphylococcus aureus* in a body cavity or on a foreign object in a body cavity. The strain of *S. aureus* that causes TSS makes an epidermal toxin, TSST-1. This toxin and staphylococcal enterotoxin B (SEB), and possibly other toxins, cause clinical symptoms.

Toxic shock syndrome may occur with menstruation, particularly when tampons are used, and has also been associated with vaginal infections, vaginal delivery, cesarean section, spontaneous abortion, diaphragm and sponge contraceptive use, CO_2 laser treatment of condyloma acuminatum, salpingitis, and postoperatively.

Diagnosis In 1980 the CDC compiled the following diagnostic criteria. The patient should have the first four of the following criteria and three or more organ system criteria:

- Temperature >38.9°C (102°F)
- Erythematous rash
- Hypotension
- Desquamation of palms and soles 1 to 2 weeks after illness onset

Three or more of the following systems:

- Gastrointestinal: Vomiting or diarrhea
- Muscular: Myalgia or elevated creatine phosphokinase (2 × upper limit of normal)
- Mucous membrane: Hyperemia of vagina, oropharynx, or conjunctivae
- Renal: Elevated blood urea nitrogen Elevated creatinine (≥ 2 × upper limit of normal) More than 5 WBC in a high-power field in urinary sediment without a UTI
- Hematologic: Low platelet count (<100,000/mm^3)
- Hepatic: Elevated SGPT ≥ 2 × upper limit of normal
- Neurologic: Disorientation or alteration in consciousness without focal neurologic signs
- Negative tests for Rocky Mountain spotted fever, leptospirosis, and measles
- Negative throat, blood, and CSF cultures[4]

The differential diagnosis includes any systemic illness associated with fever, rash, hypotension, and multi-organ system involvement.

Cultures to be obtained include those from body cavities (vagina, cervix, and throat), blood, any lesions, and wounds. Cultures of foreign objects, such as tampons, diaphragms, sponges, should be obtained when applicable.

Treatment Hospitalization is necessary. Fluid replacement is the most important aspect of supportive care. Penicillinase-resistant penicillins such as nafcillin or oxacillin are the drugs of choice.

TSS may recur in up to 30 percent of menstrual-related cases. The recurrence rates may drop to 5 percent if the patient receives β-lactamase-resistant antibiotics early in the course of the disease. Tampons should be avoided by women with a history of TSS.

References and Selected Readings

1. Centers for Disease Control: 1993 Sexually Transmitted Diseases Treatment Guidelines. *MMWR* 42, 1993.
2. Crombleholme WR, Schacter J, Grossman MA, et al: Amoxicillin therapy for chlamydia trachomatis in pregnancy. *Obstet Gynecol,* Vol 75, p 752, 1990.
3. Draper D, Parker R, Patterson E, et al: Detection of trichomonas vaginalis in pregnant women with the InPouchTV culture system. *J Clin Microbiol* 31(4):116 118, 1993.
4. Duff, P: Staphyloccal infections, in Gleicher: *Principles and Practice of Medical Therapy in Pregnancy,* 2d ed, New York: Appleton & Lange, 1992.
5. Eschenbach, DA, Hillier SL: Advances in diagnostic testing for vaginitis and cervicitis. *J Reprod Med* 34(8):555–564, 1989.
6. Eschenbach, DA: Bacterial vaginosis and anaerobes in obstetric-gynecologic infection. *Clin Infect Dis* 16(s4):S282, 1993.
7. Faro S: Infection and infertility. *Infect Dis Obstet Gynecol* 1:51–57, 1993.
8. Hill, B: Techniques for isolating pelvic bacterial pathogens, in Mead PB, Hager WD (eds): *Infection Protocols for OB/GYN.* Montvale NJ: Medical Economics Publishing, 1992, pp 265–271.
9. Mattingly RF, Woodruff JD: Surgical conditions of the vulva, in Mattingly RF, Thompson JD (eds): *Operative Gynecology.* Philadelphia: JB Lippincott, 1985, pp 694–696.
10. McCormack WM: Genital mycoplasmas, in Mead PB, Hager WD (eds): *Infection Protocols for OB/GYN.* Montvale NJ: Medical Economics Publishing, 1992, pp 217–219.
11. McCormack, WM: Current concepts: Pelvic inflammatory disease. *N Engl J Med* 330:115–119, 1994.
12. The Medical Letter on Drugs and Therapeutics. 36:113, Jan 7, 1994.
13. Piper JM, Mitchell EF, Ray WA: Prenatal use of metronidazole in birth defects: No association. *Obstet Gynecol* 82(3):348–352, 1993.

14. Thompson CD, Brekken AL, Kutteh WH: Necrotizing fasciitis: A review of management guidelines in a large obstetrics and gynecology teaching hospital. *Infect Dis Obstet Gynecol* 1:16–22, 1993.
15. Westrom L, Joesoef R, Reynolds G, et al: Pelvic inflammatory disease and fertility; A cohort study of 1,844 women with laparoscopically verified disease and 657 control women normal laparoscopic results. *Sex Transm Dis* 19:185–192, 1992.
16. Witkin SS, Jeremias J, Ledger WJ: Recurrent vaginitis as a result of sexual transmission of IgE antibodies. *Am J Obstet Gynecol* 159:32, 1988.

26 Other Disorders of the Vulva, Vagina, and Uterus

Stephen L. Curry

This chapter reviews common disorders of the vulva, vagina, cervix, and uterus, excluding infectious disorders and cancers. Of utmost importance is a careful history taken prior to a complete pelvic examination. One must question the patient regarding use of douches, deodorants, powders, and creams. Constant use of synthetic underwear, perineal pads, and tight slacks can exacerbate the symptoms of vulvar and vaginal disorders. Aggressive rubbing with toilet paper, bath towels, or wash cloths should be avoided. In carrying out the physical examination it is critically important to palpate and visualize the entire vulva and to observe carefully the entire vaginal surface as the speculum is being removed. Since the lower third of the vagina and the entire vulva have their lymphatic drainage through the groin, it is also important to evaluate all these areas during the complete examination.

Vulvar Vestibulitis

The patient with vulvar vestibulitis will present—usually in her third or fourth decade of life—complaining of the sudden onset of severe posterior vulvar burning and/or pain, which is significantly exacerbated during and immediately after intercourse. Eventually the pain becomes constant. On careful examination with the colposcope or a magnifying glass, one can see erythema around the vestibular gland openings. These glands are most prominent from approximately the four o'clock to the eight o'clock locations, just outside the hymenal ring and extending slightly down the perineum in the midline. Application of mild acetic acid used for colposcopic examination of the cervix often creates a frostlike well-circumscribed area. Many investigators have attempted to show that this inflammation is secondary to bacterial or viral infections. However, to date, no etiology is known. Some authors consider the disorder to be a combination of etiologies, including chronic yeast infection, chronic vaginitis, and atrophic vulvitis.

In many patients the condition will spontaneously regress in 6 months to 1 year. Application of diluted trichloroacetic acid every other week for 8 weeks followed by 6 weeks of vulvar rest appears to benefit a significant number of patients. Some authors recommend weekly 5-fluorouracil (5-FU) cream for 6 months. Those who do not have spontaneous regression of the problem nor respond to medical management may be treated with a vestibulectomy. This is an outpatient procedure that requires careful mapping of the involved area to ensure the best result. The patient should be warned that even under the best circumstances the response rate does not exceed 80 percent. Maximum response results from excising the posterior hymenal ring, dissecting deep into the fat to remove the glands, mobilizing the posterior vagina to bring it out to the skin, and using the finest possible suture. Laser treatment of this condition has not been successful. There is no evidence of any long-term sequelae from vulvar vestibulitis.

Vulvar Dystrophy

The classic presentation of vulvar dystrophy is the onset of vulvar pruritus and/or burning in the perimenopausal or postmenopausal period. The vulva is hormonally responsive, and one might expect that since the dystrophy appears to be due to estrogen deprivation, as is shown in other organs at or around the menopause, then estrogen replacement therapy might help, but it usually does not. Whether the failure of response is an indication that low levels of androgens produced throughout the menstrual years most affect the vulva or that the estrogen receptors in the vulva are lost is not yet well understood.

It is likely that these conditions begin with a thinning of the vulvar epithelium, which may go on to become symptomatic. This thinning of the vulvar epithelium is termed *hypotrophic vulvar dystrophy.* At the opposite end of the spectrum is the patient who, because of continuous irritation, develops hypertrophy of the vulvar epithelium. There are also those individuals who have mixed areas of hypotrophic and hypertrophic vulvar epithelium. The correct diagnosis can only be made with a biopsy. In addition, biopsy is necessary to rule out the presence of malignancy.

The most consistently successful treatment regimens are based on the biopsy results. If the epithelium is thin, treatment must be aimed at thickening it while treating the symptoms. On the other hand, if the entire epithelium is hypertrophic, then treating the symptoms and preventing the scratching and rubbing will often cause a reversion of the abnormality. Table 26-1 demonstrates the appropriate treatment in relation to the vulvar biopsy. If the patient has hypotrophic vulvar dystrophy (also called *lichen sclerosus et atrophicus*) or mixed dystrophy, in which there are areas of hypotrophic epithelium, then the aims of treatment are to thicken the epithelium and address the symptoms. Testosterone cream is utilized specifically to thicken epithelium. This cream often has to be specially prepared by the phar-

TABLE 26-1 Vulvar Dystrophy

	Diagnosis		
Treatment	**Hypotrophic**	**Hypertrophic**	**Mixed**
To produce epithelial thickening	Testosterone 2 % qhs × 8 wks	—	Testosterone 2 %, qhs × 8 wks
Of pruritus	Hydrocortisone cream, q AM	Hydrocortisone cream, bid	Hydrocortisone cream, q AM
To prevent scratching	Antihistamine, qhs	Antihistamine, qhs	Antihistamine, qhs
Healing		VULVAR DRYING REGIMEN	

macist at the request of the physician. Some investigators recommend using testosterone twice per day for 3 weeks and then reverting to once a day. A mild hydrocortisone cream may be used during the daytime to prevent vulvar burning and itching. An antihistamine may be prescribed at night to prevent itching and scratching during sleep. The patient must be cautioned that this regimen will require at least 8 weeks before significant response is noted. A 90 percent response rate is expected.

For hypertrophic vulvar dystrophy the major aim is to decrease the symptoms and allow the epithelium to heal. Thus, the patient is treated with hydrocortisone cream twice per day and an antihistamine at bedtime. For all these patients it is critically important to follow carefully the vulvar drying regimen as indicated in Table 26-2. If the condition persists after adequate and documented treatment, then second-line therapy consists of either a stronger steroid cream such as clobetasol propionate, subepithelial injections of hydrocortisone, or, rarely, surgical removal. The literature documents a high rate of recurrence with surgical removal. The patient needs to know that although vulvar dystrophies without atypia are not premalignant lesions, patients with long-term vulvar irritation may be at risk for cancer of the vulva.

Lichen sclerosis can also present in much younger women, often just after the onset of menarche. Again, the diagnosis must be confirmed with a biopsy. The first treatment which can be attempted is local progesterone cream. These patients also respond to testosterone cream. However, prior to considering testosterone cream for those young patients with lichen sclerosis who do not respond to progesterone, clobetasol propionate should be tried, thus avoiding the potential masculinizing effects of testosterone cream.

TABLE 26-2 Vulvar Drying Regimen

No unprescribed creams or medications
No douches, deodorants, or powders
Cotton underwear or no underwear
No tight slacks or pantyhose
No rubbing with toilet paper, towels, or washcloths
Liberal use of hair dryer to perineum

Vulvodynia

Chronic vulvar irritation, previous vulvar surgery, and long-term effects of vulvar viral infections, including laser treatment of the vulva, can lead to a diffuse vulvar burning or pain without any visible evidence of changes in the vulvar epithelium. Occasionally there will be a diffuse mild erythema. These patients often respond well to 3 months of treatment with low-dose amitriptyline, imipramine, or desipramine. The patients who respond most likely have a neuritis of the pudendal nerve or its branches. If the patient has not responded within 3 months, it is unlikely that she will respond to this treatment, and then local blocks or more aggressive therapy may need to be considered.

Hidradenitis

This condition occurs more commonly in the fourth and fifth decades of life. Initially presenting as small abscesses on the vulva, it eventually becomes a deep-seated inflammation of the apocrine glands. It is thought that some patients with significant hidradenitis may be unable to mobilize an appropriate immune response to staphylococcus infections of the skin. They often have lesions not only on the vulva but also in the axillary regions. Early lesions can be treated with hot soaks and regular washing with hexachlorophene soap. Deep-seated lesions should be aggressively opened and cleaned with curettage, allowing secondary healing. In the axillary regions complete removal with skin grafting may be the best treatment for some patients; however, on the vulva, patients usually respond to more conservative surgical treatment. Long-term bathing with hexachlorophene soap has been beneficial. Rarely do these patients respond to oral or local antibiotics. There is some indication that progression can be prevented by placing the patient on birth control pills until menopause, thus potentially decreasing the secretions of the apocrine glands. Obviously the patient's risk factors for use of the birth control pill and potential contraindications must be assessed.

Condyloma Acuminata

Condyloma acuminata (venereal warts) occur most commonly on the female vulva and also can be seen on the vagina, cervix, or in the perirectal area. They are a result of exposure to human papilloma virus (HPV) type 6 or 11, three months or more prior to the appearance of the warts. They can be small focal fingerlike projections or massive fungating lesions. Often in the vagina and on the cervix they present as flat white leukoplakia. The clinician must always be aware of the possibility of premalignancy or malignancy, although, following biopsy, initially conservative treatment may be appropriate, especially for the small fingerlike projections on the vulva in young women. On the other hand, in a 45-year-old woman with a large condyloma on the perineum, strong consideration should be given to complete excision in order to rule out the possibility of an underlying carcinoma.

Once it is proven that the diagnosis is condyloma, treatment should begin with the simplest and least costly regimen and then proceed, depending on response. Initially painting the external warts with 80% bichloracetic acid—or vaginal or cervical warts with 50% bichloracetic acid—would result in a response rate approaching 80 percent. Weekly applications for 4 weeks should result in the best response. If there is no evidence of regression after 4 weeks, then one must consider more aggressive therapy. The next step would be either to locally excise or freeze the warts or treat the warts with laser. All appear to be equally effective, and thus one must consider cost in choosing the most appropriate treatment.

There are two special considerations, those being massive cervical or vaginal warts during pregnancy and the very resistent warts. In the former case it is recommended that the patient be treated with 50% bichloracetic acid between 34 and 36 weeks in order to assure maximum regression at the time of delivery. Rarely is cesarean section required. In the case of very resistent warts, one must be sure that immunodeficient disorders such as acquired immune deficiency disorder (AIDS) have been ruled out, and then experimental treatments such as interferon or immunization may be considered.

Condyloma acuminata are a result of viral exposure through sexual contact, and therefore consideration should be given to having the partner evaluated and treated. Use of condoms can be effective in preventing recurrences. Rarely does this disorder result in any long-term consequences.

Other Vulvar Conditions

Hematoma of the vulva may result from either blunt trauma or spontaneous rupture of varicose veins, although such cases are rare. Treatment should be conservative unless there is evidence that the hematoma is expanding. If continued bleeding is a concern, the hematoma should be opened and packed. It is rare for the physician to find a true bleeding point.

Uncommonly, benign tumors can present as vulvar masses, including such entities as lipomas and fibromas. These lesions will usually need to be removed for cosmetic reasons and patient comfort, and to confirm the diagnosis of a benign lesion.

Gartner's Duct Cysts of the Vagina

These remnants of the mesonephric system most often present with difficulty visualizing the cervix with a speculum in a completely asymptomatic female. On palpation there is a soft, elongated cystic structure either at three or nine o'clock in the vagina, extending from the junction of the lower and middle third of the vagina up to the vaginal fornix. Rarely these can be so dilated that they obstruct intercourse or create mild pelvic discomfort. There are also reported cases of infected Gartner's duct cysts. The most appropriate management for these rare complications is marsupialization.

Nabothian Cysts of the Cervix

During the teenage years the cervix everts so that the columnar epithelium, with its glands and crypts of the endocervix, eventually is present on the exocervix. There is an aggressive attempt to cover this columnar epithelium with squamous epithelium by a process called *squamous metaplasia.* As the glandular epithelium is covered with squamous epithelium some of the glands and crypts are trapped, yet continue to secrete mucous. This becomes a nabothian cyst. It appears as a small fluid-filled cyst on the exocervix at the time of speculum examination. It is a completely benign condition without any short- or long-term risk. It does clue the clinician to the fact that this is an area of squamous metaplasia and thus the best place to take a scraping for a Pap smear. No treatment for nabothian cysts is necessary.

Endocervical Polyps

Endocervical polyps must be distinguished from pedunculated leiomyomata. The vast majority of endocervical polyps are benign; however, they should be removed and sent for pathologic evaluation. In perimenopausal women there is a potential for the endocervical polyp to be a result of prolonged unopposed estrogen, and thus consideration should be given to evaluating the endometrium to rule out adenocarcinoma. Small polyps can be removed by simply biopsying or twisting them off. Larger polyps are removed by placing a suture around the base and then cutting the stalk distal to the suture.

Leiomyomata Uteri

Leiomyomata uteri (fibroids) are the most common pathologic condition of the female genital tract. Fibroids can occur anywhere along the tract including the vulva and vagina; however, the vast majority are in the uterine fundus. One out of every five women and as many as one out of every three African American women will have a myoma in her uterus. They are classically described by their location as submucosal, intramural, subserosal, or pedunculated. Management is based on symptomology, and no longer is it acceptable to refer a patient for hysterectomy just because she has a fibroid uterus. Vaginal ultrasound can clearly differentiate uterine leiomyomata from ovarian neoplasms in the vast majority of cases.

The most common presenting complaint is that of menometrorrhagia, often secondary to either a submucosal or internally pedunculated leiomyomata. The patient may or may not be anemic. For women with abnormal bleeding that is thought to be secondary to fibroids, endometrial evaluation is essential to rule out the presence of endometrial hyperplasia or cancer. The pedunculated myoma may present as a vaginal or intracervical mass dilating the cervix. These can be removed by placing a suture around the base as high as possible and then removing the fibroid distal to the suture. This can often be done as an outpatient procedure.

The diagnosis of a submucosal myoma can be made either at the time of an endometrial biopsy, which usually has been performed to rule out uterine cancer, or by vaginal ultrasound. Occasionally a hystero-salpingogram is utilized in order to evaluate the size and location of the submucous fibroid prior to attempted hysteroscopic resection. These patients' bleeding may respond to conventional birth control pills. Depo-provera administered every 3 months also appears to be a useful conservative treatment for abnormal bleeding related to submucous fibroids, once premalignant or malignant conditions have been ruled out. If surgical removal is contemplated because of symptomatic, benign fibroids, pretreatment with a GNRH agonist may result in shrinkage of the tumor and decreased blood loss at the time of surgery.

Pain as a presenting symptom in a patient with myomas is most likely secondary to hypovascular necrosis, sometimes related to torsion of a pedunculated fibroid. This occurs most often during and immediately after pregnancy and at the time of menopause. The patient can present with the signs and symptoms of an acute abdomen, and at surgical exploration will be noted to have a necrotic myoma.

Occasionally patients with massive fibroids will present with pyelonephritis, severe constipation, or lower abdominal discomfort. These patients usually require hysterectomy based solely on the size and weight of the uterus. More than fifty percent of these patients will have a significant response to a GNRH agonist, which may allow the vaginal approach to surgery.

In the past, rapid growth of fibroids had been considered an indication for hysterectomy, with the potential of growth being secondary to leiomyosarcoma. Larger series have shown that this risk is uncommon prior to the menopause. Patients and clinicians currently more often consider myomectomy as a surgical approach to large or rapidly growing myomas in younger women. However, for some women, fibroids may recur after myomectomy and require subsequent treatment.

Adenomyosis Uteri

Also known as *endometriosis interna,* this is a condition in which the normal endometrial lining has invaded the myometrium. During the menstrual cycle this lining grows and develops in response to hormones, but at the time of the menstrual period it cannot shed and thus bleeds within itself in the myometrium. The patient will complain of central pelvic cramping and discomfort at time of the menstrual period. On examination during a menstrual period the patient may have an enlarged, boggy, tender uterus. These patients can often be treated with oral contraceptives, and surgery can be utilized if hormonal treatment fails.

References and Selected Readings

1. Kaufman RH, Friedrich EG, Gardner HL: *Benign Diseases of the Vulva and Vagina,* 3d ed. Chicago: Year Book Medical Publishers, 1989.
2. Mann MS, et al: Vulvar vestibulitis: Significant clinical variables and treatment outcome. *Obstet Gynecol,* 79:122, 1992.
3. Marinof SC, Turner ML: Vulvar vestibulitis syndrome: An overview. *Am J Obstet Gynecol,* 165:1228, 1991.
4. McKay M: Vulvodynia: Diagnostic patterns. *Dermatol Clin,* 28:123, 1992.
5. Proceedings of the 11th International Congress of the International Society for the Study of Vulvar Disease: *J Repro Med,* 38:1, 1993.
6. Ridley CM: *The Vulva.* London: Churchill Livingston, 1988.
7. Ridley CM: Genital lichen sclerosis (lichen sclerosis et atrophicus) in childhood and adolescence. *J R Soc Med* 1993; 86:69.
8. Turner ML, Marinof SC: Pudendal neuralgia. *Am J Obstet Gynecol* 165:1233, 1991.

27 Disorders of the Ovary and Fallopian Tube

David Chelmow
Kris Strohbehn
Alan DeCherney

Disorders of the ovary and fallopian tube can cause significant problems in prepubertal, reproductive age, and postmenopausal women. Many of these disorders can be managed by the primary care provider. All can be *detected* by the primary care provider, and attention should be focused during the routine history and physical exam to screen for these problems so that appropriate management or referral can be initiated. The range of possible disorders spans physiologic, infectious, anatomical, and neoplastic.

Anatomy and Physiology

The ovaries lie in the pelvis, usually immediately lateral and posterior to the fundus of the uterus. Their size varies with the stage of the woman's life. In a woman of reproductive age, ovaries each measure approximately 1.5 by 2.5 by 4.0 cm; postmenopausal ovaries measure approximately 2.0 by 2.0 by 1.0 cm. Premenopausal ovaries are frequently palpable on bimanual pelvic examination, but normal postmenopausal ovaries are seldom palpable. The ovaries are mobile, suspended from the uterus by the utero-ovarian ligaments, and from the pelvic sidewall by the infundibulopelvic ligaments. The vascular supply to the ovaries passes through these two ligaments. Occasionally, an ovary can twist on this vascular pedicle, leading to an acute emergency, ovarian torsion.

Approximately every 28 days in the reproductive age woman, the ovary will develop a single dominant follicle containing an ovum, and release it into the peritoneal cavity. It is picked up by the fimbriated end of the tube and passed down the tube into the endometrial cavity. This process of ovulation is the result of a complex combination of hypothalamic, pituitary, and ovarian interactions.

Prior to ovulation, the main steroid produced by the ovary is estradiol. Estradiol, along with two pituitary hormones, stimulates a single follicle to grow, frequently to several centimeters in diameter. In response to a surge of luteinizing hormone (LH) from the pituitary, in combination with several other factors, the follicle ruptures, releasing the ovum. For the next 14 days, the cells that originally formed the follicular cyst become a corpus luteum cyst and begin producing large amounts of a second ovarian hormone, progesterone. If the egg is not fertilized, the corpus luteum will stop producing progesterone, the corpus luteum cyst will involute, and the woman will menstruate 14 days after ovulation. As intermediates in ovarian steroid production, androgens including testosterone are made. Ovulation usually begins at around age 13 and continues on average until age 51, when the woman experiences menopause. After menopause, the ovary no longer produces significant estrogen or progesterone.

The fallopian tube, a 7- to 10-cm long tubular structure, emerges from the uterine cornua bilaterally. The distal end has frondlike, delicate fimbria, which help guide the ovum into the tube after it is released from the follicular cyst. Fertilization of the ovum by sperm occurs in the tube approximately two days after ovulation. The ovum slowly travels down the tube until it reaches the uterus approximately seven days after ovulation. Unlike the ovary, the tube is not hormonally active. Its main purpose is to facilitate egg transport and fertilization.

Physiologic Ovarian Disorders

During the reproductive age, either ovary produces an egg monthly, as well as cyclic production of estrogen, progesterone, and androgen. Most physiologic disorders are manifested by irregular or absent ovulation. In a reproductive age woman, chronic anovulation usually presents as irregular or absent vaginal bleeding, mild hirsutism, and infertility. These patients are frequently obese. Characteristically they will have ovaries with small follicular cysts visible on ultrasound, which has led to this syndrome being called polycystic ovarian disease (PCOD), formerly known as Stein-Leventhal syndrome. The name has somewhat confused understanding of this syndrome, as it implies that the ovary is the source of the syndrome. Actually, the polycystic ovary is the result of chronic disruption of androgen metabolism, and is not necessarily the cause. Such patients usually present with a long history of irregular, infrequent menses, often since menarche. Their initial complaint frequently relates to the mild androgenization—especially the hair growth and acne that often accompany the syndrome. True virilization, with temporal hair loss, voice change, and clitoromegaly is not consistent with this syndrome and requires further evaluation. The physical exam in these patients is frequently normal except for a weight in excess of ideal body weight, oily skin, and increased hair growth.

Patients fitting this description do not need an extensive work-up. The evaluation of any reproductive age woman with irregular bleeding or amenorrhea does require a pregnancy test. PCOD patients can ovulate, albeit infrequently; because many do not believe they can become pregnant, they often do not use contraception and can present with an unexpected pregnancy. Prolactin and TSH should be measured in the oligo- and amenorrheic woman to eliminate pituitary adenoma as a possible cause. The main concern in managing these patients is the protection of the endometrium from the effects of unopposed estrogen. These woman frequently have endometrial hyperplasia and are at much higher risk for the eventual development of endometrial cancer. If the patient has had more than a year of anovulation, office endometrial biopsy should be performed to evaluate for hyperplasia or cancer. The patient with anovulation and normal endometrial pathology studies should be cycled with monthly progesterone. This is frequently done by administering medroxyprogesterone acetate (Provera) 10 mg daily the first 10 to 14 days of the month. Contraception counseling should be done as well. In the patient requiring cyclic progesterone who also needs contraception, oral contraceptive pills provide a combined solution. Frequently, the patient's hirsutism also will be lessened by oral contraceptives. Patients desiring pregnancy should be referred to a gynecologist, as they will frequently need ovulation induction to become pregnant.

At around age 40, ovulation becomes less frequent, and less estrogen is produced by the ovary. Eventually ovulation ceases, with most women having their last menses between ages 48 and 55. This period is the menopause, and it is manifested by hypoestrogenic symptoms including hot flashes, vaginal dryness, sleep disturbances, and mood changes. It is a physiologic process and is addressed elsewhere in this book. Menopause is considered pathologic only if it occurs prior to age 40, when it is termed "premature ovarian failure." There are a number of causes of premature ovarian failure, including gonadal dysgenesis, especially Turner's syndrome, chemotherapy, and radiation therapy. Some autoimmune disorders including hypoparathyroidism, rheumatoid arthritis, thyroiditis, and myasthenia gravis also have been implicated, with anti-ovarian antibodies noted in some cases. The evaluation of a patient with suspected premature ovarian failure should include FSH measurement to confirm an ovarian rather than a central cause, and, if the FSH is elevated to postmenopausal levels, a karyotype and screening for autoimmune disease.

Differential Diagnosis of the Adnexal Mass

Ovarian enlargement can be abnormal at any age, and, if found, always requires further evaluation. Ovarian cancer, which has a small but appreciable lifetime risk for any woman, recently has received a large amount of media attention and is of concern to many patients. The ovaries, with their deep intraabdominal location, pose great diagnostic difficulties. Benign and malignant diseases can result in ovarian enlargement, and their location makes thorough evaluation difficult.

The routine physical examination for all women should include a pelvic examination once the woman has turned 18 or become sexually active. This examination should include careful bimanual palpation of the uterus and ovaries. Rectovaginal examination frequently is necessary to palpate the ovaries, and normal-sized ovaries cannot always be palpated, even by careful examination. As no other screening methods have been determined to be cost-effective, this examination is frequently the only opportunity a woman has for asymptomatic ovarian masses and cancers to be found.

The presence of a mass identified on pelvic examination does not ensure that the mass is gynecologic in origin. The pelvis contains a number of organs of the gastrointestinal and genitourinary systems, each of which can cause masses that are difficult to differentiate from ovarian masses. Table 27-1 lists a number of nongynecologic sources of pelvic masses. In particular, patients should be examined after emptying the bladder. In addition to making the exam more uncomfortable and the anatomy more difficult to discern, a distended bladder can mimic a pelvic mass. Chronically obstipated patients, particularly those on methadone or other narcotics, can have a stool-filled sigmoid that can mimic a pelvic mass. In these patients a rectovaginal exam is particularly important. Repeating the exam in several days or after an enema also can eliminate confusion.

Many patients are difficult to examine either because of obesity or discomfort during the exam. If the patient is asymptomatic, it is probably not cost-effective to perform ultrasound to visualize the ovaries. If the patient has pelvic symptoms and an adequate pelvic exam cannot be performed or a mass is suggested on physical exam, a pelvic ultrasound usually is performed to evaluate the pelvic anatomy.

TABLE 27-1 Pelvic Masses from Sites Other Than the Ovary or Fallopian Tube

Colon cancer
Distended bladder
Mesenteric cysts
Metastatic cancer
Omental cysts
Pelvic kidney
Stool
Diverticular abscess

A number of symptoms suggest the presence of a pelvic mass. Unfortunately, many masses including cancers can be asymptomatic, which emphasizes the importance of a pelvic examination as a routine part of the woman's physical exam. Women who have ovarian cancer often will present with feelings of pelvic pressure, bloating, dull pelvic pain, or bladder pressure. In most instances the pain begins gradually and progressively increases. Denial can be a powerful force, and in unusual instances patients can present with extremely large abdominal masses that originated in the pelvis. Advanced pelvic masses can present with increased abdominal girth, masses palpable even to the patient, or obtructed bowel or ureter.

Although most symptoms related to ovarian masses are chronic, there are two important instances in which acute events can occur which can present as acute surgical abdomens. The first is adnexal torsion. Torsion occurs when an ovarian mass rotates on its pedicle, the infundibulopelvic ligament. The fallopian tube can also torse, either with the ovary or separately. This rotation occludes the blood supply to the ovary and can lead to infarction. Commonly, bleeding occurs into the cyst and ovary, and can cause substantial blood loss.

Torsion can occur at any age, but is more common during pregnancy. It seldom occurs spontaneously and usually requires the presence of a preexisting adnexal mass to incite the torsion. Torsion presents with the sudden onset of severe abdominal pain, often with low-grade fever, nausea, and vomiting. Physical exam is usually remarkable for an enlarged, exquisitely tender unilateral adnexal mass. These patients may be so uncomfortable that adequate physical examination is impossible. Ultrasound typically shows a complex adnexal mass. Doppler ultrasound may show very reduced to absent blood flow. Torsion is a surgical emergency and requires immediate laparatomy or laparoscopy. In the reproductive age woman, conservative surgery is frequently attempted, with reduction of the torsion and cystectomy of any ovarian abnormality. If the ovary is clearly infarcted, adnexectomy is performed. After the reproductive years, torsion is usually treated by salpingoophorectomy.

The second ovarian condition that can appear as a surgical emergency is cyst rupture. Any nonsolid adnexal mass has the potential to rupture and release its contents into the peritoneal cavity. In some instances, particularly with dermoid cysts, the contents can be very irritating and can cause a severe chemical peritonitis. Most cyst ruptures occur in reproductive age women and are usually related to the midcycle rupture of follicular cysts.

Patients often will describe the sudden onset of severe abdominal pain, frequently beginning in a single location and gradually spreading. Low-grade fever is common. Physical examination can be remarkable for signs of peritoneal irritation, adnexal tenderness on pelvic exam, and cervical motion tenderness. Laboratory analysis often shows a mild elevation of the white blood cell count without a left shift. Differential diagnosis depends on the patient's age group and can be quite broad, including appendicitis, torsion, ectopic pregnancy, pyelonephritis, or gastroenteritis. Ultrasound can be helpful, revealing an adnexal mass or free fluid in the cul-de-sac. Culdocentesis, the transvaginal aspiration of fluid from the pouch of Douglas, also can be helpful, usually yielding serous or serosanguinous fluid in cases of cyst rupture.

Most cyst ruptures can be managed with pain control until the irritating fluid has been resorbed through the peritoneum. Laparoscopy is usually diagnostic if noninvasive methods are inconclusive; surgery is required when the patient's condition and differential diagnosis demand an immediate answer. Some cysts, especially corpus luteum cysts of pregnancy, can hemorrhage. Usually these are found during a surgical procedure to rule out ectopic pregnancy. If a hemorrhaging corpus luteum is suspected and intrauterine pregnancy is confirmed, the situation can often be managed by following serial hematocrits and observation, with surgical intervention reserved for the small subset of patients with a persistently falling hematocrit.

Women of Reproductive Age: The Physiologic Cyst

Among reproductive age women, the overwhelming majority of ovarian cysts are physiologic in nature, related to the normally occurring cysts of the menstrual cycle. During the early part of the menstrual cycle, a single dominant follicle is selected and progressively grows. Under normal circumstances, this cyst grows to 1 to 2 cm in diameter and ruptures approximately 14 days prior to the onset of menses, releasing an egg into the peritoneal cavity. Many women are aware of this happening, and report monthly midcycle mild unilateral discomfort as the follicular cyst expands and ruptures, a phenomenon known as "mittelschmerz."

As mentioned previously, cyst rupture can cause sudden, severe pain. The patient with suspected follicular cyst rupture can be managed conservatively, provided she is hemodynamically stable. Pain control usually can be achieved with oral analgesics. Pain from cyst rupture usually resolves over the course of 48 h. Once it has been determined that the patient is hemodynamically stable, she should be reexamined 48 h after the initial event. If the pain is not substantially resolved, further evaluation, often with laparoscopy, is warranted. A small subset of patients will have recurrent symptomatic cyst rupture. Use of a monophasic oral contraceptive pill containing at least 35 μg of ethinyl estradiol usually will suppress ovulation and give these patients relief.

Another frequently encountered problem is that sometimes either a follicular or a corpus luteum cyst may persist. In some instances this will cause discomfort, including dull abdominal pain or pressure. More frequently, a cyst or mass is noted on routine examination or as an incidental finding on a pelvic ultrasound done for other reasons. Most of these cysts are physiologic, and a careful work-up can differentiate most physiologic cysts from nonphysiologic cysts without invasive or expensive testing.

Physiologic cysts have a characteristic appearance on physical examination that usually sets them apart from a nonphysiologic cyst (Table 27-2). If the characteristics of the cyst are in doubt after physical examination, a pelvic ultrasound study should be obtained. Common ultrasonic findings more likely characteristic of benign or malignant ovarian cysts are listed in Table 27-3. Cysts that can be easily palpated on pelvic exam and meet the criteria described in Table 27-2 do not need immediate ultrasound examination. As these cysts are thought to be physiologic and related to the menstrual cycle, they can be managed by observation. Most of these cysts will resolve spontaneously over the next one or two menstrual cycles. It is a misconception that starting oral contraceptives will "treat" the cyst or hasten its resolution; however, in patients thought to be frequent cyst formers oral contraceptives do have a place in preventing the development of new cysts. The new lower dose oral contraceptives do not reliably suppress ovulation, and cysts can form in patients on these pills. Progestin-only contraceptives, particularly Norplant, may not decrease the incidence of cyst formation. The low levels of progestin do not inhibit follicular recruitment, but do inhibit the midcycle LH surge necessary for ovulation. Re-

TABLE 27-2 Typical Physical Examination Characteristics of Physiologic and Nonphysiologic Ovarian Cysts

Physiologic	Nonphysiologic
Discrete, smooth	Irregular
Simple (single cyst)	Multicystic
≤5 cm diameter	>5 cm
Fluid-filled	Solid components
Mobile	Fixed
Unilateral	Bilateral

NOTE: Presence of any of the characteristics listed under nonphysiologic makes the mass suspicious for not being physiologic.

TABLE 27-3 Typical Ultrasound Characteristics of Benign and Suspicious Ovarian Cysts

Benign	Malignant
Simple	Complex
Unilateral	Bilateral
Thin-walled	Thick-walled
Fluid-filled	Solid components
No internal echoes	Internal echoes
Smooth capsule	Papillations
	Excrescences
	Ascites

productive age patients with cysts persistent through two menstrual cycles and with ultrasonographically benign-appearing cysts need individualized management. Surgical evaluation of these cysts is usually performed, although close follow-up of benign-appearing lesions with frequent ultrasounds and pelvic exams can be done, with intervention if growth or change occurs.

Ca-125, a tumor marker, has received much recent attention. Ca-125 levels are elevated in many women who have certain histologic types of ovarian cancer, particularly serous cystadenocarcinomas. Ca-125 is also elevated with endometriosis and several bowel conditions, and varies with the menstrual cycle. Conversely, the test is not very specific and can be normal in women with early ovarian cancer and with many histologic types of advanced ovarian cancer. Given its lack of sensitivity and specificity, Ca-125 frequently is not useful in the initial evaluation of premenopausal women with adnexal masses, and often leads to diagnostic confusion. Several other tumor markers are under investigation as screening tests, but none have been found to be reliable because of poor sensitivity and specificity.

Small Ovarian Cysts Found in Postmenopausal Women

By definition, menopausal women do not have menstrual cycles, and therefore do not have physiologic cysts. Nonetheless, wider use of the new imaging modalities has shown that ovarian cysts can be quite common. Some series of transabdominal ultrasound examinations have shown cysts in 2 to 3 percent of postmenopausal women; using the more sensitive endovaginal probe, cysts have been demonstrated in 10 to 15 percent of menopausal women. This is also the age group with the highest incidence of ovarian malignancy. Adnexal masses in this age group are clearly not normal, but neither are they necessarily cancer. Attempting to detect cancer while minimizing surgery on patients with benign lesions remains one of the most challenging problems of gynecology.

As mentioned before, no effective screening modalities are available and current recommendations only include yearly pelvic exams. Unfortunately, annual pelvic exams detect most ovarian cancers at an advanced state (stage III or IV), resulting in poor five-year survival rates. The ovary normally shrinks after the menopause to approximately 1 by 2 cm. It is rarely palpable on pelvic exam in any but the thinnest, most relaxed patient. Palpable ovaries in this age group are often abnormal. Although not necessarily malignant, they do require thorough evaluation. As in premenopausal women, most small adnexal masses are not symptomatic, but others may present as bloating, increased abdominal girth, or pelvic pressure. Many are detected during the evaluation of vague urinary or gastrointestinal symptoms. If a mass is palpated, an ultrasound should be performed. Masses with any of the characteristics of malignancy noted in Table 27-3 need immediate surgical evaluation.

A diagnostic dilemma occurs when small, simple cysts are identified as incidental findings on ultrasound studies done for other reasons. Occasionally, these cysts represent early cancers, but most are benign. Close observation is reasonable if the patient is asymptomatic and if the cyst's ultrasound appearance is simple, unilateral, thin-walled, and under 5 cm in diameter without internal echoes, solid components, or ascites, and if the Ca-125 is normal. Close observation entails a repeat examination in approximately one month. If no change is detected, Ca-125 and ultrasound studies and the pelvic exam should be repeated every 3 months for 1 year and every 4 to 6 months thereafter. If at any time the cyst grows or changes characteristics, or if the Ca-125 becomes abnormal, surgical exploration is imperative. Management of these cysts with laparoscopy is advocated by some, but remains an unproven modality for this problem. Surgical excision is warranted in the patient who does not desire close observation.

Benign Ovarian Neoplasms

There are a large number of different benign neoplasms of the ovary (Table 27-4). All are of concern for several reasons. First, they can cause symptoms, including pain, pressure, and bloating. Some can grow to be quite large. Second, there is the small

TABLE 27-4 Benign Ovarian Masses

Benign cystic teratoma
Physiologic cysts (follicular and corpus luteum cysts)
Cystadenomas
Fibromas
Thecomas
Brenner tumors
Endometriomas

chance that they can cause an acute emergency either by rupturing or by inciting torsion. Third, they must be differentiated from malignancy.

Benign Cystic Teratoma (Dermoid cysts)

The most frequently encountered benign ovarian neoplasm is a mature cystic teratoma, also called a dermoid cyst. Excluding physiologic cysts, mature cystic teratomas comprise approximately 10 to 25 percent of all ovarian neoplasms. They are most frequently found in reproductive age women, but can be found in all age groups from pediatric to postmenopausal. They are often small and asymptomatic, found on routine pelvic examination, or identified because of their characteristic appearance on radiographic or ultrasound studies done for other reasons. Once they reach 6 to 10 cm in size they can cause abdominal pain, pressure, swelling, or a mass detectable by the patient.

Mature cystic teratomas are derived from germ cells; histologically, they contain mature elements derived from all three embryonic cell types: ectoderm, mesoderm, and endoderm. Ectodermal tissues predominate, and recognizable hair, teeth, cartilage, and bone are frequently found. These structures give a characteristic appearance on x-ray or ultrasound. Such cysts are surgically removed to prevent torsion or rupture (which causes a severe chemical peritonitis). In reproductive age patients, the dermoid cyst is removed by cystectomy, with preservation of the normal ovarian tissue.

Cystadenomas

Cystadenomas are the benign counterparts of epithelial ovarian malignancies. Their histology may be serous or mucinous. The serous tumor usually is uniloculated, whereas mucinous tumors frequently are multiloculated and grow to be extremely large. Rupture of a benign mucinous cystadenoma can lead to pseudomyxoma peritonei, diffuse intraperitoneal spread of the benign tumor.

Solid Benign Tumors

Fibromas, thecomas, and Brenner tumors are solid benign tumors found in women of all ages. In unusual instances, fibromas and thecomas can be associated with ascites and pleural effusions, a situation called Meig's syndrome. There are rare reports of malignant Brenner tumors.

Endometriomas

Endometriomas are found in reproductive age women. They can be associated with pelvic pain and infertility. They can be unilateral or bilateral and appear on ultrasound as complex cysts with internal echoes consistent with hemorrhage. They are discussed at length in Chap. 28.

Benign Disorders of the Fallopian Tube

The differential diagnosis of tubal disease is much more limited than ovarian disorders. Physiologic disorders are limited to structural tubal disorders preventing egg, sperm, and zygote transport. Most enlargements of the tube are benign in nature. They are in the differential diagnosis of adnexal masses, and must be differentiated from ovarian neoplasms. Primary fallopian tube malignancy is the rarest of gynecologic cancers, comprising much less than 1 percent. It is, however, a common site to which other gynecologic malignancies metastasize.

Disorders of Tubal Transport

Tubal disease is one of the most common sources of infertility, and is implicated in 25 to 40 percent of female infertility. Establishment of tubal patency is essential early in the infertility work-up, and can be done by hysterosalpingogram or by chromotubation at the time of laparoscopy. Tubal obstruction is most frequent after episodes of salpingitis. Chlamydia infection has been implicated as a source of major tubal damage after clinically asymptomatic infection. Even in cases where obstruction is not complete, damage to the ciliated lining of the fallopian tube can result in defects in the transport of gametes. The risk of ectopic pregnancy is much greater in patients with tubal damage. Kartagener's syndrome, with reversed direction of cilia movement, is a true functional disorder of the fallopian tube. Interestingly, it does not absolutely prevent fertility.

Paratubal Cysts

The fallopian tube can give rise to thin-walled, simple, clear fluid-filled cysts known as paratubal cysts. These cysts are usually quite small, but can grow as large as 20 cm. Pedunculated cysts arising from the fimbria are called hydatid cysts of Morgagni. These cysts usually are discovered as incidental findings on ultrasound study or at gynecologic surgery. They are almost without exception benign, and seldom cause problems except for rare torsions and cyst ruptures. The main difficulty is in differentiating them from ovarian neoplasms.

Ectopic Pregnancy

The fallopian tube is the most common location for ectopic pregnancy. Ectopic pregnancy should be considered first in the differential diagnosis of a reproductive age woman with an adnexal mass because it is the only part of the differential that is potentially immediately lethal apart from an actively bleeding hemorrhagic cyst. A diagnosis of ruptured ectopic pregnancy is virtually impossible in the presence of a negative sensitive urine pregnancy test. Ectopic pregnancy should be suspected in any woman with abnormal vaginal bleeding, pain, and a positive pregnancy test. It is discussed at length in Chap. 46.

Tuboovarian Abscess

Tubal abscess can result as a complication of acute salpingitis, which is discussed in Chap. 25. These masses can be quite large, as they can combine the tube, ovary, and a phlegmon of matted bowel. On physical exam they present as an enlarged, tender adnexal mass. Frequently the patient will be in such discomfort that even a large mass cannot be palpated. Ultrasound will show a complex adnexal mass, and usually the patient will be febrile and have significant abdominal tenderness. Management in the reproductive age woman is discussed elsewhere. Tuboovarian abscess is very unusual in the postmenopausal woman and merits surgical management because of the association with ovarian neoplasms.

Hydrosalpinx

Hydrosalpinx is a sequela of acute salpingitis. These are usually small, but can be as large as 5 to 10 cm and sometimes are found on pelvic exam. More frequently they are incidental findings on pelvic ultrasound study or at gynecologic surgery. On ultrasound they appear as complex multicystic masses with internal echoes. They usually are not symptomatic, and need to be removed only if necessary to differentiate them from ovarian neoplasms.

References and Selected Readings

1. DeSaia PJ, Creasman WT: The adnexal mass and early ovarian cancer, in *Clinical Gynecologic Oncology,* 4th ed. St. Louis: CV Mosby, 1993, pp 300–332.
2. Droegemueller W: Benign gynecologic lesions, in *Comprehensive Gynecology,* 2d ed. St. Louis: Mosby-Yearbook, 1992, pp 491–544.
3. Rulin MC: Controversies in the management of adnexal masses. *Clin Obstet Gynecol* 36:361–456, 1993.
4. Speroff L, Glass RH, Kase NG: *Clinical Gynecologic Endocrinology and Infertility,* 4th ed. Baltimore: Williams & Wilkins, 1989.
5. Stenchever MA: Significant symptoms and signs in different age groups, in *Comprehensive Gynecology,* 2d ed. St. Louis: Mosby Yearbook, 1992, pp 172–179.

28 Endometriosis

Kris Strohbehn
David Chelmow
Alan DeCherney

SYMPTOMS
DIFFERENTIAL DIAGNOSIS
DIAGNOSIS
Physical Examination • Laparoscopy • CA-125
AFS STAGING
PATHOLOGY
PATHOPHYSIOLOGY
TREATMENT
Medical • Surgical • Combined Therapy
SUMMARY

Endometriosis is a disease almost exclusively of reproductive age women and is defined as extrauterine growth of endometrial glands and stroma. It is a benign condition that is quite common, affecting 5 to 15 percent of all reproductive age women. Endometriosis is benign; however, it has some characteristics that are similar to those of cancer. It grows progressively while under the influence of normal ovarian function; it frequently recurs despite treatment; and it appears in sites distant from its origin.

The age at onset is usually the late twenties, but endometriosis may present in any reproductive age woman. Postmenopausal women rarely get endometriosis, even those who are receiving hormonal replacement therapy. Endometriosis has been described in male patients on high-dose estrogen agonists, such as tamoxifen, for prostate cancer. Endometriosis most frequently occurs in the pelvis and its peritoneal surfaces. It may rarely involve the lungs, brain, and prior surgical scars, such as episiotomy scars.

The regions in the pelvis that are commonly affected include the ovaries and the serosal surfaces of the uterus. The serosal surfaces of the bladder, bowel, and rectosigmoid are also commonly involved. Endometriosis can invade the stroma of the ovary, resulting in a cyst, called an "endometrioma." Endometriomas are present in approximately one-third of women surgically evaluated for endometriosis. The cysts are filled with a "chocolate" fluid composed of hemosiderin deposits, old blood, and debris. The cysts usually are lined with endometrial stroma and glands, but the normal architecture may be absent. Hemosiderin-laden macrophages may be the only histologic finding.

Symptoms

The most frequent presenting symptoms are: dysmenorrhea, pelvic pain, and infertility. Characteristically, pain from endometriosis occurs in the latter half of the cycle, usually a few days prior to the onset of the next menstrual period. The chronology of pain and other symptoms can be established by having the patient keep a menstrual calendar, recording her symptoms in relationship to her cycle. Dysmenorrhea is common, and many women have referred pain localized to the lower back. Rarely, an acute abdomen results when an endometrioma causes ovarian torsion; an endometrioma can also rupture or leak, resulting in a chemical peritonitis and acute pain.

Spotting of dark menstrual blood several days prior to the onset of the normal period is another frequent symptom. Dyspareunia often occurs and is usually associated with deep penetration. Occasionally, patients will complain of cyclical hematuria or hematochezia when endometriosis involves the mucosa of the bladder or rectum. Rarely, endometriosis occurs in other extrapelvic regions with bizarre symptoms ranging from catamenial pneumothorax or hemothorax when endometriosis involves the lung; cyclical seizures when it involves the central nervous system; or pain that mimics an inguinal hernia when it tracks along the round ligament.

The extent of visible disease often contrasts significantly with the actual symptoms. Through studies of asymptomatic patients undergoing surgery for other reasons, it has been ascertained that approximately one-third of all patients with endometriosis are asymptomatic. Frequently, the patient with extensive endometriosis will have minimal pain. Conversely, patients with minimal objective findings often will complain of severe pain.

Another common presenting symptom is infertility. Often, patients who are otherwise asymptomatic may be unable to conceive because of endometriosis. Seibel[5] suggests that the causes of infertility from endometriosis are probably multifactorial:

1. Direct tubal damage from endometriosis may result in peritubal scarring.
2. Immunologic factors, including enhanced macrophage activity in the peritoneal fluid, may prevent normal sperm function and conception.
3. Increased prostaglandin activity may inhibit the motility of the tubal cilia and smooth muscle, thus preventing normal ovum transport.

Differential Diagnosis

Endometriosis is important to consider in the differential diagnosis of several symptoms.

Among patients with pelvic pain, the differential diagnosis must include other gynecologic sources. Pelvic pain can be caused by pelvic inflammatory disease as well as by adhesions resulting from other inflammatory processes, surgery, and nongynecologic intraabdominal infections. Sexually active patients with pelvic pain should have genital cultures for chlamydia and gonorrhea.

Pregnancy should always be considered in the differential diagnosis of pelvic pain.

Many benign or maligant neoplastic processes can lead to progressive, chronic pelvic pain. Benign processes such as leiomyomata uterii may cause pelvic pain, but this presentation is rare unless the fibroids outgrow their blood supply, resulting in central tumor necrosis and pain. Ovarian neoplasms, both malignant and benign, also may present primarily as pelvic pain due to local infiltration of nerves, ovarian torsion, or chemical peritonitis. If there is any doubt regarding the diagnosis, it is prudent to rule out cancer (see Chap. 23).

Other nongynecologic sources of pelvic pain include such gastrointestinal disorders as diverticulitis, inflammatory bowel disease, appendicitis, and irritable bowel syndrome. In addition, the genitourinary system must be considered; acute cystitis should be ruled out by performing a urinalysis.

The symptoms of dysmenorrhea usually include only gynecologic sources in the differential. Most commonly, dysmenorrhea presents in patients with endometriosis or fibroids. Dysmenorrhea is particularly common with submucosal fibroids, and a hysteroscopy is advised if the patient is having irregular bleeding.

The differential diagnosis for patients presenting with infertility includes: problems with the male (abnormal semen analysis, which accounts for up to 40 percent of the problems of infertility among couples); tubal disease from causes other than endometriosis, such as infection; anovulation; cervical factors due to thick mucus, sperm antibodies, or cervical stenosis; luteal phase deficiencies due to progesterone deficiency; and, finally, endometriosis.

Diagnosis

Physical Examination

Clinical findings on physical exam that may raise suspicion include pelvic tenderness, especially in the cul-de-sac. Nodularity and tenderness may be encountered in the region of the uterosacral ligaments and posterior uterus, which are more appreciable during rectovaginal examination. The rectovaginal examination is a valuable part of the pelvic exam and can help define a retroflexed, fixed uterus. This finding is very suggestive of endometriosis although it can also be encountered with gynecologic malignancies. A palpable adnexal mass may represent an endometrioma. Any persistent palpable mass requires further evaluation with ultrasound or surgery. If the sonographic appearance is other than that of a simple cyst, surgical evaluation is warranted to rule out malignancy.

Laparoscopy

The definitive diagnosis of endometriosis is made surgically, either by diagnostic laparoscopy or by exploratory laparotomy. The characteristic endometriotic lesion is described as a "powder burn lesion," which represents a small (2 to 10 mm) collection of blood and debris, endometrial glands, and stroma within an area of fibrosis. Recently it has been recognized that there is a wide range in the gross appearance of endometriosis, and the findings are often subtle. The surgeon must be thorough in inspecting the intraperitoneal cavity when endometriosis is suspected. The spectrum of the gross appearance of endometriosis includes clear vesicles, white adhesions, red papules, and the characteristic dark purple lesions noted above. Given the wide range of gross findings, a confirmatory biopsy is often performed.

CA-125

A serum tumor marker, CA-125, is frequently elevated in patients with endometriosis. Because an elevated CA-125 level can be found in other disease processes, including infection, pregnancy, and neoplastic processes, the usefulness of CA-125 levels for the diagnosis of endometriosis is limited, and the test is not recommended at present.

AFS Staging

The staging of endometriosis is surgical, not part of an office evaluation. The staging is included for office reference, so that the extent of disease may be understood and discussed with the patient when she presents with a known history of endometriosis. Figure 28-1 outlines the current revised staging of the American Fertility Society.

Pathology

The histologic appearance of endometriosis is similar to the stromal and glandular components of endometrium. Frequently biopsies of endometriosis will fail to reveal endometrial tissue, but hemosiderin-laden macrophages usually are present.

Pathophysiology

There are many theories regarding the etiology of endometriosis. Three theories currently predominate: The first is that retrograde menstruation percolates through the fallopian tubes, leading to the deposition of endometrial tissue in the pelvis. A second theory proposes that coelemic metaplasia of "totipotential cells" of the peritoneum can differentiate into any type of tissue, including endometrial tissue. The third theory postulates that both explanations may play a role in endometriosis. Endometrial tissue and fluid settle in the cul-de-sac and pelvis, and this may lead to metaplastic changes in these inflamed regions of the peritoneum.

Patient's Name ______________________ Date ______________________

Stage I (Minimal) · 1–5
Stage II (Mild) · 6–15
Stage III (Moderate) · 16–40
Stage IV (Severe) · > 40
Total ______________

Laparoscopy __________ Laparotomy __________ Photography __________

Recommended Treatment ______________________

____

Prognosis ______________

	Endometriosis	< 1cm	1–3cm	> 3cm
Peritoneum	Superficial	1	2	4
	Deep	2	4	6
Ovary	R Superficial	1	2	4
	Deep	4	16	20
	L Superficial	1	2	4
	Deep	4	16	20

		Partial	Complete
	Posterior cul-de-sac obliteration	4	40

	Adhesions	< 1/3 Enclosure	1/3–2/3 Enclosure	> 2/3 Enclosure
Ovary	R Filmy	1	2	4
	Dense	4	8	16
	L Filmy	1	2	4
	Dense	4	8	16
Tube	R Filmy	1	2	4
	Dense	4[*]	8[*]	16
	L Filmy	1	2	4
	Dense	4[*]	8[*]	16

*If the fimbriated end of the fallopian tube is completely enclosed, change the point assignment to 16.

Additional endometriosis: ______________________

Associated pathology: ______________________

To be used with normal tubes and ovaries

L R

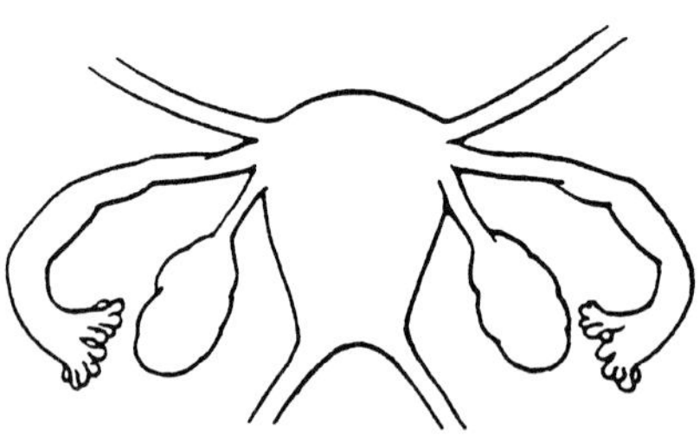

To be used with abnormal tubes and/or ovaries

L R

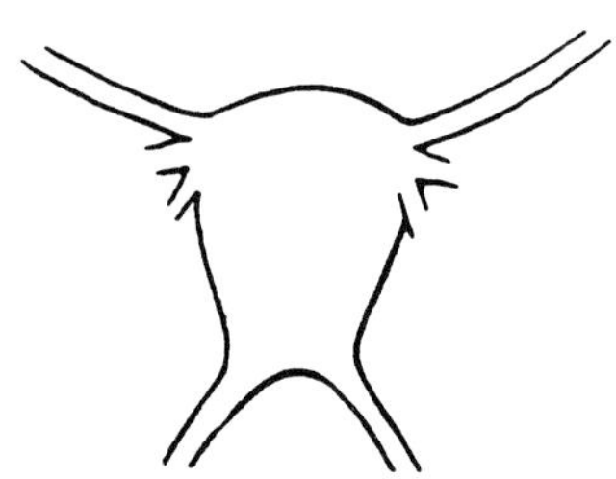

Figure 28-1 Revised staging of endometriosis by the American Fertility Society. (From the American Fertility Society. Revised American Fertility Society Classification of Endometriosis: 1985. *Fertil Steril* 1985;43-351–352. Reproduced with permission of the publisher, the American Fertility Society.)

None of the above theories explain why many patients with endometriosis have lymphatic involvement, nor how endometriosis can spread to such distant organs as lung or brain. Others have proposed that lymphatic or hematogenous transport of endometrial tissue can occasionally cause endometriosis. There is also evidence for enhanced cell-mediated activity of macrophages in the peritoneal fluid of some patients with endometriosis. This, as well as evidence for a familial predisposition for endometriosis, suggests immunologic and genetic components in the development of endometriosis.

Treatment

The goals of treatment for patients suffering with endometriosis depend primarily on reversing the presenting symptoms. When the chief complaint is pain, dysmenorrhea, or dyspareunia, the obvious goal is to alleviate this pain. Patients with infertility due to endometriosis will have treatment targeted at conception. As mentioned above, patients with an adenexal mass that is presumably an endometrioma usually require surgical evaluation and treatment. Treatment options for endometriosis range from observation, when the disease is mild, to medical and surgical options.

Patients with known mild endometriosis and infertility may be as successful in their efforts to conceive without medical or surgical intervention. Therefore, a period of 6 to 12 months without therapy usually is recommended unless the patient is approaching the end of her child-bearing potential.

Medical

If the chief complaint is pelvic pain, often nonsteroidal anti-inflammatory agents (NSAIDs) will improve these symptoms. If the goal of medical therapy for endometriosis is to halt progression, then the cyclical hormonal environment leading to proliferation of the heterotopic endometrial tissue must be stopped. This can be accomplished in two ways: by achieving a hypoestrogenic, hypoprogestational ''pseudomenopausal'' state; or by increasing the hormonal environment, causing a ''pseudopregnancy'' state. The medical options currently approved by the FDA are listed in Table 28-1.

Some suggest that pregnancy itself may palliate endometriosis. Decidualization of heterotopic endometrial tissue occurs during pregnancy, although many patients have recurrent symptoms following resumption of ovulation. Many clinicians will use an empirical trial of a pseudogestational agent such as an oral contraceptive or a progrestational agent in combination with NSAIDs without surgical confir-

TABLE 28-1 Medical Therapy for Endometriosis

Drug	Side effects
Nonsteroidal anti-inflammatory agents	Gastritis, nephrotoxicity
Ibuprofen	
Anaprox	
Pseudogestational agents	
Continuous oral contraceptive pills (must use continuous regimen with pill containing at least 30 μg estrogen)	Bloating, headaches, mood swings, weight gain, hypertension
Progestational agents	
Medroxyprogesterone (IM) (Depo-Provera)	Mood swings, weight gain, increased appetite
Medroxyprogesterone (PO)	
Pseudomenopausal agents	
Danazol	Weight gain, hot flushes, irritability, acne, ↑LDL, ↓HDL, hirsutism, deepening of the voice
GnRH agonist	
Leuprolide (Depo)	Hot flushes, vaginal dryness, depression, osteoporosis
Nafarelin spray	Hot flushes, vaginal dryness, depression, osteoporosis, nasal irritation
Goserelin	Side effects the same as Leuprolide

mation of the diagnosis. Pseudomenopausal agents are rarely used without surgical confirmation.

A "pseudopregnancy" state can be achieved by using a combined estrogen-progesterone contraceptive preparation. A low-dose combined estrogen/progesterone pill containing at least 30 μg estrogen is prescribed. The hormonal milieu should be nonfluctuating. Therefore, a continuous regimen is employed, and the placebo pills at the end of the cycle are not used. The patient is instructed to take one pill daily and to start the subsequent pack of pills after taking the first 21 pills. She should become amenorrheic on the continuous hormonal regimen, thus removing the stimulus for heterotopic endometrial tissue growth. Breakthrough bleeding is common on this regimen. If the patient has breakthrough bleeding, Droegemueller[2] recommends doubling the dose for five days to stop the bleeding and then resuming the previous dose. An alternative is to add additional estrogen for five days. Side effects are those commonly found with oral contraceptive preparations, including headaches, hypertension, weight gain, mood swings, and bloating.

A progestational agent alone can also achieve a "pseudopregnancy" state. Progesterone can be prescribed as a daily oral agent or as an intramuscular agent (see Table 28-1). Side effects include mood swings, irritability, weight gain, increased appetite, and fatigue. Breakthrough bleeding is common, and can be managed with the temporary supplementation of an estrogen. Among patients with infertility, the conception rate is approximately 30 percent after completing 6 to 12 months of the above regimens.

Two types of medication are currently available to achieve a pseudomenopausal state. Historically, this was first accomplished in the 1970s, when danazol was introduced. It is a combined androgen agonist and antagonist that causes anovulation. It affects multiple sites necessary for normal reproductive function, including the hypothalamus, pituitary gland, ovaries, endometrium, and sex-hormone binding globulin levels. The endometrial glands become atrophic, thus diminishing the symptoms.

The side effects of danazol are related primarily to the hormone's androgenic properties. These include weight gain, irregular bleeding, depression, hirsutism, acne, an adverse change in the lipid profile [increased low density lipoproteins (LDL) and decreased high density lipoproteins (HDL)] and decreased breast size. Rarely, an irreversible deepening of the voice has been described.

Gonadotropin releasing hormone (GnRH) agonists have recently been used with equal efficacy to treat endometriosis. These preparations result in a hypogonadotrophic state through the binding of GnRH receptors on the pituitary gland. After an initial stimulatory effect, the pituitary hormones FSH and LH are suppressed, leading to anovulation; amenorrhea and atrophy of the endometrial glands results.

The most common side effects of GnRH agonist are vaginal dryness, hot flushes, and progressive bone demineralization similar to that found in a menopausal woman. Because of concerns of long-term adverse effects, including osteoporosis, this type of medication has been approved by the FDA for only six months of use. Various estrogen add-back regimens to prevent osteoporosis and thus allow for long-term therapy are currently being studied.

Success rates for the two regimens are similar. Approximately 40 percent of patients successfully conceive after therapy. Pain is improved in 80 to 90 percent of patients after treatment, although the pain recurs in 15 to 30 percent of patients within two years of completing therapy.

Surgical

Historically, surgical treatment by excision or electrocautery were the only options available for treating endometriosis. Technological advances in fiberoptics, pelviscopic equipment, and laser propagation have improved surgical options for treating endometriosis. Laser vaporization offers theoretical advantages over electrocautery. The chances of damage to underlying organs are less because of decreased penetration and decreased thermal destruction. Laser has not been shown to have outcomes significantly better than electrocautery, however, and it is more costly.

Patients with suspected severe endometriosis or

an uncertain diagnosis should have a definitive diagnosis made surgically.

Patients with severe endometriosis are more likely to benefit from surgical treatment than are patients with mild or moderate disease. If severe endometriosis is encountered at the time of diagnostic laparoscopy, treatment can be performed at the time of diagnosis.

If a patient has completed her child-bearing, definitive cure is possible with hysterectomy and bilateral salpingoophorectomy. In addition, presacral neurectomy and ablation of the uterosacral ligaments has been performed to alleviate pain and dysmenorrhea successfully in some patients, while preserving fertility.

Combined Therapy

Combination surgical and medical therapy has some theoretical advantages. Because some endometriosis may be present microscopically without gross evidence of disease, these areas would be missed during surgery. Some investigators have suggested medical treatment with danazol or a GnRH agonist following surgery. One theoretical disadvantage with this approach is that the patient then must delay her attempts to conceive, with greater potential for adhesion formation from the surgery.

Summary

Patients with endometriosis present with a myriad of symptoms including pelvic pain, dyspareunia, dymenorrhea, infertility—or with no symptoms at all. Once the diagnosis is established surgically, medical treatment and follow-up in the office setting are appropriate. In selected cases, empirical medical therapy for endometriosis might be considered prior to surgical evaluation. If the diagnosis is in doubt, however, surgical evaluation is warranted.

References and Suggested Reading

1. ACOG Technical Bulletin No. 185. *Endometriosis.* American College of Obstetricians and Gynecologists, September 1993.
2. Droegemueller W: Endometriosis and adenomyosis, in Herbst AI, Mishell DR, Stenchever MA, Droegemueller W (eds): *Comprehensive Gynecology,* 2d ed. St. Louis: Mosby-Year Book, 1992, pp 545–576.
3. Loy RA, DeCherney AH: Surgery for endometriosis, in Gershenson DM, DeCherney AH, Curry SL (eds): *Operative Gynecology.* Philadelphia: WB Saunders, 1993, pp 569–584.
4. Olive DL, Schwartz LB: Endometriosis. *N Engl J Med* 328:1759–1769, 1993.
5. Seibel M: *Infertility: A Comprehensive Text.* Norwalk, CT: Appleton Lange, 1990, pp 111–128.
6. Speroff L, Glass RH, Kase NG: *Clinical Gynecologic Endocrinology and Infertility.* Baltimore: Williams & Wilkins, 1989, pp 547–564.

29 Office Evaluation of the Infertile Couple

Edward H. Illions
Robert J. Thompson

Infertility, according to American Fertility Society guidelines, is the inability to conceive within 1 year with regular coitus in the absence of any contraception. Implicit in this definition is the understanding that a monogamous relationship exists and the female is ovulatory. The rationale for waiting a full 12 months prior to initiating a complete infertility work-up is supported by known conception rates in fertile couples of 50 percent at 3 months, 75 percent at 9 months, and 90 percent at 1 year.[17] However, for older women it is not uncommon for the decision to be made to initiate the infertility work-up after six months of attempting to become pregnant. The prevalence of infertility in the general population underscores the need for the obstetrician-gynecologist and other primary care specialists to maintain proficiency in the recognition and evaluation of the infertile couple.

Approximately 12 to 15 percent of couples attempting to have children are unable to conceive. Along these lines, the demand for infertility services in this country has increased each year as women postpone attempted conception for career and other reasons. Focusing on the couple as a single unit fosters the psychological interdependence necessary for completion of the infertility work-up. With approximately 40 percent of infertile couples manifesting abnormalities in one or more of the seminal parameters, it behooves the physician to encourage and expect the full participation of the husband.

This chapter presents an approach to the office evaluation of the infertile couple. A companion chapter later in the text (Chap. 37) addresses specific office procedures for infertility patients.

Age-Related Decline in Fecundity

The delay in childbearing by many women in our society has resulted in a condensed time frame available for conception and an appropriate infertility

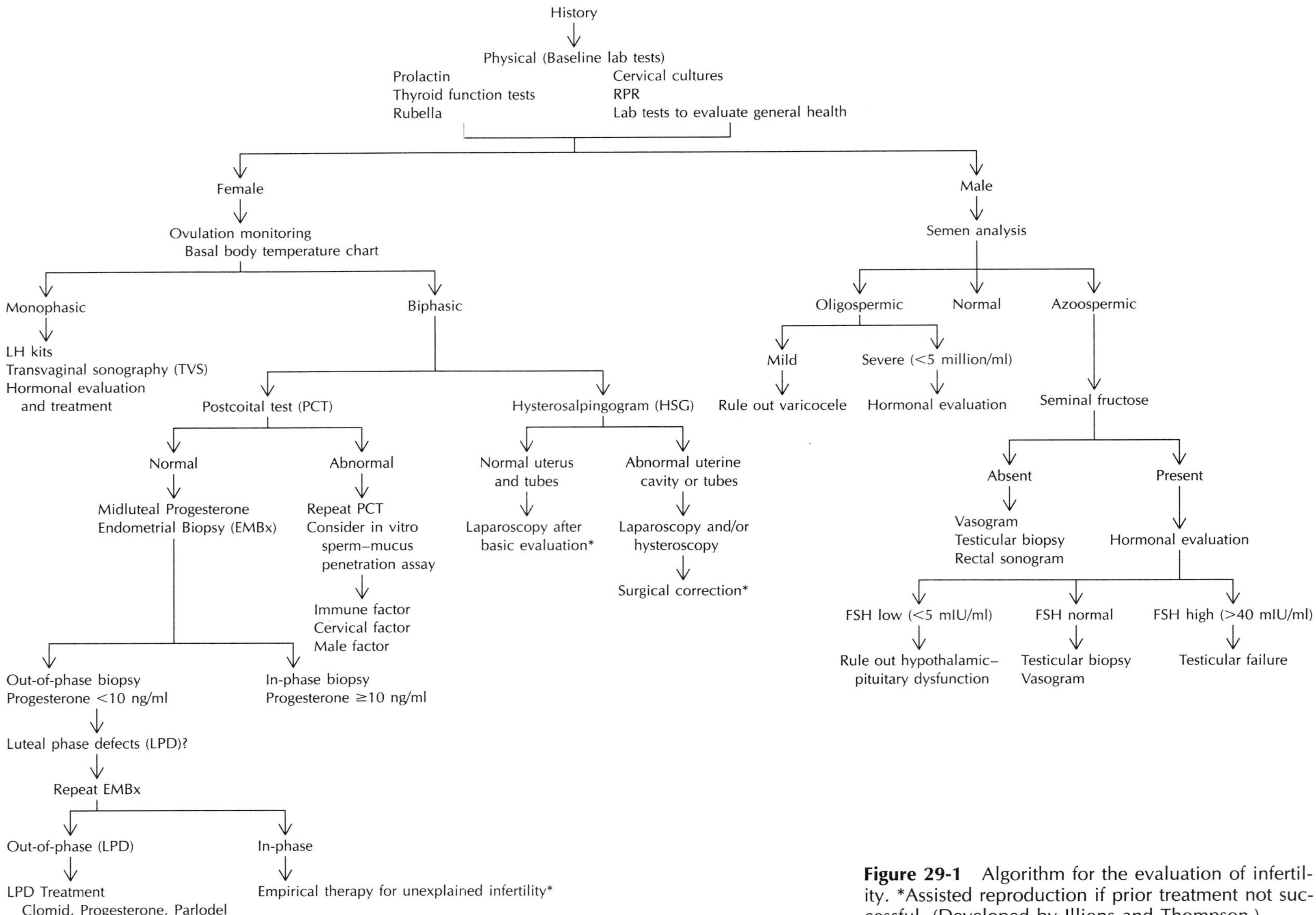

Figure 29-1 Algorithm for the evaluation of infertility. *Assisted reproduction if prior treatment not successful. (Developed by Illions and Thompson.)

work-up. A multitude of social and economic factors influence the decision for women to postpone child-bearing beyond age 35. In addition to career and financial considerations, factors associated with women in their mid-thirties have included decreased frequency of intercourse, increased reliance on contraception, and more frequent endometriosis and myoma.[9]

Fecundity is defined as the physiologic capacity of women to conceive and produce a live birth. It is often expressed in terms of a fecundability rate (observed conceptions per unit time/total number of menstrual cycles). The age-related decline in fecundity, after correcting for the previously mentioned social issues, directly relates to a diminution of ovarian function. There is abundant literature which documents a rise in FSH (follicle stimulating hormone) well in advance of the menopause.[7] Early follicular phase elevation in FSH often occurs in the early forties, whereas the average age of menopause in this country is 51.4, indicating that the ovaries are less responsive to gonadotropins well before the actual cessation of menses. Declining levels of inhibin and other gonadal peptides may be involved in the FSH rise, since LH (luteinizing hormone) levels remain relatively unchanged prior to menopause.[10]

Diminished ovarian function is further suggested by a shortened follicular phase and marked intermenstrual variability. The decrease in reproductive capabilities beyond age 35 is suggested by a 1982 study (Table 29-1) involving donor insemination of 2193 nulliparous women with azoospermic husbands. Cumulative pregnancy rates were analyzed with 12 donor insemination cycles after establishing normal ovulation and tubal patency:[4]

Pregnancy rates in IVF treatment cycles illustrate an age-related decline in clinical pregnancy rates per transfer, most notably beyond age 40.[11] Superimposed on this decline is the high abortion rate (60 percent) in this age group resulting in exceedingly low on-going pregnancy rates after age 40.[18] Data from egg donation programs suggest that declining oocyte and hence embryo quality, as opposed to decreased uterine receptivity, is responsible for low implantation rates and high loss rates in this age group.[12]

TABLE 29-1 Decrease in Fecundity with Age

Age (years)	Cumulative Pregnancy Rates (%)	Fecundability Rates (%)
Less than 30	74	10.5
31–35	61	9.1
Over 35	54	6.5

The Initial Visit

Both partners should be present at the initial infertility appointment. The physician's schedule should allow ample time for in-depth history, physical exam, and the final consultation with the couple that details the overall direction of the impending infertility work-up. An initial visit so constructed will greatly mitigate the anxiety experienced by most infertile couples. Implicit in the successful outcome of this initial office visit is the philosophy that infertility is a "couple's disorder." Combined male and female factors are often found in approximately one-third of infertile couples, documenting the multiplicity of causes and the necessity for a thorough evaluation.

Evaluation of the Female

History

Ovulatory dysfunction is suggested by irregular menses and the absence of premenstrual moliminal changes, whereas the presence of regular menses and molimina indicates ovulation in approximately 98 percent of patients. More than 60 percent of individuals with complete amenorrhea fail to ovulate. In addition, patients with infrequent menses (i.e., three to four per year) are similarly oligoovulatory. A six-month period of medical ovulatory assistance is prudent prior to beginning a lengthy work-up. Age of menarche and thelarche should be elicited in addition to current cycle characteristics (duration and flow). Psychological stress, excessive weight loss from dieting, and strenuous exercise affect ovulation, ostensibly through altered GnRH and LH pulsatility. Headaches and visual complaints occasionally accompany a pituitary tumor, especially if galactorrhea exists. Hirsutism, acne, and oily skin indicate androgen excess that can affect ovulation.

Distorted peritoneal and tubal anatomy may result in altered ovum pick-up and hinder tubal transport of gametes. A history of prior abdominal surgery (or a ruptured appendix) may indicate significant pelvic adhesions. Episodes of sexually transmitted diseases may render fallopian tubes nonfunctional owing to endosalpingeal damage or peritubal adhesions. Complaints of dysmenorrhea, dyspareunia, chronic pelvic pain, and premenstrual spotting may suggest endometriosis or adhesions.

Cervical factors account for only 3 to 5 percent of all infertility cases and may be found in patients with a history of a cone biopsy, cryosurgery, LEEP, or multiple D & Cs. In addition, the DES-exposed individual is at risk for anatomical and functional anomalies of the cervix. Prior surgical procedures on the cervix may result in cervical stenosis or decreased cervical mucus production.

Irregular vaginal bleeding may point to abnormalities within the uterine cavity. A careful history involving menstrual cycle irregularities may indicate the presence of submucosal myomas or intrauterine polyps. In addition, hypomenorrhea or amenorrhea occurring after a curettage of an infected uterus may identify the patient with intrauterine synechiae (Asherman's syndrome). DES-exposed individuals may have structural anomalies of the uterus that result in T-shaped or hypoplastic cavities.

Although many environmental toxins are implicated in reducing fertility rates in laboratory animals, obtaining a history that supports significant human exposure is often quite difficult. However, the physician should ascertain the frequency, amount, and duration of cigarette smoking, drinking of alcohol, and use of illicit drugs. Ample data exist to support detrimental reproductive effects of nicotine and other toxic metabolites found in cigarettes.[15]

A sexual history should include coital frequency and technique. In general, coitus occurring 2 to 3 times per week is adequate for conception. Too frequent ejaculation can deplete the sperm numbers, whereas infrequent ejaculation may adversely affect sperm motility. In addition, the couple should be carefully questioned regarding the use of vaginal lubricants and/or postcoital douching, because both practices potentially are spermicidal. Prior reproductive performance, particularly spontaneous or induced abortions, mid-trimester losses, and postpartum complications, should be elicited.

The Physical Exam

The general physical exam allows additional time to gain personal history by separating the couple. Such delicate topics as prior relationships may be explored at this time. A detailed physical exam should be performed early and may influence the direction of the work-up.

The physician should evaluate overall body dimension and limb length to identify the eunuchoid body habitus or short stature characteristic of genetic abnormalities. Signs of androgen excess are suggested by hirsutism, temporal balding, a male escutcheon pattern, acne, oily skin, and clitoromegaly. Careful palpation of the thyroid gland for enlargement is essential. Evaluation of breast size and shape may indicate inadequate sexual development. One should test for galactorrhea. Surgical scars on the abdomen may suggest underlying intra-abdominal adhesions that might hinder tubal and ovarian reproductive function. Evidence of hypercortisolism should be sought.

External genitalia should be evaluated for developmental abnormalities and clitoromegaly. A blind vaginal pouch in an individual presenting with primary amenorrhea may indicate either müllerian agenesis or complete androgen insensitivity. Cervical abnormalities may be the first clue to DES exposure, prompting additional studies to evaluate the uterine cavity and fallopian tubes. Painful adnexa to lateral cervical motion is suggestive of salpingitis, especially if an odiferous cervical discharge is present. A retroverted or immobile uterus and uterosacral nodularity suggest endometriosis. Ovarian enlargement, especially if associated with menstrual irregularities, may indicate polycystic ovarian syndrome. An enlarged tender uterus and hyperpolymenorrhea is often associated with leiomyoma uteri or adenomyosis. A neurologic exam is useful when screening for the CNS abnormalities that may accompany pituitary tumors.

Evaluation of Ovulation

Ovulatory dysfunction accounts for approximately 25 percent of all instances of reproductive failure. The initial evaluation should determine ovulatory status prior to performing more invasive tests. A history of cyclic menses with premenstrual molimina is indicative of ovulation in 95 to 98 percent of patients. However, since this scenario fails to predict ovulation in all patients, further tests are necessary to evaluate both the presence and quality of ovulation. An understanding of the regulation of the menstrual cycle is essential to appreciate the numerous tests available that predict ovulation.

Regulation of the Menstrual Cycle The typical menstrual cycle consists of three phases: namely, the follicular; ovulatory; and luteal phases. Each segment is characterized by a unique hormonal milieu reflected in peripheral measurements of gonadotropins and gonadal steroids as well as alterations in the female genital tract.

Regulation of the menstrual cycle results from a complex interplay of hypothalamic releasing factors that act on the anterior pituitary, resulting in the pulsatile release of gonadotropins, namely, follicle stimulating hormone (FSH) and luteinizing hormone (LH). These glycoproteins in turn direct ovarian follicular development and stimulate steroidogenesis. Gonadotropin releasing hormone (GnRH), as the hypothalamic releasing factor responsible for gonadotropin production and secretion, is similarly released in a pulsatile fashion every 60 to 90 min in the follicular phase. Control of GnRH release from the median basal hypothalamus is regulated through neuroendocrine input from higher CNS centers, with further refinement by gonadal steroid feedback on both the hypothalamus and pituitary.

Follicular development in the primate is initiated at the completion of the preceding cycle concomitant with an intercycle rise in FSH. Recruitment of a cohort of follicles occurs in the early follicular phase until selection of a dominant follicle by days 5 to 7 of the cycle. Selection is followed by dominance (cycle days 7 to 11) of a single follicle while the remaining cohort of follicles undergo atresia. The dominant follicle is successful in converting its microenvironment from an androgen to an estrogen one. FSH interacts at the level of the ovary to increase its own receptor content (via granulosa cell proliferation) in addition to increasing LH receptor levels in theca and granulosa cells under the combined synergistic influence of estrogen. Although FSH levels actually decrease in the late proliferative phase as estrogen levels rise, the dominant follicle continues to grow, presumably by retaining a higher FSH receptor content, and hence an augmented ability to respond to the lower FSH levels.

The periovulatory period is marked by an abrupt rise in serum estradiol levels to approximately 200 pg/ml for 48 h, which initiates the onset of the gonadotropin surge. The LH surge extends over 48 h, resulting in a sequence of events that culminate in ovulation. The interaction of LH with its receptors in granulosa cells causes resumption of meiosis in addition to luteinization of theca-granulosa cells. The LH surge is also associated with intraovarian elevations of prostaglandins and hyaluronic acid as well as activation of various proteolytic enzymes (collagenase and plasmin). With separation of the oocyte-cumulus mass from the remaining granulosa cells and proteolytic disruption of the follicular wall, ovulation occurs approximately 32 h after the initiation of the LH surge. Extrusion of the oocyte from the ovary coincides with initiation of the luteal phase marked by formation of a corpus luteum and progressive production of progesterone and 17-alpha hydroxyprogesterone. Although estradiol levels rise in the early luteal phase, attaining a peak on postovulatory day 7 to 8, this is less significant than the corresponding progesterone rise, which also peaks on cycle day 21 to 22. Hormonal production by the corpus luteum decidualizes the endometrium in preparation for implantation. Failure to conceive effectively withdraws support from the corpus luteum, and luteolysis ensues approximately 12 to 16 days after the LH surge. The duration of the luteal phase in primates is constant, and its continuation depends on adequate LH support. With the decline in both gonadotropin and gonadal steroid levels in the late luteal phase, endometrial vascular changes and sloughing occur, marking the onset of menstruation. Inhibin and various other gonadal peptides also participate in regulation of the menstrual cycle.

Many of the commonly utilized tests for ovulation reflect adequacy of progesterone secretion and luteinization. Progesterone levels above 3 ng/ml coincide with a temperature elevation of 0.5°F in the luteal phase and form the basis for interpretation of the basal body temperature chart.

Etiologies of Ovulatory Dysfunction The initial concern of the clinician centers around the ovulatory status of the female. Cyclic menses with premenstrual molimina suggest ovulation in the vast majority of cases. An inexpensive initial screening test for ovulation is monitoring the basal body temperature. Although not as precise as more sophisticated tests in determining the periovulatory period, the test does suggest ovulation when a biphasic temperature pattern exists. This test will be covered in detail in the chapter on infertility testing. The BBT chart is examined by the physician usually after two menstrual cycles; however, the infertility work-up is continued by the physician during this time. Since 30 percent of couples have multiple causes for infertility, it is imperative to proceed with associated testing while awaiting completion of the BBT. Obviously, the amenorrheic patient or the individual experiencing infrequent menses is usually anovulatory and need not undergo an initial evaluation with a BBT chart. Some common manifestations of ovulatory dysfunction include amenorrhea, signs of androgen excess, galactorrhea, and a variety of metabolic disorders including thyroid and adrenal dysfunction and weight alterations.

Amenorrhea is classified as either primary or secondary. Primary amenorrhea is the failure to undergo menarche by age 14 in the absence of any secondary sexual development, or by age 16 regardless of the status of secondary development. Secondary amenorrhea is defined by the absence of menses for 6 months in a previously menstruating female. The single most common disorder associated with primary amenorrhea is gonadal dysgenesis secondary to a genetic defect. Classically, patients with Turner's syndrome have a 45,X karyotype, although mosaicism can occur. These women usually present with primary amenorrhea and sexual infantilism; the ovaries typically appear as streaks, presumably secondary to accelerated follicular atresia. Other associated abnormalities include short stature, webbed neck, high-arched palate, epicanthal folds, low-set prominent ears, an increased carrying angle of the arms (cubitus valgus), wide-set nipples, and coarctation of the aorta. Infrequently, patients with Turner's syndrome may menstruate and occasionally conceive, depending on the rate of follicular atresia and/or the presence of mosaicism.

The second most common condition causing primary amenorrhea is müllerian agenesis characterized by the congenital absence of some or all of the gynecologic organs of müllerian origin (vagina, cervix, uterus, or fallopian tubes). Ovarian function is normal; thus, secondary sexual development occurs. The third most common etiology is complete androgen insensitivity characterized by a 46,XY karyotype and a functioning testes. Defects in the androgen receptor result in inability to virilize, yielding a female phenotype and absent or sparse body hair. This disorder should be suspected in any individual with a blind vaginal pouch, absent uterus, and a testosterone level in the normal male range (300 to 900 ng/dl).

Evaluation of secondary amenorrhea includes initially ruling out pregnancy followed by a systematic work-up that examines patency of the genital outflow tract and the integrity of the hypothalamic-pituitary-ovarian axis. Besides amenorrhea, various other conditions are associated with anovulatory cycles and deserve special attention.

Hyperprolactinemia, an elevated pituitary secretion of prolactin, is discovered in 20 percent of amenorrheic patients and may be present in menstruating infertile patients. Hyperprolactinemia alters GnRH pulsatility. Physiologic conditions other than pregnancy that may result in an elevated prolactin include exercise and stress. Medications such as phenothiazines, haloperidol, Aldomet, reserpine, metoclopromide, and estrogens also may result in elevated prolactin levels. Pathologic causes of hyperprolactinemia include pituitary adenomas, hypothalamic lesions, chest wall lesions, renal failure, and hypothyroidism.

In addition to ovulatory disturbances, prolactin excess can result in galactorrhea and, less frequently, signs and symptoms of hypoestrogenism. Deranged GnRH pulsatility can manifest as frank anovulation, oligoovulation, or merely altered luteal function. The vast majority of patients respond well to a change in life-style or medical therapy with bromocriptine (a dopamine agonist).

Androgen excess can occur from increased ovarian or adrenal production rates in addition to any condition that lowers sex hormone binding globulin (SHBG) levels. The decreased androgen binding sites associated with lowered SHBG elevates free androgen levels, thereby effectively increasing availability of the metabolically active androgens for intracellular use. Markedly elevated testosterone (over 200 ng/dl) or dehydroepiandrosterone sulfate (DHEAS) levels (over 700 μg/dl) suggest an androgen-producing tumor in the ovary or adrenal, respectively.[14] Signs of virilization such as deepening of the voice, change of body habitus, clitoromegaly, and temporal balding suggest an androgen-producing tumor.

Polycystic ovarian syndrome (PCO) is a state of chronic anovulation resulting from hypothalamic-pituitary, ovarian, and adrenal dysfunction. Approximately 75 percent of patients with PCO are infertile, and 70 percent are hirsute.[3] Additional symptoms include amenorrhea, obesity, and dysfunctional uterine bleeding. Tonic elevations of LH often result in marked ovarian stromal production of androgens. PCO patients frequently have hyperinsulinemia, reflecting increased insulin resistance.

Diagnosis of PCO is suggested when these symptoms occur in patients with elevated LH/FSH ratios (greater than 2:1) and moderate elevations of serum androgens (frequently high-normal levels). A more exaggerated form of ovarian androgen excess is termed stromal hyperthecosis.

Treatment of these androgen excess disorders in the infertility population consists of inducing ovulation. Androgen excess secondary to ovarian or adrenal tumors is best treated surgically. PCO patients generally respond to ovulation induction with clomiphene citrate but occasionally require gonadotropin therapy. Patients with stromal hyperthecosis frequently fail to respond to conventional medical therapy for ovulation induction.

Luteal Phase Defect accounts for 3 to 5 percent of all causes of female infertility. Corpus luteum function is vital for proper uterine receptivity and embryo implantation. Inadequate preparation of the endometrium from deficient progesterone production characterizes luteal phase defects. Luteal phase defects arise from either subnormal progesterone levels (inadequate luteal phase) or shortened duration of action on the endometrium with normal progesterone levels (shortened luteal phase). Abnormal corpus luteum function can arise from aberrant folliculogenesis, elevated prolactin levels, or hypothalamic dysfunction secondary to weight loss, stress, exercise, or hyperandrogen states.

Shortened luteal phases are suggested when luteal phase temperature elevations (BBT) are less than 11 days. When midluteal serum progesterone levels fall below 10 ng/ml, inadequate luteal phases may exist, and both entities need confirmation by endometrial biopsy. Currently, endometrial biopsy performed in the late luteal phase represents the gold standard for diagnosis of luteal phase dysfunction and is confirmatory when there is more than a 2-day lag in histologic development. A second late luteal biopsy is necessary to confirm the diagnosis. Whereas a midluteal progesterone level of 3 ng/ml corresponds with an elevation of the basal body temperature, recent studies indicate that levels over 10 ng/ml are necessary to rule out luteal phase defects.[5] The controversy involving interpretation of midluteal progesterone levels, however, precludes using this test as the sole determinant for diagnosis.

Treatment of luteal phase defects involves correction of the underlying disorder. In euprolactinemic patients with normal androgen levels, clomiphene citrate or progesterone administration is utilized. Clomiphene citrate (50 to 100 mg) is administered on days 5 to 9 of the menstrual cycle to stimulate an elevation of FSH to improve folliculogenesis. Pregnancy rates with clomiphene usage are reported between 25 and 75 percent. Pregnancy rates are highest when repeat biopsy confirms correction of the histologic lag.[2] Clomiphene used at high dosage may actually cause or worsen luteal phase dysfunction. Progesterone therapy yields similar results, but its use is limited by the required intramuscular or vaginal (or rectal) routes of administration. Refractory cases occasionally respond to gonadotropin therapy, whereas hyperprolactinemic individuals are best treated with bromocriptine.

Hypothalamic dysfunction is a common cause of deranged ovulation and in severe form may result in amenorrhea. Over 50 percent of all causes of secondary amenorrhea can be traced to the hypothalamus. In general, hypothalamic amenorrhea can be categorized as organic or functional. Congenital gonadotropin deficiency and destructive lesions of the hypothalamus represent organic causes (rare), while various physiologic states, medication usage, hyperprolactinemia, and psychogenic causes comprise the functional category (common). Stress, weight loss, exercise, and medications can disrupt GnRH pulsatility as reflected in abnormal LH pulses. Since serum estradiol levels often exceed 40 pg/ml, one can elicit a withdrawal bleed to progesterone administration that has clinical utility in the diagnostic work-up and indicates a good prognosis for ovulation induction with clomiphene therapy.

No identifiable cause for hypothalamic dysfunction is found in most individuals. However, the vast majority of these patients will respond to ovulation induction with clomiphene citrate. Hypoestrogenic patients and those failing clomiphene therapy often benefit from gonadotropins or pulsatile GnRH administration.

Endocrine dysfunction: the three most common endocrine disorders manifesting as ovulatory dysfunction include hypothyroidism, uncontrolled diabetes mellitus, and hypercortisolism (Cushing's syndrome). Although thyroid abnormalities are rare, a few simple blood tests will uncover this correctable condition. Patient complaints of weight gain, lethargy, decreased energy level, constipation, and cold intolerance should alert the physician to pursue a work-up for hypothyroidism. Similarly, approximately 75 percent of individuals with cortisol excess have menstrual irregularities. Cushing's syndrome should be considered in any patient manifesting the typical stigmata of hypercortisolism; namely dorsocerival hump, supraclavicular fat pads, hirsutism, truncal obesity, moon facies and facial plethora, proximal muscle wasting, easy bruisability, hypertension, glucose intolerance, and violaceous striae.

Initial Evaluation of Peritoneal and Tubal Factors

Abnormalities in this category comprise 22 to 25 percent of all causes of female infertility. The dramatic rise in the incidence of sexually transmitted diseases in the last two decades has contributed to a concomitant increase in tubal pathology. The three- to four-fold rise in the incidence of ectopic pregnancy during the same period is directly attributed to marked increases in the incidence of *Neisseria gonorrhoeae* and Chlamydia infections. The available tests to evaluate patency of the female genital tract, however, often yield little information regarding the overall reproductive function of these structures. In short, while luminal patency is demonstrated, these tests cannot reliably predict either ability of the fimbria to complete ovum capture or adequacy of tubal transport mechanisms. A hysterosalpingogram (HSG) is often used as the initial screening test for tubal evaluation with laparoscopy serving a back-up role and representing the "gold standard" for evaluation of tubal and peritoneal factors. Abnormalities of the uterine cavity alone comprise only 3 to 5 percent of all causes of female infertility but are included in this section since the HSG represents an important screening test for both the uterus as well as tubal and peritoneal factors. The HSG is performed fairly early in the work-up of the infertile couple but is often preceded by a semen analysis and tests to determine ovulatory status in the female.

Evaluation of the Uterine Cavity

While abnormalities of the uterine cavity are rare causes of infertility, they are nonetheless common in the general population. Myomas and endometrial polyps are most frequently encountered, though intrauterine adhesions, congenital anomalies of the uterus, and foreign bodies within the cavity may be found.

Hysterosalpingography is often used as one of the initial screening tests for most infertile patients. The HSG is less sensitive for uncovering polyps and adhesions than for diagnosing myomas and congenital defects in the uterine cavity. There is a 1 to 3 percent chance of pelvic infection associated with an HSG; therefore, it should be avoided in patients considered to be at high risk: namely, patients with a history of salpingitis or tuboovarian abscess and/or recent pelvic pain.[16] High-risk patients should be screened with hysteroscopy to avoid this complication. Similarly, any patients with an abnormal uterine cavity by HSG should undergo hysteroscopy for a definitive diagnosis. Visualization of large fundal filling defects suggests congenital anomalies such as a bicornuate or septate uterus. Intrauterine pathology may cause infertility by hindering implantation or sperm ascent, or by obliteration of the tubal ostia. In addition, intrauterine synechiae (Asherman's syndrome), which often arise from postpartum curettage of an infected uterus, may cause infertility and may result in hypo- or amenorrhea.

When lysis of intrauterine synechiae or removal of space-occupying lesions is warranted, operative hysteroscopy is the treatment of choice. In general, since intrauterine abnormalities are a rare cause of infertility, their operative correction is undertaken only after ovulatory disturbances are corrected and any significant male factor is excluded.

Evaluation of Tubal Patency

Patients with tubal pathology on HSG should undergo laparoscopy, which confirms tubal disease in two-thirds of cases. Proximal tubal disease may cause unilateral or bilateral cornual occlusion. The most common etiologies of proximally obstructed tubes include salpingitis isthmica nodosa (SIN), inflammatory changes from ascending infection, cornual myomas, endometriosis, and tubal diverticuli. SIN has a characteristic "fingerprint" pattern in the isthmus on HSG, reflecting the underlying histologic abnormality of this entity: namely, multiple luminal diverticuli throughout the tubal muscularis layer.

Distal tubal disease is the most frequently encountered tubal abnormality and arises from ascending infection or prior surgery. Distal disease includes a wide range of abnormalities, from tubal phimosis to complete obstruction with loss of all normal tubal mucosal folds (hydrosalpinx). Pregnancy rates following surgical therapy in patients with distal disease are uniformly poor, but correlate with tubal diameter, tubal wall thickness, presence of peritubal adhesions, and the presence of ampullary mucosal folds on HSG.

Surgical correction may involve hysteroscopic tubal cannulation for proximal occlusions, laparoscopic adhesiolysis and neosalpingostomy for distal occlusions and laparotomy for tubocornual anastomosis or tubal reimplantation. Patients with evidence of proximal and distal disease (bipolar tubal disease) are not surgical candidates because pregnancy rates are exceedingly low and these women are better served by in-vitro fertilization. Of course, many women with single site tubal disease are also treated with in-vitro fertilization.

Evaluation of Peritoneal Factors

Laparoscopy is the definitive diagnostic modality to evaluate peritoneal factors. Laparoscopy affords direct visualization of the pelvis, enabling the diagnosis and location of adhesions and a definitive diagnosis and staging of endometriosis.

Peritubal adhesions may restrict tubal motility and hence prevent ovum capture and inhibit embryo transport. The incidence of pelvic adhesions is not insignificant, for approximately one-third of "normal" women who have laparoscopy have adhesive disease. The incidence rises to 76 percent in infertile women with a history of pelvic surgery or pelvic pain.[1] Endometriosis occurs in 5 to 10 percent of the general population and in up to 25 percent of infertile women.

Severe endometriosis causes marked distortion of pelvic anatomy through the formation of ovarian endometriomas and dense pelvic adhesions. Minimal and mild disease is characterized by peritoneal implants without extensive ovarian involvement or pelvic scarring. In this setting, infertility may result from subtle ovulatory dysfunction and/or alterations in the peritoneal fluid environment.

Treatment is based on the severity of the condition (see Chap. 28). Minimal and mild disease can be managed expectantly, as recent studies have demonstrated equal pregnancy rates when compared to laparoscopic ablation of the lesions or medical management.[13] Moderate and severe disease is best treated surgically. Pregnancy rates are dramatically increased when either a laparoscopy or laparotomy is successful in restoring normal pelvic anatomical relationships.

Laparoscopy may serve both a diagnostic and therapeutic role. Aside from confirming pathology, the surgeon has the capability to perform adhesiolysis, resect and ablate endometrial implants, and reestablish tubal patency. Pregnancy rates are determined by the extent of preexisting disease and the surgeon's ability to restore normal tuboovarian relationships.

Evaluation of Cervical Factors

The cervix acts as a conduit and reservoir for sperm transport, a biological filter for microorganisms and unfit sperm, and a source of nutrients and capacitation for mature sperm. A history of DES exposure, prior surgery on the cervix (cone biopsy, cryotherapy), or cervical infection all may diminish mucus production and hinder sperm transport. The high estrogen levels at midcycle stimulate cervical mucus production. Midcycle mucus is acellular, nonviscous, watery, and abundant. Sperm transport through mucus is maximal under these conditions and is initially assessed with a postcoital test. This is generally evaluated prior to performance of invasive procedures such as laparoscopy. Lack of motile sperm during this test may indicate inappropriate timing, poor cervical mucus production, or sperm antibodies that inhibit proper sperm motility.

In vitro sperm-mucus penetration tests may be done utilizing a column of bovine donor mucus. Sperm penetration through this column is compared with the sperm–mucus interaction in a column of the woman's cervical mucus.

Sperm-directed antibodies represent 3 percent of all causes of infertility. Antibody-bound sperm may exist when a postcoital test (PCT) reveals nonmotile or shaking sperm. Antibodies (IgG, IgM, or IgA) secreted in the genital tract may bind to the head, tail, or midpiece of the sperm membrane, causing agglutination, immobilization or impairment of either capacitation or the acrosomal reaction.

Treatment for antisperm antibodies is limited by difficulty in removing membrane-bound antibodies. Attempts at therapy continue to result in poor fertilization rates. Glucocorticoid immunosuppressive therapy is still utilized, but has now largely been replaced by enzymatic digestion of the antibodies, intrauterine insemination of washed sperm, or in-vitro fertilization. The definitive test for detection of membrane-bound sperm antibodies is the immunobead test (IBT).

Male Factor Infertility

Male factor is found in 30 to 40 percent of infertile couples. This statistic underscores the importance of interviewing both the man and the woman at the initial interview. Too often, men are reluctant to participate in the infertility work-up and assume the female to be solely responsible for any inability to conceive. The physician must actively solicit the male's participation when initiating an infertility work-up.

Anatomy and Physiology of the Male

The testes are both sites of steroidogenesis and sperm production. These processes involve a coordinated effort of the entire hypothalamic-pituitary-testicular axis and—unlike the female—allows the male to constantly produce mature gametes. Normally, 72 days are required for an immature germ cell to develop into the mature spermatozoan, with 5 additional days allotted for epididymal maturation.

GnRH is secreted from the hypothalamus in a pulsatile fashion and results in synthesis and release of gonadotropins (FSH and LH) from the anterior pituitary. LH binds to receptors on the Leydig cell in the testis, causing testosterone production. FSH stimulates Sertoli cells and, with high intratesticular testosterone levels, generates spermatogenesis.

Normal testicular size depends directly on seminiferous tubule volume and therefore reflects the presence of a functioning germinal epithelium. A testicular length less than 4 cm or inadequate volume (less than 18 cc) may suggest a volume of seminiferous tubules inadequate for normal sperm production.

After ejaculation, mature sperm undergo various surface changes called capacitation. These changes can also be artificially induced in vitro. Spermatozoa, upon reaching the zona pellucida, undergo an acrosomal reaction, allowing release of various enzymes from the acrosome of the sperm head. These enzymes enable the sperm to effectively penetrate the oocyte via digestion of the zona pellucida. Fertilization occurs in the distal oviduct once fusion of the two pronuclei is completed.

Evaluation of the Male

History The male should be questioned on coital technique, timing, and frequency. Symptoms of inadequate androgen are suggested by decreased libido, history of cryptorchidism, decreased frequency of shaving, hypospadias, lack of pubertal development, and erectile and ejaculatory dysfunction. Recent drug usage (sulfasalazine, nitrofurantoin, ethanol, and chemotherapeutic agents) and exposure to environmental toxins must be ruled out. Excessive cigarette smoking and marijuana usage are associated with subnormal spermatogenesis. Heavy metals and ionizing radiation are often deleterious to spermatogenesis, as is testicular exposure to excessive heat. Pubertal or postpubertal mumps orchitis often results in irreparable testicular damage. A history of surgery (abdominal or genital) or genital injuries is elicited, as is a medical history of any systemic illness. Subfertile males with a history of chronic sinusitis and/or respiratory infections may have concomitant sperm motility disorders. In addition, liver disease and chronic renal failure adversely affect Leydig cell function and seminiferous tubule function. Diabetes mellitus, spinal cord injuries, and retroperitoneal lymph node dissection may result in retrograde ejaculation, as evidenced by a small semen volume and the presence of sperm in a post-ejaculatory urine. A past history of genital infections or recent testicular pain, dysuria, and penile discharge must be elicited and may indicate an active prostatitis, urethritis, or epididymitis.

Physical A complete physical exam should be performed. The physician must carefully note any signs of hypogonadism, namely, decreased facial and body hair, eunuchoid body proportions, underdevelopment of the external genitalia, and gynecomastia. The external genitalia should be evaluated for evidence of hypospadias and testicular size and consistency. Testicular dimensions are normal when linear length exceeds 4 cm and testicular volume is at least 18 cc measured with a Prader orchiometer. Presence of the vas deferens is confirmed by careful palpation of the spermatic cord while a Valsalva maneuver aids in detection of a varicocele.

The Semen Analysis

Regardless of the history and physical, all males should undergo a semen analysis as the initial screening test. The male should be carefully counseled regarding a proper collection technique. After abstaining from ejaculation for at least 48 h (longer than 72 h is not necessary) a masturbated specimen is collected in a wide mouth jar. Ideally the semen should be analyzed within 30 to 45 min of collec-

TABLE 29-2 Etiologies of Male Infertility

Etiology	Frequency (%)
Idiopathic	70–75
Testicular disorders	10–13
Genital tract obstructions	8–10
Sperm autoimmunity	4–6
Endocrine disorders	1
Coital disorders	1

tion. Any semen specimen transported to the laboratory must be kept at body temperature.

The semen is evaluated for volume, sperm concentration, viscosity, pH, sperm motility, and morphology. The normal parameters are listed in Table 29-3.

Owing to marked variability between semen specimens, it is customary to obtain at least two separate specimens 2 to 4 weeks apart.

Consistent volumes below 2 ml should prompt an investigation for ductal obstruction, absence of the seminal vesicles, and retrograde ejaculation. A combination of the physical exam, rectal probe sonography, and seminal fructose will delineate an obstruction or absence of the seminal vesicles. Retrograde ejaculation is suspected in individuals with low seminal volumes and postejaculatory urine specimens containing many sperm. Persistent oligospermia with normal collection techniques may indicate the need for an endocrine evaluation of the male.

When overall motility and/or directional motion is diminished, the physician should consider the possibility of either genital infection or varicocele. Leukocytospermia and a seminal culture will confirm the presence of bacteria and infection; a genital exam by palpation evaluates for varicocele. Scrotal Doppler studies may be needed to uncover subclinical varicoceles. Cigarette smoking, marijuana, environmental toxins, and androgen-deficient states may also decrease sperm motility, as can epididymal dysfunction. The role of antisperm antibodies as a cause of asthenospermia has been discussed previously. Rarely, a hereditary disorder in ciliary action can result in poor sperm motility along with chronic pulmonary problems (immotile cilia syndrome).

TABLE 29-3 Normal Semen Analysis

Volume	2 to 6 ml
Concentration	Greater than 20 million/ml
Viscosity	Liquefaction in under 30 min
pH	7.2 to 7.8
Motility	Over 50% (initial and 1-h)
Morphology	Over 50 to 60% oval (normal forms)
Cellularity (leukocytes)	Less than 1 million/ml

Evaluation of sperm morphology is somewhat subjective, relying on the expertise of the technician. Overall, normal forms exceeding 50 percent is considered adequate. In recent years, Kruger has developed strict criteria for sperm morphology.[6] Under his system, adequate in-vitro fertilization rates exist when at least 14 percent of sperm have normal morphology. IVF success rates fall drastically when strict criteria grading indicate less than 4 percent normal morphology.

Endocrine Evaluation of the Male

An endocrine evaluation should be done in cases of severe oligospermia (less than 5 to 10 million/ml) or azoospermia. FSH, LH, TSH, prolactin, testosterone, and estradiol levels should be obtained. An elevated TSH suggests hypothyroidism, which is easily treated. FSH and LH values that exceed 40 mIU/ml indicate primary testicular failure, which is refractory to treatment. Low FSH and LH are associated with hypothalamic-pituitary dysfunction, and further evaluation is necessary. Radiographic imaging with MRI or CT in conjunction with a GnRH stimulation test often aid in delineating hypothalamic from pituitary disorders. Gonadotropin or pulsatile GnRH therapy may be successful. Rarely, FSH may be normal while LH and testosterone levels are high, suggesting partial androgen resistance. Skin fibroblast cultures for androgen receptors are necessary to confirm the diagnosis. Occasionally, only FSH is elevated and may indicate germinal cell failure (Sertoli-cell only syndrome).

However, the vast majority of men have a normal endocrine profile. In such cases, additional studies to exclude ductal obstruction are indicated. Since fructose is produced in the seminal vesicles, its presence in semen excludes ductal obstruction or absence or atresia of the seminal vesicles. In males with azoospermia or severe oligospermia (less than 1 million/ml), a testicular biopsy may be indicated once obstruction is excluded (fructose-positive). Testicular biopsy can distinguish between disorders of sperm maturation and an acquired, proximal ductal obstruction. A vasogram combined with the biopsy further delineates the cause.

Unexplained Infertility

When the studies outlined above in the woman and the man are normal, their infertility is said to be unexplained. Approximately 10 to 15 percent of infertile couples will have no discernible cause demonstrated.[8] Obviously there is an explanation for a couple's inability to conceive, but neither medical knowledge nor the fertility investigation is sophisticated enough to find the cause. Second-level testing may define abnormalities in sperm function [sperm antibody testing, sperm penetration assay (SPA), and the hemizona sperm binding assay (HZA)], oocyte quality, and sperm–oocyte interaction. Subtle infections or autoimmunity may be present. However, spontaneous pregnancies have been reported, with an average cumulative pregnancy rate of 60 percent within 3 years without therapy.

Therapy may allow pregnancy to happen sooner and may be beneficial in correcting undefined causes.

Certainly any life-style that may have a deleterious effect on fertility should be modified. The use of alcohol and tobacco should be curtailed. Diet and exercise should be adjusted for a normal weight.

A 4- to 6-month trial of therapy may be recommended to include controlled ovarian hyperstimulation and intrauterine insemination (IUI), in-vitro fertilization-embryo transfer (IVF-ET) and/or gamete intrafallopian tube transfer (GIFT).

Summary

Primary and secondary infertility are not infrequent findings in the general population. The clinician should have a keen understanding of the various etiologies of infertility in the male and female. A simple and cost-effective work-up for the evaluation of infertility has been suggested; it includes an initial evaluation of the ovulatory status of the female combined with the evaluation of a semen analysis. Evaluation of tubal and peritoneal factors are likewise performed early in the work-up of the couple. Ovulatory dysfunction can be evaluated further by such specialized tests as urinary LH monitoring, transvaginal sonography, and late luteal endometrial biopsies. Secondary testing may include evaluation of sperm–mucus interactions and specialized tests of sperm function. A small subset of patients will have completely normal testing and are best treated by superovulation and intrauterine insemination for a few cycles. Some peritoneal and tubal disorders require surgical correction; others may require assisted reproductive technology.

In spite of a detailed work-up and advanced therapeutic modalities, some patients still fail to conceive. Owing to the intense psychological stress, these couples may be offered no treatment for a few cycles. Spontaneous pregnancies have been reported in such individuals. Finally, adoption should be discussed as a viable alternative for patients failing to conceive with assisted reproduction. Intense counseling is often required for such individuals.

References and Selected Readings

1. Collins JA: Diagnostic assessment of the infertile female partner. *Curr Probl Obstet Gynecol Fertil* 11:11, 1988.
2. Daley DC, Walters CA, Soto-Albors CE, Riddick DH: Endometrial biopsy during treatment of luteal phase defects is predictive of therapeutic outcome. *Fertil Steril* 40:305, 1983.
3. Falcone T, Bourque J, Granger L, et al: Polycystic ovary syndrome. *Curr Probl Obstet Gynceol Fertil* 16:69, 1993.
4. Federation CECOS, Schwart D, Mayaux NJ: Female fecundity as a function of age: Results of artificial insemination in 2193 nulliparous women with azoospermic husbands. *N Engl J Med* 306:404, 1982.
5. Johansson EDB: Progesterone levels in peripheral plasma during the luteal phase of the normal human menstrual cycle measured by a rapid competitive protein binding technique. *Acta Endocrinol (Copenh)* 61:592, 1969.
6. Kruger TF, Acosta AA, Simmons KF, et al: Predictive value of abnormal sperm morphology in in vitro fertilization. *Fertil Steril* 49:112, 1988.
7. Lee SJ, Lenton EA, Sexton L, et al: The effect of age on the cyclical patterns of plasma LH, FSH, oestradiol and progesterone in women with regular menstrual cycles. *Hum Reprod* 3:851, 1988.
8. Lobo RA: Unexplained infertility. *J Reprod Med* 38:241, 1993.
9. Maroulis GB: Effect of aging on fertility and pregnancy. *Semin Reprod Endocrinol* 9:165, 1991.
10. Mars R, Lobo R, Campeau J, et al: Correlation of human follicular fluid inhibin activity with spontaneous and in-

duced follicle maturation. *J Clin Endocrinol Metab* 58:704, 1984.

11. Padilla SL, Garcia JE: Effect of maternal age and number of in vitro procedures on pregnancy outcome. *Fertil Steril* 52:270, 1989.
12. Rotsztejn DA, Asch RH: Effect of aging on assisted reproductive technologies (ART): Experience from egg donation. *Semin Reprod Endocrinol* 9:272, 1991.
13. Schenken RS, Malinak LR: Conservative surgery versus expectant management for the infertile patient with mild endometriosis. *Fertil Steril* 37:183, 1982.
14. Speroff L, Glass RH, Kase NG: Hirsutism, in *Clinical Gynecologic Endocrinology and Infertility,* 4th ed. Baltimore: Williams & Wilkins, 1989, p 233.
15. Stillman RJ, Rosenberg MJ, Sachs RP: Smoking and reproduction, in Wallach EE, Kempers RD (eds): *Modern Trends in Infertility and Contraception Control.* Chicago: Year Book Medical Publishers, 1988, p 31.
16. Stumpf PG, March CM: Febrile morbidity following hysterosalpingography: Identification of risk factors and recommendations for prophylaxis. *Fertil Steril* 33:487, 1980.
17. Tietze C, Guttmacher AF, Rubin S: Time required for conception in 1727 planned pregnancies. *Fertil Steril* 1:338, 1950.
18. Warburton D, Fraser F: Spontaneous abortion risks in man: Data from reproductive histories collected in a medical genetics unit. *Hum Genet* 16:1, 1964.

30 Chronic Pelvic Pain and Dyspareunia

John F. Steege

The problems of chronic pelvic pain and dyspareunia are among the most challenging faced by the primary care physician. Women so affected are often frustrated by the chronicity of the problems and the apparent lack of clear solutions. The complexities of psychosocial and sexual factors as well as the frequent involvement of nongynecologic organ systems in symptom production may make it difficult for the clinician to help to address the problem. The concepts presented here are a brief summary of clinical guidelines for the evaluation and treatment of these problems.

The General Approach

When evaluating these problems, it often serves the patient best to maintain a careful balance between pursuit of physical factors and consideration of psychological concerns. Given the usual constraints of time, skill, and inclination, clinicians sometimes either pursue organic therapies beyond the limits of their utility, or prematurely assume that psychological factors are responsible for the problem if a clear organic etiology is not evident. Examples of the former include the repeated prescription of various vaginal medications for vaginal symptoms occurring in the absence of pathology or pathogens, or the repeated lysis of adhesions in the chronic pain sufferer. An example of the latter is immediately referring the patient with dyspareunia for psychotherapy upon learning of her past history of being sexually abused.

These approaches spring from our traditional Western cultural predilection to separate mind and body. Recent theories of pain perception and sexual function attempt to integrate psychological and physical processes very closely. The scientific underpinnings of this approach lie in our expanding understanding of the biochemical pathways involved in the regulation of mood, libido, and pain perception. Although our understanding of these pathways remains primitive, the field has progressed to the point that clinical evaluation and treatment should take its findings into account. For example, it no longer makes sense for the gynecologist to describe a "negative laparoscopy" and conclude therefore that no physical cause for pain exists. At the same time, the mental health clinician should not ask for the patient to be "cleared gynecologically" before beginning psychotherapy or other forms of counseling. Rather, the evaluation and treatment should be interactive and collaborative in an ongoing fashion.

Recognizing the Problem

Chronic pain is best viewed as a rather different illness from acute pain. It is by nature multifactorial, making it necessary often to treat with several modalities at once. For example, one might simultaneously offer suggestions for improving chronic constipation, diminishing the frequency of postcoital urinary tract infections, and resolving depression by taking a serotonergic antidepressant. One surrenders the intellectual satisfaction of figuring out which component is the most significant, but the chance of a good outcome is enhanced.

When dealing with chronic pain, the clinician also must recognize that pain will not necessarily be proportional to the amount of organic disease present. This absence of correlation has now been documented for both endometriosis and pelvic adhesions, the two forms of organic pathology most frequently present in cases of chronic pelvic pain. The clinical query must be rephrased to ask whether or not treatment of visible organic changes will be sufficient therapy, or whether the patient will need other treatments for other components of her chronic pain syndrome.

How can the clinician recognize when a patient has developed a chronic pain syndrome? While there are exceptions to every generalization, some reliable hallmarks appear to include:

1. Duration of pain longer than six months.
2. Incomplete relief by medical or surgical therapies.
3. Discontinuation of some physical function (e.g., athletics, coitus, household tasks).
4. Signs of depression (sleep disturbance, weight loss, loss of appetite).
5. Significant alterations in family roles (e.g., emotional support of children or extended family, financial decision-making). Basically, if the patient or her family considers her problem to be the most significant problem the *family* faces, then family dynamics have likely changed in important ways. Questions that might be included in the history to bring out these issues are listed in Table 30-1. Recognizing this pattern impels a shift to a multifactorial diagnostic and treatment approach.

Educating the Patient

With rare exceptions, the patient with chronic pain or dyspareunia believes—or at least strongly wishes—that a single diagnosable and treatable cause must exist. Once a patient's problem is recognized as being complex and chronic, it is worth taking the time to educate her and at least one member of her family about the nature of chronic pain. Expectations should be made more realistic, and their participation solicited in the development of a management plan to treat whatever portion of the pain cannot be resolved. This goes beyond suggesting that she must "learn to live with it," and might include the notions that: 1. no single cause is likely to be found; 2. several contributing factors may need simultaneous treatment; 3. it probably will not be possible to tell how much of the problem is physical and how much is psychological; and 4. regardless of how a problem has started, when it becomes severe, mental health help often aids the patient and her family in the effort to reduce both the discomfort itself and its impact.

With this background in mind, the following sections will summarize the historical questions, physical examination findings, and treatment suggestions appropriate for various factors commonly involved in chronic pelvic pain and dyspareunia.

Factors That Can Be Diagnosed by Physical Examination and/or Laparoscopy

Endometriosis

The severity of pain associated with endometriosis does not correlate (either directly or inversely) with the amount of endometriosis present when one com-

TABLE 30-1 Questions Relevant to the Hallmarks of a Chronic Pain Syndrome

1. Duration >6 months	How long has the pain been present? How long (months) did it take to get to its worst level? What was going on in your life when it got worse?
2. Incomplete relief by medical/surgical treatments	On a scale of 1–10, how much did each treatment help? For how long after surgery did the pain remain lessened? When the pain returned, what did you notice first? Next?
3. Discontinuation of some physical functions	What have you stopped doing because of the pain? When? What activities have you continued despite the pain? On the 1–10 scale, what happens to the pain when you do (some activity)? Are you considering stopping work? (. . . applying for disability?) Regarding sex, has frequency decreased? Is there more pain than pleasure? What were things like sexually before the pain?
4. Signs of depression	Does the pain wake you up? Do you wake up early and then can't get back to sleep, not particularly because of the pain? Do you have crying spells? Feelings of great sadness? Loss of appetite? Gain or loss of weight? Loss of sexual interest? Suicidal feelings?
5. Altered family dynamics	Who disciplines the kids? (. . . helps with their homework, pays the bills, makes vacation plans, decides what to buy)? How this changed because of the pain? Is your pain the biggest problem the family faces?

pares one patient with another. Within the experience of an individual patient, increased pain often means increased disease, with the site of the pain usually corresponding fairly accurately to the location of the disease. However, in the patient who starts to show the hallmarks of a chronic pain syndrome, the pain may progress when the organic pathology is stable. Questions aimed at diagnosing a chronic pain syndrome become appropriate (Table 30-1).

A typical historical scenario for a person who develops symptoms due to endometriosis might include a gradual increase in the duration of the strongest menstrual cramps (e.g., increasing from one to three or four days), appearance of premenstrual pain, and cylic dyspareunia that gradually becomes continuous but remains worst perimenstrually. Painful defecation is less common, as is a more internal, visceral discomfort on urination.

Another very important set of factors may increase the pain associated with endometriosis. Understanding that pelvic examinations (as well as ultrasound and other scans) are at best a crude indicator of the extent of disease, the woman with known endometriosis is left with her pain as the only real indicator of the extent of her disease. She also understands that it may require uncomfortable and expensive hormornal therapies, multiple surgeries, possible infertility, and may ultimately require hysterectomy and the removal of both ovaries. All these events may occur rapidly or may extend over many years. In fact, the clinical course of most cases of endometriosis is rather indolent, but this is scant comfort to the affected woman and her partner who understand the disease. Fear, anxiety, and a sense of helplessness may contribute to pain intensity, depression, and sexual dysfunction.

Physical examination findings are most often entirely lacking in early cases, or may be limited to cul-de-sac tenderness without palpable nodularity. In the nulliparous woman, when oral contraceptives and prostaglandin inhibitors are either ineffective against pain or if their impact diminishes over time, endometriosis must be suspected even in the absence of palpable pathology. (Other forms of intrinsic uterine pathology such as adenomyosis become more likely in the multiparous woman in her thirties or older.) While the possibility of endometriosis should certainly be reviewed when appropriate, expensive and difficult hormonal treatments (medroxyprogesterone, danocrine, gonadotropin-releasing-hormone agonists) should not be initiated in the absence of a firm diagnosis. Laparoscopy offers the opportunity for diagnosis as well as treatment in the form of laser ablation, electrocautery, or excision. Given the highly variable progression of endometriosis over time, when symptoms persist or worsen despite treatment, a repeat laparoscopy a year or more later will clarify how aggressive the disease is in a particular patient. Most often, indolent disease does not change its behavior and become rapidly aggressive. This information is often invaluable for realistic planning of childbearing attempts and treatment, and serves to adjust vigilance and anxiety to appropriate levels. When more advanced disease is discovered, stronger hormonal regimens should be started, and advanced laparoscopic surgery for reduction of the bulk of the disease should be considered.

The couple struggling with this disease also has to deal with the discomforts sometimes experienced during sexual intercourse. Dyspareunia is associated primarily with cul-de-sac disease, but also may occur when an ovary is adherent to the cul-de-sac or posterior broad ligament, especially in the case of a retroverted uterus. A woman experiencing this pain, and her partner, may understandably feel anxious about its recurrence, and may fear that the pain signals further tissue damage or progression of the disease. Sexual response may diminish as a result, which only aggravates the discomfort. Vaginal lubrication may then decrease or stop, and the normal physiologic vaginal expansion that occurs with sexual arousal may cease, leaving the tender cul-de-sac closer to the vaginal introitus, and thus more easily struck during coitus. The more pain, the less sexual response—and the less response, the more pain. Counseling suggestions appropriate for this problem will be discussed below.

Pelvic Adhesions

Since the beginnings of abdominal surgery, postoperative adhesion formation has been a problem. Many have questioned the idea that adhesions cause pain, noting that the degree of adhesive disease does not correlate with pain intensity. However, recent studies suggest that, as in the case of endometriosis, the location of pain often corresponds well to the location of adhesions. Given the complexities of pain perception described above, this allows the possibility that in cases of chronic pain, adhesions may be an important component of the problem in many individuals. Comprehensive treatment should certainly include attention to as many factors in the pain problem as possible, sometimes including attempts at adhesiolysis.

The pain associated with adhesions often starts within weeks of the physical insult responsible (e.g., pelvic infection, surgery). In most instances, pain duration varies from moments to an hour or so, and may be related to physical activity. Over time (beyond three or four months after its beginnings), pain episodes may progress in severity and duration, even if the physical pathology remains stable. Such a pattern should prompt careful inquiry regarding other factors, such as constipation, muscular deconditioning, and the development of a chronic pain syndrome as described above. When one is involved in the ongoing care of such a problem from its start, the transition to a chronic pain syndrome can be subtle. When years separate the suspected insult from the beginning of the pain, factors besides adhesions must be investigated.

Physical findings are often limited to pain roughly corresponding to the site of the adhesions (right, left, or midline). Over time, pain originating with adhesions may spread, as intestinal, muscular, and chronic pain syndrome factors are added to the mix. Depression and chronicity of pain, with a resultant lower pain threshold, serve to make the physical findings less distinct and treatment necessarily more complex. The inability to diagnose pelvic or abdominal adhesions accurately by ultrasound or other imaging techniques makes laparoscopy essential to the diagnosis and treatment of the problem in many cases. Preoperative laboratory screening should include studies to exclude more acute causes of pain, such as inflammatory conditions (e.g., sedimentation rate, cervical cultures for Chlamydia and gonorrhea, urine culture). Bowel studies such as endoscopy or barium enema should be limited to those women exhibiting *signs* (i.e., hematochezia, mucus), as opposed to only *symptoms,* of bowel disease.

Laparotomy for pain attributed to adhesions should continue to be reserved for cases of intestinal obstruction refractory to medical management. However, a number of studies of laparoscopic adhesiolysis suggest that pain relief may be obtained in 70 to 80 percent of patients.

Pelvic Support

Pelvic relaxation commonly occurs in the fifth and sixth decades of life or later, while most chronic pelvic pain problems occur in the third and fourth decades. Nevertheless, in some women pelvic relaxation may be accompanied by feelings of heaviness, pressure, dropping sensations, aching, etc. Treatment is primarily surgical, ideally employing preoperative estrogen replacement in the case of the postmenopausal woman.

Levator Spasm

Levator muscle spasm may develop by itself or, more commonly, in reaction to another pelvic discomfort. Along with occasional pain with defecation or during intercourse, the patient may note a sense of pelvic heaviness or the sensation of something ''falling out'' even when pelvic support is normal. Such sensations often resolve promptly upon reclining, worsen during the course of the day, and are frequently accompanied by progressive loss of sexual response.

Diagnosis of this problem is made primarily by the history described above and corroborated by pelvic examination demonstrating levator plate tenderness. Kegel exercises, consciously ''letting it all fall out,'' reclining at intervals during the day, and hot baths may help. Muscle relaxants are helpful in duress, but physical therapy approaches such as those mentioned above should be attempted first. Of course, relief of the primary pelvic pathology may result in spontaneous resolution of the spasm, but it can remain as an ongoing problem in some cases even when the precipitating cause is successfully treated.

Miscellaneous Causes

Other clinical problems, such as undiagnosed ovarian cysts, may also cause chronic pain and dyspareunia.

Causes of Pain in the "Laparoscopy-Negative" Patient

A variety of other etiologies (Table 30-2) for pelvic pain may occur in the absence of any laparoscopically observable cause. Of course, any of these disorders may occur in the presence of visible pathology as well. In fact, in many instances the musculoskeletal and urinary tract problems listed may accumulate over time, as a person's distress over such problems as endometriosis or adhesions increases. A careful chronologic history of the vari-

TABLE 30-2 Possible Causes for Pelvic Pain in "Laparoscopy-Negative" Patients

Gastrointestinal tract	
	Constipation
	Irritable bowel syndrome
	Inflammatory bowel disease
	Diverticulitis
Urinary tract	
	Urethral syndrome
	Interstitial cystitis
Musculoskeletal, neurologic	
	Pelvic floor tension myalgia (levator spasm)
	Piriformis syndrome
	Nerve entrapment
	Ventral hernia
	Rectus tendon strain
	Myofascial pain
	Back/pelvic postural changes
Gynecologic	
	Pelvic vascular congestion
	Cervical stenosis
	Endometritis

ous pain components may shed light on this pattern. These contributory syndromes are reviewed in detail elsewhere.

Dyspareunia (Painful Coitus)

As is the case with chronic pelvic pain, dyspareunia is a lengthy and complex topic in itself. Some of the more common contributing factors are listed in Table 30-3. An individual may certainly be afflicted with more than one cause, given that many of the problems listed are quite common.

Further, the presence of one problem may predispose a woman to the development of others on the list. For example, vaginitis may recur often enough to create anxiety, which alters sexual response often enough to diminish vaginal lubrication during coitus. The resulting vaginal dryness may cause coitus-related urinary tract infection, leading to treatment with antibiotics that bring on more episodes of vaginitis. As this unhappy scenario unfolds, deep dyspareunia begins as diminished sexual response eliminates the vaginal expansion and uterine elevation that usually accompany sexual response, allowing previously asymptomatic cul-de-sac endometriosis to be more easily struck during intercourse. These discomforts (or similar ones due to different types of pelvic pathology) and the anticipation of their regular recurrence cause a protective contraction of the vaginal introital muscles at the start of a coital attempt, resulting in involuntary spasm (vaginismus) over time.

TABLE 30-3 Factors Contributing to the Development of Dyspareunia

Vulvar
Vulvar vestibulitis syndrome
Chronic monilial vulvitis
Vaginal
Repeated or chronic vaginitis
Urethritis/urethral syndrome
Interstitial cystitis
Cervicitis
Diminished lubrication due to insufficient arousal
Levator spasm
Deep pelvic
Uterine retroversion (rare cases)
Pelvic relaxation
Endometriosis
Adhesions
Adenomyosis
Pelvic congestion syndrome
Lack of vaginal expansion due to insufficient arousal

To follow our prototypic patient a bit further, let us suggest that the stress of these problems aggravates a previously mild case of irritable bowel syndrome. Loss of orgasmic response may add to the problems by adding symptoms of chronic pelvic heaviness attributed to venous over-filling, or the pelvic congestion syndrome. Over time, levator spasm may begin, adding to the ''falling out'' sensation she experiences. Laparoscopy then reveals her endometriosis, and, since child-bearing is complete, she undergoes laparoscopically assisted vaginal hysterectomy and laser treatment of the endometriosis.

Postoperatively, some tender granulation tissue at the vaginal apex requires several treatments with silver nitrate cautery. The emotional environment surrounding attempts at intercourse has become understandably strained. Her sexual response fails to return, helping to perpetuate the vicious cycle of pain–decreased sexual response–more pain.

After this problem has continued for a total of six months to a year, she begins to note some trouble sleeping. She has some difficulty getting to sleep, but also notes that she sometimes wakes up at 4 A.M. and can't get back to sleep. Fatigue increases, and she stops exercising. Some low back pain starts, and she wonders if the endometriosis has recurred . . .

Every practicing gynecologist has seen patients with at least some portion of this story. The situation may seem hopeless and overwhelming for patient and physician at its end-point. Nevertheless, significant help often can be rendered, with time and patience, by the primary physician either alone or in collaboration with a skilled counselor. History-taking should emphasize the chronology of events, in the hope of understanding a sequence such as that described above. Interpreting this to the patient will help make it seem more manageable by breaking it down into a sequence of smaller problems. Indeed, understanding the chronology of events and each of the sequentially contributing factors may improve the physician's ability to address and alleviate the problems.

A brief listing of useful office counseling suggestions is given in Table 30-4. More complete discussions of the topic are in the references cited.

TABLE 30-4 Counseling Suggestions for Dyspareunia

Introital dyspareunia
(First eliminate tissue conditions such as vestibulitis, vaginitis)
Supplemental lubrication
Vegetable oil (don't use with latex contraceptive products)
Commercially available lubrications
Vaginal relaxation exercises
Demonstrate during pelvic examination first; patient practices contraction-relaxation cycles (Kegel exercises) alone, then with partner present, then with partner's finger inserted; then "bridge over" into intercourse, doing only what is comfortable (the "no pain" contract)
Position changes
Suggest cross-wise position for intercourse (which allows careful vaginal entry and allows the woman to have control over degree of vaginal penetration)
Deep dyspareunia
Correct pelvic pathology to the degree clinically possible, but try to avoid extirpative surgery as much as possible unless otherwise clinicially indicated
Suggest "no-pain contract," i.e., "don't do anything that hurts," proceeding with deeper entry only if sexual arousal is present and deeper entry is comfortable
Suggest cross-wise position
Supplemental lubrication, as needed
General considerations
Refer for professional counseling if:
• More than one sexual dysfunction is present (e.g., vaginismus and premature ejaculation)
• Significant marital discord is present
• The dysfunction has been present for over a year before help is sought
• The suggestions made seem difficult to implement

References and Selected Readings

1. Bachmann GA, Leiblum SR, Grill J: Brief sexual inquiry in gynecology practice. *Obstet Gynecol* 73:425–427, 1989.
2. Fedele L, Parazzini F, Bianchi S, et al: Stage and localization of pelvic endometriosis and pain. *Fertil Steril* 53:155–158, 1990.
3. Lamont JA: Female dyspareunia. *Am J Obstet Gynecol* 136:282–285, 1980.
4. Reiter RC: Occult somatic pathology in women with chronic pelvic pain. *Clin Obstet Gynecol* 33:154–160, 1990.
5. Reiter RC, Gambone JC: Demographic and historic variables in women with idiopathic chronic pelvic pain. *Obstet Gynecol* 75:428–432, 1990.
6. Sinaki M, Merrit JL, Stillwell GK: Tension myalgia of the pelvic floor. *Mayo Clin Proc* 52:717–722, 1977.
7. Steege JF, Ling FW: Dyspareunia: A special type of chronic pelvic pain. *Obstet Gynecol Clin North Am* 20:779–793, 1993.
8. Steege JF, Stout AL: Resolution of chronic pelvic pain following laparoscopic adhesiolysis. *Am J Obstet Gynecol* 165:278–283, 1991.
9. Steege JF, Stout AL, Somkuti S: Chronic pelvic pain: Toward an integrative model. *Obstet Gynecol Survey* 48:95–110, 1993.
10. Stout AL, Steege JF, Dodson WC, et al: Relationship of laparoscopic findings to self-report of pelvic pain. *Am J Obstet Gynecol* 164:73–79, 1991.
11. Stovall TG, Ling FW, Crawford DA: Hysterectomy for chronic pelvic pain of presumed uterine etiology. *Obstet Gynecol* 75:676–679, 1990.
12. Walker EW, Katon W, Harrop-Griffiths J, et al: Relationship of chronic pelvic pain to psychiatric diagnoses and childhood sexual abuse. *Am J Psychiatr* 145:75–80, 1988.

31 Menopause

R. Edward Varner
J. Benjamin Younger

Physiology of Menopause

Menopause refers to the cessation of menstruation due to the depletion of ovarian follicles. Most definitions require that women be amenorrheic for at least six months with physical or laboratory evidence of estrogen depletion before they are termed "menopausal." Prior to actual ovarian failure there is a decline in ovulatory function with fewer follicles present. Thus, there is a decline in ovarian estrogen and inhibin production. With falls in ovarian hormones there is less negative feedback on the pituitary and hypothalamus and there is a detectable rise in follicle stimulating hormone and luteinizing hormone. A serum follicle stimulating hormone (FSH) level is the most sensitive test to confirm menopause.

The physiologic period of waning ovarian function is called the *climacteric*. This period is variable in length but generally lasts for several years before atresia of all estrogen producing follicles has occurred. During the climacteric, noncyclic uterine bleeding due to anovulation or to sporadic ovulation may occur.

In the United States normal menopause is said to occur between ages 45 and 55 (95 percent confidence interval), with the median age being 51. Menopause prior to age 40 and after age 55 is termed premature and late menopause, respectively. The age of menopause is primarily genetically related; contrary to myths, it is not related to age at menarche, number of pregnancies, age at last pregnancy, or oral contraceptive use. It is also not related to race, socioeconomic status, height, or weight. The age may be lowered somewhat by smoking.

Ovarian failure and its sequelae recently have gained much attention in this country primarily because, today, one-third of all United States women are postmenopausal. The average female lifespan will approach 85 in the year 2000, in contrast to an average lifespan of 50 in 1900 (Fig. 31-1).

Changes Associated with Estrogen Decline

Vasomotor Symptoms

Vasomotor symptoms, or hot flushes, are the most common perimenopausal symptoms that compel women to seek medical attention. Seventy-five percent of women experience hot flushes. The average duration of these symptoms is 2 to 3 years. Eighty percent of women who experience the symptoms complain about them for more than one year, and 25 percent for up to 5 years.

These symptoms, which include sudden increases in central skin temperature as well as perspiration, are apparently due to deregulation of the central temperature regulating center in the hypothalamus. Both peripheral vasodilation (a sympathetic adrenergic inhibitory action) and perspiration (a sympathetic cholinergic stimulatory action) occur. The flush, which generally lasts from a few minutes to 20 min, typically is preceded by a premonition—a flash.

Although the precise etiology of vasomotor symptoms is unclear, it is apparently related to decreases in estrogen and inhibin levels, not to absence of estrogen. It is theorized that a decline below a certain level exerts more effect on the hypothalamic thermostat, thus affecting autonomic nervous system control of peripheral vasculature. Once the central nervous system has adjusted to decreased estrogen levels, vasomotor symptoms cease.

About one-third of women with vasomotor symptoms find these symptoms severe enough to require medical assistance. The symptoms, which may occur up to 15 times daily, may awaken the individual, producing sleep deprivation, and may cause sweating, necessitating a change of clothing. Hot

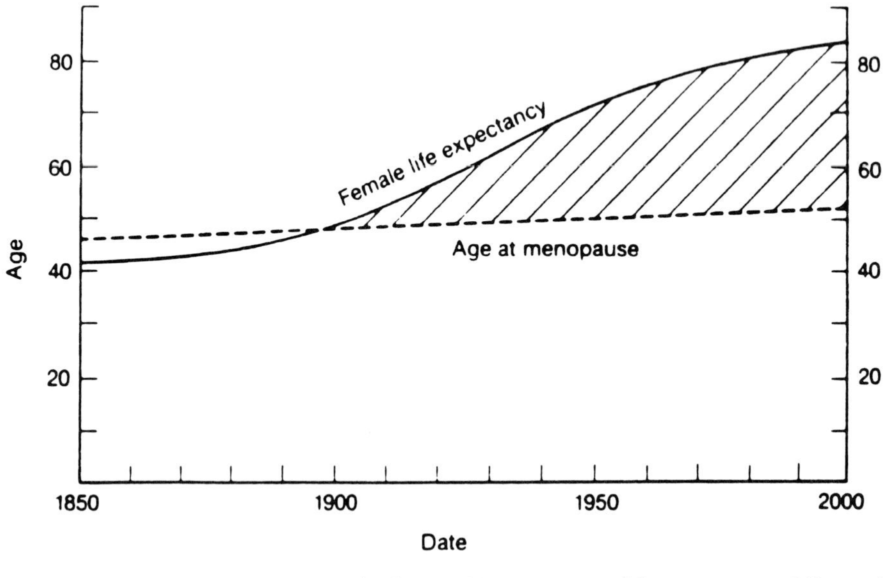

Figure 31-1 Female lifespan. [From Cope E: Physical changes associated with the postmenopausal years, in Campbell S (ed): Management of the Menopause and Postmenopausal Years. Lancaster, England, MTP Press, 1976, p 33, reprinted with permission.]

flushes may begin before menopause, but generally are more severe after cessation of menses.

Exogenous estrogen therapy,[3] progestogen therapy,[14] and, to a lesser extent, vasodilator therapy have been shown to decrease the incidence of vasomotor symptoms. Flushes may not respond optimally to estrogen replacement therapy for up to one month (Fig. 31-2); however, there is usually some decrease in frequency within the first few days of use.

Genital Atrophic Changes

Genital atrophic changes associated with hypoestrogenism are a significant problem for many women. Clinically, the atrophic vagina has a pale appearance and loses its elasticity. The epithelium is thin and friable, and with the lack of colonization by acidophilic bacteria it no longer produces glycogen. The vagina, vulva, and external urethra may become colonized by gastrointestinal bacteria and develop an inflammatory response causing tissue erythema and denudation, a purulent discharge, and bleeding. Intercourse may aggravate these inflammatory changes. At times the vaginal walls actually may agglutinate, thereby making intercourse very uncomfortable. The symptoms related to genital atrophy include vaginal and vulvar itching and burning, dyspareunia, vaginal bleeding, dysuria, urinary frequency, and urinary urgency. The sexual dysfunction, which many women do not report, may lead to decreased sexual activity and thus a psychological effect on both partners. The most effective therapy for atrophic vaginitis or urethritis is estrogen (see Individualization of Care).

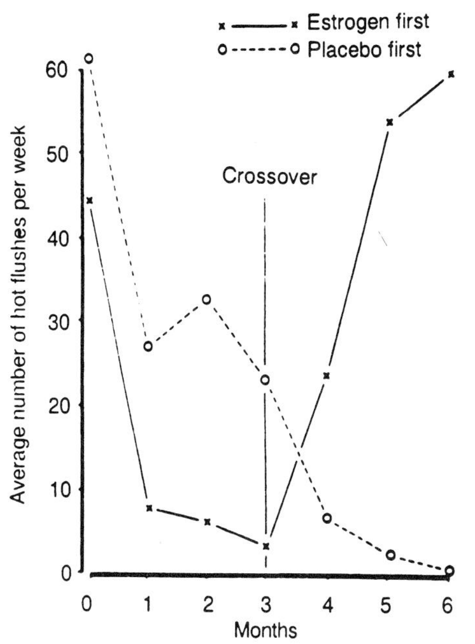

Figure 31-2 Vasomotor symptoms. The average number of hot flushes per week in a random double-blind, 6-month crossover study of estrogen and placebo therapy. Solid line (—): estrogen first; dashed line (----): placebo first. (From Coope,[3] reprinted with permission.)

Osteoporosis

Osteoporosis, defined as a reduction of bone mass per unit volume, significantly affects more than one-third of older women. This often leads to fractures, which, in addition to causing pain and disabilities, results in a direct and indirect cost of over 7 billion dollars annually in the United States.

Bone strength or bone mineral content is a function of numerous factors (Table 31-1) that, when deficient, may predispose one to develop osteoporosis. Osteoporosis is rare in African American women,[7,16] and it is more common in thin Caucasian or Asian women than in large, muscular women. Osteoporosis may be somewhat less common in

TABLE 31-1 Factors Contributing to Bone Strength

Heredity
Activity (weight-bearing exercise)
Race
Dietary intake of calcium, vitamin D, and other nutrients
Good general health
Normal functioning endocrine glands (thyroid, parathyroid, and ovaries)
Normal functioning kidneys and GI tract
Estrogen status of the woman

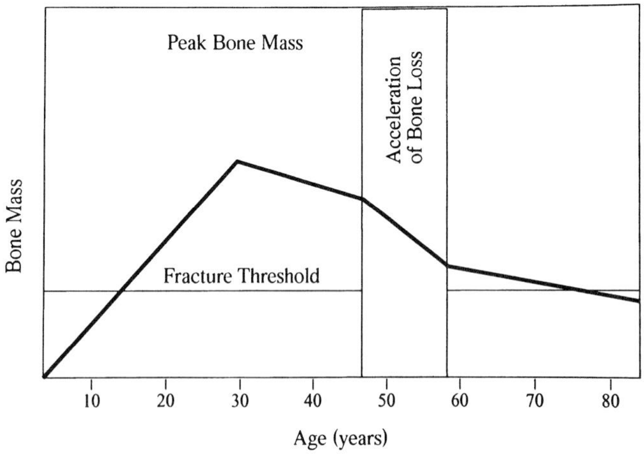

Figure 31-3 Relationship of bone mass to age in women.

women who have maintained healthy life-styles. Smoking, excessive alcohol use, sedentary life-style, as well as steroid use appear to be contributing factors for some women. Figure 31-3 illustrates the relationship between bone calcium content (bone strength) and age in women. All of the above mentioned factors appear to affect the slopes of the lines of increase and decrease in bone calcium content. They affect the peak calcium content, present in the mid-thirties, and affect the likelihood of the individual's bone calcium content reaching the "fracture point" later in life.

There is well-documented accelerated bone calcium loss beginning prior to the time of ovarian failure. This calcium loss is primarily from the trabecular (spongy) bone of the vertebral bodies, long bone shafts and heads, and the pelvis. There is now abundant evidence indicating that exogenous estrogen therapy will reduce the risk of postmenopausal (Type I) osteoporosis and fractures. Numerous studies have shown decreased fracture rates in estrogen-treated compared with untreated women. Increased calcium and hydroxyproline urinary excretion occurring after menopause have been shown to be normalized by estrogen treatment. In addition, serial bone densitometry studies have shown a halt in bone density loss in estrogen-treated patients but not in untreated controls. Other therapies, including high-dose calcium, have not been shown to affect this early postmenopausal loss of bone mass.[12]

Menopausal Skin Changes

The skin changes associated with aging include increased fragility and wrinkling, as well as some changes in sensation. These changes may increase around the time of menopause. A decline in skin collagen content parelleling the decline in bone density in postmenopausal women has been illustrated.[1] In addition, there is evidence that skin cells (at least in some areas of the body) contain estrogen receptors. Although it has not been proven, it is believed by many that menopausal women treated with estrogen may have skin that is thicker and less prone to wrinkling.

Cardiovascular Disease

In the United States, heart disease—specifically coronary artery disease—is the leading cause of death for postmenopausal women. Although the disease tends to strike men earlier in life, the overall chance of dying from heart disease is essentially equal in women and men (37.7 percent vs. 36.3 percent in 1985). The primary risk factors for coronary artery disease are tobacco use, hypertension, and elevated serum cholesterol or unfavorable lipoprotein profiles. Secondary factors include diabetes mellitus, obesity, and sedentary life-style. The modification of these risks through education, life-style changes, and medical therapy appears to reduce the incidence of the disease.

Ovarian failure may also be an important determining factor in coronary artery disease in women. The incidence of the disease in women prior to menopause is much lower than that in men of the same age. Surgical removal of the ovaries has been shown to produce an increase in coronary artery disease similar to that seen in men. This increase in oophorectomized patients may be prevented by administration of exogenous estrogens.[9] It also appears that natural menopause may increase a woman's susceptibility to the disease. The incidence of coronary artery disease in women clearly increases with age after menopause, whereas little to no increase is seen prior to ovarian failure.

Numerous epidemiologic studies indicate that hormone replacement, particularly estrogen replacement, after ovarian failure substantially reduces the incidence of coronary artery disease (Table 31-2). Metaanalyses of these data have shown relative risk of myocardial infarction (fatal and nonfatal) in ever-users of postmenopausal estrogens to be between 0.55 and 0.65.[5] The mechanisms by which estrogen may affect coronary artery disease include its favorable effect on cholesterol and lipoproteins and also its local relaxing effect on vascular smooth muscle. In theory, there appears to be some attenuation of both of these favorable effects of estrogen by synthetic progestogens administered with estrogen; however, the actual impact of the commonly used progestogens is unknown.

There remains more to be learned about hormone replacement therapy and heart disease. For example: what are the optimal regimens, doses, and administration routes of both estrogen and progestogen? Will there be a protective effect in obese women who have higher levels of endogenous estrogens after menopause and are not likely to need hormone replacement therapy for other reasons?

Symptoms Not Directly Related to Estrogen Depletion

A number of symptoms (anxiety, depression, irritability, fatigue, insomnia, emotional lability, and changes in libido) may occur around the time of menopause. Whether a person will exhibit the symptoms is variable; some individuals will show minimal or no symptoms, while others will have symptoms which they find disabling. The etiology of these symptoms is incompletely understood and appears to be multifactorial. In addition to the hormonal and metabolic changes that occur with menopause, age-related social and economic changes may affect an individual's life-style and self-image (Table 31-3). A great deal of variability exists among both men and women in the ability to withstand these changes. Estrogen decline may indirectly cause or worsen the symptoms by increasing sleep disturbances and adversely affecting overall feelings of well-being.

The management of patients with these symptoms will vary. Disorders such as thyroid disease, other chronic disease states, and clinical depression should be considered as possible causes of the symptoms; when indicated, investigational studies should be undertaken. Women having mild symptoms with no obvious organic cause should be well counseled and made aware that these symptoms generally resolve with time as long as the patient maintains a healthy life-style. Those whose symptoms affect their ability to function and to maintain a healthy life-style frequently will benefit from psychological counseling, antidepressant therapy, and, rarely, other psychiatric care.

Hormone Replacement Therapy

It is apparent from the previous discussion that estrogen deficiency may produce numerous adverse effects. Some of these, such as urogenital atrophy, vasomotor symptoms, loss of skin thickness and elasticity, and sleep disturbances may affect quality of life. Others, such as osteoporosis and coronary artery disease may affect not only quality of life, but also longevity. Since women live much longer today and spend at least one-third of their lives after menopause (Fig. 31-1) estrogen deficiency and its treatment have become much more significant issues than they were in the early 1900s.

Although the idea of "glandular therapy" can be

TABLE 31-2 Postmenopausal Hormone Use and Coronary Heart Disease

Reference (number of subjects) (year)	Unopposed estrogen			Estrogen and progestin[g]
	Ever use relative risk	Duration of use		Ever use relative risk
		Years of use	Relative risk	
Case-control				
Rosenbert (238) (1976)	1.0[a]			
Talbott (83) (1977)	0.3[a,b]			
Jick (70) (1978)	4.2[a,b]			
Pfeffer (237) (1978)	0.9			
Rosenberg (113) (1980)	1.0[a]	≥5	0.6[a]	
Adam (77) (1981)	0.6[b]	>4	1.0[b]	
Bain (229) (1981)	0.8			
Ross (81) (1981)	0.5[b,c]			
Szklo (241) (1984)	0.6			
La Vecchia (233) (1987)	3.0[a]			
Beard (230) (1989)	0.6			
Croft (231) (1989)	0.8			
Thompson (114) (1989)	1.1[d]			1.2[d]
Cross-sectional				
Gruchow (96) (1988)	0.6[c,e]			
	0.4[c,f]			
Sullivan (240) (1988)	0.6[c]			
McFarland (235) (1989)	0.5[c]			
Uncontrolled cohort				
Byrd (61) (1977)	0.4[b,c]			
MacMahon (234) (1978)	0.3	≥15	0.8	
Hunt (63) (1990)	0.4[c]			
Cohort				
Hammond (117) (1979)	0.3[b,c]			
Lafferty (204) (1985)	0.2[b]			
Wilson (73) (1985)	1.9[c]			
Bush (78) (1987)	0.4[c]			
Petitti (80) (1987)	1.3			
Criqui (79) (1988)	1.0[a]			
Avila (228) (1990)	0.7[a]	≥1	0.3[a]	
Persson (101) (1990)	0.8[c]			0.5[c]
Sullivan (82) (1990)	0.2[a,c]			
Henderson (76) (1991)	0.7[b,c]	≥15	0.5[c]	
Stampfer (85) (1991)	0.6[a,c]			
Wolf (84) (1991)	0.7[c]			
Randomized, controlled trial				
Nachtigall (64)(1979)				0.3[b]

[a]Current estrogen use.

[b]The relative risk or *P* value or both are estimated from data provided in the published study.

[c]$P \leq .05$.

[d]End points include both stroke and myocardial infarction.

[e]Moderate versus low coronary occlusion score.

[f]Severe versus low coronary occlusion score.

[g]Now called progestogen.

SOURCE: From Grady et al.,[5] with permission.

TABLE 31-3 Life Events That Often Occur around the Time of Menopause and May Affect Mental Status

Family structure changes (children leaving home)
Interpersonal changes (changes in friends)
Work changes (retirement or no further chance for advancement)
Marital status changes (divorce or marriage of child)
Relocation (e.g., couple moving to smaller home)
Educational changes (realization that one's knowledge has not kept up with new advances)
Changes in finance
Loss of family or friends
Legal concerns
Health concerns

traced back to Egyptian times, the first real attempts to treat symptoms of ovarian failure with "ovarian secretions" did not occur until 1885. It was not until the 1920s and 1930s that estrogens in the urine of pregnant mares were discovered to be active when given to humans and that estrogens could be produced synthetically in forms that could be absorbed and remain active when given orally (diethylstilbestrol and ethinyl estradiol). Although the pharmacologic development of estrogen and progesterone preparations has proceeded rapidly, it may still be in its adolescence.

Benefits

It is now clear that estrogen given to postmenopausal females in doses that produce serum levels of active estrogens (estrone or estradiol) biologically equivalent to the lowest levels seen in women of reproductive age will effectively treat vasomotor symptoms and genital atrophy, will prevent up to one-half of cases of osteoporosis, and will possibly decrease mortality from coronary artery disease by 40 to 50 percent.

Endometrial Effects—Rationale for Progestogen Therapy

Numerous epidemiologic studies have shown an increase in adenocarcinoma of the endometrium with use of exogenous estrogens without progestogen after menopause (Table 31-4). This increase appears to be related to potency, dose, and duration of use. Careful analysis of some of these studies reveals that the risk is probably overestimated, owing to more aggressive diagnosis and to the fact that, like prostate cancer in men, many women may harbor low-grade, somewhat dormant endometrial cancers that become apparent when stimulated by estrogen. Studies have not shown an increase in death from endometrial cancer in estrogen users, presumably because most of these cancers are low grade and confined to the uterus when diagnosed. There is a high cure rate with hysterectomy.

Experimental evidence indicates that administration of estrogen without progesterone to postmeno-

TABLE 31-4 Risk Estimates from Case Control Studies of Estrogen Replacement Therapy and Endometrial Cancer

Study		Relative risks[a]	
Author	Year	Ever users	Long-term users
Smith	1975	4.5	—
Ziel	1975	7.6	13.9
Mack	1976	5.6	8.8
Gray	1977	3.1	11.6
McDonald	1977	2.0	7.9
Wigle	1978	2.2	5.2
Horwitz	1978	12.0	—
Hoogerland	1978	2.2	6.7
Antunes	1979	6.0	16.0
Weiss	1979	7.5	8.2
Hulka	1980	—	4.2
Shapiro	1980	3.9	6.0
Jelovsek	1980	2.4	4.8
Spengler	1981	3.2	8.6
Stavraky	1981	4.2	14.4
Kelsey	1982	—	8.2
LaVecchia	1982	2.7	—
Henderson	1983	1.4	3.1

[a]Risk relative to never users.
SOURCE: From Peterson et al.,[10] with permission.

pausal women, even in low doses, will produce early forms of hyperplasia in 20 to 35 percent within a year's time.[13,17]

Like progesterone production in ovulatory women, exogenous progestogens will prevent hyperplasia in postmenopausal women receiving estrogens. In addition, administration of progestogens will decrease the incidence of endometrial cancer. This protective effect also appears to be related to progestogen dose, potency, and duration of use (see Hormone Replacement Regimens).

Breast Cancer

Cancer of the breast is the most frequent cancer in women and the second leading cause of cancer death. The median age at which breast cancer develops is 69, and 80 percent of breast cancers occur in women over 40.

There is an abundance of indirect evidence that estrogen and/or progesterone have roles in breast cancer etiology. Most breast cancers occur in women who have had ovarian function. Early menarche, low parity, and late menopause increase breast cancer risk, whereas early removal of the ovaries decreases it. Breast glandular tissue has estrogen and progesterone receptors that have a proliferative effect when stimulated. Ductal breast carcinoma also may exhibit receptors. Cancers exhibiting receptor activity respond favorably to oophorectomy and to therapy aimed at decreasing ovarian estrogen production. From these observations one might expect that prolonged exposure to estrogen would increase the risk of the disease.

Surprisingly, the data available on breast cancer and menopausal hormone replacement have not clearly defined an association. Numerous epidemiologic studies show varying results; however, the majority show a relative risk no greater than 1.5, and most show a relative risk very close to 1 or 1.1. Several metaanalyses suggest that the risk may be related to dose and duration of use and is possibly increased when hormone replacement is given to patients with additional risk factors for breast cancer (e.g., strong family history, which in itself gives a relative risk from 2.5 to 3.5). Data from a meta analysis by Dupont and Page of epidemiologic studies are presented in Fig. 31-4.[4]

The FDA Advisory Committee has agreed that long-term use of estrogen is associated with a mod-

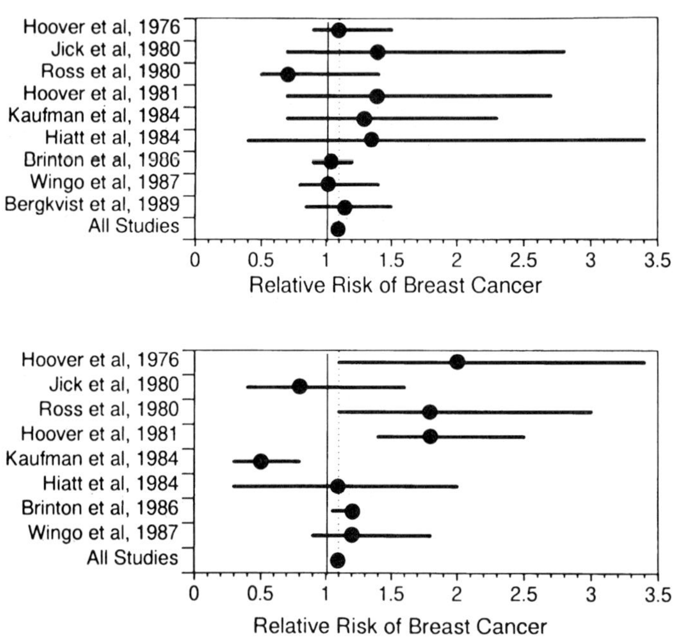

Figure 31-4 Relative risk of breast cancer with conjugated estrogen therapy by dosage. *A.* Patients treated with 0.625 mg conjugated estrogens. *B.* Patients treated with 1.25 mg conjugated estrogens. (From Dupont and Page,[4] reprinted with permission.)

est increase in breast cancer risk of a magnitude of 1.3 to 1.5; however, the risk may be significantly lower if lower doses of estrogen are used consistently. Higher doses and longer durations of exogenous estrogen use may be associated with increased breast cancer risk. In addition, the risk may increase further when women already at high risk for breast cancer take exogenous estrogen.

The association of the progestogen component of estrogen-progestogen use and the risk of breast cancer is not clear from the available data. Progesterone and progestogens cause glandular proliferation in normal breast tissue and could theoretically increase the risk of carcinogenic events. However, high-dose progestogen therapy may suppress the growth of some breast cancers. With incomplete data on how progestogens affect breast cancer risk, and since progestogens adversely affect the favorable effect of estrogen on lipoproteins and cause most of the side effects associated with hormone replacement, we favor not administering progestogens to patients without uteri solely for their presumed protective effect on the breast. However, if a woman has a uterus and is receiving hormone replacement therapy, most clinicians believe that a progestogen is required.

Benign Breast Problems

Fibrocystic breast changes respond variably to menopausal hormone replacement. The presence of premenopausal fibrocystic changes or cyclic mastalgia does not always indicate that the problem will be exacerbated by postmenopausal hormone replacement. However, some women with previous breast symptoms and a few who have never had breast symptoms will develop mastalgia and/or fibrocystic changes when treated. As with other hormone-related effects, breast symptoms usually are dose-related, and mastalgia frequently worsens during the estrogen/progestogen days of cyclic therapy.

Other Cancers

There are no known relationships between menopausal hormone replacement therapy and cervical, lung, gastrointestinal, hematologic, nor lymphomatous malignant neoplasms. A few epithelial (especially endometroid) ovarian cancers and osteoblastic sarcomas may have estrogen receptors, which would contraindicate estrogen therapy. There is some debate as to whether such therapy is contraindicated in patients with melanomas, since estrogen may stimulate melanocytes.

Other Effects (Coagulation, Hypertension, Vascular Disease, and Gallbladder Disease)

By directly or indirectly stimulating liver enzymes, estrogen may increase the production of serum globulins, including angiotensinogen, sex hormone binding globulin, and others. It favorably affects fat and cholesterol metabolism in the liver, tilting the balance toward increases in high-density lipoprotein-cholesterol and triglycerides, and decreases in total cholesterol and low-density lipoprotein-cholesterol, including apolipoproteins. It decreases antithrombin III activity, but apparently has little effect on other clotting factors. Progestogens exert no effect on clotting factors, but act against the beneficial effect of estrogens on cholesterol and lipoproteins. Estrogen also increases the cholesterol content of bile and may increase the incidence of cholesterol-containing gallstones in some individuals.

All of these effects appear to be related to hormone dose, potency, and route of administration. The formulations generally recommended for postmenopausal replacement today produce blood levels of biologically active estrogen at or below those seen in the follicular phase of reproductive-aged women. All orally administered compounds tend to exert more effect on the liver because of their entry through the portal circulation. However, there is apparently little clinical significance of this effect with doses equivalent to 0.625 mg of conjugated estrogens in women with normal hepatic and renal function. No epidemiologic study has shown an increase in thromboses, thromboemboli, cerebrovascular accidents, hypertension, or other vascular disease. The low-dose regimens used in hormone replacement therapy apparently produce a greater beneficial effect by favorably affecting cholesterol and lipoproteins and by directly causing vasodilation. There does appear to be a rare susceptible individual who will develop coagulation problems; however, there is no laboratory test known to recognize which individuals might have this increased susceptibility. Transcutaneous and premucosal administration of estrogen have less effect on liver metabolism, and antithrombin III activity has not been shown to change with therapy. However, there is not enough evidence as yet to say that the presently available patch and creams are totally safe in these susceptible individuals.

Hormone Replacement Regimens

Although there is not sufficient information regarding which treatment regimens produce the maximum benefit with minimal side effects, several regimens have emerged that, based on current experience, should be beneficial to most women. As discussed previously, unopposed estrogen therapy appears to be the optimal regimen for patients who have undergone hysterectomy, but for women with a uterus, a progestogen is important to reduce the risk of endometrial hyperplasia and cancer. Figure 31-5 represents the blood levels produced by daily administration of two doses of oral conjugated estrogens, one dose of oral micronized estradiol, and two estradiol transdermal patches.[2,11] The estradiol and estrone levels produced by most of these regimens as well as equivalent doses of other oral medications either are actually lower than or biologically equivalent to blood levels seen in reproductive-aged women. Intramuscularly administered estrogen and once a week oral estrogens produce higher peak blood levels of estrogen than do the above-mentioned regimens and probably should be avoided.

In the United States the progestogen used in most low-dose hormone replacement therapy regimes is medroxyprogesterone acetate (MPA). This progestogen is less potent than nortestosterone derivatives. It is available in 2.5 mg, 5mg, and 10 mg doses. The 10-mg dose is adequate for endometrial suppression when given cyclically for 12 days monthly with doses equivalent to 1.25 mg of conjugated estrogens or less. Five milligrams of MPA given cyclically with 0.625 mg of conjugated estrogens does not always produce histologic evidence of endometrial suppression, but in one study was shown to prevent the development of hyperplasia.[6] Doses of 2.5 mg and 5 mg of MPA and less than 1 mg of norethindrone have been shown to produce endometrial suppression when given daily combined with oral estrogen regimes. Five milligrams of norethindrone or norethindrone acetate given cyclically will suppress the endometrium and may produce fewer progesterone-related side effects than MPA. Unfortunately,

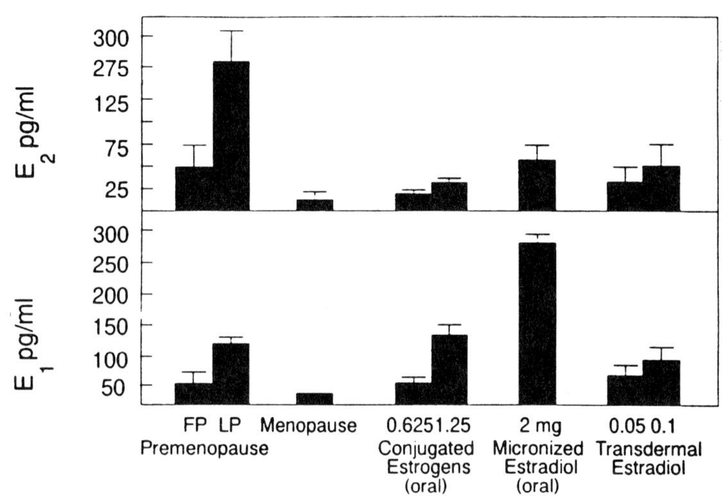

Figure 31-5 Serum estradiol and estrone levels as affected by menopause and estrogen replacement. FP, follicular phase; LP, luteal phase. (From Chetkowski et al.[2] and Powers et al.,[11] reprinted with permission.)

5 mg of norethindrone acetate may have a more pronounced adverse effect on cholesterol and lipoproteins than MPA.

Figure 31-6 provides a schematic depicting the most frequently used estrogen/progestogen regimens. The rationale for cyclic therapy is based on a normal reproductive cycle. During the estrogen-only days the endometrium is shown to exhibit some proliferative effect. When the progestogen is added, the endometrium is suppressed; when withdrawn, if adequate endometrial build-up is present, bleeding will occur. Administration of estrogen every day with no days off may produce less withdrawal bleeding and may possibly have a more beneficial effect on bone and heart. The advantage of cyclic regimens relates primarily to predictability of uterine bleeding. Absence of withdrawal bleeding does not signify a lack of endometrial suppression by the progestogen, but usually implies a lesser response of the endometrium to estrogen. The disadvantages of cyclic therapy include both bleeding and the progestogen-related side effects of bloating, GI disturbances, and premenstrual symptoms.

Continuous combined regimens utilize the same estrogen doses, with 2.5 mg of MPA or a nortestosterone derivative (generally 1 mg or less). The advantages of these regimens include absence or very low incidence of progestogen-related side effects and the potential for amenorrhea due to the progestogen's ability to inhibit endometrial proliferation. Unfortunately, more than 50 percent of women will experience breakthrough bleeding during the first four to six months on these regimens. The breakthrough bleeding decreases with time, and fewer than 10 percent will have breakthrough bleeding after six months.

Numerous other treatment plans have been used in clinical practice. Although most of these regimens should produce beneficial effects, no specific advantages of any one regimen over those mentioned above have been demonstrated in controlled clinical trials.

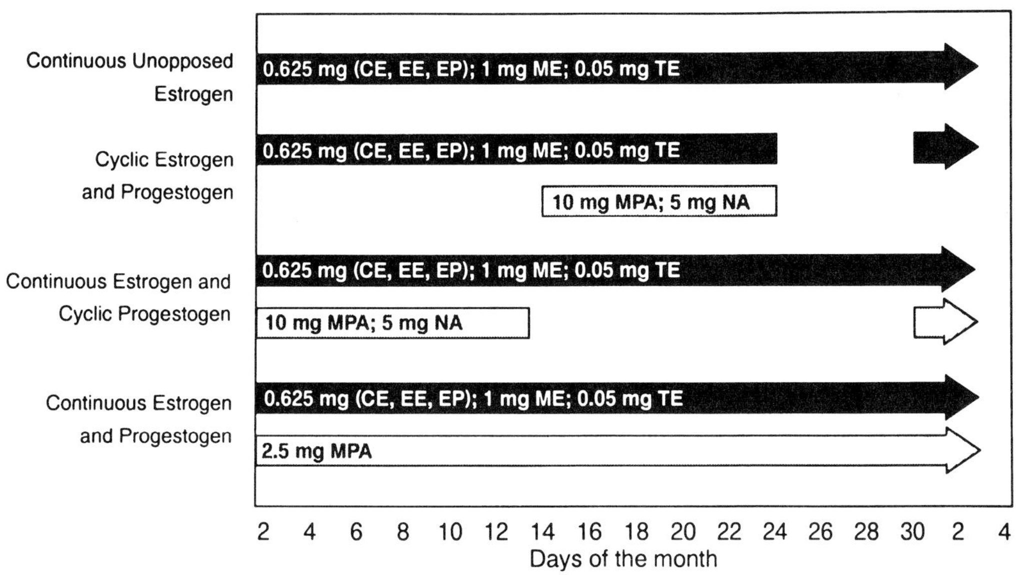

Figure 31-6 Hormone replacement regimens. Filled bars (■): estrogen. CE, conjugated estrogens; EE, esterified estrogens; ME, micronized estradiol; EP, estradiol pipate; TE, transdermal estradiol. Clear bars (□): progestogen. MPA, medroxyprogesterone acetate; NA, norethindrone. Dosages are those most commonly recommended and have been shown to inhibit bone calcium loss or to suppress endometrium. Continuous unopposed estrogen is used in women who have had a hysterectomy.

Individualization of Care

All women should be counseled or given information regarding diet, nutrition, exercise, weight control, smoking, certain drugs, excess alcohol intake, and such safety factors as seat-belt use. This emphasis on preventive care is an important part of the primary care physician's relationship with patients. This counseling should be reinforced when women are in their forties and emphasized further as they approach their menopausal years (Table 31-5). Most women want and should be given information about ovarian failure and the climacteric. It should be emphasized that the menopause does not signify a change from "young" to "old" but is simply an event—that there are many productive years ahead. The psychosocial aspects of the climacteric should be discussed, depending on the patient's symptoms, and psychological treatment or referral should be considered when indicated. Sexuality should also be discussed, emphasizing both physical and psychological factors, and emphasizing that ovarian failure does not imply sexual decline. Lastly, hormone replacement should be discussed with each patient, presenting the perceived benefits in her case and the potential risks or side effects. Primary care providers should be well informed about hormone replacement and should try to present the facts with as little bias as possible. The following paragraphs include these authors' perceptions regarding to whom, how, and when hormone replacement should or should not be recommended.

TABLE 31-5 Preventive Care of the Perimenopausal and Postmenopausal Woman

Proper dietary habits (including calcium supplements and adequate vitamin intake)
Appropriate exercise
Weight control
Avoidance of tobacco and toxic substances
Maintenance of mental activity
Consider hormone replacement
Consider low-dose aspirin
Screening studies
Appropriate immunizations
Safety counseling (e.g., seat-belts, balance, and falls)

Who Should Receive Hormone Replacement?

When absolute contraindications do not exist, all women who present with vasomotor symptoms or genital atrophic symptoms, all women with documented osteoporosis, all women with risk for osteoporosis, and women at risk for coronary artery disease should be considered as potential candiates for hormone replacement. For each individual a pro and con list should be constructed. This should include her potential benefits, potential risks, and the presence or absence of side effects once therapy is begun. From this list, individual decisions can be made.

Contraindications

Absolute contraindications to maintenance hormone replacement are uncommon, but include active or recent history of breast cancer or endometrial cancer, active liver or gallbladder disease, and active thrombophlebitis or a history of recurrent thrombotic events. Women with these problems may occasionally be candidates for temporary treatment with low-dose estrogen cream for symptomatic atrophic symptoms, since other treatments usually are ineffective for this problem. A prior breast cancer is considered a contraindication for estrogen replacement therapy, although if a patient is severely symptomatic, some physicians will prescribe replacement with a patient's thorough, informed consent. Women with a strong family history (numerous direct family members) of breast cancer should be considered at increased risk and should be given hormone replacement only when its therapeutic benefits are indicated. A prior good prognosis endometrial cancer (low-grade with minimal invasion and negative nodes) is not considered a contraindication to hormone therapy by most experts, although the PDR may still list it as an absolute contraindication. If a patient who has been treated for endometrial cancer is severely symptomatic and wishes to receive estrogen replacement, thorough informed consent is important, as it is for all patients.

It is doubtful that women who have had previous thromboses related to a fracture or a temporary stasis condition have any contraindication to low-dose hormone replacement. Since the transcutaneous administration route has no apparent effect on antithrombin III activity, it may be the best option for these patients.

There is little evidence that most benign breast disease when exposed to exogenous estrogen increases the risk of cancer. However, women who have biopsy-proven premalignant breast lesions may increase their breast cancer risk by taking estrogen. The presence of fibrocystic changes or previous mastalgia are not contraindications to hormone replacement. Some women with mastalgia on cyclic combination therapy will benefit from a continuous combined regimen utilizing a lower progestogen dose.

Women receiving hormone replacement, like all women, should receive thorough surveillance for breast cancer.

How Should Hormone Replacement Be Administered?

Generally, doses of 0.625 mg conjugated estrogens or equivalent oral doses of other estrogens or 0.05 mg of estradiol per transcutaneous patch should be given for prophylaxis against osteoporosis, cardiovascular disease, and vaginal atrophic symptoms. These dosages are also effective for vasomotor symptoms in most patients. However, if women continue to have vasomotor symptoms on these regimens, the estrogen dose may be temporarily increased incrementally or the route of administration may be changed. If vasomotor symptoms are not improved after these changes, other causes of vasomotor symptoms should be considered (e.g., dysautonomia, thyroid disease, or infectious diseases). For reasons discussed, unopposed estrogen preferably should be given only to women who have undergone hysterectomy.

Vaginal estrogen cream should be reserved for acute treatment of women with symptoms related to vaginal atrophy. Doses of 0.5 to 1 g of estrogen cream daily will reverse atrophy within one to three months' time. Estrogen cream in these doses used once or twice weekly can prevent atrophic symptoms or their recurrence. This regimen may be useful for the patient who has had previous problems with atrophy but has contraindications to or side effects from other maintenance therapies. In our experience this approach rarely causes endometrial proliferation and does not require supplemental progestogen. However, it will probably not benefit the bones or the heart.

The previously mentioned oral or transcutaneous regimens with a progestogen given either cyclically or continuously should be optimal for a woman with a uterus. Which regimen to initiate will depend on the patient's and the physician's preference (see Hormone Replacement Regimens).

We believe that the administration of unopposed estrogen to a woman with a uterus may be indicated in rare instances when the perceived benefit from estrogen is high and the woman cannot tolerate any progestogen. In such a patient it is advisable to use the lowest effective dose and to monitor the endometrium at regular intervals—initially semiannually, then annually. Monitoring should include endometrial biopsy sampling, which may at times be replaced by endometrial sonography (see Endometrial Surveillance). The same surveillance policy should be applied to women on estrogen/progestogen regimens that have not yet been proven to produce endometrial suppression. New estrogen/progestogen combination regimens and new routes of administration that will minimize side effects, suppress the endometrium, and maximize benefit may make selection of therapy easier in the future.

When and For How Long Should Hormone Replacement Be Administered?

For those at low risk for osteoporosis and those who have no worrisome vasomotor symptoms, waiting six months after the last menstrual period before initiating therapy is appropriate. By then, sporadic ovulation and its resultant bleeding is less likely to occur. For women with worrisome vasomotor symptoms that start before the last menstrual period and for those at significant risk for osteoporosis, earlier hormone replacement may be preferred. Since the low-dose regimens do not prevent ovulation, early initiation may be accompanied by what is perceived as abnormal uterine bleeding. One proposed option for these women is the very low-dose oral contraceptive (for those women for whom it is not contraindicated) containing 20 to 30 μg ethinyl estradiol and a relatively low potency progestogen. The oral contraceptive can be stopped one to two weeks before each physician visit, at which time a symptom diary can be reviewed and a serum FSH can be measured. An FSH greater than 50, although not absolutely specific, generally suggests ovarian failure; thereafter, a lower dose replacement regimen may be substituted. Smokers, women with hypertension or vascular disease, and women who do not tolerate oral contraceptives may possibly be candidates for and tolerate cyclic therapy or very low-dose (0.3 mg conjugated estrogens) estrogen replacement prior to their last menstrual period. Evaluation of the bleeding that may occur when low-dose therapy is given prior to menopause should be individualized.

We believe that when hormone replacement is given to retard osteoporosis or heart disease, the therapy should be continued as long as the prophylactic benefit is desired.

Bone Density Assessments

Several measurement techniques for bone density have been advocated to determine when or if patients will develop significant osteoporosis, and whether interventional or prophylactic therapy is indicated. Dual energy x-ray absorptiometry (DEXA) may be used to measure local bone density in the vertebral bodies, hips, radius, and elsewhere; with a special set-up, the technique may be used to interpret total bone content. DEXA appears to be as accurate or more accurate than previously recommended nuclear dual photon absorptiometry (DPA) and computed tomography (CT) interpretations. The DEXA scans also are less expensive and can be performed more rapidly than CT or DPA studies. Single photon absorptiometry is also easy to perform; however, it can only be used to measure the density of structures containing primarily cortical bone in the distal axial skeleton. It is thus not recommended for screening the early menopausal patient who is likely to lose trabecular bone first. The cost-effectiveness of bone density measurements is doubtful in women at low risk for osteoporosis who are compliant with preventive measures. Should a relatively healthy, active, early menopausal female with minimal family history of osteoporosis who eats a well-balanced diet with a gram of calcium daily and who takes estrogen replacement undergo bone density measurements? Probably not! Her risk of developing osteoporosis is low and it is unlikely that the test will influence her management. Assessment of bone density does appear to be reasonable in patients at high risk for osteoporosis or in patients who are at minimal risk and are trying to make a decision whether or not to use hormone replacement solely as prophylaxis against osteoporosis. It is debatable whether to recommend serial bone density studies in high-risk patients who are on maximum prophylactic therapy (diet, calcium, exercise, and hormone replacement). A few of these patients may benefit from slightly higher doses of estrogen or progestogens than are usually suggested, or they may be candidates for diphosphonate therapy if they do develop significant bone loss. The cost-effectiveness of performing serial studies on all patients at increased risk is doubtful; therefore, recommendations should be individualized.

Side Effects of Hormone Replacement Therapy and Their Management

Uterine bleeding is the most common side effect of hormone replacement in menopause. Withdrawal bleeding after the progestogen days of a cyclically administered estrogen/progestogen regimen occurs in 60 to 90 percent of women on these treatments. Bleeding is more common in younger menopausal women and when higher-dose estrogen regimens are used. Because cyclic menses are not acceptable to many menopausal women, continuous combined estrogen/progestogen regimens have been introduced to maintain constant endometrial suppression. However, a significant number of women (40 to 60 percent) will experience varying degrees of bleeding for several months after initiation of continuous combined therapy. This is apparently due to an abnormal endometrial response to the hormones. Endometrial histologic evaluation of these patients usually reveals small amounts of tissue with inconsistent microscopic findings, and no evidence of neoplasia or hyperplasia. Management of this problem may require only simple observation, as the bleeding will usually resolve with time (several weeks to several months) or changes in therapy.

In the protocol we utilize, we believe that endometrial evaluation usually is not indicated prior to hormone therapy, in patients with withdrawal bleeding after cyclic therapy, or in patients having breakthrough bleeding the first few months after initiating continuous combined therapy. A screening biopsy should be strongly considered before initiating therapy if a patient has a long history of anovulation or other risk factors for endometrial cancer. Likewise, patients with bleeding other than the normal withdrawal bleeding, those with an unexplained increase in bleeding that continues for several months, and those with persistent bleeding (greater than 4 to 6 months duration) on continuous combined therapy should undergo endometrial sampling. Transvaginal sonography may help with endometrial evaluation in patients on the continuous combined therapy. A thin appearing endometrium (less than 5 mm total thickness) has been shown in almost all cases, when biopsied, to represent atrophic or suppressed endometrium, but this does not totally rule out the presence of a small neoplasm as a cause for the bleeding. A few cases of carcinoma have been found within atrophic endometrium. Therefore, persistent bleeding after 4 to 6 months of combined therapy indicates the need for biopsy regardless of sonographic findings. A sonographically depicted endometrial stripe greater than 5 mm diameter usually represents estrogen-stimulated endometrium, and warrants histologic evaluation. Hyperplasia and neoplasia cannot be ruled out sonographically.[15] Sonograms may be useful in managing the patient on continuous combined therapy to exclude the possibility of excess estrogen stimulation or the presence of a large intrauterine abnormality, thus allowing one to avoid biopsy when breakthrough bleeding occurs early in the therapy.

Fluid retention, gastrointestinal symptoms, psychological effects, or other side effects may occur in 10 to 20 percent of postmenopausal women placed on hormone replacement. Bloating and a feeling of fluid retention are not uncommon complaints. These symptoms are most likely to occur during the estrogen/progestogen days of cyclic therapy and are, for the most part, progestogen dose related. Gastrointestinal dysfunction (flatulence, constipation, and diarrhea) are rare complaints that may be due to the effect of the progestogen on gastrointestinal motility. Finally, a few patients will develop depression and a premenstrual-like syndrome. Psychological symptoms may occur with estrogen alone, but are most frequently seen during the estrogen/progestogen days of cyclic therapy. The above side effects may not be related to therapy, and other causes should be considered. If the symptoms are felt to be due to cyclic progestogen use, continuous combination therapy or other therapeutic regimens with lower progestogen dosage may be useful.

Alternatives to Estrogen Replacement Therapy

Tamoxifen, a weak estrogen agonist used as therapy for breast cancer, has been shown to effectively decrease bone calcium loss when given to early postmenopausal women. There are also data to indicate some protection against heart disease. On the other hand, tamoxifen does very little for vasomotor symptoms, and may actually worsen atrophic symptoms in a few individuals. It also may increase a woman's risk of developing endometrial cancer.

Progestogen therapy given alone in doses higher than are normally used when the progestogen is given with estrogen (e.g., medroxyprogesterone acetate, 20 mg daily; Megace, 20 to 40 mg; or Depomedroxyprogesterone acetate, 150 to 300 mg IM every three months) has been shown to effectively ablate hot flashes[14] and may provide some prophylaxis against osteoporosis. However, these medications may increase the risk of heart disease and also may adversely affect atrophic symptoms.

Vasodilator antihypertensive agents such as clonidine and alpha-methyldopa have shown some effectiveness against vasomotor symptoms. The side effect of these medications is hypotension, and blood pressure should be monitored. A belladona alkaloid (Bellergal) has been used for vasomotor symptoms; however, there are no good controlled studies to document effectiveness.

As mentioned earlier, there is no very good substitute for estrogen for the reversal or prevention of vaginal atrophy. However, vaginal acidification or creams containing antimicrobial agents such as sulfa or clindamycin may decrease vaginal itching and burning.

Patients who are not receiving estrogen replacement therapy—as well as those who are—should be counseled regarding the importance of a well-balanced, low-fat diet, calcium supplementation, exercise, alcohol use only in moderation, and not smoking.

Premature Ovarian Failure

Cessation of menses due to depletion of ovarian follicles prior to the age of 40 is termed premature ovarian failure. While causes for the disorder (Table 31-6) are variable, most cases are idiopathic, with the ovaries exhibiting the same anatomical and functional appearance seen with natural menopause. Patients with premature ovarian failure exhibit the same symptoms and physiologic changes as those undergoing age-appropriate ovarian failure. Diagnosis is made by: 1. a negative pregnancy test; 2. a negative progesterone withdrawal test; and 3. an elevated FSH level (greater than 30 to 50, depending on the laboratory). The progesterone withdrawal test involves intramuscular injection of progesterone in oil, or seven to ten days of oral progestogen. Bleeding thereafter suggests estrogen production and endometrial stimulation. No bleeding implies hypoestrogenism. A few patients with a presumed diagnosis of ovarian failure will periodically experience ovulation. Therefore, reproductive failure is not absolute. In addition, some patients (particularly young patients) who have physical and laboratory evidence of ovarian failure after chemotherapy will regain ovarian function.

TABLE 31-6 Causes of Premature Ovarian Failure

Gonadotropin-resistant follicles
Autoimmune disorder
Postchemotherapy
Postovarian radiation
Ovarian sclerosis—follicular depletion
Idiopathic

Hormone replacement appears to be quite important in patients with premature ovarian failure. There is a substantial increase in coronary artery disease and osteoporosis in these patients that is preventable by estrogen administration. Patients who experience ovarian failure secondary to chemotherapeutic regimens should receive replacement therapy if not contraindicated, but probably should have their hormone therapy stopped periodically in order to remeasure FSH levels. If a patient has ovarian failure secondary to chemotherapy for breast cancer, tamoxifen therapy may be the best choice. However, it may be wise to monitor the endometrium as proliferative disorders, including endometrial cancer, may occur.

References and Selected Readings

1. Brincat M, Kabalan S, Studd J, et al: A study of the decrease of skin collagen content, skin thickness, and bone mass in the postmenopausal woman. *Obstet Gynecol* 70:840, 1987.
2. Chetkowski RJ, Meldram DR, Steingold KA, et al: Biological effects of transdermal estradiol. *N Engl J Med* 314:1615, 1986.
3. Coope J: Double-blind crossover study of estrogen replacement therapy, in Campbell S (ed): *Management of the Menopause and Postmenopausal Years*. Lancaster, England: MTP Press, 1976, p 167.
4. Dupont WD, Page DL: Menopausal estrogen replacement therapy and breast cancer. *Arch Intern Med* 151:67–72, 1991.

5. Grady D, Rubin SM, Pititti DB, et al: Hormone therapy to prevent disease and prolong life in postmenopausal women. *Ann Intern Med* 117(12):1016, 1992.
6. Luciano AA, DeSouza MJ, Roy MP, et al: Evaluation of low dose estrogen and progestin therapy in postmenopausal women. A double-blind prospective study of sequential versus continuous therapy. *J Reprod Med* 38(3):207, 1993.
7. Lucky MM, Meier DE, Mandelie JP: Radial and vertebral bone density in white and black women: Evidence for racial differences in premenopausal bone homeostasis. *J Clin Endocrinol Metab* 69:762, 1989.
8. Nactigall LE, Nachtigall RH, Nachtigall RD, et al: Estrogen replacement therapy II: A prospective study on the relationship to carcinoma and cardiovascular and metabolic problems. *Obstet Gynecol* 54:74, 1979.
9. Oliver MF, Boyd GS: Effect of bilateral ovariectomy on coronary artery disease and serum lipid levels. *Lancet* 2:690, 1959.
10. Peterson HB, et al: Genital neoplasia, in Mishell D (ed): *Menopause: Physiology and Pharmacology*. Chicago: Year Book Medical Publishers, 1987.
11. Powers MS, Schenkel L, Darley PE, et al: Pharmacokinetics and pharmacodynamics of transdermal dosage forms of 17-B estradiol: Comparison with conventional oral estrogens used for hormone replacement. *Am J Obstet Gynecol* 152:1099, 1985.
12. Riis B, Thomsen K, Christiansen C: Does calcium supplementation prevent postmenopausal bone loss? A double-blind controlled study. *N Engl J Med* 316:173, 1987.
13. Schiff I, Komarov H, Cramer D, et al: Endometrial hyperplasia in women on cyclic or continuous regimens. *Fertil Steril* 37:79, 1982.
14. Schiff I, Tulchinsky D, Cramer D, et al: Oral medroxyprogesterone in the treatment of postmenopausal symptoms. *JAMA* 244:1443, 1980.
15. Varner RE, Sparks JM, Cameron CD, et al: Transvaginal sonography of the endometrium in postmenopausal women. *Obstet Gynecol* 78:195, 1991.
16. Weinstein RS, Bell NH: Diminished rates of bone formation in normal black adults. *N Engl J Med* 319:1968, 1988.
17. Woodruff JD, Pickar JH, for The Menopause Study Group: Incidence of endometrial hyperplasia in postmenopausal women taking conjugated estrogens (Premarin) with medroxyprogesterone acetate or conjugated estrogens alone. *Am J Obstet Gynecol* 170:1213–1223, 1994.

32 Urogynecology

Jeffrey L. Cornella
Henry A. Thiede

Anatomy

The Lower Urinary Tract

Important clinical generalizations which apply to an understanding of urogynecology and urinary continence include the following:

1. The female bladder and urethrovesical junction are supported by the anterior vaginal wall. Anatomical relaxation and its surgical correction involve vaginal weakness, detachment, and resultant descent. Routine operations for female stress urinary incontinence

elevate the vagina at the urethrovesical junction.
2. Postoperative traction placed on one anatomical portion of the vagina may cause relaxation in other anatomical areas. Excessive elevation of the anterior vaginal wall may predispose the patient to subsequent enterocele formation. Similarly, excessive traction of the posterior vagina by fixation to the sacrospinous ligament may increase the propensity for cystocele formation.[50]
3. Anatomical relaxation does not necessarily translate to symptoms. Patients may have significant prolapse and still be asymptomatic. Other patients may be free of vaginal relaxation, yet experience sensations of pressure, urgency, and frequency of urination.

The Urinary Bladder

The wall of the bladder consists of an outer adventitial layer of connective tissue, a smooth muscle layer, and an inner layer of mucous membrane that lines the interior. The detrusor comprises a single unit of large-diameter, interlacing, smooth muscle cells. Contraction results in a reduction of all dimensions of the bladder lumen.

The bladder neck consists of muscle that is histologically, histochemically, and pharmacologically distinct from the detrusor proper. Although the human female bladder neck does not have a true anatomical sphincter, there is a functional contribution to the maintenance of continence.

The Urethra

DeLancey reviewed 22 paraurethral anatomical dissections and 1500 slides to identify structures that influence urethral position and resistance.[14] The position of each of these structures along the urethra was determined. Two anatomical areas appear to make the most salient contribution to urinary continence:

1. The midurethra extends for approximately 20 to 60 percent of total urethral length and includes the region of the striated urethral sphincter (rhabdosphincter) and muscular attachment of urethral supports.
2. The urogenital diaphragm with the deep transverse perineal musculature (urethrovaginal sphincter muscle and compressor urethrae muscle) are found from 54 to 76 percent of the urethral length.

The smooth muscle of the urethra is found throughout its length without specific condensations. The majority of these slender muscle bundles are oriented obliquely or longitudinally and may serve to shorten or widen the urethra during micturition. It is unlikely that the competence of the female bladder neck and proximal urethra is solely the result of smooth muscle activity.[26]

The striated internal urethral sphincter wraps around the urethra as a 1.5-cm band, extending from the 18th to the 64th percentile of urethral length. This rhabdosphincter is anatomically separate from the adjacent periurethral striated muscle of the anterior pelvic floor. The muscle fibers are of the slow twitch variety, able to exert tone upon the urethral lumen over prolonged periods of time. The internal sphincter is the site of maximal resting urethral pressure.

The maximal dynamic (during coughing) urethral pressure in the normal female corresponds to the area of the deep transverse perineal musculature. Pressure increases in this area are partially reflexive and may precede transmitted abdominal pressure by 200 to 300 ms.[11] This area may be considered the external striated sphincter of the female.

The upward and downward motion of that portion of the urethra which lies above the urogenital diaphragm is under voluntary control. Jeffcoate and Roberts have ascribed this mobility to connections of the vagina to the levator ani muscles. DeLancey has described this as the vaginolevator attachment or muscular attachment of the urethral supports.

Muscular Attachment of the Urethral Supports (Paravaginal Attachment)

Fibers connect the vagina to the pubococcygeus portion of the levator ani muscle and its fascia. As the urethra and vagina are intimately connected at this point, this vaginolevator attachment significantly affects the urethra. At the upper end of the vaginolevator fibers, the direct interdigitation of collagen and smooth muscle from the vaginal wall with levators is no longer present, but the connection of the vagina with the superior fascia of the levator ani continues as the arcus tendineus fasciae pelvis. This paravaginal attachment can be disrupted at vaginal delivery, resulting in a paravaginal defect and anterior wall descent. The reattachment of this defect is called a paravaginal defect repair.

Neurology

Innervation of the Detrusor and Urethral Smooth Muscle

The sympathetic innervation of the bladder and the associated thoracolumbar visceral afferent fibers are concerned with the filling and storage phases of micturition. The parasympathetic innervation and accompanying sacral afferent fibers are important for normal voiding.

The pelvic and hypogastric nerves supply the bladder and urethra with efferent parasympathetic and sympathetic neurons, and both convey afferent sensory neurons from these organs to the spinal cord. The parasympathetic efferent supply is classically described as originating in the intermediolateral region of the gray matter of the sacral spinal cord segments S2 to S4, and is ultimately conveyed by the pelvic nerve. The efferent sympathetic nerves to the bladder and urethra are thought to originate in the intermediolateral nuclei of spinal cord segments T11 to T12, and are ultimately conveyed by the hypogastric nerves.

Ganglia that innervate the bladder and urethral smooth musculature generally lie close to or within these structures, and give rise to "short neurons," which comprise the bulk of the nerves that actually innervate these structures.[17] The innervation of the bladder is thus remarkably complex, with reflexes that not only travel to and from the spinal cord, but also to and from individual ganglia at a subspinal level.

There is clear evidence that acetylcholine acting as a transmitter from parasympathetic efferents is responsible for detrusor contraction during micturition (Kuru). It is suggested that sympathetic mediated inhibition of the bladder depends not on direct effects from noradrenergic fibers on the detrusor, but on indirect inhibition of excitatory parasympathetics within the ganglia of the pelvic plexus.

Sacral visceral afferents have been shown to be evenly distributed throughout the bladder. They appear to convey touch, pain, and bladder distention and are essential to complete micturition.

Innervation of Urethral Striated Muscle

Somatomotor innervation of the rhabdosphincter traditionally has been believed to be conveyed exclusively by the pudendal nerves. This concept may need some revision in view of accumulating data that this structure may be partially innervated autonomically.

Pathophysiology of Stress Urinary Incontinence

The Role of Partial Denervation of the Pelvic Floor

In a remarkable study performed in 1953 by Berglas and Rubin, x-ray myography showed that, at rest, the levator plate has an almost horizontal course.[5] The uterus and vagina are situated over the levator plate posteriorly, and not over the levator hiatus as had been deduced previously by examination of cadaveric specimens. During a sudden rise of the intra-abdominal pressure in a normal patient, the thrust is directed backward and downward, which pushes rectum, vagina, and uterus against the levator plate. Adequate function of the levator plate depends on the proper activity of the nervous system. Impairment of the structural and functional integrity of the levator plate allows it to sag downward. This correlates directly with the resultant prolapse, as the total area of the muscular hiatus increases with levator inclination.

Histochemical studies of pelvic floor muscle biopsies and pelvic floor single-fiber electromyography have demonstrated evidence of muscle fiber damage in the pelvic floor of women suffering from genital tract prolapse and stress urinary incontinence.[51] There is evidence of local partial denervation accompanied by reinnervation of the posterior pubococcygeus muscle.[24] Smith performed single fiber electromyography of the pubococcygeus in 69 asymptomatic women and 105 women with stress incontinence or genitourinary prolapse.[51] These studies suggest that partial denervation of the pelvic floor is a normal accompaniment of aging and is increased by childbirth. Women with stress incontinence or genitourinary prolapse have a significant increase in denervation of the pelvic floor compared with asymptomatic women.

In a separate study, Smith evaluated the terminal pudendal nerve conduction in asymptomatic and stress incontinent women.[52] Women with stress incontinence of urine had delayed conduction to both the striated urethral muscle and the pelvic floor muscle, indicative of denervation injury. Women with normal urinary control and genitourinary prolapse had similar conduction times to the urethral sphincter striated muscle as normal women, but showed clear evidence of denervation damage to the pelvic floor muscle.

Proposed Continence Mechanisms

Continence in the female is maintained by a summation of several factors or mechanisms that act in concert. As these factors diminish the patient may reach a threshold at which pressure acting on the bladder results in loss of urine. Treatment attempts to add or restore factors to the point of patient satisfaction with symptoms.

The following factors contribute to continence in the female:

1. Proper innervation of the urethra, maintaining striated muscle function and viscoelastic properties
2. Proper innervation of the bladder neck, maintaining the function pressure of the urethrovesical junction
3. A supported urethrovesical junction which, upon straining, arrests the descent of the urethrovesical junction
4. Proper innervation and muscular function of the deep transverse perineal musculature, which acts as an external sphincter and provides reflexive increased pressure coincident with coughing
5. Submucosal vascularity of the urethra and surface tension of the mucosa
6. A stable and properly functioning detrusor

Under normal conditions, continence is maintained as a result of efficient transmission of intraabdominal pressure rises to the proximal three-quarters of the urethral length. Factors that may predispose to failure of adequate pressure transmission include: a low resting urethral closure pressure (i.e., urethral pressure minus bladder pressure), urethral pressure instability, extreme abdominal pressure variations, excessive sustained response to stress, and a shortened dysfunctional urethra.

These, in turn, may be directly affected by the levator muscular support and function. Impaired mechanical function due to loss of anatomical connections or neurologic function may result in defective pressure transmission and resultant urine loss.

Therefore, a lack of these factors can contribute to incontinence in the female. Additional conditions that contribute to incontinence include:

1. Chronic serial coughing, with resultant serial lowering of urethral pressure
2. Obesity, with presumed resultant increased abdominal pressures
3. Denervation of the pelvic floor and pudendal nerve compromise
4. Damage of the pelvic plexus secondary to pelvic surgery or pelvic mass
5. Anatomical abnormalities, such as fistulas or diverticula
6. Urinary tract infection (cystitis)

Differential Diagnosis of Female Urinary Incontinence

1. Stress urinary incontinence
2. Bladder instability or detrusor instability
3. Mixed urinary incontinence
4. Detrusor hyperreflexia (neurologic in etiology)
5. Overflow incontinence

6. Vesicovaginal, urethrovaginal, or ureterovaginal fistula
7. Urethral instability
8. Pharmacologic incontinence
9. Spurious incontinence

Office Evaluation of Incontinence

History

The evaluation of urinary incontinence, and other urogynecologic problems involves the assessment of multiple symptoms and objective findings with subsequent formation of an overall impression. The more complex the problem, the more important objective testing becomes in the evaluation of the patient. While symptoms alone are a poor predictor of the type of incontinence, objective testing should include a thorough and detailed history. As our methods of testing become more precise in the future, the predictive validity of some aspects of the medical history may improve.

The historical data should include the following as a minimum:

1. The impact of the urine loss upon the patient's life, socially and personally
2. Indicators of stress incontinence or bladder instability
3. Past urologic evaluations, treatment measures, and previous pelvic surgery
4. Medical diagnoses or medications that may be affecting the urinary tract
5. Cognitive level and capacity

If the patient feels her urine loss is a significant problem, additional evaluation and treatment are appropriate. An equal amount of urine loss in a patient who does not perceive it as a problem would most likely not receive further evaluation and therapy. Education about incontinence allows patients to make informed choices when options are presented.

Symptoms of only stress incontinence or only urge incontinence (bladder instability) are more predictive than a mixture of symptoms. However, the vast majority of patients present with mixed symptoms, especially patients beyond the fifth decade of life. The physician must then rely primarily on objective parameters for a diagnosis.[59] The pure symptoms of nonsustained, immediate urine loss with coughing, laughing, and sneezing is predictive of stress incontinence. The same symptom with a background of mixed symptoms can be found with a final diagnosis of detrusor instability or mixed incontinence.

Most patients will give a history of en route urine loss (a symptom usually associated with control loss or bladder instability). The majority of these patients will not have bladder instability on routine multichannel urodynamic testing. This is partially explained by the fact that detrusor instability may not show up on a given cystometrogram, but may be demonstrated objectively by other means, such as ambulatory urodynamic monitoring or a repeat cystometrogram on an alternate day.[67] Spontaneous complete bladder emptying and true nocturnal enuresis are rare and more predictive of bladder instability. There is a difference between awakening and subsequent urine loss in bed and urine loss in bed when asleep. Only the latter should be considered as true nocturnal enuresis.

It is important to ask the patient about previous evaluations and treatment successes or failures. Some medications previously found unsuccessful may be successful when given at different dosages. Unsuccessful pelvic floor exercise may become successful with proper instruction. Patients with failed previous operations should be considered in a complex group and should undergo urodynamic evaluation. Previous operative notes should be reviewed for technique and suture type.

Medical problems may affect a patient's tendency to experience incontinence. Diabetes may result in a propensity to develop urinary tract infections or in sacral neuropathy with resultant bladder effects. Chronic coughing may cause asymptomatic patients to become symptomatic. Multiple sclerosis, Parkinson's disease, or cerebral vascular accidents may result in incontinence. Medications such as alpha blockers may decrease urethral resistance and make an asymptomatic patient experience incontinence. Anticholinergic agents may inhibit bladder emptying and result in overflow incontinence.

Physical Examination

The office examination is a very important objective assessment in the formation of an overall diagnostic impression. The examination should be thorough, consistent, and accompanied by discussion emphasizing the reproduction of symptoms. If the office examination is inconsistent with the patient's description of symptoms, additional evaluation is indicated. If the patient's symptoms are consistent with the findings on physical examination, the practitioner has, at his or her discretion, additional testing, if it is felt to be beneficial to form the best and most accurate impression. The physician may choose to repeat portions of the vaginal examination on an alternate day, as relaxation may vary depending on activities.

Physical examination should include the following assessments as a minimum:

1. Degree of pelvic floor and vaginal descent and relaxation
2. Degree of urethrovesical junction descent with straining
3. Vaginal integrity and estrogenization
4. Bimanual and rectal examination to rule out pelvic mass and to assess anal sphincter tone
5. Neurologic examination of the perineum and lower extremities
6. Amount of urine loss on stress testing

Standing Examination The patient is asked to present with a subjectively full bladder. The physical examination begins in the standing position. The patient stands over a pad with a wide stance as the examiner looks for evidence of prolapse with straining and coughing. The labia are then separated and the patient asked to give a single, hard cough. If urine loss is absent, coughing is extended to two hard coughs, then three in a row. If urine loss is noted, a distinction is made between an immediate, nonsustained urine loss, and a loss that occurs after a one- to three-second delay and is somewhat sustained. The latter is suggestive of bladder instability and the former of stress urinary incontinence. These impressions should almost always be confirmed by additional objective testing prior to any consideration of surgery.

If prolapse is present, an additional standing examination with fingers in the rectum and vagina is repeated at the time of bimanual examination.

Sitting Examination The neurologic examination starts with the patient in the sitting position. The spinal center for micturition is in sacral segments 2, 3, and 4. (This can be considered subservient to the pontine micturition center.) The lower extremities are mainly innervated by the lower lumbar segments; therefore, it is possible to have a lesion in this area and preserve the sacral area, giving a lower motor neuron lesion picture to the extremities and an upper motor lesion picture to the bladder. The patellar reflex arc involves the second to fourth lumbar segments. The ankle reflex involves the lumbar 5 and sacral 1 and 2 segments. Extension, flexion, abduction, and adduction of the legs, and inversion, eversion, dorsiflexion, and extension of the feet are tested.

Supine Examination The patient is then sent to empty her bladder; on return she is asked to assume the dorsal lithotomy position. Attention is directed to the perineum. A cotton swab is used to test fine-touch sensation in the saddle area. Pin-prick response and dullness are also tested in the same area. Reflexes, which involves S2, 3, and 4, are the "anal wink" or anocutaneous reflex and the bulbocavernosus reflex. The former is tested by stimulating the perianal skin with the swab or a pin-prick to the mucocutaneous junction of the anus. The bulbocavernosus reflex involves visualizing or palpating lightly with a finger in the vaginal introitus; a contraction of the bulbocavernous muscle is stimulated by tapping or squeezing the clitoris, or, if these measures fail, by stimulating the bladder base with gentle traction on a Foley balloon. Bulbocavernosus reflexes should be tested bilaterally, as a unilateral lesion may exist. Local damage to the anal sphincter from surgery or childbirth may influence interpretation of the response to stimulus.

The patient is then asked to contract her anal sphincter (corticoregulatory tract) and to contract the circumvaginal muscles. The latter is assessed manually with a finger in the vagina, noting the appropriateness of response and the strength and symmetry of contraction. It is essential that the speculum used for the examination can be taken apart to form a retracting blade (Sims), which can be used to examine the anterior and posterior walls separately. The intact speculum is used initially to examine the vaginal apex or cervix for descent. The patient is asked to strain, and the speculum is withdrawn slightly. While observing the response of the apex, the examiner grades the amount of descent. The speculum is then taken apart, and the anterior vaginal wall is retracted while the examiner observes the posterior wall's response to straining. A bulge and descent in the superior aspect of the posterior wall could be termed a rotation rectocele, which involves detachment from the upper sidewall of the pelvis. Relaxation due to thinning of the posterior wall is also termed a rectocele. The amount of relaxation is graded. The speculum is then used to retract the posterior wall of the vagina. It should be noted that this compromises one of the continence mechanisms. One should test for coughing loss with the patient in a supine position without the speculum in place. The patient is asked to cough and strain; relaxation and descent are noted.

There are three areas of relaxation which may involve the anterior wall.[2] The anterior wall may be detached from the area of the cervix or high apex (cervicovaginal detachment or level I detachment).[13] The anterior wall may be detached paravaginally (lower vaginal lateral detachment or level II detachment), and elevation of the anterior lateral sulci with a forceps results in full correction or partial correction of this relaxation. The anterior wall may be thinned in the midline above the urethrovesical junction, forming what is termed a transverse cystocele. In addition, a small but important relaxation may result in midline rotation of the urethrovesical junction without any of the defects described above. The physician notes and grades the defects and judges the degree of urethrovesical junction rotation. The latter is best accomplished by insertion of a sterile cotton swab into the urethra, which has been lubricated with xylocaine jelly. Degrees of rotation are measured from a horizontal reference of zero. Rotation of greater than 30 degrees with straining is considered abnormal.

There are different grading systems for vaginal relaxation, and an effort is underway to standardize such grading. One system grades a bulge that presents to the introitus as grade III. A bulge that passes through the introitus is grade IV. A bulge halfway to the introitus is grade II, with grade I as an intermediate relaxation. Paravaginal defects are grade IV when they reach the introitus (full rotation of the anterior wall) with lesser degrees of rotation given the remaining designations. If the anterior lateral sulci are completely elevated and a bulge is noted above the urethrovesical junction (often accompanied by loss of vaginal rugae), this is termed a transverse cystocele.

A bimanual examination is then performed. First, the vaginal mucosa is carefully palpated to rule out any vaginal lesions not observed on speculum examination, and the urethra is palpated to rule out any overt tenderness or abnormality, such as a diverticulum. A bimanual exam of the pelvis is done. The rectal finger is then added to the exam. The patient is then asked to stand, and the rectovaginal exam is repeated to assess the components of relaxation.

Before proceeding, it is important to educate the patient about how incontinence is evaluated. She should understand the purpose of testing and its impact on future management decisions.

Simple Office Testing In general, the value of simple office filling tends to be underestimated and the sophistication of formal urodynamic testing tends to be overestimated. Simple office filling is extremely valuable in forming the overall impression or diagnosis. Additionally, it offers an examination on an alternate day of formal testing, and this may increase the sensitivity of diagnosis. Often, simple office testing shows a residual urine that more truly reflects the patient's status, as compared with residual examinations at cystoscopy or multichannel testing, which may be spuriously elevated.

The patient is asked to empty her bladder and the amount voided is recorded. If the patient has no need of SBE prophylaxis, a sterile catheter is used for a residual urine determination. The urine obtained can be used for urinalysis and, if indicated, culture and sensitivity testing. The physician may reflect upon the summation of the voided urine and residual amount against the background of urine loss demonstrated during initial examination. A catheter-tipped syringe minus the plunger is then attached to the catheter, and simple office filling of the bladder follows, using sterile water and filling at a rate between 75 and 100 ml per min. Urine cytologic studies may be indicated in patients over 50, especially if they have symptoms of urgency. In this case the bladder is filled with normal saline instead of water. The volumes at first sensation, fullness, and maximum fullness are then recorded. The last value is referred to as the maximum cystometric capacity on a simple office filling. This may exceed that demonstrated later at urodynamic testing—again demonstrating the value of this separate examination. The patient is then asked to give a single cough, then to add coughs incrementally to the number five or to the point of urine loss. Whether the patient loses urine with a single cough or multiple coughs, is recorded as a rough indicator of severity, at a given bladder volume. Immediate, nonsustained, or projectile loss is suggestive of stress incontinence. Delayed loss that is sustained or cannot be volitionally inhibited is suggestive of control loss or an uninhibited detrusor contraction. Throughout this process it is important to ascertain from the patient whether or not the observed losses are representative of her symptoms. The patient may give no history of stress incontinence symptoms, yet demonstrate significant loss with straining on office testing. This allows an opportunity to educate the patient regarding this component of loss and its contribution to her overall incontinence.

Patients with prolapse should be further stress-tested in the supine and standing positions with the prolapse reduced. Care must be taken not to press on the anterior vaginal wall with prolapse reduction, but rather address pressure to the vaginal apex or high posterior wall. Stress incontinence may be masked by the vaginal relaxation pressing on or kinking the urethra at the time of straining. When the relaxation is surgically corrected (or elevated with a pessary), urine loss is unmasked and becomes symptomatic. If surgery is considered, it is incumbent on the examiner to perform this aspect of testing. If incontinence is not addressed at surgery, the patient may have immediate stress incontinence, either postoperatively or within several months of surgery. Incontinence and vaginal relaxation are interrelated and must be addressed concomitantly in patient assessment and treatment. Similarly, if a small enterocele is noted at examination and not corrected at incontinence surgery, the patient may return several months later with a large, symptomatic enterocele. The best patient care dictates that *all* vaginal relaxation should be corrected at incontinence surgery to avoid this occurrence.

Urodynamic Testing

Urodynamic testing refers to multichannel pressure testing, uroflowmetry, sphincter electromyography, and cystourethroscopy. Multichannel pressure testing includes cystometrogram testing, pressure-flow studies, Valsalva leak-point pressures, and urethral profilometry. Descriptions of these techniques can be found in a separate part of this book on common tests performed in the office. The following discussion is concerned with the indications, benefit, and meaning of urodynamic testing.

The Significance of Urodynamic Testing

Urodynamic testing is technician-dependent. The skill of the examiner and the quality of the interaction with the patient are of paramount importance. It is incumbent upon the referring physician to find practitioners who have significant training in the performance of urodynamic testing and dependable knowledge of female pathophysiology. A given gynecologist or urologist may not have this training and knowledge. Experience and knowledge are more important than the particular specialty.

Urodynamic testing is technician-dependent because the patient's symptoms must be reproduced during the testing in order to arrive at a conclusion. The symptoms are temporally related to the findings on the recording. In this way, an impression is reached regarding the pathophysiologic occurrence responsible for the symptoms. If the symptoms are not reproduced, data may be reported that are not relevant or are, in fact, misleading. All symptoms may not be reproduced at the time of testing. As an example, a given cystometrogram may not demonstrate detrusor instability in a patient, but it may be demonstrated on a repeat cystometrogram or ambulatory testing.

Cystourethroscopy is also observer-dependent. A dysfunctional bladder neck may or may not always be evident to a given observer. Borderline impressions often require other testing for confirmation, such as a standing, at-rest cystogram, to rule out a severely dysfunctional or type III urethra.

Indications for Urodynamic Testing and Cystourethroscopy

The following are indications for urodynamic testing:

1. Neurologic conditions, such as multiple sclerosis or Parkinson's disease
2. Symptoms of urge incontinence suggestive of severe bladder instability or detrusor hyperreflexia
3. Urinary retention with or without a history of detrusor hyperreflexia

A case can be made for routine performance of urodynamic testing prior to surgery. The purpose is to rule out occult detrusor instability and to assess bladder contractility, both of which have prognostic implications. Some patients will also demonstrate cough-induced bladder instability on testing. These patients would be at risk for continued incontinence following operation. However, if one does not wish to perform urodynamic studies on all preoperative patients undergoing an incontinence procedure, the following should be considered as imperative indications:

1. Any patient who has had a previous incontinence operation, vaginal colporrhaphy, or radical pelvic surgery
2. Any patient with a history of pelvic irradiation
3. Any patient who does not demonstrate urethrovesical junction rotation greater than 20 degrees in the presence of stress urinary incontinence signs and symptoms
4. Patients who have a urethral diverticulum
5. Patients with equivocal findings on simple office testing or significant postvoid residual volumes (> 100 ml)
6. Elderly patients, because of the prevalence of detrusor instability and low urethral closure pressure
7. A history of multiple vaginal surgeries and/or vaginal prolapse

Cystourethroscopy also should be performed on all preoperative patients to assess the urethra and to rule out a lesion of the bladder mucosa. It is further indicated for:

1. A history of recurrent pyuria
2. A history of asymptomatic hematuria
3. New onset of bladder irritation symptoms
4. History suggesting interstitial cystitis, painful bladder syndromes, or chronic infectious cystitis

Treatment of Stress Urinary Incontinence

Education of the incontinent patient is extremely important, but its importance and benefit to the patient often are underestimated. Education can make the patient an informed partner in her care. This fosters additional motivation and understanding, which aid the success of the conservative approach. If additional testing is required, patients who know what to expect in the urodynamic laboratory feel more comfortable. Studies have also suggested that patients feel better knowing that there are options, possible improvements through therapy, and that they are not alone in their problem.

Any practitioner who has a coworker interested in educating the incontinent patient has an opportunity to add a new dimension to the practice. Education, itself, can result in improvement through bladder retraining, description of timed voiding, reemphasis of pelvic floor exercises, and adjunctive therapy measures. The use, benefits, and untoward symptoms of medications can be discussed. Patients feel that they have an opportunity to express their feelings and frustrations more fully and to have questions answered.

If patient numbers warrant, it is highly beneficial to establish a weekly or biweekly class about incontinence. Ideally, a follow-up class also may be established. If a physical therapist is not available, nurses can work with patients one-on-one to insure that they are performing circumvaginal exercises appropriately.

Conservative Treatment of Urinary Incontinence

The conservative treatment of incontinence has experienced a resurgence of interest in the last several years. As methods of performing and investigating conservative methods have improved, it has become evident that they are more beneficial than previously appreciated.

As an example, for years patients were told to perform pelvic floor exercises without testing to see whether that patient knew how to do them or which muscles to contract. The number of contractions performed each day also was often inadequate. Bump, in a recent study, demonstrated that 25 percent of uninstructed patients actually produce a reaction that may increase urine loss (such as Valsalva) when asked to contract the pelvic floor muscles.[7] If conservative methods are to be successful, a motivated and properly instructed patient is essential.

Pelvic Floor Exercises Pelvic floor exercises were performed as early as the mid-nineteenth century, although Kegel, reporting in 1948, was the first to investigate the long-term effects, utilizing somewhat objective methods with the aid of a perineometer. The results of past studies are variable, with poor follow-up, infrequent urodynamic testing, and lack of standardized methods and terms. In the late 1980s, additional studies were published that utilized more objective methods. It appears that pelvic floor exercises, when properly performed, are a useful adjunct in mild to moderate incontinence.

Mouritsen studied the long-term effect of pelvic floor exercises on female incontinence.[41] Seventy-six women underwent a 3-month exercise program and were followed for 1 year. At the 12-month evaluation, 30 percent were considered cured, 17 percent were improved. Patients with severe incontinence did not benefit from the therapy, while 72 percent of patients with mild incontinence experienced a cure. Patients in this study were instructed in digital biofeedback.

Some studies have suggested that formal biofeedback increases the success rate of pelvic floor exercises. Burgio studied a group of 11 women treated with digital biofeedback, compared with a group of 13 women with bladder-sphincter biofeedback. The latter group had a 76 percent decrease in incontinence, compared with a 51 percent decrease in the former group.[8]

The more enthusiastic and involved the instruction, the greater the success. However, it is not possible to have intensive, recurrent biofeedback sessions for all patients.

The following recommendations and interventions, which increase in scope, should be considered:

1. Assessment of circumvaginal muscle contraction during physical examination for strength and the absence of improper contraction of surrounding muscle (such as the gluteal and rectus muscles)
2. Feedback to the patient during physical examination regarding her ability to contract appropriate muscles
3. Written instructions given to the patient on the proper performance of pelvic floor exercises, including frequency and number of contractions; the patients should be instructed to perform four sets of 20 contractions per day, consistently, for at least 8 weeks
4. Follow-up visitation with the patient regarding compliance, benefit of digital pelvic floor exercise biofeedback, and changes in symptoms
5. Instruction by a therapist on biofeedback and the proper performance of circumvaginal exercises
6. Continued biofeedback with a home unit, symptom and therapy diary over weeks to months

7. Continued biofeedback with visitations to a therapist biweekly for single or group sessions over months
8. Weekly sessions with a therapist for biofeedback over months

Functional Electrical Stimulation Electrical stimulation has been used throughout the last three decades in the treatment of stress urinary incontinence. It has been employed either to aid in the treatment of bladder instability or to increase sphincteric/outlet resistance. Devices have included implanted electrodes, electronic pessaries, anal electodes, and intravaginal electrodes of various types.

The goal of electrical stimulation in the treatment of stress urinary incontinence is to increase the strength of the pelvic and periurethral muscles. Animal studies have shown that urethral pressure increases with intravaginal probes are secondary to direct stimulation of efferent motor axons. Electrical stimulation of the pelvic floor muscles results in reflexive contraction of paraurethral musculature and reflexive detrusor inhibition. There is unproven speculation that electrical stimulation may result in enhanced sprouting of previously damaged axons or a conversion of fast to slow twitch axons in paraurethral muscles. Patients with stress incontinence may benefit from the feedback of electrically induced muscle contractions, thus learning how to contract the appropriate muscles when performing pelvic floor exercises.

Studies on humans and animals have shown detrusor inhibition with electrical stimulation. A study by Bent and coworkers of patients with stress, urgency, and mixed incontinence groups has shown significant subjective patient improvement (52 percent in mixed, 70 percent in urgency, and 71 percent in pure stress incontinence), while objective parameters of improvement have remained unchanged. Additional studies are needed to determine success rates and physiologic effects.[4]

Surgical Treatment of Stress Urinary Incontinence

A number of features of urethral function distinguish symptom-free women from patients with genuine stress urinary incontinence. These include: maximum urethral pressure at rest or closure pressure, intraabdominal pressure variations, sustained response to stress (drop in urethral pressure from sustained coughing), and pressure-transmission ratios.

The aims of incontinence surgery have been variously defined as: tightening of the pubocervical fascia, elevation of the bladder neck, increasing urethral functional length, and increasing urethral resistance. Postoperative urodynamic studies have not shown consistent increases in urethral pressure or functional length in patients cured of incontinence. In fact, most studies have shown that there is no increase in urethral resting or closure pressure. Surgical success does appear to be urodynamically associated with increased pressure transmission to the urethra. These studies may also be suggestive of the duration of surgical success.[46]

It appears that the pressure-transmission ratio has an all-or-none effect in the determination of stress incontinence. The exact cause of the impairment in a given woman may not be completely apparent. The ability to maintain positive pressure in the urethra during stress may represent multiple factors acting in concert. These include a functional rhabdosphincter, anatomical support of the urethrovesical junction, a healthy estrogenized urethral lumen, and proper function of the levator musculature, as described earlier.

Surgery for urinary incontinence results in support to the urethrovesical junction, arrest of downward descent with straining, and increased pressure transmission to the urethra. The classic pubovaginal sling causes obstruction to the urethra coincident with coughing and increased pressure transmission to the urethra. Recent modifications in the procedure result in less obstruction.

The distribution of pressure transmission along the urethra following successful colposuspension is quite different from that seen in healthy women.[28] In healthy women, the maximum transmission ratios are at or just distal to the resting profile peak, which is at the middistal urethra. In women made continent by colposuspension, maximum transmission is achieved within the proximal half of the functional urethra. Thus, most incontinence operations do not restore a woman to a fully physiologic state.

The Paravaginal Defect Repair The paravaginal defect repair, or vaginolevator shelf procedure, by virtue of its close reapproximation to normal anatomy, may restore the extrinsic continence mechanism to a degree somewhat comparable to that of the normal female. Support of the urethrovesical junction is reestablished and attachment to the levator musculature may again allow movement and increased function. In most cases, patients can void almost immediately following surgery. Full function may be subclinically compromised in patients who have sustained significant damage to the pudendal nerve.

Shull and Baden reported a 6-year experience with the paravaginal defect repair for stress incontinence. Of 149 patients treated, 97 percent were reported as having excellent results with no further subjective stress incontinence.[49]

The Marshall-Marchetti-Krantz Procedure The Marshall-Marchetti-Krantz (MMK) procedure has been shown to be successful in the treatment of urinary stress incontinence as a primary operation and in patients with failure of previous surgical treatment.[36]

Considering the limitation of mobility following this procedure, and the high position of the anterior wall, it is unlikely that the continence mechanism is commensurate with that of the normal female. The MMK may work by a combination of slight obstruction, creating positive pressure transmission by an unknown mechanism, and additional features that act at the urethrovesical junction subsequent to its elevation.

The Burch Colposuspension The clinical effects of the Burch colposuspension and anterior vaginal repair for correction of stress urinary incontinence were assessed by Van Geelen in a superbly performed prospective study.[62] A full clinical examination, including simultaneous urethrocystometry, was performed with patients in the supine, sitting, and standing positions. This objective testing was accomplished preoperatively 3 months, 12 months, and 24 months after operation. Total follow-up of patients was 5 to 7 years. Neither surgical anterior repair nor Burch colposuspension affected the resting variables of the urethral sphincter mechanism. After Burch colposuspension, the transmitted intra-abdominal pressure to the urethra significantly increased in all recording positions in all women who were successfully treated. After successful anterior colporrhaphy, the increase in pressure transmission from the abdomen to the urethra was less prominent. The objective success rate of the Burch procedure was 85 percent at 2 years, compared to anterior colporrhaphy, which was 45 percent. At 5 years, the subjective cure rate for the Burch procedure was 76 percent and 31 percent for the anterior colporrhaphy. This and other studies support the belief that anterior colporrhaphy (Kelly-Kennedy type) should not be used as the primary operation for stress incontinence.

It is possible that bladder neck elevation not only allows improved pressure transmission, but also promotes greater efficiency of the pelvic floor reflex with accentuation of urethral closure by active means. Downward pressure on coughing from abdominal viscera may compress the urethra. Slight obstruction also may occur with a Burch procedure, as urodynamic studies have shown increased urethral resistance with a reduction in peak flow rate and an increase in voiding detrusor pressure.[27]

The Pubovaginal Sling Procedure The classic pubovaginal sling procedure results in obstruction at the urethrovesical junction, with descent of the bladder neck on coughing. Slings placed distal to this site will result in failure, even though the urethra is compressed with coughing. This transient obstruction results in increased pressure transmission to this area with stress. Beck reported that in 97.4 percent of 151 patients cured by fascia lata sling procedures the pressure-transmission ratio was greater than 100 percent.[3]

The Modified Pereyra Procedure (Raz, Needle Suspension Procedure) This procedure provides support to the urethrovesical junction and allows compression of the urethra with stress. There is no attachment to levator musculature or restoration of reactive function. This procedure does result in positive pressure transmission to the urethra. A recent prospective study comparing the modified Pereyra procedure to the Burch procedure revealed 70 and 87 percent cure rates, respectively.[6] Additional studies in the early 1990s have shown significantly decreased cure rates of the Raz procedure in comparison to reported cure rates of the Burch procedure and MMK procedure.

Operative Recommendations

Preoperative testing and assessment are described in the text above. The minimum preoperative evaluation of an incontinent patient includes: history, physical examination, urinalysis, urine culture, residual urine determination, and objective demonstration of stress urinary incontinence.

Stress Urinary Incontinence (Immediate, Nonsustained Objective Loss with Pure Symptoms)

I. Rotational descent of the urethrovesical junction
   A. No previous operations for urinary stress incontinence = retropubic urethropexy
   B. Previous operation for stress urinary incontinence

      Urodynamic testing, cystourethroscopy

      Nondysfunctional urethra; pressures ≥ 20 cmH_2O
      - Normal urethral coaptation = retropubic urethropexy
      - Abnormal urethral coaptation suggesting a severely dysfunctional or type III urethra; perform standing rest cystogram, if positive for type III urethra = pubovaginal sling procedure
      - Obvious scarred urethra = pubovaginal sling procedure

II. No rotational descent

   Multichannel urodynamic testing, cystourethroscopy

   Low urethral pressure dysfunctional urethra = consideration of pubovaginal sling, if mobility can be developed at operation or consideration of artificial sphincter (rare).

Stress Urinary Incontinence with Symptoms of Detrusor Instability Conservative treatment (e.g., oxybutynin, imipramine, probanthine)

I. Unstable bladder symptoms respond
   A. Persistent genuine stress incontinence: Obtain urodynamic testing and utilize algorithm above
   B. Patient satisfaction without wish for further evaluation

II. Unstable bladder symptoms do not respond
   A. Obtain multichannel urodynamic testing and cystourethroscopy
      1. Severe detrusor instability = conservative treatment with medication, bladder retraining, timed voiding, biofeedback, circumvaginal exercises, and functional electrical stimulation.
      2. No evidence of detrusor instability or other pathology = repeat cystogram on alternate day; if negative, consider ambulatory testing, if available, or consider GSI algorithm.

Severe Vault Prolapse without History of Stress Incontinence Obtain residual urine determination and test full bladder for stress incontinence in standing position with manual prolapse reduction

I. Genuine stress incontinence demonstrated with vaginal route of repair indicated = modified Pereyra procedure at time of vault repair

II. Genuine stress incontinence demonstrated with abdominal route of repair indicated = retropubic urethropexy and paravaginal repair at the time of vault repair

Bladder Instability

The most common cause of urinary incontinence in elderly women is an unstable bladder, the result of uninhibited bladder contractions. It is also a significant contributor or the second most common cause of urinary incontinence in younger women of the fifth, sixth, and seventh decades. Symptoms suggesting possible bladder instability, such as en route urine loss, frequency, urgency, nocturia, and urgency incontinence are common components of the patient's complaints. Rare components of the history suggestive of detrusor instability are true nocturnal enuresis and spontaneous complete bladder emptying. It is important for the physician who takes care of women to have an understanding of this condition. The reader is referred to an excellent review of bladder instability by L. Lewis Wall.[63]

Urinary urgency is a strong desire to void. Urgency incontinence is loss of urine (without straining) accompanied by a sensation of urgency. Detrusor instability refers to contractions noted at cystometry that are coincident with the reproduced symptoms of urgency. If control loss is secondary to a neurologic condition, it is referred to as detrusor hyperreflexia. Unstable bladder is usually used to describe the nonneurologic condition of presumed detrusor instability that may be demonstrated on a given cystometrogram.

Patients experience symptoms coincident with increased tone and pressure of the bladder. The patient may have a feeling of urgency without urine loss. As the pressure of the uninhibited contraction increases, the outlet resistance is overcome and the patient loses urine. This may or may not be preceded by relaxation of the urethral sphincter.

The pathophysiology of detrusor instability is poorly understood. Outlet obstruction is very rare in the female (although it can be induced by urethropexy), and the vast majority of patients with urgency incontinence have no evidence of abnormal outlet resistance. Neurologic examination of the S2-3-4 area is unremarkable. Cystourethroscopy is usually negative or may show mild to moderate trabeculations. A single cystometrogram may or may not show evidence of uninhibited contractions. The sensitivity of testing is increased with provocative maneuvers such as periodic heel bouncing and coughing during cystometry and the use of ambulatory monitoring. Patients who have low-level contractions ($<15\ cmH_2O$) are more likely to have symptoms of urgency and frequency without urine loss, while patients with higher level contractions ($>15\ cmH_2O$) have a greater tendency to experience incontinence.

Patients who have objectively demonstrated mixed urinary incontinence are at risk of continued bladder instability when treated surgically. Uncontrolled moderate to severe detrusor instability may preclude the option of urethropexy.

Behavioral Therapy of Detrusor Instability

One of the most underestimated and poorly utilized beneficial forms of treatment in routine practice is bladder retraining. A significant percentage of patients experiencing urgency and frequency symptoms may benefit from changes in voiding habits. The goal of bladder retraining is to suppress micturition until a set time, thus regaining control of the inhibitory reflexes or abilities.

The patient voids at regular intervals and avoids entering the bathroom in the interim. The time intervals are gradually increased to a goal of 2 or 2½ h. When the patient reaches the given time interval, she enters the bathroom and attempts to void (whether or not she has the urge to void or can void). The important considerations are attempting micturition and avoiding the restroom at unassigned times, even if it results in urine loss. With time, most patients will experience less frequency, less urgency incontinence, and more control of micturition. At night, the patient attempts to sleep as much as possible or to void once per night. The frequency of changing the time intervals can vary. Most workers recommend voiding at a set interval for 1 week before increasing the time between voids.

Gradual increases in time intervals are important for success as well as for motivation and confidence in the therapy. Occasionally, a patient will state consistently and more emphatically than most, that she will not be able to control the bladder. If the patient continues with this attitude, it will often become a subconscious self-fulfilling prophecy.

Pharmacologic Treatment of Detrusor Instability

Pharmacologic therapy for bladder instability relates to four classes of medication: anticholinergics, antispasmodics, tricyclic antidepressants, and calcium antagonists.[65] The last class has not been commonly used in the United States for this purpose.

Anticholinergics or antimuscarinics are better utilized initially at lower dosages than those commonly prescribed. This will reduce the frequency of such untoward symptoms as dry mouth and blurred vision. It is important to combine these medications with timed voiding in order to achieve the highest success. The medications allow the bladder to fill fuller before reaching the trigger volume of urgency loss. Once this volume is reached, the patient will have the same tendency for uncontrolled loss (unless retarded with concomitant bladder retraining). If the patient voids every 2 h, the higher trigger volume is not reached and the patient reduces or eliminates the episodes of detrusor instability loss.

Antispasmodics have a direct relaxant effect on the bladder in addition to anticholinergic and anesthetic properties.

Tricyclic antidepressants have some bladder anesthetic properties, anticholinergic effects, and also stimulate alpha receptors in the region of the bladder neck. The medication most commonly used has been imipramine hydrochloride. The dosage used in adults is 10 to 25 mg three times per day. This may produce sedation in some patients. The medication works especially well for nocturnal enuresis or nocturia/nocturnal en route loss. In this setting, it would be used as a one-time bedtime dosage of 25 mg. The elderly are sensitive to medication, and an initial 10-mg nightly dose should be used for several days in this group to note tolerance. It should be stressed to patients that the medication is in the antidepressant class, but that larger doses are required when used for depression. Imipramine should not be used in conjunction with monoamine oxidase inhibitors.

Some recommended drugs and dosages are recorded below.

Class	Drug	Dosage
Anticholinergics	Propanthelene	15 mg po qid
	Hyoscyamine	0.125–0.25 mg q 6 h
Antispasmodics	Oxybutynin	2.5 mg po bid—5 mg po qid
	Dicyclomine	20 mg po qid
	Flavoxate	200 mg po qid

Urinary Retention

Acute urinary retention is defined as an acute inability to void. It is rare except in patients in the immediate postpartum or postoperative state. Causes include pelvic mass, acute presentation of neurologic events, and psychogenic reactions. This discussion is limited to chronic urinary retention.

Chronic urinary retention is often insidious, usually becoming apparent during investigation of urgency incontinence symptoms or in patients later discovered to have overflow incontinence. Most females with retention have no evidence of obstruction, but rather have decreased contractility of unknown etiology. Residual urine testing reveals a significant amount of urine remaining in the bladder after voiding. A value greater than 100 ml is considered abnormal by many investigators. Evaluation to rule out any neurologic contribution is essential.

Differential Diagnosis

The differential diagnosis of chronic urinary retention includes: nonneurogenic hypocontractility of unknown etiology; detrusor hypocontractility with concomitant detrusor instability (often noted in the elderly); neurogenic causes, such as multiple sclerosis and Parkinson's disease; conditions that damage the pelvic plexus (radical pelvic surgery, pelvic masses, anterior-posterior resections); conditions that affect the spinal cord area of S2-3-4 (nerve compression or tumor); and conditions that result in neuropathy, such as diabetes. Cystoceles may cause retention from kinking of the urethra secondary to prolapse. This must be documented objectively, because many patients with complete vault prolapse and severe cystocele are able to empty their bladders to a normal residual volume (without such maneuvers as prolapse reduction).

History and Physical

Patients with chronic urinary retention may present with decreased force of stream, frequency of urination, urinary incontinence, recurrent urinary tract infections, or nocturia. Most who present with frequency and a sensation of not emptying completely are found on objective examination to be emptying their bladder well. The residual urine determination becomes important, not only in determining if the patient has true retention, but also in reassuring those who are emptying their bladder normally, before recommendations of bladder retraining.

On examination, the patient may or may not have a palpably distended bladder. A neurologic examination of the lower extremities and perineum is accomplished (see section on physical examination).

An absent bulbocavernosus reflex or decreased saddle sensation would suggest a possible neurologic lesion. A bimanual examination, including rectal examination, is carried out to detect any suggestion of a pelvic mass. This may be repeated after voiding depending on difficulty of examination. A sterile catheter is then placed for residual urine determination. A value less than 100 ml is considered essentially normal. The urine is sent for urinalysis and culture, as cystitis can result in retention. If the residual determination is abnormal, bladder filling is then done to detect any change in bladder sensations. If the bulbocavernosus reflex was absent or equivocal, a Foley catheter is used for the residual determination so that tension can be placed on the bladder base with the Foley balloon to increase the likelihood of obtaining the reflex.

Urodynamic Testing

Urodynamic testing should be considered in any patient who has evidence of a neurologic basis for retention (in addition to a complete neurologic evaluation). The factors to be assessed include normal relaxation of the pelvic floor musculature with voiding, normal coordination of the external sphincter with voiding (lack of dyssynergia), the lack of outlet obstruction, and the true detrusor pressure at the time of voiding. The lack of a detrusor contraction in the urodynamic setting is common in normal patients and cannot be equated with acontractility. Many patients are unable to generate a contraction in this setting secondary to stress or the presence of even a small urethral catheter. If the patient can generate a contraction and a significantly elevated detrusor pressure is noted in the presence of a low urinary flow rate, obstruction is suggested.

Treatment

Treatment of chronic retention is directed toward the inciting disorder or condition. Often it will not be possible to reverse the conditions causing retention, and intermittent self-catheterization becomes the therapy of choice. If the patient is able to catheterize herself, this often becomes readily acceptable despite early reservations in some patients. Catheterization often immediately reduces or eliminates symptoms of frequency, incontinence, nocturia, and problems related to urinary tract infections from stasis of urine. A clean method is utilized, the patient washing the catheter in soap and water after each use, followed by intermittent boiling of the catheter.

At this time, there are no pharmacologic agents available that can reliably increase bladder contractility. Cholinergic agents are not efficacious and often have side effects. The patient is better served with a trial of an alpha-blocking agent, such as prazosin. This results in relaxation of the bladder neck and upper urethra and aids some patients in bladder emptying when they can generate a partial contraction. An example would be a patient with chronic urinary retention following radical pelvic surgery.

Urethral dilatation is not helpful when there is no evidence of stenosis (a rare condition in the female). Many patients with retention have been treated with multiple urethral dilatations without success. If a sterile lubricated cotton swab can be passed easily through the urethra, any significant stenosis is extremely unlikely. Patients in whom this situation is questionable can be evaluated by cystourethroscopy in order to fully visualize the urethra and bladder neck.

In the past, sphincterotomy occasionally was performed for retention in females. This often resulted in urinary incontinence. Patients who suffer from a combination of detrusor instability and retention are best treated with a combination of intermittent self-catheterization and an antimuscarinic agent to suppress incontinence.

Patients with neurogenic retention should be followed by a specialist. As an example, patients with multiple sclerosis often experience a combination of detrusor hyperreflexia and detrusor external sphincter dyssynergia. Detrusor external sphincter dyssynergia is an uninhibited bladder contraction combined with an uninhibited sphincter contraction. The latter may result in retention and high bladder pressures. Other multiple sclerosis patients may demonstrate hypocontractility and retention without dyssynergia. If some of these patients are treated with anticholinergic agents without proper assessment, symptoms may improve in the face of silent increased bladder pressures that may result in reflux and upper tract damage. After proper assessment, patients may benefit from a combination of intermittent catheterization and an anticholinergic agent.

Steps in the Evaluation of Urinary Retention

1. History and physical examination (including careful neurologic examination)
2. Residual urine determination (obtained in a relaxed office setting—this may need to be repeated on more than one occasion)
3. Rule out urethral stenosis or obstruction (rare)
4. Rule out other conditions or medications associated with retention
5. Obtain urinalysis and culture (respond as indicated and reassess)
6. Consider cystourethroscopy and urodynamic testing
7. In the absence of a neurologic condition or other GU overt pathology requiring treatment, teach intermittent self-catheterization
8. In the presence of a neurologic condition, refer to a GU specialist for outline of treatment and evaluation schedule following full assessment
9. Avoid cholinergic agents and unnecessary dilatation
10. When indicated, consider a trial of alpha-blocking agent and double voiding

Incontinence in the Elderly

Incontinence is not only more prevalent in the elderly, it may have characteristics different from those seen in younger patients. These characteristics are just beginning to be recognized, and additional studies are needed to compare symptoms and pathophysiology in patients of different ages. This will allow more appropriate treatment of elderly patients and will further emphasize the importance of addressing multiple factors that, added together, can increase the margin of continence.

The percentage of patients with mixed incontinence increases as the population ages. Some workers give percentages of 55 percent mixed, 20 percent pure stress, and 15 to 20 percent pure urgency loss. This reflects a decreasing incidence of pure stress incontinence in comparison with younger age groups and transition to higher incidences of mixed and pure urgency incontinence. The elderly also manifest a condition described by Resnick as detrusor hyperactivity with impaired contractility.[44] Elderly patients also tend to have incontinence of multifactorial etiology.

History in an elderly incontinent patient must include a list of medical problems, medications, and past pelvic operative history. Bowel history also is important; previous colorectal surgery or chronic constipation can contribute to urinary symptoms. Nocturia increases with age and is related to changes in fluid hydrostasis, cardiac function, and renal filtration.

Physical examination should include pelvic examination to rule out a pelvic mass, rectal examination to rule out constipation or impaction, and neurologic examination to rule out spinal or pelvic floor abnormalities.

Urine culture results should be interpreted with urinalysis to detect pyuria or hematuria in the absence of infection or to suggest contamination. Cytology should be accomplished in patients with asymptomatic sterile hematuria, pyuria, or recurrent urinary tract infections.

Urodynamic and office testing should be sensitive to the high incidence of detrusor hyperactivity with impaired contractility in the elderly.

Urethral Diverticulum

It is important for the generalist to have a working understanding of this condition, which can be present more commonly than recognized. Diverticula may be multiple or single, with an average size of two to three centimeters in diameter. The wall of the sac is fibromuscular; its lining consists of granulation tissue or squamous/transitional epithelium. The exact prevalence rates are unknown, but reports have ranged from 1.8 to 4.7 percent.[57] The incidence appears to be higher in individuals of African descent, at a possible ratio of 6:1. Reports in the literature have been few, with some of the largest series appearing from the Mayo Clinic and Johns Hopkins.

It is postulated that acquired urethral diverticula are secondary to obstructed and infected paraurethral glands that subsequently rupture into the lumen. Congenital diverticula may be secondary to remnants of Gartner's ducts. Diverticula usually are located in the middle third of the urethra, with the neck or mouth of the diverticula connecting dorsolaterally. Tender cystic swelling may or may not be palpated in this area.

Symptoms

Symptoms are often nonspecific and may contribute to the difficulty of diagnosis if the diverticulum is not considered part of the differential. The most common complaints are frequency of urination and dysuria. Also commonly associated with diverticula are recurrent and refractory cystitis, dyspareunia, urgency, and incontinence. Postmicturition dribbling and expression of fluid on palpation of a suburethral swelling would be highly suggestive. Ten to 20 percent of patients with diverticula may be asymptomatic.[35]

Diagnosis

Suspicion of the entity is one of the most useful adjuncts in diagnosis, since the diverticulum may or may not be palpable. Diverticula can be missed on laboratory evaluation and may require more than one test to visualize. A significant percentage are missed on cystourethroscopic examination owing to the location of the orifice, the folds of the urethra, and the fact that most scopes do not balloon or distend the urethra on examination. Properly performed dye tests with the use of a Davis or Tratner catheter are valuable because the diverticulum may have more than one connection to the urethra. This becomes important when considering repair. Contrast is injected under pressure, filling the urethra and diverticulum. More recently, vaginal ultrasound appears to be more sensitive than many diagnostic modalities. MRI is another excellent method of diagnosis and may show greater involvement by the diverticula than seen by other testing methods. Although MRI may be precluded by expense, it could be considered cost-effective to prevent a diverticulum from being incompletely removed at operation. The voiding cystourethrogram is a useful adjunct. Urethral profilometry is less helpful, because pressure diminutions correlate poorly with the location of the diverticulum.

Treatment

The treatment of urethral diverticula is either observation in asymptomatic patients or surgical removal in symptomatic patients. The proper surgical removal of urethral diverticula is challenging and carries risks of local complications such as fistula formation, recurrence, and urinary incontinence. The challenge is to avoid these complications while removing all of the diverticulum wall, closing all ostia, and preserving surrounding tissue to aid in a multilayer closure. The repair is made additionally difficult by the surrounding inflammation and the friability of the tissue. Marsupialization is useful only for the distal aspect of the urethra owing to risks of urethral damage and subsequent incontinence.

One of the largest recent series was reported by Lee, consisting of 85 patients approached via an anterior vaginal wall incision.[35] Two additional supporting layers can be provided by imbricating the pubocervical fascia with a side-to-side (vest-over-pants) repair. A personal examination was accomplished in 76 patients, with a follow-up period of 2 to 15 years. The remaining nine patients were contacted by telephone or letter. Eighty-two percent of patients experienced immediate relief of symptoms. One patient experienced a postoperative fistula, two patients experienced urinary incontinence, two patients experienced urethral pain syndromes, and eight patients experienced a recurrent diverticulum.

Urethral Syndrome and Painful Bladder Syndrome

Urethral syndrome is a term used to describe chronic symptoms of urethral pain, urgency, dysuria, and frequency of urination without pathologic findings.[47] These symptoms may be present separately or in combination. Patients whose condition is described by this term are usually in the third to fourth decades of life. Similar reversible symptoms in postmenopausal patients responsive to estrogen administration are not termed urethral syndrome.

The etiology of the condition is not apparent, with studies focusing on urethral spasm, irritation, infection, and allergic causes. The vast majority of patients have no evidence of overt infection, although *Chlamydia trachomatis* has been isolated in a small percentage. Other proponents of an infectious etiology have suggested that low-count bacterial infections may be responsible. The majority of studies have shown no increased incidence of infection in urethral syndrome patients when compared to controls.

Objective studies to date have not supported the concept of spasm or urethral striated muscle hypersensitivity. The internal sphincter is relatively small and difficult to study without precise needle electrode studies. Studies can be difficult to interpret, especially considering that recent ambulatory monitoring has shown that urethral pressure variations are normal in the female and vary throughout the day.

Physical examination and office assessment include pelvic examination, wet preparation of vaginal secretions, and urethral palpation.

The diagnosis of urethral syndrome is currently a diagnosis of exclusion. Tests include urinalysis, urine culture, and consideration of urethral cultures for Chlamydia and/or gonorrhea. Cystourethroscopic examination is also helpful in reassuring the patient and enables the physician to rule out occult cystitis or interstitial cystitis. If a urethral diverticulum is suspected, additional testing can be considered, as described in this chapter. An additional consideration would be skin testing to rule out unrecognized allergies. This is similar to comparable testing in the vulvar vestibulitis syndrome.

Treatment is difficult and often centers on attempting to make individual symptoms better. Several treatments have arisen that do not have a solid pathophysiologic basis, yet may result in improved symptoms in a significant percentage of patients. As an example, empirical gentle urethral dilatations (a series of three over several weeks to months) have reduced symptoms in many patients. Regardless of the treatment, a significant percentage of patients continue to experience symptoms for months to years. Other patients experience spontaneous resolution of symptoms without therapy. Treatment also has included empirical doxycycline treatment, urethral estrogen administration, diazepam for spasm, and psychiatric evaluation in selected patients.

Some workers feel that the symptoms of urethral syndrome are actually a manifestation of painful bladder syndrome.[56] This term refers to painful conditions of the bladder when no abnormality is apparent on investigation. Patients complain of a combination of urgency, vague suprapubic discomfort, nocturia, and frequency of urination. Cystoscopic examination should be performed by a urologist to rule out interstitial cystitis. A much better understanding of interstitial cystitis and other painful bladder syndromes is needed.

Interstitial Cystitis

Interstitial cystitis describes a painful condition of the bladder of unknown etiology occurring mainly in women. Symptoms may include frequency of urination, urgency, and discomfort in the suprapubic area. Associated conditions of perineal discomfort, pain relieved by urinating, pain increased by stress factors, or vulvar vestibulitis may be present.

Pathogenic factors that have been postulated include mast cell activation with associated histamine release, abnormal bladder surface glycosaminoglycans, autoimmune abnormalities, decreased bladder blood perfusion at capacity, and altered metabolism of neuronal polypeptides. The pathogenesis of interstitial cystitis remains unclear, with published reports inconclusive and conflicting. Symptoms of persistent frequency and urgency in the absence of infection often precipitate investigation. The diagnosis of interstitial cystitis is observer-dependent as it lacks universal objective findings. Diagnosis is made by cystoscopy or cystoscopic hydrodilatation under anesthesia. Findings that suggest cystitis include glomerulations or submucosal petechial hemorrhages. In severe cases, an ulceration of the urothelium or Hunner's ulcer may be evident. Bladder biopsy may reveal marked inflammatory changes, granulation tissue in the lamina propria, suburothelial hemorrhages, and mucosal denudation.

Therapy includes self-help strategies, medication, bladder hydrodistention, intravesical pharmacotherapy, and, in some select patients, surgical intervention. Self-help strategies include bladder retraining, behavior modification, voiding diaries, stress reduction, and avoidance of dietary factors that may be exacerbating for a particular patient. Medications utilized in the treatment of interstitial cystitis include amitriptyline, hydroxyzine, nifedipine, and pentosanpolysulfate sodium (Elmiron).

Intravesical therapies have included: dimethyl sulfoxide, silver nitrate, sodium oxychorosene, heparin, Elmiron, and lidocaine. Intravesical pharmacotherapy is one of the mainstays of treatment of interstitial cystitis, and dimethyl sulfoxide (DMSO) is the only drug approved by the FDA for this entity. DMSO's properties include membrane penetration, enhanced drug absorption, anti-inflammatory and analgesic effects, collagen dissolution, and mast cell release. Healed bladder biopsy sites, and sterile urine are prerequisites for DMSO instillation. These instillations usually are given every 1 to 2 weeks for four to eight treatments. Some patients may experience a temporary worsening of their symptomatology after the initial one to two treatments.

Patients who fail to respond to therapy are considered for DMSO combination therapy, with the addition of steroids and/or heparin installation. Other intravesical therapies in addition to DMSO include silver nitrate and chloropactin (sodium oxychlorosene).

A minority of patients may fail to respond to nonsurgical modalities; if symptoms warrant, they may be considered for operation. Major surgery should be limited to patients with severe and unremitting, debilitating symptoms that have not been controlled by other measures.

Asymptomatic Hematuria

This discussion is limited to asymptomatic microhematuria in the nonadolescent patient. Numerous studies have documented the necessity for urologic investigation of patients with asymptomatic hematuria. Howard and coworkers reported an experience in 1980 with 246 patients with asymptomatic hematuria.[25] A urologic neoplasm was noted in 10 percent of patients;, an additional 12 percent had other significant urologic lesions. In a recent 10- to 20-year follow-up assessment of 191 patients. Howard and coworkers noted that all patients were free of genitourinary malignancies.[29] Of these patients 78 percent had persistent microscopic blood cells in the urine throughout their follow-up. This suggested low yield for routine IVP and cystourethroscopy, which was supported by three additional major series totaling 428 patients with a 2- to 20-year follow-up and no evidence of upper tract malignancy appearance.[29]

The urologic investigation of asymptomatic hematuria by urinalysis, urine cytology, IVP, and cystoscopy has been challenged. Kolin and Silverstein suggested that the initial diagnostic approach to asymptomatic hematuria should include cystoscopy and renal ultrasound. Some workers have suggested diagnostic follow-up only in patients who demonstrate gross hematuria, recurrent urinary tract infections, or changes in voiding characteristics.

Mariani and coworkers evaluated 1000 consecutive adults with asymptomatic hematuria in the absence of proteinuria. Some of these patients had one episode of gross hematuria in the absence of diagnostic symptoms, such as cystitis. The majority of patients received IVP, serum creatinine, culture, cytology, and cystoscopy. Lesions that could account for hematuria were detected in 88.3 percent of patients, with life-threatening lesions diagnosed in 9.1 percent. In 22.8 percent, lesions required minimal observation. The incidence of life-threatening lesions was noted to increase with age and was more common in men.[40] In the patient group with life-threatening lesions, 18.6 percent had at least one urinalysis with less than three red blood cells per high-power field within 6 months of diagnosis.

The incidence of low-grade microscopic hematuria (fewer than two red blood cells per high-power field) ranges from 9 to 18 percent. In a population-based study performed at the Mayo Clinic, 13 percent of patients were noted to have some degree of hematuria without statistically significant differences between various population groups.[53] Most investigators may not evaluate patients who have less than three red blood cells per high-power field. Measures taken to define a safe and acceptable lower limit of hematuria have not been successful.

The practitioner should consider three red blood cells per high-power field on two to three properly collected specimens as asymptomatic hematuria. Higher levels of red blood cells on one urinalysis also would be acceptable for this diagnosis. Urine cytology is performed along with screening studies for bacteria or infection. In the absence of infection, the practitioner proceeds with cystoscopy and ultrasound of the urinary tract. Additional follow-up the practitioner might consider would be urinalysis and urine cytology every 6 to 12 months, depending on the index of suspicion. Patients are instructed to return if such symptoms as gross hematuria or irritation on voiding appear. A creatinine study and IVP would be considered within the current standard of care, although in the future additional parameters may need to be present in order to indicate cost-effectiveness and the desirability of radiologic contrast studies. This also reflects a 0.03 percent incidence of life-threatening anaphylactic contrast medium reactions with excretory urograms.

Some workers have suggested that asymptomatic microhematuria may warrant investigation for parenchymal renal disease. Smith reviewed the records of 125 patients with isolated asymptomatic hematuria and elevated serum creatinine, and 83 comparison patients with no hematuria but elevated serum creatinine from a previous population-based study.[53] The results showed that disease was detected no more frequently in patients with elevated creatinine in asymptomatic hematuria that in those with elevated creatinine without asymptomatic hematuria. The investigators concluded that exhaustive diagnostic testing to detect renal parenchymal disease cannot be advised in asymptomatic elderly patients with low-grade (grade 1) microhematuria unless more specific indications are present. The degree of microhematuria in this particular study was the presence of one or more erythrocytes per high-power field.

Vesicovaginal Fistula

Vesicovaginal fistulas are rare in affluent societies where they occur most commonly following operation or irradiation. In developing countries, obstetric fistula secondary to prolonged labor is more common. In the United States, approximately 5 percent of fistulas result from obstetric situations. An additional 10 percent are from irradiation, and 85 percent are related to pelvic operative procedures.[60] Symmonds, in a large referral practice at the Mayo Clinic, noted an unchanging rate of 25 to 30 fistulas per year. The majority of these were complex, with 10 percent involving ureters or bladder, 10 percent noted in conjunction with additional ureteral or bowel fistulas, and 52 percent in patients who had at least one previous attempt at operative repair. In a Mayo Clinic experience of 600 fistulas, 75 percent occurred after hysterectomy, with more than 50 percent following a simple total abdominal hysterectomy.

The office practitioner may encounter a fistula in a postoperative patient less than 30 days from operation, in a previously operated patient who presents with incontinence and occult fistula, or a patient who has had radiation therapy months to years in the past. The majority of early postoperative patients will demonstrate urinary leakage per vagina in the first two weeks following surgery, although an additional group of patients will first demonstrate urine loss several weeks after operation.

Diagnosis

The patient with a vesicovaginal fistula describes urine loss per vagina following operation. Alternatively, the patient may present with a long-standing history of urinary incontinence and previous operation. In these patients, bona fide urinary stress incontinence may be present, but is augmented by a small amount of urine loss from an occult fistula. Patients have received operations for incontinence with elevation of the urethrovesical junction, but the presence of a small communication between the bladder and vagina was not recognized. In order to avoid incorrect diagnosis, a tampon dye test should be considered part of the evaluation in patients who describe a constant small leakage, patients with previous history of irradiation, or patients with a history of incontinence and no overt evidence of loss per urethra on stress testing.

Although cystoscopy is an important part of fistula evaluation, the absence of a fistula on visual inspection does not rule it out. Patients with occult fistulas have had negative cystoscopic examinations performed by very skilled endoscopists. Most fistulas that follow total abdominal hysterectomy tend to be high in the apex of the vagina in a supratrigonal location. A lack of surrounding inflammation in folds may make the small defect difficult to find on cystoscopic inspection.

The tampon dye test is accomplished in the following manner: The patient is assessed by speculum visualization of the vagina and pelvic examination. Colposcopic examination of the vaginal apex may be helpful in the detection of a small occult fistula as it provides magnification and improved lighting. A small fistula may have erythema surrounding the vaginal opening, which aids in detection. Approximately 300 to 350 ml of methylene blue stained saline is placed within the bladder after initial drainage with a catheter. Three separate gauze 4 × 4s or pledgets are then placed in the vagina. The patient is then asked to walk, do deep knee-bends, go up and down stairs, and finally to void after approximately 20 to 30 min. The patient is examined immediately after voiding by removal of the gauze pledgets. The first gauze pledget will be stained from urination; however, the voiding contraction may increase the sensitivity of fistula detection. The successive gauze pledgets are then examined for evidence of dye. An occult fistula often presents at the apex, and thus the second gauze pledget is free of dye, with the final pledget being stained.

It should be understood that this does not rule out a ureterovaginal fistula. Ureterovaginal fistulas can be detected by giving the patient indigo carmine dye with a concomitant tampon test over a longer time or by retrograde contrast studies. The latter studies are often helpful, even when a vesicovaginal fistula has been detected, to rule out a secondary ureterovaginal fistula.

If a vesicovaginal fistula is evident on vaginal examination or tampon testing, the timing of cystoscopy depends on consideration of operative repair. If the patient is several weeks postoperative, additional weeks to months may be needed before repair. The cystoscopy is best done just prior to the operative repair to note the position of the ureteral orifices relative to the fistula and to rule out any additional abnormalities. If the ureteral orifices are 0.5 cm from the edge of the fistula or if the communication is noted lateral to the ureters, ureteral catheters may be considered at the time of operation.

Management

Surgeons have different opinions concerning the timing of operative repair. Most small fistulas benefit from an initial trial of bladder catheter decompression to allow the possibility of spontaneous healing. Some studies have suggested a benefit from low suction applied to the catheter drainage. Fifteen to 20 percent of small posthysterectomy vesicovaginal fistulas may heal spontaneously with prolonged catheter drainage of the bladder. If spontaneous healing of the fistula has not occurred by six to eight weeks, the possibility of healing is remote and the urinary catheter should be removed.[60] The "classic" timing of repair is after a waiting period of 2 to 6 months to allow tissues to become less inflamed and edematous. Other workers have suggested that this delay is not required. The exact time for repair depends on the size of the fistula and the integrity of surrounding tissues. Symmonds advocated that a definitive repair should be deferred for 2 to 4 months, depending on the quality of tissues and the condition for which the initial operation was accomplished. In-dwelling catheterization during this time should be avoided, as it may promote infection and further delay operative repair. In addition, social pressure to repair a fistula prematurely should be resisted. Postradiation fistulas are at significant risk of recurrence owing to poor vascularity of the tissues. The surgical delay in these instances may approach 1 to 2 years to ensure the integrity of surrounding tissue.

Urinary Tract Infections

This discussion is limited to acute, sporadic urinary tract infections. Consultation should be considered in selected patients with a history of diabetes, vesicoureteral reflux, renal calculi, obstructive uropathies, immunocompromise, parenchymal renal disease, a chronic indwelling catheter, current pregnancy, severe acute pyelonephritis, and documented recurrent infections without prior history of urologic investigation.

The primary practitioner may find that 2 to 5 percent of female office appointments are related to symptoms suggesting bacteriuria, as acute uncomplicted urinary tract infections are responsible for 6 to 7 million office visits per year in the United States.

Adult women as a group experience the majority of urinary tract infections in the population at large, with related health expenditures exceeding 1 billion dollars. Approximately 43 percent of females age 14 to 61 claim to have experienced a bladder infection. In addition, the tendency for reinfection may increase with increasing age. Evans noted a 3.5 percent incidence of significant bacteriuria in teenagers, which rose to 10 percent in patients over 70.[20] Higher rates are noted in nursing home populations. Mabeck reported that 85 percent of patients experience 0.32 infections per year, while 15 percent experience two per year. He also noted that treated patients will experience recurrence at the same rate as patients whose symptoms resolve without treatment.

Evans reported that 5.7 percent of abacteriuric women complained of dysuria.[20] It may be important to document infection by culture in patients who experience recurrent infections. Many asymptomatic younger women may have periods of occult significant bacteriuria that subsequently resolve without consequence. "Significant bacteriuria" is common in females, yet the meaning of this term is complex. The amount of bacteria that should be considered "significant" varies depending on the organism, concurrent use of antibiotics, and associated pathology. Coagulase-negative staphylococcis grow slowly, and counts of 10,000 to 100,000 cfu/ml are considered significant. Gram-negative enteric bacteria and enterococci grow rapidly and more commonly fit the Kass criteria of 100,000 cfu/ml as diagnostic of infection. A small percentage of patients with true infections will have very small organism counts. This indicates that, in addition to host defenses, the characteristics of the organism and not just its presence are important in overall virulence. Fimbriae allow enteric gram-negative bacteria to have increased adherence to mucosal surfaces.

Recurrent infections are usually from different strains of bacteria. Recurrent significant bacteriuria with the same strain would suggest persistence of infection, not true recurrent infection. This is rare, and the vast majority of infections encountered in practice are recurrent.

There is evidence that vaginal colonization of enteric pathogens is a significant factor in patients with a history of recurrent infectious cystitis.[54] Fecal bacteria colonize in an ascending fashion; in sexually active individuals who experience recurrent infections, this may be intercourse-associated, although the magnitude of this association is unclear. In most women, intercourse results in the transfer of bacteria into the bladder, but this takes on greater significance in patients predisposed to vaginal colonization and/or decreased host defense factors. Diaphragm-spermicide use appears to markedly affect vaginal flora and may increase the tendency to develop infections.[55]

It is unusual for long-term, recurrent urinary tract infections to cause renal damage. High-risk groups include patients who are elderly or have diabetes, vesicoureteral reflux, immunosuppression, or are pregnant.

Diagnosis

Diagnosis includes history, microscopic examination of the urinary sediment, and quantitative urine culture. The presence of one bacterium in each high-power field of an uncentrifuged specimen corresponds to 100,000 cfu/ml of urine. Approximately 30 percent of patients with bacteriuria based on symptoms and microscopy will have sterile urine cultures.[23]

The reliability of cultures from the female is 80

percent, and this is the most accurate reflection of the amount and type of bacteriuria. Twenty percent of patients with significant Enterobacter-bacteriuria will have fewer than 1000 organisms on culture. An equal percentage of patients with sterile urine may show up to 10,000 organisms in a voided specimen. If the patient is asymptomatic and bacteriuria is detected, two to three consecutive cultures are desirable. However, a single catheterized specimen showing 100,000 organisms is considered diagnostic in an asymptomatic individual. Two consecutive specimens in a symptomatic individual are considered desirable by some experts, but this is not done commonly in most practices. Most vaginal and periurethral organisms are gram-positive, and their isolation suggests contamination. Contamination is also suggested in the absence of pyuria by isolation of unusual or multiple organisms in a voided specimen.

Pyuria reflects an inflammatory response in the genitourinary system. Associated causes are infection (typical and atypical), foreign bodies, stones, trauma, neoplasms, contamination, glomerulonephritis, and tubulointerstitial disease. Pyuria in the absence of infection requires urologic investigation to rule out these associated causes. Some patients demonstrate pyuria from vaginal leukocyte contamination in a voided specimen. A wet preparation of the vaginal secretions shows a significant number of white blood cells. A catheterized specimen may be free of pyuria in these patients and unnecessary urologic testing can be avoided.

Clean-catch specimens are the standard office sampling method, although some workers have suggested that this technique may not reduce contamination over voided, non-clean-catch specimens. Leisure and coworkers made the comparison in 100 asymptomatic women; 64 total contaminants were noted in each of the groups. In addition, 10 women had sterile non-clean-catch cultures and contaminated clean-catch cultures.[38] Regardless of the method, urine specimens should be promptly cultured or refrigerated to avoid false-positive results.

Treatment

The microorganism most commonly responsible for uncomplicated infections is *E. coli,* with six serotype strains predominating. *Staphylococcus saprophyticus* is the second most common pathogen in young women of childbearing age. Five to 10 percent of cases will involve *Proteus* or other gram-negative bacteria or enterococci.[33] Kunin notes that enteric gram-negative rods and enterococci take on a greater role in complicated infections although *E. coli* is still commonly present.

The efficacy and benefit of an antimicrobial drug depends on: ability to concentrate at the site of infection, bacterial effects (organism susceptibility), frequency of resistance, side effects, and cost.[33] Bacteriostatic agents are acceptable for uncomplicated infections, while bacteriocidal drugs may be needed in complicated cases. Individuals predisposed to the latter condition are those with congenital abnormalities, foreign bodies, diabetes, or neurologic afflictions.

The object of management in uncomplicated infections is to avoid persistence of significant bacteriuria or infection and eradicate reversible bacteriuric-related symptoms. The importance of clearing low levels of bacteriuria depend on the age of the patient, associated medical conditions, and individual history. There appears to be no definite advantage in treating asymptomatic bacteriuria in the nonpregnant female. In addition, in some groups, such as the elderly, it may be difficult to clear the bacteriuria.

Recommendations for the office practitioner would include the following as minimal treatment:

1. Three-day treatment with nitrofurantoin (Macrodantin), trimethoprim/sulfamethoxazole, or agents that concentrate primarily in the urinary tract, have excellent efficacy, and are relatively low cost.
2. Single dose therapy only in uncomplicated infections, in nonpregnant patients, and those without diabetes or history of acute pyelonephritis.
3. Office microscopy or other methods to detect pyuria, bacteria, and microscopic hematuria. Pyuria is defined as 10 leukocytes per milliliter and is present in the vast majority of women with urinary tract infections.

If the patient has acute symptoms of infection with pyuria and bacteria, the practitioner may choose not to obtain a culture. This should be considered only in the patient with less than two infections per year or the patient who has been thoroughly investigated and is under close urologic follow-up. Anatomical abnormalities of the urinary tract detected by cystoscopy and excretory urography are found in less than 5 percent of young women with recurrent uncomplicated cystitis.[55]

Recently, such considerations as cultures for patients suffering from infrequent sporadic episodes, urinalysis, susceptibility testing, the indications for urologic investigation, treating for greater than 5 days, and posttreatment cultures have been challenged.[23]

Fowler recommends the following in uncomplicated infections:

1. Treatment for 3 to 5 days with nitrofurantoin (Macrodantin), sulfamethoxazole, or penicillin-G
2. Avoidance of susceptibility testing
3. Posttreatment cultures in urologic referral practices, patients with *Proteus mirabilis* as the cause of bacteriuria, or in patients with complicated infections
4. Avoiding prophylactic treatment until the frequency and bacteriology of the infections have been determined
5. Initiating treatment in symptomatic patients with pyuria before urine culture results are known
6. Awaiting culture results before initiating treatment in symptomatic patients who do not manifest pyuria (the majority of patients without pyuria do not have infection)

Some recommended drugs and dosages for 3- to 5-day therapy of uncomplicated urinary tract infections are listed below.

Drug	Dosage
Nitrofurantoin	50–100 mg q 6–8 h
TMP-SMX	1 to 2 tabs q 12 h
Noroxin	400 mg q 12 h
Floxin	200–300 mg q 12 h
Ampicillin	250–500 mg q 6–8 h
Cephalexin	250–500 mg q 6–8 h
Tetracycline	250–500 mg q 6–8 h

Single-dose therapy can be considered for trimethoprim/sulfamethoxazole, trimethoprim, sulfonamide, and tetracyclines at increased dosage.[23] Fihn noted higher failure rates at 13 days with single dose trimethoprim/sulfamethoxazole.[22]

Prophylactic therapy can be utilized in patients with a chronic history of recurrent (nonpersistent) urinary tract infections. Low-dosage antimicrobials are utilized that lack deleterious effects on the bowel flora. Agents include nitrofurantoin (100 mg), trimethoprim/sulfamethoxazole (1 tab), trimethoprim (50 mg), cephalexin (250 mg), and cinoxacine (250 mg) in daily use. If efficacious, alternate day therapy may be considered for a trial period.

References and Selected Readings

1. Andersen MJF: The incidence of diverticula in the female urethra. *J Urol* 98:96–8, 1967.
2. Baden WF, Walker TA: Physical diagnosis in evaluation of vaginal vault relaxation. *Clin Obstet Gynecol* 15:1055, 1972.
3. Beck RP, et al: Intra-urethral-intravesical cough-pressure spike differences in 267 patients surgically cured of genuine stress incontinence of urine. *Obstet Gynecol* 72:302–306, 1988.
4. Bent AE, Sand PK, Ostergaard DR, Brubaker LT: Transvaginal electrical stimulation in the treatment of genuine stress incontinence in detrusor instability. *Int Urogynecol J* 4:9–13, 1993.
5. Berglas B, Rubin IC: Study of the supportive structures of the uterus by levator myography. *Surg Gynecol Obstet* 97:677, 1953.
6. Bergman A, Koonings PP, et al: Primary stress urinary incontinence in public relaxation: Prospective randomized comparison of three different operations. *Am J Obstet Gynecol* 166:97, 1989.
7. Bump RC, Hurt WG, et al: Assessment of Kegel pelvic exercise performance after verbal instruction. *Am J Obstet Gynecol* 165:322–329, 1991.
8. Burgio KL, et al: The role of biofeedback in Kegel exercise training for stress urinary incontinence. *Am J Obstet Gynecol* 154:58, 1986.
9. Burgio KL, et al: Urinary incontinence in the elderly. *Ann Intern Med* 104:507–515, 1985.
10. Constantinou CE: Resting stress urethral pressures as a clinical guide to the mechanism of continence in the female patient. *Urol Clin North Am* 12:247–258, 1985.
11. Constantinou CE, et al: Spacial distribution and timing of transmitted and reflexly generated urethral pressures in healthy women. *J Urol* 127:964–969, 1982.
12. Corwin HL, Silverstein MD: The diagnosis of neoplasia in

patients with asymptomatic microscopic hematuria. A decision analysis. *J Urol* 139:1002, 1988.
13. DeLancy JOL: Anatomic aspects of vaginal eversion after hysterectomy. *Am J Obstet Gynecol* 166:1717–1724, 1992.
14. DeLancey JOL: Correlative study of paraurethral anatomy. *Obstet Gynecol* 68:91, 1986.
15. DeLancey JOL: Structural aspects of the extrinsic continence mechanism. *Obstet Gynecol* 72:296, 1988.
16. DuBeau CE, Resnick MM: Evaluation of the causes and severity of geriatric incontinence: A critical appraisal. *Urol Clin North Am* 18:243–256, 1991.
17. Elbadawi A: Neuromorphologic basis of vesicourethral function. I. Histochemistry, ultrastructure, and function of intrinsic nerves of the bladder and urethra. *Neurourol Neurodynamics* 1:3, 1982.
18. Elkins TE, et al: Transvaginal mobilization and utilization of the anterior bladder wall to repair vesicovaginal fistulas involving the urethra. *Obstet Gynecol* 79:455–460, 1992.
19. Elkins TE, et al: Vesicovaginal fistula revisited. *Obstet Gynecol* 72:307–312, 1988.
20. Evans DA, et al: Bacteriuria in a population-based cohort of women. *J Infect Dis* 138:768–773, 1978.
21. Fall M, et al: Electrical stimulation. *Urol Clin North Am* 18:393–407, 1991.
22. Fihn SD, et al: Trimethoprim-sulfamethoxazole for acute dysuria in women: Double blind, randomized trial with single dose versus ten day treatment. *Ann Intern Med* 108:350, 1988.
23. Fowler JE: Urinary tract infection in women. *Urol Clin North Am* 13:673–683, 1986.
24. Gilpin SA: The pathogenesis of genitourinary prolapse and stress incontinence of urine. A histological and histochemical study. *Br J Obstet Gynaecol* 96:15, 1989.
25. Golin AL, Howard RS: Asymptomatic microscopic hematuria. *J Urol* 124:389, 1980.
26. Gosling JA: Structure of the lower urinary tract and pelvic floor. *Obstet Gynecol* 12:285, 1985.
27. Hilton P, Stanton SL: A clinical and urodynamic assessment of the Burch colposuspension for genuine stress incontinence. *Br J Obstet Gynaecol* 90:934, 1983.
28. Hilton P, Stanton SL: Urethral pressure measurement by microtransducor: The results in symptom-free women and in those with genuine stress incontinence. *Br J Obstet Gynaecol* 90:919–933, 1983.
29. Howard RS, Golin AL: Long term follow up of asymptomatic microhematuria. *J Urol* 145:335–336, 1991.
30. Karram MM: The urethral syndrome. *Am Urogynecol Soc Q Report* 8:3, 1990.
31. Karram MM: Lower urinary tract infection, in Ostergard DR, Bent AE (eds): *Urogynecology and Urodynamics,* 3d ed. Baltimore, MD: William and Wilkins, 1991, p. 306.
32. Keettel WC: Surgical management of urethrovaginal and vesicovaginal fistulas. *Am J Obstet Gynecol* 131:425, 1978.
33. Kunin CM: Detection, prevention, and management of urinary tract infections. Philadelphia: Lea & Febiger, 1987.
34. Langer R, et al: The value of simultaneous hysterectomy during Burch colposuspension for urinary stress incontinence. *Obstet Gynecol* 72:866–869, 1988.
35. Lee RA: Diverticulum of the female urethra: Postoperative complications and results. *Obstet Gynecol* 61:52–58, 1983.
36. Lee RA, Symmonds RE: Repeat Marshall-Marchetti Krantz procedure for recurrent stress urinary incontinence. *Am J Obstet Gynecol* 122:219, 1975.
37. Lee RA, Symmonds RE: Ureteral vaginal fistula. *Am J Obstet Gynecol* 109:1032–1035, 1971.
38. Leisure MK, et al: Does a clean-catch urine sample reduce bacterial contamination? *N Engl J Med* 328:289, 1993.
39. Mabeck CE: Treatment of uncomplicated urinary tract infection in non-pregnant women. *Postgrad Med* 48:69–75, 1972.
40. Mariani AJ, et al: The significance of adult hematuria: 1000 hematuria evaluations including a risk, benefit, and cost effective analysis. *J Urol* 141:350–355, 1989.
41. Mouritsen L, et al: Long-term effect of pelvic floor exercises on female urinary incontinence. *Br J Urol* 68:32–37, 1991.
42. Murakima S, et al: Strategies for asymptomatic microscopic hematuria: A prospective study of 1034 patients. *J Urol* 144:99–101, 1990.
43. Ostergard DR, Bent AE (eds): *Urogynecology and Urodynamics,* 3d ed. Baltimore, MD: Williams & Wilkins, 1991.
44. Resnick NM, Yalla SV: Detrusor hyperactivity with impaired contractile function: An unrecognized but common cause of incontinence in elderly patients. *JAMA* 257:3076, 1987.
45. Resnick NM, Yalla SV, et al: The pathophysiology of urinary incontinence among institutionalized elderly persons. *N Engl J Med* 320:1, 1989.
46. Rosenzweig BA, Bhatia NN, et al: Dynamic urethral pressure profilometry, pressure transmission ratio: What do the numbers really mean? *Obstet Gynecol* 77:586–590, 1991.
47. Schmidt RA: The urethral syndrome. *Urol Clin North Am* 12:349–354, 1985.
48. Scotti RJ, Ostergard DR: The urethral syndrome. *Clin Obstet Gynecol* 27:515–529, 1984.
49. Shull BL, Baden W: A six-year experience with paravaginal defect repair for stress urinary incontinence. *Am J Obstet Gynecol* 160:1432–1440, 1989.
50. Shull BL, et al: Preoperative and postoperative analysis of site-specific pelvic support defects in 81 women treated with sacrospinous ligament suspension and pelvic reconstruction. *Am J Obstet Gynecol* 166:1764–1771, 1992.
51. Smith ARB, et al: The role of partial denervation of the pelvic floor and the etiology of genitourinary prolapse and stress incontinence. A neurophysical study. *Br J Obstet Gynaecol* 96:24, 1989.

52. Smith ARB, et al: The role of pudendal nerve damage in the etiology of genuine stress incontinence in women. *Br J Obstet Gynaecol* 96:29, 1989.
53. Smith RF, et al: Renal insufficiency in community patients with mild asymptomatic microhematuria. *Mayo Clinic Proc* 64:409–414, 1989.
54. Stamey TA, et al: The role of vaginal colonization with enterobacteriaceae in recurrent urinary infections. *J Urol* 113:214–217, 1975.
55. Stamm WE, et al: Urinary tract infections: From pathogenesis to treatment. *J Infect Dis* 159:400–406, 1989.
56. Stone AR: Treatment of voiding complaints and incontinence in painful bladder syndrome. *Urol Clin North Am* 18:317–325, 1991.
57. Summitt RL: Urethral diverticula. *Am Urogynecol Soc Q Report,* 1993; 11:3.
58. Summitt RL, et al: The pathophysiology of genuine stress incontinence. *Int Urogynecol J* 1:12–18, 1990.
59. Summitt RL, et al: Urinary incontinence: Correlation of history and brief office evaluation with multichannel urodynamic testing. *Am J Obstet Gynecol* 166:1835–1844, 1992.
60. Symmonds RE: Prevention and management of genitourinary fistula. *J Obstet Gynecol* 21:13–24, 1979.
61. Tancer ME: The post total hysterectomy vesicovaginal fistula. *J Urol* 123:839–840, 1980.
62. Van Geelen JM, et al: The clinical and urodynamic effects of anterior vaginal repair in Burch colposuspension. *Am J Obstet Gynecol* 159:137–144, 1988.
63. Wall LL: Diagnosis and management of urinary incontinence due to detrusor instability. *Obstet Gynecol Survey* 45:15–475, 1990.
64. Wall LL: The management of detrusor instability. *Clin Obstet Gynecol* 33:367–377, 1990.
65. Wall LL: The unstable bladder. *Te Linde's Operative Gynecology Updates* 1:1–13, 1992.
66. Wall LL, Davidson TG: The role of muscular re-education by physical therapy in the treatment of genuine stress urinary incontinence. *Obstet Gynecol Survey* 47:322–331, 1992.
67. Webb RJ, et al: Ambulatory monitoring and electronic measurement of urinary leakage in the diagnosis of detrusor instability and incontinence. *Br J Urol* 68:148–152, 1991.

33 Other Pelvic Floor Dysfunctions

James P. Youngblood

In any discussion of pelvic floor dysfunction it must be emphasized that a careful medical history is paramount. A woman may be uncomfortable volunteering the information that she has severe leakage of urine on straining or coughing and must wear a pad, either socially or continuously when active. She also may be hesitant to volunteer that she must use vaginal digital pressure to empty a large cystocele or that she must use digital pressure on the posterior vagina in order to evaculate a large rectocele. A woman is often embarrassed to relate that she has, at the worst, fecal and gas incontinence or, at the least, severe fecal urgency. She may be hesitant to say that sexual intercourse is uncomfortable because of a protruding cervix or that coitus is unsatisfactory because of lack of sensation due to a relaxed introitus. Direct questioning is of great importance, and many of these maladies will not be brought out unless the physician asks specific questions.

Almost all pelvic floor dysfunction is related to childbirth trauma, and frequently is progressive with age. A very small percentage of these problems may be congenital and/or hereditary.

A brief description of each anatomical defect will be presented as well as its major symptoms, the physical findings, and the possible treatment regimen(s).

Cystocele

This is a herniation of the posterior bladder into the anterior vagina. It may be minimal, moderate, or extremely large in size. By itself it seldom causes genuine stress urinary incontinence, but may contribute to it. It may be completely asymptomatic, but the large cystocele may cause an inability to empty the bladder, therefore requiring digital pressure on the anterior vaginal wall to empty. Stasis of urine is not uncommon in the presence of a large cystocele, and this may lead to chronic or recurrent cystitis. Frequent episodes of cystitis in a patient with this anatomical problem usually is an indication for anterior colporrhaphy.

Paravaginal Defect

This defect has been well described by A. Cullen Richardson,[4] and may involve the right, left, or both anterior paravaginal sulci. If a paravaginal defect exists, the urethra will descend and rotate anteriorly when there is increased intraabdominal pressure, as with severe coughing, sneezing, or straining. Genuine stress urinary incontinence may then result. Milder forms of stress incontinence may be treated with pelvic floor and perineal exercises, such as Kegel's exercises. More severe stress incontinence may require surgical intervention, such as paravaginal defect repair, retropubic urethral suspension, or one of the various types of needle suspensions. Stress incontinence is more completely addressed in the previous chapter.

Rectocele

A rectocele is an outpouching of the anterior rectal wall into the posterior vagina. It too, may be minimal, moderate, or very large. The major symptom associated with a rectocele is an inability to evacuate the contents of the rectum, even with straining. Unfortunately, hard straining causes the rectocele to become larger; the larger the rectocele becomes, the more difficult evacuation becomes—a vicious cycle. In the larger rectocele, the patient may need to resort to using pressure with her fingers on the posterior vagina in order to evacuate. The need to use this maneuver is rarely volunteered by the patient and must be elicited by careful questioning. The severely symptomatic rectocele requires surgical intervention with a posterior colporrhaphy.

Enterocele

An enterocele is a herniation of the peritoneum of the posterior cul-de-sac that dissects down the rectovaginal septum, often far enough to protrude through the vaginal introitus. This is a true hernia, lined by peritoneum, and often containing small bowel. A smaller enterocele may be asymptomatic and also difficult to detect. Frequently, it is detected only at the time a patient is having a posterior colporrhaphy. A large enterocele may be difficult to distinguish from a rectocele, but careful rectovaginal examination while the patient is straining may reveal its existence. Incarceration or strangulation of bowel is seldom encountered with an enterocele, but its existence almost always requires surgical intervention.

Uterine Prolapse

The cause of uterine prolapse is still not clearly and completely understood, but certainly has to do with childbirth trauma, which relaxes the cardinal and uterosacral ligaments, allowing descent of the uterus. Aging and atrophy contribute to the problem, and therefore it may progress with age. Symptoms in a milder prolapse may be minimal, but the patient with significant prolapse who is still menstruating may have a wide range of complaints. These may include low back pain both premenstrually and during menstruation, as well as dysmenorrhea and dyspareunia. Uterine prolapse is usually described as first-degree when the cervix descends nearly to the introitus; second-degree when the cervix descends and protrudes through the introitus; and third degree, or total procidentia, when there is a complete evagination of the cervix and uterus. Frequently, procidentia afflicts the elderly and, in the nursing home setting, becomes a very serious care problem.

Symptomatic uterine prolapse may be treated simply with the placement of a pessary. The author has had the greatest degree of success with the use of a simple ring pessary, which is fitted to the individual patient. However, especially in the elderly, this requires an intact perineum to retain the pessary. A pessary is most satisfactory when the patient is able to care for it herself by removing, cleaning, and replacing it. If necessary, periodic visits to the gynecologist will accomplish the same thing. The patient should be routinely examined within 2 or 3 days of initial placement to make certain that the pessary has not caused vaginal ulceration or other problems, and she should be examined regularly thereafter. In addition to the simple ring, a wide variety of other types of pessaries can be used; these should be suited to the individual anatomical requirements.

For the patient who is in appropriate medical condition for a surgical procedure, vaginal hysterectomy and careful culdoplasty usually are indicated for the severely symptomatic uterine prolapse. In the very elderly, poor-risk patient with procidentia who is unable to retain a pessary, a Le Fort colpocleisis under local anesthesia may still be an option.

The Relaxed Introitus

Sexual dysfunction is a frequent complaint with this finding. Counseling alone may obviate the problem; however, surgical intervention may be indicated in a patient who is having an unsatisfactory sexual experience because of excessive vaginal introitus relaxation. Generally speaking, a carefully done perineorrhaphy will alleviate the problem. It should be emphasized, however, that this procedure probably should not be done in the relatively satisfied patient, as many women with what appears anatomically to be an extremely relaxed introitus will have a very satisfactory sexual relationship.

Anorectal Incontinence

Often in a multiparous woman a history of fecal or gas incontinence may be elicited. Not so often recognized is fecal urgency, which may occur in up to one-third of multiparas who have not experienced obvious birth injury.

Usually, chronic anal sphincter separation is readily obvious, but not so obvious may be a small rectovaginal or rectoperineal fistula. These problems require surgical intervention.

Recent literature indicates that fecal urgency is a much more common problem than previously recognized. Often physical therapy and/or other bowel training are necessary to alleviate these symptoms. Fortunately, considerable research is ongoing regarding the dysfunctions of the posterior compartment of the female pelvis, and it is hoped that effective therapies will continue to evolve.

It should be emphasized that any or all of these pelvic floor defects may occur singly or in combination with any other. It is not uncommon for them to all be present in the same patient, requiring a total vaginal hysterectomy, careful culdoplasty, anterior and posterior colporrhaphy and perineorrhaphy, as well as a retropubic, paravaginal, or periurethral operation. Again, it must be emphasized that careful history and physical examination are of paramount importance in restoring pelvic floor anatomy. This will enable the physician to determine the type and extent of the defect(s) so that the ideal surgical repair can be performed to address the individual woman's problem.

References and Selected Readings

1. Crawford LA, Quint, EH, Pearl ML, DeLancey JOL: Incontinence following rupture of the anal sphincter during delivery. *Obstet Gynecol* 82(4):527–531, 1993.
2. DeLancey JOL: Functional anatomy of the female lower urinary tract and pelvic floor. Review article. *CIBA Found Symp* 151:57–69, 1990.
3. Madoff RD, Williams JG, Caushaj PF: Fecal incontinence. Review article, current concepts. *N Engl J Med* 326(15): 1002–1007, 1992.
4. Richardson AC, Edmonds PB, Williams NL: Treatment of stress urinary incontinence due to paravaginal fascial defect. *Obstet Gynecol* 57(3):357–363, 1981.
5. Shull BL: Clinical evaluation of women with pelvic support defects. *Clin Obstet Gynecol* 36(4):939–951, 1993.
6. Sultan AH, Kamm MA, Hudson CN, et al: Anal sphincter disruption during vaginal delivery. *N Engl J Med* 329(26): 1905–1911, 1993.

Part IV

Office Gynecologic Procedures

34 Office Use of Endovaginal Ultrasound

Steven R. Goldstein

Initially, real-time ultrasound equipment had barely enough resolution to do little more than identify a breech versus a vertex presentation, measure a biparietal diameter, and localize a placenta. A complete exam was extremely limited, consisting only of two to three Polaroid pictures. Office nurses were sent to various short courses to learn obstetric scanning. Gynecologic imaging, however, first with static arm scanners, and later with small-headed sector scanners, seemed more complex. The equipment was large and expensive.

Over time, obstetric scanning has become increasingly more sophisticated. The standard obstetric exam now mandates an understanding of cross-sectional anatomy; the gynecologic ultrasound exam mandates a complete understanding of the anatomy, histology, and physiology of the pelvic organs. Since this book addresses primary ambulatory health care for women exclusive of obstetric care, only office endovaginal ultrasound is discussed here. Obviously much obstetric ultrasound is performed in the Ob/Gyn's office, and some primary care physicians may perform transabdominal pelvic sonography as well.

An important advance in gynecologic imaging has been the introduction of vaginal probes. They are smaller and less expensive than earlier equipment, and are very adaptable to use by the physician at the time of the bimanual exam, mainly because the urinary bladder is empty and because the procedure requires very little time once the operator is adequately trained. Obviously, some clinical situations will mandate full bladder transabdominal views.

It is often helpful to enhance the overall bimanual exam by using vaginal probe assessment. Furthermore, there are times when the physiologic information obtained by office vaginal probe will allow the physician to make the diagnosis on the spot. This can eliminate referring for a radiographic exam, then later receiving a report of anatomic findings, and subsequently attempting to finalize the diagnosis. Consider this example: a 46-year-old woman, P3003, status post-tubal ligation, who usually has regular menses, presents with eight weeks of amenorrhea. The 2-min pregnancy test in the office is negative. Palpation reveals a top normal size, parous, anteverted uterus and a 4- to 5-cm right adnexal mass. The physician sends her for a transabdominal pelvic ultrasound and the report's impression (2 days later) reveals: 1. normal sized uterus with thickened endometrial echo (11 mm), 2. 5.4 × 4.1 cm complex right adnexal mass. The differential diagnosis includes endometrioma, neoplasia, or hemorrhagic cyst. An endovaginal sonogram performed in the office at the time of the pelvic exam would have revealed her obvious secretory endometrium (Fig. 34-1) coupled with a hemorrhagic corpus luteum cyst showing classic clot retraction (Fig. 34-2), and this would have allowed a diagnosis of delayed ovulation. Depending on the physician's comfort level, this might have been verified with a serum progesterone, and the patient would be told to expect her menses within a maximum of two weeks. Furthermore, once normal menses did ensue, the patient could return in the proliferative phase of her second cycle to document a normal right ovary (Fig. 34-3).

The technical considerations that lend themselves to such an approach are an empty urinary bladder and higher frequency equipment used in closer proximity to the structures being studied. This results in excellent resolution, not lost with magnification. The drawbacks to the vaginal probe, compared with traditional transabdominal scanning, are the short field of view, the lack of sound enhancement that a filled urinary bladder affords, the limitations of the probe by the confines of the vagina, new orientation for those familiar with traditional transabdominal panoramic views, and the presence of loops of bowel and the confusing echoes they generate throughout the pelvis. The advantages are that the procedure is very simple once the operator has been adequately trained; further, it is time-efficient because it can easily be done by the clinician while the patient is still in the lithotomy position for the bimanual exam. The probe adds very little time to the overall binmanual exam and has very high patient acceptance.

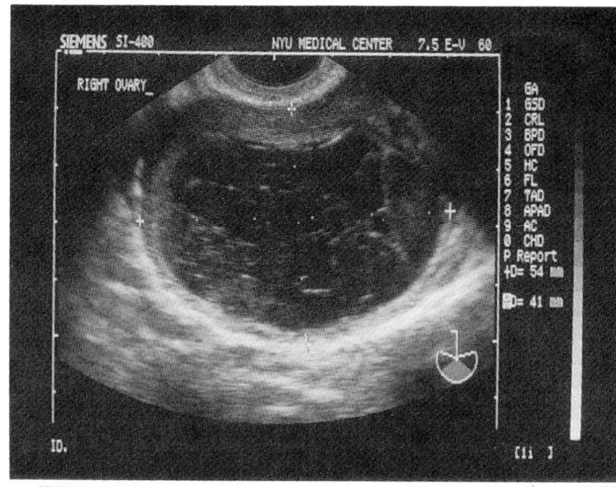

Figure 34-2 5.4 × 4.1 cm right adnexal mass. This is a cystic structure with complex features (internal echoes). However, such a picture is classic for hemorrhage into a follicle at the time of ovulation. This "cobweb"-like appearance is typical of clot retraction. It can and should be easily distinguished from endometriosis or frankly neoplastic processes.

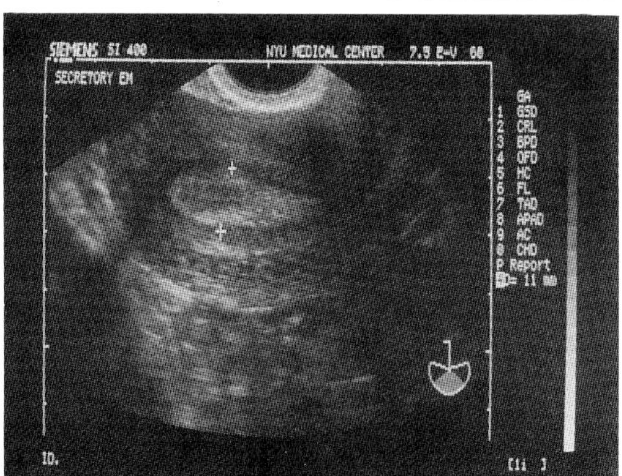

Figure 34-1 Long-axis view of the uterus depicting homogeneous echogenic endometrium (white calipers) typical of the secretory phase.

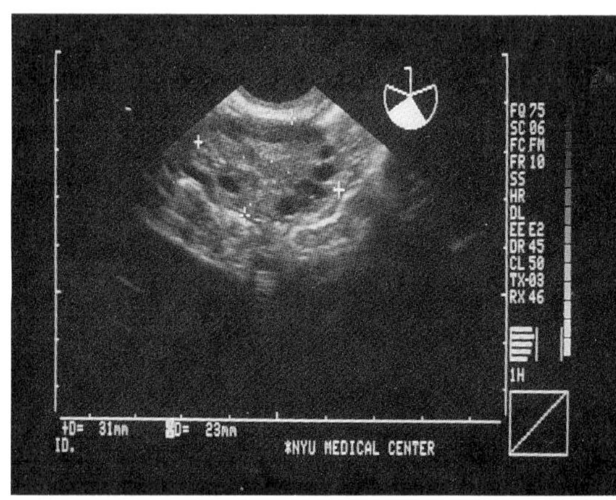

Figure 34-3 A normal ovary in the early proliferative phase displaying numerous small follicles prior to the establishment of a dominant follicle. The entire ovary measures 3.1 × 2.3 cm.

Technique of Endovaginal Sonography

The probe is covered with a clean (not sterile) condom or the finger of a glove. Ultrasound coupling gel is placed inside the condom. Outer lubricant is generally not necessary, since speculum examination and bimanual exam (with lubricant) have preceded the sonography. The pelvic organs are imaged to confirm or deny impressions obtained during palpation. Frequent use of the hand on the abdomen brings structures closer to the probe tip and will improve results.

Once the probe is inserted into the vagina it is manipulated posteriorly, anteriorly, and obliquely to the right and left, in order to image recognizable anatomical structures. The uterus in long axis (Fig. 34-1) serves as a basic anatomical landmark from which to orient one's eye and hand. One looks for a recognizable endometrial echo surrounded by typical myometrium. The contour of the myometrial border, the homogeneity of the myometrium itself, and a characterization of the endometrium both subjectively and by measurement should be determined. The transducer is then turned 90 degrees to view the uterus in a semicoronal plane. By moving one's hand in an anterioposterior direction, one will see this plane from cervix to fundus.

Returning to the long axis view, one then moves in a sagittal-oblique direction looking for ovarian structures. These are recognized in part by their location (in premenopausal patients) immediately adjacent to the iliac vessels. Remember that the iliac artery is smaller and can be seen to pulsate; the iliac vein often can be seen to have flow on real-time. Premenopausal patients who do not have significant pelvic adhesions will have ovaries that, by gravity, in the lithotomy position, can be located immediately adjacent to the iliac vessels. Ovaries are also recognized by their appearance. There is a typical gray pattern to the stroma, and the ovary contains numerous follicles at various stages of development, depending on what phase in the menstrual cycle the patient is, and whether the patient is taking oral contraceptive pills. When either ovary is found in this long axis orientation, the transducer handle once again is turned 90 degrees. Assessing the ovary in two planes at right angles to each other allows three-dimensional assessment of the structure. The method used to find the contralateral ovary is exactly the same.

Complete pelvic ultrasound examination should include assessment of the cul-de-sac and the region anterior to the uterus, where the bladder often will be seen to start to fill with a small amount of sonolucent urine. Characterization of the cervical region can be carried out as well.

Traditional transabdominal pelvic ultrasound makes use of multiple two-dimensional images (tomograms) to recreate three-dimensional anatomy. In vaginal sonography such concepts as longitudinal and transverse lose their meaning. Rather, what one is interested in obtaining is ''anatomy-derived orientation.'' A view of a structure and then a corresponding right angle view will allow three-dimensional appreciation of that structure.

Office Applications

One application for the vaginal probe by the office practitioner can be to confirm what seemed to be a normal exam by palpation. The uterus is seen in long axis and is normal in size, shape, and contour. The endometrial echo is visualized and can be correlated physiologically to the findings within the ovary. This will be reassuring. Some healthy patients do not lend themselves to meaningful palpation, especially those who may be tense and thus voluntarily guard, or those who are obese.

Conversely, we are often confronted with definitive or suspected abnormal findings by palpation. The uterine contour may be irregular in shape, suggesting the presence of intramural or subserosal myomas (Fig. 34-4). A ''fullness'' in the adnexa, when imaged, may be seen to represent a hydrosalpinx or a prominent loop of bowel. What seemed to be on bimanual pelvic examination an enlargement in the adnexa, the vaginal probe may distinguish as a prominent ovary or an actual cystic enlargement. On palpation these might have had similar size, but ultrasound demonstrates internal characteristics that are extremely divergent. This would be true of a

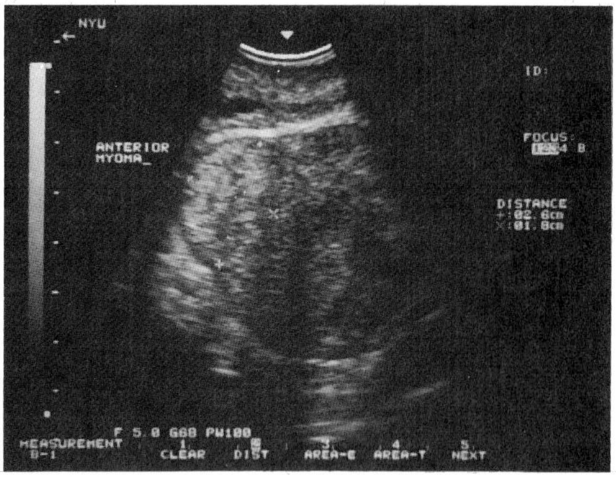

Figure 34-4 This patient, by bimanual palpation, seemed to have an irregularity to the uterine contour. Long-axis vaginal ultrasound here clearly demonstrates an anterior fundal myoma (calipers) measuring 2.6 × 1.8 cm.

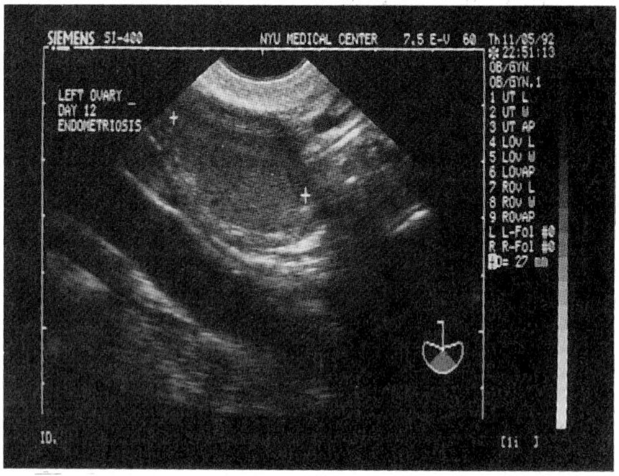

Figure 34-5 Grossly normal left ovary at the time of bimanual palpation. This sonogram clearly depicts a 2.7 cm endometrioma wholly contained within the normal ovarian contours.

prominent ovary of normal sonographic texture and appearance versus a thick-walled ovarian cyst containing debris.

At other times, findings can be imaged with a vaginal probe that either were missed by bimanual exam (small subserosal myomas, adnexal findings) or that one might not expect to find by palpation. Such would include abnormal endometrial findings or small dermoids or endometriomas (Fig. 34-5), which are almost totally contained within the body of the ovary.

In the past, ultrasound was used in early pregnancy for such indications as bleeding, size-date discrepancy, previous ectopic pregnancy, patients requesting termination of pregnancy, and to evaluate any coexisting adnexal masses. Consider the patient who is pregnant and bleeding with a closed cervical os. All such patients represent "threatened abortion," but at the same time, until proven otherwise, they also may have an ectopic pregnancy. Use of the vaginal probe can help to distinguish the patient with an obvious intrauterine pregnancy failure (Fig. 34-6) from one with a normal-appearing gestation but areas of subchorionic hemorrhage versus a patient with no evidence of a gestational sac. This can be especially valuable in a patient with severe abdomi-

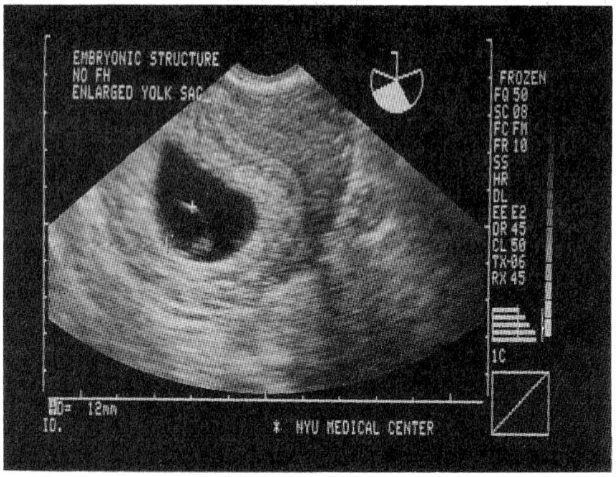

Figure 34-6 Definitive case of intrauterine pregnancy failure. This patient presented at seven weeks from her LMP with a closed cervical os and vaginal spotting. Thus, she is considered to have a "rule out ectopic" until proven otherwise. Vaginal probe ultrasound exam reveals an abnormally enlarged yolk sac (calipers) measuring 12 mm. Along one border there is an amorphus embryonic structure with no cardiac activity. Definitive diagnosis of intrauterine pregnancy that has failed is thus made.

nal pain and guarding that prevents any meaningful traditional bimanual evaluation. One can differentiate the patient with an intrauterine pregnancy and pain from a ruptured corpus luteum cyst from a patient with an obvious ectopic pregnancy. Significant size-date discrepancies often can be resolved in a matter of moments by using the vaginal probe. A gestational sac coexisting with fibroids can easily be distinguished from the uterine enlargement one sees with multiple gestations, even in the first trimester.

Routine use of the vaginal probe can help document an intrauterine location as well as identify a pregnancy that may not be developing normally. A normal gestational sac grows approximately 1 millimeter per day and a normal embryo grows 1 millimeter per day. In pregnant women who have had bleeding or other problems, once ectopic pregnancy is ruled out, serial ultrasound examinations can be carried out to verify normal continued growth. By the time a gestational sac is 8 to 10 mm, a yolk sac should be visualized. By the time an embryo reaches 5 mm, cardiac activity should be seen.

In postmenopausal patients with bleeding or palpable adnexal masses, vaginal probe sonography can be extremely helpful. In the presence of postmenopausal bleeding, an endometrial echo less than 5 mm (Fig. 34-7) has almost always been shown to be associated with lack of significant tissue. In the face of postmenopausal bleeding, an endometrial thickness greater than or equal to 6 mm has been shown to be associated with virtually all pathology tissue types. Routine use of the vaginal probe may show cystic adnexal masses (Fig. 34-8) in as many as 10 to 15 percent of postmenopausal patients; when these are small, unilocular, and unilateral, they will almost never be malignant. However, such findings should be followed at close intervals, particularly initially, to be certain that there is no progression, enlargement, or development of septation or ascitic fluid.

Use of the vaginal probe as part of screening for ovarian cancer is another area of great interest. Debates exist about both the cost and the lack of demonstrated effectiveness of such screening. It is this author's contention that our current screening for ovarian cancer with palpation alone is totally inadequate and that incorporation of the vaginal probe

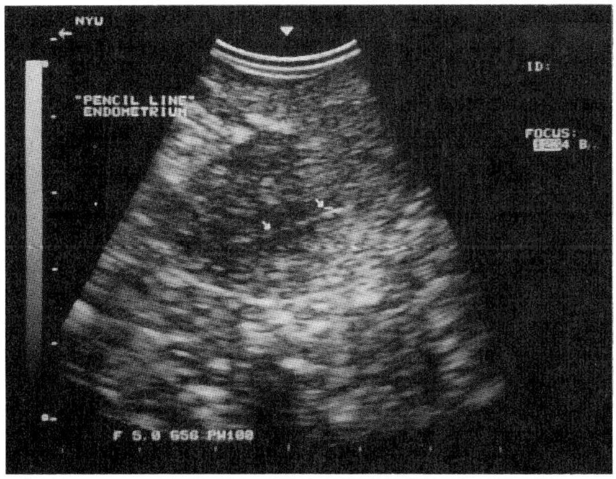

Figure 34-7 This long-axis view of the uterus was obtained in a postmenopausal patient who complained of vaginal staining. This thin "pencil line" endometrium (white arrows) has almost consistently been shown to be associated with lack of significant tissue at the time of endometrial sampling.

into the overall bimanual exam would allow more effective evaluation of the adnexa in a more sensible and less costly fashion than setting up separate ultrasound screening facilities. Any screening program that looks for ovarian cancer in this age group also

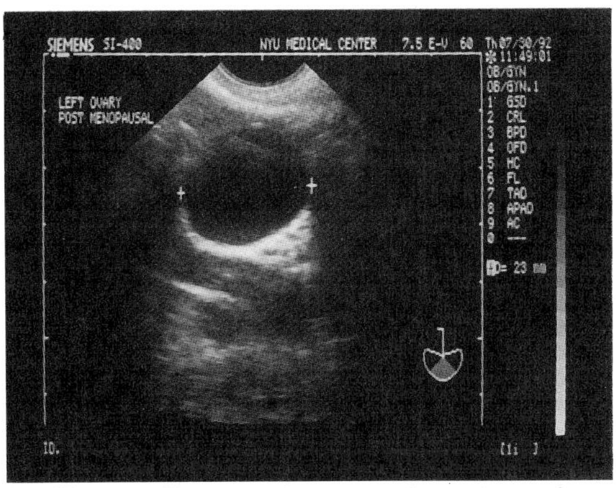

Figure 34-8 Postmenopausal ovary depicting a unilocular, smooth-walled cystic structure whose maximal diameter is 2.3 cm. There have been almost no reported cases of malignancy or borderline malignancy in unilocular, unilateral cystic structures seen with vaginal probe ultrasound measuring less than 3.0 cm.

should be looking at the size and texture of the endometrium and should correlate this with whether or not the patient is on hormone replacement therapy. At present, normative data for endometrial thickness (mean and two standard deviations around the mean) for various hormone replacement regimens have not been established. Still, there will often be instances where obvious abnormal endometrial findings can be discerned.

It is almost impossible to take care of infertility patients—and certainly impossible to properly utilize various assisted reproductive technologies—without vaginal probe ultrasound. It has revolutionized follicle surveillance and oocyte retrieval for various assisted reproductive technologies.

Other useful applications of the vaginal probe include finding the lost IUD (Fig. 34-9), which can easily be imaged in a matter of seconds. Postoperative cervical stenosis is also easily seen with the vaginal probe.

The use of vaginal ultrasound may be able to refine noninvasive diagnosis further, and thus may allow fewer diagnostic operative procedures (e.g., laparoscopy, hysteroscopy, and D&C), thus preventing further diagnostic work-up in some cases or allowing appropriate operative triage in others. Consider the following examples:

Vaginal ultrasound often can reliably distinguish the hemorrhagic corpus luteum cyst (Fig. 34-2) (no therapy or "diagnostic" laparoscopy needed) from an endometrioma (Fig. 34-5), in which case diagnostic laparoscopy can be avoided and the patient scheduled for a more definitive operative procedure. This allows proper triage for amount of OR time, equipment needed, and varying levels of operator skill.

Or, consider the patient with abnormal endometrial findings and/or abnormal uterine bleeding. Vaginal ultrasound and, more recently, fluid-enhanced endometrial assessment can help to distinguish dysfunctional bleeding (Fig. 34-10) or polyps (Fig. 34-11) from submucous myomas (Fig. 34-12). Once again, OR triage for amount of time, necessary

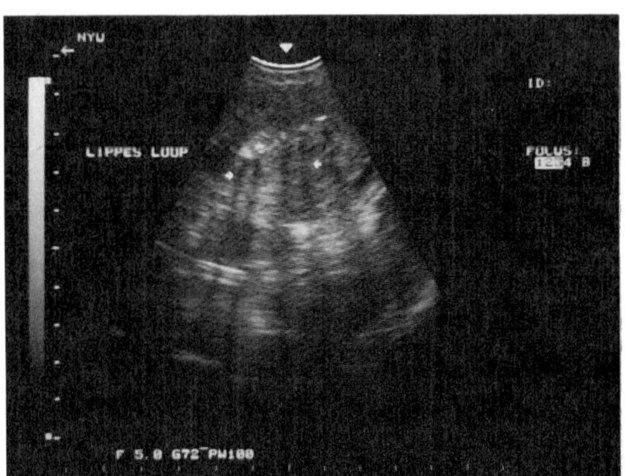

Figure 34-9 Long-axis view of the uterus in a patient with a history of use of an intrauterine device. No string could be seen coming from the cervical os. In a matter of seconds, endovaginal ultrasound revealed this Lippes loop to be centrally located. The acoustic shadowing caused by the device (white arrows) is pathognomonic.

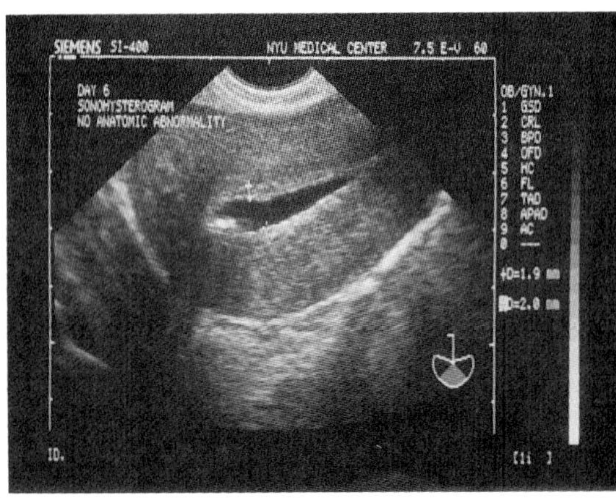

Figure 34-10 Sonohysterogram, whereby sterile saline is infused through an intrauterine catheter on day 6 of the cycle in a perimenopausal patient with menometrorrhagia; the sonohysterogram depicts no anatomical abnormality. The endometrium (calipers) measures 1.9 and 2.0 mm, respectively. Realize that these endometrial measurements, because of the distention of the fluid, are half-thickness when compared with full-thickness measurements done without fluid enhancement. Such a picture is compatible with dysfunctional uterine bleeding. A biopsy was subsequently performed that revealed early proliferative change.

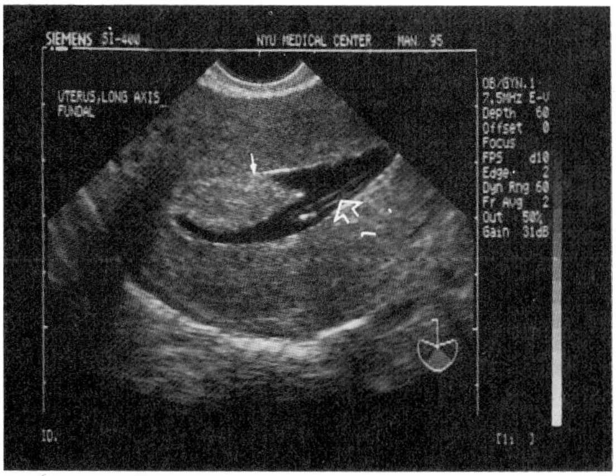

Figure 34-11 Sonohysterogram, in a patient with a similar history of abnormal bleeding, reveals an anterior fundal polyp that measured 21 mm. The endometrial layer surrounding the fluid is seen to be thin (white arrow). In addition, the intrauterine insemination catheter is clearly visible (open white arrow).

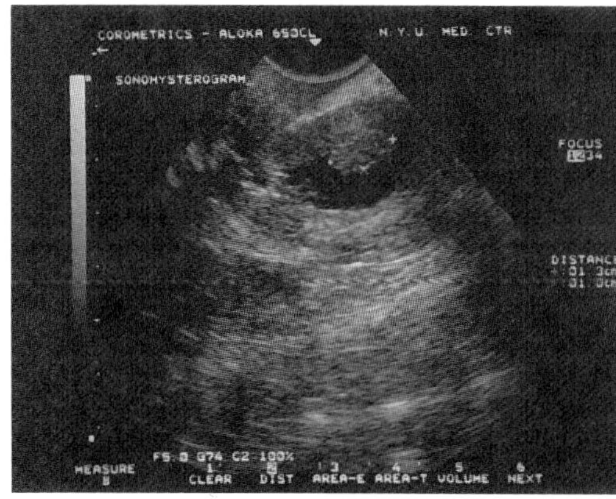

Figure 34-12 Sonohysterogram clearly depicts a submucous myoma (calipers). Approximately 50 percent of this myoma is seen extruding into the endometrial cavity. Such a patient can be offered resectoscopic myomectomy. Preoperative evaluation with this technique allows for more appropriate operative triage in terms of amount of time, instruments, and necessary skill level of the operator.

instruments, and necessary skill level of the operator can be appropriately made.

Summary

The use of vaginal ultrasound by the office practitioner can have tremendous benefits. Often diagnoses can be made on the spot, assisting the physician in providing more timely therapy or, in the case of normal findings, relieving patient anxieties. It will save time for both the physician and the patient. Vaginal scanning in the office can reduce the need to refer patients elsewhere, except when further consultation is needed. This will reduce the potential for the errors that can occur when information must be transmitted from one source to another. Most patients prefer vaginal scanning because of the annoyance of the full bladder needed when the transabdominal approach is used. Sonography also helps patients to better understand their care. The pictures generated on the screen are very helpful in discussing pathology with the patient. In addition, they can be a very powerful teaching tool of normal anatomy and physiology. Finally, vaginal scanning allows instant confirmation of the primary physician's findings at the time of the pelvic examination.

References and Selected Readings

1. Goldstein SR, et al: Very early pregnancy detection with endovaginal ultrasound. *Obstet Gynecol* 72:200–204, 1988.
2. Goldstein SR: Early pregnancy ultrasound: A new look with the endovaginal probe. *Contemp Obstet Gynecol* 31:54, 1988.
3. Goldstein SR: Incorporating endovaginal ultrasonography into the overall gynecologic examination. *Am J Obstet Gynecol* 162:625–633, 1990.
4. Goldstein SR, Nachtigall M, Snyder JR, et al: Endometrial assessment by vaginal ultrasonography before endometrial sampling in patients with postmenopausal bleeding. *Am J Obstet Gynecol* 163:114–123, 1990.
5. Goldstein SR: Significance of cardiac activity on endovaginal ultrasound in very early embryos. *Obstet Gynecol* 80:670–672, 1992.
6. Letourneau J: Gynecologic sonography: Report of the ultrasonography task force. *JAMA* 265:2851–2855, 1991.
7. Mendelson EB, Bohm-Velez M: Transvaginal sonography assessed early pregnancy. *Diagn Imaging,* November 1987.
8. Silva P, Platt L, Yee B: Transvaginal ultrasound in the infertility workup. *Female Patient* 12:14–24, 1987.
9. Timor-Tritsch IE, et al: Review of transvaginal ultrasonography. *Ultrasound* 6:1, 1988.
10. Timor-Tritsch IE: Is office use of vaginal sonography feasible? *Am J Obstet Gynecol* 162:983–985, 1990.

35 Colposcopy and the Evaluation and Treatment of Abnormal Pap Smears

Mark Spitzer

Squamous cell cancer of the cervix is the most common female genital malignancy. Worldwide, it is currently the greatest cancer killer in women under the age of 40. Cervical cancer is less frequent in countries where women have good access to health care, and it is more frequent in underdeveloped countries. This is because the premalignant phase of cervical cancer is well-recognized, easily detectable, and easily treated. This chapter will focus on the detection and treatment of premalignant lesions of the cervix, vagina, and vulva.

Squamous cell cervical cancer is considered by many to be a sexually transmitted disease. Early age at first intercourse, multiple partners, and partners who have multiple partners are all well-documented risk factors for the development of cervical cancer. In recent years, it has been well recognized that human papilloma virus (HPV) is a likely candidate as the sexually transmitted carcinogen. There is much epidemiologic, histologic, and microbiologic evidence linking HPV to cervical cancer. However, it is also quite evident that HPV infection alone will not lead to cancer. Several factors—the HPV subtype, certain cofactors such as smoking, the host-immune response, and the time in a woman's life at which she is infected—influence the potential progression to cervical cancer. Further, the colposcopic and histologic appearance of HPV infection (condyloma) and cervical intraepithelial neoplasia (CIN) are very similar and difficult to distinguish. Since

HPV infection and milder forms of CIN do not invariably progress to cervical cancer, a rational approach to the diagnosis and treatment of these lesions is essential.

The Evaluation of the Abnormal Pap Smear

Because of the high false-negative rate of Pap smears, negative Pap smears should be repeated annually for at least three years before one can be reliably reassured that no disease is present.

Since 1988, the Bethesda Classification System has been used for the reporting of cervical cytology in the United States. The Bethesda System divides epithelial changes found on cytology into several categories. A summary of these categories and their approximate equivalents in the World Health Organization (WHO) and Papanicolaou systems can be found in Table 35-1.

TABLE 35-1 Comparison of Three Classification Systems Historically Used to Report the Results of Cervical Cytology

Papanicolaou System	Descriptive System	Bethesda System[a,b]
Class I	*Negative* Negative with inflammation	*Within normal limits* Infection (specify type)
	Inflammatory atypia	Epithelial changes related to inflammation
Class II	Squamous atypia	Atypical squamous cells of undetermined significance
	Condylomatous (Koilocytotic) atypia	Low grade squamous intra-epithelial lesion (SIL) with or without cellular changes associated with HPV
	Minimal or Mild Dysplasia (CIN-1)	
Class III	Moderate Dysplasia (CIN-2) Severe Dysplasia (CIN-3)	High grade SIL
Class IV	Carcinoma-in-situ (CIN-3)	
Class V	Positive for malignant cells	Squamous cell carcinoma

[a]The Bethesda System incorporates into each report a statement on specimen adequacy.

[b]The Bethesda System incorporates a separate statement about glandular cells, atypical glandular cells, adenocarcinoma, or other malignant neoplasms when appropriate.

NOTE: It is important to note that the three classification systems overlap each other and that one cannot extrapolate results from the Papanicolaou System to the Bethesda System. To do so would be misleading and may result in errors in patient management.

The Atypical Pap Smear

Historically, the "atypical" category has included a wide range of abnormalities ranging from milder forms of inflammatory atypia, likely to be caused by infection, through squamous atypia and condylomatous atypia likely to represent low-grade intraepithelial lesions (condyloma, mild dysplasia, CIN 1). In the Bethesda classification system, the cytologist is asked to predict the etiology of the cytologic changes. Changes most likely related to inflammation with no premalignant potential are called epithelial changes related to inflammation. More marked epithelial changes are called atypical squamous cells of undetermined significance. The cytologist is asked to classify these as likely to be etiologically related to either inflammation or dysplasia.

The incidence of atypical smears has been reported as being in the range of 2 to 10 percent, with some reports indicating an incidence as high as 30 percent or more. The reported incidence of dysplasia in patients with atypical smears also varies widely. Dysplasia has been reported in 15 to 25 percent of patients with atypical smears. A variety of approaches have been suggested in the management of atypical Pap smears; however, none of these has been universally accepted as the only correct approach.

The traditional approach in the management of atypical Pap smears is to treat based on the presumed cause of inflammation and to repeat the Pap smear at a later date (commonly between 1 and 6 months). Patients whose repeat Pap smear is again atypical would undergo evaluation with colposcopy and biopsies, while patients with negative follow-up smears are returned to the regular screening pool. The problems with this traditional approach are that the interval for repeat cytology was never standardized and that the large incidence of false-negative smears may lead to misdiagnosis. Studies have shown that treatment prior to repeat cytology did not improve the rate of reversion to normal cytology. Finally, the protocol of "treat and repeat" required patience and reliability on the part of the patient. No amount of reassurance will completely allay the fears of a woman who has been told that her "cancer test" was not normal but that she merely needs to have it repeated in four months.

Other approaches have been suggested in the management of atypical Pap smears. Colposcopy of all patients with atypical Pap smears is an effective method of identifying patients with dysplasia; however, because of the significant investment required in time, resources, and trained personnel, this approach often is impractical. The Bethesda classification system attempts to identify a subset of patients with atypical Pap smears who are at greater risk of cervical dysplasia. This is the category of atypical squamous cells of undetermined significance suggestive of dysplasia. There are insufficient data currently available to indicate that this method is uniformly effective.

Intermediate triage tools also have been used to determine which patients need evaluation with colposcopy. The most successful of these tools is cervicography, a photographic method that provides a "colposcopic-type" view of the cervix, which is then interpreted for the practitioner by an expert in colposcopy. Cervicography has been shown to be effective in distinguishing atypia caused by dysplasia from other types of atypia. However, the initial experience with this method indicated that it had a high false-positive rate.

Patients with atypical smears should be considered at high risk for CIN. Since no single method of triage is perfect, further study is necessary to find the best alternative. Until the best system is found, the evaluation of patients with atypical smears should not be considered complete until they have had a negative colposcopy, three consecutive negative Pap smears, and/or a negative cervigram.

Pap Smears Suspicious for Squamous Intraepithelial Lesions

These smears must be evaluated on the assumption that the patient has a premalignant condition. The instrument used for this evaluation is the colposcope. It is a stereoscopic binocular microscope with illumination.

Colposcopy

The ultimate goal of colposcopy is to establish the severity of the patient's disease while determining that there is no evidence of microinvasive or invasive cancer. If these facts can be established, then the patient can be managed with conservative forms of treatment, and more radical approaches can be avoided. This can be accomplished by evaluation of the transformation zone. The transformation zone is the area of the cervix and occasionally the vagina that originally was covered by columnar epithelium and through a process called squamous metaplasia has changed to squamous epithelium. It extends outward from the squamocolumnar junction. The importance of the transformation zone is that almost all squamous cell carcinomas of the cervix begin in the transformation zone. If the entire transformation zone has been visualized and evaluated, the area at risk has been evaluated and the most severe lesion has been seen.

The technique of colposcopy involves washing the cervix with 3 to 5 percent acetic acid. After treatment with acetic acid, areas with a greater nuclear density, such as benign metaplastic epithelium and dysplastic epithelium, will reflect light rather than transmitting it to the underlying stroma, and will therefore appear white rather than pink or red. Neovascularization will cause vascular changes of mosaic patterns, punctations, and atypical vessels in some lesions. These changes, taken together and graded for their severity, can be used to predict which areas have the most significant histologic abnormality, and will help to direct the colposcopist's decisions regarding the optimal locations for colposcopic biopsies. A good colposcopist should be able to recognize colposcopic patterns and to predict the histologic equivalents of these patterns.

Mature squamous epithelium remains pink after the application of acetic acid. It is covered by a fine network of uniformly thin and evenly distributed subepithelial blood vessels. Certain benign changes such as inflammation and mucosal thinning due to inadequate estrogen stimulation may make the vascular markings appear more pronounced. However, these are easily distinguished from the bizarre vascular patterns of early carcinoma. The endocervical mucosa around the external os appears red prior to the application of acetic acid, and has been called eversion, ectropion, or ectopy. Its surface presents longitudinal ridges and multiple villus-like projections. After the application of acetic acid, the tips of these villi may turn white, indicating the earliest manifestations of metaplasia.

The squamocolumnar junction is the line separating these two types of epithelial cells. It is frequently identified by a thin rim of acetowhite epithelium. The acetowhiteness seen at the squamocolumnar junction and in the remainder of the transformation zone is less intense and more translucent than acetowhiteness seen in dysplastic and neoplastic lesions, and it has a less distinct border. Other manifestations of the transformation zone seen during colposcopy include endocervical gland openings and Nabothian cysts, which present as domelike structures raised above the surface and which are filled with a mucinous content behind a thin semitransparent wall, giving the cyst a yellow color. Large blood vessels found over the dome of the cyst are arranged in a characteristic branching pattern. It is this branching pattern that distinguishes these benign vessels from neoplastic atypical vessels (Fig. 35-1).

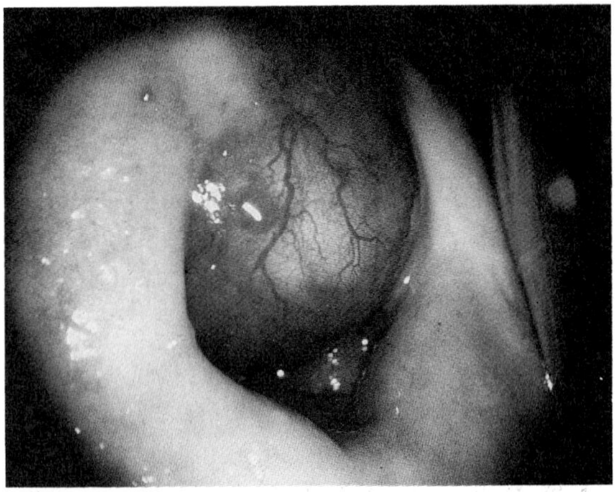

Figure 35-1 Nabothian cyst. Note the large blood vessels over the dome of the cyst. These can be distinguished from neoplastic vessels because they branch.

Abnormal Epithelial Changes

Colposcopy identifies the area of cervical epithelium with the most advanced histologic abnormality. By noting the colposcopic features characteristic of these lesions, each characteristic can be judged and graded based on the likelihood that it represents a high-grade versus a low-grade lesion. The individual criteria used to distinguish low-grade from high-grade are the epithelial thickness, its contour, the degree of acetowhiteness, the presence of vascular changes, and the border of the lesion.

The most common colposcopic manifestation of CIN is acetowhiteness. Acetowhiteness must be distinguished from leukoplakia, which appears white before the application of acetic acid. Leukoplakia is caused by hyperkeratosis and is important only because it obscures the underlying epithelium. Because it is impossible to evaluate the underlying epithelium colposcopically, leukoplakia always should be biopsied.

Acetowhiteness can range in intensity. Metaplastic epithelium is semitransparent. A snow-white shiny epithelium is found in low-grade lesions. Intermediate lesions have a grayish-white but still shiny epithelium, and high-grade lesions have a dull grayish to oyster-shell white epithelium (Fig. 35-2).

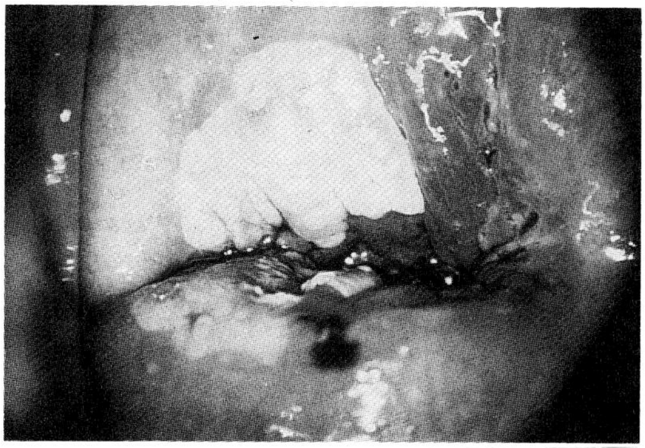

Figure 35-2 Acetowhite epithelium. This is a well-demarcated, dense acetowhite epithelium on the anterior lip of the cervix. Note the straight edges of this high-grade lesion. Also there is dense acetowhite epithelium extending into the endocervical canal on the posterior lip of the cervix.

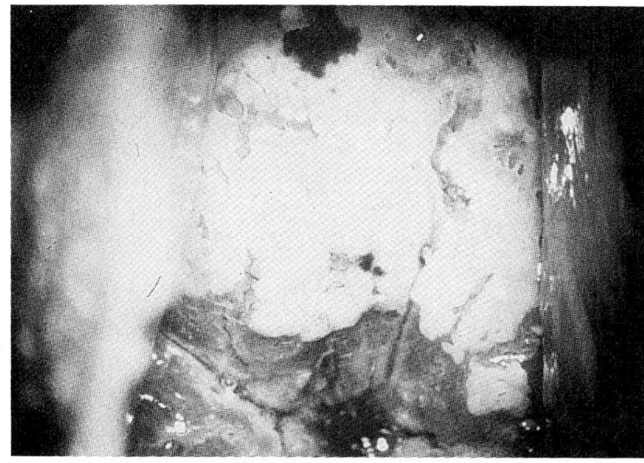

Figure 35-3 Acetowhite epithelium. Biopsies should be taken from the inner margin of this dense acetowhite lesion. This is the most immature area and likely to be the highest-grade lesion.

The sharpness of the peripheral margin is another feature used to grade epithelial abnormalities. Squamous metaplastic lesions turn white after the application of acetic acid, but their borders tend to be diffuse and to blend into the adjacent squamous epithelium. True dysplastic lesions have a sharp and well-demarcated border. In low-grade lesions, this border may be feathered or finely scalloped or may be angular and irregularly shaped, similar to geographic features on a map. Significant satellite lesions, not contiguous with the rest of the transformation zone, are most commonly low-grade lesions. Intermediate and high-grade lesions usually have straight and sharp peripheral margins. The highest grade lesions have edges that detach from the underlying stroma and curl back upon themselves. This is due to the poor cell-to-cell cohesiveness in these lesions (Fig. 35-3). Lesions that show an internal margin between two different colposcopic patterns almost always are high-grade, with the peripheral area representing a minor-grade lesion and the central area a high-grade.

Another colposcopic feature to consider when grading lesions is the epithelial thickness and contour. Condylomatous lesions have a micropapillary contour, while dysplastic lesions are more likely to be flat. Low-grade lesions are flat, with their surface at the same level as the adjacent squamous epithelium. Lesions with a definite thickness above the adjacent squamous epithelium are more likely to be high-grade.

The final colposcopic feature used to grade epithelial abnormalities is the vascular pattern. Vascular patterns in benign epithelium are seen when the hairpin capillary at the core of an endocervical villus which is undergoing metaplasia has not completely regressed. Abnormal vascularity, punctations, and mosaic patterns occur when the stromal papilla and their blood vessels persist in the neoplastic epithelium with neovascularization. Persistent blood vessels reach the epithelial surface and then become visible as colposcopic abnormalities. Punctation is seen as multiple red dots spaced over a demarcated area of white epithelium. A true punctation has an acetowhite background with well-demarcated borders. Red dots on a pink or red mucosa usually are manifestations of an inflammatory condition such as Trichomonas or some other type of vaginitis. Mosaic patterns are characterized by round or polygonal, tile-like fields of acetowhite epithelium, each encircled by a blood vessel. Mosaic patterns develop when the persistent superficial vessels run horizontally, forming a honeycomb pattern, and enclose islands of white epithelium between their anastomotic branches. A true neoplastic mosaic pattern is always associated with well-demarcated acetowhite epithelium, just as in true punctations.

Mosaic patterns and punctations may be fine or coarse. Fine punctation patterns are distinguished from coarse ones by the caliber of the vessels, the intercapillary distance, and the regularity of the pattern. Fine punctations appear as small red dots closely and regularly spaced in the field of acetowhite epithelium. In coarse punctations, the individual vessels may be dilated, the distance between the dots is increased, and the pattern is irregular (Fig. 35-4). In extreme cases, the punctations may be seen to rise above the surface epithelium, and they may begin to take on bizarre appearances (Fig. 35-5). Fine punctations and fine mosaic patterns are associated with low-grade lesions, while coarse punctations and mosaic patterns are associated with high-grade lesions. Fine mosaic patterns are characterized by thin vessels separating small, regularly spaced acetowhite tiles. The pattern may be poorly developed. In a coarse mosaic pattern, the vessel caliber is large. The acetowhite tiles frequently are raised above the surface epithelium. In the highest-grade lesions, there is frequently a punctation in the center of the mosaic tile. This pattern is almost always indicative of a high-grade lesion (Fig. 35-6).

The most extreme form of abnormal vascular pattern is the presence of atypical vessels. Atypical vessels may be comma-shaped or may have other bizarre appearances such as sharp bends, turns, or spirals. The vessel caliber may suddenly constrict or dilate, or the vessel may change course abruptly. Vessels are sometimes seen to plunge beneath the surface of the epithelium only to resurface in a serpentine manner (Fig. 35-7). Most characteristically, these vessels do not branch. Atypical vessels are the earliest colposcopic manifestation of invasive cancer (Fig. 35-8).

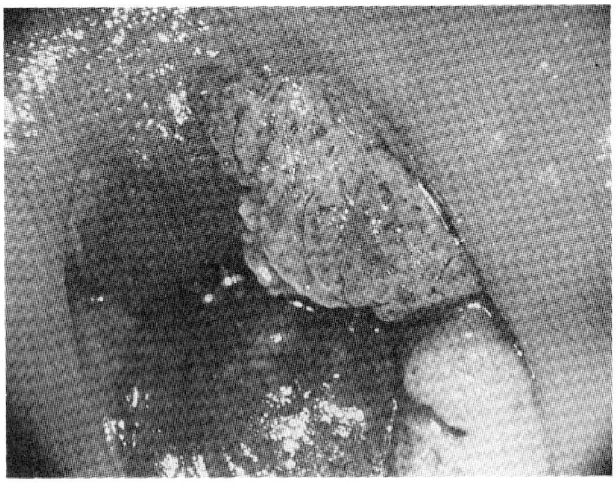

Figure 35-5 Coarse punctations. In addition to having a large caliber and large intercapillary distances (distance between punctations), these punctations rise above the surface epithelium and are beginning to take on comma shapes suggestive of atypical vessels.

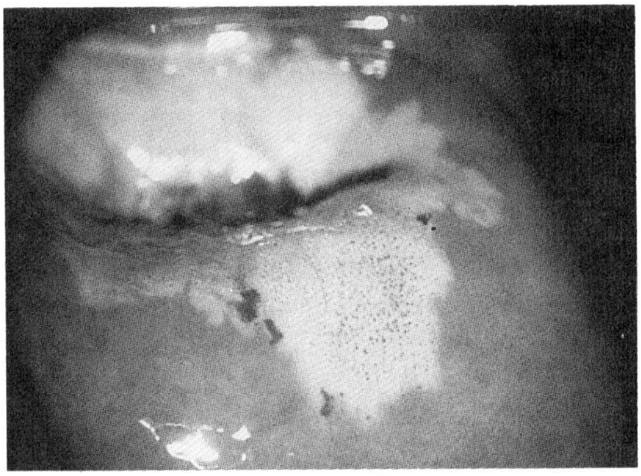

Figure 35-4 Punctation. Acetowhite epithelium with a coarse punctation pattern. Note that the dots vary in size and intensity and their pattern is irregular. This is typical of a high-grade lesion.

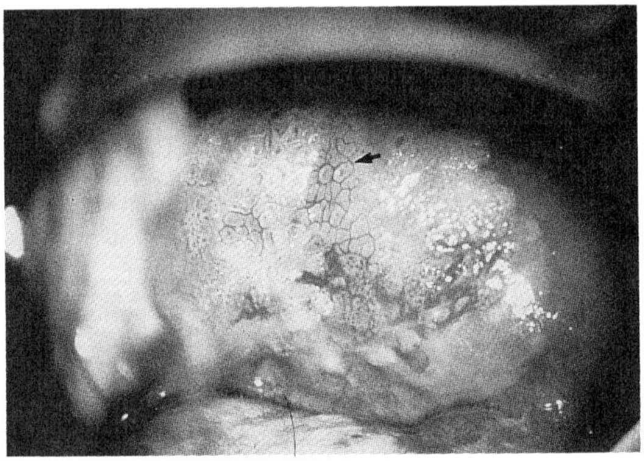

Figure 35-6 Mosaic. Acetowhite epithelium with a coarse mosaic pattern. Note that the mosaic tiles are large and irregular in size and shape. The vessels surrounding the mosaic tiles have large caliber. In several areas the mosaic tiles have a central vessel (arrow). This is highly suggestive of a high-grade lesion.

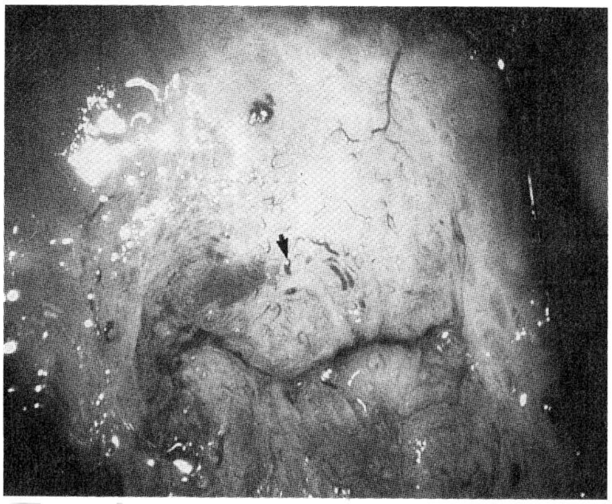

Figure 35-7 Atypical vessels. Atypical vessels have a variety of bizarre patterns. Sharp turns, comma-shaped vessels, and other bizarre patterns are seen in this colpophotograph. Several serpentine vessels are seen (arrow) which rise above the epithelium and then plunge below it only to resurface again.

The Colposcopic Diagnosis of Invasive Cancer

The colposcopic diagnosis of invasive cancer is the most important and frequently the most difficult diagnosis to make. While low-grade and high-grade intraepithelial lesions show distinctive colposcopic patterns, the colposcopic appearance of invasive cancer may be nonspecific and may resemble benign conditions such as chronic cervicitis. Because early invasive cancer is seen infrequently, even by experienced colposcopists, it is a very easy diagnosis to miss. Some features of invasive cancer are atypical vessels, a yellow color, markedly irregular contour, and multiple areas of superficial bleeding. There may be surface hemorrhages and atypical vessels. Because the intense inflammatory response may obscure the cytologic diagnosis of cancer, colposcopic recognition of these lesions is important and may be the only opportunity the clinician has to make the diagnosis. For this reason, biopsy of any suspicious areas is essential.

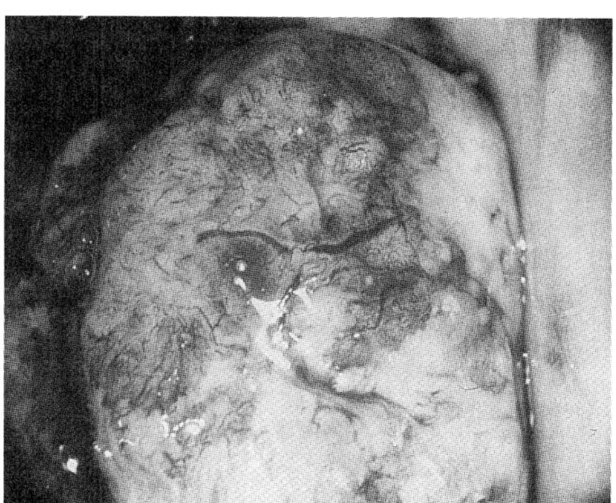

Figure 35-8 Atypical vessels. The prominent vessel in the center of the colpophotograph is one of several atypical vessels on this cervix. Note the varying caliber of this large vessel. Another characteristic of atypical vessels is that they do not branch.

Criteria for a Satisfactory Colposcopy

Colposcopy is a tool used to establish the location of the patient's most significant disease while excluding the possibility of invasive cancer. A directed biopsy (or more commonly, multiple biopsies) should be taken to establish the diagnosis. If the diagnosis can be established and cancer can be ruled out, the patient can be managed with conservative forms of treatment, and more aggressive treatment can be avoided. To avoid delays in the diagnosis of invasive cancer, certain criteria have been established to define a satisfactory colposcopy. Rigid adherence to these criteria will help avoid delay of the diagnosis and inadequate treatment of invasive cancer. In order to be certain that the worst lesion has been seen, the entire transformation zone must be visualized, and the entire lesion must be visualized. Endocervical curettage (ECC) should be done unless the patient is pregnant, and should not demonstrate any evidence of neoplastic tissue. Finally, the biopsy findings should not be significantly less severe than the cytologic and colposcopic findings. Such a discrepancy would imply that the biopsy may not have been taken from the worst lesion. When all these criteria are met, and invasive cancer has been ruled out, the colposcopy is deemed to be satisfactory, and the patient can be treated with a conservative modality such as cryotherapy or laser vaporization. If these criteria are not met, then invasive cancer has not been definitively ruled out, and the patient must undergo a cone biopsy. A cone biopsy removes the entire transformation zone, which can then be submitted for histologic evaluation to definitively rule out invasive cancer. Excision of the transformation zone will also serve to treat the disease.

Colposcopy of Vulvar and Vaginal Lesions

The colposcopic features of vulvar and vaginal intraepithelial lesions are similar to those on the cervix. Because metaplasia is uncommon on the vagina, except in DES-exposed women, mosaic and punctation patterns are almost always indicative of condyloma or intraepithelial neoplasia. Because of the large surface area of the vagina and its many folds, colposcopy of the vagina is difficult. Mulicentric disease is common on the vulva. Because dysplastic lesions of these areas are uncommon, colposcopy for disease of the vagina and vulva may need to be referred to an expert, unless the primary care physician has experience with these problems.

Treatment of Cervical Intraepithelial Neoplasia

Once the diagnosis has been established and colposcopy is satisfactory as outlined above, the patient's disease may be treated by ablation or excision of the transformation zone. If the colposcopy is not satisfactory, the transformation zone must be excised in order to establish the diagnosis and to exclude the possibility of invasion.

Whether treating the patient with ablation or excision, it is important to treat the entire transformation zone and to treat it to a depth of 7 to 10 mm so that all of the endocervical glands or crypts that may be involved with disease will be treated. None of the treatments are 100 percent effective, but any of them, properly applied, will provide cures in 90 to 100 percent of patients. Treatment of just the lesion without the remainder of the transformation zone, or treatment of the transformation zone, but to an inadequate depth, will result in significantly diminished cure rates. The techniques commonly employed in the United States are cryosurgery, laser surgery, loop electrosurgical excision, and cold knife conization. For a single small, low-grade lesion, some physicians will remove the lesion entirely by colposcopically directed biopsy, and not treat the remainder of the transformation zone.

Cryosurgery freezes the transformation zone with a liquid nitrous oxide or carbon dioxide probe. Most authors report cure rates in excess of 90 percent following one treatment. Cyrosurgery can be done on an outpatient basis and requires no anesthesia. Cryosurgery does, however, have some limitations. Since the probe size and shape need to approximate the size and shape of the lesion and the transformation zone, women who have a very large lesion, a very large transformation zone, or whose cervix is significantly distorted after obstetric trauma may be poor candidates for cryosurgery.

Several technical points must be kept in mind to obtain an optimal freeze. After insertion of an adequately sized speculum, including a vaginal sidewall retractor to prevent the vagina from making contact with the cryosurgery probe, a water-soluble lubricant jelly is applied to the probe to allow for efficient heat transfer. The probe is then applied to the cervix and the freezing initiated. The freeze should continue until an ice ball forms and its margin extends 5 mm beyond the edge of the lesion. Two freezes, each 3 min long, with a 3-min wait in between usually is sufficient. The pressure gauge on the nitrous oxide tank must be observed to insure that the gas pressure is adequate to chill the probe sufficiently at all times. A tank of adequate size should be chosen to insure that adequate pressures are maintained throughout the procedure. Because the actual depth of destruction is usually only between 2 and 5 mm, cryosurgery may be less effective in ablating lesions that extend to the endocervical glands or into the endocervical canal. For this reason, cryosurgery may be less effective in curing CIN-3.

Carbon dioxide laser surgery is probably the most versatile of the treatment modalities. Large lesions, irregular cervices, and high-grade lesions can all be managed by this modality. As experience with the laser increases, there is evidence that it can be done safely in an outpatient setting and under local anesthesia with minimal discomfort to the patient and with excellent cure rates. The disadvantages of laser surgery include a small but significant incidence of bleeding associated with the procedures, expensive equipment, and the significant amount of training and experience required to achieve good results, especially in an outpatient setting.

Loop electrosurgical excision, also known as large loop excision of the transformation zone (LLETZ), is becoming increasingly popular in the United States. A large unipolar electrocautery wire loop is used to excise the transformation zone. The procedure can be used in place of ablative techniques such as cryosurgery and laser vaporization and can be tailored as an alternative to excisional cone biopsy. It can be done under local anesthesia in an outpatient setting and has the major advantage of providing a specimen for histologic evaluation. Because LLETZ provides a histologic specimen, some practitioners use it instead of punch biopsy during colposcopic examination of patients with cytologic evidence of CIN. The use of this approach in women whose cytologic results are only mildly abnormal may result in many unnecessary excisions.

The technique of LLETZ is as follows: A wire loop is chosen of a shape and size that will excise the entire transformation zone, preferably in one pass. The loop is attached to an electrosurgical generator, and the patient is grounded to that generator. A large speculum is placed in the vagina and attached to a smoke evacuation device. Lateral side-wall retractors are placed to avoid injury to the vaginal wall. A local anesthetic is injected into the cervix. The wire loop is then slowly plunged into the cervical stroma 3 to 5 mm lateral to the edge of the transformation zone on one side of the cervix to a depth of 7 mm. It is then slowly passed under the transformation zone until it is removed 3 to 5 mm lateral to the transformation zone on the other side of the cervix. The electrosurgical generator power setting should be set with sufficient power to allow the probe to pass easily without drag but not so high that the specimen will be damaged. Approximately 30 watts of power is sufficient in most cases. One disadvantage of this procedure is the possibility of bleeding, which usually is minimal and can be controlled with electrocautery using a ball electrode or thickened ferric subsulfate solution. Also, there is a small incidence of thermal damage to the cone specimen.

Cold knife conization, which is an alternative method for cervical conization, is not discussed in this chapter because it is usually performed in the operating room, not in the office.

Who Should Be Treated?

After a complete colposcopic examination and biopsy, patients with high-grade squamous intraepithelial lesions (CIN-2 and -3, moderate to severe dysplasia, carcinoma-in-situ) should be treated. Patients with satisfactory colposcopy and negative ECC may be treated by ablation of the transformation zone. Cryosurgery, laser vaporization, and LLETZ are all good alternatives for this treatment, although cryosurgery may be slightly less effective in CIN-3. When the colposcopy is not satisfactory, a cone biopsy should be performed. This acts as a combination of diagnosis and treatment. Techniques for cone biopsy that can be utilized in an office setting include laser excisional conization and LLETZ.

When the colposcopically directed biopsy shows a low-grade lesion (condyloma, CIN-1, mild dysplasia), the alternatives are expanded. When the colposcopy is satisfactory, cryosurgery, laser vaporization, and LLETZ are all viable alternatives for treatment. However, because the vast majority of these lesions will never progress to invasive cancer and many will regress, close observation with cytology and colposcopy without treatment is another alternative. When deciding whether or not to treat such patients, some of the factors to take into consideration include the woman's age and parity, the size of the lesion, whether the lesion has persisted for a long time or whether it is newly discovered, previous treatment, her immune status, and the patient's reliability. While there is no evidence that cryosurgery, laser surgery, or LLETZ adversely affect fertility or the ability of a woman to carry a pregnancy, in cases of young nulliparous women, the alternative of watchful waiting should be favored in reliable patients who do not have other adverse factors. In patients with large or persistent lesions and in patients who cannot be relied on to continue close follow-up, the alternative of treatment should be favored. Also, in patients with a history of in utero DES exposure, therapy should be avoided when possible because of the great risk of cervical stenosis following treatment in such patients. If the colposcopy is not satisfactory, a cone biopsy should be performed. In young and nulliparous women, referral for colposcopy by an expert colposcopist should be considered prior to conization.

It is important to remember that the goal of treatment for women with intraepithelial disease of the cervix is the prevention of cancer, not the treatment of a viral infection. No treatment currently available is capable of eradicating the viral presence from the lower genital tract. Therefore, it is expected that viral presence will persist despite treatment and that flat condylomata may reappear on the mature squamous epithelium of the cervix following treatment. This does not necessarily represent a treatment failure. Once the transformation zone has been destroyed, reappearance of flat condylomata on the cervix does not necessarily need to be retreated. Such patients can be managed by careful cytologic and colposcopic follow-up. However, if the recurrent lesion is a high-grade intraepithelial lesion, these patients must be retreated, preferably using an excisional technique to assure that the margins are negative and that the lesion has been completely excised.

Treatment of Vulvar and Vaginal Lesions

Because the progressive potential of low-grade vulvar and vaginal intraepithelial lesions and condylomata is so low, once high-grade premalignant lesions in these areas have been ruled out, excessively aggressive treatment of these lesions to prevent cancer usually is not warranted. Because the disease is often multifocal and because colposcopy of the vagina and vulva are more difficult than cervical colposcopy, such patients should be evaluated by an expert colposcopist to confirm that there is no disease that is more advanced. After such an evaluation, patients with low-grade disease may be followed carefully with colposcopy and cytology. High-grade lesions should be treated. The most effective therapeutic modality for this treatment is the carbon dioxide laser. The laser can eradicate the disease with excellent precision while preserving the adjacent tissue. Loop electrosurgical excision is effective, but depth control is more difficult, and proper depth control is crucial to avoid scarring in deep excision. Unless invasive cancer has been ruled out, it is essential that therapy be by excision rather than ablation, so that the pathologist can evaluate the entire specimen.

Summary

The evaluation of women with abnormal Pap smears should follow a careful, stepwise approach. By using the protocols outlined above, significant disease can be recognized and treated and unnecessary treatment can be avoided.

Finally, the beginning colposcopist should always continue to obtain consultation from more experienced colleagues whenever difficult or unusual cases present themselves.

References and Selected Readings

1. Cartier R: *Practical Colposcopy,* 2d ed. New York: Fisher, 1984.
2. Coppleson M, Pixley E, Reid B: *Colposcopy: A Scientific and Practical Approach to the Cervix, Vagina, and Vulva in Health and Disease,* 3d ed. Springfield, IL: Charles C Thomas, 1986.
3. Follen MM, Levine RU, Carillo E, et al: Colposcopic correlates of cervical papillomavirus infection. *Am J Obstet Gynecol* 157:809–814, 1987.
4. Giuntoli RL, Atkinson BF, Ernst CS, et al: *Atkinson's Correlative Atlas of Colposcopy, Cytology, and Histopathology.* Philadelphia: JB Lippincott, 1987.
5. Kolstad P, Stafl A: *Atlas of Colposcopy,* 3d ed. Baltimore: University Park Press, 1982.
6. Spitzer M, Krumholz BA, Seltzer VL: The multicentric nature of disease related to human papillomavirus infection of the female lower genital tract. *Obstet Gynecol* 73:303–307, 1989.
7. Spitzer M, Krumholz BA: Human papillomavirus related diseases in the female. *Urol Clin North Am* 19:71–82, 1992.
8. Spitzer M, Chernys AE, Seltzer VL: The outpatient use of large loop excision of the transformation zone in an inner-city population. *Obstet Gynecol* 82:731–735, 1993.
9. Spitzer M, Krumholz BA: Intraepithelial neoplasms of the lower genital tract, in Jacobs AJ, Gast M, (eds): *Practical Gynecology: A Clinical Manual.* Connecticut: Appleton & Lange, 1994, pp 135–147.

36 Endometrial Sampling and Hysteroscopy as Office Procedures

Mark Spitzer

CYTOLOGIC SCREENING DEVICES
HISTOLOGIC SAMPLING
HYSTEROSCOPY

The need for a safe, accurate, and simple method of sampling the endometrium has become increasingly important. Financial constraints, patient demands, and advances in technology have all pushed endometrial sampling from a procedure that usually was performed in the hospital to one now commonly performed in the office. Much of the literature regarding office endometrial sampling focuses on the ability of this technique to screen and accurately detect endometrial hyperplasia and carcinoma. However, there are many other indications for endometrial sampling in the office. These include evaluation of infertility, menstrual disorders, cytology suggesting endometrial pathology, follow-up of patients receiving hormonal therapy, and the evaluation of postmenopausal and perimenopausal bleeding.

The ideal technique for endometrial sampling should be safe and easy to use. It should be well tolerated by the patient, preferably with either local anesthesia or no anesthetic at all. It should have minimal limitations on its use and should provide a diagnostic specimen in the vast majority of cases.

The most common indication for office endometrial sampling is to screen for or to diagnose endometrial carcinoma or hyperplasia. The gold standard for the diagnosis of these lesions has always been a dilatation and curettage (D&C) done in the operating room under general anesthesia. However, the sensitivity and specificity of a D&C are difficult to assess without comparing the results to the histology in a subsequent hysterectomy specimen. In one such study, endometrial lesions were missed in 10 percent of preoperative D&Cs. In some instances a curettage will sample less than half of the endometrial cavity. Nevertheless, the D&C is the standard to which the endometrial biopsy must be compared.

Two of the basic indications for endometrial sampling are screening for endometrial carcinoma or hyperplasia and for the diagnosis of other endometrial pathology. Different devices have been developed for each indication and must be considered separately.

Cytologic Screening Devices

The simplest screening device for endometrial carcinoma is the Pap smear. However, while the Pap smear is a relatively sensitive screen for early cervical cancer, it detects endometrial cancer in only 25 to 67 percent of women in whom the disease is present and detects endometrial hyperplasia in as few as 20 percent of women in whom the disease is present. Therefore, as many as 75 percent of women with endometrial cancer will have completely normal Pap smears, and the presence of a normal Pap smear is obviously not sufficient evaluation to rule out endometrial cancer in a woman with abnormal bleeding.

Other devices that have been used for cytologic screening of endometrial cancer include the Endocyte, Accurette, and the Mi-Mark sampler. These also are less than ideal. The Endocyte and Accurette devices are inserted into the endometrial cavity through a protective sleeve, which is then partially retracted. The specimen is collected and then withdrawn through the sleeve. With the Mi-Mark sampler, a plastic helix is inserted into the endometrial cavity and then withdrawn.

While cytologic devices are easy to use, inexpensive, and cause minimal discomfort to the patient, their effective use is dependent on the availability of cytologists with expertise in evaluating endometrial cytologic samples. They tend to underdiagnose hyperplasia, usually by about 20 percent. Furthermore, endometrial polyps, which can be a significant cause of abnormal bleeding, usually go undetected. Finally, the utility of screening for endometrial cancer in the absence of irregular bleeding has been questioned. Because of their limitations in diagnosing endometrial pathology other than carcinoma, cytologic devices are not ideal tools in such diagnosis.

Histologic Sampling

Histologic sampling of the endometrial lining is more accurate than is cytology in detecting endometrial hyperplasia, uterine polyps, and other endometrial pathology, and may also be therapeutic in some instances. Newer devices have greatly reduced the discomfort associated with the procedure and have increased patient acceptance.

Most descriptions of office D&Cs include the use of paracervical blocks, analgesics, and tranquilizers when deemed appropriate. Although the instrumentation and technique of office D&C is similar to a D&C done in the operating room, patient discomfort may limit one's ability to do an adequate curettage. Therefore, the vast majority of office endometrial sampling does not use this technique.

The earliest endometrial sampling tools were reusable stainless steel curettes. The Novak and Randell curettes are prototypes of this instrument. These instruments are 3- to 4-mm tubes with an opening near the distal end and an attachment for a suction apparatus at the proximal end. The Novak curette uses a syringe to provide suction and has a saw-tooth arrangement at the distal opening. This was a source of patient discomfort and the syringe was inconvenient to use. The Vabra aspirator uses a rigid plastic tube instead of stainless steel and a suction pump rather than a syringe. The Vakutage uses a preevacuated glass collection bottle instead of the suction pump and therefore is entirely self-contained.

All of these techniques obtain adequate tissue for histologic diagnosis in more than 90 percent of cases. Their diagnostic accuracy is greater than 95 percent in detecting endometrial carcinoma and 90 percent in detecting degrees of endometrial hyperplasia compared with D&C. They also are able to detect polyps in more than 75 percent of cases. Disadvantages include the need to use a tenaculum to stabilize the cervix so that the instrument can be passed through the cervical canal, failed procedures when cervical stenosis is encountered, and some degree of patient discomfort necessitating analgesia or paracervical block in certain patients.

The newest and most commonly used endometrial sampling devices are the Pipelle and the Z-sampler. These flexible polypropylene sheaths are approximately 3 mm in diameter with a 2.4-mm perforation near their distal end. Within the cannula is an internal piston that creates the suction necessary to sample the endometrial cavity. The advantages of the Pipelle are that it can pass through most endocervical canals without dilatation or the use of a tenaculum and that paracervical block and analgesia are not needed, since there is less discomfort associated with its use than with the rigid devices. Also, studies have shown that the Pipelle obtains more tissue than the Vabra. Finally, the Pipelle is more convenient to use and costs less than the Vabra.

The indications for endometrial biopsy were mentioned briefly above and will be covered in detail in another chapter on menstrual abnormalities.

Endometrial biopsy should not be done in an office setting when the patient has severe clotting disorders. Salpingitis, endometritis, and acute PID may be exacerbated by endometrial biopsy. Relative contraindications or limitations to endometrial biopsy include cervical stenosis and extreme anteflexion or retroflexion of the uterus. Also, in a patient who is bleeding heavily, it may be difficult to obtain an adeaquate endometrial sample because the Pipelle will fill with blood rather than endometrial curettings. Finally, in a patient with a large fibroid uterus, the size of the cavity or the presence of submucous myomas may impede one's ability to sample the cavity adequately.

The technique for endometrial biopsy or cytologic aspiration is essentially the same regardless of which sampling device is used. Informed consent should be obtained prior to the procedure. A prostaglandin inhibitor such as ibuprofen may be given prior to the procedure; however, when using a device such as the Pipelle this usually is not necessary. It is also usually not necessary to use a paracervical block. The patient is placed on the examination table in the dorsal lithotomy position. A recent pap smear report should be available. If it is not, one should be performed. A bimanual examination is done to assess the uterine size, position, and axis. A bivalve speculum is inserted. The cervix is cleaned using an antiseptic solution. The anterior lip of the cervix is grasped with a single-tooth tenaculum for stabilization. This is necessary when using the more rigid sampling devices, although it may not be necessary when using the more flexible Pipelle. Injecting 1 ml of 1% lidocaine into the anterior lip of the cervix may reduce the discomfort associated with this part of the procedure. If an endocervical curettage is planned, it is done at this point. A Kervorkian curette is often used to sample the endocervix.

The endometrial sampling is then performed. The sampling device is inserted through the endocervical canal and into the uterus. Although the patient may feel a cramping sensation when the instrument passes through the internal os, it usually is not necessary to dilate the cervix when using the Pipelle. It is also usually not necessary to sound the uterus prior to biopsy because most of the newer sampling devices are marked along their length so that they may also function as uterine sounds. If the cervix is stenotic and needs to be dilated, a paracervical block may be used. The block is done by injecting 2 to 3 ml of 1% lidocaine without epinephrine in three to four sites just below the mucosa at the junction of the uterine reflection and the posterior vaginal vault. The sampling instrument is then passed all the way to the fundus and suction is applied. When using the Pipelle, this is done by withdrawing the piston to its full length. The suction device is then rotated inside the endometrial cavity while it is slowly withdrawn. It usually is not necessary to repeat the procedure. If the sample seems inadequate, the procedure may be repeated; however, the second sample is usually not as good as the first.

The lower abdominal cramps experienced during the procedure usually pass within several minutes. If pain persists after a few minutes, prostaglandin inhibitors may be given. The patient should be instructed not to engage in intercourse for several days—at least as long as any bleeding persists. Infection or perforation associated with office endometrial biopsy is rare; however, the patient should report any symptoms of fever, chills, increasing pain, significant bleeding, or other problems to the physician.

Hysteroscopy

Hysteroscopy allows direct visualization of the endometrial cavity, and has been used for the evaluation and treatment of endometrial lesions for many years. Recently, improved technology including fiberoptics has allowed hysteroscopy to move from the operating room to the office. Because hysteroscopy is frequently associated with some degree of patient discomfort, its use in the office probably should be restricted to physicians who have already gained sufficient experience in the operating room. The experienced hysteroscopist can complete a diagnostic hysteroscopy using CO_2 gas in less than 10 min.

Some indications for office hysteroscopy include abnormal uterine bleeding, postmenopausal bleeding, suspected leiomyomata with bleeding, bleeding in patients who have IUDs, the evaluation of infertility with bleeding, patients in whom uterine anomalies may be suspected, patients with suspected endometrial polyps, and women who have abnormal uterine bleeding and a negative D&C, where hysteroscopy may relieve anxiety for both the patient and physician.

The most commonly used and most versatile hysteroscope for office use is a rigid, panoramic hysteroscope with a 30-degree viewing angle and a sheath measuring 3 to 5 mm in diameter. The procedure described here assumes the use of this instrument. The light source is a 100- to 300-watt halogen or xenon lamp. Office hysteroscopy usually uses CO_2 gas as a distention medium. Low molecular weight distention media such as lactated Ringer's solution are far too messy for office use because they require such large volumes of fluid. High molecular weight distention media such as Dextran 70 require significantly less volume; however, they are also messy and difficult to use in an office setting. The flow rate for CO_2 should not exceed 100 ml per min, and the pressure should remain below 100 mmHg. The total volume of CO_2 used in a patient with patent fallopian tubes should be below 600 to 700 ml CO_2. The total volume of Dextran 70 needed is rarely more than 100 ml, and should never be more than 300 ml because of the risk of pulmonary edema and blood dyscrasia.

Prior to hysteroscopy, the patient should be assessed as to her ability to cooperate during the procedure. A pregnancy test and cervical cultures for gonorrhea and Chlamydia should be checked. Premedication with a prostaglandin inhibitor 30 min prior to the procedure is helpful. The procedure is done with the patient in the dorsal lithotomy position. A paracervical block is administered. The cervix is dilated if necessary, and the hysteroscope inserted into the cervical canal. The flow of the distention medium is started and the hysteroscope is advanced slowly, allowing the distention medium to dilate the internal os.

When the hysteroscope enters the uterus, the cavity should be inspected to assess its general shape, the presence of any foreign bodies, synechiae, polyps, myomas, or septa. The appearance of the endometrium should also be checked, looking for irregularities suggestive of hyperplasia or cancer. The anterior and posterior walls of the uterus can be inspected by rotating the hysteroscope clockwise and counterclockwise. The left and right cornua and tubal ostia are examined by rotating the hysteroscope into the proper position at the fundus. If no lesions are seen, the hysteroscope is slowly removed so that the cavity can be reexamined on the way out; then the endometrium is sampled, using an endometrial sampling device as described earlier. If a lesion is seen, it can sometimes be removed through the hysteroscope; however, operative hysteroscopy requires a larger diameter hysteroscope, operative instruments, and possibly anesthesia. It may be beyond the skill level of many office practitioners. Postoperatively, the patient is given a prostaglandin inhibitor for any mild cramps that may follow the procedure and is told to avoid intercourse for several days—at least until any bleeding stops. She should call the physician if she experiences any fever, severe pain, heavy bleeding, or other problems. Potential complications of operative hysteroscopy are the same as those for D&C. They include bleeding, infection, and perforation. However, these complications are rare.

References and Selected Readings

1. Apgor BS, Dewitt D: Diagnostic hysteroscopy. *Am Fam Physician* 46:19S–36S, 1992.
2. Brown FH, Kammeyer SE: Office gynecologic procedures. *Primary Care* 13:493–511, 1986.
3. Chambers JT, Chambers SK: Endometrial sampling: When? Where? Why? With what? *Clin Obstet Gynecol* 35:28–39, 1992.
4. Gimpelson RJ: Office hysteroscopy. *Clin Obstet Gynecol* 35:270–281, 1992.
5. Goldchmit R, Katz Z, Blickstein I, et al: The accuracy of endometrial sampling with and without sonographic measurement of endometrial thickness. *Obstet Gynecol* 82:727–730, 1993.

37 Office Procedures for Infertility Patients

Edward H. Illions
Robert J. Thompson

Much of the basic infertility evaluation can be performed with simple office tests and procedures. The clinician should have a good understanding of the basic tests needed to evaluate ovulatory dysfunction, abnormal sperm-mucus interactions, intrauterine pathology, and tubal and peritoneal disease.

Basal Body Temperature Graph

Four basic office tests can be utilized to evaluate ovulation. A basal body temperature graph is the initial screening test for ovulatory dysfunction. Some controversy exists regarding the interpretation of this test; however, a sustained luteal temperature elevation is indicative of ovulation. The test is not useful in determining the quality of ovulation. The couple should be advised to initiate basal body temperature charts on the first day of a menstrual cycle. The patient should record her temperature each morning before consuming any liquids or foods and prior to any physical activity. In fact, it is helpful if patients keep their basal body thermometer by the bedside as a reminder to record their temperature at the same time every morning. The temperature will typically rise as much as 0.5°F within one to three days after ovulation and remain elevated for the duration of the luteal phase. Typical luteal phase elevation in primates is 14 days plus or minus 2 days. A biphasic elevation is indicative of ovulation in most patients, whereas an adequate luteal phase is demonstrated when the temperature rise persists for at least 11 or more days. There is some variation in the patient population as 10 percent of ovulatory patients will have a monophasic basal body temperature chart.

Urinary LH Kits

Many commercially available kits exist on the market to measure urinary LH elevations. Since the onset of the LH surge occurs 32 to 36 h prior to ovulation, these tests enjoy great clinical utility in: 1. timing coitus; 2. artificial insemination; 3. scheduling postcoital tests; 4. scheduling endometrial biopsies; and 5. performing embryo transfers of frozen-thawed embryos. The patient should be instructed to start checking the urine on day 10 or 11 of her cycle. The scheduling of these tests varies during the day, depending on the kit utilized; however, a late-afternoon or early-evening measurement usually is quite accurate. OvuSTICK and OvuQUICK utilize a control surge guide on day 1 or daily, respectively, increasing the accuracy of the tests. A significant LH surge is noted when the daily test turns bluer than the control surge guide. This indicates the onset of the LH surge as measured by levels in the urine greater than 40mIU/ml, with ovulation occurring the following day. Although ovulation occurs 32 to 36 h from the actual onset of the surge, LH kits detect urinary LH levels in their rising phase; therefore, ovulation occurs approximately 12 to 24 h after detection (if used on a daily basis).

Transvaginal Sonography

Transvaginal sonography of the female pelvis affords the physician great accuracy when evaluating folliculogenesis and predicting ovulation. Daily scanning may commence on day 12 of a normal cycle or a single scan can be performed one day after the LH surge. Follicular size typically is measured in at least two diameters, with the periovulatory follicles measuring in excess of 18 mm. The patient should be positioned in stirrups at the end of the exam table. A high-resolution vaginal probe is covered with a sterile condom and gel is applied to enhance resolution and visualization of pelvic structures. Transvaginal sonography also allows for the determination of the luteinized unruptured follicle (LUF) and is a necessity in ovulation induction cycles.

Endometrial Biopsy

The endometrial biopsy is currently the gold standard for diagnosis of luteal phase defects. The couple should utilize barrier contraception during this cycle or have a sensitive quantitative beta HCG performed one day prior to the endometrial sampling. The biopsy should be performed between the 10th and 12th postovulatory day as determined by urinary LH kits. After appropriate counseling, the patient should be placed in stirrups at the end of the exam table. A pelvic exam is necessary to ascertain uterine position. A description of the technical aspects of office endometrial sampling is found in Chap. 36. The histologic specimen should correlate with the cycle day (+/−2 days). Failure to do so may indicate the presence of a luteal phase defect.

Cervical Factor Testing

The postcoital test and in vitro sperm-mucus penetration assays are essential parts of the basic infertility evaluation. Postcoital tests (Sims-Huhner Test) are performed the morning after an LH surge. The couple should be instructed either to have intercourse the night before the test or at least 4 h prior to the postcoital test.

After placing the patient on the exam table, a speculum is inserted to allow visualization of the cervix. An attempt is made to quantitate both the amount and viscosity of the cervical mucus as this is a direct reflection of estrogen effect on the cervix. Cervical mucus is obtained from the external os utilizing an 18-gauge angiocath on a 1-ml tuberculin syringe. Recovery of cervical mucus in the syringe allows for accurate determinations of its amount. Cervical mucus elasticity (spinnbarkeit) may be determined by slowly moving the syringe away from the external os. Periovulatory cervical mucus should allow for at least 8 to 10 cm of spinnbarkeit. Cervical mucus is placed on two glass slides. A cover slip is placed over one of the specimens; the other is allowed to air-dry. The air-dried specimen is evaluated for the presence of ferning indicative of an adequate estrogen effect on cervical mucus. The other slide is microscopically analyzed for the presence and number of motile sperm per high-power field. Although much controversy exists as to normal threshold values, visualization of more than five motile sperm per high-power field is reassuring.

Slides with absent sperm should alert the physician to possible problems with coital technique, whereas the presence of shaking and immobilized sperm may indicate immunologic disorders. Periovulatory cervical mucus is relatively acellular; therefore, the presence of many leukocytes or red blood cells (RBC) may indicate a cervicitis.

In vitro sperm-mucus penetration tests are clinically useful in patients with normal semen analyses and poor postcoital test results in the presence of good cervical mucus. The timing of this test is identical to that of the postcoital test; however, the couple is instructed to refrain from intercourse for approximately 48 to 72 h prior to predicted ovulation. The couple is seen in the office 1 day after the LH surge, at which time a semen specimen is obtained. A cervical mucus specimen is similarly obtained, as previously described, and is then allowed to fill a column (maximum capacity 0.2 ml cervical mucus) in a commercially available test kit. A second column on the same slide is filled with donor cervical mucus (commonly bovine mucus). The husband's semen specimen is placed in wells at the end of each column, and mucus penetration by the sperm is measured after 30 min. Alternatively, the husband's sperm-mucus interaction may be compared against the results of a penetration assay utilizing sperm from a known fertile donor (control). Sperm penetration beyond 30 mm is considered reassuring. Values below 20 mm suggest abnormal sperm-mucus interaction.

Tubal and Peritoneal Factors

Hysterosalpingogram (HSG)

Hysterosalpingography is a fluoroscopic examination which allows assessment of the uterine cavity and tubal patency. An HSG should be performed in the midproliferative phase of the patient's cycle immediately after cessation of her menses. Contraindications to performing an HSG include dye allergy, active pelvic infection, or a past medical history of pelvic inflammatory disease. Patients with a prior history of genital infections may undergo an HSG if recent WBC, erythrocyte sedimentation rate (ESR), and cervical cultures for GC and Chlamydia are normal. Antibiotic prophylaxis may be indicated in these patients to prevent the 1 to 3 percent incidence of HSG-associated infections. No premedication is required, and the patient is positioned on the exam table in stirrups. A pelvic exam is useful to ascertain uterine position; then a speculum is placed intravaginally. A tenaculum is applied to the anterior cervical lip to stabilize the uterus during the exam. An intrauterine catheter is placed in the lower segment to allow injection of radioopaque dye with concomitant image intensification fluoroscopy. Typically only 2 to 3 ml of dye is necessary to fill the uterine cavity, and a slow injection technique aids in demonstrating intrauterine pathology. Fallopian tubes are then assessed for patency, and a final post-injection film is obtained to document free intraperitoneal spillage of dye. Most HSG studies can be completed with as little as 10 to 12 ml of contrast material. Failure to visualize either tube may indicate tubal spasm and is usually treated with intravenous administration of 1 mg of glucagon followed by reinjection of the radioopaque dye. Post-glucagon visualization of the fallopian tubes confirms a diagnosis of tubal spasm. Most contrast media are water-based and allow for better mucosal detail than the oil-based dyes previously used. Oil-based dyes, in addition, have been implicated in granuloma formation and oil embolization. Studies have suggested increased pregnancy rates after oil contrast HSGs; however, this has not been confirmed.

Office Hysteroscopy

Hysteroscopic evaluation of the uterine cavity is indicated in patients with prior abnormal HSGs as well as in DES-exposed patients. Carbon dioxide (CO_2) is the usual distension medium and allows for good visibility during these diagnostic procedures. The patient is examined during the midproliferative phase of her cycle. The technical aspects of office hysteroscopy are discussed in Chap. 36. Office CO_2 hysteroscopy allows for a diagnosis of intrauterine congenital anomalies, polyps, myomas, and intrauterine synechiae while avoiding the expense of an operating room and anesthesia. Operative hysteroscopy for correction of these defects is best performed in an operating room with adequate anesthesia available.

Endocrine Testing

Two endocrine tests may be easily performed by the clinician in the office and allow assessment of the hypothalamic-pituitary-ovarian axis.

Clomid Citrate Challenge Test (CCCT)

This test is an indirect measure of ovarian reserve. It is easily performed in the office and may predict a patient's response to ovulation induction as well as fertilization rates in upcoming IVF cycles. The patient is instructed to obtain an FSH, LH and estradiol level on day 3 of her next cycle. This test is then repeated on day 10 of the cycle after receiving Clomid 100 mg from days 5 to 9 of that same cycle. Gonadotropin levels are increased transiently after Clomid administration; however, rising estradiol levels as well as elevations in other gonadal peptides (inhibin) have a negative feedback effect on the pituitary to prevent FSH elevations by day 10. Normal values for this test vary with the gonadotropin reference preparation utilized; however, FSH values below 25 mIU/ml are considered normal in most centers.

GnRH Stimulation Test

Administration of a small intravenous dose of synthetic gonadotropin releasing hormone (GnRH) will allow assessment of the status of gonadotropin secretion by the pituitary gland. This test has great clinical utility in the diagnostic evaluation of patients with hypothalamic amenorrhea and those with known pituitary disorders. It is also of great diagnostic value when evaluating pubertal disorders in children. Patients should be instructed to be NPO after midnight, and they should be kept at bed rest during the examination. Patients are given an intravenous dose of 100 μg of GnRH over a 30-s period. Baseline determinations of FSH and LH as well as appropriately timed serial determinations are obtained. Although individual responses may vary, the usual LH and FSH peaks occur 30 and 45 min, respectively, after GnRH injection. Failure to achieve these levels may indicate pituitary dysfunction or a complete lack of GnRH priming by the hypothalamus.

Summary

The simple office tests and procedures reviewed in this chapter will assist in the accurate assessment of ovulatory status, sperm-mucus interaction, and the tubal and peritoneal factors involved in infertility. Office endocrine testing may aid in uncovering hypothalamic or pituitary dysfunction.

References and Selected Readings

1. Seibel MM: Workup of the infertile couple, in Seibel MM (ed): *Infertility: A Comprehensive Text.* East Norwalk: Appleton & Lange, 1990, pp 1–21.
2. Shane JM: Evaluation and treatment of infertility. *CIBA Clinical Symposia* 45:1–33, 1993.

38 Cystourethroscopy and Urodynamics

Jeffrey L. Cornella
Henry A. Thiede

Cystourethroscopy

Since Philipp Bozzini developed the first instrument to inspect the bladder in 1806, endoscopy has been a cornerstone of urinary tract assessment. Today, endoscopic visualization allows examination of the lower and upper urinary tracts. Cystoscopic assessment of subtle lesions requires a significant amount of experience and is beyond the scope of this section. The purpose of this discussion will be to instruct in basic cystourethroscopic technique and to familiarize the office practitioner with common terms and findings, since urogynecologic problems are such a frequent and important problem for women and one for which they are often evaluated in the primary office setting with the studies described below.

Dynamic Urethroscopy

Dynamic urethroscopy refers to visualization of the urethra during maneuvers to reproduce symptoms. Robertson has emphasized the benefit of assessment during bladder filling and stressful maneuvers in making accurate diagnoses.[2] Robertson describes the use of a zero-degree 24 French direct endoscope. Carbon dioxide or water can be used for distention with careful visualization of the urethra on initial insertion. During visualization of the urethrovesical junction, the patient is asked to cough, execute a Valsalva maneuver, and contract the pelvic floor musculature. The response of the junction is noted, including ''telescoping'' or inappropriate opening and descent of the junction with coughing. Normally the endoscopist will see gradual closure of the junction and vesical neck with bladder filling and increased muscular tone. This correlates with increased EMG activity (Fig. 38-1). The pink mucosa is examined for erythema, atrophy, and the ostia of urethral diverticula. A dysfunctional urethrovesical junction and bladder neck may be noted in the patient who has had multiple operations or in those who have experienced neurologic damage of the pelvic plexus. The junction may have a scarified appearance or an open flaccid appearance at rest.

The normal urethra may balloon during visualization if the patient experiences a detrusor contraction. This gives a sharp circular appearance to the lumen.

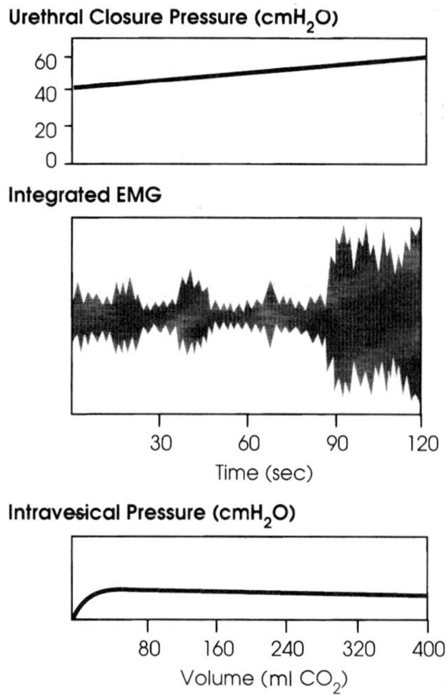

Figure 38-1. In this normal individual, urethral closure pressure and pelvic floor EMG activity gradually increase with bladder filling as intravesical pressure remains stable. [Adapted with permission of the editor, *Urogynecology and Urodynamics.* Ostergard DR, Bent AE (eds). Williams and Wilkins.]

Cystoscopy

Cystoscopy is generally performed only after acute cystitis or significant bacteriuria has been excluded. Anesthetic jelly is placed into the urethra and left in place for 5 to 10 min, but is not essential in most patients. A cystoscope (8 to 24F available) is inserted after removal of the obturator, followed by systematic bladder inspection. A 70-degree lens is used to examine the bladder mucosa throughout 360 degrees, noting vascularity, underlying muscular patterns, and trigonal appearance.

The smooth wall of the bladder may be affected by changes in the underlying musculature. Hypertrophy results in muscle bundles creating an impression beneath the mucosa resembling a cord or trabeculation. There may be an interwoven pattern of ridges. Pockets may form between the trabeculations called cellules. If cellules penetrate the underlying musculature completely they form sacculations called diverticula.

The mucosa of the bladder may be inflamed secondary to infection. Often a similar appearance is noted in carcinoma in situ and may require repeat cystoscopy after antibiotic therapy to confirm resolution of the abnormal appearance. The vascularity of the bladder may show submucosal homorrhages or glomerulations suggesting cystitis or the possibility of mild interstitial cystitis. Classic Hunner's ulcers may be seen, with cracks in the mucous membrane and stellate scarring in more advanced cases.

Examination of the trigone notes the position of the ureteral orifices, efflux of urine, the absence of ureteroceles, and the underlying trigonal mucosal appearance, which often varies from the appearance of the other mucosal areas. The bladder is examined at various stages of filling. In the half-filled state, the configuration of the ureteral orifices are noted. Interstitial cystitis may require filling to capacity or hydrodistention for diagnosis.

Urodynamic Testing

Pertinent considerations regarding urodynamics in the office setting will be discussed here. The reader is referred to the chapter on urogynecology for indications for urodynamic testing and its significance and for instruction on methods of simple office filling of the bladder. The goal of urodynamic testing is to reproduce urologic symptoms during physiologic monitoring of bladder emptying and storage. Only in this manner can conclusions be reached that have clinical implications for patient treatment.

Uroflowmetry

Flowmetry must also reproduce the normal voiding experience of the patient. If the flow rate and pattern are normal, it is unlikely that a significant emptying abnormality exists.[9] Peak flow rates and flow times depend on the volume voided. It is important that the patient has at least 150 ml within the bladder to aid interpretation, because it is unclear whether lesser volumes can be interpreted. Volume-rate nomograms aid this interpretation. Flow patterns can suggest obstruction, decreased contractility, or decreased outlet resistance. Maximum flow rates in females are 20 to 25 ml/s, as described in the literature. Measured parameters include peak flow rate, average flow rate, time to peak flow, voiding time, flow time, residual urine determination, and voided volume. Urethral relaxation is noted to precede detrusor contraction by one to two seconds (Fig. 38-2). Flow rates can vary in an individual from one episode to another, especially at different starting volumes. It is also important that the patient assume the sitting position, and she should be so instructed.

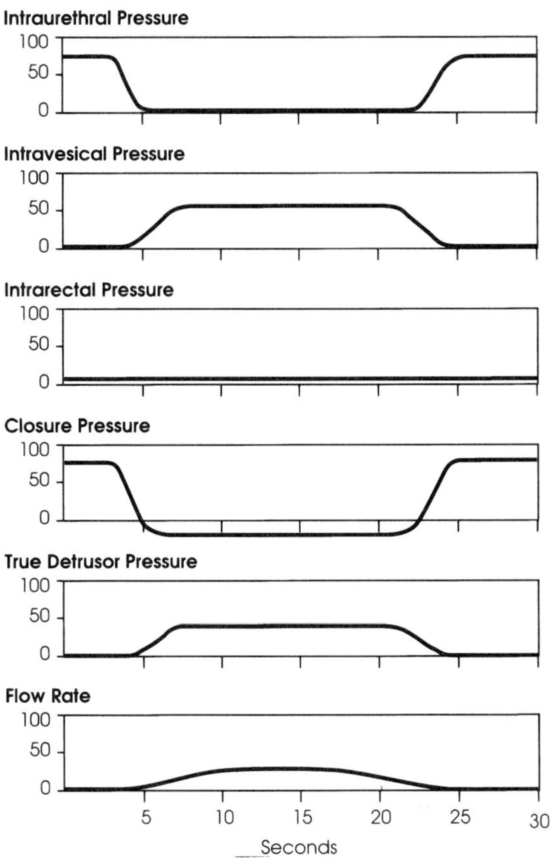

Figure 38-2. In this normal female, urethral relaxation precedes vesical contraction. [Adapted with permission of the editor, *Urogynecology and Urodynamics.* Ostergard DR, Bent AE (eds). Williams and Wilkins.]

Cystometry

Cystometry is utilized to assess bladder sensation, capacity, activity, and compliance. Filling cystometry refers to changes in bladder pressure during filling. The normal bladder shows little pressure change during most physiologic filling. The qualitative classification of bladder abnormalities is not significantly different, regardless of whether carbon dioxide or water is used as the distending medium.[9] There are quantitative differences noted between the two media in assessing sensation of the bladder. Quantitative capacities are reduced when gas is used. Fluid is administered at body or room temperature via a small catheter and at a constant rate to reduce artifact. Medium-fill cystometry refers to a filling rate of 80 to 100 ml/min. The bladder capacity of the average female is 350 to 500 ml of fluid.

Filling cystometry thus demonstrates a low pressure plateau in the normal state, which is referred to as the tonus limb of the cystometrogram. Artifacts can be created by filling the bladder too quickly, which can result in a spurious recording not reflective of the normal physiologic state. This affects the viscoelastic properties of the bladder and raises the pressure early in the cystometrogram. This is followed by the flat tonus limb of the pressure curve, but at a higher artifactual pressure.

Communication between the technician and the patient is essential in the interpretation of the tracing. A volitional contraction may be identical in appearance to a nonvolitional contraction the patient is unable to inhibit. It is only with honest communication that the tracing can be interpreted during reproduction of symptoms. First sensation of filling, fullness, and the feeling of strong desire to void (imminent micturition) are recorded. Increases in intravesical pressure may be reflective of detrusor contractions or increased muscular wall tension. The patient is asked to describe any concomitant sensations to aid in interpretation and diagnosis. The normal rise in bladder pressure during filling is less than 6 to 10 cmH_2O. The final phase of bladder filling occurs when the elastic properties of the wall have reached their limit.[9] In order for this fully to have meaning, the bladder must be filled at a standardized rate. The patient should be able to inhibit contractions at this volume (Fig. 38-3). Uninhibited spontaneous contractions at any pressure level are significant if symptoms are reproduced (Fig. 38-4). Some studies have elicited greater numbers of high-threshold contractions (>15 cmH_2O) when diuresis cystometry is utilized (physiologic filling combined with a diuretic).[5] Often, provocative maneuvers such as heel bouncing, testing in the semistanding position, and coughing are used to stimulate the appearance of symptomatic bladder instability or uninhibited detrusor contractions (Fig. 38-5). A small uninhibited phasic rise in true detrusor pressure accompanied by urgency or incontinence as a reproduction of symptoms suggests bladder instability. This may or may not be preceded by a decrease in urethral closure pressure.

Abnormalities are suggested by a reduced bladder capacity in the presence of increased pressure, or an increased bladder capacity in the presence of extremely low pressures. The latter may suggest a flaccid bladder or a sensory neuropathic condition. The former may suggest an inflammatory condition or severe bladder instability.

The second portion of cystometry is voiding cystometry. Care should be taken to avoid compromise of pressure-flow studies by the size of the intravesical catheter. A smaller catheter can be placed for this portion of the study (<8F). The patient may or may not be able to generate a void at the end of filling. Stress or discomfort may result in central inhibition of the void. The measurement of true detrusor pressure at maximum flow is evaluated on the pressure flow study. This is helpful in determining outlet resistance and strength of detrusor contractions during a volitional void.

True detrusor pressure is determined by subtracting abdominal pressure measurements from bladder pressure measurements. The former are obtained from rectal or vaginal catheters. Urethral closure pressure is determined by subtracting bladder pressure from urethral pressure. This is best measured by a single small-lumen catheter with two sensors, 6 cm apart. When both transducers are placed within the

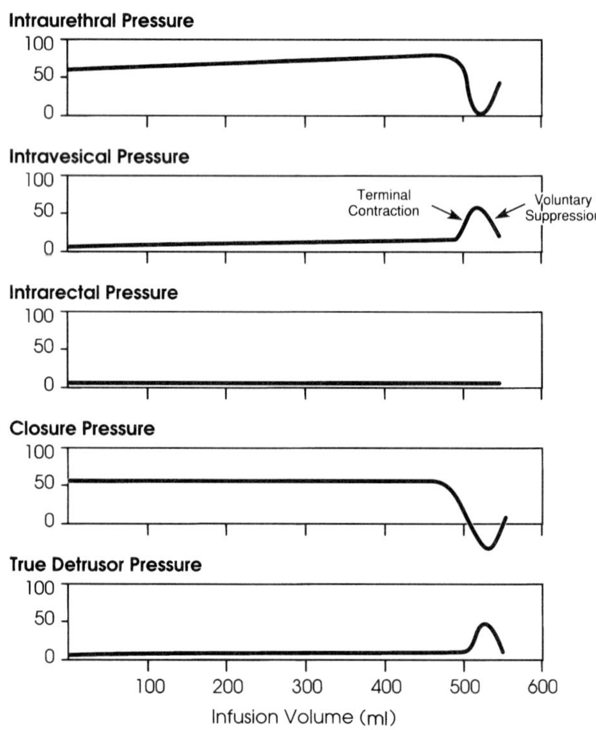

Figure 38-3. This normal female is able to inhibit the terminal contraction during cystometry. The intraabdominal pressure when subtracted from the intravesical pressure gives true detrusor pressure. The closure pressure is determined by subtracting intravesical pressure from intraurethral pressure. [Adapted with permission of the editor, *Urogynecology and Urodynamics.* Ostergard DR, Bent AE (eds). Williams and Wilkins.]

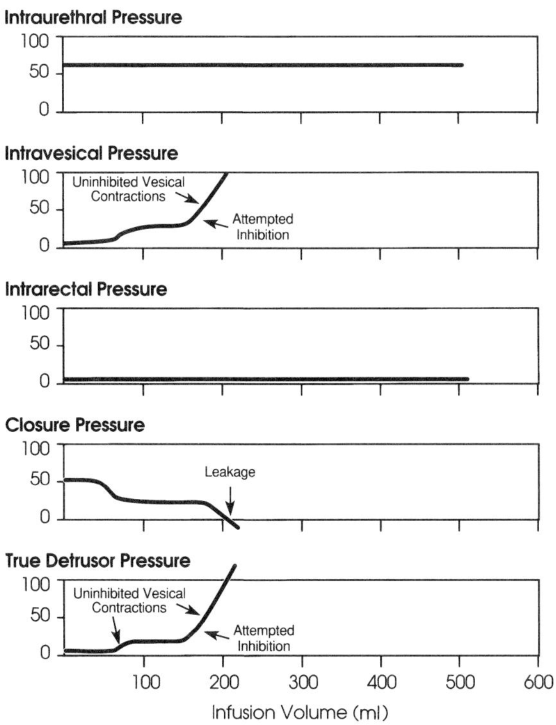

Figure 38-4. Uninhibitable bladder contractions at relatively low bladder volumes. A drop in urethral closure pressure precedes the detrusor contraction. [Adapted with permission of the editor, *Urogynecology and Urodynamics.* Ostergard DR, Bent AE (eds). Williams and Wilkins.]

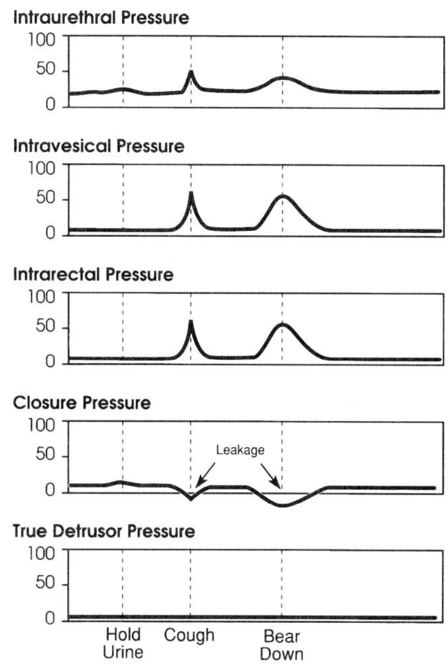

Figure 38-5. Dynamic evaluation of the urethral sphincter with negative closure pressure and resultant stress incontinence demonstrated on provocative coughing. [Adapted with permission of the editor, *Urogynecology and Urodynamics.* Ostergard DR, Bent AE (eds). Williams and Wilkins.]

bladder, coughing should result in equal pressure excursions on the graph. The catheter is then withdrawn at a constant rate (profilometer-controlled) of 1 mm/s, and the pressure differential is measured at rest and during coughing.

The EMG combines with the cystometrics to aid in diagnosis. In the normal patient, detrusor contraction is accompanied by coordinated relaxation of the urethral sphincter (Fig. 38-6). Some patients exhibit discoordination of this mechanism. As an example, patients with severe multiple sclerosis often have detrusor external sphincter dyssynergia as a component of their urologic picture. This discord between the external sphincter and the detrusor results from an uninhibited bladder contraction accompanied by an uninhibited urethral sphincter contraction. Increased EMG activity is inappropriately noted at the time of increased true detrusor pressure. Dyssynergia may result in increased intravesical pressure when sustained throughout the void (Fig. 38-7).

Urethral Profilometry

Urethral profilometry consists of static and dynamic urethral pressure profiles. The latter refers to pressure-transmission ratios (maximum urethral pressure divided by bladder pressure × 100). A discussion of pressure-transmission ratios and their meaning can be found in the chapter on urogynecology under surgical treatment of stress urinary incontinence. This discussion will be limited to resting or static urethral pressure profiles.

The urethral closure pressure is the urethral pressure that exceeds the bladder pressure. The normal value in the young female is 60 cmH_2O. Urethral

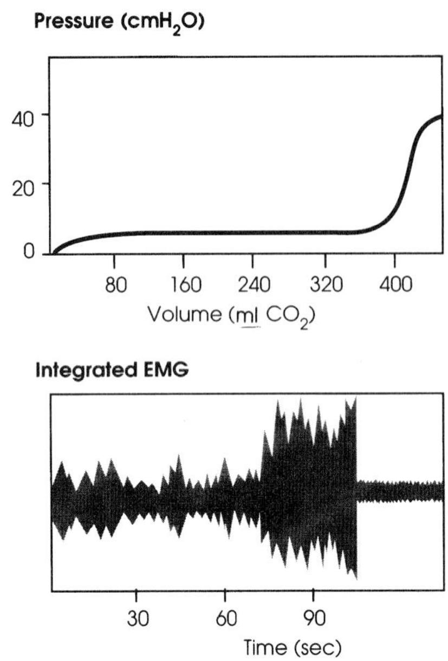

Figure 38-6. EMG activity during a normal cystometry. There is a gradual increase in activity due to increased sphincter tone during filling. Note quiescence of EMG activity coincident with bladder contraction. [Adapted with permission of the editor, *Urogynecology and Urodynamics.* Ostergard DR, Bent AE (eds). Williams and Wilkins.]

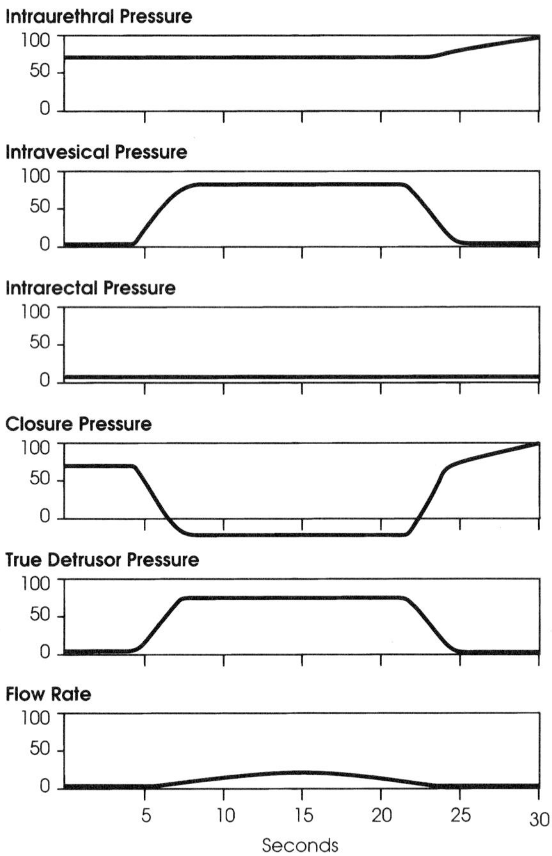

Figure 38-7. Obstruction on voiding is noted with increased intravesical pressure. This outlet obstruction may result from stenosis or if EMG activity shows an uninhibitable external sphincter contraction, from neurogenic dyssynergia. [Adapted with permission of the editor, *Urogynecology and Urodynamics.* Ostergard DR, Bent AE (eds). Williams and Wilkins.]

closure pressures decrease with age. Abnormally decreased urethral closure pressures are noted in stress incontinent patients. Pressures decrease in these patients with standing, filling of the bladder, and serial coughing.

Resting urethral pressure profiles are measured with a microtransducer catheter oriented to the three- or nine-o'clock position of the urethra (Fig. 38-8). Perfusion catheters also may be used, although some investigators would state that more artifacts are produced with perfusion measurement.

Many authors have studied the results of incontinence operations on resting closure pressures. The vast majority of the studies show no evidence of significant restoration of resting urethral pressure following retropubic urethropexy. The clinical utility of the study is low in females, and much overlap exists between continent and incontinent patients with given urethral closure pressures.

Some authors have suggested that low urethral closure pressures are predictive of increased risk of failure after retropubic urethropexy. Less than 20 cmH_2O was selected as the cut-off point in the definition of low urethral pressure by Sand.[3] He noted that in patients under 50, there was a 54 percent failure rate following Burch colposuspension in patients with low urethral pressures compared with an 18 percent failure rate in patients with >20 cmH_2O. Richardson performed Burch colposuspension in 29

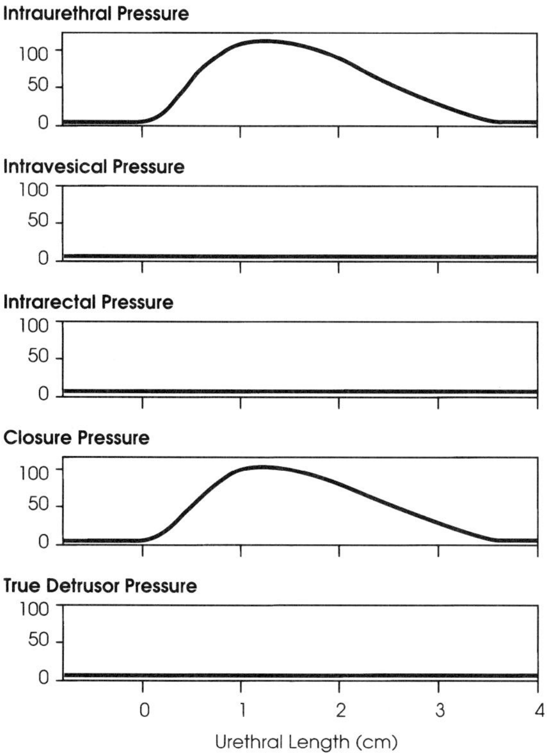

Figure 38-8. Urethral closure pressure tracing in the normal female. [Adapted with permission of the editor, *Urogynecology and Urodynamics.* Ostergard DR, Bent AE (eds). Williams and Wilkins.]

patients with low urethral pressures evaluated by preoperative and postoperative urodynamic testing. The success rate was 78 percent cured and 7 percent improved, with a 15 percent failure rate. Richardson noted that if urethral mobility is present, urethropexy is a reasonable alternative in low urethral pressure patients.[1]

Sand also reported on uninhibited urethral relaxation as a cause of incontinence.[4] Uninhibited urethral relaxation is a sudden drop in urethral pressure resulting in leakage in the absence of detrusor contraction or provocative maneuvers. Its existence as a pathologic entity is debated. Normal women on ambulatory testing have demonstrated urethral pressure variations throughout the day. Versi stated that urethral pressure variations greater than one-third the resting pressure fall outside the 99 percent confidence limit in studied patients and should be considered abnormal.[6]

Cystograms and Videocystourethrography

The static cystogram provides information about the bladder neck and urethra. This is especially helpful in the patient with a questionable dysfunctional or type III urethra. Contrast is placed within the bladder and the patient is radiographed in the standing, at-rest position. A type III urethra is suggested by a square, wide column of dye filling the upper urethra in the absence of a bladder contraction. Versi demonstrated that the prevalence of bladder neck incompetence (opening with coughing) was approximately 48 percent.[7] In a related study the incidence of open bladder neck at rest was 21 percent in patients presenting to a urodynamic clinic.[8]

Videocystourethrography combines pressure testing and fluoroscopy to assess bladder and urethral function. This can be extremely helpful in understanding complex pathologic conditions.

References and Suggested Readings

1. Richardson DA, et al: Surgical management of stress incontinence in patients with low urethral pressure. *Gynecol Obstet Invest* 31:106–109, 1991.
2. Robertson JR: Dynamic urethroscopy, in Ostergard DR, Bent AE: *Urogynecology and Urodynamics,* 3d ed. Philadelphia: Williams & Wilkins, 1991.
3. Sand PK, et al: The low pressure urethra as a factor in failed retropubic urethropexy. *Obstet Gynecol* 69:399–402, 1987.
4. Sand PK, et al: Uninhibited urethral relaxation: An unusual cause of incontinence. *Obstet Gynecol* 68:645–648, 1986.
5. van Venrooij GE, et al: Urodynamics and incontinence II: The diagnostic value of diuresis cystometry. *Int Urogynecol J* 1:191–195, 1990.
6. Versi E, Cardozo L: Urethral instability: Diagnosis based on variations of the maximum urethral pressure in normal climacteric women. *Neurourol Urodyn* 5:535–541, 1986.
7. Versi E, et al: Distal urethral compensatory mechanisms in women with an incompetent bladder neck who remain continent, and the effect of the menopause. *Neurourol Urodyn* 9:579–590, 1990.
8. Versi E: The significance of an open bladder neck in women. *Br J Urol* 68:42–43, 1991.
9. Wein AJ, et al: Office urodynamics. *Urol Clin North Am* 15:609–623, 1988.

Part V

Psychiatric and Psychosocial Issues and Societal Violence

39 Psychiatric and Psychosocial Issues in Primary Care for Women

Nada L. Stotland

It has been estimated that up to 50 percent of all patient visits regarding psychiatric illness are to primary care physicians.[58,63] The diagnosis and treatment of psychiatric illness or psychiatric complications of nonpsychiatric illness occupy a large portion of the primary care physician's time.[27] Nevertheless, there is a tendency among nonpsychiatric physicians to regard these problems as annoyances that drain time and energy from the "real" mission of care rather than as legitimate medical issues in their own right. This attitude is reinforced by the misperception that psychiatric symptoms are voluntary and manipulative and/or bizarre and frightening—neither deserving of nor responsive to primary care intervention.

Practitioners may fall back on assumptions about psychiatric conditions that they acquired in childhood or during their medical training. Most of these assumptions are not only incorrect but also deleterious to the understanding and care of the patient. Mental illness has been stigmatized for millennia; interestingly enough, it has been linked historically in women to reproductive functions and events. "Hysteria" is so termed because ancient Greek physicians believed that unexplained physical symptoms in women were caused by migrations of the uterus out of the pelvis to the afflicted areas of the body. Relationships between psychiatric illness and female reproductive events are still being explored. For instance, "Premenstrual dysphoric disorder" is described among the "Disorders Requiring Further Study" in the Appendix of the official American Psychiatric Association *Diagnostic and Statistical Manual (DSM), 4th ed.*

Many people still believe that psychiatric illness is a product of weakness and general inferiority: that patients are either incurable or undeserving of treatment. The public in general has not been adequately informed about the mechanisms of action and effectiveness of psychopharmacologic agents. Lay persons and policy makers alike tend to perceive the "talking therapies" as indulgences for worried or bored well persons, rather than as interventions whose efficacy and cost-effectiveness have been demonstrated repeatedly in the scientific literature and which compare favorably with many common and well-accepted medical treatments.[2]

Often, primary care patients do not complain of problems with their emotions, thinking, or behavior, but of physical symptoms.[63] Their psychiatric problems are manifested in somatic form or as noncompliance with the primary physician's recommendations. Therefore, the primary care physician must not only be familiar with the criteria for diagnosing common psychiatric disorders, but also must possess the interviewing skills and psychological expertise necessary to understand the patient in context and in some depth, to uncover the relevant signs and symptoms, to help the patient accept the reality of her psychiatric or psychosocial difficulty, and either to perform office therapy or to facilitate an effective referral to a mental health professional. Because psychiatric illnesses so infrequently present in the primary care setting with signs and symptoms that the physician can usefully look up in a table of contents or index, and are so frequently missed in medical evaluation and treatment, this chapter dwells extensively on diagnostic technique before describing illnesses and treatments.[54] Both sophisticated interviewing skills and the understanding of psychosocial issues and their implications are central to the ability to identify, diagnose, and treat psychiatric disorders. These skills are important for the primary care practitioner because psychiatric disorders are common; often cause serious impairment, suffering, complications in medical treatment and recovery, and even mortality; and often can be identified by the astute primary care provider and treated promptly.

While social context has always been a central factor in susceptibility to disease, in illness behavior, and in the use of medical care, physicians of the past could and frequently did take the social context for granted. The physician was familiar with the milieu from which the patient came or was able to infer it from her address, name, dress, or manner. Such assumptions, if they ever were reliable, are so no longer. Not only have there been major changes, but the change in women's roles and expectations vary among social subgroups and age groups, from woman to woman, and over the course of a given woman's lifetime. The physician must obtain specific, relevant information from each patient.

Failure to address these issues has direct medical consequences. Stereotypes may prevent physicians from identifying instances of domestic violence and other abuse, situations precipitating depressive reactions, and psychosocial etiologies for pelvic pain and infertility, as well as many other conditions.

This chapter offers an overview of the interviewing skills necessary to obtain essential data and to establish an effective working relationship with patients in a variety of primary care settings. It includes information about the prevalence and distribution of psychiatric and psychosocial problems in the female patient population. It addresses the psychology of women and psychosocial issues as they present in and complicate primary care. It covers diagnosis, triage, and outpatient management of the major psychiatric illnesses; it suggests criteria and techniques for referring patients to psychiatrists and other mental health professionals with ongoing interdisciplinary collaboration.

The Psychology of Women

Through most of Western history, male psychological development was assumed to be normative; women were conceptualized as relatively less fully developed and/or deviant versions of "human beings."[74] Sigmund Freud's work followed this pattern.

Freud believed that male and female children developed similarly until a point in toddlerhood when they first became aware of the gender differences in external genitalia. This recognition precipitated in the boy the fear that competition with his father for his mother's affection would lead his father to cut off his penis: "castration anxiety." The fear of retributive castration led to the development of the boy's moral sense. The girl, on the other hand, became enraged and resentful that her mother had not provided her with a penis, and attempted to substitute the fantasy of having a child by her father: "penis envy." Since she had no penis to protect, her conscience did not develop so fully as a boy's. Freud admitted, however, that his theory, which derived substantively from self-analysis, explained male psychology much more accurately than female.[31]

Researchers and clinicians in the century following Freud's made many observations that disprove or call into question many of his theories. Girls' envy may well have derived from their observation of the dominant position of men in Freud's turn-of-the-century Vienna rather than from their observation of anatomical differences. Recent evidence indicates that infant girls do not experience themselves as deficient boys.[52] They have a positive awareness of their internal genital structures, and their feelings about them are directly related to their parents' reactions to their sex. Insofar as their pride in their femaleness and individuality is mirrored by their parents, and they have positive female role models to admire and emulate, their being girls does not constitute a developmental problem.

Women's development has almost always been construed in terms of reproductive milestones: menarche, first intercourse, childbearing, and menopause. There is no doubt that the rhythms of reproductive physiology exert tangible and visible effects on women's development. Puberty brings with it not only increased libido and the capacity for intercourse, but the possibility of pregnancy. Bleeding connotes injury and can be very frightening to the girl who is not prepared and supported. At first intercourse, the girl or woman chooses, allows, or is forced to undergo, bodily penetration, which may be both frightening and painful. Upon becoming heterosexually active, a girl or woman must be able to address delayed consequences and to negotiate protective measures with her partner and/or a health care provider—or accept the risk of pregnancy.

Pregnancy requires that a woman literally make room for another human being in her body, her emotions, and her plans, and that she tolerate major changes in her body shape and function. During the first trimester, the woman's developmental tasks are to recognize the signs and symptoms of pregnancy, accept its reality, and, in many societies, decide whether to continue or terminate it. Again, these tasks precipitate and facilitate her assessment of her life plans, capacities, resources, and other commitments. Does she see herself as a mother, does she actively reject that possibility, or does she put the problem out of her awareness while nature takes its course?

Childbirth confronts a woman with a powerful, demanding, inexorable, concentrated anatomical and physiologic process of opening, expulsion, and separation. Simultaneously, she must form an intense relationship with a new, unique, and helpless human being. A new mother may be astounded by the strength of her attachment to the infant; she may be terrified, surprised, ashamed, and guilty because she does not feel as loving as she expects—or each, at various times. There is evidence that the parents and infant are particularly alert and attuned to one another during the period immediately after birth. Normal mothers and normal infants with good social support networks can overcome the impact of separation at this time, but those at medical, psychological, and/or social risk may require supportive professional interventions to forestall significant difficulties in parenting.[7]

Breastfeeding extends the healthy bodily symbiosis between mother and child into the child's infancy. It requires sharing of one's time and one's body with the baby while managing other tasks and the feelings of others within and without the family. The birth of each subsequent child exerts all the physical and psychological demands of the birth of the first, along with the need to integrate the new baby's needs with those of the other children. Becoming a mother invariably provokes a woman's comparison of herself with her own mother and changes her relationship with her parents.

The next reproductive life stage for women is menopause. The developmental task of menopause is the change to a self-image that does not involve the capacity for childbearing. In Western society, menopause for mothers generally coincides chronologically with the maturation of a woman's children and their financial and social independence from the family. For women who have not borne children, menopause constitutes the end of the life stage during which childbirth has been at least theoretically possible.

The Social Context of Women's Development: Relevance to Medical Care

There is no such thing as ''natural'' human behavior or emotions outside a social context. Human beings are social creatures; few have survived, and none have been considered normal, among those who developed away from other people. Specifically feminine developmental tasks involve identifying oneself as a female in relation to a particular society that defines femaleness in particular ways. Reproductive events have central social significance in all cultures; again, it is difficult and perhaps meaningless to differentiate some sort of innate, inevitable biopsychological sequence from the influences of family and culture. It is impossible to isolate ubiquitous developmental realities from the social context. What affects a woman psychologically is not so much the physiologic processes that take place in her body, but the meanings society attaches to them and the ways in which those meanings change her options and experiences. For example, menopause may be regarded as a loss of a central life function or a relief from the burdens of bleeding, contraception, childbearing, and childrearing. Even its association with aging, experienced as negative in Western societies, has very different connotations in cultures that accord women increasing respect, autonomy, and power as they grow older.[25,34] Primary care physicians can have a positive effect on the way a woman approaches and experiences particular ''milestones'' in her life.

Care providers must bear in mind the central impact of cultural expectations, attitudes, and practices on their patients' development. In most subgroups of society, girls are socialized to be submissive and agreeable. In contrast with the rearing of boys, girls may be actively discouraged from manifesting assertiveness. Following recent social changes, some families, toy manufacturers, and schools have deemphasized the gender-specificity of children's attire, playthings, and activities. However, thoroughgoing neutrality is exceedingly rare. Girls and boys are usually treated differently from birth: dressed in different clothing, surrounded by different schemes of interior decoration and different toys, subjected to different expectations by their families. Girls are usually described in terms of physical appearance, boys in terms of physical strength.

In the early years of elementary school, girls' relative passivity and conformity tend to be rewarded by teachers. Girls and boys achieve approximately equivalent self-esteem. However, things change during the preadolescent, junior high school years. At this point, some girls retreat from academic excellence and athletic achievement to become cheerleaders for boys' activities. Their self-esteem, self-assertion, and self-confidence often fall significantly. This regression may be facilitated by teachers who differentially recognize and reward male students. Though girls have entered and completed higher education in ever-increasing numbers and proportions, women do not achieve equivalent pay or leadership roles in jobs and professions.[23,28,51]

It is important for the primary care physician to recognize that milestones commonly construed as ''male'' pertain to women as well: athletic and academic achievements, first job, promotions, retirement. These milestones may provide important opportunities for the physician to play a positive and supportive role for the patient, particularly if other aspects of her social context are not supportive.

In many spheres women continue to be characterized by their domestic—and men by their employment—status. The factors contributing to this differential are complex and interwoven. A recent survey of the paid workforce again demonstrates that the employment status of the wife has little effect on the distribution of domestic tasks between marital partners.[39] Men have increased their involvement in domestic duties, but it is as helpers to their wives. At the same time, women's domestic managerial obligations are not accorded the social respect and support that accrue to organizational roles in the workplace. Despite the stresses inherent in coping with two or more demanding roles, evidence indicates that paid employment is associated with improvement in women's mental health status.[60] It is important for the primary care physician to understand the home and work dynamics of an individual woman's life—particularly since these dynamics will often impact her medical care. For instance, these dynamics may affect her ability to be appropriately involved in preventive health measures or to follow a treatment regimen.

Women's experiences of menopause may be largely dependent on the role that fertility and childbearing have played and continue to play in their valuation of themselves and others. Menopause may be quite a different experience for a nonemployed woman whose husband leaves her for a much younger rival than for a woman whose menstrual bleeding has interrupted the executive board meetings she chairs. Menopause, often associated with the departure of children from home, can signal uselessness or freedom, a decrease in youthful attractiveness or an opportunity to take care of one's self—and be taken care of—in ways difficult for women with children at home to achieve. The physician may have the capability to some extent to have a positive role in the woman's transition through the menopause.

A group whose health care issues have not been fully addressed are lesbian women. They are usually ignored in discussions of normal development, and often experience their own development as problematic and deviant because it does not conform to the behaviors and expectations of their families and cultures.[32] Now that more lesbians have dared to ''come out of the closet,'' and have revealed the psychic and social stresses to which their sexual orientation has subjected them, it is clear that the psychic conflicts described by past theorists may have been the result of social ignorance and prejudice about homosexuality.

Another social reality of women's lives is victimization. Victimization is the result of direct assaults on girls' and women's bodies and personalities; it includes incest, rape, child and elder abuse, and other forms of domestic violence. These all-too-common events cause injuries to the individual women who experience them, the children who observe them, and to women in general, whose social and physical environment may include secrecy, danger, and discrimination.[37] Despite recent increases in social awareness and responsiveness to the victimization of women, strong cultural and intrapsychic factors continue to prejudice us to blame or ignore the victim. Victimization is grossly underdiagnosed in the health care setting.[4] This is particularly ironic in view of the fact that this setting may be the only one to which the victimizer allows the woman access.

In conclusion, it is essential to recognize that

health care providers are members of society who can have a profound impact on women's experience of themselves and of their physiologic functions and illnesses. As individuals, primary care providers inevitably have experiences with and attitudes toward women, their development, place in society, and health care needs. It is essential that physicians and other members of the medical care team make themselves aware of their own attitudes and how they affect the provision of care.

Physicians today are sometimes frustrated by the many psychological and social factors that confound the effective diagnosis and treatment of disease, occasionally feeling that their opinions and statements have little weight. However, for most patients, the real—or perceived—judgment of a physician, especially theirs, is indeed important, remembered, and influential. The physician has the opportunity to have a substantial and positive impact on the patient's psychological as well as physical well-being.

Interviewing Techniques for Primary Physicians

General Interviewing Techniques

The profound impact of her cultural milieu on a woman's development and health underscores the importance of interpersonal skills and psychosocial expertise to primary health care providers. The ability to encourage patients to explain their complaints and concerns—and to ask the right questions in the right way—is also essential to the identification of psychiatric disorders and psychosocial problems that can complicate the care of other medical problems. Finally, effective communication with the patient is the only way to enhance compliance with the diagnostic and treatment approach adopted by the primary health care provider.

The exponentially increasing wealth of medical information and technological tools sometimes overshadows the ongoing critical role of the live doctor-patient interaction in medical care. In the rush to obtain diagnostic data and outline the plan of treatment, it is easy to forget that the essence of the dialogue is in listening rather than talking. A primary care provider must create an atmosphere in which the patient feels comfortable revealing intimate, sometimes frightening, often embarrassing problems. The barriers to this cornerstone of medical tradition include the pressure of time and the physician's own anxieties about the material to be discussed. Fortunately, each of these barriers can be readily addressed.

Data indicate that the average medical interviewer interrupts a patient with specific questions before a minute has elapsed, presumably with the expectation that focused questions will provide a short-cut through the patient's uninformed verbal meanderings.[14] Allowing a patient several uninterrupted minutes to present her symptoms is time-effective. It both conveys a sense of genuine interest and gratifies the patient's legitimate need for the doctor's attention. In those few minutes, the patient will reveal how she thinks, especially about her medical condition. The physician will be able to amass considerable information about her mental status in a more cogent, natural, efficient way than a formal mental status examination can provide. The need for data may lead to a more formal inquiry later in the interview. The physician can take the opportunity to observe the patient's appearance, dress, verbal facility and style, and body language. Does she appear tense, frightened, angry, embarrassed, depressed?

Those uninterrupted moments not uncommonly allow the diagnosis of a psychiatric disorder, even a serious one, which otherwise would be missed or perceived only as a puzzling distraction from the purpose of the history. For example, a frankly psychotic patient may appear only "odd" in the context of a rapid-fire exchange of questions and answers, but quickly will reveal delusional thinking in a few spontaneous sentences. A patient may forcefully deny signs and symptoms of depression, but convey clues to the diagnosis in her slumped posture, slow responses, and negative thought content. A patient with delirium and/or dementia can often give amazingly convincing "yes or no" answers while completely unaware of where she is and what is happening to her. She may nod compliantly at the recommended treatment, though unable either to comply effectively or to report on her treatment and progress at the next appointment.

Having encouraged the patient to present her concerns in her own words, the primary physician will have significant clues to the diagnosis that will help focus the questions that follow. The patient's spontaneous verbalizations also will inform the physician about verbal skills, vocabulary, and attitudes toward illness and medical treatment. Most physicians have had experiences in which a particular patient, entirely preoccupied with herself and her complaints, monopolized the physician's time and attention both in her visits to the doctor and on the telephone between visits. These experiences, combined with the overwhelming demands on physicians' time in general, make physicians wary of open-ended dialogue with patients. Caught between their sensitivity to patients' feelings and their time concerns, a physician may resort to the prescription pad as their only tool for ending the interview. A prescription for psychotropic medication, too often without benefit of accurate psychiatric diagnosis or treatment plan, is meant to address the patient's psychological distress, to give her something to carry away, and to signal that it is time for her to leave.

However, the fact is that most patients are overly worried about being too demanding and asking "silly" questions. The physician can put knowledge of each patient's style to good use in designing the course of treatment and also in formulating informed responses to patients' complaints between appointments. A call from a patient who minimizes all her symptoms and is loath to disturb the doctor, for example, may signal an unusually severe or worrisome symptom, and likely warrants an immediate and serious intervention.

It is possible to control the flow and length of a patient interview without resorting to check-off lists or unnecessary prescriptions. It is helpful to inform the patient at the outset approximately how much time has been allotted. Having this information in advance allows and encourages the patient to focus her history on the issues of most concern to her. She will generally recognize and report the most medically urgent ones. Without this guidance, she may assume it is best to "work up to" the most pressing problems—and then be forced to squeeze them in as the doctor becomes increasingly more impatient. The appointment can always be expanded if absolutely necessary. If there is not time to cover all the concerns, and the remaining issues are not urgent, the physician can offer to take them up at a subsequent visit.

Alert primary care providers will be aware of their vulnerabilities to embarrassment and will not unwittingly discourage patients from presenting concerns in those areas. When a patient is clearly embarrassed or afraid, it is helpful to acknowledge her feelings—"It seems that's hard for you to talk about"—and offer to help—"Is there any way I can make it easier?"—or to postpone the subject to the next visit.

Increasing Comfort with Uncomfortable Topics

Certain topics engender discomfort in nearly all people, including physicians. Many physicians fear that certain topics will enrage, embarrass, or alienate a patient, or, perhaps worse, precipitate the enactment of ideas that would have remained latent if not brought into the interview. We are also understandably reluctant to elicit information or problems when we doubt that we will know what to do with them. Typical topics of concern include sexuality, insanity and other kinds of incapacity, and death. Unfortunately, unspoken collusion between doctor and patient to avoid those areas entirely can result in serious medical omissions. Fortunately, there are relatively straightforward techniques for addressing these areas of doctor-patient concern.

There is no evidence that asking a patient about suicidal or homicidal ideas or intent increases the likelihood of dangerous behavior.[27] On the contrary, the physician who brings these areas into the doctor-patient dialogue is in a position to save the life of a patient, a patient's victim, or both. Similarly, there is no evidence that patients change physicians because their sexual and psychiatric histories and concerns are elicited. Patients unhappy with their physicians are far more likely to complain that a full history was not taken, that they did not feel comfortable bringing some questions to the doctor, or that their questions were not answered.

Many physicians are astonished at the straightforwardness with which patients answer straightforward questions which the physicians expected to provoke resentment. Our astonishment frequently reveals our preconceptions about the occurrence of behaviors in particular groups of patients. In the unlikely event that a patient does bristle at a question, the physician need only explain that the purpose of the question is to open the area of inquiry as widely as possible, so that patients will feel comfortable giving whatever answer is accurate and bringing up any problems that concern them. Persistent patient resentment after this explanation (which is even more uncommon) is a clue either that the physician asked the question in a provocative manner or that the patient is extraordinarily repressed or deeply ashamed of past or ongoing behavior.

The Sexual History

The primary care provider can be expected to address issues of sexual function and dysfunction. The sexual history in general is a part of the initial history, and sexual adjustment should be addressed routinely at postpartum and postoperative visits. Since society is full of sexual taboos, and sexual taboos were even more frequent when many patients were growing up, it is best to phrase questions in such a way that sexual activities are assumed. The patient can simply correct this assumption when it is not appropriate. For example:

- What are the earliest sexual experiences you can remember?
- What is the nature of your current sexual activity, by yourself or with one or more partners? (This phraseology avoids the pitfalls of assumptions about the patient's sexual orientation, marital fidelity, etc.)
- What sexual problems and questions have you encountered since your delivery/surgery?

It is helpful to have a sense of the sexual attitudes with which the patient was brought up: "How were sexual and reproductive matters handled in your family?" Always bear in mind the possibility that the patient is homosexual or bisexual, even if she is or has been either married or in some other heterosexual relationship. Lesbian women have legitimate complaints about the attitudes and behaviors of some of the physicians they encounter. They may well incur added medical risks because they avoid the medical setting or avoid sharing the realities of their sexual behavior.[42] The same may be true of women engaged in prostitution. Further discussion regarding the sexual history can be found in the section on the assessment and treatment of sexual complaints.

Suicide and Homicide

Inquiries about suicidality and homicidality can proceed logically from discussions of feelings of frustration, rage, and despair, whether precipitated by particular stressful events or arising of their own accord. It is easy to explain that everyone, or nearly everyone, entertains such thoughts at one time or another—that no longer being alive would be a relief, and the wish to "murder someone." Alternatively, such inquiries can be included and explained separately as part of a formal mental status examination. Most patients will acknowledge having had these thoughts and feelings at one time or another, and will explain spontaneously that they were not serious. Perhaps they also will say why they would not engage in that kind of behavior: "My religion is against suicide," "It would hurt my family." Should a patient vigorously deny having had either feeling, the physician will want to know why it is necessary for her to do so. It may be a clue to a very rigid system of beliefs and/or to mental efforts to suppress a suicidal or homicidal wish so strong that it threatens to become irresistible.

After the (usual) patient admits to having had fleeting thoughts of suicide or homicide, the next appropriate questions are whether the patient has been tempted to act upon them, and whether she has engaged in suicidal or homicidal behavior in the past. If there have been attempts, it is important to know whether they were planned or impulsive, and whether the situation(s) and feelings that provoked them are likely to recur. Some patients engage in such behavior impulsively because of organic brain damage or personality disorders. The degree of impulsivity or planning in past behavior that was dangerous to the self or others is an important clue to the predictability of such behavior in the future.

For the patient with a history of suicidal ideation or attempts, the following inquiry will ensue:

- How many times did this behavior occur?
- When was the last time?
- Were you hospitalized? If so, what was the nature of the hospitalization?
- Did the consequences of your self-destructive behavior require medical intervention? If so, what was it?
- If there was psychiatric hospitalization and/or outpatient treatment, what was the diagnosis and the nature of the intervention?
- Does the patient now feel that she could recognize the signs and symptoms of a similar episode and seek appropriate care earlier, before she felt desperate and hopeless?

Additional risk factors for suicide include a family history of suicide, alcoholism and/or other substance abuse, psychosis, serious recent loss, and serious, disabling, or chronic illness.[38]

When a patient describes a history of physically harming others, the inquiry is similar:

- What was the nature of the harm you did?
- Did the victim die or require medical intervention?
- When and how often did this behavior occur?
- What were the consequences for you?
- How do you explain what happened?
- Are you convinced that the problem that caused this behavior has been resolved? How?

It is generally believed that patients tell the truth in response to these questions, so long as they are confident that the information is being elicited in the interest of their care and safety. Obviously the physician must also determine whether the patient is acutely suicidal or homicidal:

- Are you having those thoughts/feelings recently? Now?
- Do you feel you can and want to resist them? Why and how?
- Do you have a plan for carrying out this behavior?
- Do you have the means for carrying out your plan?

When a primary physician discovers that a patient is experiencing suicidal or homicidal ideation, he or she must consider very seriously the need to obtain a psychiatric consultation before ending the immediate doctor-patient contact. If the physician has any reason whatsoever to suspect that the danger may be imminent, it is appropriate to summon aid in the form of the police or a security guard. The nature of medical dedication, training, and practice tends to make physicians believe they can and should handle all emergencies and to discourage them from asking for help. This well-meaning self-reliance is tragically fatal for the patient and/or physician in some clinical situations. When a patient or someone accompanying her is acutely threatening to the physician or to others, the physician must not respond with anger and confrontation; such a response escalates the situation and has been shown to correlate with tragic outcomes. It is better to leave the room—and to take other care staff along.

On the other hand, A PATIENT WHO IS ACUTELY SUICIDAL MUST NOT BE LEFT ALONE. Unused to such intrusions on a patient's privacy—and to the degree of vigilance necessary in such a situation—members of the patient's family and her care providers alike may allow the patient to go to the bathroom alone or may leave her briefly to make a telephone call or get a drink of water. Suicidal patients can be extremely fast and ingenious, crashing through upper-story windows and using medical equipment to harm themselves. If there is no telephone where the dialogue is taking place, it is best to step to the door and call calmly but firmly for help. Should it be necessary to go beyond the door for help, the physician will have to decide whether to bring the patient along, weighing the risk of her flight against the risk of leaving her alone. Inform the patient calmly of the basis for your concern and of the actions you will take: "What you have just told me makes me concerned for your/my safety. In order not to take chances, I have called for help. You will not be left alone/you must remain here until we are sure things are safe.''

Eliciting Psychotic Symptoms

Asking a patient about psychotic symptoms (hallucinations, delusions, ideas of reference) seems like suggesting that she is crazy—certainly an insult in our society. Nevertheless, this inquiry is a necessary component of the mental status examination, and is perfectly well tolerated by patients. Patients who have not suffered these symptoms answer ''No'' with relief. Patients who have chronic psychotic symptoms are used to the questions. Patients with acute psychotic symptoms tend to be frightened by them and are aware of their need for help. Paranoid ideation is often apparent in the patient's explanation of the problems that brought her to the doctor: the relatives or neighbors are plotting against her, the water is poisoned, and so forth. Nonverbal cues to acute psychotic symptoms, described as ''attending to internal stimuli,'' include fixing one's gaze at some point where there does not appear to be anything to see, and the appearance of listening to an inner dialogue rather than attending to the interview with the doctor.

Since 1 percent of the world population suffers from schizophrenia, and since many others have psychotic episodes complicating alcohol and substance abuse and other forms of metabolic, infectious, and other pathologic toxicity, the acquisition of this history can enable the physician to intervene early and effectively at the first sign of a recurrence.[48] At the same time, mindful of the profound social stigma of psychosis, the physician will not intervene prematurely or needlessly. The fact that a patient recounts a history of psychotic symptoms should not be used to undermine her standing as a historian or as an individual competent to make decisions about her own life and care.

Possible wordings for the inquiry about psychotic symptoms include:

- Have you ever seen things that other people couldn't see or heard things that other people couldn't hear?
- Who or what did you see? What did they do?
- Was it your own voice, or someone else's?
- Whose? One or more than one person?
- What did they say?
- Have you ever had the feeling that a book, magazine, or newspaper article, radio or television program, or movie was directed particularly at you, conveying a special message to you?
- What do you do when these things happen?

Some patients with schizophrenia experience ''command hallucinations,'' voices that order them to do things; sometimes they are ''ordered'' to harm themselves or others. This symptom, and the patient's past and immediate ability to resist the ''order,'' may indicate a risk of suicidal or homicidal behavior.

Death and Dying

There has been a considerable literature recently on physicians' failure to discuss issues of death and dying with their patients.[35] Patients' fears of being subjected to painful, humiliating, expensive, and ultimately useless medical interventions when they are helpless to refuse fuels much of the current preoccupation with physician-assisted suicide, durable powers of attorney, living wills, and other means of extricating dying patients from complex, invasive, and unwanted technological medical care. It is generally physicians, not patients, who are reluctant to discuss the possibility of death.[35] It is not the prospect of death itself which terrifies most people, but the prospect of pain, disability, helplessness, and loneliness. Avoidance of the subject exacerbates those fears.

How should the subject be broached? Often a patient is much more aware of the possibility of a fatal outcome than her physician and family may realize. The same is true of an elderly and/or chronically ill patient. The absence of this subject in the doctor-patient dialogue may well indicate that the patient senses the discomfort of family members or her physician. The topic probably will arise naturally when the physician corroborates with the patient her understanding of her medical condition and her expectations for the future, and elicits her questions and concerns, with a specific focus on what kinds of support and intervention she will need from the medical team.

The patient should be reassured that the primary physician will remain available and on duty to coordinate her care, even if other specialists assume a major role. It is easy for the seriously ill patient to get ''lost'' among the many subspecialists, house staff, and technicians in a tertiary setting; it is common for her to hear conflicting opinions from the same staff and to have difficulty identifying who is in charge. The primary physician is invaluable as the medical expert the patient knows and trusts to be her mediator, advocate, and interpreter. The patient must never get the message, ''There is no more we can do.'' Inability to effect a cure or to prolong life significantly should never suggest abandonment of the patient, who will continue to need support, advice, and symptom-relief until the moment of death. The knowledge that the primary physician will ''be there'' will reduce symptoms, facilitate compliance, and decrease anxiety.

Religious faith and the support of her religious community are crucially important to many critically ill patients who face painful, disfiguring, or disabling procedures, or who must make major life decisions.[41] Religion is another intimate, personal, and highly emotionally-charged area that doctors understandably may fear. It is possible to elicit information about the patient's religious beliefs, practices, and community and to apply this understanding to her care without violating her or one's own personal religious boundaries. The faith with which the patient identifies herself demographically is less important. One can ask, ''Are you a religious person?'' or ''Does your religion play a role in your ability to cope with illness?''

When specific religious beliefs, such as the Jehovah's Witnesses' refusal to accept blood and blood products, interfere with the medically indicated course of treatment, the situation is painful for both patient and physician. One must determine whether the patient's convictions are longstanding and freely held, and what implications violating them would have for her future social relationships and peace of mind. Refusal to accept any or all medical treatment, even when the refusal may result in death, is not synonymous with suicidality, which denotes an active wish to kill oneself.

Some values are more important to people than life itself, and these values must be respected. Sometimes physicians jump to the conclusion that a patient who refuses to accept a seemingly crucial medical recommendation must be psychotic. Such refusals happen, and can be expressed in religious terms. It is appropriate to ask the patient to help you understand her decision. Idiosyncratic, psychotic mentation, if present, will be revealed when the patient is allowed to expound on her position. The Jehovah's Witnesses produce educational literature for physicians to explain their beliefs, and maintain lists of physicians who are willing to treat members with respect.

Domestic Violence

One last area of avoidance, and of life-and-death concern, is domestic and nondomestic violence. Generally, patients are more likely to reveal violence perpetrated upon them by strangers than by people they know.[37] When a person you know commits a violent act against you, your very relationship with that person taints you as well. In addition, most societies, and the individual men and women who comprise them, tend to blame women for their own victimization: ''She asked for it''; ''she put up with it.'' Rape in particular is misperceived as an act of sexuality, rather than one of power and violence. The investigation of rape tends to focus on the past sexual behavior, attire, and carelessness of the victim; women already traumatized by the assault itself are understandably reluctant to have to defend themselves once again and to undergo any further humiliation.

The primary care relationship may create paradoxical difficulties for the practitioner in inquiring about domestic violence. The patient has an investment in appearing ''normal'' to her physician, who often is one of the few people outside the household she is allowed by her abuser to see. Often women are not able to reveal domestic violence for weeks, months, or years into the doctor-patient relationship—even with a skilled mental health professional. It is embarrassing for both doctor and patient to uncover the reality under the pretext they have accepted. As with sexual assault, society has a tendency to blame the victim. It is difficult to comprehend the sense of helplessness—in fact, paralysis and self-blame—which the abuser engenders in the victim. Why doesn't she leave? Why does she forgive the abuser time and time again?

The reality of domestic violence threatens us all. It cannot be ignored. Demographics indicate clearly that high socioeconomic class is not a barrier to victimization.[59] Abuse is a high-risk situation. Abused persons are likely to be abused again and to be victims of murder. Nevertheless, excellent studies demonstrate that the vast majority of cases are not diagnosed in the primary care setting.[56] Questionable explanations for injuries are accepted at face value. Often the abuser hovers over the patient, seemingly solicitous and protective, but insuring that the patient and the physician have no opportunity for private discussion of the injury. Routine screening should—and the history of injuries must—include questions about domestic violence—in the absence of persons accompanying the patient:

- Do arguments in your house sometimes get physical?
- Show me where on your body you have been hurt.

Knowledge of community resources available to victims of domestic violence lessens the doctor's psychological barrier to making the diagnosis. No one wants to know about something awful that he or she can do nothing about. Opening the subject with the patient lets her know that you are ready to hear it when she is ready to discuss it. Brochures from women's shelters and hot-lines can be displayed in the waiting area along with other resource materials that patients can select unobtrusively, or may be placed in the women's restroom where patients can select them in private.

Achieving Doctor-Patient Consensus

It is essential to learn in the interview the patient's assumptions about the cause, diagnosis, and expected work-up and therapy for her symptoms. These too-seldom articulated opinions can sabotage the finest plans for evaluation and treatment. A patient who believes that her abdominal pain results from an ulcer like her mother's 30 years ago—that her diagnosis must involve swallowing some chalky fluid and her treatment drinking lots of cream—may keep searching for a physician who will proceed in the expected manner, despite the most eloquent explanation of a proposed evaluation and treatment by the physician unaware of her beliefs. She may attempt to implement her preferred approach on her own, or may become disabled after abandoning attempts to relieve her symptoms.

If she returns for further visits, the physician may again make the unwarranted assumption that the patient has complied; again she will seldom expose herself to the doctor's criticism by revealing her noncompliance. At follow-up visits, it is best to ask the patient what she understood from the previous visit, and what she did to address her symptoms. Doctors must understand—and must communicate to patients—that patients cannot be expected to comprehend, absorb, and integrate sophisticated medical information in a single visit. Questions must be actively invited. Significant noncompliance is difficult to detect in the primary care outpatient setting. The gap between the patient and the doctor must be exposed and discussed before it can be bridged. The only way to learn whether the patient is now convinced and likely to be compliant is to hear her explain the regimen and rationale briefly in her own words, or to hear her frame a question that reflects understanding. Too many patients nod passively, make agreeable inchoate conversational responses, and ignore the doctor's advice!

Mental Status Examination

The mental status examination is an effective and verifiable technique for determining a patient's level of awareness and ability to take in, process, retain, and respond to information. There is some debate about the usefulness of the full-scale mental status examination because of its susceptibility to culture and education bias, to anxiety, and to the significance of the questions and answers for the particular patient. A patient with a distressing diagnosis, physical symptoms, or family situation may have little or no interest in what she did or did not eat for breakfast in the morning, and the physician generally has no way of corroborating her account. The proverbs used in the examination for many years were common aphorisms in the culture when they were first employed, but they are so no longer.

Performing and recording a mental status examination provide a vital component of the baseline medical evaluation. This record will be especially valuable when a patient is noncompliant or refuses to give consent for a medical intervention, leading to a question of competence. It is also essential in the detection of a delirium in the acutely ill or postoperative patient.[70] Waiting until a patient pulls out her intravenous and other connections, attempts to leave the unit, and/or harms staff or other patients, is inconvenient and medically and legally dangerous. Despite its usefulness, the mental status examination is often overlooked, possibly because primary care providers are uncomfortable about confronting a patient's possible defects in cognitive function. It is helpful to inform the patient that some questions are asked routinely to determine how she is thinking at the present time.

The so-called "mini mental state exam" is an excellent primary care screening technique:

1. What is your name?
2. What is the day? date? month? season? year? (Note: Hospitalized patients may lose track of the exact date without external cues such as newspapers and television news.)
3. Where are you/we right now? hospital? city? state? county?
4. What is your age? When were you born?
5. Can you name the President of the United States? the previous President?
6. How many nickels are there in a dollar? Or, count backwards from 100 by 7.
7. What is this? (show a watch, pen)
8. Please repeat: "No ifs, ands, or buts"
9. Hand the patient a piece of paper and instruct her: "Take this in your right hand, fold it in half, and set it on the table."
10. Read this and do what it says. CLOSE YOUR EYES
11. Write a sentence.
12. Copy this design. (interlocking pentagons)
13. Please repeat these three items: red balloon, New York, yellow pencil. I will ask you about them in about five minutes. (Ask.)[29]

Note that psychiatric disorders, notably depression, can lead to false-positive results on the mental status examination. Even in these cases, such results may predict onset of dementia in the future. A neuropsychological test battery may be indicated.

Psychosocial and Sexual Aspects of Medical and Obstetric/Gynecologic Conditions

The psychosocial impact of a physiologic condition or disease process cannot be measured or predicted solely by laboratory values, pathology reports, or physical findings; it is mediated through its meaning to the patient, her significant others, and the institutions of society. The availability of help with responsibilities and other resources, the reactions of family members and sexual partners, financial constraints, and employment implications interact with the patient's beliefs, values, and feelings.

Emotional Responses to Medical Illness

Chronic and/or severe illness is associated with a heightened risk of clinical depression. Depressive symptoms must not be confused with a patient's acute response to bad news about diagnosis or prognosis, to pain, or to adverse developments in her life and relationships. Nor may the primary physician dismiss signs and symptoms of depression on the grounds that they are inevitable responses to illness or life situations—no more than the need for medical treatment of a broken limb can be ignored because it is an inevitable response to an encounter between a pedestrian and a speeding truck.

The vegetative signs and symptoms of medical illness, such as loss of energy, appetite, and sleep may confound the diagnosis of depression. Medically ill patients without clinical depression do not tend to feel guilty, worthless, or suicidal. When clinical depression complicates a medical illness, it causes needless suffering and interferes significantly with physical recovery, motivation, and compliance with the medical regimen. It can be diagnosed using the standard criteria. Diagnosis according to these empirically validated criteria predicts a successful response to antidepressant treatment. These criteria are discussed in the next section.

Anxiety is the other common emotional complication of medical illness. Anxiety and depression may result from a patient's (or her family's) misunderstanding of the nature of her illness, treatment, and/or prognosis. It is best to elicit their beliefs before launching a new explanation. Often, small adjustments in the treatment approach can make a big difference to the patient. For example, she might choose to use an alternate route for anesthesia, to have mild sedation before a frightening procedure, or to have a comforting significant other accompany her during a test or treatment. Undue anxiety associated with a medical condition constitutes a diagnosable psychiatric disorder.

Reproductively related conditions tend to carry a special emotional meaning, and obstetric events specifically concern the possibility of the addition of a new and dependent person to the family. Because of their prevalence and the publicity about female reproductive malignancies and sexually transmitted diseases—and because of the stress on the gynecologic examination as a screening procedure—gynecologic symptoms and pelvic examination are fraught for many women with an imminent possibility of receiving distressing news. Perhaps that is one reason so many women fail to obtain regular check-ups.

Rape

One condition, or event, that may fall through the cracks between medical and mental health care is rape. Rape constitutes both a physical and an emotional trauma. When the psychological aspects are not addressed, the patient is at significant risk for the development of sexual dysfunction. Because rape is a crime that usually leaves the victim feeling sullied and ashamed, she finds it difficult to discuss and to work through. If she does attempt to find support among her friends and relatives, the discussion will likely provoke their anxiety and defensiveness, which will result in avoidance or blame. The responses of the men in her life are particularly important. At worst, they may see the victim as a "slut" or as "damaged goods." At best, they can help to restore her faith in her goodness, safety, and continued sexual and personal desirability.

Typically, a rape victim discards clothing or other items soiled in the assault, and attempts to cleanse her body of its after-effects by douching and bathing. Paradoxically, these activities often destroy the legal evidence most crucial to the conviction of the rapist. She may sacrifice a successful career and a satisfying living arrangement to remove herself from the places and routines that remind her of the rape, or which she fears may expose her to a second assault. Her sleep will be disrupted by nightmares and her relationships, especially with men, by difficulties with intimacy and trust.

The primary care provider must actively inquire about symptoms of sleep or appetite disturbances, difficulties with concentration, flashbacks and nightmares about the assault experience, social withdrawal, and sexual disturbance. The patient/victim, anxious to put the rape behind her, may tend to deny ongoing psychological difficulties. Whether or not the patient complains of psychiatric symptoms immediately after the rape, brief counseling is advisable. The primary practitioner will have to balance the need to convince the patient to enter psychotherapy with the risk of intruding on her sense of autonomy, already threatened by the assault.

Primary Care Presentations of Psychosocial, Sexual, and Psychiatric Problems: Explicit, Implicit, and Somatic

Unlike problems in dermatology, for example, psychosocial, sexual, and psychiatric problems are not always apparent. In the primary care setting, the patient may present with psychiatric complaints attributable to other systemic illness, may mention life problems tangentially, or may develop somatic symptoms derived primarily from psychiatric disease. The primary care challenge is to be aware of the criteria for psychiatric diagnoses, alert to the possibility of psychiatric disorders masked as other complaints, and observant of indications of mental status in the patient's appearance, speech, and behavior. Familiarity with the patient's baseline personality style and previous interactions with physicians is also extremely useful.

A patient may come to the primary practitioner suspicious or convinced that she has a psychiatric illness. She may have been told that she was "crazy," read an article in a magazine, or learned that a friend or relative with similar symptoms has been diagnosed as psychiatrically ill. Her views must be taken seriously, but corroborated with specific findings. The physician's observations about the patient's life circumstances, appearance, and social status should not confound that process. Wealthy and well-loved women can become depressed; successful women can be psychotic. Disadvantaged women are not necessarily depressed; if they are, they deserve and respond to treatment. If the primary physician does not agree with the patient's impression and cannot convince the patient, a referral for psychiatric evaluation or a consultation between the primary provider and a psychiatrist may be necessary to allay the patient's concerns.

Rather than complaining of psychiatric symptoms per se, a patient may allude to adverse family or work events. A patient bereaved, in the throes of divorce, subjected to a natural or human disaster, harassed or fired by an employer, and/or responsible for the care of dependent relatives, should be queried about symptoms of anxiety, depression, post-traumatic stress, or eating disorders. Her level of coping, ability to carry on with her responsibilities and with the functions of eating, sleeping, concentrating, and relating to people, must be ascertained.

A number of psychiatric illnesses can present with somatic symptoms. Conversion disorder, hypochondriasis, and somatization are classic examples, but depression may present as tiredness, psychosis as somatic delusions ("my insides are rotting"), eating disorders as infertility, panic as palpitations and dyspnea, domestic violence as pelvic pain. These presentations are common, and the diagnosis is often missed.

Psychiatric Illnesses: Recognition, Diagnosis, and Interventions

The Diagnostic System

Modern psychiatry is informed by a valid and reliable nosological system, a system whose validity and reliability compare favorably with diagnostic criteria in other areas of medicine. Diagnostic categories are described in the *Diagnostic and Statistical Manual of Mental Disorders* (DSM), the fourth edition of which was published in 1994 (DSM-IV). The Manual is researched and published by the American Psychiatric Association, is compatible with the International Classification of Diseases (ICD) #10, and is used officially in most health care settings in North America and all over the world. Its validity and reliability have been achieved by the use of observable behaviors—rather than imputed intrapsychic memories, motivations, and conflicts—as diagnostic criteria.[74] Field trials have served to further refine and confirm the diagnostic categories. DSM IV's empirical approach makes the system more accessible to the nonpsychiatrist physician. The American Psychiatric Association is also in the process of developing therapeutic guidelines for each diagnostic category. To date, the guidelines for depression and for eating disorders have been released.

Diagnoses in DSM IV are classified along several "axes." Axis I comprises disorders with acute episodes or exacerbations and which cause the patient direct distress.

Axis II consists of personality disorders—chronic disorders in which many or most of an individual's ideas and behaviors derive from a skewed inner experience and view of the world. The manifest behaviors of a person with a personality disorder provoke responses in others which often corroborate and exacerbate this world view. For example, the excessive demands of a person with a dependent personality disorder cause those on whom the demands are made to pull away, deepening the patient's feelings of helplessness and loneliness. She attributes her feelings to the behavior of others, however, not to her own.

Axis III contains the patient's nonpsychiatric medical diagnoses.

DSM IV axes IV and V have to do with the level of stressors in the patient's life and her level of functioning. As with other medical illnesses, the diagnosis of a psychiatric illness influences, but does not completely determine, a patient's ability to relate to others, carry out family, social, and domestic responsibilities, or care for herself.

It is very useful clinically and prognostically to categorize the patient's highest level of functioning during the past year. Similarly, the psychosocial stresses under which she must function will have played a role in the genesis of her psychiatric illness and will go on to figure in the chances for functional recovery.

DSM IV categories are used throughout this chapter. Since some terms are used differently in everyday speech and in psychiatry, and because others are peculiar to psychiatry, a short glossary follows, including terms used in this chapter and others which the primary practitioner may encounter or use.

Affect: Subjective experience of emotion accompanying an idea or mental representation. The word *affect* is often used loosely as a generic term for feeling, emotion, or mood. Affect and emotion are commonly used interchangeably.

Agitation: Excessive motor activity, usually nonpurposeful and associated with internal tension. Examples: Inability to sit still, fidgeting, pacing, wringing of hands, or pulling of clothes.

Ambivalence: The coexistence of contradictory emotions, attitudes, ideas, or desires with respect to a particular person, object, or situation. Ordinarily, it is not fully conscious and suggests psychopathology only when present in an extreme form.

Anhedonia: Inability to experience pleasure from activities that usually produce pleasurable feelings.

Anniversary reaction: An emotional response to a previous event occurring at the same time of year. Often the event involved a loss and the reaction involves a depressed state. The reaction can range from mild to severe and may occur on any anniversary after the event.

Anxiety: Apprehension, tension, or uneasiness from anticipation of danger, the source of which is largely unknown or unrecognized. Anxiety is primarily of intrapsychic origin, in distinction to fear, which is the emotional response to a consciously recognized and usually external threat or danger. Anxiety may be regarded as pathologic when it interferes with effectiveness in living, achievement of desired goals or satisfaction, or reasonable emotional comfort.

Association: Relationship between ideas and emotions by contiguity, continuity, or similarity.

Behavior therapy: A mode of treatment that focuses on modifying observable and, at least in principle, quantifiable behavior by means of systematic manipulation of the environment and behavioral variables though to be functionally related to the behavior.

Character: The sum of a person's relatively fixed personality traits and habitual modes of response.

Compulsion: An insistent, repetitive, intrusive, and unwanted urge to perform an act that is contrary to one's ordinary wishes or standards. Since it serves as a defensive substitute for still more unacceptable unconscious ideas and wishes, failure to perform the compulsive act leads to overt anxiety.

Conflict: A mental struggle that arises from the simultaneous operation of opposing impulses, drives, external (environmental) or internal demands; termed intrapsychic when the conflict is between forces within the personality; extrapsychic, when it is between the self and the environment.

Conversion: A defense mechanism, operating unconsciously, by which intrapsychic conflicts that otherwise would give rise to anxiety are, instead, given symbolic external expression. The repressed ideas or impulses, and the psychological defenses against them, are converted into a variety of somatic symptoms involving the nervous system. These may include such symptoms as paralysis, pain, or loss of sensory function.

Defense mechanism: Unconscious intrapsychic processes serving to provide relief from emotional conflict and anxiety.

Delusion: A false belief firmly held despite incontrovertible and obvious proof or evidence to the contrary. Further, the belief is not one ordinarily accepted by other members of the person's culture or subculture.

Denial: A defense mechanism, operating unconsciously, used to resolve emotional conflict and allay anxiety by disavowing thoughts, feelings, wishes, needs, or external reality factors that are consciously intolerable.

Dysphoria: Unpleasant mood.

Empathy: Insightful awareness, including the meaning and significance of the feelings, emotions, and behavior of another person.

Euphoria: An exaggerated feeling of physical and emotional well-being, usually of psychological origin.

Hallucination: A sensory perception in the absence of an actual external stimulus; this may occur in any of the senses.

Ideas of reference: Incorrect interpretation of casual incidents and external events as having direct reference to oneself.

Loosening of associations: A disturbance of thinking in which ideas shift from one subject to another in an oblique or unrelated manner; the speaker is unaware of the disturbance.

Mood: A pervasive and sustained emotion that, in the extreme, markedly colors one's perception of the world.

Obsession: A persistent, unwanted idea or impulse that cannot be expunged by logic or reasoning.

Panic: Sudden, overwhelming anxiety of such intensity that it produces terror and physiological changes.

Paranoid ideation: Suspiciousness or nondelusional belief that one is being harassed, persecuted, or unfairly treated.

Personality: The characteristic way in which a person thinks, feels, and behaves; the ingrained pattern of behavior that each person evolves, both consciously and unconsciously, as the style of life or way of being in adapting to the environment.

Pressured speech: Rapid, accelerated, frenzied speech.

Psychomotor: Combined physical and mental activity.

Psychosis: A major mental disorder in which a person's ability to think, respond emotionally, remember, communicate, interpret reality, and behave appropriately is sufficiently impaired so as to interfere grossly with the capacity to meet the ordinary demands of life.

Secondary gain: The external gain derived from any illness, such as personal attention and service, monetary gains, disability benefits, and release from unpleasant responsibility.

Thought disorder: A disturbance of speech, communication, or content of thought, such as delusions, ideas of reference, loosening of associations.

Disorders Usually First Diagnosed in Infancy, Childhood, or Adolescence

Mental Retardation Mental retardation is characterized by the onset before age 18 of intellectual function significantly below average (Intelligence Quotient below about 70) that significantly interferes with the individual's performance in her life situation.

This chapter will not discuss the causes, diagnoses, and management of developmental disorders. It is important to note, however, that most medical care requires that a patient, at the very least, have an average capacity to retain, process, and act upon information. The possibility that an adolescent or adult patient is mentally retarded often is overlooked. The diagnosis of mild-to-moderate mental retardation is much more common in the school-age population than in adults, but not because the patients disappear or improve. Once free of the intellectual demands of the academic environment, individuals with mental retardation often find a niche in the family and society and blend into the general population.

An undiagnosed below-average general intelligence and/or specific deficits in cognition can lead to major disruptions in the primary care relationship. The physician is bewildered, frustrated, and angry because the patient fails to follow up on a diagnosis or therapeutic regimen that the physician assumes she understands. The highest level of education the patient attained is a useful piece of information—although patients may inflate the level, may have been unable to finish school despite a normal intelligence, or may have been allowed to continue in mainstream or special classes despite serious disability.

The intelligence relevant to clinical care is that required to comprehend, agree to (or disagree with), and implement medical recommendations, and also to take care of oneself in a general way—to obtain food, clothing, and shelter. Therefore, while specialized intelligence or neuropsychological testing may be necessary in complex situations, a practical assessment performed during the clinical interview is all that is necessary in most cases. The care provider must ask for detailed, practical, and verifiable information directly relevant to the clinical issues at hand: "Tell me how you get pregnant," "How do you get groceries?" "What do you eat for dinner?" "How do you cook that?" "What do you do if your blood sugar is 200?" The same approach is applicable to patients diagnosed with, or suspected of having, dementia or another psychiatric illness that might interfere with self-care or consent capacity.

The needs of the primary care patient with mental retardation extend beyond the evaluation of her ability to understand, consent to, and comply with medical treatment. These needs vary according to the patient's degree of impairment and the circumstances in which she lives. A severely retarded patient is unable to carry out basic self-care. If society or the extended family are not able to provide the resources to maintain the patient, the nuclear family may be severely stressed. The primary practitioner may be called upon to advise, support, and refer the mother or other female relative of a severely retarded person.

The gynecologic and other health care needs of the retarded patient are also at issue. Her intellectual deficits affect her ability to perceive and communicate symptoms of significant disorders. If unable to understand the purpose of physical and laboratory examinations, she is likely to be terrified and uncooperative. Special efforts must be made to prepare and support her. Menstruation can pose challenges of hygiene. Patients with intellectual deficits are at high risk of emotional, physical, and sexual abuse, unable to protect themselves, recognize standards of behavior, and to communicate convincingly in order to obtain help. Parents often seek the expertise of the physician in educating their intellectually impaired daughters about sexuality and making decisions about contraception, sterilization, and pregnancy. Collaboration with specialists in developmental disabilities is essential.

The impact of mild-to-moderate intellectual deficits is largely a factor of the fit between the individual and her environment. A relatively slight degree of retardation may be experienced as a disaster in a subculture of competition and high achievement. On the other hand, an easygoing society may easily accommodate the affected individual in roles consonant with her abilities. The primary practitioner can be of enormous help to the patient and family in accepting and adapting to her limitations and recognizing and employing her strengths.

Attention Deficit/Hyperactivity Disorder Another childhood dysfunction that sometimes persists into adult life is *attention deficit/hyperactivity disorder (ADHD)*. This disorder hampers the patient's ability to pay and sustain attention, follow through, organize, remember, and ignore ordinary distractions. Patients with ADHD encounter a great deal of difficulty in school situations, where they are required to sit, prepare, pay attention, and follow instructions for extended periods. All children must attend school, but adult life offers more options and styles. Some patients develop other psychiatric problems, but others either "grow out of" ADHD or adapt their lifestyles to it. Problems may recur if they are faced in adult life with situations similar to school.

For example, a patient with a placenta previa was hospitalized on bed rest, but often was noted to be up and moving around her hospital room, precipitating episodes of vaginal bleeding. The staff repeatedly explained the dangers of ambulation for the patient and her unborn infant and could not understand what could motivate her to violate such well-reasoned advice. The psychiatric consultant learned that the patient had been constantly "in trouble" in school because she did not sit still, and that prior to her complicated pregnancy she had been extremely active physically. The patient genuinely desired to do what the doctor ordered, but could not comply. She had never enjoyed passive activities such as reading or watching television. The diagnosis of adult ADHD was made. The hospital activity therapist was able to provide the patient with crafts activities she could complete in bed. There were no further psychiatric or obstetric difficulties. The patient was delivered uneventfully and readily adapted to the physical demands of motherhood.

One additional psychiatric disorder of childhood and adolescence may come to the attention of the primary practitioner. *Conduct disorder* is a constellation of dangerously destructive, antisocial behaviors. Since sexual behavior may be one of these, parents may bring a daughter with a conduct disorder to the physician for reproductive education and/or care. It is appropriate to attempt to provide the requested care, but it is not realistic to assume that the young woman will cooperate. Conduct disorder can lead not only to health complications, but to legal problems, and the family is best dealt with by a specialist.

Many other kinds of disorders are manifest early in life, but they are beyond the scope of this chapter. Questions mothers may have about their children are best referred to the pediatrician or to a child and adolescent psychiatrist. The mother's primary practitioner should be alert, when a child exhibits behaviors of concern to the family, for signs and symptoms of stress in the mother. Useful parameters are changes in sleep, appetite, mood, and perceived effectiveness in her various social roles. The primary physician may ask the patient to call or to come for brief visits at shorter intervals than would otherwise be necessary for her care and advise her that s/he is available for counseling or referral if she desires.

Affective or Mood Disorders

The affective disorders include depression and mania, which are unipolar mood disorders, and combinations of the two (manic-depression), which is a bipolar disorder, and variants of these. Ups and downs in affective state are normal. The universality of sad and happy affects help others to understand something of the experience of depression and mania. By the same token, it is difficult for others to understand that depression, mania, and bipolar disorder in which the two alternate, are diseases, not mere variations of mood and not susceptible to cheering up or calming down by the usual means. The failure by family and friends, and by primary physicians, to recognize these conditions for the diseases they are results in unnecessary morbidity and mortality.

Manic-Depression or Bipolar Illness Manic-depression may begin at any time from adolescence through adulthood. The episodes tend to become more frequent and more severe over time; in some patients, cycles are shortened to as little as days or hours. Unipolar mania is quite uncommon; bipolar illness is more frequent, and depression affects up to one-fifth of the population at least once in their lives.[3]

Mania: Mania is a condition that was life-threatening before the advent of effective pharmacologic interventions. Untreated patients can die from the lack of food and rest.

Mania is characterized by:

1. Elevated, expansive, and/or irritable mood
2. Grandiose ideas and behaviors
3. An excess of energy, with reduced sleep
4. Pressured speech
5. Racing thoughts/flight of ideas
6. Excessive involvement in pleasurable activities with high risk for adverse consequences: e.g., reckless expenditures and ill-planned ventures
7. Distractibility
8. Increase in goal-oriented activity or psychomotor agitation

Mild hypomania may be chronic or episodic. The hypomanic individual is full of energy, confident, and intolerant of waiting. Although the excess vitality may be wearing, the hypomanic's zest is somewhat infectious, and her energy and accomplishments may be the envy of both peers and exhausted physicians. The hypomanic patient is also loath to "come down." This disinclination stems both from poor judgment and from the enjoyable quality of the hypomanic state, often making it difficult for the patient with prodromal mania to seek and comply with medical advice during the period when a full-blown episode could be averted. The patient's family may watch helplessly while the patient squanders her own and shared family assets, and embarrasses family and friends by her grandiose, flamboyant, inappropriate behavior.

The primary physician who is alert to the signs and symptoms of mania can make sense of the problem to the family and assume the delicate burden of intervening with the patient. The suspicion of bipolar illness demands timely consultation with a psychiatrist; interventions including neuroleptics, lithium, electroconvulsive treatment, and voluntary or involuntary hospitalization, may be indicated.[49]

Depression: Clinical depression is a common disorder, as mentioned above, and more common in women in most demographic groups.[38] Depression has been accurately diagnosed as early as toddlerhood and throughout the remainder of the life span. Young, unmarried mothers with young children are at highest risk.[22] While marriage decreases the risk for men, married women are at higher risk for depression than are unmarried women.[45] The illness, depression, is characterized by at least five of the following signs and symptoms, which must have persisted for at least two weeks:

1. Sad or irritable mood
2. Decreased energy
3. Decreased interest in usual activities
4. Decreased pleasure
5. Difficulty concentrating
6. Withdrawal from social relationships
7. Thoughts of death or suicide
8. Slowing of thought and action (psychomotor retardation)
9. Changes in sleep
10. Changes in appetite and weight
11. Loss of libido
12. Feelings of worthlessness and guilt
13. Helplessness and hopelessness

In addition to at least five of the above being present, at least one of the symptoms must be either a depressed mood and/or decreased interest or pleasure.

Typically, depression causes decreased sleep, especially early morning awakening. Anxiety, in contrast, results in difficulty falling asleep. Depression also typically decreases appetite, though "atypical depression," more common in younger patients, is associated with increased sleep and increased food intake.

Depression exists along a broad spectrum of clinical severity. The determination whether to treat a depressed patient, to seek consultation, and/or to refer to a mental health professional depends on the interests and competence of the primary physician, the response to a trial of treatment, the availability of psychiatrists, the interest of the patient in primary or specialty care, the existence of diagnostic uncertainty, and the clinical state of the patient. It is extremely unwise for a nonpsychiatrist to assume responsibility for a patient with active suicidal ideation of any kind, unless there is no alternative. The assessment of suicidality is discussed under interviewing techniques. Active delusions and/or hallucinations also demand psychiatric evaluation. (Visual or tactile hallucinations, and auditory hallucinations experienced for the first time after age 40, are often associated with metabolic, infectious, circulatory, degenerative, or neoplastic central nervous system pathology.)

Full-blown clinical depression can be treated in two-thirds of cases with antidepressant medication and/or psychotherapy. Table 39-1 is a chart of antidepressant drugs. Drugs are chosen largely on the basis of their side effects, expense, and convenience of administration, with the newer serotonin reuptake inhibitors requiring only one daily dose. It is not yet clear whether there are significant differences among agents or classes of agents in speed of therapeutic response.

The psychotherapeutic modality that has proven effective on its own is called cognitive therapy.[2] In cognitive therapy, the therapist helps the patient to identify thought patterns of hopelessness, helplessness, and self-reproach, and systematically and willfully to interrupt them and replace them with thoughts of competence, confidence, self-acceptance, and hope. Cognitive therapy requires specific training. Less specific supportive and/or insight-oriented psychotherapy is an important adjunct to pharmacotherapy. The medication reduces or elimi-

TABLE 39-1 Antidepressant Medication

Drug (brand names)	Side Effects	Comments
Tricyclics	All: Quinidine-like slowing of cardiac conduction, weight-gain, impotence	Avoid in patients with heart block
Amitriptyline (Endep, Elavil)	Moderate orthostatic hypotension, sedation, anticholinergic effects	
Desipramine (Norpramin, Pertofrane)	Mild sedation, mild insomnia, mild orthostatic hypotension, mild anticholinergic effects	Also used in bulimia; good for patients with associated panic or anxiety
Doxepin (Adapin, Sinequan)	Sedation, mild anticholinergic effects, orthostatic hypotension	Approved for use in anxiety; used for insomnia
Imipramine (Tofranil, Janimine, SK-Pramine, Tofranil PM sustained release)	Moderate sedation, moderate orthostatic hypotension, moderate anticholinergic effects	Also used in bulimia; good for patients with associated panic or anxiety
Nortriptyline (Pamelor, Aventyl)	Moderate sedation, moderate orthostatic hypotension, moderate anticholinergic effects	
Protriptyline (Vivactil)	Mild sedation, moderate insomnia, moderate anticholinergic effects, mild orthostatic hypotension	
Trimipramine (Surmontil)	Sedation, anticholinergic effects, orthostatic hypotension	
MAOIs	All: Weight-gain, possible impotence, delay in cardiac conduction (rare)	May be better than TCSs in atypical refractory, or bipolar depression
Isocarboxazid (Marplan)	Moderate orthostatic hypotension, moderate insomnia	
Phenelzine (Nardil)	Mild sedation, mild insomnia, orthostatic hypotension	Approved for OCD
Tranylcypromine (Parnate)	Moderate insomnia, mild nausea, orthostatic hypotension	Possible toxic effects: altered mental status, hyperpyrexia, hyperreflexia
Newer Agents		
Amoxapine (Asendin)	Generally less dangerous in overdose, moderate sedation, mild anticholinergic effects, moderate orthostatic hypotension, low delay in cardiac conduction	
Bupropion (Wellbutrin)	Moderate insomnia, low delay in cardiac conduction	
Fluoxetine (Prozac)	Moderate insomnia, moderate nausea, low delay in cardiac conduction	Also used for OCD
Maprotiline (Ludiomil)	Moderate sedation, mild anticholinergic effects, moderate orthostatic hypotension, delay in cardiac conduction	
Trazodone (Desyrel, generic)	Sedation, moderate orthostatic hypotension, mild nausea, low cardiac conduction delay, priapism (rare)	

NOTE: Anticholinergic effects include: dry mouth, constipation, urinary hesitance, blurred vision, confusion.

SOURCE: Adapted from Schatzberg and Cole,[62] Potter et al.[57]

nates the signs and symptoms of clinical illness, while the talking therapy helps the patient to understand how her history and circumstances affect her susceptibility to depression, to improve her personal relationships and effectiveness, and to decrease the likelihood of recurrence.

Mood Disorders Limited to Women *Premenstrual Dysphoric Disorder:* Some menstruating women complain of irritability and transiently depressed mood premenstrually, or "premenstrual syndrome," "PMS." Physical symptoms of breast tenderness, bloating, headache, etc., are even more common premenstrually. Studies estimating the number of women with symptoms of PMS report from 5 to 95 percent.[73] Many of these retrospective accounts of psychological changes cannot be corroborated by prospective daily ratings. Most interventions tested, including hormone, antianxiety, and antidepressant medications, exercise regimens, and dietary changes, have been reported to be effective. Since there has been no scientific agreement on criteria for the diagnosis of "PMS," the older and much of the current literature can be difficult to analyze and compare.

Beginning with the publication of DSM III-R in 1987, the American Psychiatric Association has sought to differentiate a diagnosable mental illness from the more common "PMS," in hopes of standardizing research and improving knowledge about etiology and treatment. It is believed that approximately 4 to 7 percent of menstruating women suffer from this condition. No specific hormonal concomitants have yet been identified. DSM IV lists "Premenstrual Dysphoric Disorder" (PMDD) as an example of an otherwise unspecified depressive disorder and enumerates the diagnostic criteria in the Appendix of Disorders Requiring Further Study as follows:

The confirmation by two months of prospective daily ratings of the following signs and symptoms, occurring premenstrually, remitting menstrually, interfering markedly with domestic, educational, and/or work responsibilities, and not caused by another psychiatric disorder:

1. Irritability
2. Mood lability
3. Difficulty concentrating
4. Anxiety
5. Decreased interest in usual activities

The following is a suggested protocol for the evaluation and treatment of a woman who complains of premenstrual psychological symptoms:

1. Perform a complete physical examination to rule out pelvic and/or systemic causes of malaise.
2. Take a careful and thorough history, including past psychiatric history, past sexual, physical, and psychological abuse, and current living circumstances. PMDD is associated with an increased lifetime, but not current, diagnosis of major depressive episodes, and with a history of abuse. The patient may fail to note a chronic depression, dysphoria, and/or personality disorder, because of lack of insight, fear of stigma, or acceptance of the disorder as a fact of life. It has also been postulated that the premenstruum merely mobilizes feelings and behaviors appropriate to adverse circumstances that are suppressed during the remainder of the cycle.
3. Instruct the patient to begin charting her symptoms on a prospective, daily basis. The use of a calendar with an individual sheet for each day is preferable. The menstrual cycle should be charted separately.
4. Inquire about the patient's life situation, life stressors, and coping techniques.
5. Suggest that the patient decrease or eliminate her use of caffeine, nicotine, and alcohol.
6. Help the patient to establish regular and health-promoting exercise, sleep, and dietary habits.
7. Continue to follow and get to know the patient over time. Symptoms of abuse, personality disorders, and/or depression may become apparent only on longer acquaintance and when she feels more at ease in the doctor-patient relationship. If another discrete disorder is identified, treat or refer as outlined in the relevant section of this chapter. If no other diagnosis is identified, and the symptoms do not respond to the lifestyle changes suggested, the patient may

respond to fluoxetine or another antidepressant, in the usual doses.

Postpartum Psychiatric Symptoms: As mentioned above, there is ongoing scientific dispute about the existence of a discrete postpartum psychiatric disorder, whether depression or psychosis. Evidence for the efficacy of hormonal treatment is problematic, but some clinicians do treat patients with progesterone. The practical problems for the primary practitioner, especially one who is an obstetrician, are: the fact that patients are now discharged from the inpatient setting very soon after delivery, the universal stress of adjusting to life with a newborn, and the subsequent difficulty of differentiating a normal reaction from the prodrome or onset of a serious psychiatric illness.

Fifty to 80 percent of U.S. women manifest a brief, self-limited, period of affective lability within a few days of delivery.[61] Though crying is very common, new mothers often report that sadness is not precisely what they experience, but rather a globally heightened emotionality. Probably hormonal changes, physical exhaustion, psychological adjustment, and social factors all figure in the etiology of this benign disturbance. Perinatal customs in the United States, unlike those in many other societies, provide for increasingly intense monitoring of a woman through pregnancy and delivery, with an abrupt fall-off at hospital discharge. This sequence derives from custom and from assessments of obstetric risk, but does not correspond to the psychological experience and needs of many patients. During pregnancy, there are multiple anxieties, adjustments, and discomforts, but the fetus is cared for more or less automatically. In Chinese and Nigerian societies, care for the mother is focused heavily on the postpartum rather than the antepartum period.[12] Psychiatric sequelae of childbirth in those cultures may be less frequent and most often is attributable to the family's reaction to the failure of the mother to produce a healthy infant of the desired sex.

Frank depressive or psychotic illness may manifest gradually or suddenly within days or weeks of delivery. The newly delivered mother who has the psychiatric illness typically is sleepless, agitated, increasingly inattentive to nutrition and personal hygiene, and preoccupied with concerns or delusions about the newborn. Psychosis may exist on its own or as a concomitant of depression. The delusional postpartum patient can pose mortal risk to her infant. Depression alone impairs the woman's ability to develop affection for her child and confidence in her maternal role. Friends and relatives may make matters worse by reminding the woman how lucky she is to have a healthy child and how this period should be the happiest of her life. She feels increasingly inadequate and guilty about her inability to react as they—and she—expect. Many cases of postpartum depression go undiagnosed and untreated, leaving women with a lifelong sense of fear, guilt, loss, and inadequacy associated with the delivery. The clinical approach to psychological symptoms following childbirth should take into account both the frequency of benign reactions and the risks of severe psychiatric illness:

1. Information about the possibility of a period of emotional lability should be part of the routine postpartum education of every newly delivered woman.
2. Since patients leave the hospital soon after childbirth, routine telephone contact by a member of the primary care team can provide support, information, and monitoring for obstetric, pediatric, and psychiatric complications.
3. When a patient complains of, or a family member observes, symptoms including sleeplessness (even when the infant is asleep), weeping, agitation, sadness, guilt, and/or obsessive thoughts, explain that transient psychological changes after birth are common, but that on rare occasions there are more serious complications.
4. Advise the patient, and the family, with her permission, to call immediately if there is an abrupt change, and daily to advise you about her condition.
5. Obtain psychiatric consultation if the patient's symptoms do not improve or grow worse. Obtain immediate consultation for patients with psychotic symptoms or ruminations about harming the infant.

6. Women who have experienced episodes of postpartum depression/psychosis are at increased risk for repeated episodes after subsequent deliveries. Their postpartum care should be comanaged with a psychiatrist, whom the patient may want to meet prior to delivery so that they know and feel comfortable with each other. They can be reassured that psychiatric complications, if detected early, respond well to treatment.

Anxiety Disorders

Anxiety, as defined above, consists of a feeling of dread, with accompanying somatic manifestations, in the absence of a stimulus or situation indicating realistic danger (the response to such a situation is fear). The anxiety disorders comprise panic disorder, agoraphobia, specific phobias, social phobia, obsessive-compulsive disorder, post-traumatic stress disorder, acute stress disorder, generalized anxiety disorder, and anxiety disorders secondary to a general medical condition or substance use.

Panic attacks occur in several anxiety disorders, and are of particular importance to the primary practitioner because they often lead patients to seek care in the emergency room or clinic, convinced that they are suffering from a life-threatening cardiac or respiratory disorder. A panic attack is a discrete period of intense fear or discomfort, with the abrupt onset of four or more of the following additional symptoms:

1. Palpitations, increased heart rate, a sense of pounding
2. Diaphoresis
3. Trembling
4. Shortness of breath
5. Choking feeling
6. Thoracic discomfort
7. Nausea or gastrointestinal upset
8. Dizziness, lightheadedness, unsteadiness
9. Feelings of unreality
10. Fear of going crazy, losing control
11. Fear of dying
12. Paresthesias
13. Chills or hot flushes

The diagnosis of *panic disorder* requires: recurrent panic attacks without a specific trigger situation, and a month or more of concern about future attacks or deleterious consequences of attacks, or behavioral changes related to the attacks. *Agoraphobia* consists of anxiety about the prospect of being in a situation where symptoms of panic might occur, and anxiety that the patient will be unable to escape or obtain help. This anxiety leads the patient to avoid those situations, to enlist the presence of a companion, and/or to endure the situations despite the discomfort. Panic disorder and agoraphobia can occur separately or in combination.

Specific phobias are unreasonable fears of specific objects or situations, despite the patient's recognition that there is no real danger, eliciting avoidance or discomfort that interferes with relationships and normal functioning. Phobias particularly likely to become evident in the primary care situation include fear of blood or injections and fear of vomiting. Social phobia is a chronic, severe fear of situations where the patient will encounter and be observed by others; she imagines that she will humiliate herself in some way. Although she realizes that her fears are out of proportion to the situation, she either endures the pain of social situations or avoids them, causing deterioration in her relationships or normal performance.

Obsessive-compulsive disorder is characterized by *obsessions*—irrepressible, recurrent thoughts, impulses, or images that the patient recognizes as products of her own mentation but cannot obliterate. These may occur with *compulsions*—pointless, repetitive behaviors she feels driven to perform to forestall some dreaded events with which they have no causal relationship, and that significantly intrude upon her life. The disorder can be utterly disabling, with the patient spending nearly all her waking hours in various rituals. The natural course for over half the patients is chronic. The psychodynamic etiologies and treatments of past decades have been largely superseded by neurobiological explanations, centering especially on disregulation of serotonin. The most promising treatment for obsessive-compulsive disorder is psychopharmacologic. Clomipramine, a tricyclic antidepressant that blocks

5-HT reuptake more effectively than other tricyclics, is effective in a majority of cases.

Post-traumatic stress disorder (PTSD) results from a traumatic event that confronts the individual with actual or threatened death or serious injury to herself or others, resulting in terror, horror, and/or a sense of helplessness at the time of the occurrence. Afterward, the individual psychologically reexperiences the event through intrusive thoughts, upsetting dreams, "flashbacks" in which the event seems to be recurring, and subjective distress or physiologic reactivity in response to reminders of the event. As a result, the patient feels emotionally numb, disinterested, or detached, and makes efforts to avoid situations that recall the event. She may be unable to remember some aspects of the trauma. At the same time, she is hyperarousable, with irritability, difficulty concentrating, and/or sleep disturbance. PTSD was first noted in veterans of military combat, but is not limited to that group. The clinician should be alert for signs and symptoms of this disorder in victims of domestic and nondomestic violence, disasters, war, and other traumatic events.

A patient with generalized anxiety disorder suffers from chronic, irrational, excessive nervousness or worry not caused by any other psychiatric or medical disorder that causes her significant distress or loss of function. Associated with the anxiety are three or more of the following symptoms: restlessness, fatigability, difficulty concentrating, irritability, muscle tension, or sleep disturbance. One antianxiety agent, Buspirone, has been introduced specifically for use in patients with chronic anxiety. Reports of its efficacy are contradictory.

There are specific diagnostic designations for anxiety resulting from a general medical condition or substance use. Anxiety is a common human experience, especially among a population seeking medical attention. Pharmacologic agents, notably the benzodiazepines, are effective anxiolytics. However, these medications are among the most commonly prescribed drugs in the United States, raising concern that they are used too often as a first or only approach.[11] When a patient is in distress, it is often difficult for her physician to conclude the medical visit without providing something tangible—and this something is often a prescription for a minor tranquilizer.

Some physicians have too little confidence in the power of their listening, talking, and caring, and feel concern that they have too little time for them in today's busy practices. If medication is prescribed after the first interview, the physician never has the opportunity to observe the effectiveness of the doctor-patient interaction itself on the patient's anxiety, and may leave the patient with the impression that medication is thought to be the answer to all problems. Other physicians are reluctant to use any "mind-altering" medications, urging upon patients a stiff-upper-lip mentality regardless of the circumstances. Anxiety, like any other symptom, is optimally explored before or while being treated:

- When did it begin?
- Under what circumstances?
- What is it that you're nervous about?
- Is it getting better or worse?
- What brings it on and/or alleviates it?
- How is it affecting your life?

Allow the patient some time to explain and explore her anxiety. You may discover misconceptions about her symptoms, diagnosis, or treatment that can readily be allayed with accurate information. See the patient for a follow-up visit in a few days and ask her how it felt to talk about her feelings. Although the treatment of anxiety can often be accomplished without medication, and the medications that are used are always evolving, some medications that may be helpful for patients with anxiety disorders are listed in Table 39-2.

Panic disorder, agoraphobia, obsessive-compulsive disorder, generalized anxiety, PTSD, and specific phobias have been treated successfully both with behavioral psychotherapy and with antianxiety and antidepressant medications. Any of these diseases can be utterly crippling for a patient and tremendously disruptive to her family. Because the treatments are specialized, and because new approaches are rapidly evolving, it is probably best to consult with, or refer the patient to, a psychiatrist

TABLE 39-2 Compounds Used for Anxiety

Medication	Trade Name	Rate of Absorption[a]	Half-Life[b]	Active Long-Acting Metabolite	Comments
Benzodiazepines					Metabolism of benzodiazepines is inhibited by cimetidine, disulfiram, isoniazid and oral contraceptives Metabolism of benzodiazepines is enhanced by rifampin
Alprazolam	Xanax	Intermediate	Intermediate	No	Preferred in elderly patients of patients with poor hepatic function
Chlordiazepoxide	Librium, others	Intermediate	Intermediate	Yes	
Clonazepam	Klonopin	Long	Long	No	
Clorazepate	Tranxene, others	Short	Short	Yes	
Diazepam	Valium, others	Short	Long	Yes	Half-life increased three or four times in elderly patients
Lorazepam	Ativan, others	Intermediate	Intermediate	No	Preferred in elderly patients or patients with poor hepatic function
Oxazepam	Serax	Long	Intermediate	No	Preferred in elderly patients or patients with poor hepatic function
Prazepam	Centrax	Long	Short	Yes	
Atypical agent					
Buspirone	BuSpar				Not effective in panic disorder, little sedation, little risk of dependence/tolerance

[a]Long ≥2 h; Intermediate = 1–2 h; Short ≤1 h.

[b]Long >20 h; Intermediate = 6–20 h; Short <6 h.

SOURCE: Adapted from Gilman AG, Rall TW, Nies AS, Taylor P (eds): *The Pharmacological Basis of Therapeutics,* 8th ed. New York, McGraw-Hill, 1990.

who specializes in anxiety disorders. Many academic departments of psychiatry offer clinics and new research protocols for these illnesses. The primary practitioner will want to remain involved, to coordinate the patient's psychiatric care with other aspects of her health care, and to offer support and interpretation to her family.

Psychotic Illness

Psychotic illnesses include schizophrenia, paranoia, brief reactive psychoses, and psychotic symptoms secondary to other systemic and/or central nervous system diseases. Despite immense recent strides in the understanding and treatment of psychosis, the stigma is little changed from decades ago. Psychotic patients are frequently impoverished and medically ill, but lack the skills and the advocates to access what meager social and medical services are available without continuing care and support. We see untreated psychotic citizens on our streets and in our prisons, which have dramatically increased their capacities just as the psychiatric hospitals have shrunk and closed or reduced their capacities.

Although psychotic illness is the most florid psychiatric condition, and the one most caricatured in folklore and the arts, it can actually be overlooked in the primary care setting, particularly if open-ended questions are not asked by the physician.

Schizophrenia occurs in 1 percent of the world population. Especially since the "deinstitutionalization" of the chronically psychiatrically ill in the 1960s and 1970s, affected individuals can be expected in every primary practice setting. Derived from the Greek for "split mind," schizophrenia originally referred to the patient's emotional distance from his/her own behaviors and to the preservation of cognitive functions such as orientation and memory despite the intrusion of hallucinations and delusions.

The etiology of schizophrenia includes biological and environmental components. Current research implicates disruptions in neurodevelopment as a contributing factor.[48] The likelihood of the disease is increased in relatives of those with schizophrenia. The signs and symptoms generally manifest in adolescence or early adulthood; onset in the 30s or later is rare. First-onset psychosis in middle age or later should prompt the physician to initiate an investigation for systemic and/or central nervous system disease. Patients who become schizophrenic may have been considered perfectly normal as children; some are described as having been distant and "odd." Onset may be insidious, with gradual withdrawal from social contacts, deterioration in functioning (schizophrenia was once called "dementia praecox"), neglect of personal hygiene, and increasingly bizarre ideas and behavior. Sometimes onset is more abrupt; frantic patients will call the primary care physician because their late adolescent/young adult child is flagrantly psychotic and out of control.

The diagnostic criteria for schizophrenia include positive symptoms of delusions, hallucinations, disorganized speech or behavior, and negative symptoms of affective flattening and diminished speech and activity. These symptoms must persist for six months or more and markedly worsen the patient's social and/or occupational functioning. They must not be the result of a mood, substance use, or some other medical disorder. There are many subcategories and degrees of severity of schizophrenia.

Many patients with schizophrenia, properly treated and followed, can live in the community and support and care for themselves. Schizophrenia in and of itself is not grounds to deny a patient care or the right to make decisions about that care. Patients who have not required hospitalization ever, or for some years, can be cared for by an interested primary care practitioner in close collaboration with a psychiatrist. In most cases of schizophrenia, the psychiatrist will need to assume direct responsibility for the care of the mental disorder while the primary care provider oversees other aspects of medical care.

Paranoid schizophrenia: "Paranoid" is yet another misused term, often applied to situations in which one feels more or less rightly resentful or suspicious. Genuinely paranoid ideation connotes not only the fear that something bad is likely to happen, but the conviction, in the absence of logical evidence, that others are consciously and purposely plotting to inflict harm in some way. Paranoid disorders may present in primary care setting as persons with seemingly rational complaints about past medical care, or with somatic symptoms for which they blame conspirators in the home, neighborhood, work place, or major institution (e.g., the Federal Bureau of Investigation). Since family members, employers, coworkers, and neighbors can and do harass, torment, and injure people at times, and since such treatment can result in direct or psychologically mediated physical symptoms and illness, such complaints must not be discounted out of hand. The following points are often helpful in differentiation. The paranoid patient is more likely than the abused patient to volunteer her story, to tell it repeatedly and insistently, and to attribute all her troubles to mistreatment by others.

Schizoaffective disorder includes signs and symptoms of schizophrenia concurrent with those of a depressive or manic episode. A *brief psychotic disorder* consists of psychotic symptoms lasting at least one day but not meeting criteria for schizophrenia. Patients with *delusional disorders* not infrequently present in primary care settings. Their symptoms do not meet criteria for schizophrenia, but are limited to nonbizarre delusions—delusions that could be true: for example, being poisoned, deceived in love, having a disease. Aside from the effects of these unfounded beliefs, the patient's functioning does not deteriorate. Patients may present to their primary physicians convinced that they have a sexually transmitted disease, that they emanate an unpleasant odor, or that a famous person is in love with them. The primary practitioner need neither attempt to disprove the delusion nor pretend to believe it. The focus should be on the patient's distress. High-potency neuroleptics such as trifluoperazine and haloperidol may be useful.

Somatoform Disorders

Patients with somatoform disorders experience and manifest psychological distress in the form of somatic pains and disabilities rather than in disturbances of thought, feeling, or behavior. This substitution is completely unconscious; that is, the patient does not consciously create, mimic, or manipulate physical signs of illness. Somatoform disorders include somatization disorder, conversion disorder, undifferentiated somatoform disorder, and ''somatoform disorder not otherwise specificed.''

Somatization disorders begin before the age of 30 and extend over several years, with many physical complains resulting in a search for health care and/or in impairment of life functioning. Either the symptoms cannot be explained by a known medical condition or the complaints and impairment exceed what seems to be justified by objective findings. Some time during the course of the disorder, the patient will have manifested each of the following:

1. Pain related to four different anatomical sites or physiologic functions
2. Two gastrointestinal symptoms
3. One sexual or reproductive symptom
4. One pseudoneurologic symptom or deficit other than pain

The precise incidence of somatization disorder is not known, since the patients visit many physicians, each of whom may not be aware of the full spectrum of complaints and history. The patients' own perceptions are that they are the unfortunate victims of general ''sickliness'' and/or a host of physical illnesses which their physicians are not always able to diagnose and treat effectively. Although they do not hide their history, their preoccupation with a current complaint may overshadow it; careful inquiries about the listed criteria must be made. An abdomen crisscrossed with surgical scars is an ominous sign.

Unfortunately, the diagnosis of a somatoform disorder, in and of itself, can never rule out the possibility of a somatic disorder that requires medical intervention. However, invasive procedures and potent medications should be contemplated with caution. Neither is it effective to insist that the symptoms are baseless. This is a chronic illness. The best management approach is to sympathize with the patient about the vexing nature of her symptoms, minimize complex diagnostic and therapeutic procedures, offer psychological support through frequent but short outpatient visits, and encourage and applaud her ability to fulfill her responsibilities despite her suffering.

A *conversion disorder* consists of voluntary motor or sensory complaints or loss of function that do not result from diagnosable medical illness, are not deliberately produced by the patient, and that seem to be related to psychological conflicts and/or stress. This is the disorder historically known as ''hysteria.'' The disorder is diagnosed more often in women, often in less socially and psychologically sophisticated patients.[30] The psychological etiology may be complex or relatively transparent. Medical illness must be carefully ruled out; patients with such disorders as multiple sclerosis not uncommonly are painfully dismissed as ''hysterical'' for some interval before the correct diagnosis is made. Prognosis is directly related to the length of time the symptom has been present. In an acute situation, a 45-min interview can, not infrequently, reveal the source of the problem to the physician and the patient and alleviate the symptoms. *Pain disorder* is a related condition in which pain with a significant psychological etiology disrupts the patient's life and brings her to medical attention.

The medical staff may be tempted to trick a patient with an obvious conversion disorder into revealing the normality of the affected body part. Superficially, such maneuvers can be effective. For example, the patient with a conversion paraplegia will manage to ambulate if someone yells "Fire!" However, this crude duplicity ultimately backfires; the source of the patient's distress is not illuminated, the patient is humiliated, and the doctor-patient relationship is ruptured. It is preferable to design a face-saving, step-wise course of treatment for the patient, described with reassurance and confidence by the primary physician. For example, the dysphagic patient may be prescribed a dietary regimen beginning with liquids and progressing incrementally to pureed foods, soft foods, and finally a regular diet. The paralyzed patient can progress from wheelchair to crutches to cane. The family should be instructed to facilitate the course of treatment but to avoid structuring their lives around the patient's illness.

Hypochondriasis often is confused with somatization disorder. The hypochondriacal patient's preoccupation is not with physical symptoms per se, but with a nondelusional fear or conviction that she has a serious disease, despite medical reassurance. She overinterprets normal bodily sensations as omens of disaster. Treatment, as with somatization, is aimed at restoring function rather than eliminating symptoms.

A patient with *body dysmorphic disorder* is preoccupied with some imagined or trivial defect in appearance. When there is any hint of this disturbance, a patient should be referred for a full psychiatric evaluation before undertaking cosmetic surgery.

Factitious Disorders

This is a complex and mysterious group of disorders in which the patient actively causes or consciously feigns her own somatic damage. It is easy, and has been traditional, to ascribe these disorders to patients' enjoyment of the invalid role.[72] However, everyone wants attention, care, and freedom from onerous responsibilities; but few are willing to harm and hospitalize themselves to obtain them. These patients are extraordinarily adept at producing medical histories and physical examinations that assure them hospital admission. They willingly submit themselves to painful and dangerous diagnostic and therapeutic procedures. They do not, however, submit themselves to psychiatric examination; few of them have been studied in depth. Patients with factitious disorders often are very winning with medical staff, mobilizing whole units to worry about them. When the true diagnosis begins to be suspected, staff are conflicted and enraged. Not uncommonly, the condition is brutally revealed when staff search the patient's room without her knowledge or consent (despite the fact that this is unethical), finding medical equipment or medications. At this point she leaves the hospital abruptly, only to take her story to another facility.

Persons who feign illness to gain specific, realistic ends such as release from prison or military service are *malingerers.*

Dissociative Disorders

Dissociative experiences and disorders do not present frequently in primary practice. Dissociation is a process in which some aspect of the patient's behavior or experience is rendered inaccessible to the rest of her consciousness. The disorders include amnesia, fugue (sudden travel away from home, with inability to recall the past), identity disorders ("multiple personality disorders"), and depersonalization (feeling "outside oneself").

Sexual and Gender Identity Disorders

Each category of sexual dysfunction can be classified as to whether it is due to a combination of factors or to psychological factors alone, whether it is lifelong or acquired, and whether it occurs in all situations or only particular ones. Disorders correspond to the stages of genital arousal—disorders of desire, arousal, and orgasm. There are also sexual pain disorders and sexual dysfunctions secondary to a general medical condition or substance use. Little is known about what makes a particular level of sexual interest or activity "normal." At best, we may have an idea of what is normative and/or expected in a given subculture. There are no sexual equivalents to caloric or nutritional requirements. One can live without conscious sexual feelings or behavior, but not without food. On the one hand, sexual activity may be extremely difficult to suppress, even under the most adverse circumstances; on the other, sexual feelings and activity are very susceptible to psychological conflicts and social context. Assessment and treatment of sexual complaints are discussed below in the section of the same name.

Homosexuality is no longer considered to be an illness.

Gender identity disorders are those in which the patient does not feel comfortable with her own gender. This disorder is more common in men.[13]

There are a variety of "paraphilias," or perversions, classified in DSM IV: exhibitionism, fetishism, pedophilia, sexual sado-masochism, voyeurism, and transvestic fetishism. Diagnosis and treatment of these disorders is best performed by subspecialists.

Disorders of Cognition: Delirium, Dementia, Amnesia

Delirium consists of decreased orientation and ability to initiate and sustain attention, with changes in memory, language, and/or perception, developing over hours to days, fluctuating during the course of the day, and not due to a preexisting dementia. Delirium is caused by a general medical condition that interferes with brain function, and/or by the use of a substance. In the context of an acute care environment, the onset of a delirium may go unnoticed. Despite the fact that a postoperative or otherwise ill patient may appear lucid, make appropriate brief social responses, and make no objections to ongoing treatment, her mental status cannot be assumed without a specific determination. Routine "mini" mental status examinations can provide a baseline if there are problems later, and can prevent situations in which the patient suddenly removes access lines, hurts or frightens herself or others, and/or attempts to leave the hospital.

Dementia is characterized by multiple cognitive deficits including memory (registration and recall) and aphasia, apraxia, agnosia, or disturbance in organizing or abstracting. The course of dementia is determined by its underlying cause. The Alzheimer's type, in which no specific etiology can be identified, has an insidious, gradual onset and a progressive course. Vascular dementia is associated with focal neurologic signs and symptoms. Dementia also can be caused by a wide variety of general medical and central nervous system diseases and by the abuse of substances.

Since women live longer than men, and are much more likely to assume responsibility for dependent family members, women are doubly affected by dementia.[40] Patients seen in primary care may be suffering from a dementia and/or caring for someone else with dementia. Caring for a spouse afflicted with dementia is a grinding, draining task. The primary physician can help the patient who is providing care locate helpful resources. It is important to monitor her condition—her ability to care for herself and her dependent relative—and to encourage her to allow herself to relax. Decisions about overriding a patient's wishes and autonomy are among the most ethically complex and painful in medical practice. The primary practitioner can draw on essential knowledge about a patient's baseline level of function, supports, philosophy of life, and previously expressed wishes.

The physician's task is more complicated when the patient herself is suspected of having a dementia. As with delirium, patients may retain the ability to make appropriate brief social responses in the face of substantial cognitive impairment. They are generally terrified and humiliated by memory and other lapses, and make great efforts to hide or compensate for them. Again, formal assessment of cognition must be performed. What is particularly important is the patient's ability to keep herself safe, fed, clothed, and housed. The physician may have to decide to contact family members, even over the patient's objections.

Eating Disorders

Women's preoccupation with slenderness and food intake is endemic in most subcultures in our society. In the middle classes, only a minority of women do not report that they are heavier than they would prefer. Physicians may unwittingly reinforce this preoccupation by praising slim patients and scolding heavier ones.

Eating disorders involve other signs and symptoms in addition to changes in eating habits. The syndrome of *anorexia nervosa* includes an intense fear of becoming fat, amenorrhea, the use of body size as an indicator of one's self-worth, and refusal to acknowledge and address dangerously low body mass. Weight loss may be achieved by food restriction or by purging with laxatives or inducing vomiting after eating. The patient with *bulimia nervosa* has episodes in which she experiences her eating as out of control. She eats inordinate amounts of food during discrete "binges," and then compensates by fasting, excessive exercise, vomiting, and/or using diuretics or laxatives. She also measures her self-esteem, chronically low, by her weight.

Overeating is an eating disorder that is often overlooked, even though obesity is a major public health problem. Obese patients, unlike those with other eating disorders, are ostracized by society. They are often the butt of jokes, and they are discriminated against in all kinds of competitive situations. While underweight patients are viewed as victims of illness, overweight patients are considered infantile and self-indulgent. Unless the patient's weight has put her at medical risk, the best approach may be to ask her how she feels about her weight, to assure her that she will not be lectured about it, and to let her know that the physician will offer advice if and when she wants to deal with the problem. Patients who are morbidly obese are in serious medical danger and this must be addressed. Some patients do not do well psychologically if forced to lose weight.[36]

Eating disorders may present directly or indirectly in primary care. In the gynecology setting, anorexic patients may complain of amenorrhea, and childless patients of infertility, without recognizing the connection between their inadequate food intake and these gynecologic signs and symptoms. Dentists and physicians who examine the oral cavity sometimes make a presumptive diagnosis of recurrent self-induced vomiting on the basis of a characteristic pattern of erosion of dental enamel. Anorexia and bulimia can cause grave metabolic disturbance, and can be associated with serious psychiatric conditions such as depression. They may be fatal. They are best treated by a team of primary physician and psychiatrist.

Substance-Related Disorders

The psychiatric nomenclature includes categories for syndromes associated with alcohol, amphetamines, caffeine, cannabis, cocaine, hallucinogens, inhalants, nicotine, opioids, phencyclidine, sedative/hypnotic/anxiolytics, and polysubstances. The primary practitioner responsible for triage in an emergency room or a similar setting will be familiar with the signs of acute intoxication and withdrawal from each of these agents. For office and inpatient primary practice, the critical issues are alertness to the possibility of substance use and abuse in every patient and awareness of the association between substance use and other psychiatric and medical disorders. While the questions may seem intrusive, irrelevant, or tactless, they may be literally lifesaving.

The use or non-use of substances cannot be inferred, but must be specifically inquired about: What alcoholic beverages/cigarettes/prescription medications/other drugs do you use? How often? How much? Do you use it to the point of intoxication? Does the use of the substance cause concern or friction with significant others? Have you had episodes in which you could not remember afterwards what had happened while you were using the substance?

The general categories of substance-related disorders are substance dependence, substance abuse, substance intoxication, and substance withdrawal (DSM IV Draft Criteria, H:5 and H:6). Substance dependence consists of a pattern of use that causes distress and life impairment, with three from among the following findings seen during one year: tolerance, withdrawal, increasing and prolonged use, inability to control the use, continued use despite known adverse physical or psychological sequelae, the consumption of substantial amounts of time around substance use, and the loss or reduction of significant life activities because of the use. Substance abuse consists of a pattern of substance use causing significant distress or life impairment manifested by the use of the substance under at least one of the following circumstances during a year: failure to fulfill major role obligations, physical hazard, legal problems, or continued use despite social and interpersonal problems.

The diagnosis and treatment of substance abuse disorders in women is complicated by discriminatory societal attitudes that stigmatize women who abuse alcohol and other substances as "immoral." There is a traditional assumption that the consumption of substances is associated with promiscuous sexual behavior.[53] Substance use puts women at greater risk for sexual victimization; when sexual assaults occur, the male perpetrator who is intoxicated may be viewed as less culpable, while the female victim is considered more guilty.[16] Women addicts may resort to prostitution rather than more violent criminal activity to obtain money for drugs. Women in relationships with substance-abusing men may be pressured to use those substances, and often suffer a host of medical, psychiatric, and social consequences, regardless of socioeconomic class.

Given a dose of alcohol standardized for body weight, women's blood alcohol levels are higher than men's. Social custom dictates that women consume less alcohol than men, but alcohol intake, especially among younger women, has been rising steadily. Approximately 5 percent of the adult female population is estimated to suffer from either alcohol dependence or alcohol abuse. The male-to-female ratio is 2:1. Inner-city, criminal justice, and military populations are reported to be at higher risk; patients with family histories of alcoholism may be as well.[16] There are strong associations between substance abuse and low self-esteem, depression, and a history of victimization. Since women are more likely to be prescribed sedatives and minor tranquilizers, they are at risk for overlapping dependencies and addictions.

Sleep Disorders

Sleep disorders are also termed dyssomnias. Disturbances of sleep are frequently caused by general medical conditions and psychiatric illnesses. Primary sleep disturbances include insomnia, hypersomnia, narcolepsy (irresistible attacks of sleep, with brief episodes of sudden loss of muscle tone), breathing-related sleep disorder ("sleep apnea"), and disorders of circadian rhythm, which may be spontaneous or secondary to changes in time zone or work schedule. Entrenched sleep disorders can be evaluated in a sleep laboratory, where sleeping electroencephalograms and other parameters are measured. Short-term sleep disturbances are best approached with "sleep hygiene." Many patients do not realize that their life-styles are causing sleep problems. Suggestions include:

1. Decrease or stop caffeine intake
2. Regular exercise
3. Nutritious diet
4. Calming activities in the hour before bedtime: warm bath, low-key reading material, music, television program
5. Regular bedtime routine
6. Removal of anxiety-producing items (bills, work) from the bedside

Hypnotic agents can be useful in the short term after a traumatic experience or to break the wakefulness cycle. However, there is some question as to whether they continue to be useful. Patients tend to become psychologically and physiologically dependent on them with long-term use.[9]

Impulse Disorders

This is a group of conditions in which the patient experiences increasing tension which is relieved abruptly by the performance of a behavior dangerous to herself or others. Impulse disorders include intermittent explosive disorder (outbursts of aggression without reasonable precipitants), kleptomania (stealing), pyromania (fire-setting), pathologic gambling, and trichotillomania (pulling out one's hair). These diagnoses may be made by a primary physician to whom the patient confides, or after apprehension by the police. These conditions, however, are not usually treated by primary physicians. The existence of a diagnosable psychiatric disorder does not exonerate the patient from legal culpability.

Adjustment Disorders

Many of the psychiatric symptoms brought to the attention of the primary practitioner are the result of adjustment disorders. An adjustment disorder occurs in response to a specific stress, within three months after its onset, and ceases spontaneously within six months after the stress ends. The stress may cause depressed mood, anxiety, behavioral disturbances, or any combination, that cause the patient distress and/or interfere with her normal functioning. The symptoms must not be the result of any other psychiatric disorder or of *uncomplicated bereavement.* Adjustment disorders are treated with brief outpatient psychotherapy, augmented with psychopharmacologic agents to relieve specific symptoms if necessary.

Bereavement leads to signs and symptoms much like a psychiatric disorder: sleep and eating disturbances, preoccupation with the person who has died, loss of interest and pleasure in usual activities and relationships. Both clinicians and our society in general tend to underestimate the length and severity of normal reactions to the loss of an important person or function in a patient's life. The grief reaction need not follow any regular sequences, and may recur on anniversaries of the death or of special occasions with the loved one. However, if a patient does not begin to feel better after six months and is unable to go on with her life—even sadly—office counseling is in order. The patient may be experiencing guilt, conscious or unconscious, over her interactions with the person who died. A protracted grief reaction that does not respond to office counseling requires psychiatric consultation.

Personality Disorders

Personality or character disorders, comprise Axis II of DSM IV. These disorders do not cause symptoms, per se; patients do not usually complain of them, but rather of the complications they cause in relationships with others. However, personality disorders can cause aggravation and sometimes havoc in the primary care setting, as well as significant complications in the patient's health and health care. Personality disorders are to be differentiated from personality styles, which are normal and do not cause significant personal unhappiness or social dysfunction. The distinction is sometimes a matter of judgment.

Personality disorders are persistent, problematic, pervasive disturbances in a patient's perception of and relation to the world. The patient sees her problems as originating outside herself. The world and other people are unreliable, fearsome, dismissive, all-powerful. She experiences herself as helpless, justifiably outraged, all-important, and/or unimportant. Unfortunately, the behavior she exhibits in response to these perceptions often confirms them. For example, a person who fears abandonment will cling desperately to important others, causing them to run away.

Personality disorders are organized into clusters. Very often patients manifest some signs and symptoms from more than one diagnostic entity in the cluster. Diagnostic criteria are as follows:

Cluster A: Paranoid personality disorder involves a world view in which other people are perceived as exploiting, maligning, and abusing the patient. The patient is unable to confide in, trust, or forgive others. The patient with *schizoid personality disorder* appears detached with little interest in activities, relationships, and the opinions of others, whereas the *schizotypal personality disorder* causes cognitive distortions and eccentric behaviors as well.

Cluster B: Antisocial personality disorder begins with a conduct disorder before age 15. It progresses to a life-style lacking in respect for the rights and feelings of others, and is manifested in illegal activities, aggressiveness, irresponsibility, lying, and/or lack of remorse. *Borderline personality disorder* is perhaps the single greatest challenge for the physician. "Borderline" patients are unstable in their relationships, affects, impulse control, and self-image. Their attitudes toward others are extreme, and may alternate toward one person or fix upon some as benign and others as malignant. This can wreak havoc in a medical setting with several providers (e.g., doctors, nurses, aides). These individuals are impulsive in potentially self-damaging ways and are recurrently self-destructive. Their anger is intense and inappropriate. They feel empty, and respond to terror of abandonment with frantic efforts to maintain contact. Under stress, they may experience short-lived paranoid ideation and/or dissociative symptoms. A patient with *histrionic personality disorder* tries to be the center of attention, using physical appearance, theatricality, shallow emotional displays, and provocative behavior. She exaggerates the intimacy of her relationships and is highly suggestible. *Narcissistic personality disorder* is associated with grandiosity and grandiose fantasies, a sense of uniqueness and entitlement to special treatment, exploitation, envy, arrogance, and lack of empathy.

Cluster C: A patient with an *avoidant personality disorder* believes that she is inferior or inept; she avoids situations and relationships in which she might be unsuccessful, ashamed, disliked, or criticized. *Dependent personality disorder* causes submissiveness and an excessive need to be taken care of. The patient relies on others for decisions, opinions, and the initiation of activities; fearful of being alone, she clings to others and seeks immediate replacements when a relationship ends. *Obsessive-compulsive personality disorder* is characterized by preoccupation with details, routine, and perfection. Patients have difficulty parting with possessions and money, and are inflexible in routines and values. They do not delegate readily, and devote themselves exclusively and unnecessarily to work activities to the exclusion of relationships and relaxation.

At present, personality disorders are difficult if not impossible to cure. A sincerely motivated patient can make major strides in long-term psychotherapy with a dedicated, gifted, and well-trained therapist. It is inadvisable to shelter patients who engage in antisocial behaviors from the logical consequences of them. What the primary physician must remember is that patients tend to induce in others the feelings they themselves are experiencing; the angry patient makes others angry; the depressed patient, depressed; the victim, victimized. Patients with personality disorders tend to arouse strong feelings that make care providers uncomfortable. When a patient's dependence, grandiosity, indignation, or admiration consistently exceeds that appropriate to the situation, the physician must carefully review his/her own behavior and responses. It is extremely helpful to inquire about the nature of the patient's experience with other physicians; these disorders are chronic and pervasive. Especially dangerous is the situation in which the patient extols the virtues of a new doctor in contrast to the failings of all previous doctors. The new doctor, perhaps seduced by the praise, should expect the same fate. The primary physician must determine what can reasonably, justly, and ethically be offered to the patient, maintaining a steady posture despite the patient's emotional demands. It is often useful to consult or collaborate with another physician or member of the medical team in order to obtain corroboration, support, and relief.

Assessment and Treatment of Sexual Complaints

Sexual complaints are quite common in primary care practice. However, medical school education and residency training often are insufficient to make physicians knowledgeable about sexual diagnosis and treatment—much less comfortable with them. Layers of social mores, religious beliefs, family values, and personal experiences are mentally piled atop a small modicum of information and skills in the area of human sexuality. This may impair the physician's ability to obtain accurate and useful diagnostic information, to set the patient appropriately at ease, and to help her resolve the problem. Resolving the physician's discomfort and professional dysfunction need not entail a personal psychosocial metamorphosis, but it does require honest self-appraisal, the acquisition of basic information, and practice.

Recognizing and Addressing Obstacles to Care

Sexuality is emotionally the most heavily weighted of human physiologic functions. Fueled by a poorly understood but necessary and extremely powerful drive to perpetuate the species, it is universal but often shrouded in mystery, ignorance, and shame.

Sexual functions in every culture are subject to a wide variety of regulations and taboos. Almost all of the rules apply considerably more stringently to women's sexual behavior; it is women who risk sexual attack if not modestly dressed, and who are ostracized or worse in many societies when it occurs. The Victorian tradition still influences Western mores to some extent. The so-called "sexual revolution" was associated with many changes in sexual rules and behaviors, but deep-seated attitudes require many generations to change. For example, it is not uncommon in both the lay and the medical community for people to assume incorrectly that women have little sexual interest or capability after menopause.

Female genitalia, unlike those of the male, are not easily seen. Women's generative organs are internal, and the external genitalia are not visible in the usual postures of everyday life. Many women are extremely reluctant to touch or inspect the sexual parts of their own bodies. They have little or no opportunity to compare their genitalia with those of other women and may feel that their appearance is ugly or even abnormal.

These issues are important because they contribute to a situation in which many women are neither knowledgeable nor comfortable with their own anatomy and physiology. Few women could draw an accurate diagram of the external and internal genitalia, and many have major misconceptions about the mechanisms of menstruation and reproduction. Of particular significance in the medical setting is the lack of language through which women can think about and describe sexual concerns; further, they have sometimes well-founded fears that their sexual functions or behavior will elicit negative judgments from the physician. All this historical, psychological, and social baggage burdens the woman patient who has sexual concerns.

The anatomical charts and models that many physicians keep in their offices are excellent basic tools for providing patients with this missing knowledge and language. Installing a mirror over the examining table will allow the patient to participate visually in the pelvic examination, and often is instructive to both the patient and her physician. The physician may be surprised to learn of patients' reluctance to look at their own bodies, and patients will have an opportunity to see what the doctor sees—to learn the names of body parts and to associate the physical sensations of the examination with those names.

An informative commentary during the examination is likely to be preferable to frozen silence or irrelevant small talk. Such discussion increases the likelihood of effective compliance with therapeutic and contraceptive techniques that require the patient to touch her reproductive organs. It also conveys to the patient, in the most convincing possible way, the doctor's attitude that it is permissible and indeed desirable to speak openly of sexual parts and functions.

General History and Examination

The clinician needs to determine the general state of the patient's health, the conditions of the external and internal sexual organs in particular, and any specific disorders or treatments that might be interfering with her sexual functioning. The pelvic examination may disclose painful foci (see Chap. 30). Debilitating conditions such as anemia may decrease the patient's energy level so severely that there is no energy left for sexual activity after the routines of daily life are accomplished. Disease such as diabetes may affect nervous system functions related to sexual gratification. Medications prescribed for medical or psychiatric conditions may cause iatrogenic sexual dysfunction (see Table 39-3). Gynecologic procedures or surgery may cause psychological and physical changes that interfere with sexuality. Infertility treatment often is associated with changes in sexual function secondary to feelings of inadequacy, to medical intrusions on intimacy, and to the need to have intercourse under prescribed conditions.

The Sexual History

As with most areas of primary care, the key to the diagnosis and treatment of sexual complaints is a good history. Most physicians share with the rest of the population a burden of some discomfort in talking about sexual matters. It is extremely helpful

TABLE 39-3 Medications That Cause Sexual Dysfunction

Loss of libido (decreased responsiveness and interest)
Adrenal steroids
Alcohol
Analgesics (narcotics)
Antiandrogens
Hallucinogens (chronic use)
Sedative-hypnotics (e.g., barbiturates)
Stimulants (chronic use, e.g., cocaine, amphetamines)
Impotence
Alcohol
Antiandrogens
Anticholinergic drugs (e.g., atropine, probanthine)
Antihypertensives (especially guanethidine, rauwolfia alkaloids, and methyldopa)
Antipsychotics (especially thioridazine, haloperidol)
Tranquilizers
Increased Libido
Hallucinogens (e.g., marijuana, LSD)
Hormones (androgens)
L-dopa
Stimulants (acute use, e.g., cocaine, amphetamine)
Retrograde Ejaculation
Phenothiazine (thioridazine)
Retarded Ejaculation
Butyrophenone (haloperidol)
Orgasmic Dysfunction
MAOIs
Tricyclic antidepressants

SOURCE: Adapted from Dubovsky and Weissberg,[27] p 227.

to prepare for this aspect of practice by making a personal appraisal of the sexual attitudes with which one was raised, and one's sexual experiences, beliefs, and knowledge. If, after honest effort the physician cannot approach sexual diagnosis and treatment with some degree of equanimity, she/he ought either to undertake specialized training or to refer patients to a specialist. Most clinicians will be able to proceed, but perhaps not without some vestiges of discomfort.

Some physicians fear that inquiries about sexual behaviors not generally condoned socially will insult and alienate their patients. However, most patients welcome the idea that the physician's mission is to help and not to judge. Specific questions, or the history as a whole, can be prefaced with an explanation that the physician's aim is to address a range of issues to obtain needed information relevant to the understanding and amelioration of the patient's problems.

The primary care physician asks the patient whether she has any concerns, problems, or questions relating to sexuality and whether there is anything that she would like to discuss. If the answer is no, the fact that her doctor has opened the subject will greatly increase the likelihood that she will be able to discuss it at a subsequent visit. If the answer is yes, the physician can either focus totally on the current problems or obtain a detailed chronological sexual history, depending on what is appropriate under the circumstances.

The complete sexual history begins in childhood, with the patient's first sexual education, family attitudes, and masturbatory experiences. It is best to phrase questions in terms that assume the behavior or experience did occur, since this often puts the patient more at ease. If she has not engaged in a behavior asked about, she has only to say "no." Obtain a chronological sense of the patient's sexual life. An open-ended question will yield the most information: "Tell me about your sexual experiences, by yourself and/or with one or more others." "Tell me about the problem you are having." Rapid-fire, specific questions introduced too early into the dialogue are likely to interrupt the flow of information central to diagnosis and treatment. A few minutes of spontaneous communication represent an excellent investment of time. Experiences of sexual abuse and assault are extremely important, and may not be volunteered.

Inquire into the stages of sexual interest, arousal (lubrication), and orgasm, and dysfunctions in any or all of them. Be sure to determine under what circumstances the patient's sexual complaint began and in what circumstances it now occurs. Is the complaint lifelong (primary) or of later onset (secondary)? What is the nature of her relationship with and feelings toward the partner with whom the problems occur? If she has ever had a satisfactory experience, what was it, and how did it come about? What techniques do the sexual partners use, and under what circumstances does sexual activity occur? What approaches has she already tried? What is her opinion about the cause of the problem and the appropriate treatment? How does she expect the physician to proceed?

Sexual Disorders: Nosology

As classified by DSM IV, all the sexual dysfunctions listed below are: 1. due to psychological factors, or due to combined psychological factors and a general medical condition (although sexual dysfunction can also be secondary solely to a medical condition); 2. lifelong (since the onset of sexual activity) or acquired; 3. generalized or situational. The types of sexual dysfunction are disorders of desire, or arousal, or of orgasm, as well as disorders in which sexual activity is associated with physical pain. Intoxication with and withdrawal from substances of abuse also can cause sexual dysfunction. The psychiatric diagnosis of a sexual disorder requires that the condition cause marked distress or interpersonal difficulty for the patient and that the dysfunction not be exclusively secondary to another psychiatric (major depression, for example) or medical disorder.

Disorders of sexual desire include hypoactive desire and active aversion to genital contact with a partner. Sexuality is one of many human factors/behaviors for which there is no scientific definition of the boundaries of normal. Sexual interest, desire, and activity are normal from birth to death. It is left to the clinician and the patient to determine how much desire and how many sexual episodes per day, week, or month are acceptable, satisfactory, or deficient. There is little reason to label sexual experience that does not trouble the patient as pathologic; if her partner(s) is (are) the source of the complaint, the clinician will need to determine whether the relationship is the source of the problem.

Female sexual arousal disorder is a condition in which the patient does not lubricate and become aroused despite sexual interest/desire. Orgasmic disorders exist when the patient does not reach orgasm despite normal sexual excitement. There is wide variation among human beings in the amount of sexual stimulation required for desire, arousal, and orgasm. Responses also depend on the circumstances: for example, mood, distractions, energy level, previous experience, age, and privacy.

Sexual pain disorders include dyspareunia, or pericoital pain, and vaginismus, a condition characterized by involuntary spasm of vaginal musculature preventing intromission.

Management

A careful history and physical examination will elucidate some sexual complaints well enough to make it evident to the patient and physician how to proceed. It may be clear that a particular relationship is not gratifying. Sometimes simple reassurance is enormously relieving—for example, with the exhausted woman four weeks postpartum who is afraid that her sexual feelings will never return, or the 70-year-old woman who is surprised at her continued interest in sexual activity. Some patients will be found to be victims of domestic abuse, and others of common psychiatric illnesses like depression, which require interventions discussed elsewhere in this chapter. Some patients will have gynecologic or general medical conditions that interfere with sexual function. The fact that a patient is chronically ill, that she is recovering from serious illness, or has had surgery on her sexual organs is not an indication for dismissing consideration of her sexual functioning and pleasure.

Techniques for the treatment of disorders of arousal and orgasm utilize behavioral desensitization, sensate focus, and improvements and practice in sexual technique. Patients learn to pay attention to their own preferences and responses, to give and receive pleasurable stimulation, and to relax. Some women are uncomfortable with their sexual fantasies and inhibit them. They need permission and recognition of the central normal role of fantasy in sexual life. The pressure for sexual performance may be decreased by the suggestion that intercourse itself be postponed for some weeks until the partners have gained more experience with other aspects of sexual interaction. If there is a steady sexual partner, he/she and the patient may be educated/treated together. A patient who has never experienced an orgasm is generally advised to begin with private self-stimulation. The primary clinician may wish to study these therapeutic techniques or to refer patients to a specialized sexual disorders program.

The Homosexual or Bisexual Patient

Lesbian and bisexual patient groups have been increasingly vocal in recent years about their negative experiences with physicians. Unwarranted assumptions about such issues as the nature of sexual activity and contraceptive needs may make the lesbian patient conclude that the physician is ignorant, prejudiced, or both, thereby undermining her trust that the medical interaction will be respectful and beneficial. Sexual orientation can provoke intense emotional reactions if either or both patient and physician are uncomfortable or unaccepting. These reactions can negatively impact medical care. One cannot determine sexual orientation on the basis of any parameter other than straightforward, unprejudiced inquiry of the patient as a part of the routine history. The same is true for the specifics of sexual practices.

Conclusion

Psychosocial and psychiatric issues are ubiquitous, pervasive, and critical in primary care. The ability to elicit the patient's story and perspectives, to listen nonjudgmentally and thoughtfully, to monitor one's own reactions, and to tolerate powerful feelings and awkward topics is critical to accurate diagnosis, patient satisfaction, and compliance.

Knowledge about women's psychology, women's experience and roles in society, and the psychosocial impact of medical disorders can help the primary physician to put behavioral and emotional findings in context. Lastly, frank psychiatric disorders are common, are often overlooked, and cause tremendous suffering and disability in patients and pain for their loved ones. Informed treatment by the primary physician, a consulting psychiatrist, or the two in collaboration, can almost always alleviate the patient's symptoms.

Acknowledgments

The author gratefully acknowledges the expert research and technical assistance of Bryna Harwood (coordinator), Amy Ravin, and Deepa Rao.

References and Selected Readings

1. American College of Obstetrics and Gynecology: *The Obstetrician-Gynecologist and Primary-Preventive Health Care.* Washington: ACOG, 1993.
2. Andrews G, Harvey R: Does psychotherapy benefit neurotic patients? A Reanalysis of the Smith, Glass and Miller data. *Arch Gen Psychiatr* 38:1203–1208, 1981.
3. Angst J: Epidemiology of depression. *Psychopharmacol* (suppl) 106:71–74, 1992.
4. American Medical Association Council on Scientific Affairs: Violence against women: Relevance for medical practitioners. *JAMA Council Reports* 267(23):3184–3189, 1992.
5. American Psychiatric Association: *Diagnostic and Statistical Manual of Mental Disorders,* 4th ed. Washington: American Psychiatric Press, 1994.
6. American Psychiatric Association, Task Force on DSM-IV: Diagnostic and Statistical Manual of Mental Disorders, 4th ed, draft criteria. Washingon: American Psychiatric Press, 1993.
7. Apfel RJ, Handel MH: *Madness and Loss of Motherhood: Sexuality, Reproduction and Long-Term Mental Illness.* Washington: American Psychiatric Press, 1993.
8. Arms S: *Immaculate Deception: A New Look at Women and Childbirth in America.* Boston: Houghton Mifflin, 1975.
9. Ashton H: Psychotropic-drug prescribing for women. *Br J Psychiatr* 158(Suppl 10):30–35, 1991.
10. Association of University Women: *How Schools Shortchange Girls: A Study of Major Findings on Girls and Education.* Washington: American Association of University Women Education Foundation and the National Education Association, 1992.
11. Baldessrini RJ: Drugs and the treatment of psychiatric disorders, in: Gilman AG, et al: *Goodman and Gilman's The Pharmacological Basis of Therapeutics,* 8th ed. New York: McGraw-Hill, 1990.
12. Bagedahl-Strindlund M: Postpartum mental illnesses: Cross cultural and social anthropological aspects—a review, in Wijma K, von Schoultz B: *Reproductive Life: Advances in*

Research in Psychosomatic Obstetrics and Gynecology. Trenton, NJ: Parthenon, 1992.
13. Becker, JV, Kavoussi RJ: Sexual disorders, in Talbott JA, Hales RE, Yudofsky SC (eds). *Textbook of Psychiatry.* Washington: American Psychiatric Press, pp 587–604, 1988.
14. Beckman HB, Frankel RM: The effect of physician behavior on the collection of data. *Ann Int Med* 101:692–696, 1984.
15. Bleier R: Gender ideology and the brain: Sex differences research, in Notman MT and Nadelson CC (eds): *Women and Men: New Perspectives on Genera Differences.* Washington: American Psychiatric Press, 1991.
16. Blume SB, Russell M: Alcohol and substance abuse in the practice of obstetrics and gynecology, in Tewart DE and Stotland NL (eds): *Psychological Aspects of Women's Health Care.* Washington: American Psychiatric Press, pp 449–470, 1993.
17. Blumenthal SJ: Psychiatric consequences of abortion: Overview of research findings. In Stotland N (ed): *Psychiatric Aspects of Abortion.* Washington: American Psychiatric Press, 1991.
18. Boston Women's Health Collective: *The New Our Bodies, Ourselves: A Book By and For Women.* New York: Simon & Schuster, 1992.
19. Boston Women's Health Collective: *Changing Bodies, Changing Lives.* New York: Simon & Schuster, 1989.
20. Boston Women's Health Collective: *Ourselves and Our Children.* New York: Simon & Schuster, 1988.
21. Boston Women's Health Collective: *Ourselves, Growing Older.* New York: Simon & Schuster, 1991.
22. Brown G, Harris TO: *Social Origins of Depression: A Study of Psychiatric Disorder in Women.* London: Tavistock, 1978.
23. Calandra B: Closing the gap. *Scott Levin's Pallas Athena* 1(1):27–30, 1992.
24. Cramer DW: Epidemiology and biostatistics, in Berek JS, Hacker NF (eds): *Practical Gynecologic Oncology.* Baltimore: Williams & Wilkins, 1989.
25. Datan N: Aging into transitions: Cross-cultural perspectives on women at midlife, in Formanek R (ed): *The Meanings of Menopause: Historical, Medical and Clinical Perspectives.* Hillsdale, NJ: The Analytc Press, pp 117–132, 1990.
26. Dreifus C (ed): *Seizing Our Bodies: The Politics of Women's Health.* New York: Vintage Books, 1978.
27. Dubovsky SL, Weissberg MP: *Clinical Psychiatry in Primary Care,* 3d ed. Baltimore: Williams & Wilkins, 1986.
28. Faludi S: *Backlash: The Undeclared War against American Women.* New York: Crown Publishers, 1991.
29. Folstein MF, Folstein SE, McHugh PR: Mini-mental state, a practical method for grading the cognitive state of patients. *Psychiatry Res* 12:189–1948, 1975.
30. Ford CV, Folks DG: Conversion disorders: An overview. *Psychosomatics* 26(5):371–382, 1985.
31. Freud S: Feminity, Lecture 33 (1931), in *The Standard Edition of the Complete Works of Sigmund Freud,* vol 22. London: Hogarth Press, 1961.
32. Gartrell N: The lesbian as a ''single'' woman. *Am J Psychother* 35(4):502–516, 1981.
33. Gilligan C: *In a Different Voice.* Cambridge: Harvard University Press, 1982.
34. Greene JG: Psychosocial influences and life events at the time of the menopause in Formanek R (ed): *The Meanings of Menopause: Historical, Medical and Clinical Perspectives.* Hillsdale, NJ: The Analytic Press, pp 79–116, 1990.
35. Hales RE: Dying patients: A challenge to their physicians and consultation psychiatry. *Milit Med* 145:674–680, 1980.
36. Halmi KA: Eating disorders, in Talbott JA, Hales RE, Yudofsky SC (eds): *Textbook of Psychiatry.* Washington: American Psychiatric Press, pp 753–766, 1988.
37. Hamilton JA: Emotional consequences of victimization and discrimination in ''special populations'' of women. *Psychiatr Clin North Am* 12:35–5, 1989.
38. Hirschfeld RMA, Goodwin FK: Mood disorders, in Talbott JA, Hales RE, Yudofsky SC (eds): in *Textbook of Psychiatry.* Washington: American Psychiatric Press, pp 403–441, 1988.
39. Hochschild A: *The Second Shift: Working Parents and the Revolution at Home.* New York: Viking Press, 1989.
40. Horton JA (ed): *The Women's Health Data Book: A Profile of Women's Health in the United States.* Washington: The Jacobs Institute of Women's Health, 1992.
41. Jacobsen DM: Religious experience and the biopsychosocial model, in Browning DS, Jobe T, Evison IS (eds): *Religious and Ethical Factors in Psychiatric Practice.* Chicago: Nelson–Hall, 1990.
42. Johnson SR, Guenther SM, Laube DW, Keettel WC: Factors influencing lesbian gynecologic care: A preliminary study. *Am J Obstet Gynecol* 140(1):20–25, 1981.
43. Kirkpatrick M, Smith C, Roy R: Lesbian mothers and their children: A comparative survey. *Am J Orthopsychiatr* 51(3):545–551, 1981.
44. McEwen BS: Sex differences in the brain: What they are and how they arise, in Notman MT and Nadelson CC (eds): *Women and Men: New Perspectives on Gender Differences.* Washington: American Psychiatric Press, 1991.
45. McGrath E, Keita GP, Strickland BR, Russo NF (eds): *Women and Depression: Risk Factors and Treatment Issues.* Washington: American Psychological Association, 1990.
46. McKinlay SM: The Massachusetts Women's Health Study: A longitudinal study of the health of mid-aged women and the epidemiology of the menopause. *Psychol Women* 16:1–4, 1989.
47. Mendelsohn R: *Male Practice: How Doctors Manipulate Women.* Chicago: Contemporary Books, 1982.
48. Michels R, Marzuk PM: Progress in psychiatry (first of two parts). *N Engl J Med* 329(8):552–560, 1933.
49. Michels R, Marzuk PM: Progress in psychiatry (second of two parts). *N Engl J Med* 329(9):628–638, 1933.

50. Mullen PE, Romans-Clarckson SE, Walton VA, et al: Impact of sexual and physical abuse on women's mental health. *Lancet* 1(8590):841–845, 1988.
51. Nadelson CC: Professional issues for women, *Psychiatr Clin North Am* 12(1):25–33, 1989.
52. Okey JL: Is psychoanalytic theory relevant to the psychology of women? *J Am Acad Psychoanal* 19:396–402, 1991.
53. Oppenheimer E: Alcohol and drug misuse among women: An overview. *Br J Psychiatr* 158(suppl 10):36–44, 1911.
54. Pierce C: Failure to spot mental illness in primary care is a global problem. *Clin Psychiatr News* 21(8):5, 1993.
55. Platt FW, McMath JC: Clinical hypocompetence: The interview. *Ann Int Med* 91:898–902, 1979.
56. Post, RD, Willett AB, Fransk RD, et al: A preliminary report on the prevalence of domestic violence among psychiatric inpatients. *Am J Psychiatr* 137:974–975, 1980.
57. Potter WZ, Rudorfer MV, Manji H: The pharmacologic treatment of depression. *N Engl J Med* 325(9):633–642, 1991.
58. Regier DA, Goldberg ID, Taube CA: The de facto US mental health services system: A public health perspective. *Arch Gen Psychiatr* 35:685–693, 1978.
59. Rose DS: Sexual assault, domestic violence, and incest, in Tewart DE, Stotland NL (eds): *Psychological Aspects of Women's Health Care.* Washington: American Psychiatric Press, pp 447–483, 1993.
60. Rosenfeld S: The effects of women's employment: Personal control and sex differences in mental health. *J Health Soc Behav* 30:77–91, 1989.
61. Rosenthal M, O'Grady P: Affective anxiety disorders, in O'Grady JP (ed): *Obstetrics: Psychological and Psychiatric Syndromes.* New York: Elsevier, 1992.
62. Schatzburg AF, Cole JO: *Manual of Psychopharmacology,* 2d ed. Washington: American Psychiatric Press, 1991.
63. Schurman RA, Kramer PD, Mitchell JB: The hidden mental health network: Treatment of mental illness by nonpsychiatrist physicians. *Arch Gen Psychiatr* 42:89–94, 1985.
64. Stevens PE, Hall JM: A critical historical analysis of the medical construction of lesbianism. *Int J Health Serv* 21(2):291–307, 1991.
65. Stewart DE, Stotland NL (eds): *Psychological Aspects of Women's Health Care.* Washington: American Psychiatric Press, 1993.
66. Stewart DE: Psychiatric admission of mentally ill mothers with their infants. *Can J Psychiatr* 34:34–37, 1989.
67. Stotland NL: The myth of the abortion trauma syndrome (commentary). *JAMA* 268(15):2078–2079, 1992.
68. Stotland NL (ed): *Psychiatric Aspects of Abortion.* Washington: American Psychiatric Press, 1991.
69. Stotland NL (ed): *Psychiatric Aspects of Reproductive Technology.* Washington: American Psychiatric Press, 1990.
70. Stotland NL, Garrick TR: *Manual of Psychiatric Consultation.* Washington: American Psychiatric Press, 1990.
71. Stotland NL: *Social Change and Women's Reproductive Health Care: A Guide for Physicians and Their Patients.* New York: Praeger, 1988.
72. Stoudemire GA: Somatoform disorders, factitious disorders, and malingering, in Talbott JA, Hales RE, Yudofsky SC (eds): *Textbook of Psychiatry.* Washington: American Psychiatric Press, pp 533–556, 1988.
73. Tavris C: *The Mismeasure of Women: Why Women are Not the Better Sex, the Inferior Sex, or the Opposite Sex.* New York: Simon & Schuster, 1992.
74. Williams JH: *Psychology of Women: Behavior in a Biosocial Context,* 2d ed. New York: WW Norton, 1983.

40 Sexual Assault

Helen Greco

Sexual assault occurs when any sexual act is performed by one person on another without that person's consent. The U.S. Department of Justice has indicated that the annual incidence of sexual assault is 73 per 100,000 females, accounting for approximately 6 percent of all violent crimes.[6]

Rape is defined as sexual intercourse without the consent of one party, whether from force, threat of force, or incapacity to consent due to a physical or mental condition. Acquaintance rape is a variant of sexual assault and is more widespread than previously realized. The age group with the highest rates of acquantance rape in the United States is 16 to 24 years.[4] Studies report estimates of violence ranging from 17 to 52 percent among college students and from 12 to 27 percent among high school students.[1] There is concern throughout the country regarding the substantial number of adolescents who have experienced some form of violence in a dating relationship.

Sexual assault can occur in any age, socioeconomic, or racial group. The very young, very old, and handicapped are particularly vulnerable. Statutory rape is defined as sexual intercourse with a person under a specified age. Even if such a person gives consent it is illegal because, by law, the person is defined as being incapable of consenting.

It is very important for the health professional caring for a victim of sexual assault not only to comprehend their medical and legal responsibilities, but also the psychological and emotional stresses of the "rape-trauma" syndrome. When a woman is sexually assaulted she has lost control of her life, and may have experienced the threat of losing her life. Fear and anxiety may render her helpless. This acute phase may last for hours or days, with loss of the woman's usual coping mechanisms. Her responses may range from complete loss of control to outwardly well-controlled behavior. The signs vary in each individual and may include the following: eating and sleep disorders; physical symptoms such as vaginal itch, pain, discharge, headaches, and gastrointestinal disturbances; generalized body aches and pains, such as chest pain, backaches, or pelvic pain; and mood swings, such as anxiety and depression.

The acute phase usually is followed by a reorganization phase that may be characterized by phobias, flashbacks, and nightmares. In addition, there may be gynecologic complaints. This phase may be delayed, occurring months or even years after the event. Therefore, it is imperative that the victim receive appropriate psychological and emotional support and counseling, regardless of the extent of her injuries or her apparent emotional control at the time. The victim's defense mechanisms should not be misinterpreted as indicating that she is able to cope with the particular circumstance. It should always be anticipated that she will demonstrate one or more aspects of the rape-trauma syndrome. In addition, arrangements should be made for immediate family counseling, if appropriate, as well as for follow-up treatment.

Medical Assessment

The physician's medical and legal responsibilities are outlined in Table 40-1.

Informed consent must be obtained prior to any examination, collection of specimens, or taking of photographs. After the acute injuries have been addressed, a thorough history and physical examination should be performed. As many as 40 percent of victims sustain injuries, the severity of which will vary according to the violent nature of the attack and how the patient has attempted to protect herself.[2] Approximately 1 percent of injuries require hospitalization and major operative repair; about 0.1 percent are fatal.[2]

All examinations must be performed in the presence of a female chaperone, even if the health care provider is female. This person can also reassure the victim, provide support, and help her gain control of her situation. A history and physical examination with collection of indicated data must be done in a compassionate manner; otherwise, the patient may feel victimized again and may experience feelings of guilt and self-deprecation.

The patient should be asked to state in her own words a history of the events that occurred. She should be asked to identify her attacker(s), if possible, as well as the date, time, place, and to describe the specific act(s) performed. The victim should also be asked if she bit, scratched, or pulled the hair of the assailant. This may aid in his/her identification.

Also important is the patient's previous gynecologic history, including her last menstrual period, contraceptive use, last consensual sexual activity, preexisting pregnancy, and sexually transmitted diseases. Few studies are available to predict the actual risk of acquiring a sexually transmitted disease (STD) as a result of sexual assault, but *Chlamydia trachomatis* is the STD organism most likely to be acquired.[3] The current risks of acquiring the human immunodeficiency virus (HIV) in this circumstance do not appear to be very high, but obviously this is a serious concern. A study from the Centers for Disease Control found that the chance of victims acquiring gonorrhea ranges from 6 to 12 percent, and the chance of acquiring syphilis is up to 3 percent.[3]

A thorough physical examination of the entire body should be performed. Pertinent drawings should be made, or photographs taken. Any evidence of abrasions, lacerations, and bruises (especially of the neck, back, buttocks, genitalia, and extremities) should be noted. It is important to examine the vaginal vault completely for lacerations or possible rupture into the abdominal cavity. A flat and upright abdominal radiograph may aid in the latter diagnosis. This can be particularly useful in a young child, a woman who has never before had sexual intercourse, or an elderly woman.

Assessment of the reproductive organs and collection of samples and cultures from the cervix and vagina are very important parts of the physical examination. Baseline serologic tests should be done as outlined in Table 40-2. Appropriate slide preparations should be performed to identify any preexisting or recently acquired infections, such as the human papillomavirus, Candida infections, and trichomoniasis.

TABLE 40-1 Physician's Responsibilities

Medical
Obtain thorough gynecologic and medical history
Assess and treat physical injuries
Obtain appropriate cultures
Provide counseling and prophylaxis for sexually transmitted diseases
Provide preventive therapy for unwanted conception
Assess psychological and emotional status
Provide crisis intervention
Arrange for follow-up medical care and psychological counseling
Legal*
Obtain consent for treatment, collection of evidence, the taking of photographs, and the reporting of the incident to the authorities
Provide accurate recording of events
Provide accurate description of injuries
Collection of appropriate samples as well as clothing
Report to authorities, with the victim's consent to do so
Label photographs, articles of clothing, and specimens with the patient's name; seal and store safely

NOTE: Various jurisdictions have different legal requirements for evidence, with which the physician should be familiar. Most emergency rooms have written protocols for handling evidence.

TABLE 40-2 History and Physical Examination

History
Complete sexual, gynecologic, and general medical history
Pertinent "positive and negative" account of the event
Thorough and objective documentation
Any loss of consciousness at any time during the assault
Has the victim changed clothes, voided, defecated, and/or douched since the incident?
Condom use or ejaculation by the assailant
Physical Examination
General appearance
Assessment of psychological and emotional status
Assess entire body for signs of trauma such as bruises, bites, lacerations, abrasions
Photographs, if appropriate
Condition of external genitalia
Speculum examination of cervix and vagina
Oral and rectal assessment for injury
Collection of samples, as indicated, that include the following:
Oral cavity—secretions and culture for *Chlamydia* and gonorrhea
Genitalia—hair combings, hair sample, vaginal secretions, cultures for *Chlamydia* and gonorrhea
Fingernail scrapings
Rectal cultures for *Chlamydia* and gonorrhea
Baseline serology tests for syphilis, hepatitis B antigen, herpes simplex virus, cytomegalovirus, and human immunodeficiency virus (if appropriate), as well as a urine pregnancy test
Search for foreign bodies
Evaluation of all pertinent areas for sperm and acid phosphatase
Collect pertinent clothing
Arrange for follow-up of repeat cultures and serology in 4–6 weeks
Tests for HIV serology repeated in 3–6 months

Prophylaxis against infection should be offered (Table 40-3). If appropriate, prophylaxis against unwanted pregnancy (Table 40-4) should be offered as well. Hormonal postcoital contraception is extremely effective, with a failure rate of 1.6 percent or less when administered within 72 h of sexual intercourse. Treatment is useless after implantation. The patient should be warned to expect severe nausea and told that she will have vaginal bleeding within 21 to 30 days after treatment. Follow-up must be arranged to detect any treatment failures. This treatment should be offered no matter where the patient is in her menstrual cycle, although it should be determined that the victim was not already pregnant prior to the attack.

TABLE 40-3 Prophylaxis against Infection

Prophylaxis
Gonorrhea, *Chlamydia,* and incubating syphilis
Ceftriaxone 250 mg IM, plus doxycycline 100 mg orally twice daily for 10–14 days
Alternate therapy
Spectinomycin 2 gm IM, plus doxycycline 100 mg orally twice daily for 10–14 days
If the patient is pregnant: Use erythromycin, to substitute for doxycycline, 500 mg orally 4 times daily for 10–14 days
Tetanus Diphtheria Toxoid To Be Administered when Indicated

Medical and Legal Responsibilities

Sexual assault is a legal term and not a medical diagnosis. However, the medical report should document, when present, all signs consistent with the use of force.

Documentation of the complete history, physical examination, and emotional condition of the patient is extremely important. Evidence collection should be labeled and sealed. It is also particularly important to make written notes of whether the victim has bathed, brushed her teeth, used mouthwash, defecated, voided, or douched prior to examination. When possible, patients must be encouraged to go immediately to a health care facility. Evidence of coitus may be present in the vagina for up to 48 h

TABLE 40-4 Postcoital Regimen

Ovral: 2 tablets orally stat, then 2 additional tablets 12 h later
Nordette or Lo/Ovral: 4 tablets stat, then 4 additional tablets 12 h later
Ethinyl estradiol (Estinyl): 2.5 mg orally twice daily or 5.0 mg daily for 5 days.

SOURCE: Adapted from Schnare.[3]

after an assault. However, other orifices may retain such evidence for only up to 6 h.

Vaginal secretions (and other appropriate areas, as indicated by history) should be investigated for motile sperm, and samples collected for the presence of acid phosphatase. Acid phosphatase is present in high concentration in seminal fluid. Motile sperm may be present in the vagina for up to eight h after intercourse, but may be present in cervical mucus for as long as two to three days. Nonmotile sperm may be noted in the vagina for up to 24 h and in the cervix for up to 17 days.[7] Even if no sperm are noted, evidence for acid phosphatase should be obtained, since the assailant may have had a vasectomy. Motile sperm may be present in the rectum for an undetermined amoung of time. However, nonmotile sperm can be found for up to 24 h. Acid phosphatase may also be detected in the rectum.[7]

Secretion of a major blood group antigen is found in the saliva of 80 percent of people. Saliva should be obtained from the patient to assess whether she is a secretor, thus aiding in the differentiation of her secretions from those of the assailant.

Fingernail scrapings should be obtained to look for possible skin or blood from the assailant. DNA fingerprinting and specific blood from these materials may assist in the identification of the assailant.

Seminal fluid is rapidly destroyed by salivary enzymes and makes identification difficult after several hours. Staining of clothes and skin by seminal fluid and/or blood may be noted several hours after a crime. Skin washings and clothing should be examined for acid phosphatase.

Psychological and Emotional Support

At all times during the examination and collection of medical and legal evidence, the victim's emotional status should be of foremost concern. Questioning should proceed in a compassionate manner. Although this statement should be obvious, it does not always occur, especially if the woman is drunk, a prostitute, or claiming spouse/date rape. A nonjudgmental manner must be assumed during the examination.

The patient should not be discharged from the health care facility without proper psychological and emotional counseling from health personnel specifically trained to help victims of sexual assault. In addition, follow-up counseling should be scheduled, and an emergency resource made available, should the patient require acute care for psychological symptoms prior to the counseling visit. The latter should be scheduled within one to two weeks after the medical assessment.

References and Selected Readings

1. Koval JE: Violence in dating relationships. *J Pediatr Health Care* 3:298–304, 1989.
2. Marchbanks PA, Lui KJ, Mercy JA: Risk of injury from resisting rape. *Am J Epidemiol* 132:540–549, 1990.
3. Schnare S: Postcoital contraception. *Contemp Ob-Gyn* 1(1):4, 1993.
4. Schwarcz SK, Whittington WL: Sexual assault and sexually transmitted diseases; detection and management in adults and children. *Rev Infect Dis* 12 (suppl b):5682–5689, 1990.
5. U.S. Department of Justice: *Uniform Crime Reports for the United States, 1987*. Publication No. 14. Washington: U.S. Government Printing Office, 1987.
6. Ward SK, Chapman K, Cohn E, et al: Acquaintance rape and college social scene. *Fam Relations* 40:65–71, 1991.
7. Warner CG: *Rape and Sexual Assault; Management and Intervention*. Germantown, MD: Aspen Publications, 1980, Chapter 4.

Part VI

General Health

41 Cardiovascular Disease

Judith Hsia

Cardiovascular disease is by far the leading cause of death among women in the United States; more women die from cardiovascular disease—predominantly heart attacks, congestive heart failure (CHF), and strokes—than from all other causes combined.[20] The opportunity for screening and prevention lies in the hands of the primary care physician. In the office, efforts should focus on prevention of cardiovascular disease through risk factor reduction and on identification of cardiovascular disease in patients with symptoms.

Cardiovascular Risk Factors: Screening and Modification

Public education efforts have led to a fairly precipitous decline in cardiovascular mortality since the 1960s; however, the rate of decline among women has lagged behind that of men. Despite significant public education efforts, cancer, specifically breast cancer, is widely viewed by women as their greatest health threat, and most women do not have a sufficient understanding of their risk related to cardiovascular disease. Consequently, behaviors such as smoking, sedentary life style, inadequate attention to blood pressure (BP) control, and consumption of a high-fat diet—all of which confer added cardiovascular risk—remain widespread.

Traditional cardiovascular risk factors—hypertension, diabetes mellitus, hypercholesterolemia, smoking, and a family history of premature atherosclerosis—are predictive of subsequent myocardial infarction (MI) and stroke. In addition to identification and modification of risk factors, promotion of healthful activities such as regular exercise, attainment of ideal body weight, and consumption of a high-fiber, low-fat diet should be encouraged.

History

At the woman's initial visit, a history of hypertension, treated or untreated; smoking, past or current; and family history of premature atherosclerosis (that is, a parent or sibling with heart attack or stroke before age 55 for men or 65 for women) should be obtained (Table 41-1). Patients should be asked if they have been told of hypercholesterolemia. A history of glucose intolerance, whether treated or not, and symptoms of diabetes mellitus such as polydipsia and polyuria should be ascertained. Especially in patients who are middle-aged or older, they must be asked about additional evidence of cardiac disease such as chest discomfort, particularly when exertional in nature, dyspnea, syncope, known heart murmurs, and hospitalization for MI or other heart disease. It may also be useful to determine whether previous cardiac evaluation, such as exercise testing, has been performed. Patients should also be asked if they get any regular exercise as a prelude to exercise promotion.

During follow-up visits, a simple query, "Have you developed any problems with high blood pressure, diabetes, or chest discomfort?" is important. Because women often view coronary disease as a problem limited to men, their discounting of cardiac symptoms is commonplace and underscores the necessity for the physician to prompt them in revealing symptoms that may reflect coronary insufficiency and/or cardiac risk.

Physical Examination

Recording of weight and blood pressure (BP) is appropriate at every visit. For risk factor screening, observation of body habitus to encourage weight control and exercise is desirable. Xanthomas (cholesterol-filled nodules) may be found on the eyelids or extensor tendons of the extremities of patients with familial hyperlipidemias. Funduscopic examination may reveal retinal arteriopathy in patients with hypertension or beading of the retinal artery in those with hypercholesterolemia. Auscultation of the chest for rales or diminished breath sounds due to pleural effusion may provide evidence of CHF.

Cardiac examination should start with palpation of the chest to locate the point of maximum impulse (PMI), which should normally be in the midclavicular line of the fifth intercostal space. Lateralization of the PMI may indicate cardiomegaly. Palpation over the sternum will identify a right ventricular lift, characteristic of right heart dilation and failure, which may be due to pulmonary disease, primary pulmonary hypertension, or intrinsic cardiac disease. Systematic auscultation of the heart will assess the splitting of S_2, which may permit identification of heretofore undetected atrial septal defects in which splitting of S_2 is fixed rather than narrowing during expiration. An S_4 may be heard in older patients or those with hypertension; an S_3 may be normal in young patients but reflects left ventricular dysfunction in older patients. Murmurs, both innocent and pathologic, should be recorded.

Assessment of the waist-to-hip ratio permits risk stratification, since upper body fat distribution has been associated with a number of cardiovascular risk factors including elevated systolic BP, total cholesterol, low-density lipoprotein (LDL) cholesterol and triglyceride levels, as well as lower high-density lipoprotein (HDL) cholesterol.[24] Examination of the abdomen may reveal hepatomegaly due to right heart failure or other causes such as primary liver disease or a pulsatile abdominal mass in patients with abdominal aortic aneurysms. Flank bruits may also be audible in those with renal artery stenosis.

Peripheral edema may be evident in patients with CHF, and peripheral pulses should be checked to document the condition of the peripheral arteries.

Laboratory Evaluation

Laboratory screening for cardiac risk factors should include a fasting glucose and lipid profile, i.e., total cholesterol, total triglycerides, low-density lipopro-

TABLE 41-1 Obtaining a Cardiac History

Cardiovascular risk factors
Hypertension
Diabetes mellitus
Hypercholesterolemia
Family history of premature atherosclerosis
Cigarette smoking
Obesity
Cardiovascular symptoms
Chest discomfort
Shortness of breath
Palpitations/syncope
Claudication
Past hospitalization or evaluation for cardiovascular disease
Regular exercise
Medications

tein cholesterol (LDL-C), and high-density lipoprotein cholesterol (HDL-C). Glucose and lipid abnormalities are commonly related, with about half of non-insulin-dependent diabetics manifesting lipid abnormalities.

A 12-lead electrocardiogram (ECG) may be obtained as a baseline study for future reference or for prognosis. The yield in normal subjects varies with their age. Among 67,375 young U.S. Air Force personnel, electrocardiographic abnormalities were detected in 3.8 percent.[2] Among 2940 women over 65 years of age abnormal ECGs were found in 23 percent.[7] Data from the Framingham Study suggest that the development of ECG abnormalities has predictive value for coronary heart disease[12] and sudden death.[14] The relative risk of MI during 12 years of follow-up among women with nonspecific ST segment abnormalities was 1.5 for women younger than 65 years and 1.7 ($p < .05$) for older women. The presence of MI, left ventricular hypertrophy, intraventricular conduction delay, heart block, or nonspecific ST changes on a 12-lead ECG was highly associated with sudden death ($p < .0001$). Therefore, a periodic electrocardiogram in older women appears justified provided that interpretation of the tracing will be performed by a knowledgeable physician. Detection of new abnormalities should trigger further evaluation for ischemic heart disease such as exercise thallium testing.

Hypertension

In the United States 57.5 million residents were estimated to be hypertensive by the National Health and Examination Survey. By the age of 60, about half the population will have a diastolic pressure ≥ 90 mmHg and/or a systolic pressure ≥ 140 mmHg. The incidence and severity of hypertension is greater among African Americans than Caucasians at all ages after adolescence. In the Framingham Study—a large, longitudinal population-based study in Framingham, Massachusetts—increased risk of stroke or coronary heart disease was associated with diastolic pressures exceeding 90 mmHg. Since most hypertensives are asymptomatic, blood pressure screening should be undertaken at every opportunity.

The Joint National Committee on Detection, Evaluation, and Treatment of High Blood Pressure classification of adult blood pressure is shown in Table 41-2. The classification is based on an average of two or more BP readings on two or more occasions.

Once a patient has been identified as hypertensive, what is the significance of this finding? A number of studies have demonstrated increased cardiovascular risk in patients with mild hypertension as well as the protective benefit conferred by antihypertensive therapy against strokes and probably CHF (Table 41-3). Demonstration of protection against MI is less well established. In general, treatment of all patients with diastolic pressures > 100 mmHg, many with a diastolic pressure of 95 to 100 mmHg, and some with a diastolic pressure of 90 to 95 mmHg, is indicated. The threshold for pharmacologic therapy will depend, in part, on the presence of other risk factors.

TABLE 41-2 Classification of Blood Pressure in Adults

	Systolic Pressure (mmHg)	Diastolic Pressure (mmHg)	Follow-up
Normal	< 130	< 85	Check in 2 years
High normal	130–139	85–89	Check in 1 year
Hypertension			
Stage 1 (mild)	140–159	90–99	Confirm within 2 months
Stage 2 (moderate)	160–179	100–109	Refer or Rx within 1 month
Stage 3 (severe)	180–209	110–119	Refer or Rx within 1 week
Stage 4 (very severe)	≥ 210	≥ 120	Refer or Rx immediately

NOTE: When systolic and diastolic blood pressures fall into different categories, the more severe category applies.

SOURCE: From the National High Blood Pressure Education Program. National Institutes of Health. NIH Publication No. 93-1088, January 1993.

TABLE 41-3 Antihypertensive Medications

	Side Effects
Diuretics Hydrochlorothiazide—inexpensive Chlorthalidone (Hygroton)—inexpensive Furosemide (Lasix)—inexpensive Bumetanide (Bumex)	Hypokalemia
Beta-adrenergic blockers Nonselective Propranolol (Inderal) short-acting, inexpensive Nadolol (Corgard)—1 time daily	Bronchospasm, depression, negative ino- and chronotrope; masks hypoglycemia in diabetics.
Beta-selective Metoprolol (Lopressor)—1 time daily Atenolol (Tenormin)—1 time daily	Bronchospasm, negative ino- and chronotrope; masks hypoglycemia.
With intrinsic sympathomimetic activity Acebutolol (Sectral)—2 times daily Pindolol (Visken)—2 times daily	Like other beta blockers, may cause less bradycardia.
Alpha-beta-adrenergic blockers Labetolol (Normodyne)—2 times daily Trandate—2 times daily	Orthostatic hypotension.
Alpha, receptor blockers Prazocin (Minipress)—2–3 times daily, inexpensive Doxazosin (Cardura)—2–3 times daily	Orthostatic hypotension.
Central $alpha_2$ antagonists Clonidine (Catapres)—2 times daily or TTS patch once per week Alphamethyl dopa (Aldomet)—2 times daily, inexpensive	Rebound if abruptly withdrawn; impotence.
Calcium channel blockers Diltiazem (Cardiazem)—1 time daily	Usually well tolerated in older patients; can cause bradycardia, heart block; mild negative inotrope.
Verapamil (Calan, Verelan, Isoptin)—1 time daily	More likely to cause heart block than diltiazem; moderate negative inotrope.
Nifedipine (Procardia)—1 time daily; Nicardipine (Cardene)—2 times daily; Isradipine (Dynacirc)—2 times daily; Amlodipine (Norvasc)—1 time daily	More potent vasodilators than diltiazem or verapamil; can cause edema, headache, dizziness.
Angiotensin-converting enzyme (ACE) inhibitors Captopril (Capoten)—2 times daily Enalapril (Vasotec)—1–2 times daily Lisinopril (Zestril)—1–2 times daily Benazepril (Lotensin)—1–2 times daily Fosinopril (Monopril)—1–2 times daily Ramipril (Altace)—1–2 times daily Quinapril (Accupril)—1–2 times daily	Potent antihypertensives; commonly cause cough, hyperkalemia, rise in creatinine; hypotension if volume-depleted.
Direct vasodilator Hydralazine—2–4 times daily Minoxidil—1–2 times daily	Fluid retention (need concurrent diuretic); reflex tachycardia which can aggravate angina.

Treatment of isolated systolic hypertension—i.e., systolic blood pressure ≥ 160 mmHg with diastolic pressure < 90 mmHg—is indicated in the elderly in whom the risk of stroke was reduced 36 percent by diuretic treatment in the Systolic Hypertension in the Elderly Program (SHEP).

Following identification of hypertension, patients should be evaluated for causes of hypertension such as renal failure, renal artery stenosis, coarctation of the aorta, endocrinopathies, and for end-organ damage. Funduscopic examination and urinalysis should be performed on all hypertensive patients. A baseline 12-lead electrocardiogram to document the presence or absence of evidence of left ventricular hypertrophy may be warranted, particularly in African Americans, who have a higher prevalence of left ventricular hypertrophy, a higher incidence of stroke, and a higher mortality rate than Caucasian hypertensives.

Renovascular hypertension is often severe, abrupt in onset, and prevalent in smokers and Caucasians. The prevalence in large series has been about 3 percent, although estimates as high as 43 percent have been reported in patients with accelerated or malignant hypertension with marked retinopathy. In young women, fibromuscular dysplasia is the usual cause; in older patients, the cause is usually renal arterial atheroma. Abdominal bruits will be audible in about 40 percent of patients and are moderately specific indicators of renal artery stenosis. Elevated blood urea nitrogen (BUN) or serum creatinine suggests renal parenchymal, rather than renovascular, disease. Asymmetric renal uptake and retention of radioisotopes during a captopril renal scan suggests renovascular hypertension; arteriography is the definitive test. Treatment involves either percutaneous or open angioplasty.

The objective when treating patients with hypertension is to achieve a sustained BP below 140/90 mmHg (Fig. 41-1). In patients with stage 1 or 2 hypertension, lifestyle modification should be attempted for 3 to 6 months before instituting drug treatment. During this interval, close follow-up is warranted to vigorously reinforce the necessity of lifestyle modification and to ensure that hypertension is not progressing to stage 3. Initial steps to lower BP in patients with essential hypertension include weight reduction and dietary sodium restriction. If these are ineffective, drug therapy should be instituted, usually with a single agent. Diuretics and beta-adrenergic blockers have established efficacy in large clinical trials and are comparatively inexpensive. Calcium channel antagonists and ACE inhibitors are reasonable alternatives. If, after 1 to 3 months, adequate response has not been obtained, the dose may be increased or a different agent tried. A second drug may be added if minimization of side effects by using lower doses of two drugs is desired.

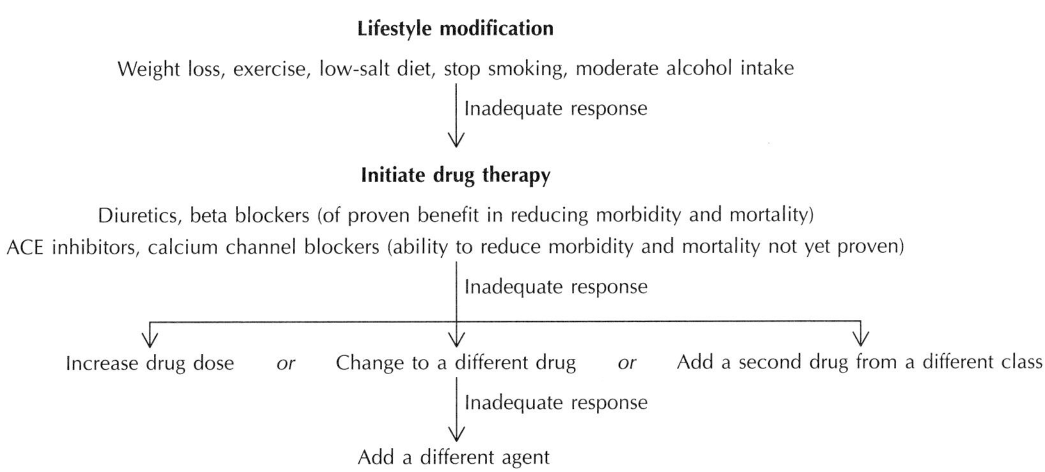

Figure 41-1 Treatment of hypertension.

For stage 3 or 4 hypertension, chances are slim that BP will be controlled by lifestyle modification alone. Therefore, drug therapy should be instituted earlier and with the understanding that single-drug therapy is less likely to be sufficient.

An ever-growing armamentarium of antihypertensives is available, including diuretics, adrenergic blockers, calcium channel blockers, angiotensin converting enzyme (ACE) inhibitors, and direct vasodilators. Trials have used antihypertensives from a variety of classes, all of which appear to be effective. Cost, dosing convenience, and side-effect profile will influence the choice of an agent. These are particularly important issues since treatment is often lifelong.

Patients with hypertensive emergencies have acute end-organ sequelae of hypertension, such as encephalopathy, acute heart failure with pulmonary edema, or dissecting aortic aneurysm. These situations require prompt hospitalization for parenteral antihypertensive therapy.

Diabetes Mellitus

The prevalence of diabetes mellitus in the United States is 2 to 6 percent, with impaired glucose tolerance in as much as 20 percent of the population. Diabetes is clearly associated with increased risk of cardiovascular disease; mortality from coronary disease among diabetics is twice that of nondiabetics. Recent data from the Diabetes Control and Complications Trial[19] suggest that intensive treatment of insulin-dependent diabetes with three or more daily injections of insulin or using an infusion pump can reduce end-organ damage. A similar study of intensive therapy of noninsulin-dependent diabetics is in the planning stages. In the meantime, diabetics should be identified and receive aggressive weight control, dietary education, and in many instances drug therapy. Diabetes is discussed in depth elsewhere in the book.

Hyperlipidemia

The prevalence of hypercholesterolemia has fallen in recent years; however, the proportions of women with elevated (> 240 mg/dl) or borderline (200–239 mg/dl) total cholesterol are still estimated at 20 and 30 percent, respectively.[18] Hyperlipidemia usually causes no symptoms until coronary, cerebral, or peripheral vascular insufficiency develops. Physical manifestations are comparatively infrequent, so the diagnosis is usually made through blood screening.

The lipid profile generally includes total cholesterol, triglycerides, HDL, and calculated LDL. Nonfasting patients can be screened with random glucose and total cholesterol. Since the triglyceride level depends on recent dietary intake, this value as well as the LDL level, which is calculated using the triglyceride level, is inaccurate in nonfasting patients. The total cholesterol, however, is not influenced much by food consumed during the preceding few hours and thus may be measured in the nonfasting state.

The National Cholesterol Education Program classification and guidelines are summarized in Table 41-4. Patients with undesirable total cholesterol or LDL levels should receive lipid-lowering management, including education in the NCEP "Step One" diet (Table 41-5). Counseling in the Step One diet can be carried out by physicians or their office staff; education in the Step Two diet often requires the assistance of a registered dietician. After 6 weeks of dietary therapy, the fasting lipid profile should be repeated. If lipids are still above the desirable range, drug therapy is indicated. NCEP guidelines call for pharmacologic therapy in women if the LDL level remains > 190 mg/dl on a diet, or > 160 mg/dl on a diet in the presence of two other risk factors (hypertension, diabetes, obesity, HDL

TABLE 41-4 National Cholesterol Education Program Guidelines

	Total Cholesterol (mg/dl)	Low Density Lipoprotein Cholesterol (mg/dl)
Desirable	< 200	< 130
Borderline	200–239	130–159
Elevated	≥ 240	≥ 160

TABLE 41-5 National Cholesterol Education Program Dietary Recommendations

	Step One Diet	Step Two Diet
Total fat	< 30 % of total calories	< 30 % of total calories
Saturated fatty acids	< 10 % of total calories	< 7 % of total calories
Polyunsaturated fatty acids	Up to 10% of total calories	Up to 10% of total calories
Monounsaturated fatty acids	10–15% of total calories	10–15% of total calories
Carbohydrates	50–60% of total calories	50–60% of total calories
Protein	10–20% of total calories	10–20% of total calories
Cholesterol	< 300 mg/day	< 200 mg/day
Total calories	To achieve and maintain desirable weight	To achieve and maintain desirable weight

< 35 mg/dl, or a family history of coronary disease).

Patients with desirable cholesterol levels should have them repeated at 5-year intervals. Management of those with borderline cholesterol levels is discretionary; lipid profiles should be repeated in a fasting state. Patients with known coronary disease should be referred for dietary education and, if necessary, drug therapy to achieve an LDL level ≤ 100 mg/dl.

A wide range of cholesterol-lowering drugs are available including niacin, resin agents (cholestyramine, colestipol), and HMG Co-A reductase inhibitors (lovastatin, simvastatin, pravastatin). Niacin is inexpensive and raises HDL as well as lowering LDL, but patients often dislike and will not tolerate the flushing that is common even when niacin is titrated up from a low dose. Resin agents' ability to prevent MI and cardiac death are well established, as is their safely record. Patients frequently complain of constipation and dislike consuming quantities of granules suspended in liquid several times a day. The HMG Co-A reductase inhibitors have greater LDL-lowering capability and are well tolerated. Unfortunately, they lower HDL as well as LDL and are expensive. Myolysis with marked elevations of CPK may necessitate discontinuation. Hepatitis is more common, with asymptomatic transaminase elevation exceeding three times the upper limit of normal in 3 percent of patients taking lovastatin for at least 1 year. Therefore, transaminase should be monitored at baseline, every 6 weeks during the first 3 months, every 8 weeks for the remainder of the first year, and periodically—e.g., semiannually—thereafter.

Cigarette Smoking

Cigarette smoking is the foremost factor associated with a preventable cause of death in the United States. The risk of coronary disease among smokers is twice that of nonsmokers; cardiac risk is directly related to the number of cigarettes smoked each day. Secondary exposure to cigarette smoke through passive inhalation by nonsmokers increases risk as well. Cigarette smoking also enhances the risk of stroke and peripheral vascular disease.

Smoking cessation should be universally encouraged. Among 35-year-old women, cessation is expected to prolong life expectancy by more than 3 years; 55-year-old women may expect to live 2 extra years. Physician advice to discontinue smoking will induce about 5 percent of patients to stop. Other interventions such as referral to smoking cessation programs increase the likelihood of success. Smoking cessation programs often use aversive techniques such as rapid puffing in combination with steps to enhance recognition of situations provoking a desire to smoke as well as behavioral modification techniques.

Management of physical nicotine dependence in smokers may include prescription of nicotine patches or chewing gum. Transdermal nicotine patches are usually applied daily using the 21-mg size for the first 6 weeks, followed by the 14-mg patch and the 7-mg patch for 2 weeks each. Nicotine chewing gum (Nicorette, 2 mg nicotine polacrilex each) may be prescribed as needed, up to 30 doses per day, although the average consumption is 10 doses daily. Patients usually reduce their use of nicotine chewing gum over several months. Persistent gum use for more than 6 months suggests that the gum dependency has replaced cigarette dependency.

Exercise

Physical activity reduces cardiovascular risk, lowers BP, improves glucose tolerance, assists with maintenance of ideal body weight, and may improve the lipid profile. Any amount of aerobic activity appears preferable to no exercise. The American Heart Association recommends three 20-min sessions per week, each preceded by a warm-up and followed by a cool-down period. Patients with previously sedentary lifestyles should start slowly and gradually increase the intensity of their exercise.

For exercise programs to be successful, patients must realize that exercise is a lifelong commitment and thus should choose types and intensities of exercises that are enjoyable or, at least, tolerable. A variety of different exercise activities is desirable to prevent injury from repetitive stress, provide seasonal adaptability, and maintain interest. Women with known coronary disease or suggestive symptoms such as exertional chest discomfort or dyspnea should be evaluated for cardiac ischemia before initiating an exercise program. Such evaluation may also be warranted in some asymptomatic patients with cardiac risk factors.

Aspirin

In the Physician's Health Study, aspirin, 325 mg every other day, was found to provide cardiovascular protection in middle-aged and older men. No women were included in that study. A similar placebo-controlled randomized trial in women is currently in progress, but the results will not be available for a number of years. In the meantime, no blanket recommendation is appropriate regarding aspirin for cardiovascular prophylaxis in women. On an individualized basis, physicians may choose to recommend aspirin for women with cardiac risk factors.

Exogenous Hormone Replacement

Long-term follow-up with users of oral contraceptives has indicated that there is no increased risk of cardiovascular disease from oral contraceptive use. Nevertheless, it seems prudent to use those preparations with progestins, such as norgestimate or desogestrel, which are least likely to alter lipoprotein profiles adversely. In general, women over 35 years who smoke should be counseled against oral contraceptive use, unless they can stop smoking. In one paper, the risk of MI was stated to be increased 30-fold in women over age 35 who use oral contraceptives and smoke.[22]

The relationship between menopause and cardiovascular disease is undergoing extensive evaluation. The Framingham Study identified a striking increase in coronary artery disease (CAD) in postmenopausal compared with premenopausal women. Since 1970, a number of large cohort and case control studies and one small randomized trial have examined estrogen's role in the prevention of cardiovascular disease among postmenopausal women. A recent meta-analysis of these studies found the relative risk for coronary heart disease in women who have ever used estrogen compared to those who have never used estrogen to be 0.65. Among women with angiographically documented coronary disease, the protective benefit of estrogen appears even more striking. Although there is a substantial amount of evidence regarding the cardiovascular benefits of estrogen replacement therapy (ERT), some believe that definitive evidence of cardiovascular protection conferred by estrogen is not yet available. However, such evidence should become available in the future from the Heart & Estrogen/Progestin Replacement Study (HERS), in women with preestablished coronary disease, and from the National Institutes of Health (NIH)–supported Women's Health Initiative.

Evaluation of Signs and Symptoms during Routine Office Visits

Women are less likely than men to seek medical attention for potential cardiac complaints, and they are less likely to be referred for diagnostic testing once they do seek medical attention, despite the fact that cardiovascular mortality in older women actually exceeds that in men of the same age. Gender bias in evaluation as well as treatment of coronary heart disease should be avoided.

Chest Pain

Chest pain is a common complaint, the differential diagnosis of which is summarized in Table 41-6. The quality, location, and duration of chest discomfort should be elicited, along with precipitants and factors providing relief. An antecedent viral illness and positional quality to the chest pain suggest pericarditis. Association of chest discomfort with upper extremity and perioral paresthesias in high-stress situations suggests hyperventilation. Greater age and the presence of cardiac risk factors should increase one's suspicion of coronary disease.

On examination, costochondritis may be diagnosed if chest wall tenderness is present. A pericardial or pleural friction rub suggests pericarditis or pleuritis. A midsystolic click should be audible in patients with mitral valve prolapse and possibly a holosystolic murmur at the apex as well. Epigastric tenderness suggests gastrointestinal disease.

In the Framingham Study, angina pectoris rather than MI was the predominant presenting symptom for women with coronary heart disease. Classic angina is characterized as substernal heaviness or pressure radiating to the neck, left arm, or jaw and lasting minutes; brought on by exercise and relieved by rest. The character of chest symptoms should be ascertained, bearing in mind the lack of specificity of a diagnosis of coronary disease based on patient history alone. Since the history in both men and women who have coronary artery disease may be rather nonspecific, the decision regarding the need for further evaluation should be as aggressive for women as it is for men. Usually no specific physical findings will be apparent.

A 12-lead ECG may be helpful in identifying pericarditis (Fig. 41-2) or previous MI. Evidence of ischemia is unlikely unless the patient is having symptoms at that time. Echocardiography will identify mitral valve prolapse.

Treadmill testing, nuclear imaging, and coronary angiography remain the mainstays for the diagnosis of CAD. Treadmill testing is well established as a valuable, safe, and comparatively inexpensive means for diagnosing coronary heart disease in men (Fig. 41-3). Its value in women, however, is less certain. In one comparison of treadmill testing in men and women in which one third of patients in each group had angiographically documented coronary disease, the false-positive rate in men was 7 percent compared with 22 percent in women ($p <$ .05). The false-negative rate—i.e., negative tread-

TABLE 41-6 Differential Diagnosis of Chest Pain

	Location	Quality	Duration	Provoked by	Relieved by
Angina pectoris	Substernal; radiating to arm, neck, jaw	Pressure	Few minutes	Exertion, stress	Rest, NTG*
Pericarditis	Substernal, can radiate	Sharp	Hours	Lying down, inspiration	Sitting forward
Esophageal reflux, spasm	Substernal, epigastric	Pressure	Variable	Recumbency, food or spontaneous	NTG
Gastritis, peptic ulcer	Epigastric	Burning	Hours	Food or lack of food	Antacids
Pulmonary (embolism, tumor, pneumonia)	Can be substernal, with dyspnea	May be pleuritic	Hours	Inspiration or spontaneous	Specific therapy
Costochondritis	Costosternal joints	Tenderness	Variable	Palpation	Analgesics
Mitral valve prolapse	Left chest	Sharp	Variable	Spontaneous	Beta blockers
Hyperventilation	Precordial	Pressure	Minutes	Emotional stress	Relief of stress

*NTG = sublingual nitroglycerin.

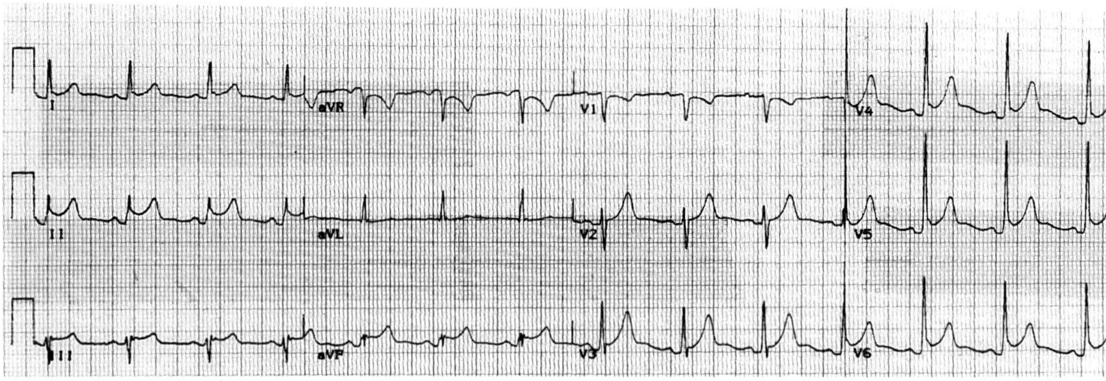

Figure 41-2 Twelve-lead electrocardiogram (ECG) in pericarditis. Electrocardiogram of a young woman with positional chest pain. Diffuse elevation of the ST segments is present as well as depression of the PR segment in relation to the TP segment.

mill tests in patients with angiographic coronary disease—was 13 percent for men and women. Overall, treadmill results were misleading in 35 percent of women, severely limiting the utility of this approach for screening of a very common disease. False-positive exercise tests have been related to phases of the menstrual cycle and to oral contraceptive use, suggesting a relationship between sex hormones and ECG responses to exercise.

Fortunately, nuclear imaging has provided a more accurate noninvasive means of diagnosing coronary heart disease in women (Fig. 41-4). For patients unable to achieve a reasonable exercise level, pharmacologic stress using either dipyridamole, adenosine, or dobutamine appears to have similar diagnostic accuracy to exercise. Using thallium 201 in conjunction with exercise or pharmacologic stress, diagnostic accuracy is comparable in men and women when valve plane, breast artifacts, and diaphragmatic attenuation are taken into account by experienced interpreters. Newer technetium 99m–based imaging agents may prove to be as useful as thallium.

Stress echocardiography, using either exercise or dobutamine, is also an effective approach to evaluation of patients with suspected coronary disease, provided the quality of the echocardiographic images acquired is adequate. Pulmonary disease and unsuitable body habitus may limit the necessary visualization of the endocardium.

Coronary angiography remains the gold standard for diagnosis of coronary heart disease but does involve ionizing radiation and a small risk of MI,

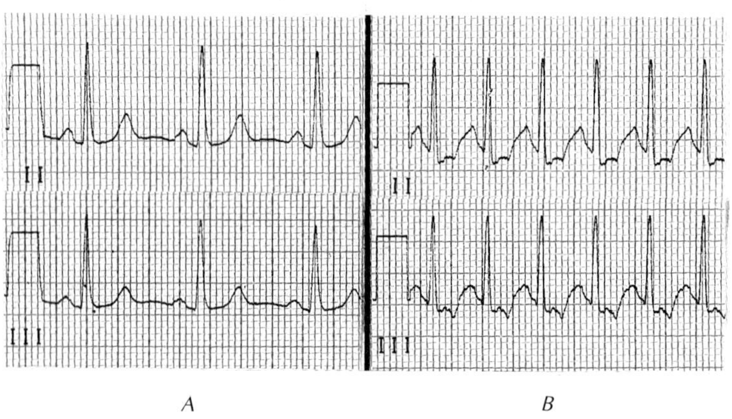

Figure 41-3 False-positive treadmill test. Electrocardiographic tracing of leads II and III from a 50-year-old woman with exertional chest discomfort. At baseline (*A*), ST segments are normal; at peak exercise (*B*), significant horizontal ST depression is apparent. Thallium images were normal.

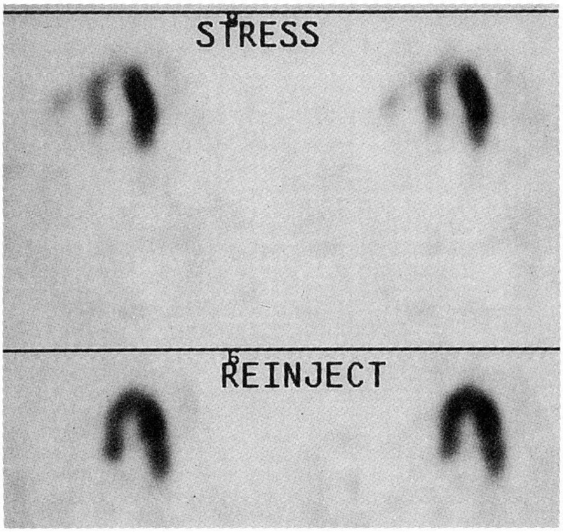

Figure 41-4 Abnormal thallium-201 scintigraphy. Short-axis tomographic images obtained immediately after peak stress and following reinjection of thallium after 2 h of rest in a 60-year-old woman with typical angina. Thallium uptake in the septum and anterior wall is reduced at peak exercise but is restored following rest, consistent with stress-induced myocardial ischemia.

stroke, hemorrhage, vascular damage, or allergy to the contrast medium. Therefore, unless the a priori suspicion of coronary disease is high, noninvasive evaluation should precede angiography. Patients with Prinzmetal's variant angina—i.e., coronary artery spasm—may have normal exercise tests, nuclear imaging studies, and coronary angiography. Administration of ergonovine during angiography often induces spasm in such patients, provided they are not receiving vasodilators such as nitrates or calcium channel blockers at that time.

Some types of coronary disease warrant more urgent evaluation. Patients with new-onset angina or crescendo angina—i.e., increasing frequency and/or severity of angina which may be provoked at a lower level of exertion—should be seen by a specialist that day. Those with unstable angina—i.e., pain at rest, including nocturnal angina—should be hospitalized that day. Those with suspected MI—i.e., severe chest pain with or without associated dyspnea, diaphoresis, nausea, vomiting, or syncope—should be brought to the closest emergency room by ambulance.

Treatment of chronic coronary disease consists of medical therapy and/or revascularization. Revascularization can be performed percutaneously by balloon angioplasty or through coronary artery bypass grafting. Medical therapy options include aspirin, beta-adrenergic blockers, calcium channel blockers, and nitrates, singly or in combination.

Aspirin for primary and secondary prevention of MI and stroke has been studied predominantly in men. Women with documented coronary disease should take aspirin, 325 mg every other day, in the absence of any specific contraindication such as peptic ulcer disease, gastritis, concurrent warfarin therapy, or known aspirin allergy. In other women, prescription of aspirin for primary prevention is discretionary.

Beta-adrenergic blockers (also known as "beta blockers") are highly effective in the treatment of chronic stable angina and have the added benefit in hypertensives of lowering BP concurrently. Beta blockers are categorized by their specificity for beta receptor subtype 1 or 2. Beta$_1$ receptors predominate in the heart, where stimulation of them increases heart rate and contractility. Stimulation of beta$_2$ receptors induces vasodilation, bronchodilation, and glycogenolysis. The clinical efficacy of beta blockers in angina patients is attributable to these agents' negative chronotropic and inotropic effects. In titrating the dosage of a beta blocker, the treatment goal of freedom from angina or control of BP should be kept in mind; a reasonable starting point is to aim for a resting heart rate of 50 to 60 beats per minute. Once-a-day formulations of beta blockers are available and represent a tradeoff between cost and convenience. The common adverse effects of beta blockers include

- Increased plasma triglyceride levels by as much as 50 percent and lowering of HDLs by 15 percent
- Exacerbation of heart block in patients with conduction abnormalities
- Bronchoconstriction
- Nightmares, depression, fatigue

Beta blockade permits unopposed alpha-adrenergic stimulation, which is undesirable in patients with coronary spasm. Patients taking ophthalmic preparations of timolol commonly manifest systemic effects of beta blockade such as bradycardia and bronchospasm. $Beta_1$ selective agents such as atenolol and metoprolol are somewhat less likely to cause bronchospasm than nonselective agents such as propranolol and nadolol. Lipid-soluble beta blockers such as propranolol and metoprolol are more likely to cross the blood-brain barrier and cause central nervous system (CNS) side effects such as nightmares, fatigue, and depression.

Calcium channel blockers impede the influx of calcium into cardiocytes and vascular smooth muscle cells. Vasodilation and negative inotropic and chronotropic effects contribute to the efficacy of these agents and also to the profile of adverse effects. Predominant vasodilators such as nifedipine have vasodilation-related effects including peripheral edema, reflex tachycardia, headache, and hypotension. Verapamil and diltiazem are negative inotropes and can also cause atrioventricular (AV) block, which makes them effective for the treatment of some arrhythmias but disadvantageous in patients with conduction abnormalities.

For treatment of angina and/or hypertension, long-acting nifedipine is very effective with a starting dose of 30 mg/day, increased to 60 or 90 mg/day as tolerated. The combination of nifedipine with a long-acting beta blocker is particularly good. Long-acting diltiazem is another reasonable alternative, particularly well tolerated in older patients, with a starting dose of 180 mg/day of the sustained release formation, increased to 240 mg/day as needed. Caution is warranted when prescribing the combination of diltiazem with a beta blocker, as excessive bradycardia may ensue. Other calcium channel blockers include verapamil, isradipine, bepridil, nicardipine, nisoldipine, and amlodipine. Calcium channel blockers are effective antianginals in conjunction with nitrates, although the combination of preload and afterload reduction can lead to hypotension.

Nitrates are predominant venodilators and have been the mainstay of antianginal therapy since the nineteenth century. Acute anginal episodes are treated with sublingual nitroglycerin, 0.3 mg, repeated if necessary. Sublingual nitroglycerin is also effective when taken prophylactically before planned angina-provoking activities. Adverse reactions to nitrates are related to its vasodilating effects and include flushing, hypotension, headache, and dizziness. Patients should be instructed to be seated or supine when taking sublingual nitroglycerin to avoid abrupt hypotension with loss of consciousness.

Long-acting nitrate preparations can be oral or topical. Nitrate tolerance will develop in most recipients unless a nitrate-free interval is provided. Nitroglycerin patches in doses ranging from 2.5 to 15 mg/24 h should be applied in the morning and removed at night to avoid tolerance. Oral nitrates are available as isosorbide dinitrate or isosorbide-5-mononitrate. Isosorbide dinitrate is susceptible to substantial first-pass hepatic metabolism and thus should be prescribed in fairly high doses to ensure adequate bioavailability—e.g., 30 to 40 mg two or three times daily. Isosorbide-5-mononitrate is somewhat longer-acting and may be prescribed as 10 to 40 mg twice daily. A 10- to 12-h drug-free interval will prevent tolerance to oral nitrates.

Combination therapy with aspirin and antianginals from one, two, or three other classes provides effective treatment for most patients.

Dyspnea

Dyspnea can be attributed to a wide variety of causes (summarized in Table 41-7). Distinguishing among these causes may be aided by a determination of the acuteness of dyspnea onset; precipitants; asso-

TABLE 41-7 Causes of Dyspnea

Noncardiac causes
Deconditioning
Anxiety
Pulmonary disease
Parenchymal disease, pulmonary embolism, obstructive airway disease, pulmonary interstitial disease
Anemia
Cardiovascular causes
Congestive heart failure
Aortic or mitral valvular disease
Pericardial tamponade

ciated cough, fever, chest pain; orthopnea; paroxysmal nocturnal dyspnea; peripheral edema; a history of past heart or lung disease; cardiac risk factors; and medications.

On physical exam, tachycardia suggests a problem with delivery of oxygenated blood to end-organs, because of either pulmonary or cardiac disease or anemia. The presence of a pulsus paradoxicus exceeding 10 mmHg suggests either pulmonary disease or pericardial tamponade. Pulsus paradoxicus is an exaggerated effect of respiration on the arterial pulse, detectable by inflating a blood pressure cuff to suprasystolic level, then deflating slowly. The difference between the pressure at which Korotkoff sounds first become audible and the pressure at which they are audible throughout the respiratory cycle is the pulses paradoxicus, normally < 10 mmHg.

Fever, cough, and localizing pulmonary signs suggest pneumonia. The presence of jugular venous distension, rales, and an S_3 suggests cardiomyopathy. A delayed arterial upstroke, single or narrowly split S_2, and midpeaking systolic ejection murmur are consistent with aortic stenosis. A diastolic rumble and opening snap in early diastole may be heard in mitral stenosis. A blowing decrescendo diastolic murmur along the upper right or left sternal border with a wide pulse pressure suggests aortic insufficiency, and a holosystolic murmur at the apex radiating to the axilla suggests mitral insufficiency. A harsh systolic ejection murmur that gets quieter with squatting and louder with Valsalva maneuver suggests obstructive hypertrophic cardiomyopathy. Swollen, red, warm, or tender legs raises the possibility of deep venous thrombosis with subsequent pulmonary embolization.

If deconditioning is a consideration, a treadmill test will quantify exercise capacity to a much greater extent than will history. A treadmill test may also provide an opportunity to encourage regular exercise. Pulmonary disease may be evident on chest roentgenography or pulmonary function testing. If pulmonary embolism is suspected, a scintigraphic ventilation/perfusion scan should be obtained promptly. Cardiac diagnoses such as valvular disease or cardiomyopathy are usually confirmed by echocardiography.

Congestive heart failure (CHF) is defined as cardiac function inadequate to meet the metabolic needs of peripheral tissues, most commonly because of valvular disease or ventricular dysfunction. Dyspnea, either exertional or at rest, cough, orthopnea, paroxysmal nocturnal dyspnea requiring a patient to arise from bed to aid breathing, and peripheral edema are characteristic symptoms in CHF. Physical findings may include tachycardia, hypotension, jugular venous distension, hepatojugular reflux, hepatomegaly, rales, pleural effusion, an S_3 gallop, and peripheral edema. The severity of CHF is often characterized by the New York Heart Association functional class (Table 41-8). Annual mortality among patients with class III heart failure is about 20 percent, rising to 60 percent in class IV.

Valvular disease Recommendations for antibiotic prophylaxis of patients with valvular disease and congenital cardiac malformations are summarized in the preoperative evaluation section of this chapter.

Mitral stenosis in adults results from previous rheumatic fever. Patients commonly present with fatigue and exertional dyspnea or with atrial fibrillation, which exacerbates their difficulty filling the left ventricle through a stenotic mitral valve because of loss of the atrial contraction. Physical findings (diastolic rumble and opening snap) may be subtle, but mitral stenosis is readily diagnosed by echocardiography. Treatment is surgical.

Mitral insufficiency may also be a sequela of rheumatic fever, but it also results from

- Papillary muscle ischemia or infarction
- Ruptured chordae tendinae
- Endocarditis
- Mitral valve prolapse

TABLE 41-8 New York Heart Association Functional Classification

Class I	No limitation; ordinary activity does not cause fatigue, dyspnea.
Class II	Slight limitation of physical activity; ordinary activity results in fatigue, dyspnea.
Class III	Marked limitation of physical activity; modest activity results in fatigue, dyspnea.
Class IV	Dyspneic and fatigued at rest.

- Mitral annular calcification (in older patients)
- Dilatation of the mitral annulus in dilated cardiomyopathy

Mitral insufficiency may present as an asymptomatic holosystolic apical murmur, as atrial arrhythmia, or as CHF. Serial echocardiography will provide a record of changes in ventricular and atrial dimensions over time. The regurgitant volume assessed by color flow Doppler ultrasound will vary with loading conditions. Medical therapy includes afterload reduction (ACE inhibitors or nifedipine) to improve forward flow and diuresis to reduce pulmonary congestion. In chronic mitral insufficiency the left ventricle must pump both the cardiac output to the aorta and the regurgitant fraction into the left atrium, resulting in chronic volume overload, which will lead to irreversible ventricular damage. Thus, surgical valve repair or replacement should be undertaken before the development of cardiomyopathy. Determining the optimal time for surgery can be tricky since left ventricular emptying into a low-pressure chamber, the left atrium, can present a misleading appearance of normal intrinsic ventricular contractility.

Mitral value prolapse (MVP) is a common congenital abnormality in which the mitral valve leaflets are myxomatous, redundant, and prolapse into the left atrium during systole. MVP may occur sporadically or through autosomal dominant inheritance and can be associated with the Marfan syndrome, Ehlers-Danlos syndrome, and other connective tissue diseases. Symptoms that can be associated with MVP include chest pains, palpitations, and sometimes neuropsychiatric complaints. Classic physical findings include one or more mid- to late systolic clicks with or without a murmur of mitral insufficiency.

Over the years, many patients were erroneously diagnosed with MVP on the basis of physical findings and/or M-mode echocardiography. Although the prevalence of MVP has been reported to be as high as 6 percent, that estimate will fall with application of stringent two-dimensional echocardiographic criteria for diagnosis. Adverse outcomes associated with MVP include infective endocarditis, severe mitral insufficiency requiring mitral valve replacement, arrhythmias, and cerebral embolic events.

Asymptomatic patients with MVP have an excellent prognosis and require only periodic echocardiography (every 2 to 4 years) and endocarditis prophylaxis. Patients with palpitations, dizziness, or chest pain should be evaluated to exclude ischemic heart disease or significant arrhythmia with treadmill testing, with or without nuclear imaging and Holter or event monitor recording. Beta-adrenergic blockade is the treatment of choice for chest discomfort. Patients with documented arrhythmias may need to be referred to a cardiologist. Those with mitral insufficiency should be followed with more frequent echocardiography. Afterload reduction may be warranted to enhance forward flow, and a proportion of patients will eventually require mitral valve repair or replacement. Patients with cerebral ischemic events should be evaluated for other causes of cerebral ischemia and may require antiplatelet therapy or anticoagulation.

Aortic insufficiency may result from rheumatic fever, congenital malformation of the leaflets including a bicuspid valve, endocarditis, trauma, or aortic annular dilation due to aortic root disease (Marfan syndrome, Ehlers-Danlos syndrome, hypertension). Patients with acute aortic insufficiency will develop CHF. Those with chronic aortic insufficiency are often asymptomatic for years. Eventually they may develop exertional dyspnea, orthopnea, and fatigue. Physical examination may reveal a wide pulse pressure, systolic ejection murmur, and blowing diastolic murmur along the right or left sternal border in the third or fourth intercostal space. Echocardiography is helpful in determining the number of aortic cusps and aortic root dimension as well as quantifying the severity of aortic insufficiency and left ventricular dimensions. Afterload reduction will improve forward flow. Timing of aortic valve replacement to precede irreversible ventricular dysfunction from chronic overload should be undertaken with cardiology consultation. Patients with aortic root disease may require beta blockade and earlier surgical intervention to prevent aortic rupture.

Aortic stenosis may also be rheumatic in origin but is usually due to degeneration of either a normal or congenitally malformed aortic valve. Patients may present with asymptomatic murmurs but more often have angina, heart failure, or syncope. The angina may be due either to coexisting coronary disease or to subendocardial ischemia in a hypertrophied heart. Heart failure may reflect ventricular failure, a poor prognostic indicator. Syncope caused by inadequate cerebral perfusion during exertion results from peripheral vasodilation and the inability to increase the cardiac output to meet demand during exercise. Physical findings include a blunted arterial upstroke, harsh systolic ejection murmur, S_4, and, in severe aortic stenosis, a single S_2. Occasionally an ejection click may be audible shortly after S_1. Signs and symptoms of heart failure may be apparent.

Echocardiography will estimate the pressure gradient across the stenotic aortic valve and the cross-sectional valve area. Afterload reduction is of no value in aortic stenosis since the afterload is fixed by the stenotic valve. Preload-reducing agents, such as nitrates, are contraindicated since preload must be adequate to generate the interventricular pressures (as high as 300 mmHg) necessary to force blood through the narrowed valve orifice. Once symptomatic, mortality is about 25 percent per year. Valve replacement should be carried out in all symptomatic patients and in asymptomatic patients developing ventricular dysfunction.

Tricuspid and *pulmonic insufficiency* can be congenital or caused by endocarditis, trauma, carcinoid syndrome, or annular dilation. Pulmonary hypertension, either primary or secondary to parenchymal disease or recurrent pulmonary embolism, leads to dilation of the right heart, including the tricuspid annulus. Tricuspid insufficiency due to failure of the tricuspid leaflets to coapt may result, with subsequent development of right heart failure with peripheral edema, jugular venous distension, hepatic congestion, and right-sided S_3 (louder with inspiration). Echocardiography will identify the lesion, estimate the severity, and shed light on the etiology. Treatment may include diuretics, digoxin, and afterload reduction.

Ventricular dysfunction As a practical matter, *ventricular dysfunction* can be categorized as due to systolic dysfunction (that is, impaired emptying) or diastolic dysfunction (impaired filling). These may be present concurrently.

Systolic dysfunction may be ascribed to

- Ischemic cardiomyopathy due to prior myocardial infarction
- Cardiomyopathy due to long-standing hypertension or diabetes
- Alcoholic cardiomyopathy
- Peripartum cardiomyopathy
- Other causes

The patient history may provide insight into the etiology of systolic dysfunction; symptoms do not distinguish between causes. The severity of ventricular dysfunction and the presence of associated abnormalities such as mitral or tricuspid insufficiency due to cavity and annular dilatation can be assessed by echocardiography. Coronary angiography is required to confirm the diagnosis of CAD.

Treatment should initially be directed at the underlying cause; e.g., alcoholics should stop drinking, and the management of hypertension and diabetes should be optimized. Risk factors for CAD such as smoking and hyperlipidemia should be addressed. In symptomatic patients, restriction of physical activity to reduce cardiac work is appropriate. Dietary sodium restriction will attenuate salt and water retention. Pharmacologic therapy with inotropic agents (digoxin), vasodilators, and diuretics will usually improve functional status. Afterload reduction in particular appears to prolong life. Cardiomyopathy patients are also prone to thrombus development in hypokinetic ventricles with subsequent embolization and thus are frequently anticoagulated with warfarin. Patients should also be evaluated for risk of arrhythmic death, which is markedly increased in this population as a whole.

Diastolic dysfunction is less commonly identified as a cause of heart failure, but it may be due to

- Restrictive/constrictive cardiomyopathy due to amyloidosis, hemochromatosis, or chronic pericardial disease

- Hypertrophic cardiomyopathy
- Hypertensive cardiomyopathy

Restrictive and constrictive cardiomyopathies often present with signs of right heart failure (i.e., edema), jugular venous distension, and hepatomegaly. The liver may be pulsatile. In constrictive pericardial disease, a pericardial knock may be audible early in diastole. Echocardiographic signs of restrictive myocardial disease may include marked biatrial enlargement, thickened ventricular walls, ventricular dilatation, and Doppler evidence of impaired ventricular filling. Amyloidosis is confirmed by biopsy of subcutaneous fat, rectum, or endocardium. Hemochromatosis is suggested by elevated plasma iron and serum ferritin levels and by elevated transferrin saturation. Constrictive pericardial disease may be difficult to identify by echocardiography, but a thickened pericardium might be evident by computed tomographic radiography.

Hypertrophic cardiomyopathy is a hereditary disease with autosomal dominant transmission. Occurrence in about half of patients, however, is spontaneous. The left ventricle is abnormally thickened, with the ventricular septum often disproportionately so. This asymmetric septal hypertrophy can cause dynamic outflow obstruction, particularly when left ventricular filling is impaired by dehydration, diuresis, nitrates, upright posture, or arrhythmias. Microscopic examination reveals hypertrophied muscle cells with marked architectural disarray. Dyspnea is the most common symptom, but patients may present with asymptomatic murmurs, angina, or sudden death. Murmur may be absent in patients without outflow obstruction. The presence of a harsh systolic ejection murmur at the lower left sternal border, which is quieter upon squatting, with handgrip or passive leg elevation and louder upon standing or during Valsalva maneuver, should raise the possibility of hypertrophic cardiomyopathy. The diagnosis is readily confirmed by echocardiography. Because this is a potentially life-threatening disease, these patients should be referred for negative inotropic therapy (calcium channel blockers), management of arrhythmic risk, and genetic counseling. Volume management is a particular cause for concern in this population. Because of the high blood flow velocity across the left ventricular outflow tract, patients with hypertrophic cardiomyopathy are at risk for infective endocarditis and should receive appropriate prophylaxis.

Management of CHF Appropriate management of CHF will depend on etiology, which is why it is important to determine the underlying cause of heart failure. Some of these causes and their treatment are summarized in general terms in Table 41-9.

The common types of heart failure will vary from community to community. Physicians seeing predominantly older patients may be faced with a pre-

TABLE 41-9 Management of Congestive Heart Failure

Etiology of Congestive Heart Failure	Management
Transient ischemic mitral insufficiency or systolic dysfunction	Nitrates, calcium channel or beta-blockers, revascularization.
Ruptured chorda tendina	Afterload reduction (nitroprusside, ACE, inhibitor), valve repair or replacement.
Infectious endocarditis	Antibiotics, afterload reduction, valve replacement.
Other mitral or aortic insufficiency	Afterload reduction, diuretics, valve repair-replacement.
Mitral or aortic stenosis	Valve replacement or mitral commissurotomy.
Cardiomyopathy with systolic dysfunction	Afterload reduction, inotropic support (digoxin), diuretics, sometimes warfarin.
Diastolic dysfunction	Avoid diuretics; use negative inotropes (verapamil, beta blocker, disopyramide).
Atrial fibrillation	Rate control with digoxin, diltiazem, beta blocker; conversion to sinus rhythm.
Other atrial and ventricular tachycardias	Antiarrhythmic therapy, ablation.
Bradyarrhythmias	Pacemaker.

ponderance of ischemic, dilated cardiomyopathies, which can be treated with maintenance digoxin, 0.125 to 0.25 mg/day (with normal renal function); afterload reduction such as enalapril titrated to systolic blood pressure or symptoms of hypotension (bearing in mind that enalapril causes cough, renal failure, and hyperkalemia, thereby affecting digoxin levels); with or without diuretics.

In other communities with a high proportion of hypertensives, CHF may be due predominantly to diastolic dysfunction, in which case inotropic agents such as digoxin are deleterious, and diuretics, by reducing preload, may aggravate left ventricular outflow obstruction. Drugs of choice for diastolic dysfunction are negative inotropic agents such as verapamil, beta-adrenergic blockers, and disopyramide, titrated to symptoms and outflow obstruction assessed by echocardiography. It is worth bearing in mind that for patients with structurally abnormal hearts, drugs are double-edged swords and often have a narrow therapeutic window.

Palpitations

Palpitations are variously described as skipped beats, pounding, or racing of the heart. They may represent paroxysmal atrial tachycardia (Fig. 41-5) or any other type of tachycardia, premature atrial or ventricular beats, atrial fibrillation (Fig. 41-6), compensatory or sinus pauses, sudden onset of sinus bradycardia (Fig. 41-7), complete heart block (Fig. 41-8), or may not be associated with any rhythm disturbance at all. In evaluating patients with palpitations, past cardiac history including MVP and MI should be obtained, and questions should be asked regarding any symptoms suggesting thyrotoxicosis. Physical examination may reveal evidence of MVP, i.e., a midsystolic click with or without a holosystolic murmur.

If MVP is suspected, an echocardiogram will confirm the diagnosis. Thyroid function tests will assess the possibility of thyrotoxicosis. A 12-lead electrocardiogram may reveal evidence of an accessory atrioventricular pathway such as a delta wave slurring the upstroke of the R wave. Patients with Wolff-Parkinson-White syndrome who note palpitations should be referred for electrophysiologic study whether or not arrhythmia is documented by other means because of their increased risk of sudden death. Documenting the presence or absence of arrhythmia is important for other patients. This can be undertaken either through Holter monitoring if the palpitations occur daily or event monitoring if they are less frequent. Event monitors record brief intervals of heart rhythm selected by the patient because of symptoms. These recordings are transtelephonically transmitted for interpretation. This approach enhances the possibility of capturing infrequent arrhythmias.

Syncope

Syncope is loss of consciousness, usually due to inadequate cerebral perfusion. Syncope may be caused by

- Vasomotor instability
- Drug effects
- Cerebrovascular disease
- Cardiac outflow obstruction
- Brady- or tachyarrhythmias

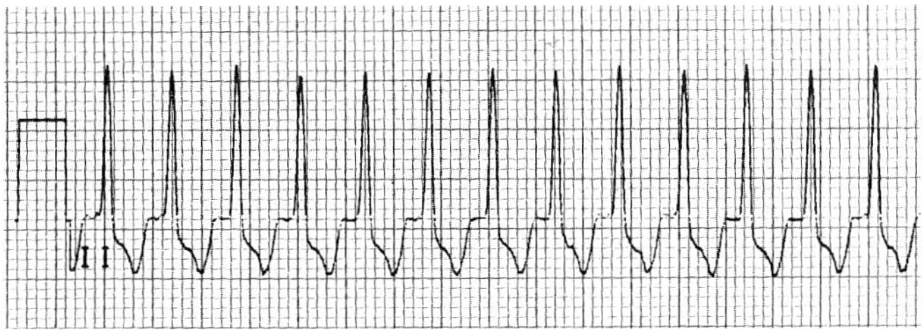

Figure 41-5 Electrocardiographic recording of paroxysmal atrial tachycardia with regular rate of 180 beats per minute, narrow complex, and absence of P wave preceding QRS complex.

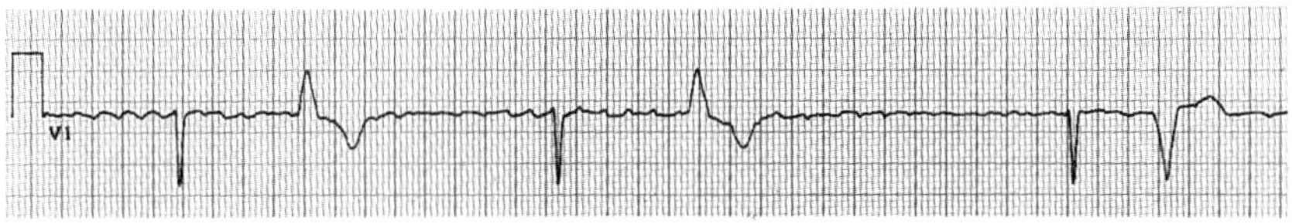

Figure 41-6 Electrocardiographic recording of atrial fibrillation with slow, irregular rate, narrow complex, and absence of P waves. Ventricular beats are interpolated.

Vasomotor syncope is common, particularly in young people. Patients may report many past syncopal episodes, which may be precipitated by prolonged standing, fear, heat, the sight of blood, perceived threat, or pain. The autonomically mediated vasodilation with subsequent fall in blood pressure is usually associated with other vagal symptoms such as diaphoresis and nausea. If this diagnosis is suspected, referral for tilt table testing is appropriate. During tilt testing, patients are maintained upright with arterial pressure and ECG monitoring, with or without intravenous isoproterenol provocation. The upright posture provokes gravitational pooling of blood, reducing venous return to the heart and thereby reducing stroke volume. In patients with abnormal compensatory responses, bradycardia, hypotension, and syncope may ensue, supporting the diagnosis of vasomotor syncope. Pharmacologic therapy with beta-adrenergic blockers, disopyramide, or other agents may be initiated, with repeat tilt testing on treatment to confirm efficacy.

Drug effects may cause syncope as well. In cardiac patients, syncope can be induced by vasodilation following sublingual nitroglycerin consumption, particularly in older patients taking several sequential doses of nitroglycerin. Proper instruction to use this agent while seated or supine usually solves the problem. Other antihypertensives may cause excessive hypotension, leading to dizziness or syncope as well. Digoxin toxicity may cause any type of brady- or tachyarrhythmia, leading to syncope.

Syncope due to *torsade des pointes,* a life-threatening form of ventricular tachycardia, is usually a result of toxicity from quinidine, procainamide, flecainide, bepridil, disopyramide, propaphenone, encainide, or, rarely, amiodarone. Recently antihistamines such as terfenadine (Seldane) and astemizole (Hismanal), particularly in conjunction with erythromycin, have been associated with torsade des pointes as well. Patients taking these histamine H_1 receptor blockers should be warned not to exceed prescribed doses, and such drugs should *never* be prescribed in combination with erythromycin. Overall, in 2 to 9 percent of patients with syncope, the problem is caused by drug toxicity.

Cerebrovascular disease may lead to syncope. Transient ischemic attacks (TIAs) of the vertebrobasilar system may infrequently cause syncope. Carotid sinus syncope is a form of carotid sinus hypersensitivity leading to loss of consciousness when pressure is applied to the carotid sinus, as when turning the head or wearing a tight collar. Carotid sinus hypersensitivity occurs predominantly in men.

Cardiac outflow obstruction can lead to inadequate cerebral perfusion with loss of consciousness.

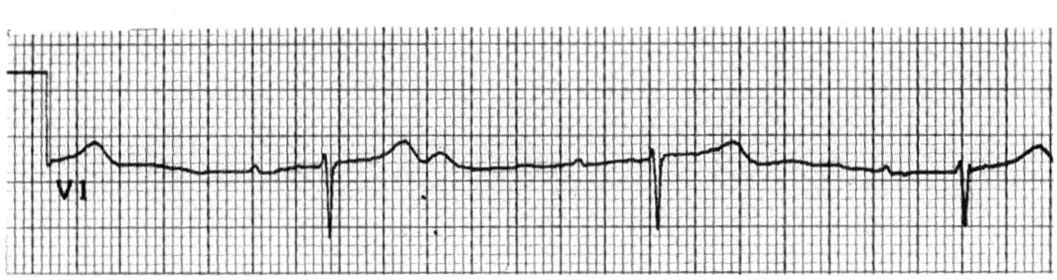

Figure 41-7 Electrocardiographic recording of marked sinus bradycardia with first-degree atrioventricular block. Note regular rate about 40 beats per minute; P wave precedes each narrow QRS complex, conducting with PR interval of 0.36 s.

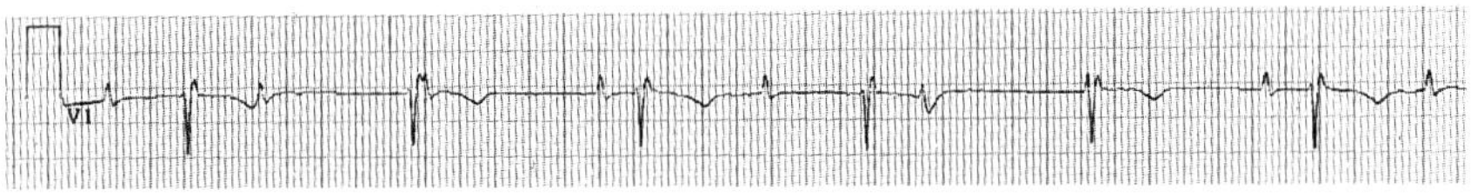

Figure 41-8 Electrocardiographic recording of complete heart block with dissociation between P waves and QRS complexes.

Characteristically, the cardiac output fails to rise in response to exertion because of fixed outflow obstruction such as aortic stenosis or dynamic outflow obstruction such as hypertrophic cardiomyopathy. In general, syncope is a poor prognostic sign in such patients, and should serve as an indication for intervention.

Syncope due to brady- or tachyarrhythmias may be difficult to diagnose since rhythm disturbances are often intermittent. Among patients with cardiac syncope, about 30 percent will die suddenly within 3 years of follow-up; thus, referral for further evaluation is appropriate. The specifics of the workup will depend on indications from history, physical examination, and a 12-lead ECG, but they may include echocardiography to evaluate for structural heart disease, signal-averaged electrocardiogram to assess the potential of the myocardial substrate for ventricular tachycardia, tilt table testing to exclude vasomotor syncope, Holter monitoring, event recording, coronary angiography if ischemia is implicated, and/or electrophysiologic testing to assess sinus node, atrioventricular node, and His bundle conduction studies as well as the inducibility of atrial and ventricular arrhythmias.

In obtaining a history from patients with syncope, a description of events leading up to the syncopal episode, concurrent symptoms, drug regimen, past MI, valvular disease, and past cardiac evaluation may be helpful. Physical examination should include measurement of supine and upright pulse and blood pressure. Attention should be given to signs of aortic stenosis or hypertrophic cardiomyopathy (systolic ejection murmur which gets softer with squatting and louder with upright posture). Electrocardiography may reveal evidence of prior MI, conduction abnormalities, or left ventricular hypertrophy (which may indicate aortic stenosis or hypertrophic cardiomyopathy).

Whether the presenting symptom is syncope or palpitations, the presence of an arrhythmia must be sought and documented either by telemetry, Holter monitoring, event recording, or during electrophysiologic testing. Once a rhythm abnormality has been identified, specific treatment may be instituted for relief of symptoms or for prognosis. Bradyarrhythmias requiring treatment include high-grade heart block [i.e., complete heart block or distal second-degree atrioventricular block (Mobitz II)] and sick sinus syndrome. Symptoms are often iatrogenic sequelae of beta-adrenergic or calcium channel blockade, in which case discontinuation of the offending medication will suffice. Otherwise, placement of a permanent transvenous pacemaker may be indicated.

Common *supraventricular tachyarrhythmias* include atrial fibrillation and flutter, ectopic atrial tachycardias, and reentrant supraventricular tachycardias. Patients with new-onset atrial fibrillation/flutter should be evaluated for causes such as mitral stenosis, pulmonary embolism, thyrotoxicosis, and coronary disease if none is readily apparent. The objectives of treatment are (1) control of ventricular rate, (2) conversion to sinus rhythm, and (3) prevention of thromboembolism.

Ventricular rate, assessed by electrocardiography or apical (not peripheral) pulse, can be controlled in stable patients using oral or intravenous digoxin, a calcium channel blocker such as diltiazem or verapamil, or a beta-adrenergic blocker such as esmolol. Unstable patients should be electrically cardioverted without delay. Patients should be electrocardiographically monitored during this interval. Either electrical or chemical cardioversion to sinus rhythm may be attempted once the ventricular rate is controlled. Patients with atrial fibrillation of less than 3 days duration may be cardioverted to sinus rhythm without prior anticoagulation, according to guidelines suggested by the American College of Chest Physicians. Those with atrial fibrillation of longer duration should be anticoagulated for 3 weeks before cardioversion and for 2 to 4 weeks afterwards. Electrical cardioversion is usually carried out with short-acting anesthesia. Chemical cardioversion and attempted maintenance of sinus rhythm may be attempted with class 1A agents such as quinidine and procainamide, class IC agents such as flecainamide, and class III agents such as amiodarone and sotalol. All of these drugs have serious side effects, including sudden death, and should be administered with monitoring by physicians experienced with their use. Some patients cannot be converted into or maintained in sinus rhythm. Rate control and long-term prophylaxis against thromboembolism are the mainstays of therapy in that group.

Other atrial tachycardias, including *paroxysmal atrial tachycardia,* may be treated with calcium channel or beta-adrenergic blockers if clinically warranted. Transvenous ablation of reentrant pathways or automatic foci may be performed by an electrophysiologist as an alternative to drug therapy. Patients with Wolff-Parkinson-White syndrome conduct electrical impulses from the atrium to the ventricle faster than usual by conducting down an accessory pathway, so-called preexcitation. These patients are susceptible to reentrant supraventricular tachycardias and to atrial fibrillation that may be life-threatening if ventricular fibrillation is precipitated by rapid stimulation of the ventricle via the accessory pathway. Drugs that may shorten refractoriness of the accessory pathway, such as digoxin and intravenous verapamil, are thus relatively contraindicated in patients with preexcitation. Patients with symptomatic preexcitation should be referred for electrophysiologic testing and possible accessory pathway ablation.

Ventricular arrhythmias vary in severity from isolated premature ventricular contractions to sudden death. In general, isolated premature ventricular contractions do not require treatment. Indications for treatment of ventricular tachycardia depend on the substrate; patients with normal ventricles and no coronary disease may not need treatment. If the underlying precipitant for ventricular arrhythmia is myocardial ischemia, treatment should be directed accordingly. On the other hand, cardiomyopathy patients at high risk for sudden death may require aggressive arrhythmic therapy and/or implantation of an automatic pacer-cardioverter-defibrillator. The latter devices can be placed transvenously and no longer require thoracotomy.

As indicated above, cardiac arrhythmias vary in severity and certain arrhythmias can result in sudden death. Many of the arrhythmias are not commonly treated in the office as a component of primary care, and therefore a more detailed discussion regarding this management is beyond the scope of this book.

Claudication

Most leg cramps are not claudication, yet claudication is important to identify, in part because of its close association with CAD. Of patients with peripheral vascular disease but no symptoms referable to the heart, half will have coronary disease, and all should be evaluated for this possibility. *Claudication* is the peripheral vascular equivalent of angina, characterized as crampy pain in the buttocks, posterior thigh, or calf, brought on by exertion and relieved by rest. Cardiovascular risk factors, particularly smoking, should be carefully assessed. Physical exam should include palpation of femoral, popliteal, dorsalis pedis, and posterior tibialis pulses bilaterally. Ischemic foot ulcers may be apparent.

Initial management is conservative, with good control of hypertension, diabetes, and hyperlipidemia. Patients must stop smoking. Modest exercise training is sometimes helpful, enabling muscles to make efficient use of the blood flow that is available. Most patients will improve with conservative management. If patients have pain at rest or persistent claudication after a trial of conservative management, they should be referred to a vascular surgeon.

Peripheral Venous Disease

Venous thrombophlebitis is prevalent following gynecologic surgery. Some studies report that 40 percent of deaths following pelvic surgery are attributable to venous thrombosis and pulmonary embolism. Not surprisingly, the frequency of these adverse events increases with the age of the patient, the duration of the surgery, and in those immobilized for prolonged intervals. Other risk factors for venous thrombosis include obesity, malignancy, and hypercoagulable states. Estrogen has also been suggested as a possible risk.

Clearly, prophylaxis against deep venous thrombosis or pulmonary embolism is preferable to treatment after the problem has arisen. Prophylaxis using either compression stockings such as TEDS (thromboembolic deterrent stockings) or intermittent pneumatic compression will reduce the risk of thromboembolic events originating in the lower legs. A variety of pharmacologic regimens for prophylaxis against venous thrombosis have been recommended, including low-dose warfarin and intravenous or subcutaneous heparin. The suitability of any of these approaches depends on the clinical setting.

Characteristic physical findings of deep venous thrombosis include localized warmth, redness, tenderness, and swelling of the extremity. Tenderness over the femoral veins is more suggestive of proximal venous thrombosis. Clinical signs are not especially specific so that patients in whom venous thrombosis is suspected should have noninvasive testing.

Impedance plethysmography is widely available and inexpensive. Venous outflow from the leg is occluded with a cuff inflated to 45 to 60 mmHg. Arterial inflow is not affected, so blood accumulates distal to the cuff. When the cuff is suddenly released, blood flows out of the leg. In the presence of venous obstruction, the venous outflow will be impaired. This diagnostic test is particularly helpful in patients with proximal vein thrombosis; it is less sensitive for distal thrombosis. Two-dimensional ultrasound (duplex) scanning is even more sensitive and specific than impedance plethysmography; it is noninvasive and comparatively inexpensive as well. Venography is the gold standard. If embolization of a thrombus from the leg to the pulmonary circulation is suspected, ventilation-perfusion lung scanning is recommended. Usually pulmonary angiography can be avoided.

Once proximal deep venous thrombosis or pulmonary embolism has been confirmed, patients should be given a bolus of intravenous heparin and a heparin infusion begun at about 1000 IU/h, adjusted to maintain an activated partial thromboplastin time 1.5 to 2 times the control value. Anticoagulation should be transitioned to warfarin, adjusted to maintain the protime at 1.5 times the control and maintained for at least 3 months. Pregnant women who cannot take warfarin may be transitioned to subcutaneous heparin, adjusted to achieve an activated partial thromboplastin time of 1.5 times the control when measured 6 h after subcutaneous administration.

Calf vein thrombosis is generally associated with a good prognosis even when treated conservatively. However, over 10 to 14 days, about 6 percent of affected individuals will develop abnormal impedance plethysmographic studies, indicating extension into the popliteal vein. Therefore, either conventional anticoagulation with heparin and warfarin or serial noninvasive evaluation for 10 to 14 days is recommended.[11]

Superficial phlebitis can be managed conservatively with analgesics or anti-inflammatory agents, heat, and elevation.

Aortic Disease

Aortic disease is generally structural, since the aorta predominantly functions as a conduit from the left ventricle to end-organs. Structural aortic disease can be categorized as congenital or acquired.

Coarctation of the aorta is a congenital malformation. It is associated with a bicuspid aortic valve and with Turner's syndrome. Coarctation is usually identified during childhood because of the loud murmur, unequal extremity blood pressures, and hypertension. The presence and severity of the coarctation and any associated anomalies can be readily confirmed by echocardiography, and the aorta either dilated by balloon angioplasty or surgically repaired. Restenosis occurs in a proportion of patients using either of these treatment approaches. During pregnancy, placental blood flow may be inadequate due to aortic obstruction, and aortic rupture has been reported.[21] Additionally, women with coarctation have increased likelihood of having offspring with congenital heart disease. Genetic counseling and, if desired and available, fetal echocardiography at 16 to 17 weeks gestation are appropriate.

The other comparatively common group of congenital diseases with aortic manifestations is connective tissue diseases such as Ehlers-Danlos and Marfan syndromes. In Ehlers-Danlos syndrome, echocardiography for detection of associated mitral valve prolapse and appropriate antibiotic prophylaxis usually suffice. Genetic counseling is indicated, and women with subtype IV should avoid pregnancy because of enhanced risk of spontaneous, catastrophic arterial rupture.[17] Mitral valve prolapse is also common in Marfan syndrome. In addition to echocardiography for mitral valve evaluation, all patients with Marfan syndrome should have serial echocardiographic follow-up of their aortic root dimension and should be seen periodically by a cardiologist. Prophylactic aortic surgery is usually carried out to prevent rupture once the aorta reaches 60 mm in diameter. Aortic dissection is a prominent cause of death in patients with Marfan syndrome, and may occur without marked aortic root dilatation. Inheritance of Marfan syndrome is autosomal dominant, thus affected women have a 50:50 chance of transitting the disease to their offspring. Further, the risk of aortic rupture or dissection is augmented by pregnancy.

The two most common acquired structural abnormalities of the aorta are aortic aneurysm and dissection. Although the differential diagnosis of thoracic or abdominal aortic aneurysm is extensive, in the current era, most cases are due to atherosclerosis. Abdominal aortic aneurysms are usually detected as asymptomatic, pulsatile abdominal masses. Aneurysm size is readily quantified by abdominal ultrasound, and surgical repair recommended for aneurysms exceeding 6 cm in diameter. Aneurysms less than 6 cm should be followed with serial ultrasound studies.

Thoracic aneurysms are more frequently symptomatic due to compression of intrathoracic structures, leading to cough, hoarseness, stridor, hemoptysis, and obstructive pneumonia. Diagnosis of thoracic aneurysms may be confirmed by MRI, CT scan, or transesophageal echocardiography. Surgical repair is recommended for thoracic aneurysms producing symptoms or for asymptomatic aneurysms exceeding 7 cm in diameter because of the risk of rupture.

Aortic dissection is a dramatic event, presenting with severe, knifelike back or chest pain, hypotension, and at times a sensation of impending doom. In contrast to aortic aneurysms, in which the vessel wall remains intact, aortic dissection is caused by a tear in the intima or hemorrhage into the media with immediate propagation of the dissection along the vessel wall. Upper extremity pulses may be absent, and congestive heart failure may result from acute aortic insufficiency. Since the pleura and pericardium enwrap the ascending aorta, aortic rupture can lead to pleural and pericardial effusions. If the dissection extends into the carotid arteries, localizing neurologic signs may be present. Dissection is more common in patients with Marfan syndrome and those with hypertension. When aortic dissection is suspected, the patient should urgently be transported to an emergency room for diagnosis and management.

Myocarditis, Pericarditis, and Endocarditis

Dilated cardiomyopathy can present as new-onset congestive heart failure or with atrial or ventricular arrhythmias. As many as 10 percent of patients with dilated cardiomyopathy have otherwise structurally normal hearts and normal coronary arteries. In one large series of such dilated cardiomyopathy patients, 12 percent had endomyocardial biopsy-proven myocarditis.[13] In contrast to idiopathic cardiomyopathy, patients with myocarditis often recover. Congestive heart failure and arrhythmias in myocarditis are responsive to conventional treatment; immunosuppressive therapy has not proved efficacious.

Pericarditis usually presents as substernal or left precordial chest pain, often relieved by leaning forward and exacerbated by cough, deep inspiration, or supine posture. A pericardial friction rub may be audible. A sequence of characteristic electrocardiographic changes includes sinus tachycardia, diffuse ST elevation, and PR depression followed several days later by return of ST and PR segments to baseline with T wave inversion. Echocardiography may reveal a pericardial effusion. Pericarditis may be idiopathic, infectious, malignant, uremic, or associated with collagen vascular diseases such as systemic lupus erythematosus or rheumatoid arthritis. Idiopathic pericarditis, a self-limited disease, is treated with nonsteroidal anti-inflammatory agents. Patients with bacterial, tuberculous, or fungal pericarditis are acutely ill, and require prompt diagnosis, pericardial drainage, and specific antibiotic therapy. Malignant effusions occur most commonly in patients with known breast or lung cancer, lymphoma, or melanoma. Pericardial effusion with or without symptoms is also prevalent in human immunodeficiency virus infection, occurring in 17 percent of patients during 2-year follow-up.[10]

Pericarditis due to any etiology may result in pericardial tamponade. Patients with tamponade are severely dyspneic, with tachycardia, jugular venous distension, and a pulsus paradoxicus; they may be hypotensive. Characteristic echocardiographic findings confirm the diagnosis of pericardial tamponade, which may be relieved by either percutaneous or open pericardial drainage.

Bacterial endocarditis is an infection of a native or prosthetic heart valve, usually with characteristic organisms such as Staphylococci, Streptococci, or Enterococci. Patients commonly present with fever and a new heart murmur. Individuals with structural heart abnormalities, such as mitral valve prolapse or ventricular septal defect, have increased susceptibility to endocarditis, as do the elderly, diabetics, and intravenous drug users. The responsible pathogen is identified by blood culture; vegetations and paravalvular abscesses may be identified by echocardiography. Antibiotic therapy is tailored to the specific organism. Indications for valve replacement include persistent sepsis despite adequate antibiotics, embolization, paravalvular abscess, and congestive heart failure due to valvular insufficiency.

Preoperative Evaluation

Antibiotic Prophylaxis

The American Heart Association recommends antibiotic prophylaxis in patients with

- Prosthetic heart valves
- Most congenital cardiac malformations (except ostium secundum atrial septal defects)
- Rheumatic and other acquired valvular disease
- Hypertrophic cardiomyopathy
- Mitral valve prolapse with mitral insufficiency

Prophylaxis is recommended for the following obstetrical and gynecologic procedures:

- Vaginal hysterectomy
- Vaginal delivery in the presence of infection
- Urethral dilatation
- Urethral catheterization or urinary tract surgery in the presence of a urinary tract infection
- Incision and drainage of infected tissue

Prophylaxis is generally not recommended for low-risk procedures such as uncomplicated vaginal delivery or dilation and curettage when there is no evidence of infection. In patients with prosthetic heart valves or previous endocarditis, however, physicians may elect to provide antibiotic prophylaxis even for low-risk procedures. In addition, many physicians utilize antibiotic prophylaxis for all patients having any one of the five aforementioned cardiac problems, even when performing procedures which are considered "low risk" since there may be a transient bacteremia even in these so-called low-risk situations. In addition, many physicians utilize antibiotic prophylaxis when performing procedures on women with MVP, even when mitral insufficiency is not present.

In the presence of infection, antibiotic therapy should be directed against known or suspected pathogens in addition to providing the standard prophylactic regimen for genitourinary and gastrointestinal procedures, summarized in Table 41-10. Recommendations for prophylaxis during dental, oral, or upper respiratory tract procedures are summarized in Table 41-11.

Assessment of Operative Cardiac Risk

Cardiac ischemia during the perioperative period is a primary determinant of operative morbidity and mortality. The objectives of preoperative cardiac evaluation are (1) to assess the risk of MI or cardiac death during and immediately following surgery,

TABLE 41-10 American Heart Association Guidelines for Antibiotic Prophylaxis in Genitourinary and Gastrointestinal Procedures

Standard regimen
Ampicillin, 2 g IV or IM + gentamicin, 1.5 mg/kg IV or IM (not to exceed 80 mg), 30 min before procedure; followed by amoxicillin, 1.5 g orally, 6 h after the initial dose.
Alternatively, parenteral regimen may be repeated once 8 h after initial dose.

For amoxicillin-ampicillin-penicillin–allergic patients
Vancomycin, 1 g IV, administered over 1 h + gentamicin, 1.5 mg/kg IV or IM (not to exceed 80 mg), 1 h before procedure; may be repeated once 8 h after initial dose.

Alternate oral regimen for low-risk patients
Amoxicillin, 3 g orally, 1 h before procedure; then 1.5 g 6 hours after initial dose.

(2) to develop a management plan intended to minimize cardiac operative risk, and (3) to evaluate the risks and benefits of surgery and make an assessment regarding the risk/benefit ratio. In carrying out this assessment the following factors should be kept in mind:

1. The type of operation
2. Whether it is an emergency or an elective procedure
3. The patient's underlying health status

Intraabdominal operations are associated with increased risk, in part because of the comparatively prolonged postoperative course associated with such operations and the fluid and electrolyte shifts that often accompany them. Cardiovascular risk is also related to the complexity and duration of the surgery. There is ample evidence that the likelihood of perioperative MI and cardiac death are increased 2.5- to 4-fold if the operation is performed as an emergency.

History

Age. Age is a potent predictor of operative risk, albeit one that is not susceptible to alteration.

Prior MI. Past history of ischemic heart disease predicts cardiovascular operative risk; the likelihood of intra- or postoperative myocardial infarction is 10 to 50 times greater in patients with prior MI than in those without. The 6 months following MI represent a particularly high risk interval. In general, elective surgery should be delayed until 6 months after an MI.

Angina Pectoris. In patients with stable angina—i.e., no pain at rest or crescendo anginal pattern—an objective assessment of ischemic burden can be performed prior to elective surgery. Depending on the degree of exercise achieved, blood pressure re-

TABLE 41-11 American Heart Association Guidelines for Antibiotic Prophylaxis in Dental, Oral, or Upper Respiratory Tract Procedures

Standard regimen
Amoxicillin, 3 g orally, 1 h before procedure; then 1.5 g 6 h after initial dose.

For amoxicillin-penicillin–allergic patients
Erythromycin ethylsuccinate, 800 mg, or erythromycin stearate, 1 g orally, 2 h before a procedure; then one half the dose 6 h after initial administration.

or

Clindamycin, 300 mg orally, 1 h before a procedure and then 150 mg 6 h after initial dose.

For patients unable to take oral medication
Ampicillin, 2 g IV or IM, 30 min before procedure; then ampicillin, 1 g IV or IM, or amoxicillin, 1.5 g orally, 6 h after initial dose.

For amoxicillin-ampicillin-penicillin–allergic patients unable to take oral medication
Clincamycin, 300 mg IV, 30 min before a procedure and 150 mg IV or orally 6 h after initial dose.

For patients considered to be at high risk who are not candidates for the standard regimen
Ampicillin, 2 g IV or IM + gentamicin, 1.5 mg/kg IV or IM (not to exceed 80 mg), 30 min before procedure, followed by amoxicillin, 1.5 g orally, 6 h after initial dose.
Alternatively, parenteral regimen may be repeated once 8 h after initial dose.

For amoxicillin-ampicillin-penicillin–allergic patients unable to take oral medication and considered to be at high risk
Vancomycin, 1 g IV, administered over 1 h starting 1 h before the procedure; no repeat dose is necessary.

sponse, area of ischemic myocardium, and evidence of prior MI, adjustment of the medical regimen or revascularization may be recommended. Evidence that revascularization prior to elective noncardiac surgery prevents perioperative cardiac events is scanty.

Unstable angina. Patients with unstable angina should be hospitalized and generally undergo coronary angiography before elective noncardiac surgery. Whether revascularization or medical therapy is recommended depends on the angiographic findings.

Claudication. About one half of patients with peripheral vascular disease will have coronary disease whether or not they have angina. Often such patients are unable to achieve a sufficient degree of exercise to develop angina; nonetheless, their coronary atherosclerosis contributes to their operative risk. Therefore, individuals with intermittent claudication should undergo pharmacologic stress nuclear imaging before undergoing noncardiac surgery.

Cardiac risk factors. Risk factor assessment should be included as part of the preoperative evaluation since one half of patients with MI have no premonitory angina. Individuals with several risk factors may warrant stress testing as well.

Medications. If patients will be unable to take their oral medications before or after surgery, contingency plans for alternative management of hypertension or diabetes should be developed. Lipid-lowering medications may be held during the perioperative period, but other agents such as clonidine and beta blockers need to be tapered and possibly replaced with alternatives not susceptible to rebound in advance. Reduced insulin dosing on the day of surgery should be planned if appropriate.

Physical examination Physical examination may reveal hypertension, evidence of congestive heart failure, or valvular disease. Congestive heart failure is a particularly adverse prognostic indicator.

Preoperative testing Perhaps the most common indication for preoperative cardiac evaluation is an abnormal 12-lead ECG, usually evidence of prior MI. Upon specific questioning, many patients will have had prior ECGs. With the advent of the facsimile machine, comparison of current and past tracings has been significantly facilitated. If the ECG abnormality was present at least 3, and preferably 6, months previously, operative risk is reduced. In the absence of an available prior ECG, echocardiography demonstrating normal wall motion may provide a degree of reassurance, although patients with prior MI may have normal or near-normal wall motion, particularly in the thrombolytic era.

Evaluation and optimization of preoperative status In view of known predisposing factors to cardiac events following surgery, purely elective operations should be deferred in patients with recent MI, uncompensated heart failure, or severe mitral or aortic stenosis. Beyond these few clear-cut situations, a balance must be struck between the urgency and strength of surgical indication and the estimated risk of a perioperative cardiac event. A number of studies have evaluated indices assessing risk, the best known of which may be the Goldman criteria (Table 41-12). Patients with 26 or more Goldman points have a 56 percent risk of perioperative myocardial

TABLE 41-12 Assessment of Cardiac Risk Prior to Noncardiac Surgery

Factors	No. of Points
Age > 70 years	5
Myocardial infarction within 6 mo	10
S_3 gallop or jugular venous distension	11
Significant aortic stenosis	3
Nonsinus rhythm on preoperative ECG	7
> 5 premature ventricular contractions/min documented at any time	7
$P_{O_2} < 60$ or $P_{CO_2} > 50$ mmHg, or K < 3 or HCO3 < 20 mEq/l, or BUN > 50 or creatinine > 3 mg/dl, or chronic liver disease or bedridden patient	3
Intraperitoneal, intrathoracic, or aortic operation	3
Emergency operation	4
Total possible points	53

NOTE: In Goldman's study, patients with 26 or more points had a 56 percent risk of perioperative MI, pulmonary edema, ventricular tachycardia, or death.

SOURCE: From Goldman L et al: Multifactorial index of cardiac risk in noncardiac surgical procedures. *N Engl J Med* 297:845, 1977.

TABLE 41-13 Resuscitation Cart Supplies and Equipment

Top of cart
Synchronizing defibrillator.

Side of cart
Cardiopulmonary resuscitation board.

Drawer 1

Atropine	0.5 mg/5 ml	4 prefilled syringes
Bretylium	500 mg/10 ml	2 ampules
Calcium chloride	1 g/10 ml	3 prefilled syringes
50% dextrose	25 g/50 ml	1 prefilled syringe
Epinephrine, 1:10,000	1 mg/10 ml	4 prefilled syringes 1 with cardiac needle
Heparin, 1:1000	10,000 IU/10 ml	1 vial
Isoproterenol	1 mg/5 ml	2 ampules
Norepinephrine (Levophed)	4 mg/4 ml	2 ampules
Lidocaine	100 mg/5 ml	4 prefilled syringes
Naloxone (Narcan)	0.4 mg/1 ml	3 ampules
Normal saline for infusion	500 cc	2 bags
Sodium bicarbonate	50 mEq/50 ml	6 prefilled syringes
Valium	10 mg/2 ml	2 prefilled syringes
Magnesium	1 g/2 ml	4 prefilled syringes

IV additive and blood labels, 3 rubber stoppers, 20 alcohol swabs, vacutainers, pen

Drawer 2
Subclavian catheter kit, selection of needles and syringes, five preheparinized syringes, cotton 4 × 4 s, sterile gloves, tape, scalpel handle and blades, kelly clamp, 3.0 silk suture on a needle, tourniquets, betadine and benzoin swabs, padded tongue blade.

Drawer 3
Bags of normal saline and 5% dextrose for infusion, IV tubing, premixed dopamine (800 mg/500 ml D5W) and lidocaine (1 g/250 ml D5W) infusions, IV catheters.

Drawer 4
Nasogastric tube, lubricating jelly, suction cannister and connectors, Yankauer suction tip catheter, normal saline for irrigation, laryngoscope handle and blades, copper stylet, oral airway, adult McGill forceps, assorted endotracheal tubes, batteries and replacement bulb for laryngoscope.

Drawer 5
Tracheostomy tray and tubes, cut down tray.

TABLE 41-13 Resuscitation Cart Supplies and Equipment (Continued)

Bottom of cart
Self-inflating resuscitation bag with oxygen accumulator, adult masks (large and small), oral airway, oxygen tank, tubing and flow meter.

NOTE: This list includes the items on a resuscitation cart in one university hospital. By evaluating this list, physicians can determine which items might be needed in their individual office situations.

infarction, pulmonary edema, ventricular tachycardia, or death.

Optimization of preoperative status should be undertaken in all nonemergency situations. These measures include repletion of serum potassium to > 4 mEq/dl, serum magnesium > 2 mEq/dl, insulin management, pulmonary toilet, nutritional status, intravascular and total body volume adjustment including dialysis if necessary, optimization of CHF and anti-ischemic treatment. In patients with significant cardiac history this often includes intravenous inotropic support for several days with invasive hemodynamic monitoring, diuresis, intravenous nitroglycerin, and aspirin. Usually the consulting cardiologist will assume responsibility for preoperative optimization of patients with cardiac problems with this degree of complexity.

Cardiac Life Support

Although it is extremely uncommon for a patient to require cardiopulmonary support in an office situation, so much more is being done for patients in office settings because of the mandates of managed care companies that there is the potential for its incidence to increase. The likelihood of a cardiac arrest occurring will vary depending on the patient population seen and the type of practice.

Resuscitation carts are not standardized; the contents of such carts at one university hospital are noted in Table 41-13. Cardiac life support is discussed in greater in depth in Chap. 65.

Conclusion

Cardiovascular disease is widespread, yet underdiagnosed and undertreated in women in the United States. The woman's primary care physician should use the opportunity of the office visit to screen for and identity cardiovascular risk factors and either treat or refer the woman with cardiovascular disease.

Acknowledgment

The advice of Dr. John C. LaRosa, Professor of Medicine and Dean for Research at the George Washington University, in preparation of this chapter, is gratefully acknowledged.

References and Selected Readings

1. Adesanya CO, Angorin FI, Adeoshun IO et al: Peripartum cardiac failure. A ten year follow-up study. *Trop Geogr Med* 41:190, 1989.
2. Averill KH, Lamb LE: Electrocardiographic findings in 67,375 asymptomatic subjects. I. Incidence of abnormalities. *Am J Cardiol* 6:76, 1960.
3. Bonnar J: Venous thromboembolism and gynecologic surgery. *Clin Obstet Gynecol* 28:432, 1985.
4. Dunn M, Alexander J, deSilva R, et al: Antithrombotic therapy in atrial fibrillation. *Chest* 95(suppl):118S, 1989.
5. Emergency Cardiac Care Committee and Subcommittees, American Heart Association: Guidelines for Cardiopulmonary Resuscitation and Emergency Cardiac Care. *JAMA* 268:2171, 1992.
6. Expert Panel on Detection, Evaluation, and Treatment of High Blood Cholesterol in Adults: Summary of the second report of the National Cholesterol Education Program (NCEP) Expert Panel on detection, evaluation, and treatment of high blood cholesterol in adults (Adult Treatment Panel II). *JAMA* 269:3015–3023, 1993.
7. Furberg CD, Manolio TA, Psaty BM, et al: Major electrocardiographic abnormalities in persons aged 65 years and older (The Cardiovascular Health Study). *Am J Cardiol* 69:1329, 1992.
8. Goldman L: Multifactorial index of cardiac risk in noncardiac surgery: Ten-year status report. *J Cardiothorac Anesth* 1:237, 1987.
9. Grady D, Rubin SM, Pettiti DB, et al: Hormone therapy to prevent disease and prolong life in postmenopausal women. *Ann Intern Med* 117:1016, 1992.
10. Hsia J, Ross AM: Pericardial effusion and pericardiocentesis in human immunodeficiency virus infection. *Am J Cardiol* 74:94, 1994.
11. Hyers TM, Hull RD, Weg JG: Antithrombotic therapy for venous thromboembolic disease. *Chest* 95(suppl):37S, 1989.
12. Kannel WB, Anderson K, McGee DL, et al: Nonspecific electrocardiographic abnormality as a predictor of coronary heart disease: The Framingham Study. *Am Heart J* 113:370, 1987.
13. Kasper EK, Agema WRP, Hutchins GM, et al: The causes of dilated cardiomyopathy: A clinicopathologic review of 673 consecutive patients. *J Am Coll Cardiol* 23:586, 1994.
14. Kreger BE, Cupples A, Kannel WB: The electrocardiogram in prediction of sudden death: Framingham Study experience. *Am Heart J* 113:377, 1987.
15. Liedhom H, Melander A: Drug selection in the treatment of pregnancy hypertension. *Acta Obstet Gynecol Scand* (suppl)118:49, 1974.
16. National Diabetes Data Group: Classification and diagnosis of diabetes mellitus and other categories of glucose intolerance. *Diabetes* 28:1039, 1979.
17. Rudd NL, Nimrod C, Holbrook K, et al: Pregnancy complications in type IV Ehlers-Danlos syndrome. *Lancet* 1:50, 1983.
18. Sempos CT, Cleeman JI, Carroll MD, et al: Prevalence of high blood cholesterol among US adults. An update based on guidelines from the second report of the National Cholesterol Education Program Adult Treatment Panel. *JAMA* 269:3009, 1993.
19. The Diabetes Control and Complications Trial Research Group: The effect of intensive treatment of diabetes on the development and progression of long-term complications in insulin-dependent diabetes mellitus. *N Engl J Med* 329:977, 1993.
20. U.S. Department of Health and Human Resources: Vital statistics of the United States 1983. II. Mortality, part B. Washington, DC: U.S. Department of Health and Human Services Publication, 87–1114, 1987.
21. Wachtel HL, Czarnecki SW: Coarctation of the aorta and pregnancy. *Am Heart J* 72:251, 1966.
22. Willett WC, Green A, Stampfer MJ, et al: Relative and absolute excess risks of coronary heart disease among women who smoke cigarettes. *N Engl J Med* 317:1303, 1987.
23. Williams GB, Gott VL, Brawley RK, et al: Aortic disease associated with pregnancy. *J Vasc Surg* 8:470, 1988.
24. Wing RR, Matthew KA, Kuller LH, et al: Waist to hip ratio in middle-aged Women: Associations with behavioral and psychosocial factors and with changes in cardiovascular risk factors. *Arterioscler Thromb* 11:1250, 1991.

42 The Breast

Bruce H. Drukker

Embryologic and Anatomic Characteristics

A fundamental understanding of breast embryology and anatomy is essential for understanding the clinical changes that occur in the female breast.

Embryology and Development

Embryologically, the mammary gland begins as a linear bilateral symmetric area of epidermal thickening known as the mammary ridge, seen at the sixth week of embryonic development. The ridge retains its position in the developing embryo until the third month of gestation, at which time the caudal two-thirds disappear, but at the level of the fourth intercostal space a proliferation of basal cells creates the nipple bud. At approximately the fifth month of embryonic development, squamous cells from this surface area invade down into the nipple and mesenchymal tissue, forming 15 to 20 solid cords of cells. These cords grow and proliferate with many branches, providing the genesis for the primary and secondary epithelial ducts of the breast. During the seventh or eighth month of gestation, the ducts become canalized, forming the lactiferous ducts that open in the depressed nipple area and eventually on the nipple surface.

At birth the mammary glands are not well developed. However, as an indirect effect of maternal hormones circulating in the fetal blood during gestation there frequently occurs bilateral or unilateral breast enlargement in all infants, both male and female. Secretory activity may take place, the nipple becomes slightly elevated, and there may be some pigmentation in the areola area. These changes, however, are brief and regress after the second or third week of life.

At puberty—and particularly as a result of estrogen and progesterone secretion—the dormant nipple and areolar structures become more prominent, expand, and the duct system elongates and acquires branching. With subsequent ovulation, the breast enlarges, with a significant deposition of fatty tissue and the development of connective tissue around the breast ducts.

There are three congenital abnormalities seen with some frequency. First is the *inverted* or *retracted nipple,* which is caused by a failure in the development of the nipple substance. Although not important from an anatomic point of view, it is of concern from a cosmetic standpoint and may also be associated with difficulty during breast feeding. *Polythelia* and *polymastia,* specifically accessory nipples and breasts, can also occur. These are usually found along a line corresponding to the mammary ridge, beginning in the axillary area and continuing to the groin. Pigmented areas with small central hyperpigmentation can be noted, and occasionally even a small mound of fatty glandular tissue may be present. *Athelia,* or absence of the nipple, is quite uncommon but has been reported.

Anatomic Characteristics

The breast in the adult female is located between the second and sixth rib in its vertical position and between the parasternal and midaxillary line in its horizontal configuration. The average central thickness of the breast is 7 cm. The breast weighs approximately 200 g in the nonpregnant state and may have differences in size and occasionally configuration. Often the left breast is slightly larger than the right. The weight of the breast increases dramatically during pregnancy, with increases up to 600 g being noted. With lactation there is an additional increase, with estimates of 600 to 800 g of breast tissue.

The breast appears domelike and conical in nulliparous females but tends to be pendulous in parous females. The axillary tail (tail of Spence) can be very prominent in some patients and may cause discomfort, not only at the time of menses but also when the patient lactates.

The skin of the breast has elastic tissue, which permits an increase and decrease in its size. This skin is thin and flexible with occasional hair follicles and sebaceous, as well as sweat, glands.

The nipple in the adult woman is a conical elevation generally located at the fourth intercostal space and having apertures from 15 to 25 epithelial-lined milk ducts. Sensory nerve endings are located in the chorial papillae, and although sebaceous and apocrine sweat glands may be present, there is no hair in the nipple area. The areola in the mature woman varies in size from 1.5 to 6 cm. At the periphery are Morgagni's tubercles, which are the openings of Montgomery's glands. These tubercles hypertrophy significantly in the early portion of pregnancy and often have increased pigmentation.

The substance of the breast includes stroma-containing connective tissue, fatty tissue, blood vessels, nerves and lymphatics, and, importantly, the lobe structure. There are approximately 15 to 25 lobes with 20 to 40 lobules in each lobe. Each of the lobules has 10 to 100 tubulosaccular secretory units. This ductal, lobular, alveolar structure has a characteristic tree-like branching. The distal alveoli are small, averaging 0.12 mm in diameter, and the ducts as they progress towards the subareolar area become dilated, averaging 2 mm. The lactiferous sinuses, which are just below the duct ostea, are dilated to 5 to 8 mm.

The breast also has fascia present, which includes the superficial pectoral fascia that envelopes the breast and is contiguous with the cervical and Camper's superficial abdominal fascia. Fibrous bands (Cooper's suspensory ligaments) extend down into the breast parenchymal tissue, fixing the breast to the skin. In older postmenopausal women with a decrease in glandular tissue but an increase in fatty tissue, Cooper's ligaments may produce a depression in the skin that can be noted visually, particularly when a patient is sitting and with her hands placed on her head and her chest accentuated in an anterior position.

The major arterial supply of the breast includes the internal mammary artery, which arises from the subclavian artery. The internal mammary artery passes behind the cartilage of the sixth upper ribs and has four to five anterior perforating branches. It makes up 60 percent of the arterial blood supply of the breast. The lateral thoracic artery coming from the axillary artery passes along the lateral margin of the breast and supplies the lateral component and a large portion of the upper outer quadrant of the breast with arterial blood. The third major suppliers of arterial blood are the intercostal arteries, which follow courses generally between the third, fourth, and fifth rib, supplying the lower lateral quadrant of the breast and making up 5 to 10 percent of the total arterial blood supply to the breast. Venous drainage can be both longitudinal and transverse as well as circular around the areola. It tends initially to be superficial and becomes very prominent during pregnancy. The venous drainage eventually drains into the internal mammary, intercostal, and lateral thoracic veins.

The lymphatics of the breast are prominent. Cutaneous lymphatics drain from the superior and inferior portions of the breast in the lateral projection into the axillary nodes. The medial portion of the breast will also drain into the axillary nodes but additionally has pathways to the opposite breast, and the inferior medial pathway, or Gerota's pathway, passes via subdiaphragmatic and subperitoneal channels to intraabdominal nodes and the liver. The nipple areola complex itself has a lymphatic plexus known as the *plexus of Sappey,* which drains to the anterior pectoral lymph nodes. Within the glandular substance of the breast, the superior and lateral portions drain into the anterior and central axillary nodes while the retroareolar area drains into the interpectoral (Rotter's) nodes. The medial area of the breast drains into the internal mammary and eventually mediastinal nodes, while the inferior portion of the breast follows Gerota's pathway to subdiaphragmatic channels, leading to the intraabdominal nodes as well as the liver.

In general, the nerves of the breast demonstrate an abundant sensory supply to the nipple and areola. Within the distal tubulosaccular units, there is the alveolar unit, which is made up of three types of cells: superficial or lumenal cells, which are stimulated by sex steroids; the basal or chief cells, which are the predominant cells of mammary epithelium; and myoepithelial cells of ectodermal origin, which proliferate during pregnancy and lactation but regress significantly thereafter. The tubulosaccular alveolar unit hypertrophies greatly during pregnancy and, of course, during lactation.

The physician, keeping these basic fundamental anatomic characteristics in mind, will have a much greater appreciation of the subtle and obvious changes that can occur in the breast, both as a result of lactation and normal physiologic responses and when benign or malignant breast tumors are noted.

History and Physical Examination

The History

Although detection of early breast cancer and implementation of treatment is a prime consideration for both physician and patient, benign breast problems comprise by far the more common conditions encountered in a primary care practice. The two most common breast complaints for which a woman sees a physician are breast pain or a breast mass. Appropriate historical information is critical for this and all other breast complaints.

After determining the standard information regarding age and parity, the presenting symptom should be evaluated. When was it noted? How long has it been present? Have there been any changes in the condition since it was originally noted? Was there anything like this in the patient's previous health assessment? Are there any changes related to the menses? Does the brassiere cause any discomfort, or has the patient noticed any change in the size of her breasts? Has she noted any visible changes in the breast? Has there been any recent nipple discharge? If so, what was the character of the discharge? Other pertinent areas of history to consider include: a family history of breast cancer, particularly on the maternal side and, specifically, in the mother or sister; age of the patient at the time of her first full-term childbirth experience; lactation; and medications, particularly oral contraceptives and exogenous hormones utilized for estrogen replacement therapy. A past history of pelvic surgery should be explored, particularly surgery for ovarian or endometrial cancer. Diet is also an important consideration. Is the diet high in caffeine or fats?

Significant past medical history includes a review of past problems with the breast or previous breast surgery, particularly breast biopsy. If a biopsy has been done, an attempt should be made to obtain previous pathology reports. The patient should also be questioned regarding her habit of breast self-examination and whether she has had regular screening mammography in accordance with established guidelines.

Breast Examination

Breast self-examination Breast self-examination is an integral component of a woman's breast disease awareness and offers an opportunity for the physician to help her understand changes in her breasts. It enables a woman to bring to the attention of the physician conditions that are very early in their natural history. Breast examination should be encouraged in women and is enhanced if its importance is emphasized by the health care professional. Although the benefits of breast self-examination and breast awareness have been controversial, some evaluations have been done that note a significant association between periodic examination and early disease stage at diagnosis. Patients should be advised to do breast self-examination on a monthly basis starting at age 20, and for women in the menstrual years, it is recommended that the examination be done approximately 2 to 3 days after the termination of a normal menstrual cycle. At this time physiologic changes in the breasts associated with menses have dissipated and the breast is in its classic nonhormonally stimulated form. For women who do not menstruate, a regular time each month should be recommended for the examination.

The breast examination should be completed in a comfortable, warm, private surrounding. First, the patient should observe both breasts for any physical changes, specifically spontaneous nipple discharge, changes in the skin, erythema, visible nodularity, dimpling, or ecchymoses. It is advantageous to do this portion of the examination while looking in a mirror. While the woman is looking at her breasts, she should then change her position to accentuate the prominence of the breasts. Two methods are commonly used: either placing the hands behind the head and pushing the chest cage forward or placing the hands on the hips and contracting the pectoral muscles. Another position often overlooked in breast self-examination and one which might be suggested is that the patient place her hands on her hips and lean forward toward the mirror. In this position with the shoulders and elbows pulled forward, the breasts become very dependent from the chest wall and have a different visual appearance. Again, the patient should carefully evaluate her breasts in this position to look for abnormalities of the types previously specified.

The most important part of breast self-examination, however, is breast palpation. Ideally, this should be done with the breast moistened either by a soapy solution or water. Patients often choose to do this portion of the examination while in the shower or bath. The patient should be instructed to use the sensitive areas of the second, third, and fourth fingers to gently glide over the breast in a circumferential fashion. The patient is instructed to raise her arm, and the fingers of the opposite hand are used to palpate the breast area. The patient should be advised to always follow a standard examination pattern.

Generally, it is appropriate to ask the patient to begin in the upper outer quadrant of the breast and then to move the fingers around the breast, moving initially medially, inferiorly, and then up the lateral side of the breast. Concentric circles will increase the accuracy of the examination. It is important, too, to emphasize examination of the axilla. The areola should be compressed, as should the nipple, to determine if there is a nipple discharge. After the examination in the shower or tub is completed, it is recommended that the breast be dried and that the patient assume a supine position and place a small pillow under the rib cage on the side of the breast that is going to be examined. Then, using her opposite hand, she should gently repeat the examination that has been done in the upright position.

Emphasis should be made on uniformity and a concentric circular pattern. Patients should be advised that notation of a lump which is new or unusual is of concern and should be brought to the attention of the physician.

Physician breast examination Breast examination by a physician or health care professional is an essential component of breast care and particularly in screening for breast cancer. It is not as sensitive as mammography, which will often detect cancers that cannot be palpated. However, sometimes physical examination will detect cancers that have *not* been identified on mammography.

Limitations in tactile sensitivity make it more difficult for a physician to identify nodules that are smaller and softer. Consider the study reported in 1985 by Fletcher, O'Malley, and Bunce using manufactured silicone breast models with lumps of differing size and consistency. These investigators found that a physician group could identify only 44 percent of total lumps present in such models. The physician participants were able to identify 87 percent of 1-cm masses, 33 percent of 0.5-cm masses, and only 14 percent of 0.3-cm masses. Masses which were noted to be hard were detected 56 percent of the time, but medium and soft masses were only detected 36 and 40 percent of the time. Likewise, masses located deeply or at medium depth in the silicone models were detected only 44 percent of the time. Detection was enhanced when each examiner used a consistent examination mode, when the examination duration was longer, and when only three fingers, specifically the fingertips, were used in a circumferential motion while examining the various breast quadrants. These data emphasize the importance of finger sensitivity, consistent methodology in examination, and the utilization of appropriate time.

What about the actual examination by the physician? First, the breast should be inspected with the patient sitting and with the chest accentuated. A critical visual assessment of the breast is important, in which the examiner looks specifically for

- Asymmetry
- Thickening of the skin
- Dimpling or retraction of the skin
- Nipple retraction or surface change such as redness or excoriation
- Spontaneous nipple discharge
- Erythema
- Ecchymoses
- Obvious nodularity

After completing the visual examination, the patient should lie in a supine position with her head slightly elevated. The arm on the side of the examining table that is approached by the physician should be extended over the head and the opposite hand should be placed on the hip with the elbow flexed. The examination should be conducted by the physician using the second, third, and fourth fingers of the examining hand and examining each quadrant of the breast carefully and ideally in a circumferential maneuver. When the physician has completed palpation of the breast substance the patient should gently compress the areola area and the nipple to determine if discharge can be expressed. The physician should then take the examining hand and move it up to the axilla with palpation of the medial, cephalad, and lateral portions of the axilla with the examining hand. After completion of the axillary examination, the supraclavicular nodes should also be palpated and be included as a routine part of breast examination.

Examination of the breasts can occasionally be enhanced by using a so-called wet technique that involves a water-miscible lubricating gel, a soapy solution, or ultrasound coupling gel. In theory, this enhances the opportunity to detect subtle changes in breast anatomy, but it is often quite messy and not very practical. An alternative that the physician may wish to consider employs a thin cotton, linen, or silk cloth that is placed over the breast after the visual examination has been completed. Utilizing this type of fabric and the very sensitive surfaces of the second, third, and fourth fingers of the dominant hand, the breast is carefully examined in a methodical fashion, in which the sensitive tactile surfaces of the fingers are slid over the breast and nipple with minimum pressure. This maneuver can be carried out in the supine and sitting position. In the latter position, an assistant is needed to hold the fabric so that it can be kept in a smooth fashion over the patient's breast. Obviously, examination of the breast is crucial, when performed both by the woman and by the physician. When these techniques are coupled with screening mammography, the patient is afforded the best opportunity for early diagnosis of breast cancer.

Diagnostic Techniques

Mammography

Currently, mammography is the most critical screening tool available for the diagnosis of early breast cancer. Since breast cancer is the most frequent cancer in women and the second most lethal, the utilization of mammography for appropriate health care screening in women is mandatory. Currently, it is estimated that 1 in 8 women will develop breast cancer during their lifetime and that there is a dramatic increase in the incidence of breast cancer with aging. For example, at age 40 the frequency of breast cancer is 1 in 217 women. This drops to 1 in 93 women at age 45, 1 in 50 at age 50, 1 in 33 at age 55, 1 in 24 at age 60, 1 in 17 at age 65, and 1 in 14 at age 70. The compounding factor of age is apparent.

It must also be remembered that mammography is the only method of detecting nonpalpable breast lesions that are early cancers, and at this point up to 90 percent of such cancers are curable.

The primary care physician must also note that mammography has two diagnostic components. The first is screening of the asymptomatic woman. In this situation, usually two breast views are obtained, specifically, a lateral, or oblique, and a craniocaudad film. Films are taken by a certified technician under stringent quality control standards, and most frequently screening mammograms are read in a batched fashion at the end of the day or the next day. Approximately 1 in 10 women who are screened will subsequently have to be called back for a so-called diagnostic mammography. The diagnostic mammogram is used to evaluate women who have an abnormality noted on a screening mammogram or to evaluate symptomatic women (e.g., those who have a distinct lump that was noted clinically). When diagnostic mammograms are obtained, multiple views are taken, which may include oblique, lateral, compression, cone down, and magnified views. These studies permit the radiologist a high level of sophistication in the evaluation of small, discrete lesions.

Although mammography is the most sensitive technique for breast cancer screening, physicians must note that variable factors such as breast size, consistency, and location of a potential lesion, as well as training of radiologists and quality technical factors of equipment can affect mammographic interpretation. False-negatives are known to occur with a frequency of 10 to 15 percent. *Whenever a patient has a palpable mass it must be evaluated, even if the mammogram is normal.* It is important for the primary care physician ordering screening or diagnostic mammography to be familiar with the facility used for mammographic procedures. Each facility should be certified by the American College of Radiology, which has developed a program of quality control that certifies the equipment, calibrations of the equipment, and training of the technicians. The selection of a radiologist to interpret the films is critical. It is important that the radiologist dedicate a substantial amount of time to this endeavor and employ consistent diagnostic standards and terminology when generating reports.

Although mammography has been accepted as a screening test of substantial benefit to women over the age of 50, there continues to be an ongoing dialogue relative to its benefit in women under age 50, particularly between the ages of 40 and 49. Some argue that the cost and effort are excessive, that no distinct benefit can be identified, and that the resources utilized should be diverted to other health care activities. Statements have been promulgated suggesting routine screening in ages 40 to 49 be discontinued. A more supportive stand has been taken by Dr. Steven Feig, who states, "Annual screening of all women age 40 and over by means of state-of-the-art mammography with two views per breast and physicial examination could reduce breast cancer mortality by at least 40 percent and possibly as much as 50 percent." This statement strongly argues for continuing screening mammography for women ages 40 to 49. It must be remembered that breast cancer is the leading cause of death for women in the United States between the ages of 40 and 44.

Further controversy exists regarding the appropriateness of a baseline mammogram at age 35. One of the problems with the baseline examination is that the initial mammogram may in fact not be available for comparison when subsequent mammography is done. Despite this negative observation, it would appear that patients who have substantial risk factors should begin the process of screening earlier than the standard age of 40. Patients with first-degree relatives with premenopausal breast cancer might have an advantage by beginning the screening process at 35 years of age and, potentially, age 30. For women with high risk factors who undergo the screening process between 40 and 49, annual mammograms may be more appropriate than biannual mammograms.

Another problem that has surfaced relative to mammography is the question of radiation risk. The American Cancer Society states, "Modern technology has reduced the radiation exposure of low dose mammography to the point of negligible risk, if risk exists at all, and has increased its diagnostic capabilities at the same time."[21]

The current ACOG guidelines for screening mammography for the woman who is not at high risk are

1. Mammogram every one to two years between ages 40 and 49
2. Annual mammogram from age 50 onward

Not infrequently, a mammogram report will indicate the presence of a nonpalpable occult lesion in the breast. This requires prompt and careful evaluation.

Ultrasonography

Ultrasonic evaluation of the breast is utilized for determining whether a lesion is solid or cystic. Utilization of a 5- or 7.5-MHz ultrasound linear array head is the most appropriate instrument for assessing the solid versus cystic characteristic of breast masses. Although this is a very useful tool, it may not be as cost-effective as a rapid needle aspiration. On the other hand, it can have a distinct advantage in evaluating spherical masses noted on screening mammography that are thought to be cystic but cannot be determined to be completely cystic by that diagnostic modality. This can be extremely helpful when a nonpalpable lesion found deep in the breast is demonstrated to be cystic. Ultrasonography can be done in an office setting using appropriate equipment and qualified, certified, trained technicians.

Cyst Aspiration

The finding of a dominant mass at the time of examination is disconcerting for the patient as well as the physician. Fortunately, this situation can be addressed instantaneously. A determination of the cystic or solid characteristic of the mass can be made by performing needle aspiration.

Basic office equipment such as a 5- or 10-ml syringe and a 22- or 23-gauge needle is all that is necessary. Local anesthesia is not required. After the mass has been identified and the equipment obtained, the mass should be immobilized between the index and middle finger of the nondominant hand and the skin over the mass cleansed with an alcohol or povidone iodine swab. The needle can then be gently placed into the center of the mass and the syringe plunger retracted. If the mass is cystic, fluid will appear. It can be either clear or cloudy. If fluid is obtained, it should be completely removed, and following removal, the mass should not be palpable.

If this is the situation, the patient should be reexamined in a month. If the mass recurs, it should be reaspirated, and, it is my opinion that if it recurs again after a second aspiration, the mass should be considered for excision. If the fluid removed is not clear or cloudy but actually bloody, the aspiration is of concern, and excisional biopsy of the area at a later date, but without undue delay, is important. Cyst fluid can have a variety of colors, from cloudy white to serous to dark green or even greenish black. These are the characteristic findings of fibrocystic change. It is very important to note that if the mass does not completely dissipate at the time of aspiration, further evaluation is necessary, often requiring biopsy.

The need for cytologic evaluation of cyst fluid is controversial. With respect to cyst fluid, it is my opinion that it is important to submit an initial specimen for cytologic evaluation. The reports generally indicate the presence of foam cells, which may or may not have atypical characteristics. Foam cells are quite common in fibrocystic change. The finding of malignant cells is very infrequent, approaching only 0.1 to 0.2 percent of all cyst fluid evaluations. However, it is my opinion that documentation of the characteristics of cyst fluid initially is important. Many others believe that it is not useful to send cyst fluid for cytologic evaluation.

If there is a spontaneous nipple discharge or one that can be obtained on compression, preparation of this in a standard format such as Papanicolaou immersion staining does not often yield a significant abnormality but is appropriate at the time of initial screening. Nipple discharges, which comprise 3 to 7 percent of all breast complaints, can also be evaluated for blood, utilizing a test similar to that for fecal occult blood, such as Seracult.

Fine Needle Aspiration

Fine needle aspiration is currently being used with much greater frequency in the office. Although the technique is quite basic, prior to beginning, it is important to discuss with the cytopathologist the methodologies to be followed for preparation of the slide immediately following aspiration. The most common recommendations are to place the contents of the syringe needle directly on a slide near the labeled end. A second slide is used to carefully smear the material the length of the slide. The slides are placed against each other and then separated by sliding laterally. Use of a frosted Dakin slide as one of the slides permits adherence of cells despite the occasional fatty content of the fluid. The slides are placed in an alcohol fixative. The technique itself can be carried out with a standard disposable syringe such as a 10- or 20-ml syringe. A regular syringe needle, 22- to 24-gauge, is adequate. Although local anesthesia is not utilized in routine cyst aspiration, it may be advantageous in these situations. The author prefers a small amount of 1% xylocaine without epinephrine. Once the mass has been identified, it should be localized between the index and second finger of the nondominant hand. The skin should be prepared with an alcohol or povidone iodine swab similar to cyst skin preparation. If local anesthesia is going to be used, it should be injected at this time. Following injection of local anesthesia, the needle is passed into the mass, and the plunger of the syringe is pulled back from the barrel to create negative suction. By passing the needle back and forth five to eight times in the mass, tissue fluid can be aspirated into the bore of the needle. The tissue fluid should not be withdrawn into the barrel of the syringe but allowed to remain only in the bore of the needle. After the procedure is completed, the tissue fluid should be placed on the slide and prepared in accordance with the recommendations provided by the cytopathologist or as previously described.

If a needle aspiration of this type is positive for malignant cells, it permits immediate institution of treatment planning with discussion with the patient of alternatives for treatment of breast cancer. At the time of definitive surgical intervention, initially a biopsy is done to confirm the needle aspiration findings. However, definitive treatment can continue at that time, thus having the patient exposed to only one surgical procedure.

If the specimen obtained at the time of fine needle aspiration is not positive for malignant cells, one cannot be 100 percent sure that carcinoma is not present, and further investigation may be necessary. On the other hand, a certain degree of pragmatism is necessary. For example, in a woman age 35 who has a firm, palpable 2-cm mass in the breast which is smooth and nontender and who on mammogram has the mass documented and following ultrasound examination the mass is characterized as a fibroadenoma, it is probably a fibroadenoma if the cytologic aspirate suggests cells compatible with a fibroadenoma. Despite this finding of benignity, however, it is my opinion that a fibroadenoma of this size should be removed in a patient age 35. Thus, the argument is somewhat moot, but the physician must realize that if the lesion feels like a fibroadenoma, has the mammographic and ultrasonic characteristics of fibroadenoma, and has cytologic aspirate characteristics compatible with a fibroadenoma, then one is probably dealing with a fibroadenoma. This logic may be more advantageous for a mass deeper in the breast that is evaluated by fine needle aspiration.

Stereotaxic Needle Biopsy

Stereotaxic needle biopsy, a technique that has developed over the past 5 to 8 years, is becoming increasingly more prominent in managing nonpalpable mammographic abnormalities. This procedure has reduced the number of open breast biopsies. Stereotaxic needle biopsies are done using mammographic equipment and either hollow-bore needles, which will obtain cytologic specimens, or larger hollow-bore needles, which will obtain core tissue specimens. In either situation, the needle is placed directly in the center of the occult lesion by the radiologist, using sophisticated computerized mammographic localization. A specimen should be obtained with sufficient material to make an accurate diagnosis.

If there is any question, an open surgical biopsy utilizing wire localization is necessary. In this latter situation the radiologist, under mammographic guidance, places a localizing needle with a wire obturator in the breast and advances the wire to a point immediately adjacent to, or within the area of, the occult lesion. The surgeon then carries out an excisional biopsy, following the wire to the point of its termination and excising the breast tissue in that area. If calcifications or a solid nodular area were seen on the original mammogram, specimen radiographic films using a compression container device should be taken of the specimen after it is removed to confirm that the mass in fact has been removed.

Once confirmation of removal via specimen radiography has been obtained, the tissue can be processed in a routine fashion by the pathologist. The pathology report should demonstrate, too, that the suspicious area has been removed, and inked margins should be assessed for residual marginal disease if the primary condition is found to be malignant. Residual marginal disease has been documented to be present in 10 to 15 percent of needle localization biopsies, yielding either intraductal or invasive breast carcinoma.

Breast Biopsy

Currently, excisional breast biopsy is an ambulatory surgical procedure. In selected situations with appropriate preparation and availability of sterile operative facilities, certain breast biopsies can be done in an office setting. This is particularly germane for small, superficial lesions in which only local anesthesia is needed for patient comfort at the time of surgery. The principle of excisional breast biopsy is the same whether it is done in an office setting, ambulatory surgical setting, or in a traditional surgical suite.

Many breast biopsies can be done with local anesthesia. However, for small occult lesions, lesions which are deep within the breast, or in some situations where wire utilization is necessary for localization, local anesthesia plus intravenous sedation is advantageous. Large amounts of local anesthesia, which might be necessary in certain circumstances (e.g., 15 to 20 ml of local anesthesia) may distort the breast tissue sufficiently so that it would be difficult to find small lesions. If this is considered a potential problem, general anesthesia may be considered a preferable option. However, general anesthesia is not used with the frequency it was a decade ago.

Once the decision has been made to plan an excisional breast biopsy for the patient, the site of incision is important. Most incisions in the breast should be circumferential. However, in the lower quadrants of the breast, particularly between the four and eight o'clock positions, linear incisions occasionally are used, particularly if they are hidden by the normal breast contouring. When circumferential incisions are made, they, of course, should follow the so-called skin lines of the breast. Ideally, circumferential incisions should be made at the areolar margin. However, this is only useful if the lesion to be excised is close to the areolar margin or not more than 2 to 3 cm away. Should that occur, the incision can be made and one can tunnel minimally under the skin and subcutaneous tissue to the lesion to be excised. More commonly, however, the incision needs to be made in a more lateral or cephalad or medial portion of the upper quadrants of the breast.

Locating the point of incision can be deceptive. It is helpful to have the patient sitting and to observe the normal contour of the breast as noted in that position. Once the lump has been palpated and the skin lines observed, a marking pencil can be used to draw the anticipated site of incision to be confluent with the skin lines, thus doing everything possible to make a desirable, cosmetically esthetic final surgical result. If the patient is seen in the operating room after being prepped and in the supine position, often the position of the breast is deceptive and the skin incision may not be as symmetrical, circular, or aesthetic as one would like.

It is important to remember that if a patient is going to have a breast biopsy, she has two concerns. First, what is the outcome? Is the mass which is excised going to be benign or malignant? Second, and very important, how will the breast look after the breast biopsy? Keeping these important facts in the forefront of the surgeon's mind emphasizes the importance of care and precision in incision location.

The choice of incision length, location, and direction is critically important to provide the best cosmesis and yet to provide the pathologist with an adequate portion of tissue for definitive diagnostic evaluation. The incision, generally circumferential, is carried into the subcutaneous tissue, and the area of the mass is identified. Small bleeders can be treated with pinpoint electrocautery or ligated with 000 or 0000 polygalactin-type suture. Once the area of the mass has been identified, it can be grasped with a small Allis clamp, elevated, and by sharp dissection completely removed. Hemostasis then should be obtained again, using pinpoint cautery or polygalactin sutures. The defect should be flushed with normal saline, and, if substantial, can be closed with two or three interrupted 000 polygalactin-type sutures. If the defect is minimal, no closure is necessary in the subcutaneous tissue, and the skin can be closed with a 0000 subcuticular polygalactin-type suture. Steri strips can be applied to the wound, and a small, dry sterile pressure dressing is applied, which should be changed in 48 h. The patient should be advised to wear a brassiere day and night for approximately 7 days following the procedure to give the breast good support. On occasion, if support is not provided, patients will develop a substantial ecchymosis.

Fibrocystic Change

Fibrocystic change is by far the most widely encountered nonmalignant condition of the breast. It occurs most commonly in reproductive age women between 30 and 50 years old. The condition has a number of subgroups that run the gamut from small to large cyst formation, i.e., micro- or macrocysts, ductal hyperplasia, apocrine changes in the ductal cells, ductal papillomatosis, ectasia, sclerosing adenosis, and pure stromal fibrosis. Because of the variety of conditions and the ubiquitous character of fibrosis, ductal dilation, and cellular proliferation, the American Cancer Society has recommended that this constellation of conditions be placed under the umbrella terminology of *fibrocystic change.* In an attempt to simplify the classification of histologic changes seen in fibrocystic change, three categorizations seem appropriate: (1) cystic change; (2) changes associated with ductal hyperplasia; and (3) stromal alterations, particularly fibrosis.

Histologic and Clinical Changes

Types of fibrocystic change Cystic change encompasses conditions in which the breast ducts show varying alterations in the lobular, lobe, or subareolar areas. Small cysts, generally less than 1 mm in size, are commonly called *microcysts.* They are ubiquitous and not palpable. When evaluated histologically, they are noted to be lined by a single layer of cuboidal or columnar epithelium. These ductal alterations rarely cause significant symptoms and can be considered within the realm of normality for many women. The condition, however, can progress with the development of larger ductal dilatations, specifically exceeding 3 mm. When this degree of dilation occurs, they are then generally characterized as *macrocysts.* Not all patients with microcysts will progress to macrocyst formation, although 20 to 40 percent of patients have been reported to do so.

Macrocyst as well as microcyst formation most commonly is bilateral. Macrocysts may increase in size, exceeding 1 cm, and are occasionally noted to be 2 to 3 cm. Larger cysts, between 3 to 6 cm, may also be encountered and are particularly noted in women approaching the end of their menstrual years. Thus, macrocyst formation in its largest configuration is more often found in women in their forties.

Duct ectasia *Duct ectasia* refers to a dilatation of the duct system, occurring most commonly as the ducts coalesce below the areola and approach the nipple. This condition is seen most commonly in peri- and postmenopausal women. It is noted in approximately 25 percent of patients, although certainly not that many are symptomatic from the condition. Occasionally, duct ectasia manifests itself by distention of the subareolar ducts with the development of a yellowish orange material thought to be of lipid origin. Penetration of the duct by this material can lead to a chronic inflammatory condition at the areolar margin with an associated mass that can be problematic and occasionally become infected. Although the condition may spontaneously resorb, frequent recurrences lead to the condition of recurrent periareolar abscess, requiring treatment. Recurring abscesses will eventually lead to fibrosis in the adjacent breast tissue, which can be associated with firmness and retraction of the tissue, causing a diagnostic problem, since these physical characteristics may also be associated with carcinoma. If a diagnosis of mammary duct ectasia with mass is identified, the treatment is excision of the involved ducts as well as a small portion of breast tissue surrounding the area.

Hyperplastic epithelial changes Hyperplastic epithelial changes are the second most common condition encountered, concomitant with pure fibrocystic change. The etiology of this hyperplastic condition remains obscure but in some situations can be associated with atypia and an oncogenic potential. The normal ductal epithelium, as stated, is cuboidal or cylindrical and can undergo metaplastic apocrine transformation. These cells are cylindrical and have small, round, basal uniform nuclei. The cellular cytoplasm has an acidophilic appearance and a peculiar outpouching from the lumenal surface of the cell. Apocrine metaplasia can be seen in both macrocyst and microcyst formation.

Occasionally fibrocystic change will also demonstrate a proliferation of the acini in the distal mammary lobes, forming a densely packed adenosis-type pattern. Frequently, this can be noted in multiple areas of the breast but does not distort the normal lobular architecture. In contrast to the apocrine metaplasia-type cells, these cells are small with oval nuclei and have an entirely benign appearance. Fibrosis is commonly found in and around the cells, forming a firm, hard, often irregular nodular mass. In most patients, this type of condition is without symptoms and is diagnosed only at the time of microscopic evaluation of tissue obtained when an excisional breast biopsy is performed.

Although usually asymptomatic, occasionally progression of fibrosis and ductal proliferation can develop to form a palpable firm mass that has a preponderance to create abnormal mammographic imaging findings, leading to the necessity of a breast biopsy. These changes in the stroma and glands are commonly called "sclerosing adenosis" and appear more commonly in women during the latter portion of the reproductive life. This will occasionally undergo spontaneous regression in and around the menopausal period. Because of the anatomic characteristic, sclerosing adenosis may have an appearance very similar to an early infiltrating carcinoma. Sclerosing adenosis is not malignant, and it is therefore very important that the pathologist correctly makes the distinction.

Ductal papillomatous change Ductal papillomatous change is another alteration of the ductal epithelium. Patients with these changes are generally without symptoms. The proliferation occurs in the small and medium ducts rather than the distal acini in the outer portion of the quadrants of the breast. In this situation, the cells of the papillomas are uniform in size and do not have malignant characteristics. The nuclei and cytoplasmic characteristics are clearly benign.

In some situations, papillomatous structures may undergo a degenerative process with inflammatory cells and fibrosis occurring within the papilloma. Fibrosis can develop around the group of ducts, separate the ducts, and eventually lead to a firm, small, palpable mass. Single-stalk papillomas, however, are more commonly associated with clinical symptoms, the most prominent is bleeding and the second most common is the development of a palpable mass. In contrast to multiple duct papillomatosis, these intraductal papillomas characteristically have a two-layer cell characteristic, with the inner layer small and round and the outer layer columnar with a small, round nucleus. Cytoplasm is often seen pushing out the surface, similar to that seen in apocrine metaplasia. This condition occurs more frequently in the late menstrual years but often will continue and be found in postmenopausal women, even being noted with moderate frequency in women in their sixties. Thereafter, there is some regression. Bloody or serous discharges can occur with both single or multiple intraductal papillomas in approximately 20 to 50 percent of patients. When a palpable mass is noted, most commonly it is located just at the periphery of the areola.

Fibrosis Breast fibrosis itself is much less frequent than cyst formation or ductal hyperplasia. It is noticed more commonly in the menstrual years. The characteristic lesion is a palpable, nonmobile, flat, irregular mass that may increase in size to 1 to 3 cm, although large fibrotic areas up to 5 cm have also been noted. This condition appears to be a response to alterations in the lobular or acinar system with accompanying lymphocyte infiltration concomitant with previous ductal inflammation.

Controversies Regarding the Potential for Malignancy

Fibrocystic change has frequently been an area of concern related to whether it has any bearing on the potential for developing carcinoma. Many studies have been done, but one of the most important is the one by Dr. Susan Love. She evaluated five series of patients with fibrocystic changes, including 6511 patients, and noted that only 3 percent of these patients subsequently developed breast cancer. Devitt reviewed 2161 patients with a clinical diagnosis of benign disorders of the breast and 345 patients with breast cancer. He noted that of the 345 patients who had carcinoma only 10 percent gave a history of previous breast biopsy or breast cyst aspiration. Generally speaking, it is fair to assume that women who have had a previous diagnosis of benign disease form only a small portion of those who will develop breast cancer.

Although the finding of pure fibrocystic change does not appear to increase the risk of breast cancer, the finding of fibrocystic change with atypia is a potential premalignant finding. Three atypical conditions have been identified and are problematic. They include atypical epithelial hyperplasia, atypical lobular hyperplasia, and diffuse papillomatosis with atypia. Of these conditions, atypical lobular hyperplasia has a higher predictive value than the other lesions and imparts a sixfold increased risk of breast cancer in patients, particularly those 45 years of age or younger. The risk was noted to be substantially less, only threefold for older patients. On the other hand, ductal epithelial proliferative lesions were noted to increase the risk by approximately 2.6 times in women over 45 years old.

Page and Dupont have contributed significantly to our understanding of atypia. In their study, women with atypia and a family history of breast cancer had a substantially increased risk of developing breast cancer, approaching 11 times that of a woman who had nonproliferative lesions without a family history. Patients who fell in the former group had an approximately 20 percent chance of developing breast cancer over a follow-up period of 15 years as compared to an absolute risk for those with atypia and a negative family history of only 8 percent. The findings of calcifications in breast tissue with atypia was a substantial concern. Page and Dupont demonstrated that the risk of developing breast cancer was over eight times greater in patients with proliferative fibrocystic change with atypical hyperplasia and calcification as compared to patients with nonproliferative disease, either with or without calcifications.

Another figure to keep prominently in mind is that the Page and Dupont studies demonstrate that the chance of developing an invasive cancer after a patient had been diagnosed and treated for an intraductal carcinoma was 11 times higher than that noted in the general population.

Etiology of Fibrocystic Change

The etiology of fibrocystic change remains speculative and controversial. The changes brought about by estrogen on ductal epithelium focuses a point of interest on imbalance between estrogen and progestins, leading to excessive ductal stimulation. Estrogens in their most classic form have been found to enhance development of the ductal epithelium of the breast while progestins are associated with distal lobular alveolar growth. The progestin itself may inhibit the action of estradiol on breast ductal epithelial cells by decreasing the concentration of estrogen receptors within the cell cytoplasm. Interesting studies done on castrated rats indicated that when given estrogen, the rats produced a proliferative change within the ductal epithelium, with accompanying dilation of the lobules and cyst formation and with increased connective tissue between the lobules. When progesterone was given with the estradiol, the mammary glands themselves developed normally without abnormal proliferation of ductal epithelium in connective tissue. This certainly suggests the potential for fibrocystic change to be related to estrogen and progesterone.

A high point of controversy relative to the etiology of fibrocystic change has been the influence of dietary substances and vitamins. In 1981, Minton postulated that caffeine (methylxanthine) ingestion was related to mastalgia and accompanying fibrocystic change. Minton suggested that women who reduced methylxanthine consumption in their diet had a significant resolution of the symptoms of fibrocystic change. He felt that substances such as coffee, chocolate, tea, caffeinated colas, and certain other soft drinks containing methylxanthines inhibited cyclic adenosine monophosphate and cyclic guanosine monophosphate phosphodiesterase enzymatic activity. This enzymatic inhibition led to accumulation of adenosine monophosphate and guanosine monophosphate, which was found to stimulate extant fibrocystic change. Other studies by investigators such as Hayden, and Parazzini lead to inconclusive observations related to the effectiveness of methylxanthine ingestion reduction. It has been noted that in many women who rigorously restrict methylxanthines from the diet, there is a notable 60 to 65 percent reduction in symptoms of mastalgia, reduction in nipple discharge frequently associated with fibrocystic change, and an improvement in symptoms of mastalgia. This could be a placebo effect, but the observation of improvement is intriguing. Further studies, particularly those in a hospital-based controlled situation, demonstrated that women consuming 30 to 250 mg of caffeine per day had a 1.5-fold increased potential for developing fibrocystic change, and if women consumed over 500 mg of caffeine per day, the risk increased to 2.3 times normal.

Diagnosis of Fibrocystic Change

Fibrocystic change presents most commonly as mastalgia, often noted in the premenstrual phase of a woman's menstrual cycle. The pain itself can be localized and is more commonly noted in the upper outer quadrants of the breasts. There may be accompanying nipple discharge. Pain may also extend into the lower axilla. The discomfort generally begins 4 to 7 days into the luteal phase and continues until the onset of menstruation. The pain will disappear after 1 or 2 days of menstrual flow. The pain itself is related to edema occurring in the breast stroma, and there is a concomitant breast volume increase of approximately 10 to 15 percent. Although breast pain that is cyclic carries with it a relatively high suspicion of fibrocystic change, other diagnostic considerations include intercostal neuralgia, stretching of Cooper's ligaments, costochondritis, cholelithiasis, or possibly even intermittent mild ischemia.

Treatment

Although treatment options for fibrocystic change are numerous, those that provide substantial long-term patient-satisfying results are few. Options range from dietary alterations to medications that correct symptomatology only to potent medications altering steroid hormone function. One of the most important concepts of treatment is to be sure that both the treating physician and the patient have realistic expectations relative to the outcome. It is very difficult to get 100 percent resolution, but most patients are pleased with improvements of 60 to 70 percent in their symptomatology. Following the institution of any treatment plan, a careful program of follow-up is necessary to support the patient and to assure compliance and a continued beneficial effect. I examine patients at 3- to 4-month intervals for a year after institution of treatment and as frequently or less as needed in subsequent years.

Treatment for fibrocystic change can be categorized into three major areas: those related to agents that do not alter hormonal function, those that are specific sex steroid therapy agents, and finally those that inhibit the function of sex steroids.

With respect to therapeutic modalities that do not alter hormonal function, common sense is important and must be emphasized to the patient. For example, does the patient wear a comfortable supporting brassiere during the daytime hours? This will reduce tension on supporting ligaments of the breast and reduce any concomitant inflammation that may occur. One may consider the use of a mild diuretic for 2 to 3 days prior to the onset of menses. This will reduce symptoms of edema in many patients and can be beneficial. As previously described, the dietary regimens that include a reduction in methylxanthines as proposed by Minton have been helpful in many patients, although the scientific background and substantiation of the decaffeination regimen continues to be questioned by the scientific community. Despite these findings, many patients benefit from substantial methylxanthine reductions.

Vitamins have also been utilized, specifically vitamins E and A. Vitamin A has been noted to alter proliferative change on mammography in a small series of patients, although the physiologic mechanism for this has not been well established. Studies of vitamin E have been undertaken and initially this was felt to be beneficial, but in more closely controlled studies, it was found to produce no specific significant benefit relative to the course of the problem. Interestingly, patients who took vitamin E in appropriate dosages were noted to have some reduction in dehydroepiandrosterone sulfate, but this could not be correlated specifically with any benefit. It is curious, however, that many patients who take vitamin E acknowledge some improvement—perhaps a placebo effect.

What about sex steroid therapy, particularly oral contraceptives? Without question, in many patients these have been noted to reduce the symptoms of fibrocystic change, particularly after treatment has been ongoing for a year. Maximum benefit is often not noted until 2 years of treatment with oral contraceptives. In the studies with oral contraceptives, benefit was more commonly seen when higher progesterone dose contraceptives were used than the dose of progesterone of those oral contraceptives in contemporary use. It is felt that the effectiveness of this medication is based on the reduction in ovarian estradiol production with some alteration of breast estrogen receptors by the progestin component of the oral contraceptives. Li Volsi demonstrated that women who used oral contraceptives for 4 years had an approximately 50 percent reduction in fibrocystic change and symptomatology from that condition. The effectiveness of new low-dose estrogen, phased estrogen, and progesterone dosage medications has not been specifically evaluated with respect to improvement in fibrocystic changes, but again many patients will have some benefit after a protracted period of time using the medication. If a patient has significant symptoms of fibrocystic change and has not responded to conservative dietary changes such as methylxanthine reduction, it may be worthwhile to consider the use of contemporary oral contraceptives, particularly if the patient wishes a contraceptive benefit. Even if the latter is not of interest to the patient, it is advantageous to consider the use of oral contraceptives when there are no specific contraindications and the risks and benefits have been evaluated.

Sex steroid–inhibiting substances have also been evaluated in the treatment of fibrocystic changes. The initial studies utilized danazol (17-nor-alpha-ethisterone), a synthetic androgen with greater anabolic than androgenic activity. Danazol reduced breast nodularity in almost 50 percent of patients taking 200 mg a day for 6 months and up to 75 percent of patients who took the medication at a dosage level of 400 mg a day for 6 months. Danazol's action appears to be related to its inhibition of sex steroid synthesis and its competitive inhibition of the binding of sex steroids to receptors. Additionally, the medication was noted to abolish midcycle FSH and LH surges. Essentially, a postmenopausal hormonal milieu was created with concomitant reduction in estrogen production and thus reduction in estrogen concentrations in breast tissue. It is this estrogen reduction that is felt to be the mechanism whereby danazol has been effective when treating fibrocystic change.

Despite its apparent benefit, symptoms have been noted to recur in up to 65 percent of patients when the medication is terminated. In addition, in some patients the side effects such as anxiety, nausea, headache, muscle cramps, vaginal spotting, nervousness, depression, and virilization were sufficient to cause them to stop taking the drug. Cost also is a major factor. Only a very small number of patients with fibrocystic changes will need danazol.

Another sex steroid inhibitor that has been evaluated is tamoxifen, a partial estrogen antagonist. When used in treating women with fibrocystic change, there has been an approximate 65 to 75 percent reduction of symptoms. The medication, however, is not approved for this use in the United States.

Finally, what is the place of surgical intervention with respect to fibrocystic change? The utilization of excisional breast biopsy remains the gold standard for obtaining tissue to make a definitive diagnosis or to evaluate a suspicious area that eludes precise diagnosis by needle biopsy or mammographic interpretation. It is essential to bear in mind that *all breast masses should be considered possible breast cancer unless proven otherwise.* It also is an important part of the management paradigm that a patient who has a recurring mass after multiple, specifically two, aspirations should have a biopsy. In many situations, surgical intervention cannot be avoided. Even if the pathology report is benign, the information that it yields following histologic evaluation is valuable in evaluating the patient's overall prognosis with respect to fibrocystic change.

Prophylactic mastectomy has also been considered a possible treatment for women with advanced fibrocystic change. This was particularly noted and recommended in women who have had atypia. Certainly this is controversial and needs to be carefully evaluated. When considering the place of prophylactic mastectomy, multiple factors must be evaluated, and the author believes it is important to adopt a reasonable and conservative approach toward the operation. Those patients who are at substantial risk and who have a strong family history of breast cancer as well as a known previous diagnosis of epithelial proliferation with atypical ductal hyperplasia and papillomatosis may be candidates. I would submit, however, that prophylactic mastectomy is reserved for very few patients with fibrocystic change in this high-risk category. Certainly the most appropriate treatment in these situations is still lumpectomy or cystectomy and reexamination with clinical imaging techniques on a regular basis.

Other Common Breast Problems

Adenofibroma (Fibroadenoma)

Adenofibroma (fibroadenoma) is the third most common lesion of the breast, following fibrocystic change and carcinoma. It is the second most common benign condition and makes up approximately 19 percent of benign breast biopsies. The condition can occur at any age but is more common between the ages of 20 and 45, with most lesions occurring before age 30. Fibroadenomas are derived from specialized connective tissue that is proximate to the ducts and acini of the breast, and microscopically they consist of proliferating connective tissue stroma as well as an atypical multiplication of the ducts and acini. In some patients, particularly in older women and when the adenofibroma has been present for an extended period of time, they may show calcification, which is classic for an adenofibroma. These are slow-growing tumors which may take up to 12 months to double in size and may approximate 2 to 3 cm in diameter, after which many of them will not increase further in size. They are discoid, rounded, or have been noted to be lobulated with a rubbery-type of firmness. Most commonly, they are mobile, and occasionally they can be confused with a breast cyst. Generally, adenofibromas are solitary, but multiple adenofibromas have been noted in from 13 to 20 percent of patients. Diagnosis is made on the basis of clinical awareness, and this can be augmented by ultrasound, which reveals a characteristic appearance of smooth external borders and a homogeneous echo pattern within the mass. There is no evidence of cystic change. Needle aspiration also will delineate a solid from a cystic lesion but does not provide a 100 percent accurate diagnosis of fibroma, and excision is usually the appropriate management both for diagnosis and treatment. On the other hand, if the lesion is noted in a woman particularly under age 25 and has the physical characteristics of a fibroadenoma plus confirmation by ultrasound, and if needle biopsy indicates a fibroadenoma, it can be assumed that it is a fibroadenoma with a very high degree of accuracy. Since growth is slow and the frequency of carcinoma in women 25 years of age and under is very low (only 2 percent of all breast carcinomas), these patients can be observed carefully. For women under age 25 in whom the diagnosis is apparent, it is my opinion that observation is appropriate and that the fibroadenoma does not have to be removed unless it increases in size or becomes psychologically disturbing for the patient. Palpable fibroadenomas in women over age 25 should be excised. Nonpalpable fibroadenomas found and specifically delineated on mammographic interpretation in women over age 25 can be observed if they are located deep within the breast and if there are no concomitant mammographic imaging observations suggestive of malignancy.

There are two unusual types of fibroadenomas. One is the massive fibroadenoma, commonly noted in younger women, in which there is a very large fibroadenoma that develops and must be treated by excision. A second condition is multiple sequential adenofibromas developing throughout the entire extent of the breasts. One lesion can be excised and another one will subsequently develop in another area of the ipsilateral or contralateral breast and require excision. If there are multiple resections of sequential adenofibromas that form in the breast, these will not be completely eliminated until the breast tissue has been removed. Obviously, this is a very drastic course to take in a younger woman and must be approached with great caution, understanding, and conservatism.

Cystosarcoma Phylloides

Cystosarcoma phylloides, often derived from an adenofibroma, makes up only 2 percent of all adenofibromas. It commonly occurs around age 45, but can also be found in younger women, specifically those under age 20. The lesion presents as a rapidly developing large growth in the patient's breast and may grow to 10 to 15 cm. It has a firm characteristic, may be lobulated, and can be tender to the touch. It is uncommon to see cystosarcoma phylloides as a small lesion.

Classically, the lesion is diagnosed by the pathologic characteristics that include fibroblasts forming the stroma. These cells have a benign appearance with small, elongated nuclei. Mitoses are usually not present. Except for the cellularity of the stroma, the tumor appears much like a benign fibroadenoma. Since the potential for malignancy exists and a cystosarcomatous characteristic can develop, the stroma must be evaluated very carefully. The degree of malignancy is evaluated by thorough microscopic evaluation of the stroma and inspection for evidence of subepithelial stromal cellularity and anaplasia. If a lesion has a high cellularity, the potential for malignancy and metastasis exists in 7 percent of patients.

Intraductal Papilloma

Intraductal papilloma is a benign lesion arising as a solitary proliferation from the lactiferous duct epithelium. Most commonly, it develops within a centimeter of the areola itself and rarely is more than 0.5 cm in size. At its point of development the duct is generally dilated, and there is a single attachment to the duct wall. The papilloma has a friable, delicate, villus-type structure with gland cells palisading upon a central core connective tissue network. Usually the cells are only one to two layers in thickness, are uniform in size, and without evidence of atypia. Although they can occur at any age, they are most common in a patient's fifth decade and can present with a serous, serosanguineous, bloody, or turbid-type nipple discharge. Occasionally, there may be fullness or pain beneath the areola. It should be noted that only 3 to 5 percent of patients seen for breast problems will present with a nipple discharge, and only approximately 25 percent of these patients will require a surgical procedure for this condition. Of interest, too, only 3 to 5 percent of all patients presenting with a nipple discharge will be found to have a malignant neoplasm. Despite this somewhat comforting observation, if nipple discharge is found in older women, specifically in their fifties and sixties, the possibility of malignancy increases to from 30 to 50 percent. Twenty-five percent of bloody discharges will eventually be found to be due to cancer, but also 33 percent of watery discharges may be associated with carcinoma.

The benign solitary intraductal papilloma is not premalignant but must be differentiated from a less common condition of multipapillomatosis, and also from papillary carcinoma. In this condition, there can be extensive palisading of cells, cellular atypia, and even invasion. These lesions, which are multiple, are located in the smaller ducts in conjunction with fibrocystic change, i.e., in the outer portions of the breast rather than centrally located as an intraductal papilloma. The patient does not present with a nipple discharge but rather a breast mass, and the diagnosis is most commonly made following excisional biopsy. In addition, these lesions are more common in younger women, although there is some overlap with the age of patients who have intraductal papillomas. Generally, these lesions can be excised, if they are not malignant, with a wide margin of tissue.

Traumatic Fat Necrosis

Traumatic fat necrosis is a condition that simulates carcinoma and arises following breast trauma. Clinically, a mass is formed which is firm and relatively fixed. This occurs more commonly in perimenopausal women with large breasts, and there is a history of known trauma in up to 50 percent of the patients. Ecchymoses may be apparent in 20 to 30 percent of the patients. Although one may be suspicious of this condition based on the patient's history, its appearance mandates excisional biopsy irrespective of the findings on mammography, which in and of themselves can be suspicious for carcinoma, showing calcifications and an irregular density.

Nipple Discharge

Nipple discharge is a disturbing observation for a patient and also can be perplexing for the physician. Fortunately, most nipple discharges are due to benign lesions rather than cancers. In a large series of patients studied at New York Medical College and Affiliated Hospitals, nipple discharge was the presenting symptom in 9 percent of patients with benign disease and 3.4 percent of patients with malignant disease.

There are some conditions that produce a discharge which mimics nipple discharge. These conditions include nipple inversion, eczematoid nipple lesions, traumatic erosions, and conditions with chronic stimulation of the nipple area as well as infections, particularly herpes simplex type I. Nipple discharges are also noted in women taking oral contraceptives, phenothiazines, tricyclic antidepressants, rauwolfia alkaloids, and methyldopa.

Milky discharges and multicolored, thick, sticky-type discharges often occur from multiple ducts and are frequently bilateral. Most frequently, these are greenish but can be yellowish, brown, gray, and even blackish. Purulent discharges have the characteristic appearance of pus and can be diagnosed by a Wright stain.

Serous, serosanguineous, sanguineous, or clear-watery discharges are more likely to be associated with malignancy, and biopsy is mandated when such discharges are present. Most commonly, they are unilateral, occur from a single duct, and are associated with intraductal carcinoma or papilloma. The frequency with which carcinoma is associated with these varied types of discharge has been reported as follows: watery, 33 percent; sanguineous, 27.5 percent; serosanguineous, 12.9 percent; and serous, 5.9 percent. On the other hand, the frequency with which the discharges occur is just the opposite: serous, 40.3 percent; serosanguineous, 31.7 percent; sanguineous, 25.4 percent; and watery, 2.6 percent. Obviously, a watery discharge is of substantial concern and should carry as much weight in the necessity of evaluation as a bloody discharge.

When one considers these discharges totally, the most common causes are: intraductal papilloma, 48.1 percent; proliferative papillomatosis and cystic change, 32.9 percent; and cancer, 14.3 percent. Advanced duct ectasia comprises 4.8 percent. When nipple discharge is identified and is not considered to be physiologic, the ultimate and appropriate treatment is excision of the duct segment for definitive diagnosis.

Mastitis

Mastitis commonly occurs in the puerperal state, although nonpuerperal mastitis may also occur. Puerperal mastitis generally is associated with lactation, with the development of tenderness, erythema, and a temperature elevation. Once mastitis is considered as a diagnosis, lactation should continue, usually by emptying the breast with a breast pump. The most common organism is *Staphylococcus aureus,* although streptococcal and anaerobic organisms also have been cultured. Treatment should usually be with a penicillin derivative that will cover the more resistant types of staphylococcus. Response should be noted within 24 to 48 h. However, if the patient does not respond and the mass becomes larger and more erythematous with increased tenderness, breast abscess must be suspected. Breast abscess is best treated by incision and drainage done under appropriate anesthesia with breakdown of loculations within the mass. Occasionally a drain needs to be placed in the wound and removed 24 to 48 h afterwards. It is occasionally necessary to irrigate the wound during healing. An irrigating fluid of normal saline and hydrogen peroxide is useful. Patients respond to incision and drainage remarkably well with very little eventual disfigurement of the breast.

Nonpuerperal mastitis is generally associated with squamous metaplasia of the lactational ducts close to the areola with the development of so-called periareolar abscesses. Incision and drainage will create resolution of the problem, but it will often recur, requiring definitive excision of the duct segments and drainage of the abscess for complete resolution of the problem.

It is important to make certain that inflammatory carcinoma is not mistaken for mastitis. If there is doubt, a biopsy must be performed.

Superficial Angiitis (Thrombophlebitis): Mondor Syndrome

Superficial angiitis is an uncommon condition of inflammation of major venous drainage channels of the breast, more characteristically noted on the lateral surface of the breast. It occurs most frequently in puerperal women and those having mammary augmentation or reduction. The patient presents with a firm, erythematous, linear, cordlike structure, which may or may not be associated with dimpling. This can be treated conservatively if a diagnosis can be made. Treatment includes the application of heat with the use of analgesics. Over a period of time the condition will undergo spontaneous resolution. If there is question regarding the diagnosis, excisional biopsy should be considered.

Noninvasive Carcinoma of the Breast

Noninvasive breast carcinoma, a challenging problem, is increasing in incidence. In 1975, it comprised approximately 5 percent of all new breast cancer cases; this had increased to 9 percent in 1985 and by 1990 ranged from 15 to 20 percent of all new breast cancer cases. Of these new carcinomas, about two-thirds were noted to be in situ ductal carcinoma, with the remaining being lobular carcinoma in situ. Ductal and lobular carcinoma in situ represent lesions confined to the preexisting duct system of the breast with no evidence of penetration of the basement membrane. From a diagnostic standpoint, ductal carcinoma in situ is frequently noted as an abnormal mammographic calcification, although it can present as a mass or abnormal discharge. The latter two presentations currently are less frequent than abnormal mammographic calcifications. On the other hand, lobular carcinoma in situ often does not form calcifications and is commonly diagnosed by biopsy of an occult or palpable mass or is found as an additional finding when a biopsy is done for a benign breast condition.

Ductal Carcinoma in Situ

There are a number of types of ductal carcinoma in situ, comedo-type being the most common, followed by cribriform, solid, papillary, and micropapillary. Almost 50 percent of the comedo-type may ultimately be demonstrated to have microinvasion, as compared to 14 percent for solid and 8 percent for papillary types of lesions.

Nipple changes have also been noted in patients with ductal carcinoma in situ. Generally, when lesions are detected only mammographically, there are no nipple changes. On the other hand, with non-mammographically detected lesions, up to 50 percent of patients with ductal carcinoma in situ show some type of nipple discharge and/or erythema, retraction, or excoriation. An interesting comparison can be made with invasive ductal carcinoma, which has a lower frequency of nipple change—only 20 to 25 percent. Nipple discharge has also been noted with ductal carcinoma in situ in up to 28 percent of patients but is only found in 10 to 11 percent of patients with invasive ductal carcinoma.

Treatment recommendations for ductal carcinoma in situ have changed dramatically during the past decade. When simple mastectomy was considered the standard for treatment, recurrences were infrequent, ranging from 0 to 10 percent, with a mean of 4 percent. Recurrences generally were directly related to the size of the primary lesion. As the concept of conservatism gained increased recognition, excision only was utilized to treat some patients. In a number of studies, this resulted in a substantial recurrence rate, ranging from 10 to 28 percent during a follow-up period of 1 to 8 years. The mean was noted at approximately 20 percent. Factors influencing the frequency of recurrence included the size of the primary lesion, with larger lesions obviously leading to a greater change of recurrence. Multicentricity is another compounding factor and is found with substantial frequency in intraductal carcinoma. In a variety of studies, *multicentricity* (cancer located in a quadrant separate from the quadrant where the primary tumor was found) was noted in 23 to 41 percent of patients. This problem was noted more frequently with large primary tumors. Disease was also noted to be *multifocal* (cancer in the vicinity or at least in the same quadrant as the primary tumor). This is documented by studies showing margin involvement following wide local excision in 28 to 31 percent of patients. Obviously, local segmental resection alone has a high failure rate and should not be considered standard treatment by itself, except for perhaps a very small primary lesion with no other abnormal mammographic features. Recently, wide excisional biopsy or segmental resection followed by breast irradiation has been advocated as the appropriate standard for treatment in many clinical situations.

Axillary lymph node resection or sampling is not indicated, with only 1 to 2 percent of patients reported as having axillary metastases.

Lobular Carcinoma in Situ

Lobular carcinoma in situ refers to an in situ lesion arising in the lobules and terminal ductules of the breast. In this condition, the ductal epithelial cells proliferate, becoming uniformly enlarged and appearing ovoid with pale, scanty cytoplasm surrounding a large nucleus. The cells may lose their characteristic orientation within the duct and tend to fill and pack the duct, causing distention. However, the lobule per se is not distorted. From a purely histologic perspective, this lesion is occasionally difficult to differentiate from lobular hyperplasia or so-called blunt duct adenosis. For this reason, all treatment decisions should be made only after reviews of permanent histologic sections. Because of its clinical course, lobular carcinoma in situ continues to be a controversial lesion.

This is not a common lesion but is noted more

frequently in younger women. It has been identified in about 1 percent of patients with documented benign breast conditions and in 3.5 to 6 percent of patients who have undergone mastectomy for other conditions. Lobular carcinoma in situ has no heralding sign and may be found when evaluating mammographic calcifications (50 percent), parenchymal distortion, clustered microcalcification, or benign-appearing densities. Approximately 75 percent of patients with lobular carcinoma in situ are in the premenopausal years, suggesting that the condition may be hormonally dependent. The most common age group has been noted to be between 45 and 51 years.

Lobular carcinoma in situ has a propensity for bilaterality and multicentricity, and there are substantial concerns relative to developing subsequent invasive carcinoma. Patients with lobular carcinoma in situ have seven to nine times the usual risk of developing an invasive carcinoma, either in the ipsilateral or contralateral breast. It is estimated to occur with a frequency rate of 5 percent in 5 years, 10 percent in 10 years, and 15 percent in 15 years. An overall incidence of 36 percent has been noted in one study in which patients were followed for 24 years. Overall, the lifetime cumulative risk of developing breast cancer has been estimated to be 0.9 percent per year for women diagnosed with lobular carcinoma in situ. Because of these findings, treatment options are challenging and controversial.

Treatment recommendations have run the gamut: local excision, subcutaneous mastectomy, total mastectomy, partial mastectomy, contralateral breast biopsy, modified radical mastectomy, and bilateral mastectomy. However, based on our current information, it would appear that treatment options are either local excision with careful follow-up or bilateral mastectomy.

The rationale for local excision with follow-up is based on the fact that approximately 65 to 75 percent of patients with lobular carcinoma in situ will not have a further problem. Patients opting for local excision are, however, mandated to a rigorous regimen of continuing follow-up, including monthly self-examination, physician examination every 3 to 4 months, and, of course, annual mammography. Despite this, both the patient and her physician must acknowledge that there is no foolproof method of detecting a cancer if it is present.

If mastectomy is considered, it is reasonable to suggest bilateral mastectomy since the incidence of a woman with lobular carcinoma in situ subsequently developing carcinoma is the same in either the ipsilateral or contralateral breast. On the other hand, this is a substantial recommendation since 65 to 75 percent of patients will not develop an invasive carcinoma. Because of this, some surgeons will advise a unilateral total mastectomy and low axillary lymph node dissection with a contralateral breast biopsy with the intention of performing the mastectomy on the contralateral side only if the breast biopsy is abnormal. This plan is carried out in approximately 40 percent of patients. Relying on unilateral mastectomy tends to overlook the fact that both breasts are at risk and puts a high level of reliance on the contralateral biopsy. The contralateral lesion can be easily missed because of its multicentric characteristics. Partial mastectomy itself carries no benefit greater than local excision.

If contralateral biopsy is considered, the location for the biopsy is problematic. It is based either on clinical findings or abnormal mammographic findings. If neither of these is present, it is recommended that the contralateral biopsy be in the upper outer quadrant of the breast. However, if the lesion in the breast where the condition was initially diagnosed is not in the upper outer quadrant, then not only should a mirror image biopsy be done but also a biopsy from the upper outer quadrant. The overall yield for positive contralateral biopsies ranges from 4.5 to 12 percent, and of these 43 to 46 percent of carcinomas are invasive and 54 to 57 percent are noninvasive.

In the few radiation therapy studies that have been conducted to evaluate radiation therapy after local excision for lobular carcinoma in situ, there are no definitive data at this time.

Whatever choice is finally determined by the patient and her physician, the patient must completely understand the risks and benefits of her choice of treatment. The treatment of lobular carcinoma in situ is clearly one of the most complicated issues in the care of women with breast disease.

Breast Cancer

Early Infiltrating Ductal Carcinoma

Major changes have occurred in the treatment of invasive carcinoma of the breast during the past 20 years. The traditional Halstead radical mastectomy was replaced by the modified radical mastectomy in the 1960s and early 1970s. In the early 1980s, more conservative approaches were introduced for consideration.

Segmental resection and axillary node (level I and II) sampling followed by radiation to the breast was presented as acceptable standard treatment following analysis of a series of seminal studies including the work of Veronesi et al from the National Cancer Institute of Milan, the results of a major trial from the Institute Gustave-Roussy in France, preliminary results from a National Cancer Institute trial abstracted in 1987, an additional trial from Guy's Hospital in London, and the NSABP B-06 study, published in 1989. When all of these data were put together, it led to an NIH consensus development conference on the treatment of early breast cancer and the following statement: "Breast conservation treatment is an appropriate method of primary therapy for the majority of women with Stage I and II breast cancer and is preferable because it provides survival equivalent to total mastectomy and axillary dissection while preserving the breast."

Although that is the ideal, there are some patients who are not good candidates for conservative management. This includes patients in whom the cosmetic appearance of the breast would be significantly altered and unacceptable to the patient despite attempts at breast conservation and also patients who are at high risk for local failure following a conservative procedure. Those patients who fall within the cosmetic category are those in whom the primary tumor is of relatively large size and the breast tissue small, which would result in an unacceptable cosmetic defect if wide excision and radiation therapy were used. It also should be noted that patients who have underlying collagen vascular diseases may have a poor cosmetic result with added radiation therapy. Patients at high risk for local failure include those with diffuse microcalcifications on mammography and those who have ductal carcinoma in situ, particularly with an extensive intraductal component, as well as patients with lymphatic vascular invasion or comedo necrosis.

For patients choosing a conservative approach, they should be advised of the likelihood of some slight darkening of the breast skin, a slight decrease in breast size, and possibly some increased firmness of the breast. These changes are the result of radiation. Thus, at the time of final definitive treatment planning all factors must be carefully considered with the patient and a final decision made by the patient after extensive consultation and complete understanding of her options as well as the potential risks and benefits of each option.

Invasive Lobular Carcinoma

Invasive lobular carcinoma is infrequent in comparison to invasive ductal carcinoma. It represents only 3 to 14 percent of all invasive breast carcinomas. The higher figure, 14 percent, is found only when less restrictive microscopic criteria are used.

In its classic form—using restrictive criteria—the invasive malignant cells of lobular carcinoma have small, round nuclei without prominent nucleoli. Cytoplasm is limited with the occasional occurrence of intracytoplasmic mucus-filled lumina. These mucus-filled lumina can push the nucleus to a peripheral location in the cell, creating a "signet ring" appearance. This signet type of characteristic can also be found in some invasive ductal carcinomas. The infiltrating pattern of this carcinoma is quite unique, accompanied by a prominent desmoplastic stromal reaction. The invading cells tend to form a linear arrangement or to grow circumferentially around ducts and lobules, creating a so-called targetoid pattern.

The condition can occur at any age that breast cancer occurs, although the mean is 57 years—similar to many studies related to invasive ductal carcinoma.

Since this lesion does not frequently produce calcifications, early diagnosis by mammography is thwarted. Generally, these patients will present with a palpable tumor, usually in the upper outer quadrant of the breast. Unfortunately, the lesions do not have well-differentiated margins, and often the only sign of infiltrating lobular carcinoma is a minimal thickening and induration of the breast tissue. Nipple discharge and Paget's-type change of the nipple are not encountered frequently.

From a clinical management standpoint, one of the most disconcerting problems is the frequency of bilaterality. For example, prior and concurrent carcinoma of the contralateral breast has been reported in up to 28 percent of patients. Most frequently, however, the percentage is lower. Equally of concern is the fact that 9 to 14 percent of patients with invasive lobular carcinoma will develop a subsequent contralateral breast carcinoma. These synchronous or metachronous tumors described have a pure or partial lobular component, and up to 50 percent will be invasive. Positive estrogen receptors have been reported in up to 50 percent of primary invasive lobular carcinomas. This is not significantly different from other infiltrating ductal carcinomas of the breast.

Treatment options that exist for invasive lobular breast carcinoma are similar to other breast cancers. For example, lumpectomy and radiation therapy are appropriate for selected lesions, particularly if surgical margins are clear and the primary lesion is not extensive or diffuse throughout the upper quadrant of the breast. Obviously, too, modified radical mastectomy with axillary dissection can be considered appropriate for large or diffuse tumors. Treatment must bc individualized with a clear presentation of prognosis and outcome to the patient. Because of the high incidence of bilateral disease, mirror imaging or upper quadrant biopsy of the contralateral breast has been considered. The yield, however, is low, provided lobular carcinoma in situ is excluded.

Lobular carcinoma of the breast, whether in situ or invasive, remains a perplexing problem and requires knowledge and understanding by the physician caring for the patient with breast disease.

Paget's Disease of the Nipple

Paget's disease of the nipple is an uncommon condition occurring in the ducts of the breast at the duct-skin interface. Its incidence is approximately 0.7 percent to 4.3 percent of all breast cancers, and its peak occurrence is during the sixth decade of life. Early on, the skin appears thin and reddened and may be associated with the symptoms of itching, burning, or slight pain; 40 percent of patients will eventually complain of discharge or bleeding. The classic description by Sir James Paget written in 1784 describes the lesion: "In the majority it had the appearance of a florid, intensely red, raw surface, very finely granular, as if merely the whole thickness of the epidermis were removed; like the surface of a very acute, diffuse eczema." From such a surface on the whole or greater part of the nipple and areola, there was always clear, yellowish, viscid exudation.

Histologically, Paget's disease has the classic Paget cells with large vesicular nuclei and a vacuolated cytoplasm. Recent immunohistochemical studies have confirmed that the lesion is of primary ductal origin and not related to a change in the squamous epithelium of the nipple surface. Also, the condition does occur de novo and is not an extension of an underlying invasive ductal carcinoma. On the other hand, approximately 50 percent of patients with Paget's disease will have an underlying mass below the nipple areola complex, and almost always (94 percent of the time) this is an invasive carcinoma.

Diagnosis is made on the basis of history and observation. Mammography per se does not have any specific imaging characteristic unique to Paget's disease. However, it should be done to exclude other microcalcifications or parenchymal densities that might herald the possibility of multifocal or multicentric ductal carcinoma in situ as well as invasive ductal carcinoma.

The treatment of Paget's disease is evolving, with opportunities for conservatism in specific early lesions. The decision for conservatism is based primarily on whether or not an underlying mass is present and whether mammographic evaluations are entirely normal. For patients with an underlying mass, one must assume this to be a cancer, and after biopsy confirmation, these patients are considered as having multifocal carcinoma and should be treated by modified radical mastectomy including axillary dissection. Five-year survival studies for patients with a mass in this situation have varied from 0 to 43 percent, while the 5-year survival rate of those with Paget's disease with no mass has been estimated to be 94 to 100 percent.

For patients without an accompanying mass, there is an option, as previously indicated, to be considered for conservative therapy, specifically, central segmentectomy (a cone excision of the nipple-areola complex and deeper ductal structures). This includes the resection of a generous portion of the adjacent breast parenchyma. The axillary lymph nodes should also be resected. This latter step is always indicated even in patients only with the Pagetoid characteristic of the nipple and proximal ducts of the nipple-areola complex, since approximately 13 percent of these patients will have positive lymph nodes. Despite its uncommon occurrence, the physician can make an early diagnosis of Paget's disease by careful attention and assessment of symptoms related to the nipple, specifically of an itching or burning sensation. Awareness should be heightened, particularly if the nipple has the thin reddish characteristic of the epithelial surface or if eczematoid changes are present.

Other Uncommon Types of Breast Cancer

There are a number of other types of breast cancer including malignant melanoma, basal cell carcinoma of the nipple, squamous ductal cell carcinoma, lymphoma of the breast, mesenchymal and stromal sarcomas, as well as angiosarcomas. These lesions are extremely uncommon and are mentioned for completeness but will not be described.

However, physicians dealing with patients who have been treated for breast cancer in a conservative fashion must be alert to the potential for the development of postirradiation sarcomas of the breast. Sarcomas have been described in patients who have received radiation therapy for breast cancer in the past, specifically for postmastectomy, adjuvant radiation, or if radiation therapy was utilized as palliative treatment for advanced disease. The sarcomas that have been described include not only osterosarcomas of the scapula, humerus, and the ribs, but also soft tissue fibrosarcomas that have been found within the muscle and subcutaneous fatty tissue of the breast. These conditions occur after a latency period that is variable, but they have been observed most commonly with an average latency of 10 years. With changing radiation technology and skin sparing, the potential frequency of this condition is likely to be significantly less.

On the other hand, with the emergence of a conservative view in treating early invasive breast cancer by local resection, axillary node sampling, and radiation therapy, one must be concerned about the possibility of radiation induction of sarcomas. Since there is a long latency period for development of sarcomas, the literature to date does not clearly describe this potential consequence of radiation therapy. However, anecdotal cases have been reported. Careful examination of patients treated with conservative surgery and radiation therapy plus appropriate mammography is critical for continuing patient follow-up.

Breast Cancer Associated with Pregnancy

Approximately 12 percent of all breast cancers occur in reproductive age women, and between 0.2 to 3.8 percent of breast cancers occur during pregnancy or lactation. The incidence of breast cancer in women of reproductive age changes dramatically from 0.1 per 100,000 women less than the age of 20 to approximately 103 per 100,000 women aged 40 to 44 years. In evaluations of pregnancy associated with breast cancer, the most common period of occurrence is between the age of 30 and 39, with a mean of 35 years in most series.

In the past, breast cancer associated with pregnancy was thought to have a very poor outcome. More recently others have become more optimistic when considering the condition. Although during pregnancy there are high concentrations of circulating estrogen, progesterone, and chorionic gonadotropin as well as evidence of depression of T lymphocyte function, the more critical factor affecting adverse outcome is a delay in diagnosis, with discovery of breast cancer in pregnancy often at advanced stages and with frequent delays or compromise in the onset and type of therapy due to the fetus. Current thinking is focused more on accurate and prompt diagnosis with uncompromised appropriate treatment and an overall better outcome.

Carcinoma occurring in pregnancy usually presents as a mass or, on occasion, a bloody nipple discharge. Because of the enlarged state of the breast in response to the hormonal milieu of pregnancy, masses are often not diagnosed early, leading to more advanced stages and a distinctly higher chance of axillary metastases, which have been reported in as many as 89 percent of pregnant patients with breast cancer. An additional problem is the inaccuracy of mammography, which fails to demonstrate cancer when present in up to 40 percent of pregnant patients, even when a palpable tumor is present. This mammographic deficiency is related to the dense parenchymal characteristics of the breast. Bloody nipple discharge is generally assumed to be related to ductal hyperplasia during pregnancy rather than malignancy and that this will dissipate following delivery. Although benign bloody nipple discharge is not infrequent during pregnancy, obviously great concern and care must be taken to elucidate the cause of the bloody nipple discharge.

The most common solid mass occurring in the breast during pregnancy is a lactating adenoma, but other conditions such as fibroadenoma and galactocele can also be present. Needle aspiration and biopsy are certainly feasible during pregnancy and should be encouraged when a mass of concern is present. If the diagnosis of a suspicious mass cannot be made by needle aspiration cytology, an open biopsy should be undertaken. The biopsy should be conducted in a meticulous manner, with adequate hemostasis and attempts to avoid transecting major ducts. However, if transections do occur, they should be closed with meticulous care. If a galactocele develops at a biopsy site, it can be treated with repeated aspiration and can be expected to undergo spontaneous resolution after normal completion of pregnancy.

The treatment of breast cancer during pregnancy or lactation is straightforward and should occur promptly and according to the same basic principles of treatment that apply when the patient is not pregnant. If a diagnosis of early breast cancer is made in the first trimester of pregnancy, termination is not necessary unless the patient considers a conservative treatment option or desires elective termination. Radiation is of concern, and the ability to shield completely a fetus from therapeutic radiation effects is virtually impossible because of the scatter that can occur both within the mother and by leakage from the source of the radiation.

The probability of malformation or developmental defects from radiation therapy occurring during the second to eighth week has been documented. The potential for a defect or malformation becomes significant after delivery of 10 cGy and is virtually assured if the radiation dose exceeds 100 cGy. If carcinoma is diagnosed later in pregnancy—i.e., in the second or third trimester—the enlarging fetus will become more proximate to the irradiation field and may absorb an increasing fraction of the total radiation dosage delivered to the mother's breast or chest wall.

Once again, because of the potential for radiation to the fetus, conservative treatments should not be considered unless the mother is near term and early delivery is feasible, with subsequent delivery of radiation therapy after delivery.

For those patients after treatment who require adjuvant chemotherapy, this can usually be initiated after the first trimester without incurring serious fetal abnormalities. The patient should be advised not to lactate while receiving chemotherapy since the agents are secreted in the patient's milk and may cause neutropenia in the newborn infant.

In general, today the results of treatment for patients who have breast cancer during pregnancy are more encouraging than they have been in the past. In 1991, Petrek et al. reviewed the records of 56 pregnant women with operable breast cancer and compared them to 166 nonpregnant patients of comparable age. She reported that axillary node involvement was more frequent in the pregnant group but that there were no significant differences found in the 5- and 10-year survival rates when comparing both groups, particularly when correcting for nodal status. At 5- and 10-year periods, node-negative patients had a survival rate of 82 percent and 77 percent compared to 82 percent and 75 percent of patients who were not pregnant. If lymph nodes were positive during pregnancy, the 5-year survival rate was 47 percent and 10-year survival 25 percent, while in nonpregnant women the survival rates were 59 and 41 percent at the 5- and 10-year periods.

Another study reported by Nugent and O'Connell in 1985 evaluating pregnancy in breast cancer patients under the age of 40 revealed that younger patients tended to have a higher stage of disease compared to older patients and that age affected the prognosis but that pregnancy did not. In general, the more recent reports do not show a significant correlation between prognosis and the trimester of pregnancy in which the patient was diagnosed and treated.

What about pregnancy following treatment for breast cancer? The current literature suggests that future pregnancies may not compromise the patient's chances for an ultimate cure and that adjuvant chemotherapy poses minimal to no risk to subsequent pregnancies. At what time a patient can be advised that pregnancy seems to be safe is still somewhat controversial, and arbitrary decisions of 2 to 3 years have been put forward as speculative time limits. One of the reasons to recommend a delay in becoming pregnant, particularly in patients at high risk for early recurrence, is that if treatment becomes necessary, the pregnancy may be compromised. A recommendation for delaying pregnancy 3 to 5 years has been put forth because recurrence risk is highest during that period. The risk of recurrence 5 to 10 years following treatment in women under the age of 40 ranges from 2 to 7 percent. Actually, there is no specific time delay after which one can be 100 percent certain that disease will not recur, but, of course, it must be pointed out that long waits are associated with an overall decline in fertility.

Tamoxifen and Chemotherapy

The recommendations for adjuvant therapy as presented in the St. Gallen Consensus in 1992 are shown in Table 42-1. However, it is important to note that information regarding adjuvant therapy for breast cancer is evolving rapidly, and, therefore, recommendations change frequently. Currently all node-positive women who have completed primary therapy for breast cancer and have no known residual disease receive adjuvant therapy with chemotherapy and/or tamoxifen. Many node-negative breast cancer patients who have completed initial therapy receive adjuvant therapy as well.

Tamoxifen, a nonsteroidal antiestrogen, has been found to be a very effective agent in the treatment of breast carcinoma. Clinical trials using tamoxifen were instituted in 1971. It was also postulated that as an adjuvant therapy there would be an advantage for patients who had a primary tumor of the breast removed and that this drug would control micrometastases. Tamoxifen was found to be particularly useful

TABLE 42-1 St. Gallen Consensus, 1992

Treatment for Node-Positive Breast Cancer Patients

Menopausal Status	ER (−)	ER (+)
Premenopausal	Chemotherapy	Chemotherapy +/− tamoxifen
Postmenopausal	Chemotherapy	Tamoxifen +/− chemotherapy

Treatment for Low Risk and Increased Risk Node-Negative Breast Cancer Patients

Menopausal Status	Low Risk	Increased Risk
Premenopausal	None vs. Tamoxifen	Tamoxifen
Postmenopausal	None vs. Tamoxifen	Tamoxifen

Low risk = focally invasive tumors; tubular, colloid or papillary histological type; tumor size < 1 cm; ER(+)
Increased risk = tumor size > 1 cm but < 2 cm; ER(+); good nuclear grade; diploid and low S phase

Treatment for High Risk Node-Negative Breast Cancer

Group	Treatment
Premenopausal	
ER(+)	Chemotherapy +/− tamoxifen
ER(−)	Chemotherapy
Postmenopausal	
ER(+)	Tamoxifen +/− chemotherapy
ER(−)	Chemotherapy +/− tamoxifen

High risk = any tumor > 2 cm; ER(−) tumors, even those less than 2 cm; poor nuclear grade; high S phase (aneuploid or diploid)

since it had a long serum half-life, was highly efficacious, and appeared to have a minimum number of side effects.

The initial trials suggested that tamoxifen produced a survival advantage when given to postmenopausal, node-positive, estrogen receptor–positive women. Studies of premenopausal women were instituted, and the significant National Surgical Adjuvant Breast Project (NSABP) B-14 study clearly demonstrated the value of tamoxifen when given to premenopausal node-negative women. These results were significant enough to lead to a recommendation to all oncologists that advised the use of tamoxifen as an adjuvant therapy in all patients with estrogen–receptor positive, node-negative breast carcinoma. Additional information suggests that some patients will have an improved prognosis when utilizing tamoxifen independent of their receptor status. Therefore, there is an increasing argument suggesting that tamoxifen would be advantageous for all breast cancer patients.

With a drug that appears to be so advantageous, concerns are appropriately raised regarding its ancillary effects. On the benefit side, tamoxifen decreases low-density lipoprotein cholesterol. Initially there had been concern that the antiestrogen effect of tamoxifen could increase the potential for osteoporosis. However, tamoxifen has demonstrated estrogenlike effects in bone tissue, and so far there is no evidence of significant osteoporosis in long-term tamoxifen users.

On the other hand, tamoxifen is associated with some potential adverse effects. With the use of long-term tamoxifen therapy, there have been reports of hypercalcemia, particularly in patients with breast cancer metastatic to the bone. Tamoxifen use has also been associated with retinopathy, endometrial carcinoma, and sarcomatous change in the uterus. In addition, cystic ovarian necrosis has been reported in premenopausal women being treated for breast cancer with tamoxifen.

The axillary node–negative (ANN) patient fuels the controversy regarding appropriateness of adjuvant therapy. Ever since the 1988 NCI Clinical Alert that adjuvant hormonal or cytotoxic chemotherapy can have an important impact on patients with stage I disease, this statement has led some to consider treatment for all patients, considering that 15 to 20 percent of node-negative patients relapse in the first 10 years after local-regional therapy. However, one must consider that this category, ANN, includes nonpalpable microscopic tumors detected by mammography, for example, T0 and T1ab cured by surgery alone or surgery and radiation. The category also includes patients with disease advanced to stage T2 or T3.

Various prognostic factors can be identified. Of paramount concern in node-negative cancers is tumor size: for example, the disease-free status at 7 years for a T1a (<0.5 cm) tumor has been reported as high as 98 percent while the T1b (0.5–1.0 cm) tumor is 93 percent and 86 percent for T1c (1.1–2.0 cm). This disease-free survival drops rapidly to 74 percent for T2 (2.1–5.0 cm) lesions. Other studies have reported 20-year disease-free survival rates of 86 percent for tumors less than 1 cm and 69 percent for tumors 1.1 to 2.0 cm treated by mastectomy alone. Thus, patients with minimally invasive breast cancer (<1.0 cm) are often not treated with adjuvant therapy if other parameters are also favorable.

Histologic, nuclear, and mitotic grades are also important evaluating factors. For example, well and moderately differentiated tumors have a significant disease-free survival rate (90 percent at 7 years) while poorly differentiated tumors have a disease-free survival rate of only 77 percent at 7 years.

Age is also a factor to consider. In general, younger patients have a shorter disease-free period than older patients. This observation is particularly important for patients with small tumors, e.g., those less than 1.0 cm. For women less than 50 years of age, the 7-year disease-free period has been reported as 90 percent and for those over 50 years old as high as 99 percent. By combining age, tumor size, and histologic grade, patient subsets can be developed for those patients who have a high probability of recurrence.

Estrogen and progesterone receptor status is another important prognostic factor, particularly in patients with positive nodes. However, in early breast cancer patients, specifically early ANN patients, the differences are not as great, although there is a suggestion that patients with ER-positive tumors do slightly better than those with ER-negative tumors, for example, an 82 percent 7-year disease-free period for ER positive patients and 76 percent disease-free survival rate for ER negative patients. This difference is not, however, statistically significant. These small differences may also be due to the fact that the smaller tumors in the past often had unknown receptor status.

Other prognostic indicators have become available during the past decade including evaluation of DNA variables by thymidine labeling and the determination of the percentage of cells in S and G2-M phase combined (SPF).

DNA studies showing aneuploidy have suggested some prognostic alterations; however, unfortunately results are not conclusive. Essentially, aneuploidy has been noted more commonly in large, poorly differentiated tumors, particularly in younger women—e.g., 72 percent in tumors greater than 2 cm compared to 52 percent in tumors less than 1.0 cm. Likewise, tumors with a high volume of cycling cells will be poorly differentiated. The NIH Consensus Development Conference made some important statements regarding DNA variables, specifically, "S-phase fraction by flow cytometry does correlate with prognosis, but ploidy status alone is not of clear prognostic value." In this report the NIH also noted that approximately 25 percent of specimens may not be evaluated by flow cytometry because of technical problems and that quality control must be at extremely high levels before all studies relative to flow cytometry can be accepted. The NIH panel concluded, stating, "Although SPF has been shown to be an independent prognostic factor in some studies, its clinical value is being defined."

HER-2/neu oncogene (C-erb B-2 oncoprotein) has been found to be increased from two- to twenty-fold in 20 to 30 percent of primary breast cancers. This was noted particularly in node-positive patients. However, its usefulness as a predictor of the need for adjuvant chemotherapy and of potential adverse outcome for axillary node negative patients has not been demonstrated. Similarly, cathepsin-D, a lyposomal enzyme, has been suggested as a prognostic indicator independent of traditional prognostic factors in some breast cancer patients, i.e., those with concentrations of cathepsin-D greater than 70 pmol/mg protein. Unfortunately for axillary node–negative patients, these studies are not sufficient to enthusiastically endorse this substance as useful for identifying early-stage axillary node–negative patients with good or poor prognoses.

In summary, until further data becomes available regarding which patients with node negative breast cancers should receive adjuvant therapy and what therapy is optimal, patients should be encouraged to participate in clinical trials. For those women not involved in clinical trials, clinicians can use many of the aforementioned parameters to determine which women with node negative breast cancer are most likely to benefit from adjuvant therapy.

In addition to the fact that adjuvant hormonal and chemotherapy regimens are currently being used for many subsets of node-negative breast cancer patients and for almost all node-positive breast cancer patients after the completion of primary therapy, chemotherapy and hormonal therapy clearly play a very important role in the treatment of advanced breast cancer and recurrent breast cancer. Responses to hormonal and chemotherapy in patients with advanced and recurrent disease often have a substantial impact on the duration and quality of life for these women.

The possibility that tamoxifen may prevent breast cancer has been raised. A pilot trial at the Royal Marsden Hospital using tamoxifen as a so-called chemopreventive substance in healthy women has been undertaken. This study is directed at women between the ages of 30 and 69 who have one first-degree relative—specifically, a sister, mother, or daughter—who developed breast cancer prior to the age of 40; women with a family history of bilateral breast cancer occurring at any age; and women with at least two first-degree relatives with breast cancer at any age. The final results from this intriguing study are not yet completely available. The benefits as well as the risks of tamoxifen are being evaluated.

After Breast Cancer Treatment: Long-Term Follow-Up

An important function of the physician in the management of the patient following treatment for breast cancer is for the patient to have complete confidence that the physician is there for her as a resource for questions, support, and ongoing health care. It is imperative that the physician be aware not only of the requisites of medical follow-up but also of the need for continued psychological support, particularly over the first 3 to 4 years following treatment for breast cancer.

From a purely physical standpoint, it is during this period that the major objective of follow-up, specifically, early detection of persistent or recurrent cancer, is of prime concern. To effect this, the patient should be examined every 3 months for the first 3 years following treatment. This is the period of highest recurrence, although, of course, recurrence following breast cancer can occur many years after primary treatment. This examination should be targeted to areas where recurrence might most likely be identified—specifically, supraclavicular lymph nodes, lung, axillary area, the breast which was the site of the primary lesion and treatment, as well as the contralateral breast. If the patient has had a modified radical or simple mastectomy as a part of her treatment, particular attention should be paid to the incision on the chest wall, at which time the physician gently palpates the skin adjacent to the incision to be sure that there is no evidence of local palpable recurrence. If the patient's breast has been treated conservatively, both breasts should be carefully examined according to the guidelines previously discussed. The physician must remember that the radiated breast may have a slightly increased pigmentation and be somewhat firmer than the contralateral breast. Careful palpation is undertaken to find evidence of specific nodularity, skin retraction, erythema, or nipple discharge. The abdomen must be carefully examined also to exclude hepato- or splenomegaly.

Laboratory studies are an important part of follow-up and should be considered at 6-month intervals for the first 3 years. The studies are basic, including routine liver enzymes, a plasma CEA, with additional consideration for utilizing biological tumor markers. Cathepsin-D, HER-2/neu, and EGFR have all been utilized but do not have a high specificity. With the rapid development of information, new markers can be anticipated. After a patient has had laboratory studies completed for a 3-year period, the frequency can be reduced to annually. At the end of 5 years these studies should be ordered only on the basis of changes in the patient's clinical findings.

Radiologic procedures are important in routine follow-up of patients treated for breast cancer. Mammography must not be overlooked as an important and key evaluation tool. For patients choosing a breast-conserving treatment, mammograms of the breast in which the primary tumor was located should be taken every 6 months for the first 3 years and bilateral mammography performed annually thereafter. Also, of course, for the patient with a breast-conserving procedure, the contralateral breast should be examined mammographically on an annual basis. For patients being treated by a modified radical mastectomy, mammography should be done on an annual basis. Chest x-ray should also be considered every 6 months for the first 3 years following treatment and then on an annual basis until 5 years. Thereafter, chest x-ray should be based on the clinical findings at the time of examination. Bone scans should be considered every 6 months for 3 years and then on an annual basis until 5 years in patients who are particularly suspect for recurrence, i.e., those with large primary lesions or those with positive axillary lymph nodes. The frequency of finding a positive bone scan in an asymptomatic woman is very low and has been reported in one NSABP study to be approximately 0.06 percent. It is for this reason that bone scan should be offered only to those with a high risk of recurrence. A liver scan should not be done on a routine basis during follow-up unless there is a new elevation of liver enzymes, and brain scans are not indicated unless neurologic symptoms become evident.

Psychological Support

An important part of supportive care for a woman with breast cancer encompasses understanding tangential factors that have an impact on decision making and life style, and dealing with prognostic variables. Appreciation of a woman's personality type and psychological makeup are important and significantly affect her decision making. Additionally, one must consider familial, marital, social, and economic factors. Once a diagnosis of substantial increased risk is presented to a patient—e.g., atypical ductal hyperplasia compounded by a mother or sister with a history of breast cancer—the physician must help the patient acquire and process appropriate information that will lead her to a comfortable decision regarding "watchful observation with regular screening" or mastectomy with reconstruction. Information dissemination, discussion, and gentle support by a significant partner, physician, or close friend are enriching and helpful factors during the critical decision-making process.

Once a decision has been made, continuing discussions, venting of personal feelings, and finally resolution of concerns is critical. Decisions involve critical choices, and long-range prognostic factors can be difficult to assess and are often clouded. Gentle empathetic support is a tremendous asset to share with the patient. Her life may be at an impasse. The future is unknown. Caring and concern are critical and must be shared by the contemporary physician with the patient.

Suggested Reading

1. American Cancer Society: Mammography 1982. *CA* 32:226, 1982.
2. Bogle CA, Berkowitz GS, et al: Caffeine consumption and fibrocystic disease: A case control epidemiologic study. *J Natl Cancer Inst* 72:1015, 1984.
3. Bornstein BA, Recht A, Connolly JL, et al: Results of treating ductal carcinoma in situ of the breast with conservative surgery and radiation therapy. *Cancer* 67:7–13, 1991.
4. Devitt JE: Clinical benign disorders of the breast and carcinoma of the breast. *Surg Gynecol Obstet* 152:437, 1981.
5. Drukker BH: Examination of the breasts by the patient and by the physician, in Hindle WH (ed): *Breast Disease for Gynecologists.* Norwalk, CT: Appleton-Lange, 1990, p 47.
6. Drukker BH, de Mendonca WC: Fibrocystic change and fibrocystic disease of the breast. *Obstet Gynecol Clin North Am* 14:685, 1987.
7. Feig SA: Decreased breast cancer mortality through mammographic screening: Results of clinical trials. *Radiology* 167:659, 1988.
8. Fisher B, Costantino J, et al: Lumpectomy compared with lympectomy and radiation therapy for the treatment of intraductal breast cancer. *N Engl J Med* 328:1581, 1993.
9. Fisher B, Constantino J, Redmond C, et al: A randomized clinical trial evaluating tamoxifen in the treatment of patients with node-negative breast cancer who have estrogen receptor positive tumors. *N Engl J Med* 320:479, 1989.
10. Fisher B, Redmond C, Poisson R, et al: Five year results of a randomized clinical trial comparing total mastectomy and segmental mastectomy with or without radiation in the treatment of breast cancer. *N Engl J Med* 312:665, 1985.
11. Fletcher SW, O'Malley MS, Bruce LA: Physicians' abilities to detect lumps in silicone breast models. *JAMA* 253:2224, 1985.
12. Glant MD, Clark SA: A procurement and processing system to ensure optimal definitive diagnoses in aspiration biopsy. *Acta Cytol* 28:650, 1984.
13. Glick JH, Gelfer RD, Goldhirsch A, Hans-Jorg S: Meeting highlights: Adjuvant therapy for primary breast cancer. *J Nat Can Inst* 84:1479, 1992.
14. Gump FE: Lobular carcinoma in situ: Pathology and treatment. *Surg Clin North Am* 70:873–883, 1990.
15. Kurtz JM, Jacquemier J, Torhorst J, et al: Conservation therapy for breast cancers other than infiltrating ductal cancer. *Cancer* 63:1630, 1989.
16. Lagios MD, Westdahl PR, Rose MR, Concannon S: Paget's disease of the nipple. Alternative management in cases without and with minimal extent of underlying breast carcinoma. *Cancer* 54:545, 1984.
17. Li Volsi VA, Stadel BV, et al: Fibrocystic breast disease in oral contraceptive users. A histopathological evaluation of epithelial atypia. *N Engl J Med* 299:381, 1978.
18. Love SM, Gelman RS, Silen S: Fibrocystic "disease" of the breast—a non-disease. *New Engl J Med* 307:1010, 1982.
19. Minton JP, Abou-Issa H, Reiches N, Roseman JM: Clinical and biochemical studies on methylxanthine-related fibrocystic disease. *Surgery* 90:299, 1981.
20. National Cancer Institute: Clinical Alert. Bethesda, MD: Department of Health and Human Services, May 18, 1988.
21. National Institutes of Health: *Consensus Development Conference Statement. Treatment of Early Stage Breast Cancer.* Bethesda, MD: National Institues of Health, June 18–21, 1990.
22. Nugent P, O'Connell TX: Breast cancer and pregnancy. *Arch Surg* 120:1221–1224, 1985.

23. Page DL, Dupont WD, Rogers LW: Ductal involvement by cells of atypical lobular hyperplasia in the breast: A long-term follow-up study of cancer risk. *Hum Pathol* 19:201–207, 1988.
24. Paget J. On disease of the mammary areolar preceeding cancer of the mammary gland. *St. Bartholomew's Hospital Report* 10:87, 1974.
25. Petrek JA, Dukoff R, Rogatko A: Prognosis of pregnancy-associated breast cancer. *Cancer* 67:869–872, 1991.
26. Rosen PP: The pathology of invasive breast carcinoma, in Harris JR (ed): *Breast Diseases.* Philadelphia: Lippincott, 1991, p 245.
27. Solin LJ, Recht A, Fourquest A, et al: Ten year result of breast conserving surgery and definitive irradiation for intraductal carcinoma (ductal carcinoma in situ) of the breast. *Cancer* 68:2337–2344, 1991.
28. Stockdale AD, Brierly JD, et al: Radiotherapy for Paget's disease of the nipple: A conservative alternative. *Lancet* 11:664, 1989.
29. Veronesi U, Saccozzi R, Del Vecchio M, et al: Comparing radical mastectomy with quadrantectomy, axillary dissection, and radio-therapy in patients with small cancers of the breast. *N Engl J Med* 305:6, 1981.
30. Veronesi U, Zucali R, Luini A: Local control and survival in early breast cancer: The Milan trial. *J Radiat Oncol Biol Phys* 12:717, 1986.

43 Pulmonary Disorders

David R. Dantzker
Alan S. Multz

The major function of the lung is the exchange of oxygen and carbon dioxide with the environment, and it accomplishes this effortlessly under normal circumstances. The energy cost of normal breathing is less than 10 percent of the total basal energy requirements of the body. The lung has an enormous amount of redundancy and uses barely 15 to 20 percent of its capacity at rest. Even during strenuous exercise it is rarely called upon to use more than 50 percent of its capability. For this reason there can be a considerable loss of function before a patient becomes symptomatic, and many lung diseases are, as a result, picked up late in their course. A patient may give a history of sudden onset of symptoms even when the disease has been progressing for a considerable time.

The process of respiration is intimately linked with three other organ systems: cardiovascular, nervous, and musculoskeletal. An abnormality of any of these may present initially in the form of some respiratory complaint. While it is often difficult to identify the origin of the complaint from the history and physical examination alone, simple diagnostic studies exist that can usually point in the correct direction.

This chapter cannot serve as a complete discussion of the pathophysiology, diagnosis, and treatment of pulmonary disease. The authors will, however, attempt to elucidate those factors that suggest the lungs may be the source of an observed or perceived illness and indicate steps that should be taken to confirm the supposition. We will also expand on the more common or important disorders that may be seen by the primary care provider.

Signs and Symptoms of Pulmonary Disease

General Information

The presence of lung disease is usually suspected because of some specific complaint by the patient. However, the long latency period between the beginning of disease and the onset of symptoms of many lung diseases requires alertness by the physician in ferreting out those symptoms which may be early indicators of an abnormality. Particular vigilance must be exercised in those patients whose family history, occupation, social habits, or travel make them particularly prone to the development of lung disease. Smokers should be counseled to stop and helped to do so. Patients who run the risk of environmental exposure to noxious or infectious agents should be educated about those risks, and, when indicated, proper preventative measures or epidemiologic screening should be advised as in the case of tuberculosis exposure.

While respiratory disease may present in a number of ways, there are some complaints that are common enough to be worthy of separate discussion.

Breathing is ordinarily an automatic, unconscious act, and, thus, a sensation of breathlessness or increased difficulty in breathing is often the first complaint. This awareness of difficulty breathing is termed *dyspnea.* Its pathophysiologic basis is unknown, but it probably represents an imbalance or disproportion between the perceived demand for ventilation and what is achieved. This may be due to an abnormality of the lung itself, a heightened input from receptors in the chest wall, or a change in the relationship between the respiratory center drive and minute ventilation. Occasionally, the patient's history may be helpful in clarifying the origin of the dyspnea. Episodic dyspnea associated with wheezing or cough at rest or following exercise may be an indication of bronchospasm. Dyspnea causing arousal from sleep may be due to nocturnal asthma, neuromuscular disease, sleep apnea, chronic aspiration, or congestive heart failure. Dyspnea only on exertion may represent lung, heart, or neuromuscular disease, which can often be differentiated only by cardiopulmonary exercise studies. Rarely, dyspnea on exercise, or even at rest, may be an initial clue to a slowly developing chronic anemia. While a sense of breathlessness at rest or during exercise—often described as a reduction in exercise tolerance—may be a manifestation of depression, boredom, or other functional disorders, the complaint of dyspnea should never be ascribed to this until all possible organic sources are ruled out.

Cough has been called "the watchdog of the lungs." It is usually initiated by mechanical or chemical stimulation of the upper or lower airways and serves as a reflex to protect the lungs against potentially dangerous inhalants. As with dyspnea, the development of a cough may be a manifestation of a functional problem, but ascribing it to that cause should never be done without a full exploration of potentially pathological conditions. Cough is usually indicative of the need for increased clearance of mucus from the lungs, which may result from infectious or noninfectious inflammatory conditions. The most common noninfectious inflammatory condition that stimulates the cough receptors is asthma, and episodic cough may be the first and only symptom of bronchospasm. Cough that occurs predominantly when lying down at night may be secondary to the aspiration of gastric contents or from postnasal drip. Smokers often have a chronic productive or nonproductive cough, but a change in the character of the cough should raise the suspicion of bronchogenic carcinoma. Occasionally, a cough may be due to nonpulmonary disorders. The most common of these is gastroesophageal reflux. A more unusual cause of cough is that seen secondary to tympanic membrane stimulation, often due to an impacted hair.

When cough is productive of blood, it always requires immediate evaluation. While a bleeding site in the upper airway should be excluded, the most common causes of blood-streaked sputum are chronic bronchitis, pneumonia, and (particularly in a smoker) a tumor. Rarely, hemoptysis may be the presenting complaint in a patient with pulmonary embolic disease. The diagnosis of the cause of hemoptysis can usually be made following a history and physical examination and simple chest roentgenogram, but occasionally more complex studies such as bronchoscopy may be necessary to determine the source of the bleeding.

The lung parenchyma and visceral pleura are insensitive to painful stimuli, and therefore the presence of chest pain should always indicate disease of parietal pleura, the large airways, the chest wall, or structures located within the mediastinum. Noncardiac chest pain is often difficult to differentiate from cardiac pain. Pericardial and pleural pain are also often difficult to separate from each other. Occasionally, chest pain may be referred from abdominal disease, and, not infrequently, an abnormality in the chest may present as abdominal pain.

Hoarseness indicates intrinsic or neuromuscular disease of the vocal cords. It may be due to such minor problems as overuse, cigarette smoke, or viral infection, or it may indicate more serious disease such as cancer or granulomatous disease of the vocal cords.

The Physical Examination

The physical examination of the chest should be familiar to all physicians, and we will not review it in detail here. Suffice it to say that significant pulmonary disease may be present despite a normal physical examination. On the other hand, a careful physical examination may discover an unsuspected abnormality or at least assist in directing the workup of a respiratory complaint.

Certain points about the physical examination are worth emphasizing. The normal resting respiratory rate is approximately 8 to 12 breaths per minute. A respiratory rate of greater than 20 almost always suggests some underlying cardiopulmonary disease. When lung disease is suspected, the respiratory rate is an easily obtainable variable that may be a useful confirmatory sign. Patients with obstructive lung disease may show no evidence of wheezing on normal breathing and yet have dramatically abnormal chest sounds during a forced expiration. A forced expiratory time (the amount of time that one can hear air moving during a forced expiratory maneuver) of greater than 3 to 4 s usually suggests significant airway obstruction.

Observation of the breathing pattern may also be very useful. Under normal circumstances the chest wall and abdomen move outward symmetrically during inspiration and inward during expiration. Paradoxical movement of either of these components of the chest wall may indicate the presence of underlying disease. Inward movement of the abdomen during inspiration suggests diaphragmatic dysfunction or excessive respiratory work while inward movement of the intercostal spaces is seen with marked airway obstruction. The inward inspiratory movement of the lower portions of the chest wall (Hoover's sign) is often suggestive of significant lung hyperinflation and is caused by the horizontal orientation of the depressed diaphragm.

Digital clubbing may occasionally be congenital, but it usually indicates significant underlying lung disease such as carcinoma of the lung, chronic inflammatory disease such as bronchiectasis, cystic fibrosis or lung abscess, or the presence of diffuse interstitial fibrosis. When clubbing is due to cancer or bronchiectasis, it may be accompanied by the full-blown syndrome of hypertrophic osteoarthropathy. This includes, in addition to clubbing, long-bone tenderness and pain as well as asymmetrical arthritis-like changes in the joints, increased thickness of the soft tissue in the distal third of the arms and legs, and neurovascular changes in the hands and feet. Occasionally, clubbing may be indicative of a nonpulmonary disease, as it can be seen with inflammatory bowel disease, chronic liver disease, and cyanotic congenital heart disease.

Any patient presenting with pulmonary complaints should have a thorough cardiac examination. In addition to the normal areas of attention, one should concentrate on evidence of right-sided heart disease. The presence of a pulsus paradoxus of greater than 10 mmHg often indicates significant obstructive airways disease. Increased neck vein distention, a substernal heave, the murmur of tricuspid insufficiency, or a widely split second sound may all be evidence of cor pulmonale.

Diagnostic Studies

The presence, and often the degree and specific diagnosis of, many common pulmonary diseases can be defined by a few relatively simple laboratory studies. These include spirometry, a measurement of the diffusing capacity for carbon monoxide (DLCO), arterial blood gases, and a chest roentgenogram. A patient who needs more complicated studies will usually require consultation with a pulmonologist or thoracic surgeon.

Simple spirometry is an easy-to-obtain, accurate screening test of lung mechanics. The variables that are usually measured are listed in Table 43-1. Most patients with symptomatic obstructive or restrictive lung disease will have some abnormal spirometric variable. Occasionally, as in the case of asthma, which may be asymptomatic at the time of testing, or early interstitial lung disease, the spirogram may be within normal limits.

The measurement of lung volumes is easy to obtain and an often useful adjunct to simple spirometry. A reduction in one or more of these volumes may point to restrictive or neuromuscular disease or implicate obesity as the cause of the symptoms (see Fig. 43-1).

When asthma is considered and the patient is asymptomatic at the time of testing, one of the many provocative tests meant to induce bronchospasm may be useful. A fall in the expired flow rate after methacholine or histamine inhalation or isocapnic hyperventilation of cold air are sensitive screening tests for hyperactive airways.

Measurement of arterial blood gases can be a good screening study, especially if spirometry is normal. While blood gases may remain normal in the early phases of lung disease, a widened alveolar-arterial gradient for oxygen (O_2) is almost always present in patients with symptomatic disease. O_2 saturation by oximetry may not be a useful substitute for arterial blood gases when the goal is early identification of pulmonary dysfunction. Because of the shape of the oxyhemoglobin dissociation curve, the arterial P_{O_2} must fall into the low seventies before the saturation becomes significantly abnormal, and the O_2 saturation does not provide a measurement of P_{CO_2}.

TABLE 43-1 Spirometric Variables

Variable (units)	Symbol	Change with Disease: Obstructive Disease	Change with Disease: Restrictive Disease
Forced vital capacity (liters)	FVC	D	D
Forced vital capacity in 1 s (liters)	FEV_1	D	D
Forced vital capacity in 1 s/forced vital capacity (%)	$\frac{FEV_1}{FVC}$	D	N
Maximum Midexpiratory flow (liters/s)	MMEF	D	N

Note: D = decreased, N = normal.

An easily obtainable and often useful test in the workup of the patient who complains of exercise intolerance, especially if spirometry and arterial blood gases are normal, is the diffusing capacity for carbon monoxide (DLCO). The DLCO can be looked upon as an index of the integrity of the pulmonary vascular bed. Therefore, it is commonly decreased in the setting of lung-destructive processes such as emphysema and diffuse interstitial diseases, although it is rarely the only abnormal pulmonary function study in these settings. In patients with pulmonary vascular disease, by contrast, it may be the only abnormality found during a routine pulmonary function screening. An isolated reduction of the DLCO that is found in a dyspneic patient with otherwise normal studies should raise the possibility of pulmonary hypertension, embolic disease, or vasculitis. Unfortunately, the sensitivity of the DLCO is not good enough, even with far advanced pulmonary vascular disease, to rule out the diagnosis.

The standard posteroanterior (PA) and left lateral chest roentgenograms should be a routine part of the workup for respiratory complaints. When done correctly, they allow visualization of the air-containing lung, blood vessels, large airways, heart and mediastinum, pleura, lymph nodes, and chest wall. Significant improvement in visualization of the thorax can be obtained with computerized tomography (CT). Recent improvements in technology will allow complete scanning of the chest with a single breathhold and with much less radiation exposure. This spiral CT technique may eventually replace standard roentgenograms as a screening study. High-resolution CT provides a very sensitive view of the lung parenchyma and is rapidly becoming a standard part of the workup of dyspnea that remains unexplained after more routine studies.

When all of the routine tests of lung function are normal, a cardiopulmonary exercise study may be helpful as a way of differentiating organic disease

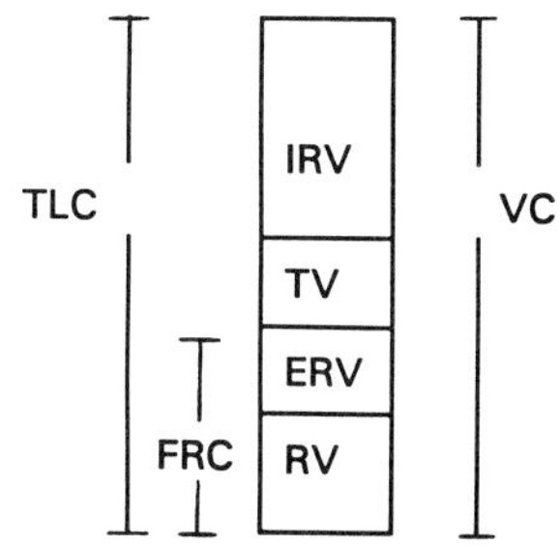

Disease	TLC	VC	FRC	ERV
Obstruction	↑ or N	↓	↑	↑ or N
Restriction	↓	↓	↓	↓
Neuromuscular	↓	↓	N	↑
Obesity	↓ or N	↓ or N	↓ or N	↓

RV = residual volume
TV = tidal volume
TLC = total lung capacity
VC = vital capacity
ERV = expiratory reserve volume
IRV = inspiratory reserve volume
FRC = functional residual capacity

Figure 43-1 Lung volume changes in various categories of lung disease. The characteristic alterations in lung volume can often be used to narrow down the differential diagnosis of a pulmonary abnormality.

from a functional complaint. By combining continuous recordings of heart rate with measurements of expired gas and minute ventilation during a progressive exercise load using a treadmill or exercise bicycle, a clear picture of both cardiac and respiratory response to stress can be assessed. It can differentiate malingering or asthenia from disease as well as separate a cardiac from pulmonary source of limitation.

Obstructive Lung Diseases

A reduction in inspiratory and expiratory flow rates is the characteristic finding in a number of common lung diseases (Table 43-2). Asthma affects as many as 5 to 10 percent of Americans, and chronic obstructive pulmonary disease (COPD) is one of the most common causes of time lost from work.

TABLE 43-2 **Obstructive Lung Diseases**

Asthma
Chronic obstructive pulmonary disease (COPD)
Bronchiectasis
Cystic fibrosis

Upper Airway Obstruction

Upper airway obstruction is a rare clinical entity associated with abnormalities in any anatomical site proximal to the major bronchi, including the nose, pharynx, larynx, and trachea. Patients usually present complaining of difficulty breathing. Important findings on physical examination include stridor, inspiratory and possibly expiratory wheezes, and necessity for use of the accessory muscles of respiration. If left untreated, respiratory failure may ensue with rapid development of cyanosis that is inevitably followed by cardiopulmonary arrest. The more serious abnormalities associated with the development of this clinical entity are shown in Table 43-3. They include pharyngeal infection; glottic obstruction due to a malignancy, foreign body, epiglottitis, or endotracheal intubation trauma; or laryngeal obstruction due to malignancy, connective tissue disorders, or involvement in neurologic disease.

Management depends on the clinical setting. Paradoxical breathing, tachycardia, and cyanosis in the presence of stridor suggest a medical emergency requiring immediate tracheostomy or cricothyrotomy. In a conscious and stable patient, a judicious search for the cause of the upper airway obstruction may be pursued. Heliox, a mixture of helium and

TABLE 43-3 Causes of Upper Airway Obstruction

Disorders of the Pharynx
Enlarged tonsils
Ingestion of corrosive material
Syphilitic gumma
Mucosal destruction
Deep neck infections
Retropharyngeal abscess
Ludwig's angina
Trauma/intubation injury
Foreign bodies
Disorders of the Glottis
Glottic obstruction from foreign body
Angioneurotic edema
Intubation trauma
External neck trauma
Epiglottitis/croup
Disorders of the Larynx
Congenital malformations
Cartilaginous tumors
Relapsing polychondritis
Arthritis of the arytenoid joint
Malignant tumors
Benign tumors
Sarcoidosis
Tuberculosis
Histiocytosis X
Vocal cord paralysis—unilateral or bilateral

oxygen, may have a role in the treatment of non-life-threatening upper airway obstruction because of its decreased density.

Asthma

Asthma is an obstructive lung disease characterized by chronic and persistent inflammation of the airways, manifested by the presence of cellular infiltrates, epithelial disruption, mucosal edema, and mucous plugging. About half of all patients will develop their first symptoms of asthma before the age of five, with many becoming asymptomatic in their late teens. However, most patients who have an apparent resolution of asthma will experience recurrences later in life, and even those who remain relatively symptom-free can often be shown to manifest bronchial hyperreactivity. These "asymptomatic" individuals often develop overt bronchospasm during episodes of infection or inhalation of environmental irritants in the air. The remaining patients with asthma develop their first symptoms as adults, and even some will show no abnormalities until their sixth or seventh decade.

Patients with asthma have episodic wheezing, cough, and shortness of breath due to the widespread narrowing of their airways. Such narrowing varies over time and can be ascribed to both inflammation and bronchospasm. The stimulus for the response is often immunologic in origin, but in many cases, there may be no clear-cut immunologic link with bronchospasm following exercise, cold air exposure, or even emotional stress.

The asthmatic response has been divided into two stages, immediate and late phase. The *immediate response* is due mainly to bronchial smooth muscle contraction initiated by exposure to some immunologic stimulus or irritant. If untreated, the bronchospasm usually goes away on its own after about 30 to 60 min. In about half of patients, with no further stimulus, airway obstruction will occur again after about 4 to 6 h. This *late phase response* is inflammatory in nature and is caused by the recruitment of inflammatory cells and release of mediators in airway walls. The late phase response may last, if untreated, for 24 h or more and makes the airways hyperreactive to a variety of stimuli, in addition to the initial offender—thus perpetrating the attack. A patient with a specific allergy to a single agent, such as pollen, who has developed generalized hyperreactivity might therefore go on to develop bronchospasm and airway inflammation in response to any sort of irritant.

Many different types of asthma have been defined (Table 43-4) based on the clinical presentation or the presumed inciting "trigger." However, there is marked overlap in these groups and since, in general, there is a common approach to treatment, differentiation of these different forms is usually important only if there is an easily identifiable extrinsic factor such as a drug or industrial substance that

TABLE 43-4 Types of Asthma

Classification	Initiating Factors
Extrinsic	IgE-mediated allergens
Intrinsic	?
Adult onset	?
Exercise induced	Change in airway temperature
Aspirin sensitivity or triad (associated with nasal polyps)	Aspirin and other nonsteroidal antiinflammatory drugs
Bronchopulmonary *Aspergillosis*	Airway colonization with *Aspergillus*
Occupational	Toluene diisocyanates (TDI) Cotton dust (byssinosis) Wood dust Animal proteins, etc.

needs to be avoided. In general, a careful identification of all substances the patient is allergic to is unnecessary since attempts at desensitization do not appear to alter the clinical course of the asthma.

The diagnosis of asthma can often be made on the basis of a history of intermittent dyspnea and wheezing in a patient with an underlying allergic diathesis. Occasionally patients will complain only of episodic cough. Pulmonary function studies in symptomatic patients will confirm the presence of airway obstruction that is usually reversible, at least in part, following acute administration of a bronchodilator. In asymptomatic patients, the diagnosis can be made by stimulating the hyperactive airways with methacholine, histamine, or cold air. Alternatively, the patient can be sent home with a peak flowmeter and asked to keep a diary of peak flows throughout the day. Marked variability in peak flow rate is also diagnostic of asthma. If a diagnosis of occupational asthma is suspected, a similar record of peak flow rates in the workplace is helpful.

An attack of asthma can vary in intensity from a mild increase in wheezing that is easily reversible with an inhaled bronchodilator to the development of severe unremitting dyspnea that requires hospitalization (status asthmaticus). Severe asthma usually develops in a patient with increased lability of expired flows that are unresponsive to gradually increasing amounts of medication, although, on occasion, the attack will arise suddenly and without warning. Death from asthma is rare and usually occurs when increasing symptoms are disregarded and the correct therapy not initiated.

The degree of physiologic disturbance can be best monitored by the measurement of expiratory flow rates in the office or emergency room. These indices are helpful in assessing the response to therapy because they provide immediate quantitative estimates of the obstruction and can be repeated at frequent intervals. Arterial blood gases correlate less well with the degree of mechanical impairment, although the presence of significant hypoxemia, especially if accompanied by hypercapnia, suggests severe obstruction and indicates the need for hospitalization. The presence of a significant paradoxical pulse is also an indicator of severe airways obstruction.

During pregnancy, patients with asthma must be carefully observed. About a third of the patients will have worsening of their asthma, in a third the asthma will remain the same, and in a third it will actually improve. Pregnant patients already have some compromise of respiratory function due to incursion of the uterus on thoracic space, and thus development of asthma may have even greater physiologic consequences in the mother as well as the fetus. Hypoxemia and a decrease in cardiac output that may accompany severe airway obstruction may potentially interfere with fetal growth and development. Thus vigorous treatment of the pregnant asthmatic is important.

On rare occasions the symptoms of asthma may be fictitious with airway obstruction produced by abduction of the vocal chords. This syndrome of "pseudoasthma" is probably a hysterical conversion syndrome and is often difficult to diagnose. Patients are typically treated with increasing amounts of medication before the true diagnosis is suspected. It may sometimes be recognized by the presence of stridor instead of true wheezing, and a diagnosis can be made if a reduction of peak inspiratory flow on the flow volume loop is seen during an attack. Speech therapy may be useful as a symptomatic therapy in these patients.

The management of chronic asthma in adults is summarized in Table 43-5.

Chronic Obstructive Pulmonary Disease (COPD)

Normal subjects have a slow decline in pulmonary function with increasing age. Patients with chronic obstructive pulmonary disease (COPD) have an exaggeration of this decline. The progressive decrease in pulmonary function in patients with COPD may also be punctuated by acute exacerbations secondary to infection, the development of heart failure, or poor patient compliance with prescribed medications.

COPD affects middle-aged and older individuals, although, on rare occasions, COPD can be demonstrated in patients by the time they reach their fifth decade. The patients are almost invariably cigarette smokers, although, under rare circumstances, patients with an inherited deficiency of α_1-antiprotease develop obstructive lung disease even in the absence of cigarette smoking.

TABLE 43-5 Management of Chronic Asthma in Adults

Type	Characteristics	Therapy	Medications[a]	Alternatives[a]
Mild	Intermittent, brief symptoms, up to 2 times per week	Inhaled beta-2-agonists, 2 puffs every 3 to 4 h prn for the duration of the episode	Albuterol MDI Metaproterenol 15 MDI Isoetharine 5 mg nebulizer Terbutaline MDI	Pirbuterol MDI Bitolterol MDI Epinephrine MDI
Moderate	Symptoms > 1 to 2 times per week; exacerbations lasting days; exacerbations affecting sleep or activity; requiring ER care	Inhaled beta-2-agonist to qid and anti-inflammatory therapy with inhaled corticosteroids or cromolyn	Triamcinolone 3 to 6 puffs BID Beclomethasone 3 to 6 puffs BID (may be increased to 8 to 10 puffs BID)	Inhaled beta-2-agonist to qid and/or sustained released theophylline; increased inhaled steroid dosage; addition of Cromolyn or Nedocromil
	Increasingly frequent symptoms	Oral corticosteroids followed by inhaled corticosteroids	Oral prednisone or Medrol in 5 or 4 mg increments respectively; inhaled corticosteroids as above	Increase prednisone dose to 40 mg or Medrol dose to 32 mg
Severe	Continuous symptoms, limited level of activity; frequent exacerbations; occasional hospitalization and ER treatment; frequent nocturnal symptoms	Inhaled beta-2-agonist qid and anti-inflammatory therapy with inhaled corticosteroids 5 to 10 puffs BID; extra prn beta-2-agonists for exacerbations and oral corticosteroids, either daily or alternate day use in a single dose	Same as above with the dosages adjusted as suggested; corticosteroids should be a large dose (i.e., 40 mg of prednisone or 32 mg Medrol) and tapered slowly as tolerated on a weekly basis	Same alternatives as suggested above with the additional suggestion of ipratropium bromide MDI, 4 puffs qid

[a]MDI = metered dose inhaler.

SOURCE: Adapted from *Advances in Asthma Care,* 1991, SCP Communications, New York; pp. 11–16.
Executive Summary: Guidelines for the Diagnosis and Management of Asthma, National Asthma Education Program, Expert Panel Report reprinted from the National Asthma Education Program, Office of Prevention, Education, and Control, National Heart, Lung, and Blood Institute, National Institutes of Health, Bethesda, MD, Publication no. 91-3042A, June 1991.

The diagnosis of COPD can usually be made on the basis of a history of cough and sputum production with gradually increasing functional impairment and dyspnea on exertion in a cigarette smoker. The physical examination is consistent with airway obstruction, and pulmonary function studies demonstrate reduced expiratory flow rates, which may or may not respond to an acute trial of bronchodilators. The degree of improvement in flow rates, however, unlike that seen with asthmatics, is usually modest—on the order of 15 to 25 percent.

Arterial hypoxemia is almost inevitable as the disease progresses, and in some patients, hypercapnia may develop as well. Patients who develop significant hypoxemia are prone to the development of pulmonary hypertension and right-sided heart failure, the constellation known as *cor pulmonale.* On occasion these patients may have acceptable oxygenation during the day but develop significant desaturation at night. The finding of cor pulmonale in a patient with good daytime oxygen saturation should lead to a sleep study in order to rule out nocturnal hypoxemia.

Patients with COPD are clinically diverse, depending, in part, on the underlying pathological changes that are present. Almost all patients with significant symptomatic COPD have *emphysema,* which is defined as an abnormal enlargement of the air spaces distal to the terminal bronchials accompanied by destructive changes in the alveolar walls. As with other forms of COPD, the major etiologic factor in the development of emphysema is cigarette smoke, which appears to work by increasing the number of inflammatory cells in the lung, enhancing the release of proteases, and impairing the activity of normally active antiproteases. However, other factors must also be operative since as few as 10 to 15 percent of smokers will develop clinical evidence of emphysema.

The earliest manifestation of COPD appears to be inflammatory changes in the small peripheral airways. These changes are also related to cigarette smoke and are probably the abnormalities most amenable to therapy.

Chronic bronchitis is a chronic inflammatory condition of the large airways characterized by cough and sputum production. As with the other two abnormalities just mentioned, cigarette smoke is the major etiologic factor in the development of chronic bronchitis, although exposure to other pollutants may play a role. While almost all heavy smokers will develop the symptom complex of chronic bronchitis, very few of them—as already mentioned—go on to develop airway obstruction. Therefore, there is a poor correlation between the presence of chronic bronchitis and the development of emphysema or small airways disease.

Bronchiectasis

Bronchiectasis is an abnormal and persistent dilatation of the bronchi due to destructive changes in the elastic and muscular walls of the airway. It may be localized or widespread depending on the underlying etiology and is found as a consequence of a variety of clinical disorders (Table 43-6). Prior to the introduction of antibiotics and immunization for common viral illnesses, infection was the most common cause of bronchiectasis. In underdeveloped countries it is still most commonly seen as a consequence of severe necrotizing lung infection, predominantly gram-negative pneumonia. In the United States bronchiectasis is most commonly associated with other systemic disorders that lead either to reduced immunologic capacity or an abnormality in lung clearance of secretions. Deficiencies in secretory IgA as well as IgG subclasses and infection with HIV are considered potential predisposing factors.

The most common abnormality of lung clearance is *cystic fibrosis,* a generalized disorder of exocrine

TABLE 43-6 Causes of Bronchiectasis

Cystic fibrosis
Hypogammaglobulinemia
Immotile cilia syndrome (Kartagener's syndrome)
Severe bacterial or viral infection
Exposure to corrosive gases
Bronchopulmonary *Aspergillosis*
Unilateral hyperlucent lung (Swyer-James-Macleod syndrome)

gland function, which also impairs clearance of secretions in a variety of other organs. Cystic fibrosis is associated with abnormal chloride transport and is one of the most common genetic disorders, occurring in about 1 in every 200 births in Caucasians. It is inherited in an autosomal recessive pattern, and the abnormal gene is located on the long arm of chromosome number 7. Infertility in men is a common manifestation with approximately 95 percent of all males affected unable to bear children. Females with cystic fibrosis have reduced fertility and the remainder have difficulty conceiving because of the thickness of the cervical mucus.

Immotile cilia syndrome, which may include, in addition to bronchiectasis, situs inversus, nasal polyps, and recurrent sinusitis, is another cause of abnormal lung clearance. It is inherited in an autosomal recessive pattern. This syndrome is noteworthy because of its association with male and female infertility.

The diagnosis of bronchiectasis is suggested by historical evidence of long-standing cough and the production of large quantities of purulent as well as, occasionally, foul and/or bloody sputum, along with the physical findings of persistent crackles over the affected lung zones. With chronic disease, clubbing and cor pulmonale may be seen. A definitive diagnosis is often made on the basis of a chest radiograph, although occasionally high-resolution CT scanning is necessary. A definitive etiology of bronchiectasis requires additional testing, looking for the presence of immunodeficiency, abnormal structure of ciliated cells, or an elevated sweat chloride in the case of cystic fibrosis.

Treatment

For the most part, specific therapy aimed at underlying pathophysiologic abnormalities are unavailable for most patients with obstructive lung diseases. The use of alpha-1-antiprotease replacement in patients who have a hereditary absence of this important antiprotease is now being studied, but its ability to prevent the development of emphysema is unknown. Immunoglobin replacement in patients with immune deficiencies is helpful in reducing the rate of infection. Gene therapy to replace the missing chloride channel, reported to be the defect in cystic fibrosis, is also under intense investigation. The best specific treatment for COPD is smoking cessation. Following cessation of smoking, the rate of decline of pulmonary function in susceptible smokers is reduced to that of a nonsmoker over a period of 3 to 4 years. Counseling by health care professionals along with the use of transdermal nicotine patches and behavioral modification increase the success of cessation attempts.

The main treatment modalities for these patients are directed at amelioration of symptoms and correction of the physiologic consequences of the various disorders that are involved.

Bronchodilators Drugs that can affect smooth muscle tone or decrease bronchial hyperreactivity may be divided into five categories (Table 43-7). The sympathomimetic drugs are the most potent bronchodilators, and the development of non-catecholamine, beta$_2$-specific agents has improved their specificity as well as increased the duration of action to 4 h or more. In general, aerosolization is the preferred route of administration because of the lower total dose required and the rapidly of onset of action. Significant side effects of these drugs are rare, but tolerance may develop with repeated and excessive use. For this reason, present recommendations require that inhaled beta agonists be used intermittently to control the symptoms of bronchospasm.

TABLE 43-7 Drugs That Decrease Bronchial Smooth Muscle Tone and Inflammation

Sympathomimetics
Epinephrine
Beta$_2$-specific agents
Metaproterenol, albuterol, fenoterol, etc.
Anticholinergic Agents
Atropine
Ipratropium bromide
Methylxanthines
Theophylline
Aminophylline
Corticosteroids
Sodium cromoglycate
Nedocromil

There appear to be minimal problems with the use of inhaled beta agonists in pregnant patients, although a higher incidence of pregnancy-induced hypertension was found with frequent use. Since the control of asthma is so important in pregnancy, inhaled beta agonists should be prescribed in the same way as for nonpregnant patients.

Anticholinergic agents were the first clinically available bronchodilators, but their use declined because of concerns about side effects, specifically, decreased lower airway secretions. This is no longer felt to be a problem, and inhaled anticholinergic agents have been shown to be quite effective in the setting of COPD and in selective patients with exacerbations of asthma. The use of the anticholinergic agent ipratropium bromide has markedly reduced anticholinergic side effects since its systemic absorption from the airways is poor. Use of ipratropium bromide in pregnancy has not been associated with a significant increase in adverse fetal outcome.

Methylxanthines, such as theophylline, are less effective bronchodilators than sympathomimetics and anticholinergic agents, but their availability as long-acting oral preparations may be useful when nocturnal symptoms develop because of the loss of activity of the more short acting inhaled bronchodilators. Because of the significant toxicity that may develop from high blood levels of methylxanthine, considerable controversy exists as to their risk/benefit ratio. In general, blood levels of 8 to 10 mg/ml are a reasonable compromise between efficacy and toxicity. In pregnancy, blood levels in the fetus are similar to those in the mother, and theophylline appears in breast milk. For all of these reasons, it is probably best to consider methylxanthine a second-line drug in most patients, and its use in pregnancy should be approached with care and careful monitoring of blood levels.

Corticosteriods are a required part of the treatment of most patients with asthma. With the exception of patients who are only intermittently symptomatic, corticosteroids are usually indicated to reduce the inflammatory phase of the disease and prevent symptoms. They are safest and most effectively used as an inhaled medication. In patients with acute exacerbations of asthma, it is usually necessary to give steroids as oral or occasionally intravenous medications in equivalent dosages of 40 mg of prednisone per day or more. Their early use in acute exacerbations can be an important way of preventing the requirement for hospitalization.

The use of corticosteroids in COPD is more controversial. In one study, corticosteroid therapy for the acute exacerbation of COPD was shown to increase the rate of improvement of airway function, although not the duration of hospitalization. However, this has been disputed by other well-controlled studies. The chronic utilization of corticosteroids for patients with COPD is even more controversial and should be reserved only for those patients who can be shown to demonstrate objectively a significant improvement in airway obstruction when they are prescribed.

Corticosteroid use during pregnancy is also controversial, although there are now numerous reports that have shown successful administration without adverse fetal effects. Because of the complications of persistent asthma during pregnancy, our opinion is that its control with corticosteroids is preferable to continuing symptoms.

Inhaled sodium cromolyn, as well as the newer drug nedocromil, have been shown to prevent bronchospasm in some asthmatics, probably due to the antiinflammatory effect of the medication. These drugs are not helpful, however, in the management of an acute asthmatic attack. Cromolyn has been used in pregnant patients, and although there are no large studies, there is currently no evidence that its use results in adverse effects.

Antibiotics Antibiotics are a mainstay in the therapy of acute exacerbations of bronchiectasis. Antibiotics are less clearly indicated in acute exacerbations of asthma or COPD since bacterial infection is rarely implicated. In patients with bronchiectasis, especially cystic fibrosis, the specific organisms responsible are usually *Staphylococcus aureus* or *Pseudomonas* spp. Antibiotics in these patients should, therefore, be chosen to cover these two organisms. In patients with asthma and COPD, antibiotics should be used when there is other evidence of infection such as the development of fever, an infiltrate that appears on x-ray, or a change in the character or quantity of sputum. In these patients it is usually difficult to identify the specific offending organism, and the empirical use of broad-spectrum antibiotics such as ampicillin, trimethoprim sulfamethoxazole, or erythromycin is appropriate. In patients with underlying obstructive pulmonary disease who have developed pneumonia, the present recommendations for community-acquired pneumonia are the use of the third-generation cephalosporin with or without the addition of a macrolide, depending on underlying clinical circumstances. In pregnant patients penicillin, cephalosporins, and erythromycin (with the exception of erythromycin estolate) are considered safe for use.

Oxygen Significant hypoxemia should always be corrected by oxygen therapy with the goal of maintaining an oxygen saturation of about 90 percent. In patients with chronic obstructive lung disease, especially those who develop hypercarbia with acute exacerbations or who have chronic hypercarbia, the use of even low concentrations of oxygen may lead to an increase in the partial pressure of CO_2 in the blood. This is an expected occurrence and is normally not a problem unless the P_{CO_2} rises progressively or signs of CO_2 narcosis develop.

In patients with COPD, chronic hypoxemia below the level of 60 torr may indicate the need for chronic oxygen therapy. This has been shown to reduce both morbidity and mortality in these patients.

Sleep Disorders

Complaints related to sleep are commonly encountered by the primary care physician because sleep is an important basic need of all human beings. There are many sleep-related disorders (Table 43-8). Those that cause sleep-related breathing disorders include obstructive sleep apnea, periodic breathing, and central sleep apnea. Abnormalities of breathing during sleep may also be seen in other diseases of the respiratory system including alveolar hypoventilation syndromes, respiratory neuromuscular disorders, chest wall abnormalities, and pulmonary diseases like asthma, COPD, cystic fibrosis, and idiopathic pulmonary fibrosis. The clinical consequences of sleep disorders are due to either a change in the quality or quantity of sleep, a change in the structure of sleep, nocturnal hypoxemia, or asphyxia. Their clinical manifestations include recurrent awakenings, unsatisfying or restless sleep, morning headaches, daytime somnolence, personality disorders, intellectual impairment, nocturnal cardiac arrhythmias, the development of pulmonary hypertension or cor pulmonale, polycythemia, or even chronic respiratory failure.

TABLE 43-8 Examples of Sleep-Related Disorders

Insomnia
Narcolepsy
Periodic limb movement disorder
Drug-dependent sleep disorder
Breathing disorders
Obstructive sleep apnea
Periodic breathing
Central sleep apnea
Hypoventilation secondary to neuromuscular, pulmonary, or chest wall disease

Of all the aforementioned disorders, obstructive *sleep apnea* is probably the most important. It occurs during the deep phases of sleep when decreased skeletal muscle tone, combined perhaps with reduced respiratory drive, allows occlusion of the pharyngeal airway. Sleep apnea represents the leading cause of daytime sleepiness and may play a causative role in automobile accidents in this group of patients because of daytime hypersomnolence. Both snoring and obstructive sleep apnea have been identified as risk factors in the development of cardiovascular morbidity.

The diagnosis should be suggested by patient history and clinical manifestations (Table 43-9). Sleep apnea is most common in obese people. Its incidence increases with increasing age and is unusual in women before menopause. Excessive daytime sleepiness is the most common complaint and may significantly limit the ability to perform activities of daily living, even to the point of disability. Snoring is the most common nocturnal symptom and indicates upper airway narrowing during sleep. Nocturnal cardiac arrhythmias are common in these pa-

TABLE 43-9 Clinical Manifestations Suggesting Obstructive Sleep Apnea

Restless sleep
Loud snoring
Daytime sleepiness
Abnormal mentation
Personality changes
Impotence
Morning headaches

tients, as is systemic hypertension. A small but significant percentage of patients with obstructive sleep apnea may go on to develop pulmonary hypertension and eventually cor pulmonale. Patients suspected of sleep apnea should be referred to a certified sleep laboratory for confirmation of the diagnosis.

The management of sleep apnea is guided by the severity of the disease. In mild to moderate cases, patients can be managed by avoidance of alcohol or other agents that depress upper airway muscle activity, by weight reduction, or by medical-surgical correction of nasal narrowing. In severe cases, more aggressive measures like nasal continuous positive airway pressure (CPAP), tracheostomy, or uvulopalatopharyngoplasty (UPPP) may be necessary in addition to supplemental oxygen therapy. Drug therapy has not proven useful.

Restrictive Lung Diseases

The restrictive lung diseases compromise a wide variety of disorders. Their common characteristic is the restrictive ventilatory defect that is seen on pulmonary function testing. The major physiologic abnormality associated with these disorders is a decreased vital capacity (VC) with normal expiratory flow rates. With time, as the underlying disease becomes more severe, all lung volumes will decrease, and the total lung capacity (TLC) will follow the trend started by the VC. Other abnormalities include a reduction in the single breath diffusing capacity (DLCO), chronic hyperventilation, and an increased alveolar-arterial P_{O_2} difference.

Interstitial lung disease is a vast topic and consists of diseases of known etiology, those due to occupational and environmental inhalants, and those of yet unknown causes. They are summarized in Tables 43-10 and 43-11. The scope of this chapter does not permit a discussion of every interstitial lung disease, but a few of "unknown etiology" merit consideration in a little more detail.

TABLE 43-10 Interstitial Lung Diseases of Known Etiology: Occupational and Environmental Inhalants

Inorganic Dusts	Drugs
Silica	Chemotherapeutic agents
Silicates such as asbestos and talc	Busulfan
Asbestos	Bleomycin
Aluminum	Cyclophosphamide
Carbon	Methotrexate
Beryllium	Nitrosoureas (BCNU)
Hard metal dusts	Procarbazine
	Mitomycin
	Antibiotics
Organic Dusts	Nitrofurantoin
	Sulfonamides
Farmer's lung	Penicillin
Bagassosis	Others
Mushroom worker's lung	Diphenylhydantoin
Humidifier lung, air conditioner lung	Drugs inducing lupus-like syndrome
Maple bark stripper's lung	Gold salts
Sequoiosis	Poisons
Bird breeder's lung	Paraquat
	Radiation
	External
Gases, Fumes, Vapors, Aerosols	Inhaled
Gases	
Oxygen	
Sulfur dioxide	
Fumes	
Oxides to zinc, copper, managanese, cadmium, iron, magnesium, nickel, brass, selenium, tin, and antimony	
Vapors	
Mercury	
Thermosetting resins	
Toluene diisocyanate	

SOURCE: From *Am J Med.* 70:542, 1981.

TABLE 43-11 Interstitial Lung Disease of Unknown Etiology

Idiopathic Pulmonary Fibrosis
Chronic interstitial disease associated with the collagen-vascular disorders
Rheumatoid arthritis
Progressive systemic sclerosis
Systemic lupus erythematosus
Polymyositis-dermatomyositis
Sjogren's syndrome
Overlap syndrome
Sarcoidosis
Histiocytosis-X
Goodpaster's syndrome
Idiopathic pulmonary hemosiderosis
Wegener's granulomatosis
Lymphocytic infiltrative disorders
Lymphomatoid granulomatosis
Immunoblastic lymphadenopathy
Vasculitides
Churg-Strauss syndrome
Hypersensitivity angiitis
Overlap
Inherited disorders
Tuberous sclerosis
Neurofibromatosis
Familial pulmonary fibrosis
Ankylosing spondylitis
Diffuse amyloidosis of lung
Chronic eosinophilic pneumonia
Lymphangioleiomyomatosis
Whipple's disease
Weber-Christian disease

SOURCE: From *Am J Med* 70:542, 1981.

Idiopathic Pulmonary Fibrosis (IPF)

Idiopathic pulmonary fibrosis (IPF) is a disorder limited to the lung. Since it has no known cause, its diagnosis is one of exclusion. Hamman and Rich initially described a group of patients who presented with interstitial infiltrates, dyspnea, and cor pulmonale and died within a 6-month period.

The disease as we have come to know it has a more variable clinical course. Patients who present with IPF are usually between 40 and 70 years of age and often exhibit dyspnea on exertion, nonproductive cough, and bibasilar end-inspiratory dry crackles on examination. It is not uncommon to find clubbing of the fingers. The chest roentgenograph commonly reveals a diffuse reticulonodular interstitial infiltrate, although in its late stages honeycombing may be seen. High-resolution chest CT may show peripheral infiltrates with central sparing and may serve to rule out other clinical entities in the differential diagnosis, like asbestosis. Pulmonary function studies reveal characteristic findings of restrictive lung disease with reduced lung volumes and a reduced DLCO. The mean survival is between 4 and 6 years.

The major pathologic abnormality of IPF is an increased amount of fibrous tissue in the alveolar septae or in the intraalveolar tissue in the septae. Depending on the type of idiopathic pulmonary fibrosis, the fibrous tissue may be present in focal parts of the lung or spread out in a diffuse pattern. There are usually increased numbers of inflammatory cells noted in the areas of fibrosis. The two most common clinical variants of IPF are *desquamative interestitial pneumonitis* (DIP) and *usual interstitial pneumonitis* (UIP). These diseases are likely to represent different stages of the same entity, with DIP being the earlier and possibly more treatable disease.

All known causes of interstitial lung disease must first be excluded before a diagnosis of IPF can be accepted. This is best done with a careful history and search for evidence of systemic disease. It may be necessary to perform a lung biopsy to make the diagnosis. Should this be required, open or transthorascopic lung biopsy is the procedure of choice so that a larger tissue specimen may be obtained. Other studies like gallium-67 lung scans or bronchoalveolar lavage (BAL) have not proven useful in the diagnosis or long-term management of IPF.

Corticosteroids are the treatment of choice in an attempt to suppress the inflammatory response and prevent progression to fibrosis. A clinical response is judged by subjective data as well as serial pulmonary function studies and exercise testing. Other immunosuppressive agents have been used to treat

IPF, with cyclophosphamide being the second line of therapy should a second agent be necessary. However, controlled studies have not clearly demonstrated their efficacy in patients unresponsive to corticosteroids. Single lung transplantation has been successfully performed in end-stage patients with IPF.

Sarcoidosis

Sarcoidosis is another disease of unknown etiology. It was first described in the late nineteenth century and was soon recognized as a multisystem granulomatous inflammatory disease. The most common organs involved are the lungs, lymph nodes, skin, eyes, and liver.

Sarcoidosis is found worldwide and is essentially a disease of young people. Seventy percent of the patients with sarcoidosis are under the age of 40 when they first become symptomatic. In the United States, sarcoidosis has a greater incidence in blacks. In the white population it has an equal gender distribution, but in the black population it predominates in females.

The characteristic histologic finding on biopsy is the presence of noncaseating granulomas, which may be found virtually anywhere in the body. Prior to a diagnosis of sarcoidosis, a variety of other diseases that may also be characterized by the presence of granulomas must be excluded, including infections with mycobacteria or fungi, malignancy, mineral dust exposures, brucellosis, hypersensitivity pneumonitis, and Wegener's granulomatosis. This is best accomplished by a thorough history, special staining of biopsied tissue, and immunologic procedures.

Sarcoidosis has many clinical manifestations, depending on which organ system is involved (Table 43-12). The lung is the most common organ involved. Frequently, the patient is asymptomatic, and the diagnosis is suspected from a chest roentgenograph obtained for some other reason. Pulmonary symptoms include dyspnea, with or without exertion, as well as a nonproductive cough and nonspecific chest pains. Laboratory evaluation may reveal hypercalcemia, hypergammaglobulinemia, abnormal liver function studies, or an elevated angiotensin-converting enzyme (ACE) level, although the latter is not specific for sarcoidosis.

TABLE 43-12 Common Manifestations of Sarcoidosis by Organ System

Nervous System	*Cardiac*
Blindness	Arrhythmias
Hypopituitarism	Conduction disturbances
Polyneuropathy	Left ventricular failure
Subacute meningitis	
	Musculoskeletal
Eye	Arthritis, tenosynovitis
Keratoconjunctivitis	Myopathy
Optic neuritis	
Uveitis	*Skin*
	Erythema nodosum
Liver-Spleen	Lupus pernio
Intrahepatic cholestasis	Lymphadenopathy
Splenomegaly	Maculopapular lesions
Upper Respiratory Tract	*Endocrine*
Laryngeal sarcoid	Hypercalcemia
Tracheitis	Diabetes Insipidus
	Panhypopituitarism
Pulmonary	
Interstitial lung disease	*Lymph Node Involvement*
Lymphadenopathy	
Airways obstruction	
Cavitation	

Radiographic manifestations are broken down into stages: Stage 0 has a normal chest roentgenograph. Stage 1 has lymph node enlargement without pulmonary parenchymal disease. Stage 2A has a combination of lymph node and diffuse pulmonary disease; stage 2B shows diffuse pulmonary disease without lymph node enlargement. Finally, stage 3 has radiographic changes indicating pulmonary fibrosis (''honeycombing''). The largest review of sarcoidosis patients suggested a distribution of 8 percent for stage 0, 51 percent for stage 1, 29 percent for stage 2, and 12 percent for stage 3.

When diffuse pulmonary disease is present, it tends to have an upper lobe prevalence. Pulmonary function studies are consistent with a restrictive ventilatory defect showing decreased lung volumes and a reduced DLCO. However, sarcoidosis frequently causes an additional obstructive ventilatory defect ascribable to granulomatous involvement of the airways. When an obstructive defect is present, it suggests a worse overall prognosis.

It is worthwhile to mention briefly some clinical manifestations of sarcoidosis in other organ systems. One common skin lesion associated with sarcoidosis is erythema nodosum. When seen in sarcoidosis, it implies a more benign clinical course. Ocular involvement is common and may present as an anterior or posterior uveitis. Myocardial sarcoidosis has become increasingly important because of its association with sudden death owing to involvement of the conduction system. Central nervous system (CNS) sarcoidosis presents most commonly as aseptic meningitis or a neuropathy and rarely as a space-occupying lesion.

The natural history of sarcoidosis is not predictable, although patients with radiological stage 3 disease or multiple system involvement have a worse prognosis. Unfortunately, there are no conventional tests that can predict its course or prognosis. Serial chest roentgenographs, ACE levels, and GA-67 lung scans have not proven to be useful prognostic tools in long-term prospective trials. Pulmonary function studies are the best test to follow in this illness. The VC correlates best with dyspnea and the response to treatment. Since sarcoidosis is usually self-limited, patients should only be treated if they have significant and symptomatic lung disease or granulomatous involvement of organs like the brain, eye, or heart where the physical presence of granulomas may lead to significant organ dysfunction. Hypercalcemia is another clear indication for treatment.

Corticosteroids are the therapy of choice in sarcoidosis, with dosage guided by symptoms and pulmonary function studies. Despite adequate treatment, a small percentage of patients will continue to deteriorate. Other immunosuppressive agents have been tried in an uncontrolled fashion in patients who fail a trial of corticosteroids, without reproducible success.

TABLE 43-13 Examples of Allergic Extrinsic Alveolitis

Disease or Occupation	Exposure Material	Specific Antigen
Farmer's lung	Moldy hay, grain, silage	Micropolyspora faeni *Thermoactinomyces* spp.
Bird breeders	Bird droppings Dander Feathers	Avian proteins Feathers
Humidifier lung	Forced air ventilation	Amebae *Thermoactinomyces* spp.
Bagassosis	Moldy sugar cane	*Thermoactinomyces sacchari*
Malt workers	Moldy sprouting barley	*Aspergillus clavatus*
Woodworkers	Moldy logs	*Alternaria* spp. *Rhizopus* spp. Saccharomonospora
	Moldy redwood sawdust	*Graphium* spp. *Aureobasidium* spp.
Mushroom workers	Mushroom compost Mushroom spores	*Actinomycetes* (?) *Pleurofus florida*
Rodent handlers	Urine, dander	Rodent protein
Chemical workers	Plastic manufacture	Methyl isocyanate, TDI

Hypersensitivity Pneumonitis

Hypersensitivity pneumonitis results from recurrent exposures and sensitization to organic dusts (Table 43-13). It results in a diffuse mononuclear inflammatory response in the alveoli, bronchioles, and interstitium, which may organize into granulomas and eventually produce fibrosis. The pathological changes are felt to result from the formation of antigen-antibody complexes in the lung.

There are two common modes of presentation. The first is an acute reaction characterized by the abrupt onset of fever, chills, malaise, cough, chest tightness, and wheezing. On examination, crackles are audible in both lungs, and cyanosis may be present. These symptoms usually subside over hours or days. Mild hypoxemia and a restrictive ventilatory defect are found, and the chest roentgenograph shows fleeting, nodular interstitial infiltrates in the lower and midlung fields. Removal from the inciting source usually leads to complete resolution of the problem. The chronic form results from repetitive acute exposures or continued subacute antigen exposure. This type is characterized by irreversible lung damage with pulmonary fibrosis. Symptoms include dyspnea on exertion and hyperventilation, with the eventual development of cor pulmonale and respiratory failure. Pulmonary function studies reveal a mixed obstructive and restrictive defect with a reduced DLCO. Arterial blood gases frequently demonstrate hypoxemia and a widened alveolar-arterial P_{O_2} gradient, while the chest roentgenograph shows progressive fibrotic disease with loss of volume, particularly in the upper lung zones, and no hilar adenopathy. The serum may be tested against known antigens, but a positive study is evidence only of exposure, not active disease.

The therapy for HP is avoidance of exposure to the antigen, since the risk of development of chronic disease increases as the number of acute episodes exceeds five. Corticosteroid treatment is rarely needed but may accelerate recovery and improve gas exchange in symptomatic individuals. The prognosis for recovery from acute episodes is usually excellent.

Connective Tissue Disorders

Connective tissue disorders frequently involve the lung and may manifest themselves roentgenographically as a chronic interstitial pattern that cannot be differentiated from IPF (Table 43-11). In addition to interstitial lung disease, these disorders may affect the respiratory muscles, predispose to infection or aspiration, involve the pleura or pleural space, or present as a pulmonary vasculitis with pulmonary hypertension.

Rheumatoid arthritis While rheumatoid arthritis (RA) has a female predominance, pulmonary disease associated with RA has a male predominance. Diffuse interstitial pneumonitis and fibrosis indistinguishable from IPF may be seen, which can progress to honeycombing. Symptoms are usually dyspnea on exertion and a dry cough. Other pulmonary manifestations of RA include pleurisy with or without effusion, necrobiotic nodules with or without cavities, pulmonary hypertension due to pulmonary vasculitis, Caplan's syndrome (rheumatoid pneumoconiosis), bronchiolitis obliterans with or without organizing pneumonitis, or upper airway obstruction from rheumatic involvement of the arytenoid cartilage.

Progressive systemic sclerosis *Progressive systemic sclerosis* (PSS), or *scleroderma,* is a systemic disease characterized by skin changes, microvascular abnormalities, and esophageal dysfunction. Interstitial pulmonary fibrosis is the most common pulmonary manifestation and has been reported in 14 to 90 percent of all clinical cases. Pulmonary function studies frequently show a restrictive ventilatory defect with a decreased DLCO in spite of a normal chest roentgenograph. A low DLCO in this disease is a predictor of mortality. Progressive asymmetric basal interstitial infiltrates spread upward and in late stages produce honeycombing. D-penicillamine may be useful in treating the interstitial lung disease associated with PSS. Other pulmonary complications described with PSS include pulmonary hypertension from medial hypertrophy of pulmonary arteries, aspiration pneumonitis due to involvement of the esophagus, increased incidence of carcinoma of the lung, and a "pulmonary-renal" syndrome. Pleural involvement due to scleroderma is very rare.

Systemic lupus erythematosus *Systemic lupus erythematosus* (SLE) is a systemic disease of unknown etiology that is characterized by autoimmune damage to tissue. Lung manifestations include pleuritis with or without pleural effusion, atelectasis, diaphragmatic dysfunction with loss of lung volume, alveolar hemorrhage syndrome, secondary pulmonary infections from immunosuppression, acute lupus pneumonitis, and bronchiolitis obliterans with or without organizing pneumonitis. Interstitial lung disease is an uncommon manifestation of this connective tissue disorder. The chronic interstitial pneumonitis, when seen, presents with nonproductive cough, dyspnea, and pleuritic chest pain. Drug-induced SLE, due most commonly to INH, procainamide, and hydralazine, may produce many of the same thoracic manifestations of SLE, although the symptoms are usually mild and reversible when the drug is stopped.

Polymyositis/Dermatomyositis Lung involvement, in the form of interstitial pneumonitis, is seen in about 5 to 10 percent of patients with polymyositis/dermatomyositis (PM/DM). The infiltrates are alveolar and interstitial in nature and start at the bases. Other pulmonary manifestations of PM-DM include hypercapnic respiratory failure secondary to muscle weakness and recurrent aspiration pneumonias.

Sjogren's syndrome *Sjogren's syndrome* (SS) is a systemic disease manifested by xerostomia, recurrent swelling of the parotid glands, and keratoconjunctivitis sicca. This disease had been associated with interstitial lung, clinically indistinguishable from IPF, but histologically it is a lymphocytic interstitial pneumonitis. This lymphocytic pneumonitis is frequently difficult to differentiate from lymphoma or pseudolymphoma.

Lymphangioleiomyomatosis *Lymphangioleiomyomatosis* (LAM) is a devastating disease that affects young women during their reproductive years. Both its etiology and pathogenesis are unknown, but it is felt to be a hormonally related disorder because it is frequently exacerbated by menses and pregnancy. Clinically, it presents with dyspnea on exertion, cough, chest pain usually due to recurrent hemoptysis, unilateral or bilateral chylous pleural effusions, or hemoptysis. Chylous pleural effusions are seen in about 75 percent of cases and hemoptysis in about 50 percent. A chest roentgenograph usually reveals a coarse reticular interstitial pattern but with normal or large-appearing lung volumes. Cystic changes and honeycombing are common findings. On pulmonary function testing, there is evidence of airway obstruction due to obstruction of air flow from smooth muscle bundles in the alveolar walls or a mixed picture of restriction with obstruction. There is almost always a reduction of the DLCO. A diagnosis requires an open lung biopsy, although CT scanning of the chest may be diagnostic if the characteristic thin-walled cystic air spaces that suggest LAM are seen. Treatment including oophorectomy, medroxyprogesterone, tamoxifen, or combination therapy have been attempted in LAM without much success.

Pulmonary Vascular Disease

The pulmonary vascular bed is normally a low-resistance, low-pressure system that receives blood from the right ventricle, predominantly due to the reciprocating change in intrathoracic pressure. The right ventricle, in turn, serves mainly as a capacitance chamber and under normal circumstances is able to generate only relatively low pumping pressure. The maximum pressure that the right ventricle can produce under normal circumstances is a mean pressure of about 40 mmHg. If the resistance in the pulmonary vascular bed goes up acutely, such that higher pressures must be generated by the right ventricle in order to permit forward flow, the right ventricle will fail and cardiac output will drop drastically. If the resistance in the pulmonary vascular bed increases gradually, as it does with chronic diseases, the right ventricle has time to hypertrophy and can eventually generate systemic pressures.

A large variety of conditions and diseases can lead to a rise in pulmonary vascular resistance and thus the development of pulmonary hypertension (Table 43-14). Many of these are discussed elsewhere in this chapter or the book; in this section we will confine our comments to two diseases that are often difficult to diagnose. One of these is relatively common, pulmonary embolic disease, and the other relatively rare, primary pulmonary hypertension.

Pulmonary Embolism

The pulmonary vascular bed acts as a filter for the circulation. Thus, any substance that gets into the venous blood will embolize to the lung. The response to this embolization depends on the composition of the embolic material. Embolization of air or amniotic fluid leads to an alteration in the alveolar capillary membrane and results in a picture typical of the adult respiratory distress syndrome. Talc granules or cotton fibers injected during illicit drug use will lead to slowly progressive inflammatory disease of the pulmonary capillaries and pulmonary hypertension. The consequence of the most commonly embolized material, thromboemboli, depends on the degree and rapidity with which the pulmonary

TABLE 43-14 Causes of Pulmonary Hypertension

Postcapillary pulmonary hypertension (increased venous pressure)
Left ventricular failure
Mitral valve disease
Pulmonary veno occlusive disease
Obliterative or obstructive pulmonary hypertension (loss of pulmonary vessels)
Pulmonary emboli
Primary pulmonary hypertension
Parenchymal lung disease
Vasculitis
Hyperkinetic pulmonary hypertension (increased pulmonary flow)
Atrial and ventricular septal defects
Patent ductus arteriosus
Peripheral arteriovenous shunt
Reactive pulmonary hypertension (vasoconstriction)
High altitude
COPD
Persistent or intermittent hypoventilation
Neuromuscular disease
Sleep apnea

vascular bed is occluded as well as the underlying cardiac status of the patient. The symptoms may vary from mild dyspnea and tachycardia to cardiopulmonary arrest.

More than 80 percent of pulmonary thromboemboli originate in deep veins of the iliofemoral system. Other sources of clot include the inferior vena cava, the right side of the heart and, less commonly, the upper extremities. The diagnosis of deep venous thrombosis (DVT) is a difficult one to make since 50 percent of the patients have neither the signs nor the symptoms of venous occlusion. On the other hand, in patients presenting with the classic findings of thrombophlebitis, pain and swelling in the legs, only 50 percent will be found on objective examination to actually have DVT. While DVT is often underdiagnosed in hospitalized patients, it is also often overdiagnosed in the ambulatory arena, where a clinical misdiagnosis can lead to inappropriate and high-risk therapy. For this reason, a diagnosis of thrombophlebitis should always be confirmed by objective study. For disease in the lower legs, the best techniques are Doppler ultrasound studies or impedance plethysmography. When these are nondiagnostic, a contrast venogram may be required. Ultrasound can also be useful in diagnosing a mural thrombus in the heart and upper extremity clots.

The diagnosis of pulmonary embolic disease can be difficult, especially in the ambulatory population, since the presenting symptoms and signs are both nonspecific and insensitive. About 80 percent of patients will complain of dyspnea, which in a slightly smaller percentage is accompanied by pleuritic chest pain. Hemoptysis is seen in less than 20 to 30 percent of patients with pulmonary emboli. While tachypnea is almost invariable and tachycardia is common, obvious thrombophlebitis, evidence of acute right ventricular strain, or positive findings during auscultation of the heart and lungs are seen in less than 40 percent of cases. However, patients who present without dyspnea, pleuritic chest pain, or tachypnea are unlikely to have acute pulmonary embolism. A low-grade fever is common, but persistent fever with marked leukocytosis is unusual in embolic disease and more likely to suggest pneumonia. Perhaps the most important clue to the presence of pulmonary embolic disease is identification of patients at high risk for a DVT. These conditions are listed in Table 43-15.

A chest x-ray and electrocardiogram (ECG) may be reasonable diagnostic aids in a patient presenting with chest pain and shortness of breath, but both of

TABLE 43-15 Patients at High Risk for Pulmonary Emboli

Prolonged bed rest
Congestive heart failure (CHF)
Malignant tumor
Postsurgery (greater than 30 min of anesthesia)
Lower extremity trauma or surgery
Pregnancy
Abnormal clotting
Antithrombin III, protein S and C deficiencies
Thrombocytosis
Heparin-induced thrombocytopenia
Anticardiolipin antibody

them serve more to rule out other causes of these symptoms than to help make a diagnosis of pulmonary embolic disease. The same thing can be said for the measurement of arterial blood gases. While studies have suggested that a patient with both normal alveolar-arterial P_{O_2} difference and a normal P_{CO_2} has less than a 5 percent chance of having had a pulmonary embolism, no pattern of blood gas abnormality is specific enough to make the diagnosis of embolic disease. Thus, clinical presentation and routine laboratory studies may suggest a diagnosis of pulmonary embolism, but confirmation will require more specific investigation.

The most important diagnostic test is the ventilation-perfusion lung scan. Patients with a normal ventilation-perfusion scan are effectively eliminated from the diagnosis while a high-probability scan, described as the presence of segmental or larger defects on the perfusion scan with normal ventilation, is virtually diagnostic. Any other combination of matched or mismatched defects should be considered an indeterminate scan and requires further diagnostic testing. If the patient is hemodynamically unstable, this test should be a pulmonary angiogram, still considered the gold standard in the diagnosis of pulmonary emboli. In all other cases, the next step is to look for the presence of DVT. Clearly, patients with objective evidence of DVT and an indeterminate scan require no further testing and can be treated for embolic disease. Unfortunately, in as many as 30 to 40 percent of patients with a pulmonary embolism, these studies may be negative because the clot has already embolized. They will require either a pulmonary angiogram or repeated noninvasive testing to look for the development of further clots in the leg. Studies have suggested that in patients suspected of having had a pulmonary embolism, repetitive negative noninvasive tests for DVT preclude the need for anticoagulation since the goal of therapy is the prevention of further clots rather than the treatment of the embolism. A schema for the diagnosis of pulmonary embolism is shown in Fig. 43-2.

The treatment of DVT and pulmonary embolism consists of anticoagulation, initially with intravenous heparin sufficient to prolong the partial thromboplastin time (PTT) to 1.5 to 2 times control values. Once the PTT is therapeutic, warfarin can be started with the goal of prolonging the prothrombin time to 1.3 to 1.5 times control or an international normalized ratio (INR) of 2 to 3. Patients who are hypercoagulable, such as those with anticardiolipin antibodies, require higher levels of anticoagulation. In pregnant patients warfarin should not be used in early pregnancy due to teratogenic effects, and it must be stopped several weeks prior to anticipated delivery due to the fetal risk of intracranial hemorrhage. These patients will therefore require heparin when anticoagulation therapy is utilized during these periods. In addition, for patients who have had serious side effects from warfarin, continued heparinization is required. This can be done on an ambulatory basis using controlled doses of subcutaneous injections.

Most patients require continuing anticoagulation for 3 months. In those patients in whom the risk for embolic disease remains at the end of 3 months or in whom recurrent embolic episodes have been demonstrated, a longer term of antiocagulation will be required.

For most patients, there is no indication for the use of fibrinolytic drugs. Extensive studies have demonstrated that the outcome of patients with pulmonary emboli treated with fibrinolytic drugs is no different from those treated with heparin, although resolution of the clot is faster. Thus, it has become common practice to reserve fibrinolytic therapy for patients with massive embolization and evidence of cardiovascular compromise since fibrinolytic therapy carries a higher risk of hemorrhagic side effects.

The best way to treat thromboembolic disease is to prevent its occurrence. Appropriate prophylaxis of high-risk patients is safe and efficient. Different patients may require different types of prophylaxis, and these are listed in Table 43-16.

Primary Pulmonary Hypertension

Primary pulmonary hypertension is a disease of unknown etiology that can occur in patients at any age

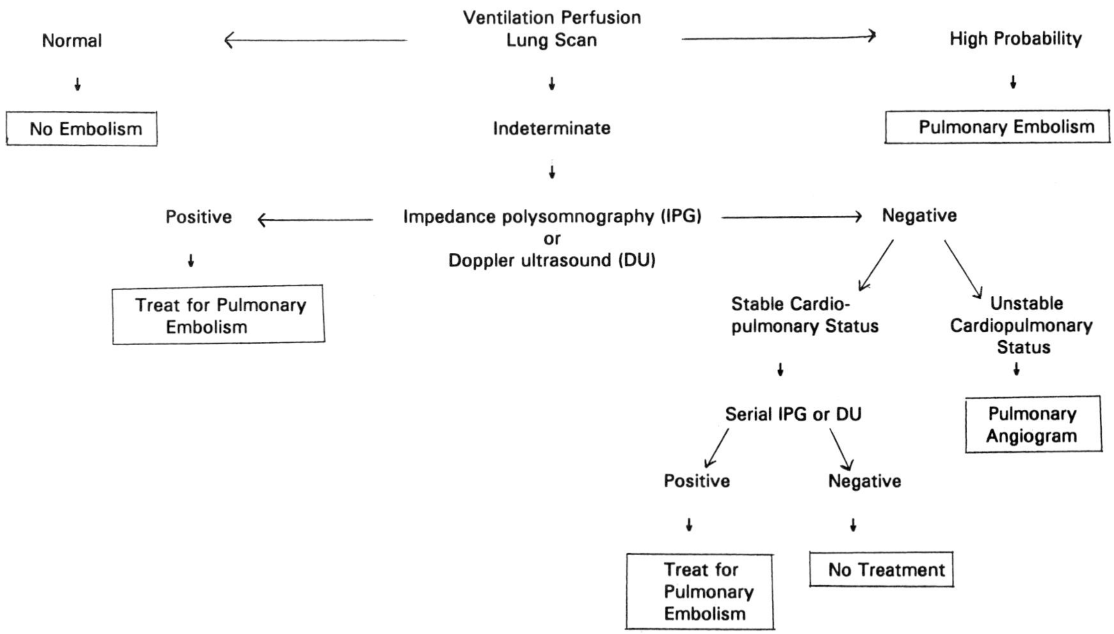

Figure 43-2 Clinically suspected pulmonary embolism.

but is most common in the third and fourth decades. In children there is no gender predominance, but in adults, the female-to-male ratio is about 2 to 1. These patients often present to the physician complaining of vague symptoms of decreased exercise tolerance or shortness of breath. Oftentimes the physical examination is normal, and, not uncommonly, the symptoms are written off initially as functional. In time the patient's complaints will progress, and chest pain, cor pulmonale, and syncope on exertion may develop. By this time the physical examination is often diagnostic of the presence of pulmonary hypertension with the development of a right ventricular heave and tricuspid insufficiency. Once the pulmonary artery pressures get high enough, the diagnosis can often be suspected by an echocardiographic assessment of the right ventricle and an estimate of a right ventricular systolic pressure. It is confirmed by right catheterization and the exclusion of other causes of pulmonary hypertension.

TABLE 43-16 Preventing Deep Venous Thrombosis

Risk Group	Recommendation
Hip or knee surgery	Low-dose warfarin or adjusted dose heparin or low-molecular-weight heparin
Neuro-, ophthalmologic, or urologic surgery	Intermittent pneumatic compression (IPC)
All others	Low-dose heparin or IPC

The prognosis for patients with primary pulmonary hypertension is dismal, with only 20 percent survival 3 years after diagnosis. In about 25 percent of patients, pulmonary vasodilation is possible using either prostacyclin or a calcium channel blocker. Chronic anticoagulation is recommended because low-grade thrombosis and small pulmonary arteritis is thought to contribute to the progressive increase in pulmonary vascular resistance. These treatment approaches, however, should only be thought of as bridges to lung transplantation, the only long-term successful therapy presently available.

Pneumonia

Pneumonia is a common cause of morbidity and mortality in women. While pneumonia can affect anyone at any age, it is more frequent in older patients and those with other comorbid conditions (Table 43-17). The diagnosis of pneumonia is relatively easy to make and confirm, but it is usually difficult or impossible to define the specific pathogen responsible for the infection. Even with extensive testing and careful pathologic follow-up, a clear etiologic diagnosis of pneumonia can be made less than 50 percent of the time. For this reason, the treatment of pneumonia is usually empiric, based on what is known about its epidemiology.

The patient with pneumonia typically has a history of cough with fever and sputum production, which may be accompanied by pleuritic or nonpleuritic chest pain. Occasionally, pneumonia may present with minimal pulmonary symptoms, the patient complaining, instead, of upper abdominal pain or diarrhea. The physical findings of crackles or consolidation on examination of the thorax are typical, although early in the course of pneumonia the physical examination may be entirely normal. Clinical features are rarely useful or reliable in trying to determine the specific etiology, although on occasion the history may be helpful. For example, a travel history to the river valleys of the Midwest or the Central Valleys of California or to Arizona may suggest a fungal disease. Occupational exposure, a recent hospitalization, or a nursing home stay may also raise the specter of an unusual infecting agent.

Once the diagnosis of pneumonia is suspected, a posterior-anterior and lateral chest radiograph should be obtained for confirmation of a pulmonary infiltrate. While the x-ray is rarely specific enough to be diagnostic, occasional findings may be useful in determining the approach to treatment. Obtaining sputum for Gram stain and culture is a common recommendation, although it is rare that either of these procedures will provide useful information leading to the diagnosis of a specific pathogen. Similarly, serologic testing may be useful from an epidemiologic standpoint, but is rarely helpful in the clinical approach to the patient, since both acute and convalescent titers are usually required to define recent infection. From a diagnostic and therapeutic standpoint, the most important considerations are the clinical severity of the illness, the presence or absence of coexistent conditions as stated in Table 43-17, and the presence of advanced age, defined in this context as being older than 65 years.

Once the diagnosis of pneumonia is made, two questions should be considered. The first of these is whether or not the patient is ill enough to require hospitalization. Table 43-18 lists some criteria that may confirm the need for hospitalization. This chap-

TABLE 43-17 Comorbid Conditions Associated with Increased Risk and Poor Outcome of Pneumonia

Chronic obstructive pulmonary disease
Diabetes mellitus
Renal insufficiency
Congestive heart failure
Chronic liver disease
Altered mental status
Postsplenectomy
Alcohol abuse or malnutrition

TABLE 43-18 Decision To Hospitalize a Patient for Pneumonia

Age over 65 y
Comorbid conditions (as defined in Table 43-17)
Physical findings suggesting sepsis or extrapulmonary spread of infection
White blood cell count of less than 4000 or greater than 30,000 or an absolute neutrophil count of less than 1000
Requirement for supplemental oxygenation or mechanical ventilation
Chest radiograph demonstrating multilobar involvement, cavitary disease, or pleural effusion
Significant anemia (a hematocrit less than 30%)

ter will not discuss the in-hospital treatment of pneumonia, which is discussed in Chap. 50.

In those patients who do not require hospitalization, a second question serves to divide the patients based on age and the presence of a comorbid illness. This differentiation will assist in selecting the most likely organism involved and, therefore, define therapy. For patients less than 65 years of age without any comorbid illnesses, the most common organisms, in order of occurrence, are shown in Table 43-19. For patients older than 65 years of age or with one of the comorbid illnesses listed in Table 43-16, a slightly different order of occurrence is found (see Table 43-20). Patients who have been in a nursing home have an increased incidence of methicillin-resistant *S. aureus, Mycobacterium* tuberculosis, and viral pneumonias.

Based on this approach, treatment of pneumonia can be initiated empirically. Our recommendations for women who will be treated for pneumonia on an ambulatory basis are discussed below. For younger patients with no comorbid conditions, treatment is started with either a macrolide or, if the patient is allergic to macrolides, tetracycline. While erythromycin is an effective initial therapy, some of the newer macrolide agents have a broader spectrum and are quickly becoming the initial choice of outpatient management of pneumonia in this group of patients. For older patients or those with comorbid illness, our first choices include a second-generation cephalosporin, trimethoprim-sulfamethoxazole, or a beta lactamase inhibitor combination. In this group of patients, the macrolide is added as a second drug if there is a significant suspicion of *Legionella.*

TABLE 43-19 Common Pathogens in Patients Less Than 60 Years of Age with No Comorbid Illnesses Who Can Be Treated in an Outpatient Setting

Streptococcus pneumoniae
Mycoplasma pneumoniae
Respiratory viruses
Chlamydia pneumoniae
Haemophilus influenza

Miscellaneous Organisms

Legionella species
Staphylococcus aureus
Mycobacterium tuberculosis
Aerobic gram-negative bacilliae

TABLE 43-20 Common Pathogens in Patients Being Treated As Outpatients for Pneumonia Who Are Greater Than 60 Years of Age or Who Have a Comorbid Illness

Streptococcus pneumoniae
Respiratory viruses
Haemophilus influenza
Aerobic gram-negative organisms
Staphylococcus aureus

Miscellaneous

Moraxella catarrhalis
Legionella species
Tuberculosis fungi

Most patients with pneumonia will continue to have fever for 2 to 3 days following therapy. However, if fever persists or symptoms do not begin to show some resolution, repeat evaluation is necessary, and hospitalization should be considered if the patient shows any signs of worsening. A total duration of therapy of 10 to 14 days is usually sufficient. A repeat chest x-ray should be taken probably 4 to 6 weeks following completion of antibiotic therapy. A persistent infiltrate this long after therapy should raise the suspicion of abnormal underlying lung pathology and lead to a more extensive workup. In particular, an obstructing bronchial lesion in patients with a smoking history should be ruled out.

Certain patients who are at high risk for pneumonia should be considered for prophylaxis. In many patients, pneumococcal pneumonia may be preventable by immunization with a polyvalent pneumococcal polysaccharide vaccine. While this has proven to be effective in normal hosts, unfortunately it is not particularly effective in immunocompromised patients. Even in patients with COPD, the efficacy of pneumococcal vaccine has been questioned. Yearly influenza vaccinations should be given to patients at high risk and to all older patients since this decreases the attack rate of influenza as well as the morbidity and mortality due to secondary bacterial pneumonia. Tuberculosis is preventable with prophylactic therapy and this should be provided for all patients who have a positive tuberculin test and an increased risk for reactivation. Indications for prophylaxis in patients with a positive skin test are shown in Table 43-21.

Lung Cancer

Although cardiac disease remains the most frequent cause of death in American women, mortality due to cancer continues to rise. Lung cancer is the most common cause of cancer mortality in both American women and men. In 1992, lung cancer accounted for about 146,000 deaths. All projections for the future suggest that lung cancer mortality will continue to rise. Although it is expected that the rate of lung cancer in men will plateau through the 1990s, it is projected that in women the rate will continue to rise into the early 2000s before a decline and plateau are seen.

Risk Factors

The cause of lung cancer is multifactorial and includes cigarette smoking, occupational exposures, environmental factors, and diet. The most important and most modifiable of these factors is cigarette smoking. Tobacco causes about 90 percent of all lung cancers. The reduction of risk in males parallels the lower rates of male smoking, as the increasing rate in women correlates with their increasing use of cigarettes. Smoking cessation decreases lung cancer risk, but there is a long latency period from cessation to normalization of risk. The risks of lung cancer are increased in cigar and pipe smokers in relation to user inhalation practices. Smokeless tobacco has not been proven to be a risk factor for lung cancer.

Occupational carcinogens have also been identified as causes of human lung cancer. The most important of these are asbestos and radon. Smoking in these cohorts, especially in those with asbestos exposure, serves to augment the carcinogenic potential of such agents. Passive smoke accounts for the major environmental factor. Studies have confirmed that there is an increased risk of lung cancer from passive inhalation of cigarette smoke which is directly proportional to the concentration of smoke in the environment.

TABLE 43-21 Indications for Antituberculosis Chemoprophylaxis in Patient with Positive Tuberculin Skin Test

Recent skin test converters
Patient less than 35 y of age from high endemic area
History of tuberculosis without adequate treatment in the past
Chest roentgenogram consistent with prior tuberculosis
High risk of activation of latent disease
HIV infection
Alcohol and IV drug abuse
Silicosis
Chronic renal failure
Malnutrition
Diabetes mellitus
Immunosuppressive therapy
Malignancy

Classification of Lung Cancer

Bronchogenic carcinoma of the lung is classified by histologic type. It is best divided into small cell carcinoma and non-small cell carcinoma, which includes squamous cell carcinoma, adenocarcinoma, large-cell carcinoma, and adenosquamous carcinoma. The most common cell types are squamous and adenocarcinoma, which account for about 60 percent of all carcinomas of the lung.

Symptoms and Clinical Features of Lung Cancer

At the time of presentation, nearly 90 percent of all patients with lung cancer are symptomatic. Symptoms like dyspnea, hemoptysis, cough, or chest pain may be related to the primary tumor while evidence of hoarseness, dysphagia, and superior vena cava syndrome are usually due to regional spread. Lung cancer not infrequently presents with complaints referable to metastatic spread, particularly to bone or the central nervous system (CNS). Constitutional complaints may be nonspecific such as anorexia, weight loss, weakness and fevers, or they may be a result of paraneoplastic endocrine or metabolic abnormalities. The more common of these paraneoplastic syndromes include Cushing's Syndrome (usually associated with small cell carcinoma), Eaton-Lambert Syndrome (a myasthenia-like syndrome associated with small cell carcinoma), hypercalcemia (due to PTH-like substance and associated with squamous cell carcinoma), and the syndrome of inappropriate ADH secretion.

Initial assessment of the patient suspected of having lung cancer should consist of a complete history and physical examination, with the review of systems focusing on symptoms and signs suggestive of metastatic disease. The most important imaging study is the standard posteroanterior and lateral roentgenogram of the chest. There is considerable overlap in the radiographic abnormalities among the various cell types of bronchogenic carcinoma of the lung. However, central lesions are more characteristic of squamous cell or small cell carcinoma, while peripheral lesions are usually adenocarcinoma, or, if particularly large in size, large cell carcinoma. Other radiologic techniques become more useful in the staging of lung cancer and include computerized tomography (CT) of the chest and brain and nuclear imaging procedures such as bone scanning.

There are two primary modalities for diagnosing the primary lesion in bronchogenic carcinoma: fiberoptic bronchoscopy and percutaneous needle biopsy. The sensitivity of bronchoscopy for central lesions is between 90 and 95 percent. For peripheral tumors of greater than 2 cm diameter, the sensitivity is between 60 and 75 percent, although some investigators have increased the yield significantly with bronchoalveolar lavage. Percutaneous needle biopsy has a greater sensitivity than bronchoscopy for solitary peripheral nodules, especially if the lesions are less than 2 cm. However, there is a significant complication rate of pneumothorax with this procedure (20 to 25 percent), and about 5 percent of these patients may require a chest tube to be placed.

Once a tissue diagnosis is made, the staging process begins. If a CT scan was not obtained as part of the initial diagnostic workup, it is essential in order to assess the mediastinum for adenopathy. If significant adenopathy is present, then either mediastinoscopy or thoracoscopy are required to determine if they are involved. The chest CT should be extended down to the level of the adrenal glands to rule out what is usually asymptomatic involvement of this site.

If the physical examination or routine laboratory studies are suggestive, the search for distant metastases may include an abdominal or a head CT scan. The presence of a pleural effusion itself does not imply metastatic disease unless the cytology is positive.

The most important determinant of survival is the extent of the disease. Seventy-five percent of patients with squamous cell carcinoma die of complications of the thoracic tumor, and only 25 percent demonstrate extrathoracic spread at autopsy. Forty percent of the patients with adenocarcinoma and large cell carcinoma die of intrathoracic complications, whereas 55 percent have evidence of distant metastases. Thirty percent of patients with small cell carcinoma die of local tumor compilations and 70 percent of disseminated carcinomatosis. Approximately 50 percent of patients with small cell carcinoma, adenocarcinoma, or large cell carcinoma have brain metastases at autopsy.

The treatment of non-small cell carcinoma depends on the extent of the disease and the physiologic ability of the patient to withstand lung resection. Surgery is the only curative method available. Patients whose disease is confined to a single lung and its regional lymph nodes and who are physiologically resectable should always be considered for surgery. If the tumor has spread to the chest wall, diaphragm, or pericardium even with ipsilateral mediastinal involvement, patients may be considered surgical candidates with the use of adjuvant or neoadjuvant therapies. Adjuvant or neoadjuvant therapies consist of chemotherapy, radiation therapy, or a combination of the two moieties. Patients with greater involvement or distant metastasis are not curable and may be treated with radiation, chemotherapy, or combination therapy or given only symptomatic treatment.

For small cell carcinoma, combination chemotherapy is the primary treatment of choice. Chest radiation has not been shown to be of benefit in extensive disease but may be of benefit to patients with limited disease in combination with chemotherapy. For those patients with very localized disease, surgery as an adjuvant to aggressive chemotherapy may be beneficial, with 5-year survival rates approaching those seen in stage 1 non-small cell carcinoma. Prophylactic whole brain irradiation has been studied and has not been proven to be of any value in reducing the number of brain metastases found at autopsy.

The Asymptomatic Coin Lesion

The *asymptomatic coin lesion* is defined as a mass up to about 6 cm in diameter. About three-fourths of these patients will be asymptomatic on presentation. Malignant disease is diagnosed in these patients about 50 percent of the time, and the likelihood of malignancy increases as age increases. A lesion greater than 3.5 cm and with a spicular contour suggests a malignant process. The pattern of calcification does not always exclude malignancy, but concentric lamellated rings, for instance, are almost always associated with benign lesions. Stability of the abnormal lesion over time, particularly 2 years or more, is more likely to be associated with a benign course and nature of disease. Unless the lesion can be shown to be stable or the pattern of calcification is clearly benign, the most expeditious approach is to remove the lesion as long as the patient is physiologically able to tolerate surgery.

References and Selected Readings

1. American Thoracic Society: Standards for the diagnosis and treatment of patients with chronic obstructive lung disease (COPD) and asthma. *Am Rev Respir Dir* 136:225–244, 1987.
2. Bone R, Dantzker DR, George R, et al. *Pulmonary and Critical Care Medicine.* St Louis, MO: Mosby; 1993.
3. Bunn PA: Lung cancer. *Semin Oncol* 15:197, 1988.
4. Cannon GW, Zimmerman G: *The Lung in Rheumatic Diseases.* New York: Marcel Dekker, 1990.
5. Cooper JAD: Drug induced pulmonary disease. *Clin Chest Med* 11:1–189, 1990.
6. Glynn TJ, Manley MW: *How to Help Your Patient Stop Smoking: A National Cancer Institute Manual for Physicians.* Bethesda, MD: Department of Health and Human Services, National Institutes of Health, National Cancer Institute, Division of Cancer Prevention and Control, Smoking, Tobacco and Cancer Program 1989; NIH Publication No. 89-3064.
7. Kales A, Vela-Buena A, Kales JD: Sleep disorders: Sleep apnea and narcolepsy. *Ann Intern Med* 106:434–443, 1987.
8. Lieberman J: *Sarcoidosis.* Orlando: Grune & Stratton, 1985.
9. Moser KM. Venous thromboembolism. *Am Rev Respir Dis* 141:235–249, 1990.
10. National Asthma Education Program: *Guidelines for the Diagnosis and Management of Asthma.* Bethesda, MD: U.S. Department of Health and Human Services, National Heart, Lung and Blood Institute 1991; Publication No. 91-3042.
11. Niederman MS, Buss JB, Campbell GD, et al: Guidelines for the initial management of adults with community-acquired pneumonia: Diagnosis, assessment of severity and initial antimicrobial therapy. *Am Rev Respir Dis* 148:1418–1426, 1993.
12. Niederman MS: Pulmonary disease in pregnancy. *Clin Chest Med* 13:555–740, 1992.
13. Occupational and environmental medicine: The internist's role. *Ann Intern Med* 113:974–982, 1990.
14. The PIOPED investigators: Value of ventilation/perfusion scan in pulmonary embolism. *JAMA* 263:2753–2754, 1990.
15. Rich S, Dantzker DR, Ayres SM, et al: Primary pulmonary hypertension: A national prospective study. *Ann Intern Med* 107:216–223, 1987.
16. Schwarz MI, King TE: *Interstitial Lung Disease.* Toronto: Decker, 1988.

44 Renal Disorders

John D. Wagner

Symptomatic Urinary Tract Disease

Urinary Tract Infections

Urinary tract infections (UTIs) are among the most common reasons women seek medical care, with many women experiencing recurrent infections. UTIs are divided into lower tract infections (cystitis/urethritis) and upper tract infections (acute pyelonephritis).

Patients with lower UTIs present with a varying combination of small volume urinary frequency, nocturia, dysuria (''internal'' dysuria), and lower abdominal discomfort. Patients with acute pyelonephritis may have some of these symptoms, as well as flank pain and fever. Depending on the severity of the infection, patients with upper tract infection may have nausea, vomiting, and prostration.

Using laboratory techniques, it is apparent that symptoms do not clearly distinguish the anatomic site of infection in all cases. However, the approach to the patient is usually predicated on the differences discussed above. In examining patients who present with lower tract symptoms, one should confirm the lack of systemic toxicity, fever, or flank tenderness. A urine reagent strip incorporating tests for nitrite and leukocyte esterase is quite reliable in confirming the presence of bacteriuria and/or pyuria in a freshly voided specimen. Another clue to infection is a urine pH greater than 7.5, found when urea-splitting organisms are the causative pathogens.

If symptoms are compelling but the dipstick testing is negative, microscopy can be performed to look for pyuria (more than five white blood cells on a high-power view of a centrifuged sediment). One should be aware that the degree of centrifugation and thickness of the urine sediment under the coverslip are subject to significant variability. Hence, pyuria defined by this technique does not correlate highly to the technique of direct quantification of urinary white cells per microliter. Nonetheless, its simplicity has established it as the conventional standard.

Additional facts worth eliciting from patients with cystitis are whether UTIs have occurred in the past, whether sexual activity seems to precipitate UTIs, whether the patient might be pregnant, whether the patient is aware of any anatomic or functional disorders of the urinary tract, and whether the patient uses a diaphragm. If the patient has no drug allergies, is not pregnant, has not had symptoms for more than 2 days, has no known urinary tract disease, and has had no prior UTIs for 6 months, therapy can be initiated without urine culture if the urinalysis is consistent with UTI. The most common organisms causing UTIs are *Escherichia coli* and other coliform bacteria. Staphylococcus saphrophyticus is another common pathogen in cases of cystitis/urethritis.

The enthusiasm for single dose therapy has waned given the significant number of treatment failures. Three- to five-day courses of oral antibiotics in uncomplicated lower tract disease offer a high cure rate. For patients who are diabetic, have had symptoms longer than 2 days, or who are pregnant, a longer course of therapy might be prudent (7 to 14 days). If not obtained initially, cultures need not be obtained unless the patient's symptoms fail to respond.

The reasons that patients fail to respond include noncompliance with medication, upper tract infection, antibiotic resistance, or incorrect diagnosis. A pelvic exam will exclude some of the other potential diagnoses. These include periurethral inflammation from vaginitis or local lesions such as herpes. The 3-day course of antibiotics chosen for cystitis will not prove effective in the treatment of gonococcal or nongonococcal urethritis. Interstitial cystitis is a noninfectious bladder disorder associated with urinary frequency, nocturia, and suprapubic discomfort as the bladder distends. Hematuria may be the predominant urinary finding, and cystoscopy usually serves to confirm the diagnosis. Occasionally, passage of urinary stones or clots will provoke urinary frequency and dysuria.

The antibiotics used for 3-day therapy include trimethoprim alone, sulfamethoxazole–trimethoprim in combination, cephalosporins (such as cephalexin), nitrofurantoin, fluoroquinolones (ciprofloxacin, norfloxacin, ofloxacin), and amoxicillin–clavulanate. Fluoroquinolones should not be used in pregnancy and sulfa drugs should be avoided late in pregnancy. Given the level of resistant organisms in the community, ampicillin is not recommended unless a sensitive organism is proven by culture. If a urine culture has been done initially or is done because of an initial lack of response, the antibiotics can be adjusted according to sensitivity.

Patients with low-grade temperature or flank pain (presumed pyelonephritis) who do not appear toxic, with good overall health, and who are reliable may also be treated with oral antibiotics. If nausea and vomiting are present, this will not be feasible. Infecting organisms are usually the coliforms responsible for cystitis, and the antibiotics chosen are the same. However, a longer course (14 days) would be prescribed. If the patient worsens on therapy or fails to respond within 3 days, parenteral therapy is advisable.

The laboratory evaluation of the patient with presumed pyelonephritis includes the urinalysis as well as urine culture, hemogram, BUN, creatinine, and glucose. Pregnancy should be excluded if appropriate. Laboratory investigations in excess of the urinalysis yield information that will prove useful should the patient fail to respond as expected to the antibiotic course.

Other disorders that can mimic acute pyelonephritis include perirenal abscess, infected renal cyst (particularly seen in patients with polycystic kidney disease), renal abscesses, nonrenal infections with musculoskeletal back pain and fever, rare presentations of acute glomerulonephritis, renal infarction from thromboembolism or renal vein thrombosis, hemorrhage into a renal cyst, renal colic or obstruction from stones, blood clots, papillary necrosis, or neoplasms. Unusual presentations of lung or intraperitoneal disorders can sometimes suggest acute pyelonephritis.

The issue for the office practitioner is whether treating pyelonephritis as an outpatient is likely to be successful. If the diagnosis is in doubt and/or if the appropriateness of oral therapy is in doubt, then an inpatient approach is preferable. Pyelonephritis can be diagnosed readily when flank pain, fever, lower tract symptoms, and pyuria are present. The urine culture and response to antibiotics will confirm the diagnosis. Some of the other disorders in the differential diagnosis will be apparent from the history and other features of the disease (for example, circulatory congestion in a patient with acute glomerulonephritis).

Patients with lower tract infections, or a single rapidly treatable episode of pyelonephritis, do not need to undergo radiologic or cystoscopic evaluation of the urinary tract unless other symptoms prompt such an investigation. These patients only rarely demonstrate anatomic disorders, and those that are found do not usually lead to a different therapeutic approach. Patients whose UTIs do not readily respond to therapy or perhaps who have had prior episodes of pyelonephritis should undergo imaging studies. If azotemia is present, it might be prudent to begin with a renal ultrasound. Urinary tract infection associated with obstruction requires prompt urological intervention, with stones, congenital abnormalities, or tumors among the causes of such obstruction. Infected renal cysts or renal or perirenal abscesses may require prolonged antibiotic therapy and drainage. Abnormalities of bladder emptying might be uncovered by additional studies.

Patients whose urological evaluation is unrevealing and whose urine cultures are negative may need to undergo evaluation for noninfectious renal parenchymal inflammatory disease (acute glomerulonephritis or interstitial nephritis) or for extrarenal disease producing the patient's symptoms. One might suspect nephritis in patients with evidence of a multiorgan disorder, whose blood tests demonstrate unexplained renal insufficiency, or whose urinalysis reveals red cell casts and proteinuria.

For patients with frequent UTIs, various strategies have been proposed to reduce the recurrence rate. Adjunctive measures include increasing fluid intake, switching from a diaphragm to another method of contraception, and avoidance of fecal contamination of the vagina. Estrogen therapy has been proposed as beneficial in preventing UTIs in postmenopausal women. Patients with recurrent cystitis might be offered the option of self-treatment at the earliest sign of a lower UTI, low-dose prophylaxis on a 3-times weekly schedule, or postcoital prophylaxis. Drugs used for prophylaxis include trimethoprim with or without sulfa.

Urolithiasis

Urolithiasis is another common disorder with clinical manifestations ranging from a patient in agony to one with an incidental finding on x-rays done for another purpose. Urolithiasis may present with colicky flank pain radiating anteriorly to the groin. Stones in the distal ureter may provoke urinary frequency and dysuria. The patient may notice hematuria. Symptoms of infection may coexist with stone symptoms.

Historical clues to the presence of stones include passage of gravel or prior stones; a family history of stone disease; a gouty diathesis in postmenopausal women; coexisting inflammatory bowel disease; or dietary habits favoring intake of large amounts of vitamin C, dairy products, or brewed tea. Failure to maintain adequate hydration (particularly women who exercise heavily or work in hot environments) is also noteworthy. The stone-forming role of high calcium intake in women who are not metabolically predisposed to stone formation is doubtful.

If the patient's pain is intolerable, the diagnosis of urolithiasis is usually made in the emergency department, since the differential diagnosis includes the multitude of causes of an acute abdomen, and the patient requires an expeditious evaluation. If the patient with urolithiasis appears relatively stable, the physician needs to identify whether fever is present, which might indicate complicating infection. Mild costovertebral angle tenderness may be present, but physical findings are usually nonspecific.

A urinalysis will reveal hematuria. The dipstick should suffice as a screen for hematuria, but microscopy is needed to confirm the presence of red cells and to allow a search for crystals. Red cell casts should not be present, and if seen, suggest the diagnosis of glomerulonephritis. Pyuria may be variably present. Concomitant urinary tract infection should be excluded by culture. While cystine crystals are diagnostic of cystinuria, an autosomal recessive disease, uric acid, calcium oxalate, or phosphate crystals may be seen in normal patients. However, marked crystalluria is suggestive of stone disease. Low urine pH favors uric acid stones; high pH favors calcium phosphate stones. A concentrated urine increases the risks of all types of stones.

Blood screening with a blood urea nitrogen (BUN), serum creatinine, potassium, chloride, total CO_2, calcium, and uric acid provides information about whether renal function is normal (obstruction may result in azotemia), and whether metabolic risk factors for stone formation are present (hypercalcemia, hyperuricemia, renal tubular acidosis). The definitive diagnosis of stone disease rests on the patient presenting the physician with the passed stone or on radiologic imaging.

A plain film of the abdomen (KUB) quickly indicates the presence of a calcium-containing stone (most stones fall into that category), while pure uric acid stones are radiolucent. Infection stones (struvite) and cystine are radiodense, but less so than calcium oxalate. In the absence of allergy, azotemia, or pregnancy, an intravenous pyelogram is usually indicated to localize the stones and to exclude obstruction. Ultrasonography and CT scanning also contribute to the evaluation of stone disease, with the former particularly useful in those with azotemia, allergy, or pregnancy in whom radiocontrast or x-rays are undesirable. Patients with elevated serum creatinine levels are at risk of acute renal failure from radiocontrast.

If radiologic imaging confirms stone disease, urologic intervention should be sought for relief of complete obstruction or when stone size greater than 5 mm makes spontaneous passage unlikely. The patient can be instructed to strain her urine. If at all possible, retrieved stones should be sent for analysis. It is helpful to learn what comprises the center of the stone as well as its outer layers.

Oral hydration and analgesic may allow outpatient management, but severe pain prompts hospitalization. Stones which are likely to be uric acid (radiolucent on x-ray) may shrink and pass if the urine is alkalinized. The alkalinizing agent of choice is potassium citrate, although some patients cannot take this drug because of gastrointestinal intolerance or hyperkalemia. Sodium bicarbonate is an alternative alkalinizing agent, but it increases calcium excretion and may predispose to calcium stone formation. If spontaneous passage of the stone is not an option, the present urological techniques of percutaneous stone extraction and lithotripsy allow stone removal with minimal patient morbidity and inconvenience.

While waiting for the stone to pass, the physician is left with the task of delineating the metabolic risk factors for stone formation, an oft-neglected aspect of stone management. Although it is simple to do the testing, one needs to interpret the results with some care. A 24-h collection of urine for volume, pH, sodium, uric acid, and calcium might serve as an initial screening test for patients with known uric acid or calcium stone disease. If a radiologically visualized but chemically unidentified stone is not densely calcified, a qualitative cystine screen can be done as well.

Depending on the results of the initial screen, one may want to measure urinary oxalate, citrate, phosphate, and magnesium as well. For hypercalciuric patients, some would proceed further with urinary testing on calcium restricted diets followed by measurement of calcium excretion after an oral load. This investigation probably lies outside the interests of a primary caregiver. Therapeutic intervention to reduce the risk for stone disease is probably best left to those with specific experience. However, in most patients, encouragement of at least 2 liters of daily water intake spread throughout the course of the day into the evening is appropriate. This will result in the passage of a dilute urine containing lower concentrations of all stone constituents. In general, in normocalcemic hypercalciuric calcium stone formers, thiazide diuretics are usually prescribed to reduce the calcium excretion rate. In uric acid stone formers one attempts to raise the urine pH to 6.5 to 7 by using potassium citrate, sodium citrate, or bicarbonate preparations. Hyperuricosuria can be treated with allopurinol.

Nonstone Causes of Renal Colic

Renal colic can also be produced by the passage of blood clots or sloughed renal papilla. The intravenous pyelogram will demonstrate papillary necrosis or may indicate tumor-associated urinary tract bleeding. Papillary necrosis is seen in patients with severe acute pyelonephritis, sickle cell disease, analgesic abuse, and diabetes mellitus. It is important to recognize when papillary necrosis is associated with infection and obstruction. Such patients require relief of obstruction and antibiotic therapy, presumably in a hospital setting. Identifying clots from a bleeding tumor will prompt a referral to the urologist. Occasionally, the upper tract bleeding site is not evident from the usual radiologic studies. Some of these patients have glomerular renal disease, some have vascular anomalies. Input from a nephrologist may be helpful.

Other causes of renal colic have been mentioned. Bleeding into a renal cyst, particularly in a patient with polycystic kidney disease, may produce flank symptoms, although one would not expect radiation to the groin. An obscure disorder, loin pain hematuria syndrome, manifests with pain and hematuria; its cause is unclear. Variable obstruction from intrinsic or extrinsic lesions of the urinary tract may cause flank pain which waxes and wanes.

Occasionally, patients present with poorly localizing symptoms of urinary tract pain that might be confused with musculoskeletal back pain, irritable bowel disease, or other nonrenal disorders. In the assessment of abdominal, back, or pelvic complaints, one must keep in mind the possibility of renal obstructive lesions. Retroperitoneal disease may result in no discernible abnormalities on urinalysis, and unilateral obstruction may not sufficiently alter renal function to produce a recognized elevation in BUN or creatinine. Occasionally, the renal etiology is inadvertently discovered during x-ray studies designed to elucidate skeletal or gastrointestinal pathology. Inflammatory masses from diverticular disease, Crohn's disease, retroperitoneal fibrosis, or metastatic retroperitoneal deposits are some of the causes of obstructive uropathy. Renal obstruction from gynecologic disorders occurs as well. By maintaining an index of suspicion, one can make the diagnosis of renal obstruction by any of a variety of imaging studies: IVP, ultrasound, CT, or nuclear renography.

Edema

Patients who complain of edema challenge the clinician to distinguish between a variety of ailments. The presence of lower extremity edema that may worsen towards the end of the day is consistent with either local anatomic disease or total body salt and water overload. Local disease may stem from chronic venous insufficiency, arthritic knee effusions, or from more ominous acute phlebitis or neoplastic lymphatic obstruction. Upper extremity, trunk, or facial puffiness should be absent; the legs may be asymmetrically edematous. Recumbency may not eliminate the edema, although the swelling may diminish. The edema of renal disease is generalized, although the total salt and water accumulation may be such that the patient notices only the effect of gravity in inducing lower extremity swelling.

The edema of renal parenchymal disease may be on the basis of intravascular congestion leading to interstitial extravasation of salt and water, or it may be on the basis of the nephrotic syndrome leading to hypoalbuminemia and a redistribution of salt and water to the extravascular space. In either case, renal sodium retention results in a period of positive sodium and water balance. An example of the former mechanism is acute post-Streptococcal glomerulonephritis. Affected patients classically have symptoms and signs of vascular congestion (dyspnea, hypertension, increased jugular venous pressure, pulmonary crackles). An example of the latter mechanism is minimal change disease which induces heavy proteinuria (more than 3.5 g/1.73 m^2 per day) and hypoalbuminemia. Diseases leading to renal failure can provoke edema by diminishing the filtered load of sodium to the renal tubules as the glomerular filtration rate falls. An incomplete ability to balance salt excretion with intake results in a positive sodium balance. The increase in total body salt and water produces edema, vascular congestion, and hypertension.

Both heart and liver failure can activate renal sodium retention. The physician should attempt to elicit historical clues pointing to these disorders in approaching the patient with edema. Stigmata of chronic liver disease and a palpably abnormal liver make the case for cirrhotic edema. Differentiating circulatory congestion on the basis of cardiac failure from renal disease can be difficult on examination, although one should take note of the history and findings of S3 gallops and significant cardiac murmurs.

Certain commonly taken medications can be associated with edema on rare occasions, notably estrogen preparations and nonsteroidal anti-inflammatory agents. An entity known as idiopathic edema or cyclic idiopathic edema is a waxing and waning sodium retentive state described only in females, some of whom took diuretics. In these women who took medication, cessation of diuretic use provoked an exaggerated renal avidity for sodium. In some of the women described, the patients took the diuretic initially not for true edema, but misused the diuretic for purposes of weight reduction.

The diagnosis of edema of a primary renal etiology gains support by the finding of elevated levels of blood urea nitrogen and creatinine, proteinuria of 200 mg/dl or more on a random urine specimen, 24-h protein excretion rates of 2 g or more (3.5 g/1.73 m^2 body surface area in nephrotic syndrome), hypoalbuminemia in association with such proteinuria, and urine sediment activity (red cells with or without white cells and cellular casts). Patients with the nephrotic syndrome classically have hyperlipidemia as well. Further evaluation of such evidence of renal parenchymal disease might benefit from the participation of a nephrologist, who might elect to do a renal biopsy. The differential diagnosis would include primary glomerular diseases, such as minimal change disease and membranous nephropathy, versus systemic diseases affecting the kidneys, such as systemic lupus and diabetes.

Nonspecific Symptoms Related to Electrolyte Disturbances and Azotemia

The symptoms associated with advanced azotemia or electrolyte disorders are numerous and nonspecific. The differential diagnosis and treatment of acute renal failure are presented in Tables 44-1 and 44-2 and of chronic renal failure in Tables 44-3 and 44-4. Blood tests incorporating a BUN, creatinine, sodium, potassium, chloride, and total CO_2 are obtained so commonly that it is probably superfluous to recommend measurement of these values in patients with somatic complaints whose etiology is unclear.

Chronic renal failure may remain asymptomatic until the glomerular filtration rate falls to less than 10 percent of normal. The degree of azotemia found at such low levels of function depends on factors such as the magnitude of dietary protein intake, but a

TABLE 44-1 Etiologies of Acute Renal Failure

Prerenal
Volume depletion
Congestive heart failure
Cirrhosis
NSAID or ACE inhibitor therapy
Renal artery stenosis
Intrinsic Renal Disease
Glomerulonephritis
Drug-induced interstitial nephritis
Acute tubular necrosis (toxin-induced, sepsis, shock)
Embolic disease
Postpartum renal failure
Postrenal
Obstruction secondary to urinary tract, retroperitoneal, or pelvic tumors
Obstruction secondary to urolithiasis
Obstruction secondary to extrinsic inflammatory masses (retroperitoneal fibrosis, abdominal abscesses)
Neurogenic bladder
Congenital obstruction diagnosed in adulthood

TABLE 44-2 Diagnosis and Treatment of Acute Renal Failure Based on Etiology

Prerenal Etiology
If related to volume depletion, restore effective arterial blood volume; hydration
If related to cardiac or liver disease, address primary problem while providing supportive therapy
If medication-induced, discontinue suspect medication
If related to renal artery stenosis, renal revascularization
Intrinsic Renal Disease
If etiology is inflammatory, identify source of the problem by extrarenal manifestations or by renal biopsy in cases of glomerulonephritis
In infected patients, antibiotics
In infected patients, immunosuppressive therapy may be indicated in certain types of nephritis
Discontinue unnecessary medications
Supportive care
Postrenal Etiology
Utilize surgical or interventional radiologic techniques to bypass or eliminate obstruction

TABLE 44-3 Etiologies of Chronic Renal Failure

Systemic Disease Affecting the Kidney
Diabetes mellitus
Hypertension
Systemic lupus
Vasculitis
HIV-associated nephropathy
Renal Parenchymal Disease
Chronic glomerulonephritis with or without specific etiology (focal and segmental glomerulosclerosis, membranous nephropathy)
Polycystic kidney disease
Chronic interstitial nephritis (analgesic abuse, chronic hypercalcemia, idiopathic)
Longstanding renal obstruction

BUN of 100 mg/dl accompanying a serum creatinine of about 8 mg/dl roughly correlates to a glomerular filtration rate (GFR) at which symptoms might develop. Diseases which cause acute renal failure may induce symptoms at lower levels of BUN and creatinine.

Features of advanced azotemia include anorexia, lassitude, weight loss, muscular cramps, hiccupping, pruritus, twitching, headache, nausea, vomiting, chest pain from pericarditis, and bone pain from renal osteodystrophy. If azotemia is moderate (BUN less than 50), and one is uncertain if vague symptoms are likely to be on the basis of uremia, a 24-h urine for creatinine and urea excretion will allow the determination of creatinine and urea clearances. As renal function approaches low levels, the creatinine clearance tends to overestimate the glomerular filtration rate. By averaging the urea and creatinine clearances, one may get a truer picture of the level of function. With clearances less than 15 ml/min per 1.73 m^2, renal failure may account for the symptoms enumerated above although they need not be present. However, because they are nonspecific symptoms, evidence of other possible etiologies should not be overlooked. Patients with symptomatic azotemia need to be referred to a nephrologist as soon as possible so that dialysis can be initiated if necessary.

TABLE 44-4 Treatment of Chronic Renal Failure

- For patients with underlying systemic disease, address systemic disease [e.g., for patients with hypertension, treat hypertension (particularly with ACE inhibitors in diabetics or patients with chronic glomerulonephritis)]
- Protein restriction (patients with glomerular disease)
- Avoid renal insults
- Dialysis or transplantation when uremic

The etiologies of azotemia can be prerenal, intrinsic renal disease, or postrenal (obstructive). The onset of these diseases can be acute or chronic. Prerenal disease may occur secondary to severe dehydration, severe liver disease, or heart failure. Intrinsic renal etiologies which are chronic include sclerosing lesions of the kidney, inflammatory glomerular disease, inflammatory interstitial disease, and small vessel disease. Acute intrinsic renal etiologies include acute tubular necrosis or acute interstitial nephritis. Acute renal failure may be caused by drugs such as antibiotics or non-steroidal antiinflammatory agents, or by radiocontrast. Postrenal etiologies include stone disease, congenital obstructive anomalies, urothelial or extrinsic tumors, and other extrinsic causes of obstruction.

Headache, anorexia, muscular twitching, somnolence, nausea, and vomiting are manifestations of hyponatremia. The degree of symptoms depends on the rapidity with which hyponatremia developed, and the absolute level of serum sodium. It is doubtful that patients with serum sodium levels greater than 130 mEq would be symptomatic from hyponatremia. Symptoms are more likely at values of 125 mEq or less. The primary care physician may wish to investigate those patients with mild asymptomatic hyponatremia before seeking nephrology consultation. However, symptomatic patients should have their hyponatremia attended to quickly.

To evaluate the asymptomatic mildly hyponatremic patient, the physician should confirm the abnormality with a repeat serum sodium, and also obtain a serum and urine osmolality. The volume status of the patient should be assessed. If she is hypovolemic from vomiting, diarrhea, or diuretics, salt and water repletion should correct the disorder.

In patients with euvolemic hyponatremia, the

physician should exclude adrenal and thyroid insufficiency, cirrhosis, and renal failure. A BUN and creatinine will exclude renal insufficiency. Additional laboratory testing can exclude the other diagnoses if necessary. Medications which can cause hyponatremia include thiazide diuretics, certain psychotropic drugs, anticonvulsants, and chemotherapeutic agents. If appropriate, medications can be changed. Certain neoplasms and lung and CNS disorders can yield the syndrome of inappropriate antidiuretic hormone. A thorough history and physical examination should direct any additional investigations for these possibilities.

Hypervolemic hyponatremia is present in patients with edematous disorders: congestive heart failure, cirrhosis, and nephrotic syndrome. Diuretics and fluid restriction may be appropriate therapy.

Although neurologic symptoms may accompany hypernatremia, the water losses that invariably account for this disorder are usually what bring the patient to medical attention. Diarrhea, vomiting, excessive diuretic use, and uncontrolled glycosuria in diabetic patients are the usual causes. Management often requires parenteral fluids in an inpatient setting.

A disturbance in thirst and renal concentration in elderly women may result in varying degrees of hypernatremia. Rarely, central or nephrogenic diabetes mellitus provokes hypernatremia when the urinary losses exceed the ability of the patient to replace fluid orally. These patients have large urine volumes (in excess of 2 liters per day). Investigation of these disorders likely requires inpatient testing and consultation.

Hypo- or hyperkalemia can lead to muscle weakness and arrhythmias, usually with values of potassium less than 3 or greater than 6 mEq/liter. Patients with these symptoms require urgent intervention to normalize potassium levels and will probably be hospitalized. Patients with mild asymptomatic hypokalemia (greater than 3.0 mEq) can be given a potassium supplement while the etiologies of their problem are sought. Diuretic use is the usual cause. Other possibilities include extrarenal losses from diarrhea or vomiting, or renal losses from osmotic diuresis from glycosuria, or from rare endocrine and renal tubular disorders. Urine electrolytes (sodium, potassium, and chloride) will help direct the diagnostic approach. For example, surreptitious vomiting or laxative abuse might be suggested by unexplained hypokalemia accompanied by a low urine chloride.

Certain drugs (potassium-sparing diuretics, angiotensin-converting enzyme inhibitors, nonsteroidal anti-inflammatory agents), renal failure, diabetes or sickle cell induced tubular defects, or renal obstruction are among the causes of hyperkalemia. Potassium levels of 6.0 mEq/liter or more require immediate hospitalization, confirmation, and treatment. Hyperkalemia can be life-threatening although potassium levels are usually greater than 5.5 to 6.0 when cardiac toxicity becomes evident. Hence, patients with hyperkalemia of this magnitude should have an electrocardiogram, in order to discern conduction abnormalities or peaked T waves related to hyperkalemia. Urgent therapies for hyperkalemia with cardiac toxicity include parenteral glucose and insulin, sodium bicarbonate, and calcium therapy with electrocardiograph monitoring in a hospital setting.

Patients with lesser values should be immediately retested and referred if the disorder is confirmed. In the meantime, if prescribed, potassium supplements should be discontinued, and dietary intake of potassium-rich foods curtailed. For elevated but not immediately life-threatening hyperkalemia patients may be treated with sodium polystyrene sulfonate (Kayexalate).

Acid-base disorders in primary care usually present in association with obvious related problems. For example, patients with uncontrolled diabetes may develop ketoacidosis, characterized by polyuria, polydipsia, malaise, and other symptoms. Occasionally, one comes across minor abnormalities in the total CO_2 content of an electrolyte profile. For example, diuretics may induce a mild metabolic alkalosis producing a slightly higher CO_2 value. Pregnancy usually results in a lower value related to a chronic respiratory alkalosis. The differential diagnosis of acid-base disorders is extensive. If the CO_2 consistently deviates from normal by more than 2 mEq/liter, one may wish to have the patient evaluated for a metabolic or respiratory acid-base disturbance of consequence, such as renal tubular acidosis, chronic respiratory alkalosis from heart failure or intrinsic lung disease, chronic hypercapnia from neuromuscular disorders, etc. Of course, pregnancy is normally associated with a low CO_2.

Urinary Frequency

Patients occasionally present with complaints of passing urine frequently. One needs to distinguish between problems of bladder function, and frequent voiding related to the passage of atypical amounts of urine. Nocturia may or may not accompany daytime frequency.

If the urinary concentrating mechanism is intact, and if patients drink less than two liters of fluid a day, urine output should also be less than 2 liters a day. If fluid intake diminishes in the evening, an intact renal concentrating mechanism will increase the urinary concentration such that the average patient should have less urine to pass during the night than during the day. Hence, patients usually do not need to urinate after retiring to sleep. The first voided urine of the morning should reflect urinary concentration (urine specific gravity more than 1.015). The need to pass larger amounts of urine obligates more frequent voiding. If large volumes of urine are passed throughout the 24-h period, nocturia will result.

In evaluating patients with urinary frequency, symptoms suggestive of local bladder problems are usually not difficult to elicit if present. Infection or inflammation, bladder outlet dysfunction, or extrinsic bladder compression may result in small-volume frequent voids, throughout the day and night. Besides the genitourinary exam, urinalysis and urine culture may be helpful. Patients whose symptoms and examination do not clearly point to a lower tract etiology may be experiencing polyuria. A 24-h urine volume should be obtained. The urine should be assayed for osmolality, protein, creatinine, and sodium. If the urinalysis indicates glycosuria or if the patient is diabetic, the 24-h urine can also be used to quantify the glycosuria.

Causes of polyuria include solute diuresis from glycosuria (diabetic patients), or diuretic use, water diuresis from increased fluid intake unrelated to renal disease, or solute diuresis consequent to kidneys that are unable to concentrate maximally to maintain fluid balance. Patients who habitually drink large volumes of fluid may be difficult to separate from those whose obligatory renal salt and water losses drive the thirst mechanism. The latter group of patients includes patients with central or nephrogenic diabetes insipidus. The search for such disorders is prompted by the finding of polyuria (more than 2 liters of urine output per day), particularly if accompanied by hypernatremia (diabetes insipidus patients), hyponatremia (compulsive water drinking patients), or a urine specific gravity less than 1.010 measured on the first voided urine of the day. The patients with urinary frequency without polyuria, infection, or known bladder pathology might be further studied with urodynamics.

Screening and Management of Abnormal Findings

Although urinalysis is one of the most frequently performed laboratory tests, its true value in altering patient outcome when used to screen truly asymptomatic patients is not known. Perhaps up to 18 percent of unselected patients will have abnormalities on reagent strip testing in a general practice setting. The ease with which such testing is done has to be compared with the difficulty in consistently obtaining the complete and accurate histories from patients which would allow one to conclude that a patient is asymptomatic. Hence, it seems reasonable to offer reagent strip testing of urine on a yearly basis, at the time of an examination being performed for other reasons, until it is shown conclusively that false positive results outweigh the benefits.

The reagent strip should include tests for pH, protein, heme pigment, nitrite, and leukocyte esterase. Strip testing of specific gravity is also available if one prefers that to the other techniques of measurement. The sensitivities of the reagent chemicals for the detection of clinically significant hematuria, pyuria, and bacteriuria are high. Microscopy can be reserved for specimens with dipstick abnormalities or for patients with symptoms.

When performing urine microscopy, the specimen examined should be freshly voided in order to preserve formed elements from degradation. Ten milliliters of urine should be centrifuged for 5 min at about 2500 rpm. The sediment should be resuspended in 0.1 ml after pouring out the remaining supernatant, and it is viewed under a coverslip. As one might imagine, the relationship of formed elements per unit volume in unspun urine to that seen per high-power field is quite variable. Despite this imprecision, the number of cells observed by this method forms the basis for determining which patients need further evaluation for hematuria and pyuria.

TABLE 44-5 Evaluation of Hematuria

1. Confirm with microscopy and repeat urinalysis (patient should submit specimen after refraining from exercise and, if feasible, when not febrile).
2. Exclude urinary tract infection with culture if pyuria is present without RBC casts.
3. (a) If RBC casts and/or more than 200 mg/dl protein, check BUN, creatinine, and electrolytes, and 24-h urine protein and creatinine. If new azotemia is present, evaluate quickly for systemic or primary renal inflammatory disease (may require renal biopsy). If patient has stable renal function, order serologic work-up and assess need for biopsy as indicated by history and physical (differential diagnosis may include vasculitis, lupus, post-Streptococcal glomerulonephritis).
   (b) Isolated hematuria without casts or heavy proteinuria: Image kidneys (IVP unless contraindicated). If anatomic or stone disease, evaluate further as indicated.
4. Normal imaging: In young patients obtain 24-h urine for calcium and uric acid. Treat confirmed hyperuricosuria (allopurinol) or hypercalciuria (thiazides) if present to remit hematuria. Obtain hemoglobin electrophoresis in patients at risk for sickle hemoglobinopathy.
5. For other than young women or those with persistent hematuria without other explanation: Cystoscopy
6. If cystoscopy is negative, consider more detailed imaging studies (such as CT, retrograde pyelography, or angiography), urinalysis of family members to exclude familial hematuria syndromes, Tb skin testing, and urine cultures for acid-fast bacilli, and renal biopsy. The order in which one chooses to do any of these studies depends on the history and physical, and one's index of suspicion.

Hematuria (Table 44-5)

Microscopic hematuria, defined as more than three to five red cells on multiple high-power views of centrifuged urine, will cause a positive dipstick reaction. Although, occasionally, ingested substances (such as phenazopyridine) will render a reddish tinge to urine and lead to patient concern, the dipstick should remain negative. If the reagent strip indicates the presence of heme, one needs to perform microscopy in order to confirm that red cells are present. False positive reactions may occur from contamination of urine with the povidone disinfectant solution used to cleanse the meatus for a urine culture.

Myoglobin released from the breakdown of muscle will also cause a positive reaction, but red cells are usually absent (unless there is accompanying renal parenchymal injury). Strenuous muscular activity such as long distance running, occasionally viral illnesses, and use of cocaine or other drugs may provoke rhabdomyolysis. One can confirm myoglobin as the cause of a positive dipstick by getting a urine myoglobin test. If myoglobinuria seems likely, one should also obtain a blood urea nitrogen, serum creatinine, and electrolyte panel. If the patient appears ill, notes a reduced urine output, or manifests azotemia, the patient will need hospitalization.

If red cell casts accompany microscopic or gross hematuria, the patient has renal parenchymal inflammatory disease until proven otherwise. Proteinuria, particularly at a level greater than 200 mg/dl is highly suggestive of renal inflammatory disease as well. In evaluating a patient who presents because of what turns out to be hematuria, one must perform a careful review of systems in search of clues to the possibility of a multisystem disorder. For example, the diagnosis of systemic lupus erythematosus might come to light because of urinary tract manifestations. Careful questioning might reveal the presence of joint, skin, and constitutional symptoms. The physical examination should be particularly thorough, with a focus on how sick the patient appears, whether hypertension or fever is present, and whether the patient manifests salt and water overload.

Laboratory evaluation should include a chemistry profile, and a complete blood count with platelet count. Results should be available in a timely fashion. One should quickly refer patients who appear sick, or who exhibit obvious multisystem disease, or who manifest renal insufficiency. Certain patients will benefit from early renal biopsy and initiation of anti-inflammatory or early immunosuppressive therapy.

If there is doubt as to the source of the urinary tract bleeding, quantification of a 24-h urine for protein is useful in identifying patients in whom glomerular disease is highly likely. More than 2 g proteinuria per 24 h is particularly suggestive of glomerular disease. Definitive diagnosis of a glomerular disease will probably require the input of a nephrologist to decide whether a renal biopsy is necessary. Furthermore, if glomerular disease is excluded, further evaluation of the etiology of hematuria by the nephrologist might be in order.

If red cell casts or heavy proteinuria are not present, then the anatomic site of urinary tract bleeding is unclear. One should exclude urinary tract infection if pyuria is present. Tuberculosis of the urinary tract may manifest as "sterile" pyuria with hematuria, although this is indeed a rare diagnosis. Mycobacterial culture of the urine should be sought if other diagnoses are not forthcoming.

In the absence of pyuria or dysuria, or if the predominant urinary finding is hematuria with or without urinary tract pain, one needs to investigate the gross anatomy of the urinary tract. Persistence of microscopic hematuria should be confirmed with additional specimens.

Neoplastic processes usually occur in middle age, but should be sought in any adult with unexplained hematuria. One should exclude renal insufficiency by chemistry profiling and then proceed to an intravenous pyelogram if not contraindicated by allergy. One may choose to substitute renal ultrasound or CT without intravenous contrast if contraindications to IVP are present (such as allergy or renal insufficiency).

If evaluation of the upper urinary tract is negative, evaluation of the lower tract with cystoscopy and cytology is usually appropriate. The discovery of primary urinary tract neoplasia prompts urologic consultation. If one wishes, the finding of nonobstructive stone disease can be evaluated further before referral as outlined above. Occasionally, one discovers previously unsuspected anatomic abnormalities such as congenital ureteropelvic obstruction or polycystic kidney disease during the course of investigation of hematuria. Anatomic urinary tract disease usually prompts urologic consultation. Polycystic disease, usually inherited as an autosomal dominant disease when diagnosed in adults, may lead to urinary tract infection, pain, hypertension, and renal insufficiency. Nephrologic input in the care of such patients is useful.

Papillary necrosis is another hematuria producing renal disorder most readily identified on intravenous pyelogram. Risk factors include sickle cell disease, diabetes mellitus, analgesic abuse, and obstructive uropathy. Infection and secondary renal obstruction from sloughed renal papillae may complicate the disease and require management. Hence, such patients often do not present with simple asymptomatic hematuria.

Occasionally, one finds patients with hematuria in whom the gross anatomy of the urinary tract appears normal and in whom the evidence for renal inflammatory disease is lacking (that is, urinary casts, heavy proteinuria, and renal insufficiency are not present). Some of these patients have occult glomerular disease such as IgA nephropathy or thin basement membrane disease that can be definitively diagnosed by renal biopsy. Applicable at-risk populations with sickle cell disease or trait can develop microhematuria from renal medullary microinfarcts. Sickle cell screening may be helpful in identifying candidates for this disorder. Hypercalciuria and/or hyperuricosuria without gross calculous disease have also been implicated in causing hematuria. Twenty-four–hour urine testing might suggest such an etiology. Angiography may indicate vascular anomalies as the cause of urinary tract bleeding.

Some of these hematuria producing conditions are not specifically treated and the probability of a yield from extensive evaluation is difficult to predict.

How aggressively to pursue a diagnosis of hematuria is usually decided on a case by case basis. Input from a nephrologist and/or a urologist may be helpful.

Proteinuria (Table 44-6)

Normal urinary protein excretion does not exceed 150 mg/day. The urinary dipstick detects albumin in concentrations from 30 mg/dl to more than 300 mg/dl. Depending on how concentrated the urine is, the dipstick might read up to 100 mg/dl on normal random specimens. In patients without renal pathology, protein excretion can increase with exercise or fever. Certain younger individuals manifest postural proteinuria, whereby the upright position is associated with increased levels of urinary protein. Recumbency returns the protein excretion to the normal range. "Overflow" proteinuria occurs when an increased production of filtered proteins overwhelms the ability of the nephron to prevent their appearance in the excreted urine. This situation occurs in patients with multiple myeloma who excrete light chains. Glomerular proteinuria occurs when the normal glomerular filtration barrier fails to restrain the free passage of serum proteins.

Patients with elevated BUN and/or creatinine, diabetes mellitus, or persistent proteinuria on reagent strip testing of more than 30 mg/dl warrant the collection of a 24-h urine for measurement of protein and creatinine. Dividing the 24-h period into daytime and recumbent collections serves to distinguish nonpathologic postural proteinuria from fixed proteinuria. Patients with orthostatic proteinuria excrete all their urinary protein when in the upright position. Such patients should have periodic assessments including measurement of blood pressure, urinalyses, and 24-h urine protein excretions. One would expect that these patients would remain normotensive, their urine sediments would stay benign, and their protein-excretion pattern would not change. If fixed proteinuria, hypertension, abnormal urinalysis, or azotemia becomes manifest, the patient has either a glomerular, vascular, or interstitial renal disorder. Some of these are related to systemic diseases while others are primary renal disease. Occasionally it is possible to make a definitive diagnosis that will dictate a course of therapy. Therefore nephrologic evaluation will be helpful.

TABLE 44-6 Evaluation of Isolated Proteinuria

1. Urinalysis indicates greater than 100 mg/dl proteinuria on random specimen or patient has any degree of proteinuria associated with azotemia.
2. Check BUN, serum creatinine, glucose, and measure 24-h urine protein, and confirm abnormal excretion. Collect specimen when patient has refrained from exercise, and, if feasible, when patient is not febrile, and does not have decompensated congestive heart failure.
3. Exclude postural proteinuria: divide 24-h collections into ambulatory versus recumbent time periods. If proteinuria is not present during recumbency, reassure patient that she has benign findings.
4. If fixed proteinuria is present and patient is not diabetic, identify abnormal proteins: Obtain urine protein electrophoresis or immunoprotein electrophoresis. If monoclonal gammopathy is present, exclude multiple myeloma, amyloidosis, other dysproteinemias by biopsy of affected organs (such as fat aspirate, bone marrow examination, rectal, or renal biopsy).
5. If less than 2 g proteinuria and no diabetes, hypertension, or azotemia, renal imaging study (such as ultrasound) to look for renal scarring or obstruction, which might give rise to small amounts of proteinuria. If normal, observe patient over time to assess whether proteinuria is increasing, or azotemia is developing. Further investigations might include renal biopsy if proteinuria becomes heavy (membranous nephropathy or focal and segmental glomerulonephritis occasionally evolve in this fashion).
6. If more than 2 g proteinuria and no diabetes, search for other features of the nephrotic syndrome (albumin less than 3.0 mg/dl, hyperlipidemia, lipiduria). Consider renal biopsy (differential diagnosis includes minimal change disease, membranous nephropathy, focal and segmental glomerulosclerosis, amyloidosis, light chain deposition disease).
7. If diabetes mellitus is present, evaluate for the presence of retinopathy. If present, proteinuria is most likely diabetic renal disease. Control blood pressure (use ACE inhibitor unless contraindicated), optimize glycemic control, offer low-protein diet (efficacy is uncertain). If retinopathy is not present, renal disease may still be diabetic, but evaluate as outlined above.

Immunoproteinelectrophoresis of blood and urine identifies those patients with overflow proteinuria related to monoclonal gammopathy and these tests might be obtained in patients with unexplained proteinuria, particularly if unexplained anemia is present. Patients with monoclonal immunoproteins in blood or urine might have multiple myeloma or amyloidosis.

Patients who do not have evidence of systemic disease and who have abnormal urine protein excretion rates less than 2 g/day as their sole urinary abnormality (no red cells, white cells, or cellular casts, no azotemia, no hypertension, no edema) can be followed with periodic surveillance for systemic disease or additional renal disorders (hypertension, edema, azotemia, active urine sediment). An increase of protein excretion into the nephrotic range or the development of additional signs and symptoms should prompt a reevaluation, and renal biopsy may be indicated.

Patients with nephrotic-range proteinuria (3.5 grams protein excretion/1.73 m^2 per day) may or may not have normal renal function, normotension, and an acellular urinary sediment. Most of these patients have some form of primary or secondary glomerular disease. Often these patients are diagnosed with the aid of a renal biopsy. Nephrologic input should be sought for such patients.

Pyuria

Patients who have no urinary tract symptoms may have pyuria. It is important to exclude vaginal contamination of the specimen. Some of these patients have silent bacterial infections; some have interstitial renal disease. Rarely, genitourinary mycobacterial disease presents as ''sterile'' pyuria. Appropriate cultures may elucidate whether infection is the cause of pyuria. One should also obtain a chemistry profile to assess whether azotemia is present. If so, one proceeds to investigate for causes of azotemia as outlined above.

The need to treat asymptomatic bacteriuria unassociated with known urinary tract disorders is unclear. Pregnant women have an increased risk of symptomatic urinary tract infection. These patients should receive antibiotics.

BUN, Creatinine, and Electrolytes

Blood testing of truly asymptomatic nonpregnant women is also an ill-defined area. In the absence of some evidence of possible urinary system disease, the outpatient determination of BUN, creatinine, and electrolytes is not clearly cost effective, but certainly any abnormalities uncovered would be meaningful. It seems reasonable to screen for azotemia or electrolyte disorders in truly asymptomatic women at least once before age 40, and perhaps every few years in women above the age of 40. Women with diseases known to affect the kidney such as systemic lupus or diabetes mellitus obviously need more frequent testing. Women who will need repetitive therapy with medications whose pharmacodynamics would either alter renal function or cause toxicity in the setting of renal disease would also benefit from blood testing. For example, chronic therapy with nonsteroidal anti-inflammatory agents might influence renal function, which should therefore be assessed.

Familial Disorders

Autosomal dominant polycystic kidney disease (ADPKD) is one of the most common genetic disorders in this country, with about 500,000 affected individuals. On average, 50 percent of offspring of an affected parent will inherit the disease. After reviewing the potential benefits of presymptomatic diagnosis versus the drawbacks, one may screen adult children by means of renal ultrasound. The characteristic cysts are demonstrable even before the kidneys are palpably enlarged. Usually, ultrasound criteria for ADPKD are met before the fourth decade, but on rare occasions they are still inconclusive at this point. Renal CT scanning may help resolve matters. If imaging studies fail, genetic linkage studies may be helpful if an aggressive diagnostic strategy is considered warranted.

Women affected by the rare familial hematuria syndromes have variable clinical manifestations. Females carrying the X-linked Alport's gene may exhibit hematuria and proteinuria, and rarely progress to end-stage renal disease. Hearing loss and lenticular abnormalities are apparent in some patients. Benign hematuria syndromes must be distinguished from Alport's syndrome, either by detailed family studies, or by renal biopsy. The screening test for this group of disorders is urinalysis.

Dialysis Patients

There are approximately 66,000 women in the United States on dialysis (1991 data), and their need for routine gynecologic care is no less than that of the population at large. Unfortunately, the overwhelming physical demands made on the dialysis patient may make it difficult for her to seek care outside the dialysis unit setting. Dialysis patients should undergo screening for breast and pelvic gynecologic neoplasms on a schedule similar to nondialysis patients. The incidence of endometrial cancer may be increased fourfold compared to nonuremic patients.

Anovulatory menstrual cycles are common. Evaluation of abnormal bleeding by endovaginal sonography and/or endometrial biopsy may be necessary at appropriate intervals. Once endometrial cancer has been ruled out, one can treat menstrual irregularities with hormonal manipulation similar to patients with normal renal function. Although secondary amenorrhea and infertility are common problems for dialysis patients, in a recent series of 1281 women of childbearing age who were on dialysis, 1.5 percent became pregnant in a 2-year period.

Hyperprolactinemia may accompany advanced renal failure, although levels are usually less than 100 ng/ml. Levels above this warrant investigation. Galactorrhea may result from hyperprolactinemia, but, as in nonuremic subjects, other causes should be sought. Bromocriptine has been used in dialysis patients, but intradialytic hypotension may make this therapy problematic. In postmenopausal women, hypertension may be aggravated by the use of estrogens.

Transplant Patients

There are approximately 20,000 women with functioning renal transplants in the United States (1991 data). Immunosuppressed transplant recipients are at heightened risk for the development of neoplasms. In situ cervical carcinoma has a 14-fold increase in incidence; vulvar and vaginal cancers are 34 times more likely than in the general population.

Infections in renal transplant recipients are a major cause of morbidity. Symptomatic urinary tract infections should be diagnosed and treated. Reactivation of genital herpes occurs and responds to acyclovir.

Fertility returns in women of childbearing age after transplantation. A high percentage of pregnancies which enter mid-trimester end successfully. However, women should enter pregnancy with an understanding of the potential risks to maternal and fetal health. In order to ensure stable graft function and to allow for minimal immunosuppressive dosing, one usually advises that pregnancy not be attempted for a 2-year period after transplant. Absence of hypertension and renal disease (proteinuria, renal insufficiency) is desirable. Preeclampsia occurs more frequently than in patients without renal disease. A variety of neonatal problems have been described including preterm delivery, growth retardation, depressed hemopoiesis, and CMV infections.

Ectopic pregnancy occurs in patients with renal transplants as in other women. Because of the pelvic location of the transplant, symptoms pointing to other pathology may be attributed erroneously to the transplant. One must remain vigilant to all possibilities.

The choice of contraceptive method is difficult for the transplant recipient. Estrogen-containing contraceptives have been used, but they may have effects on immune function, aggravate hypertension, and lead to thromboembolism. Cyclosporine levels need to be monitored because of drug interactions. An intrauterine device in an immunosuppressed host predisposes to chronic pelvic infection, hence an IUD is best avoided.

References and Selected Readings

1. Coe FL, Parker JH, Asplin JR: The pathogenesis and treatment of kidney stones. *N Engl J Med* 327:1141–1152, 1992.
2. Hayslett JP: Pregnancy complicated by renal disorders, in Reece EA, Hobbins JC, Mahoney MJ, Petrie RH (eds): *Medicine of the Fetus and Mother*. Philadelphia, Lippincott, 1992, pp 1086–1096.
3. Hou SH: Frequency and outcome of pregnancy in women on dialysis. *Am J Kidney Dis* 23:60–63, 1994.
4. Jacobson HR, Striker GE, Klahr S, (eds): *The Principles and Practice of Nephrology*. Philadelphia: B.C. Decker, 1991.
5. Kiel DP, Moskowitz MA: The urinalysis: A critical appraisal. *Med Clin North Am* 71:607–624, 1987.
6. Paller MS: Drug-induced nephropathies. *Med Clin North Am* 74:909–917, 1990.
7. Stamm WE, Hooton TM: Current concepts: Management of urinary tract infections in adults. *N Engl J Med* 329:1328–1334, 1993.

45 Gastrointestinal Disorders

Renée L. Young

Abdominal Pain—An Approach to the Differential Diagnosis

History taking remains the most important tool in the evaluation of abdominal pain. Chronic or nonacute abdominal pain is rarely immediately life threatening. Acute abdominal pain, on the other hand, may represent a situation that is an immediate threat to the woman's life. Thus, it is very important to determine the exact duration of the abdominal pain. Distinguishing features of the more important causes of abdominal pain are reviewed below.

Diseases of the Gallbladder, Biliary Tree, and Pancreas

Biliary Colic *History* Biliary colic is usually a steady, midepigastric or right upper quadrant pain that is not crampy, but rather continuous in nature. Biliary colic is more common in the evening or at night, although it is not restricted to these times. This pain is frequently referred to the back at the angle of the right scapula. Nausea and vomiting are associated with biliary colic, especially when it is related to acute cholecystitis or acute pancreatitis.

Physical examination Tenderness at Murphy's point, often accompanied by rebound tenderness and right upper quadrant spasm, is suggestive of biliary colic. Significant negative findings include absence of rectal tenderness, and absence of lower abdominal pain or tenderness.

Diagnostic studies Laboratory findings such as elevated white blood cell count and liver enzymes are suggestive of but not specific for biliary colic. Imaging studies such as ultrasound or radionuclide scanning may be helpful (see under Gallbladder Disease below).

Acute Cholecystitis Right upper quadrant pain that lasts more than 3 to 4 h accompanied by tenderness and rebound in the right upper quadrant, a rising white blood cell count, and ultrasound evidence of thickening of the gallbladder wall, all support the diagnosis of acute cholecystitis rather than biliary colic. Biliary colic usually lasts less than 2 to 3 h; the pain of acute cholecystitis persists longer than this.

Acute Pancreatitis Acute cholecystitis and biliary colic must be distinguished from acute gallstone pancreatitis (see Pancreatitis, p. 491). The most prominent symptoms in acute pancreatitis include nausea, vomiting, and epigastric discomfort which radiates to the back. Physical examination findings usually include diffuse abdominal tenderness, often extending into the lower abdomen. Patients with acute pancreatitis may also have discomfort on rectal examination. Serum levels of amylase and lipase are typically elevated, and ultrasound should depict an edematous pancreas.

Acute Appendicitis

The classic symptom of acute appendicitis is periumbilical pain which moves to the right lower quadrant, usually severe and steady, made worse with moving, especially after the appendix has ruptured. Frequently patients are constipated and anorexic. Exceptions to these classic presentatons of appendicitis include the case of a retrocecal appendix, which is usually associated with diarrhea; and situations in which an inflamed appendix is overlying the ureter, which will give rise to ureteral colic-type pain when appendicitis is present.

Physical findings of right lower quadrant tenderness at McBurney's point with rebound, and rectal tenderness on the right, are the findings most consistent with acute appendicitis.

The white cell count is usually elevated; however, in the immunocompromised patient this will not always be the case. Ultrasonography may reveal the characteristic doughnut, which represents the edematous appendix. An important condition to consider in a granulocytopenic patient with signs of apparent appendicitis during intensive chemotherapy is a typhlitis. In patients with typhlitis, ultrasound will usually show a thickened cecum, and the patient should be treated with IV antibiotics and observation.

Ischemic Bowel Disease

Acute Ischemia Ischemic bowel disease is much more common in older patients, particularly in patients over the age of 60. Classically, the patient gives a history of severe abdominal pain followed by the passage of a large bloody stool. However, the passage of the bloody stool is not essential for this diagnosis, and frequently the abdominal pain is a rather nonspecific pain, which can be diffuse or localized in the right or left lower quadrants.

It is imperative to distinguish ischemic small bowel disease, which is typically occlusive in origin, from ischemic colitis, which is typically nonocclusive. Mesenteric ischemia from occlusive disease can be related to arterial thrombus, embolus, venous thrombosis, or vasculitis. Occlusive ischemia or acute mesenteric ischemia generally present with one or a combination of the following: periumbilical pain out of proportion to tenderness, nausea, vomiting, distention, GI bleeding, or altered bowel habits. Nonocclusive ischemia, ischemic colitis, usually is related to hypotension, heart failure, or arrhythmia. It more frequently presents with severe lower abdominal pain, rectal bleeding, and hypotension.

The most impressive physical finding is the lack of an abnormal physical manifestation in the face of severe abdominal symptoms. The abdomen is soft. Plain abdominal films are helpful and can demonstrate either the absence of intestinal gas or a thickened bowel wall with thumb-printing suggestive of submucosal edema. Computed tomography of the abdomen will also show the edematous bowel wall and can also demonstrate air in the portal vein. Sigmoidoscopy will demonstrate submucosal hemorrhage, friability, and ulcerations, often with sparing of the rectum, in ischemic colitis. Full colonoscopy should not be undertaken in patients suspected of ischemic colitis, because of the risk of perforation. If embolic occlusion is suspected, early arteriography and surgical embolectomy should be considered.

Speed is of the essence when treating occlusive ischemia. Occlusive ischemia will require vascular surgery if reversible; however, when necrotic bowel is found, this requires bowel resection and often leaves the patient with short bowel syndrome. Conservative management with NPO and IV fluids, and correction of hypotension, heart failure, or arrhythmia, is the preferred approach to ischemic colitis.

Chronic Mesenteric Insufficiency "Abdominal angina" which is a dull, crampy, periumbilical pain associated with eating and lasting several hours after eating, is the hallmark of chronic mesenteric insufficiency. Patients typically have lost weight because they are afraid to eat. This type of chronic abdominal pain requires evaluation with mesenteric arteriography for possible bypass graft surgery.

Abdominal Aortic Aneurysm (AAA)

If the physician waits for the typical triad of 1. pulsating abdominal mass, 2. abdominal pain, and 3. hypotension to develop in the patient with an AAA, a good outcome is unlikely. Unfortunately abdominal aneurysms often produce no symptoms at all until they are ruptured. The chances of rupture increase with the size of the aneurysm. If a pulsatile mass in the abdomen is found on physical examination, then further diagnostic studies should be undertaken to evaluate for an aneurysm.

Plain films may show the calcified outline of an aneurysm, but ultrasound is more sensitive and specific. CT scan with contrast is also an excellent tool for diagnosing an aneurysm. Vascular surgeons should be consulted once an aneurysm is detected. Operative excision and replacement graft are indicated for AAA greater than 5 to 6 cm in diameter, as well as for rapidly expanding aneurysms regardless of the size.

Diverticular Disease

Diverticula are herniations or saclike protrusions of the mucosa through the muscularis at the points of nutrient artery penetration. The presence of diverticula is termed diverticulosis. Inflammation of these herniations leads to diverticulitis. Some patients with diverticulosis have recurrent bouts of left lower quadrant pain in the absence of diverticulitis, and this is called painful diverticular disease without diverticulitis. Diverticula tend to increase in incidence with increasing age and tend to be more common in the left colon than in the right colon. They are usually asymptomatic, but in the case of diverticulitis, present with abdominal pain, fever, and altered bowel habits.

Laboratory evaluation when diverticulitis is present reveals a leukocytosis, frequently with an increase in band forms. Although diverticular disease can be diagnosed with barium enema or with colonoscopy, neither one of these tests should be undertaken in the presence of acute diverticulitis since the rate of perforation is high when diverticula are inflamed.

If the patient is known to have diverticular disease, treatment should be started with high-fiber diet and psyllium extract (e.g., Metamucil). For acute diverticulitis, treatment is with antibiotics which cover gram-negative organisms and bowel flora. Depending on the extent of patient illness, these patients may be treated on an ambulatory basis with oral antibiotics. Diverticula can bleed, sometimes profusely. Patients suspected of diverticular hemorrhage should be admitted to the hospital. Complications of diverticulitis include pericolic abscess, perforation, fistula, and stricture.

Irritable Bowel Syndrome

This is a very common diagnosis and is more frequent in women. This syndrome is characterized by altered bowel habits, abdominal pain, and the absence of other detectable organic pathology. It is therefore a diagnosis of exclusion. There are three variants of this syndrome: 1. alternating constipation and diarrhea; 2. spastic colon which presents as chronic abdominal pain with or without constipation; and 3. chronic painless diarrhea. Frequently the patient will present before the age of 30. She may complain of bloating and diffuse abdominal pain, pasty stools, or ribbon or pencil-thin stools. Patients frequently have mucus but no blood in their stools. Since this is a diagnosis of exclusion, other organic pathology needs to be excluded. Further information regarding irritable bowel syndrome can be found in the last section of this chapter.

Intestinal Obstruction

Intestinal obstruction is generally caused by adhesions from a previous operation, but sometimes an incarcerated hernia will be the etiology. Occasionally intestinal obstruction presents in patients who have never had abdominal operations. Malignancy, both intraintestinal and extraintestinal, can cause intestinal obstruction. Occasionally an appendiceal abscess or other intraperitoneal infection will lead to obstruction. Volvulus, a twisting of the intestine (usually cecum or sigmoid), can also account for the problem.

Intestinal obstruction is generally defined as a blockage of the intestine that prevents passage of intestinal contents. When the patient presents with obstruction, this requires hospitalization and surgical evaluation. Intestinal obstruction leads to early dehydration and fluid and electrolyte loss and requires immediate medical attention and resuscitation of the patient.

The exact clinical presentation of the patient will depend upon where the obstruction is located. Higher obstructions, such as in the small intestine, frequently present with early vomiting, whereas obstructions that are more distal, such as in the colon, may present with constipation. The most classic presentation is colicky abdominal pain along with vomiting and scars from a previous operation all suggesting intestinal obstruction. Physical examination of the abdomen could reveal high-pitched abdominal tinkles or rushes. A succussion splash can frequently be heard with small intestinal obstruction; strangulation or bowel necrosis must be suspected when the abdomen becomes tender.

Diagnosis still depends on the characteristic history and physical examination providing the best clues, but abdominal X-rays provide another important diagnostic study. Radiologic films in the standing and supine and left lateral decubitus positions will show air or gas accumulation in the bowel. CT scan of the abdomen may be helpful to look for malignancy. Occasionally endoscopic exams or barium studies are performed to further define the etiology and site of the obstruction.

Management of the intestinal obstruction will depend on the etiology of the obstruction. Generally total obstruction will require surgical intervention, as will many cases of partial obstruction.

The presence of alimentary tract dilation anywhere along its course raises the possibility of obstruction or a functional hypoperistaltic adynamic state. The former is frequently referred to as intestinal obstruction or mechanical obstruction, whereas the latter is referred to as adynamic ileus or ileus. Classically, mechanical obstruction results in bowel dilation due to the accumulation of air and fluid proximal to the point of obstruction, but diminished bowel caliber occurs distal to the point of obstruction with little or no air and fluid present. Often on x-ray films there is a sharp cutoff point below which there is no air or dilation and above which there is a dilated air-filled intestine. Adynamic ileus is often metabolic or toxic in origin in which case it is global in effect, often involving both large and small bowel and resulting in dilation of both colon and small bowel with air fluid levels. Focal areas of ileus may also occur in both small bowel or colon. It is sometimes difficult to determine on x-ray films whether the condition is an obstruction or an ileus. Both conditions, however, require hospitalization, fluid resuscitation, and nasogastric tube decompression. Obstruction will more likely require surgical intervention as well.

Gynecologic Problems

Gynecologic pathology is a common cause of pelvic and, often, abdominal pain. Acute pain may be secondary to an ectopic pregnancy, a ruptured ovarian cyst, torsion of the adnexa, pelvic infection, a tubo-ovarian abscess, or an infarcted myoma. Chronic or subacute pain may be secondary to chronic salpingitis, an adnexal mass, endometriosis, pelvic adhesions, uterine leiomyomata or adenomyosis, or advanced malignancy.

Esophageal Diseases

Gastroesophageal Reflux Disease

Gastroesophageal reflux disease (GERD) is the term used to describe symptoms or damage secondary to reflux of gastric contents into the esophagus. Presentations of GERD vary widely and can be classified into typical symptoms, atypical symptoms, and complications. However, neither the severity of the symptoms nor the pattern can be used to predict the presence or absence of esophagitis.

Typical symptoms of gastroesophageal reflux disease are heartburn and regurgitation. Endoscopic evidence of esophagitis will only be found in approximately 1/3 of patients complaining of these symptoms. An increased frequency of the symptoms of heartburn and regurgitation are very common in pregnant women, and this is thought to be secondary to increased gastric pressure from increased abdominal pressure relating to the pregnancy. Another frequent, but less readily reported, manifestation of reflux in women is "reflux dyspareunia," symptomatic reflux during intercourse.

Some atypical symptoms of gastroesophageal reflux disease include angina-like chest pain, hoarseness, bronchospasm, and hiccups. Chest pain caused by GERD should be evaluated after life-threatening cardiac disease has been ruled out. Chronic hoarseness associated with reflux is secondary to posterior inflammation of the vocal cords. Nocturnal episodes of nonallergic asthma preceded by reflux symptoms is very suggestive of reflux disease. Protracted hiccups have also been reported in reflux patients.

Complications of GERD can also be a presentation of this disease. These complications include erosive or ulcerative esophagitis and dysphagia secondary to peptic strictures. Another complication is the frequent association with metaplasia of the epithelium referred to as Barrett's esophagus. Barrett's esophagus typically appears after chronic untreated reflux disease. Approximately 10 to 20 percent of patients with chronic symptoms of heartburn and regurgitation will already demonstrate changes consistent with Barrett's esophagus at time of initial endoscopy.

The pathophysiology of gastroesophageal reflux disease is a topic of ongoing investigation. The mechanisms that normally prevent damage from gastroesophageal reflux are manifold. The role that a particular defect in these mechanisms plays varies with the individual situation and is not always easily identified. However, knowledge of the mechanisms that are involved in a particular case of GERD will often be helpful in establishing a therapeutic regimen. Reflux disease is generally considered to result from prolonged contact of reflux gastric acid with the esophageal epithelium. Factors that determine reflux injury to the esophagus include both offensive and defensive ones. The principle offensive factor is potency of the refluxate, which is primarily related to its acid and pepsin concentration. Defensive factors consist of a three-tiered system including antireflux barriers, luminal clearance mechanisms, and epithelial resistance.

The anti-reflux mechanisms are not totally protective. Even normal individuals, without evidence of reflux injury, reflux approximately once per hour with increasing episodes following meals. Reflux episodes occur more frequently in patients with reflux esophagitis than in normal individuals. There is a strong correlation between the duration of contact of the acidic gastric contents with the esophagus and the extent of esophageal damage. Intraesophageal pH monitoring has shown the percentage of time below pH 4 is higher in patients with complicated esophagitis.

Mechanisms for esophageal clearance include gravity, but this is only operational in the upright position. Elevation of the head of the bed does not decrease the frequency of reflux events in the recumbent position, but it does reduce the duration of contact of acidic contents with esophageal mucosa. Esophageal peristalsis and saliva are two other factors involved in esophageal acid clearance. Gravity, peristalsis, and secretion of saliva are less operative in the recumbent position; therefore, the potential for acid contact with the epithelium is greatest during sleep.

The esophageal epithelial resistance factors provide another level of defense against the risk by limiting esophageal damage during contact with acid.

The role of hiatus hernia in gastroesophageal reflux disease is debated. Studies in the past have concluded that hiatus hernia does not play a causal role in the production of GERD. However, while only 50 to 60 percent of patients with hiatus hernia have endoscopic evidence of esophagitis, up to 90 percent of patients with esophagitis will have a hiatus hernia, implying that there is a contributing factor. The hiatus hernia may, in fact, impair lower esophageal sphincter (LES) function during straining. Displacement of the LES from the abdomen to the chest leads to mechanical alterations as well. This is an area of ongoing investigation, and there is not yet general agreement about the role that hiatus hernia plays in the pathophysiology of gastroesophageal reflux disease. A simple clinical point to remember is that most people with a hiatus hernia are asymptomatic. If the patient is having symptoms, that patient should be evaluated for gastroesophageal reflux disease.

There is also not general agreement about the role of delayed gastric emptying in gastroesophageal reflux disease; however, the greater gastric residual volumes found in patients with delayed gastric emptying does increase the number of lower esophageal sphincter relaxations, allowing further gastroesophageal reflux to occur.

Gastroesophageal reflux disease is more common in patients with Zollinger-Ellison syndrome because of the overwhelming hypersecretion of acid. The hypersecretory state, however, is not a mechanism in the great majority of patients with GERD.

Scleroderma, more common in the female patient, presents a combined alteration of the clearance mechanisms and of the anti-reflux barrier. Scleroderma patients have fewer reflux events, but the reflux events have significantly longer duration in comparison with patients who have esophagitis of similar severity and no connective tissue disease. Lower esophageal sphincter pressure is reduced and the loss of this LES barrier, along with impairment of esophageal clearance, may result in severe reflux disease.

Initial diagnosis of gastroesophageal reflux disease is made by history. A 24-h esophageal luminal pH recording is the most sensitive test to determine whether or not reflux is present. Endoscopy (esophagogastroduodenoscopy) is sensitive in detecting mucosal changes caused by reflux disease. Esophageal biopsies can be taken at the time of endoscopy; these often detect microscopic esophagitis not seen grossly. Esophageal biopsies should also be taken looking for dysplasia associated with Barrett's esophagus. Although barium swallow can detect esophageal strictures and gross esophagitis, there are frequent false positives for reflux disease, since many people reflux during barium studies and do not have gastroesophageal reflux disease.

Therapy of gastroesophageal reflux disease has multiple tiers. For mild disease, patients can be instructed in weight reduction, sleeping with the head of the bed elevated 30 to 60°, no meals taken for 1 to 2 h before recumbency, and avoidance of smoking, caffeine, alcohol, chocolates, fatty foods, spicy foods, peppermints, and specific foods that cause heartburn. The patient with documented esophagitis or any complications of GERD, will require more intensive medical therapy. Omeprazole, a sodium potassium ATPase protein pump inhibitor, is currently the best medicine available for treatment of esophagitis. This medicine should probably not be given to patients for symptoms of heartburn alone, but rather for those individuals who have documentation of reflux disease with 24 h pH probe and/or endoscopy. Acid suppression can also be obtained with the H_2 receptor antagonist, which can also be used for maintenance treatment of gastroesophageal reflux disease. A pro-kinetic agent, such as cisapride or metoclopramide, frequently needs to be added for patients with esophagitis or other complications of GERD. Cisapride is currently being marketed for maintenance treatment of gastroesophageal reflux disease without an accompanying drug such as an H_2 antagonist or omeprazole.

Other therapy to be considered for gastroesophageal reflux disease would be surgical therapy, including Nissen fundoplication. Currently this procedure is available to some patients laparoscopically. The decision regarding whether to proceed to surgical intervention should be considered carefully, putting into perspective such factors as severity of the disease, underlying medical condition, and the effect of long-term medication versus surgical intervention. Esophageal strictures related to GERD will need to be dilated.

Other Forms of Esophagitis

Not all forms of esophagitis are related to gastroesophageal reflux disease. Pill-related esophagitis can be caused by any medication; however, the most commonly offending agents include doxycycline, tetracycline, aspirin, nonsteroidal anti-inflammatory drugs, potassium chloride, quinidine, ferrous sulfate, and clindamycin. Pill-esophagitis is more commonly seen in patients who take pills with small sips of water, who recline after swallowing their pill, and in individuals with anatomic defects such as an enlarged left atrium or ectatic aorta which impinges on the esophagus and causes the pills to ''hang up'' in these areas. Pill-related esophagitis is usually diagnosed endoscopically. The primary treatment is withdrawing the offending drug and providing acid suppression with H_2 receptor antagonist, omeprazole or antacids. If this is a recurrent problem, it predisposes the patient to strictures, and if strictures are present, they need to be dilated.

Immunocompromised patients, such as patients with AIDS, are predisposed to develop other forms of esophagitis. Patients with malignancy, diabetes, hypoparathyroidism, hemoglobinopathies, systemic lupus erythematosus, and corrosive esophageal injury are also predisposed to develop infectious etiologies of esophagitis. These include both herpes esophagitis and candida esophagitis. Esophagitis can also be caused by cytomegalovirus and varicella zoster virus as well as herpes virus I or II. These patients can present with dysphagia, odynophagia, fevers, bleeding, and oral thrush (particularly in candida esophagitis). Diagnosis is generally by endoscopy with brushings for cytology or culture and/or biopsies for culture.

Herpes and varicella esophagitis are treated with acyclovir. CMV is treated with ganciclovir. Candida esophagitis can be treated with oral nystatin or clotrimazole, ketoconazole, or amphotericin, depending on the severity of the disease.

Peptic Ulcer Disease

Ulcerations most commonly occur in the duodenal bulb (duodenal ulcer) and stomach (gastric ulcer). However, peptic ulcer disease (PUD) may also occur in the esophagus, pyloric channel, distal to the duodenal bulb in the second or third portions of the duodenum, in the jejunum, or in relation to a Meckel's diverticulum. The precise mechanisms underlying ulcerogenesis are still debated, but simply stated, it results from an imbalance between ''aggressive'' factors (gastric acid, pepsin) and ''defense'' factors involved in mucosal resistance (gastric mucus, bicarbonate, microcirculation, prostaglandins, and the mucosal barrier).

There are numerous risk factors and associations with PUD: heredity, smoking, gastrinoma (Zollinger-Ellison syndrome), hypercalcemia (hyperparathyroidism), and mastocytosis. The prevalence of peptic ulcers has shifted from male predominance to comparable prevalence in both sexes. These changing trends in ulcer occurrence reflect declining rates in young men and increasing rates in older women.

Most recently, *Helicobacter pylori,* a spiral urease-producing organism that colonizes gastric antral mucosa in 90 to 100 percent of persons with duodenal ulcers and 70 to 80 percent of those with gastric ulcers has been implicated in the pathophysiology of those ulcers that are not associated with nonsteroidal anti-inflammatory drugs (NSAIDs). This organism is also found in normal individuals with increasing prevalence with increasing age. Its exact role in ulcer pathogenesis is controversial but recent literature strongly supports treatment for *H. pylori* in cases of documented peptic ulcer disease.

Nonsteroidal anti-inflammatory drug use also predisposes to PUD. Rheumatoid arthritis and degenerative joint disease predominate in women. Women with these arthritic conditions frequently develop PUD from NSAID use. Chronic salicylate or NSAID use may account for over 30 percent of gastric ulcers and is associated with an increased risk of bleeding and perforation.

The hallmark of PUD is burning, gnawing epigastric discomfort. This presentation is common in both gastric and duodenal ulcers, although the pattern can differ in each case. The classic presentation of a duodenal ulcer is that of periodic gnawing epigastric discomfort with onset 1 to 2 h after eating, usually relieved by food or antacids. Nighttime pain is common, often occurring between midnight and 4:00 A.M. Pain may also be relieved with vomiting. On the other hand, the classic presentation of a gastric ulcer is persistent epigastric pain not relieved by food, antacids, or vomiting. In fact, food frequently exacerbates the abdominal discomfort; as a consequence patients tend to lose weight.

Upper gastrointestinal hemorrhage is a less frequent but important presentation of PUD. Ten percent of duodenal ulcer patients present with bleeding without a prior history of ulcer pain. Bleeding is an especially common presentation of PUD in the elderly. Among patients with nonsteroidal anti-inflammatory drug-related ulcerations, abdominal discomfort may be minimized by the analgesic properties of the NSAID. Ulcer bleeding may present as hematemesis, melena, or if low-grade the sole manifestation may be either iron deficiency or a hematest-positive stool.

Other presentations of PUD besides pain and bleeding include gastric outlet obstruction, perforation, or penetration causing acute pancreatitis, the latter as a consequence of penetration through to the pancreas.

The diagnosis of PUD can be made either by upper gastrointestinal endoscopy or upper GI barium examination. In the past, the standard diagnostic tool for PUD was the upper GI barium study. More recently endoscopy has become an effective and commonly used tool. Endoscopy is particularly accurate and superior to the barium examination in detecting diffuse mucosal abnormaliteis such as gastritis. It is preferable to barium studies for diagnosis of gastric ulcers since endoscopy has the added benefit of allowing a biopsy to be obtained. Gastric ulcers may be malignant and therefore should always be biopsied.

The primary objectives of treatment of PUD are to relieve symptoms and heal the ulcer. Gastric ulcers need to be followed endoscopically with biopsies until healed. The previous use of dietary restrictions for treatment of PUD is unnecessary given the drugs now available. Nonsteroidal anti-inflammatory drugs should be stopped to promote healing, and smoking should be curtailed as it also prevents healing. H_2 antagonists (such as cimetidine, ranitidine, famotidine, or nizatidine) are the most widely used medications for healing PUD. Antacids are also effective in healing peptic ulcers; however, they need to be taken frequently and this decreases patient compliance. Omeprazole, the sodium potassium ATPase pump inhibitor, is the most powerful acid suppressant available and can be used to heal PUD.

Eradication of *H. pylori* from the stomach decreases the subsequent ulcer relapse rate. If *H. pylori* has been documented, then drugs to eradicate *H. pylori* should be given as well as an acid-suppressing drug. The optimum regime for the eradication of *Helicobacter* continues to undergo definition. At present the most widely accepted regimen is triple therapy consisting of a 2-week course of amoxicillin (500 mg PO QID), bismuth (Pepto-bismol 2 tabs QID), and metronizadole (250 mg QID).

A surgery referral will be necessary for complications such as persistent or recurring bleeding, obstruction, perforation, or intractability. One should always exclude gastrinoma with a serum gastrin if the patient has a history of intractable or recurrent PUD despite optimal treatment.

Pancreatitis

Acute Pancreatitis

Acute pancreatitis is an inflammatory disease that can range in severity from mild edema to severe pancreatic and peripancreatic necrosis.

There are four major theories of pathogenesis; each theory is only partly supported, however, by research and clinical data. The four major theories are: secretion against an obstructed duct, bile reflux into the pancreatic duct, duodenal reflux into the pancreatic duct, and intracellular protease activation.

The most common causes of acute pancreatitis in the United States are alcohol and cholelithiasis. In females, the most frequent cause of pancreatitis is gallstones. Less common etiologies include abdominal trauma, hereditary pancreatitis, infection (mumps, hepatitis viruses, coxsackie), medications (azathioprine, 6-MP, sulfonamides, thiazides, furosamides, estrogens, tetracycline, valproic acid, pentamidine), vasculitis (lupus, necrotizing angiitis, thrombotic thrombocytopenia purpura), penetrating peptic ulcer, obstruction of the ampulla of Vater or pancreatic duct by tumor, pancreas divisum, postoperative or postendoscopic retrograde cholangiopancreatography (post-ERCP), metabolic (hypertriglyceridemia, hypercalcemia, renal failure), and hereditary pancreatitis.

One usually diagnoses acute pancreatitis on the basis of the clinical symptoms of abdominal pain associated with chemical evidence of pancreatic inflammation in the form of elevated serum concentrations of pancreatic enzymes such as amylase and lipase. The pain is most typically epigastric in location. It is described as a steady, boring midepigastric pain often radiating to the back. Nausea and vomiting are frequent associations. Physical exam may yield a low-grade fever up to 101°F. However, if the temperature is higher than this one must consider an alternate diagnosis or complications of pancreatitis. Patients with pancreatitis may present with volume depletion, manifested as hypotension or shock. The abdomen is frequently distended and bowel sounds may be diminished or absent. Epigastric tenderness may be severe, and localized rebound may be elicited.

Less frequent physical findings associated with pancreatitis include Cullen's sign (a blue discoloration in the periumbilical area due to hemorrhage in the pancreatic bed) and Turner's sign (a blue, red, purple, or green-brown discoloration of the flanks due to tissue catabolism of hemoglobin).

The association of hyperamylasemia with acute pancreatitis has been recognized for many years but is not pathognomonic, as amylase is produced in other structures and when those structures are inflamed, they may also produce both an elevated amylase and abdominal pain. Duodenal perforation and mesenteric infarction may also give rise to abdominal pain and elevations of amylase. Hyperamylasemia is occasionally associated with salivary gland inflammation, diabetic ketoacidoses, anorexia nervosa, bulimia, HIV infection, and macroamylasemia.

In acute pancreatitis the magnitude of the amylase elevation is often three times or more greater than normal. However, a normal serum amylase does not absolutely exclude the diagnosis of acute pancreatitis and the degree of elevation does not predict the severity of pancreatitis. Amylase levels typically return to normal in uncomplicated pancreatitis in 48 to 72 h.

The serum lipase level is more specific for pancreatic disease although it is also present in other organs including the duodenum, liver, tongue, and other parts of the intestine. In patients with acute pancreatitis, lipase usually remains elevated longer than amylase, often remaining elevated for 7 to 14 days.

Radiographic imaging studies are of great value in a patient suspected of having pancreatitis. Abdominal radiographs are abnormal in about half of the patients with acute pancreatitis but they are nonspecific for pancreatitis. Common findings include total or partial ileus (sentinel loop) and spasm of the transverse colon. Abdominal radiographs are very useful for excluding other etiologies of abdominal pain associated with elevated amylase levels such as an intestinal perforation.

Ultrasonography is used to evaluate the patient with acute pancreatitis. Although it may fail to visualize the pancreas because of overlying intestinal gas, it may detect gallstones or edema or enlargement of the pancreas. It is most useful in evaluating the biliary tract and especially for identifying gallstones, but may define features such as thickening of the gallbladder wall and pericholecystic fluid collections suggestive of cholecystitis, or reveal dilation of the bile ducts suggestive of obstruction by stone or tumor.

Computed tomography (CT) scanning is superior to ultrasound in evaluating the pancreas since it is not limited by the presence of bowel gas. CT scan can often confirm the diagnosis of pancreatitis by finding an edematous pancreas and is also useful for predicting and identifying late complications.

Endoscopic retrograde cholangiopancreatography (ERCP) is not routinely indicated in the evaluation of patients during an attack of acute pancreatitis. It does, however, have an important role in specific situations. For example, endoscopic sphincterotomy and stone extraction can be performed on those patients suspected of having gallstone pancreatitis who are not clinically improving within 24 h after admission. ERCP is also used for the preoperative evaluation of patients suspected of having traumatic pancreatitis to localize the site of the pancreatic duct disruption. In patients with no identifiable cause of acute pancreatitis, ERCP may be performed once the attack of pancreatitis has subsided in order to define such causes as occult common bile duct stones, pancreatic or ampullary carcinoma, or other causes of obstruction.

The differential diagnosis of acute pancreatitis should include other causes of severe acute abdominal pain, which may or may not be accompanied by an elevation of amylase, such as intestinal perforation, especially from PUD, ectopic pregnancy, tubo-ovarian abscess, torsion of the adnexa, ruptured ovarian cyst, acute cholecystitis, acute intestinal obstruction, mesenteric ischemia, renal colic, myocardial ischemia or infarction, aortic dissection, connective tissue disorders, pneumonia, and diabetic ketoacidosis.

Treatment for acute pancreatitis generally involves hospitalization and supportive measures such as analgesia (meperidine), IV fluids and colloids, no oral alimentation (NPO), and correction of hypocalcemia. Fulminant pancreatitis requires aggressive fluid support and meticulous management of cardiovascular collapse, respiratory insufficiency, and pancreatic infection. These patients require hospitalization and usually need consultations from gastroenterologists and surgeons.

Chronic Pancreatitis

The differentiation between acute and chronic pancreatitis is based on clinical criteria. Following recovery from acute pancreatitis there is restoration of normal pancreatic function. In chronic pancreatitis there is permanent loss of function, and pain usually predominates. Chronic pancreatitis may present either as recurrent episodes of acute inflammation superimposed on a chronically damaged pancreas or as a more chronic and persistent syndrome of pain and malabsorption.

The most common etiology of chronic pancreatitis in the United States is alcoholism. Less common causes include hypertriglyceridemia, hypercalcemia, hereditary pancreatitis, hemochromatosis, and cystic fibrosis. In approximately one-quarter of patients with chronic pancreatitis no specific etiology is identified.

Pain is the cardinal symptom of chronic pancreatitis. Weight loss, steatorrhea, and other signs of malabsorption are frequent associations. Physical exam is commonly unremarkable except for signs of malabsorption. There are no specific laboratory tests for chronic pancreatitis. Both the serum amylase and lipase levels will often be normal. Steatorrhea typically occurs late in the course of chronic pancreatitis.

Abdominal x-rays can reveal pancreatic calcification, especially when the etiology of the chronic pancreatitis is alcohol abuse. Ultrasound or CT scan of the abdomen may reveal dilation of the pancreatic duct or the presence of pancreatic pseudocysts. ERCP is helpful in showing the characteristic ductal changes of chronic pancreatitis—irregular dilation of the main pancreatic duct and pruning of its branches.

It is very important but often difficult to distinguish chronic pancreatitis from pancreatic carcinoma, as both can present with recurrent attacks of abdominal discomfort.

Treatment of these patients is frequently difficult and discouraging. The main goals should be to control pain and correct malabsorption. Intermittent attacks should be treated much like acute pancreatitis. Narcotics can be given for severe pain but subsequent addiction is very common. Surgery may control pain if there is a ductal stricture. Subtotal pancreatectomy may also control pain but at the cost of exocrine insufficiency and diabetes. Malabsorption is managed with a low-fat diet and adequate pancreatic enzyme replacement.

Gallbladder Disease

Cholelithiasis

In the United States there are approximately 1 million new cases of cholelithiasis per year. There are three major types of gallstones: cholesterol, pigment, and mixed stones. In the United States 80 percent of stones are cholesterol stones or mixed and 20 percent are pigmented stones.

There is an increased incidence of gallstones in American Indians, the obese, diabetics, in relation to ileal disease or resection, during pregnancy, in association with estrogen or oral contraceptive use, in type IV hyperlipidemia, and in patients with cirrhosis. Females predominate in a ratio of 4 to 1.

In the evaluation of women for abdominal pain, gallstones are frequently found. However, gallstones are the cause of this pain only in a minority of cases.

Since most gallstones are silent, the majority will be diagnosed in asymptomatic patients undergoing ultrasound or radiographic studies for another reason. Symptoms tend to occur when the stones produce inflammation or obstruction of the cystic or common bile ducts. The major symptoms associated with cholelithiasis are: (1) nausea and vomiting, (2) biliary pain, which is usually constant rather than colicky, and (3) postprandial right upper quadrant or epigastric pain; this pain typically occurs 30 to 60 min after meals, lasts for several hours and occasionally radiates to the right scapula or back. Physical exam may be unremarkable or show epigastric or right upper quadrant tenderness.

Accompanying an attack of biliary colic there are usually mild and transient elevations in bilirubin and alkaline phosphatase. Since only 10 percent of gallstones are radiopaque, ultrasonography is the best diagnostic test. To opacify the gallbladder an oral cholecystogram requires a functioning gallbladder and is nowadays used less frequently than ultrasound.

The differential diagnosis of gallbladder pain includes PUD, gastroesophageal reflux disease, the irritable bowel syndrome, and other inflammatory processes in the right upper quadrant such as hepatitis or pancreatitis.

Since one cannot improve symptoms in asymptomatic patients, asymptomatic cholelithiasis should not be an indication for surgical intervention. Elective cholecystectomy should be reserved for symptomatic patients, those with previous complications of cholelithiasis, and those asymptomatic patients who are at an increased risk of complications. Oral dissolution agents (chenodeoxycholic acid, ursodeoxycholic acid) completely dissolve radiolucent stones in approximately half of suitable patients, but are ineffective in dissolving large radiopaque or pigmented stones. Only a small number of patients meet the four criteria and are eligible for dissolution therapy: those with radiolucent gallstones less than 20 mm in diameter, functioning gallbladder by oral cholecystogram, noncalcified gallstones and when surgery is relatively contraindicated. Unfortunately, recurrence is inevitable when these agents are stopped. Pregnancy is a contraindication for dissolution therapy.

Acute Cholecystitis

Acute cholecystitis or acute inflammation of the gallbladder usually is caused by cystic duct obstruction by an impacted stone. Over 90 percent of acute cholecystitis is associated with gallstones, with distention of the gallbladder due to obstruction of the cystic duct being the primary event. The bile may either be sterile or may become infected secondarily. Gram-negative organisms such as *Escherichia coli, Klebsiella,* and enterococcus are the most common organisms isolated in cases of acute cholecystitis. If the bile is infected, this can lead to abscess formation and perforation. Approximately 10 percent of the time acute cholecystitis occurs in the absence of gallstones (acalculous cholecystitis). This is generally associated with prolonged acute illness, prolonged fasting, or intravenous hyperalimentation that leads to gallbladder stasis. The differential diagnosis of acalculous cholecystitis includes carcinoma of the gallbladder or common bile duct and vasculitis.

The most common presenting symptoms of acute cholecystitis are abdominal pain, nausea, vomiting, and fever; usually onset of symptoms is acute. The pain is typically in the right upper quadrant with localized tenderness. In 20 percent of patients there is a palpable right upper quadrant mass which is the distended gallbladder.

Laboratory evaluation usually reveals a mild leukocytosis with increased polymorphonuclear cells and band forms. There is typically a mild elevation of bilirubin, aspartate aminotransferase (AST), alanine aminotransferase (ALT), and alkaline phosphatase.

Ultrasonography is useful for demonstrating gallstones but may not confirm the diagnosis of acute cholecystitis. Ultrasound findings suggestive of acute cholecystitis include gallbladder wall thickening, gallbladder sludge, pericholecystic fluid, marked distention of the gallbladder, and the demonstration of a positive Murphy's sign during direct probing of the gallbladder at the time of ultrasonography. Radionuclide biliary imaging (HIDA or DISIDA scans) is highly sensitive and specific in the diagnosis of cystic duct obstruction. Both radionuclide studies and ultrasonography are very accurate; however, the choice of imaging studies remains controversial. Ultrasound is often selected as the initial test because it can be performed quickly, is less expensive, and provides information about nonbiliary structures.

The differential diagnosis of acute cholecystitis should include acute pancreatitis, appendicitis, pyelonephritis, PUD, hepatitis, and hepatic abscess.

The initial management of acute cholecystitis is supportive and includes IV fluids, antibiotics, NPO, and parenteral analgesics (meperidine or other narcotics); a nasogastric tube should be inserted if the patient has nausea and vomiting. Surgical cholecystectomy, either open or laparoscopic, is the definitive treatment and should be performed as soon as is feasible, generally within 24 to 48 h of admission. Delayed surgery is reserved for patients who would be at high risk if they had emergency surgery or when the diagnosis is in doubt. Urgent surgery is indicated for patients with complications such as perforation of the gallbladder or empyema or for those patients who fail to respond to initial medical therapy or who deteriorate while receiving medical therapy.

Complications related to acute cholecystitis include empyema, hydrops, gangrenous gallbladder, perforation, fistulization, and gallstone ileus.

Chronic Cholecystitis

Chronic cholecystitis is usually caused by gallstones and this is a much more difficult diagnosis to make than acute cholecystitis. In fact, many physicians think this is a pathologic rather than a clinical entity.

Symptoms and signs are often nonspecific, including fatty food intolerance, abdominal pain, and dyspepsia. Laboratory tests are often normal. Ultrasonography usually shows gallstones within a contracted gallbladder; sometimes a thickened gallbladder wall may be demonstrated.

The diagnosis is usually made following the exclusion of other etiologies of right upper quadrant discomfort such as PUD, esophagitis, and the irritable bowel syndrome.

Inflammatory Bowel Disease

Chronic inflammatory disorders of unknown etiology involving the GI tract are subdivided into two principal categories. Ulcerative colitis is a diffuse mucosal inflammatory process generally limited to the colon. It invariably affects the rectum and may extend proximally in a symmetrical uninterrupted pattern to involve part or all of the large intestine. By contrast, Crohn's disease is a patchy transmural inflammation that can affect any part of the gastrointestinal tract from the mouth to the anus. It most commonly involves the small bowel alone, the colon alone, or both the large and the small bowel simultaneously. The peak occurrence of either of the inflammatory bowel diseases lies between ages 15 and 35, but the onset may occur at any age.

Ulcerative Colitis

This disease is characterized by inflammation which is confined to the mucosa. It is not a transmural process. The rectum is almost always involved with inflammation extending continuously. Skip areas do not occur. Typical histologic features include epithelial damage, inflammation, crypt abscesses, and loss of goblet cells.

The most common clinical manifestation of ulcerative colitis is bloody diarrhea. Other manifestations include passage of mucus, fever, abdominal pain, tenesmus, and weight loss. There is a wide spectrum of severity at presentation which may extend to toxic megacolon, a surgical emergency. Other clinical features at presentation may also include anemia, hypokalemia, hypoalbuminemia, and dehydration.

Acute colitis can be diagnosed on a limited sigmoidoscopic examination; full colonoscopy should not be undertaken during the acute phase as the risk of perforation is high. Endoscopic features of ulcerative colitis include mucosal erythema and granularity, friability of the mucosa, hemorrhage, exudate, ulceration, and pseudopolyp formation.

Complications of ulcerative colitis include toxic megacolon and colonic perforation. There is also an increased risk of colon cancer in patients with ulcerative colitis; this risk is related to the extent and duration of colitis. Patients with long-standing extensive ulcerative colitis should be enrolled in a screening colonoscopy program in which colonoscopy with multiple biopsies is performed at regular intervals to detect dysplasia, an early marker of carcinoma.

Crohn's Disease

Any part of the GI tract can be involved in this inflammatory process. However, the terminal ileum or colon are most frequently involved. Unlike ulcerative colitis this is a transmural inflammation. The bowel wall becomes very thickened. Involvement is discontinuous; skip lesions, which feature intervening segments of inflamed and normal intestine, are quite common. Characteristic histologic features include transmural inflammation, granulomas, fissures, and fistulas.

Typical clinical manifestations of Crohn's disease include fever, abdominal pain, diarrhea (often not bloody), fatigue, and weight loss. Acute ileitis can often mimic appendicitis. Other presentations of Crohn's disease include anorectal fissures, fistulas, and abscesses. If the colon is involved, the diagnosis can be made with sigmoidoscopy or colonoscopy. Often an upper GI and small bowel series is required to make the diagnosis since the small bowel is frequently involved. Complications include obstruction, fistulas (to bowel, bladder, vagina, or skin), abscess formation, bile salt malabsorption leading to cholesterol gallstones, oxalate kidney stones, amyloidosis, and intestinal malignancy.

The differential diagnosis of either ulcerative colitis or Crohn's disease should include infectious colitis, ischemic bowel disease, diverticulitis, radiation-induced colitis, bleeding colonic lesions such as neoplasm, and irritable bowel disease.

Any of the infectious etiologies of colitis can present in a manner indistinguishable from inflammatory bowel disease. These infections would include shigella, salmonella, campylobacter, *Yersinia*, gonorrhea, lymphogranuloma venereum, *Clostridium difficile* toxin, tuberculosis, and amebiasis.

There are a number of important extraintestinal manifestations of ulcerative colitis and Crohn's disease: 1. skin: aphthous ulcerations, erythema nodosum, and pyoderma gangrenosum; 2. eye: episcleritis, iritis, and uveitis; 3. joint: peripheral arthritis (monoarticular, asymmetrical, large joints; no synovial destruction, no subcutaneous nodules, seronegative), ankylosing spondylitis, and sacroileitis (associated with HLA B27); 4. liver; fatty liver, cholangiocarcinoma, and primary sclerosing cholangitis; 5. hematologic: autoimmune hemolytic anemia and a thrombotic tendency which may lead to deep venous thrombosis and pulmonary embolism.

There are several major categories of drug therapy for inflammatory bowel disease. Symptomatic agents include antidiarrheals, antispasmodics, and occasionally cholestyramine. Anti-inflammatory compounds include oral sulfasalazine, topical sulfasalazine, oral 5-aminosalicylic acid and its analogs, topical 5-ASA and 4-ASA, corticosteroids including both oral and parenteral forms, immunosuppressives such as azathioprine and 6-mercaptopurine, and antibiotics such as metronidazole. Other agents such as cyclosporin and methotrexate are currently undergoing evaluation.

Malabsorption

Intestinal malabsorption of ingested nutrients often produces diarrhea, specifically, steatorrhea, or fat in the stools. Specific deficiencies (vitamins A, D, E, and K, B_{12}, folate, and iron) are other manifestations of malabsorption. Although the three major nutrients, fat, carbohydrate and protein, may all be malabsorbed, clinical symptoms are generally recognized due to the malabsorption of either carbohydrate or fat.

Different symptoms provide clinical clues as to the substance malabsorbed. Steatorrhea means that fat is not absorbed; anemia may be a clue that iron, B_{12} or folate is not being absorbed; edema might suggest protein as the malabsorptive substance; milk intolerance suggests lactose malabsorption. Steatorrhea is the hallmark of malabsorption. These patients present with diarrhea. These stools are generally greasy, bulky, putty-like, foul-smelling stools. They are not watery nor bloody. Fat absorption requires an intact liver, pancreas, small bowel and lymphatic function. There are many intricate tests in the evaluation of malabsorption, but the most important step is to suspect malabsorption when a patient presents with diarrhea and weight loss.

The initial evaluation of a patient with malabsorption should involve documenting steatorrhea. The most cost-effective method to document steatorrhea is a qualitative fecal fat determination on a single stool collection. The qualitative fecal fat determination done on a single stool collection is about 90 percent sensitive and specific for detecting steatorrhea. The 72-h stool collection is very costly and inconvenient, and should not be included in the initial evaluation of these patients. When collecting stools for evaluation of fat, it is important to remember that the patient needs to be on a full fat diet. Collecting stools for fat from patients who are fasting or being fed intravenously could lead to false negative results.

Once significant steatorrhea has been documented, a small bowel biopsy is the most cost-effective way to proceed with the evaluation. A small bowel biopsy could be characteristic and diagnostic for celiac sprue, Whipple's disease, abetalipoproteinemia, or agammaglobulinemia. Patchy diseases that may show a normal biopsy due to sampling error include intestinal lymphoma, intestinal lymphangiectasia, amyloidosis, eosinophilic enteritis, systemic mastocytosis, or parasitic infections. These may require repeat biopsy in order to secure the diagnosis.

The D-xylose test involves D-xylose, which is a five-carbon sugar that is incompletely absorbed in the duodenum and jejunum. It is used as a small intestinal absorption test. This test is helpful in those mucosal diseases in which a patchy distribution of the histologic lesion may invalidate the endoscopic biopsy. Careful administration and collection of serum levels or 5-hour urine collections should be undertaken if this test is performed, since less than meticulous administration and collection in performing this test would result in uninterpretable results. Abnormalities could result from small bowel diseases as listed in the above paragraphs. There are other causes of an abnormal D-xylose test besides malabsorptive diseases, including abnormal renal function, bacterial overgrowth leading to breakdown of xylose in the bowel, poor hydration, congestive heart failure or the use of nonsteroidal anti-inflammatory drugs.

Other tests employed in the evaluation of malabsorption include the lactose tolerance test by breath and hydrogen analysis to diagnose both lactose intolerance and bacterial overgrowth. Small bowel x-rays may also be helpful to find defects as clues to the cause of malabsorption. The Schilling test for B_{12} absorption is another useful test and abnormalities can be seen with intrinsic factor deficiency, bacterial overgrowth or ileal dysfunction.

Protein-losing enteropathy may result from several causes of the malabsorption. It is associated with hypoalbuminemia and can be detected by measuring stool alpha antitrypsin.

These evaluations for patients with malabsorption frequently require a referral to a gastroenterologist. Many of the specific tests required for the diagnosis are not readily available at all institutions.

Therapy is directed at the underlying disease. Some of the more common etiologies of malabsorption and the appropriate therapy are presented in Table 45-1.

Motility Disorders

Gastrointestinal motility testing is a developing area of gastrointestinal investigation. Although esophageal manometry and rectal manometry are available in most institutions, small bowel motility studies are available in only a few centers. Patients with motility disturbances need to be referred to a gastroenterologist, preferably one subspecializing in motility disturbance. Some of the more common gastrointestinal motility problems are discussed below.

Esophageal Motor Disorders

These patients typically present with dysphagia. Investigation should be undertaken first to rule out other etiologies of dysphagia such as gastroesophageal reflux disease, tumor, or stricture.

Achalasia (failure of the smooth muscles of the esophagus to relax) has a number of etiologies including primary (idiopathic) or secondary causes. Secondary causes include Chagas' disease, lymphoma, carcinoma, ischemia, neurotropic viruses, drugs, toxin, post-vagotomy radiation and chronic intestinal pseudo-obstruction. The manometric findings include hypertensive lower esophageal sphincter (LES), inadequate relaxation of the LES, and loss of peristalsis in the smooth muscle portion of the esophageal body. Diagnosis can be suspected if on a chest x-ray there is absence of the gastric air bubble.

TABLE 45-1 Disease States Causing Malabsorption

Disease State	Examples	Treatment
Insufficient pancreatic enzyme activity	Chronic pancreatitis Pancreatic carcinoma Pancreatic resection Cystic Fibrosis	Low fat diet Pancreatic enzyme replacement
Insufficient intraluminal bile acid activity	Intrahepatic cholestasis Extrahepatic cholestasis Intestinal stasis syndromes Ileal resection Ileal Crohn's disease	Treat the underlying disease Antibiotics if bacterial overgrowth present Bile salt binding agents may help, cholestyramine
Intramural small bowel disease	Celiac sprue Tropical sprue Whipple's disease Intestinal lymphangiectasia Abetalipoproteinemia Eosinophilic enteritis	Gluten free diet Antibiotics and folic acid Antibiotics Low-fat diet and medium chain triglycerides Low-fat diet and medium chain triglycerides Steroid therapy
Malabsorption due to multiple defects	Zollinger-Ellison Scleroderma Postgastrectomy Radiation enteritis	Treat the underlying disease

Helpful studies include a barium swallow showing a dilated esophagus with distal beak-like narrowing and air fluid levels. Endoscopy should be done to exclude tumor. Esophageal manometry should be done to confirm the diagnosis. Treatment involves a trial of calcium antagonists, pneumatic balloon dilatation, or surgical Heller myotomy of the lower esophageal sphincter.

Patients with scleroderma may also have an esophageal motor disturbance. They are usually diagnosed with scleroderma before GI manifestations of the disease occur. These patients have gastroesophageal reflux disease and should be treated for this. Their manometric findings include incompetent lower esophageal sphincter leading to reflux esophagitis and stricture and aperistalsis due to atrophy of the esophageal smooth muscle and fibrosis of the muscle.

Gastric Motor Disorders

The most common cause of gastroparesis in the United States is diabetes mellitus. Gastroparesis generally presents with recurrent episodes of nausea and vomiting postprandially. It also can present with blood sugars that are difficult to control in diabetic patients because of the uneven emptying of the stomach and resultant highs and lows in blood sugars. Diabetic gastroparesis can also present with abdominal distention or abdominal discomfort. Endoscopy or barium studies should be done to exclude gastric outlet obstruction causing delayed gastric emptying secondary to peptic ulcer disease or malignancy. Low level intestinal obstruction or partial obstruction should also be excluded. Gastric emptying studies through nuclear medicine provide good documentation of the delayed gastric emptying. Another cause of gastroparesis is eating disorders such as anorexia nervosa. It is not unusual to see temporary gastroparesis related to a viral infection; these tend to resolve spontaneously but can be associated with permanent gastroparesis. Gastroparesis is generally treated with a prokinetic agent, metoclopramide or more recently, cisapride. It also will help to have patients eat more frequent, smaller meals.

Small Bowel Dysmotility

Ambulatory small bowel motility testing is available at a very few centers currently. Patients are generally referred for small bowel studies when they have such disease states as diabetic enteropathy, chronic idiopathic intestinal pseudoobstruction, primary pseudoobstruction from visceral myopathy or visceral neuropathy.

Anorectal Manometry

Anal and rectal motility tests are usually undertaken in the evaluation of fecal incontinence. Childbirth may sometimes result in a sphincter defect which may be detected with anal manometry. Other etiologies of fecal incontinence in which anal rectal manometry may be useful include neurologic disease; central nervous system process such as dementia, stroke, brain tumors, spinal cord lesions, Tabes dorsalis, multiple sclerosis; peripheral nervous system process such as cauda equina lesions, polyneuropathies, traumatic neuropathies, or altered rectal sensation in which the site of the lesion is not known; skeletal-muscle diseases such as myasthenia gravis; myopathies such as muscular dystrophy; smooth muscle dysfunctions such as abnormal rectal compliance and internal and anal sphincter weakness; anatomic derangement such as congenital anomalies of the ano-rectum, fistula, rectal prolapse; anorectal trauma secondary to injury, surgery, or childbirth; and miscellaneous disease (such as severe diarrhea, irritable bowel syndrome, hypoparathyroidism).

Anal manometry generally gives the measurement of basal and squeeze pressure in the anal canal. Rectal balloon manometry gives measurement of rectal sensation, compliance, inhibitory reflex, and contractile responses. Other tests to consider in the evaluation of rectal-anal function would be electromyography, nerve conduction studies, mucosal electrosensitivity, reflex or stimulation, radiographic tests (defacography, balloon proctography, anal endosonography). Often these tests are available at a motility center and often these centers provide biofeedback information as a treatment for fecal incontinence. These tests as a group can provide useful information to determine whether or not a patient would be helped by any surgical intervention as well.

Gastrointestinal Malignancies

Malignancies of the gastrointestinal tract are relatively common. Common to most of the GI malignancies are clinical presentations consisting of weight loss; iron deficiency; or gastrointestinal dysfunction such as dysphagia, altered bowel habits, or abdominal pain.

Esophageal Cancer

Common clinical features of esophageal carcinoma include progressive dysphagia (typically first with solids, followed by liquids), weight loss, hoarseness from laryngeal nerve involvement, pulmonary aspiration (either from obstruction or tracheal esophageal fistula), and occasionally chest pain from mediastinal spread of the tumor.

Esophagoscopy is the most sensitive and specific test for diagnosing tumors of the esophagus; pathologic confirmation of the tumor is performed by a combination of endoscopic biopsies and cytologic examination of mucosal brushings. Barium swallow is another tool used for diagnosis of esophageal tumors; however, esophagogastroduodenoscopy (EGD) still should be done to provide a pathology specimen. A CT scan of the chest is valuable in assessment of local and nodal spread. Endoscopic ultrasound is a new modality for staging tumors of the esophagus.

Squamous cell carcinomas are most commonly in the upper two-thirds of the esophagus; adenocarcinoma occurs more frequently in the distal third of the esophagus, often arising in a region of metaplastic columnar epithelium. Proximal gastric adenocarcinomas frequently extend directly up into the esophagus and sometimes it is difficult to judge whether the adenocarcinoma is of esophageal or gastric origin. Lymphomas and melanomas occur in the esophagus, but these are rare.

The 5-year survival is about 10 percent for esophageal cancers, and this has not changed in approximately 4 decades. Depth of penetration of the esophageal wall, lymph node involvement, weight loss, and age of the patient are major prognostic factors for patients with localized esophageal cancer.

Therapy will depend on the extent of spread of the tumor. For patients with localized cancer who are medically fit, resection is the best choice of therapy, resulting consistently in 5-year survival rates of 10 to 20 percent. Radiation therapy alone should not be recommended to patients with squamous cell carcinoma of the esophagus, since a combination of chemotherapy and radiation therapy is superior. If a contraindication to chemotherapy exists, however, radiation therapy alone can provide effective palliation for a few weeks to months. Combination chemotherapy usually involving 5FU plus cisplatin, can provide a partial response; unfortunately, these responses are short lived.

Palliative measures include laser ablation, dilation, luminal prosthesis to bypass the tumor, and gastrostomy or jejunostomy tube feedings for nutritional support.

Physicians should be aware of risk factors associated with esophageal tumors. Long-term gastroesophageal reflux disease with Barrett's mucosa is associated with an increased incidence of adenocarcinoma. Ethanol abuse and smoking (with the combination being synergistic) are major risk factors for squamous cell carcinoma of the esophagus, and physicians should counsel all their patients regarding the risks associated with the use of these substances. Other risk factors include previous lye ingestion, radiation exposure, other head and neck cancers, achalasia, tylosis, Plummer-Vinson Syndrome, and vitamin A deficiency.

Gastric Cancer

Gastric carcinoma most commonly presents with upper abdominal discomfort, frequently associated with weight loss, anorexia, nausea, and evidence of acute or chronic GI blood loss (iron deficiency anemia in two-thirds of patients; fecal occult blood in 80 percent).

The exact cause of gastric carcinoma is unknown. It is currently thought that *Helicobacter pylori* may play a role. There are several dietary factors which correlate with an increased incidence of stomach cancer including the ingestion of nitrates, smoked foods, and heavily salted foods. A genetic component is suggested by an increased incidence in relatives of affected patients. Other risk factors include atrophic gastritis, adenomatous gastric polyps, pernicious anemia, and Ménétrier's disease.

EGD is the most sensitive and specific test to diagnose gastric cancer, and it can also provide pathologic confirmation by biopsy. Barium examination of the stomach is unable to provide pathologic confirmation. Adenocarcinoma is the pathology found in approximately 90 percent of gastric carcinomas. Lymphoma accounts for about 7 percent of gastric malignancies and leiomyosarcoma is considerably less frequent.

The conventional treatment for early gastric carcinoma is resection, as it is the only potentially curative modality available. Feasibility of resection is dependent on the stage of the tumor. Adjuvant radiation therapy has been shown to improve survival in combination with adjuvant chemotherapy.

Small Bowel Tumors

Tumors of the small intestine are uncommon, and represent less than 5 percent of all GI neoplasms. They typically present with bleeding, abdominal pain, or intestinal obstruction. There is an increased incidence of lymphomas in patients with celiac sprue (gluten-sensitive enteropathy).

The barium small bowel series is the best diagnostic test, and its sensitivity in finding a tumor may be increased with the use of enterolysis, which is direct small bowel installation of contrast. CT is useful to evaluate the extent of tumor, especially in the case of lymphomas. Angiography is frequently used when there is an undetermined site of bleeding, and this can be used to detect a plexus of tumor vessels.

Most small bowel tumors are benign. These include adenomas, which are most frequently found in the duodenum; leiomyomas, which are intramural benign tumors; and lipomas, which are most frequently found in the ileum. Of the malignant tumors of the small bowel, 50 percent will be adenocarcinomas. Lymphomas are the second most frequent malignant tumors of the small intestine. Treatment usually involves surgical excision and adjuvant chemotherapy for lymphomas.

Colorectal Cancer

Adenocarcinoma of the colon and rectum is predominantly a disease of the Western world. There are approximately 70,000 deaths annually in the United States alone attributed to colorectal cancer. This tumor is common in North America and Europe and less common in developing nations. Over the past 20 years, a proximal migration of the location of colorectal cancer has been noted with an increase in frequency in the transverse and right colon, and a slight decrease in frequency in the sigmoid and rectum.

Theories explaining the high prevalence of this tumor in the Western world include: diet high in animal protein and animal fat, decreased fiber in the diet, and hereditary factors. It is increasingly clear that genetic predisposition plays a role in a substantial number of patients with colorectal cancer. Hereditary factors in colon cancer are most obviously manifested in those with inheritable polyposis syndromes (Gardner's syndrome, Turcot syndrome, and familial polyposis coli). These syndromes are inherited and are characterized by the presence of hundreds to thousands of colonic adenomas with or without extracolonic tumors. The nonpolyposis hereditary carcinoma groups (Lynch I and Lynch II) suggest the presence of a genetic predisposition among certain populations in the Western world. Lynch first described a cancer family syndrome involving a colon in which there was no familial polyposis and 75 percent of the carcinomas involved the ascending colon. He later described a second family colon cancer syndrome that included carcinomas of the breast, ovary, and endometrium in women, and bowel and urologic malignancy in both sexes. In these syndromes, discrete polyps but not polyposis may precede the cancers.

Occurrence of colorectal cancer is approximately equal in both sexes. Occurrence below the age of 40 is unusual but the incidence increases dramatically between the ages of 50 and 90. Most colorectal cancers are believed to arise from adenomatous polyps. Patients with one colorectal carcinoma have an increased risk of developing a second carcinoma either simultaneously (synchronous carcinomas) or subsequently (metachronous carcinomas). In addition to the previously mentioned risk factors, the incidence of carcinomas dramatically increases in patients with ulcerative colitis, approximately 20 percent at 20 years when pancolitis exists.

The clinical picture of adenocarcinomas of the colon and rectum is quite variable. Presentations include: occult or gross bleeding, weight loss, generalized malaise or fatigue, iron deficiency anemia, obstruction of the colon, and metastatic disease including liver metastases. A common presentation in colon cancer is change in bowel habits or change in the caliber of the stool or increasing constipation. Distal cancers are more likely to present with narrowing of the stool, whereas cancers in the right colon are more likely to present with anemia and fatigue. Rectal tumors frequently present with change in the caliber of the stool, fecal urgency, rectal bleeding, frequency, tenesmus, and occasionally tumor prolapse outside the rectum.

Bleeding from carcinomas may be slow and intermittent or profuse. In a nonacute patient who presents with occult or gross rectal bleeding, the best evaluation would be a colonoscopy; however, sometimes a proctosigmoidoscopy combined with an air contrast barium enema is performed. The advantage of colonoscopy is that it can provide important biopsies for diagnosis.

There are routine screening procedures available for the early detection of colorectal cancer including fecal occult blood testing and screening flexible sigmoidoscopy. Between the ages of 40 and 50 for the average-risk-group patient, yearly digital rectal examinations and testing the stool for the presence of occult blood should be undertaken. Although there is debate regarding when and with what frequency sigmoidoscopy screening should be utilized, one recommendation for the average risk patient is flexible sigmoidoscopy or proctosigmoidoscopy to 60 cm every three years to commence at age 50. When colorectal cancer is suspected because of clinical signs or when a screening test for occult blood is positive, prompt diagnostic evaluation should be undertaken endoscopically with colonoscopy. If colonoscopy is unavailable, refused by the patient, or technically difficult, then an air contrast barium enema and flexible sigmoidoscopy should be undertaken.

Fecal occult blood testing with a hemoccult-type guaiac test is convenient, inexpensive, and readily available, but not specific for colon cancer. Bleeding from any part of the GI tract can test positive on these cards. Other sources of GI blood loss would include epistaxis, upper GI tract bleeding, hemorrhoids, gingival bleeding, or ingestion of aspirin or nonsteroidal anti-inflammatory agents. Exogenous peroxidase activity from red meat or uncooked fruits and vegetables can also lead to false positive tests. These false positives can be avoided if the patient is instructed to avoid rare red meat and peroxidase-containing vegetables and fruits (cauliflower, radishes, cantaloupe, turnips, broccoli) for the 3 days prior to the collection of the stool for occult blood testing. Nonsteroidal anti-inflammatory drugs, aspirin, and vitamin C should also be avoided during the testing period. Two stool samples on each of three consecutive stools should be tested.

These screening recommendations are for the woman at average risk. Patients in high risk groups for colon cancer (including patients with longstanding ulcerative colitis, previous colorectal cancer, previous adenomas, familial polyposis or Gardner's syndrome, and familial colon cancers) are generally followed by a gastroenterologist with more frequent surveillance for colon cancer. The physician should also bear in mind that women who have had breast, ovarian, or endometrial cancer are also at increased risk for colon cancer.

Patients who have had a colon cancer resected should have colonscopy performed at 6 months to 1 year following surgery, followed by yearly colonoscopies for 2 years. If the results are negative then, in general, colonoscopies should be performed every 3 years. This, of course, would be combined with yearly fecal occult blood testing. In the patient who has had a preoperative elevated carcinoembryonic antigen (CEA) level, postoperative CEA levels should be followed three times at 4- to 6-month intervals, then five times at yearly intervals.

Current treatment for adenocarcinoma of the colon is surgical, either palliative or curative. Staging of colon cancer is helpful prognostically. Staging is usually done by the Duke's classification or a derivative. Duke's A tumors are limited to the mucosa; B_1 tumors have penetration of the muscular mucosa; B_2 tumors penetrate through the true muscle wall; C_1 (fewer than 4 lymph nodes), B_1 with positive nodes; C_2 (more than four lymph nodes), B_2 with positive nodes. Controlled studies showed that adjuvant therapy with 5FU and levamisole for Duke's C colorectal carcinoma and adjuvant radiotherapy for rectal cancer improved five-year survival.

Pancreatitic Cancer

Clinical features suggestive of pancreatic cancer include painless jaundice, weight loss, abdominal pain, back pain, and anorexia.

Pancreatic cancer is the fourth most common cause of cancer death in the United States and the incidence appears to be increasing, particularly in women. The peak incidence occurs in the seventh decade. 70 percent of pancreatic cancers are found in the head of the pancreas and 30 percent are found in the tail and body of the pancreas. There is a very high incidence of local invasion or metastatic disease at the time of initial diagnosis. Pathology generally shows adenocarcinoma. There are other types of pancreatic tumors, but these are significantly less common. Gastrinomas, insulinomas, and VIPomas (tumors producing vasoactive intestinal peptide) most frequently present because of the clinical effects of the hormones being secreted by these islet cell tumors.

There is a clear association between chronic pancreatitis and pancreatic cancer. In addition, alcohol consumption plays a causative role in pancreatic cancer, as does cigarette smoking.

Ultrasound is a useful screening test, and is sensitive for lesions over 2 cm in the head and body of the pancreas. CT is somewhat more sensitive, and can frequently identify lesions in the tail of the pancreas that ultrasound cannot. Endoscopic retrograde cholangiopancreatography is the most sensitive test for carcinoma in the pancreatic head; pancreatic duct abnormalities can be seen in the majority of patients regardless of the location of the tumor. Pathologic confirmation is obtained by aspiration of biliary secretions during ERCP or percutaneous needle biopsy of the mass under ultrasound or CT guidance.

Surgical resection for partial pancreatectomy or Whipple procedure is potentially curative; however, careful selection is mandatory. Primary contraindications include visceral metastases, extrapancreatic serosal implantation, periportal or periaortal adenopathy, or invasion of the superior mesenteric artery or vein. The majority of patients will have obvious metastases or micrometastasis at the time of diagnosis, and the tumor is resectable in only 10 to 20 percent of patients and curable in less than 5 percent. Palliative relief of biliary obstruction can be provided by endoscopic or transhepatic stent placement. There are ongoing trials evaluating radiation therapy and specialized radiation techniques and chemotherapy.

Biliary Tract Cancers

Biliary tract cancers are less common than pancreatic cancers and usually present with one or a combination of the following: obstructive jaundice, pruritus, right upper quadrant pain, weight loss, anorexia, nausea, and vomiting.

Cholangiocarcinoma is adenocarcinoma of the bile duct epithelium. Predisposing factors for this tumor include primary sclerosing cholangitis, ulcerative colitis, chronic *Clonorchis sinensis* infestations, and choledochal cysts. This tumor is usually unresectable at the time of diagnosis and may frequently present with obstructive jaundice, but occasionally with hemobilia. Diagnosis is made with a combination of either ultrasound or CT and ERCP. Biliary fluid can be sent for cytology and frequently CT guided biopsies are needed for tissue diagnosis.

Ampullary carcinoma is a tumor of the papilla of

Vater or ampullary involvement of duodenal adenocarcinoma. These patients present with obstructive jaundice or GI bleeding and can have silver stools as a clinical presentation. Direct visualization using EGD or a side-viewing endoscope, accompanied with biopsy, are best for diagnosis.

Gallbladder carcinoma may be found incidentally at laparotomy or autopsy. The advanced tumor usually presents in patients in the seventh to eighth decade of life, with right upper quadrant pain, a palpable mass, jaundice, and weight loss. Preoperative diagnosis can be made by ultrasound or CT.

Treatment of these biliary duct cancers is similar to treatment for carcinoma of the head of the pancreas. The cure rate of advanced or symptomatic tumors is usually less than 5 percent.

Hepatocellular Carcinoma

Hepatocellular carcinoma is one of the most common and deadly malignancies in the world. There are substantial geographic differences in its prevalence, with the highest incidence in areas where hepatitis B virus infections are endemic. In the United States the peak incidence is in the fifth and sixth decades, but in endemic areas it is often 10 to 20 years earlier than this.

There is a strong correlation with chronic hepatitis B infection, suggesting a causative role of this virus in the majority of cases. In the western world the most common associations are alcoholic cirrhosis and other forms of cirrhosis, the use of anabolic steroids, and the administration of Thorotrast (a radiologic contrast agent used in the 1940s and 1950s). Inherited hemochromatosis, hepatitis C, schistosomiasis, alpha$_1$ antitrypsin deficiency, and chronic methotrexate ingestion are all associated with hepatocellular carcinoma. Oral contraceptives, aflatoxin ingestion, and exogenous androgens have each been suggested as being associated with hepatocellular carcinoma in noncirrhotic livers. There are no data at present which have demonstrated that oral contraceptive use increases the risk of hepatocellular carcinoma.

Hepatocellular carcinoma in cirrhotic patients frequently presents as decompensation of underlying liver disease, weight loss, right upper quadrant pain, and jaundice. Physical exam can reveal a tender, enlarged liver and a palpable liver mass. Ascites may be present, and when associated with hepatocellular carcinoma it is frequently blood tinged. A bruit or hepatic friction rub may be auscultated over the liver. Besides abnormal liver function tests, an elevated serum alpha fetoprotein (AFP) is suggestive of this tumor.

A mass in the liver can be demonstrated with ultrasound, CT, or MRI. Pathologic confirmation by radiologically guided percutaneous liver biopsy is necessary. Radionuclide scanning and angiography may be undertaken in the preoperative evaluation, since the only chance for cure in patients with hepatocellular carcinoma is hepatic resection. Unfortunately, only a very small percentage of patients with hepatocellular carcinoma are candidates for resection. Cirrhosis often limits the extent of hepatic resection, because the diseased liver has limited functional reserve. A small minority of patients are actually cured by a hepatic resection, and most patients die from recurrent or metastatic disease. Liver transplantation has been tried for hepatocellular carcinoma, but this approach remains highly controversial.

Gastrointestinal Carcinoid Tumors

Carcinoid tumors are rare tumors of the gastrointestinal tract. Carcinoids are members of the neuroendocrine or amine precursor uptake and decarboxylation (APUD) tumors. This family also includes other rare tumors such as islet cell carcinoma of the pancreas and medullary carcinoma of the thyroid. These cells produce biogenic amines and polypeptide hormones, which account for the striking clinical displays of excessive hormonal production.

The carcinoid tumor has been found in almost every organ derived from the primitive entoderm as well as from teratomas. In the gastrointestinal tract 95 percent of all GI carcinoids take origin in one of these sites: the colon, the appendix, the rectum, and the small intestine. However, they have been found in such unusual locations as the esophagus, bile duct, ampulla of Vater, and Meckel's diverticulum.

Carcinoid tumors of the appendix are fairly common neoplasms. It is not known what percentage of the population have carcinoid tumors of the appendix that are asymptomatic. Frequently these tumors are not even noticed until the pathologist finds them after appendectomy. The vast majority are exceedingly small. It is generally accepted that those carcinoids of the appendix less than 2 cm in diameter can be treated with simple appendectomy. Only carcinoids $\geq$ 2 cm in their largest dimension should be considered for a more radical operation such as right hemicolectomy.

Carcinoids of the rectum are found most typically in middle aged adults, but these individuals are also the most likely people to undergo screening proctoscopic examination These carcinoids are usually not palpated by the examining finger and are generally asymptomatic. Carcinoids of the rectum less than 1 cm rarely metastasize; however, those greater than 2 cm usually have metastasized by the time of diagnosis. If the tumor is 2 cm or larger, the patient, in general, should have a cancer operation. Those carcinoids of the rectum between 1 and 2 cm will require clinical judgement based on patient age, operative risk, and the necessity for and the acceptability of a permanent colostomy.

Carcinoids of the small bowel are more common in the distal compared to the proximal small intestine. They tend to congregate in the distal ileum where almost 40 percent are located within 2 ft of the ileal cecal valve. The most common clinical presentation for small bowel carcinoids is abdominal pain that is periodic and consistent with intermittent bowel obstruction. The lack of physical signs, nondescript nature of the symptoms, negative x-ray findings, and frequently long duration of symptoms often lead to erroneous diagnosis of a psychosomatic problem. These tumors are often unresectable at initial surgery. This tumor spreads locally and can encase the mesenteric artery. The liver is another frequent site of spread. These carcinoids tend to grow slowly and the liver appears to adapt to its presence. Patients can present relatively asymptomatic with large hepatic masses and near normal liver function tests. Accepted therapy of these tumors is local resection if possible. The malignant carcinoid syndrome is a striking, unusual syndrome which is directly related to tumor bulk in an area that drains into the systemic circulation. It is common in patients with hepatic metastases and is generally a manifestation of late stage disease. Flushing is the hallmark and diarrhea is a frequent manifestation. More unusual manifestations include carcinoid asthma and pellagra.

Although its exact role in producing symptoms has been disputed, serotonin and particularly its metabolite, 5 hydroxyindoleacetic acid (5-HIAA) provides an important biological marker for this disease. 5-HIAA is measured through collection of a 24-h urine sample.

The characteristic flush of the carcinoid syndrome has the appearance of a sunburn involving the face, neck, and upper trunk. It typically lasts for seconds to minutes and can be precipitated by almost anything that changes vascular tone, such as emotional stress, exertion, a large meal, or sexual intercourse. Especially common are flushing with first morning exertions. This carcinoid flush is usually associated with carcinoids of the ileum, and has also been classified as the "midgut flush." The most dramatic manifestation of the malignant carcinoid syndrome is the carcinoid crisis. These patients have greatly elevated 5-HIAA levels and have flushes described as the "foregut flush." This is a much more intense flush than the midgut variety and it is also associated with conjunctival injection and facial edema. After repeated bouts of flushing patients may actually take on a cyanotic hue and lionesque appearance. This type of flush is usually associated with gastric or pulmonary carcinoids.

Management of the patient with advanced and metastatic carcinoid tumors usually involves a combination of chemotherapeutic agents, octreotide and in some instances, hepatic arterial infusion. It should be kept in mind, however, that this is a very indolent disease. For many patients no treatment is the best treatment.

Differential Diagnosis of Jaundice

Jaundice is an abnormal yellow discoloration in the skin, sclera, or mucus membrane developing as a result of an elevated concentration of bilirubin in the sera. The concentration of bilirubin is determined by the rate of bilirubin formation from breakdown of heme-containing compounds and the rate of bilirubin elimination via hepatic uptake, conjugation, and secretion into bile.

Generally, jaundice is not physically evident until serum bilirubin concentration exceeds 3 mg/dl. The measurement of serum bilirubin is conventionally by the diazo-reaction (van den Bergh reaction). Conjugated bilirubin will react "directly" with diazo reagents. Total bilirubin measurement requires the addition of other compounds which facilitates the reaction of unconjugated bilirubin with the diazo reagent. Indirect bilirubin fraction is calculated by subtracting the direct bilirubin concentration from the total. Direct and indirect bilirubin concentrations are not entirely equivalent to those of conjugated and unconjugated bilirubin respectively, but in general an increase in the serum concentration of conjugated bilirubin will be reflected by an increase in the direct bilirubin concentration and likewise an increase in the concentration of unconjugated bilirubin will be reflected by an increase in the concentration of indirect bilirubin. More sophisticated testing methods are used to measure the concentrations of unconjugated monoglucuronidated and diglucuronidated bilirubin as well as conjugated bilirubin-albumin complexes. These sophisticated methods may occasionally be helpful in determining isolated disorders of bilirubin and metabolism from other causes of jaundice but the conventional diazo method for measurement of serum bilirubin is what is used in the vast majority of patients.

In considering the differential diagnosis of jaundice, either an increase in bilirubin formation or a decrease in hepatic clearance may lead to jaundice. This differential can be further simplified by dividing into three broad categories: (1) isolated disorders of bilirubin metabolism, (2) liver disease, and (3) obstruction of the bile ducts. Table 45-2 reviews the more common etiologies in the differential diagnoses of jaundice. Many of the conditions listed under liver disease and obstruction of the bile ducts will be covered in other sections. Further discussion of the isolated disorders of bilirubin metabolism are included in this section.

There are isolated disorders of bilirubin metabolism that have decreased hepatic clearance leading to jaundice.

TABLE 45-2 Differential Diagnosis of Jaundice

- Isolated Disorders of Bilirubin Metabolism
  - Increased production (hemolysis, blood transfusion, hematomas)
  - Decreased hepatic clearance
    - Decreased uptake or conjugation of bilirubin—(Gilbert's syndrome, Crigler-Najjar syndrome, physiologic jaundice of the newborn, drugs)
    - Decreased canalicular secretion (Dubin-Johnson's syndrome, Rotor's syndrome)
- Liver Disease
  - Hepatocellular dysfunction—acute or chronic
    - Viral hepatitis, hepatotoxins (ethanol, acetaminophen), drugs, ischemia, metabolic disorders (Reyes syndrome, Wilson's disease, hemochromatosis), pregnancy-related (acute fatty liver of pregnancy, eclampsia), autoimmune hepatitis
  - Cholestatic
    - Primary biliary cirrhosis, graft versus host disease, drugs, infiltrative disorders (granulomatous disease such as sarcoid, lymphoma, mycobacterial infections, Wegener's), amyloidosis, malignancy, miscellaneous conditions including benign recurrent intrahepatic cholestasis, estrogens, anabolic steroids, total parenteral nutrition, bacterial infections, pregnancy-related such as hyperemesis gravidarum, intrahepatic cholestasis of pregnancy, pregnancy.
- Obstruction of the Bile Ducts
  - Choledocholithiasis
  - Bile duct disease
    - Neoplasms
    - Inflammation (primary sclerosing cholangitis, AIDS cholangiopathy)
  - Biliary compression
    - Neoplasms (pancreatic carcinoma, hepatoma, metastatic lymphadenopathy)
  - Pancreatitis

Gilbert's syndrome is a hereditary disorder of decreased hepatic clearance of bilirubin leading to unconjugated hyperbilirubinemia. It is fairly common, seen in about 5 percent of white adults in the United States. This most frequently presents in an otherwise healthy patient in the second or third decade of life, frequently presenting with mild scleral icterus. The diagnosis of Gilbert's syndrome is established by demonstration of repeated normal liver function tests in an asymptomatic patient with a mild elevation of unconjugated bilirubin and no evidence of hemolysis. Liver biopsy is unnecessary. It is most important to establish the diagnosis of Gilbert's syndrome as reassurance to the patient and also to avoid unnecessary investigations or even surgical interventions.

Crigler-Najjar syndrome, congenital nonhemolytic jaundice, is uncommon and also leads to unconjugated neonatal hyperbilirubinemia. There are two types of this syndrome. In Type I, the majority of patients develop kernicterus and die in the neonatal period. Type II Crigler-Najjar syndrome patients may reach adulthood. These patients have bilirubin concentrations between 5 to 50 mg/dl, all of which is unconjugated.

Examples of hereditary conjugated hyperbilirubinemias are Dubin-Johnson's and Rotor's syndromes. Dubin-Johnson's syndrome is uncommon, and has autosomal recessive inheritance. The plasma bilirubin concentration is usually less than 7 mg/dl and about half of this is conjugated. The bilirubin concentration frequently rises with exogenous estrogen, so some of these patients are not detected until they are placed on birth control pills. There is no specific therapy except avoidance of exogenous estrogens. A classic diagnostic test is the slow disappearance of sulfobromophthalein, with a frequent secondary rise at 1 to 2 h. Rotor's syndrome is a very rare autosomal recessive disorder of excretion or storage of conjugated bilirubin. The plasma bilirubin concentration is usually less than 7 mg/dl and about half of this is conjugated. Affected patients classically have a very slow disappearance of the plasma sulfobromophthalein without a secondary rise. There is no treatment available and affected individuals have a normal prognosis.

The most common causes of increased bilirubin production leading to jaundice are hemolysis, ineffective erythropoiesis, or resorption of a hematoma. Patients with hemolytic anemia are prone to jaundice, as are patients with hereditary or acquired megaloblastic anemia from either folate or vitamin B_{12} deficiency. Jaundice may also follow massive transfusion. Major trauma with subsequent resorption of hematomas can also cause an increase in bilirubin production.

Important clues regarding the etiology of jaundice can be obtained through the patient history and physical examination. In a jaundiced patient who is otherwise asymptomatic, has a normal physical examination, and normal serum activities of alkaline phosphatase and transaminases, jaundice is unlikely to be due to liver disease or biliary obstruction. Further testing for specific disorders such as isolated defects in bilirubin metabolism or hemolysis is warranted. On the other hand, if the history and physical examination is abnormal and laboratory studies suggest the possibility of obstruction of the biliary tree, an imaging study is appropriate either to confirm the presence of biliary tract obstruction and localize an obstruction or to exclude it. The least invasive imaging studies are abdominal ultrasound and computed tomography of the abdomen. Ultrasound has the advantage of being non-invasive, portable, and least expensive; however, bowel gas may obscure the common bile duct and it is difficult to perform in obese individuals. Abdominal CT scan is another non-invasive test with higher resolution than ultrasound, and it is also not as operator dependent as ultrasound. However, it is not available in portable form and it can only visualize calcified gallstones. Intravenous contrast is typically required for abdominal CT and this is potentially nephrotoxic. Other biliary imaging studies include endoscopicretrograde cholangiopancreatography or percutaneous transhepatic cholangiography. These permit direct visualization of the biliary tree as well as the pancreatic ducts (for ERCP). They are more invasive than ultrasound or CT and require consultation with a gastroenterologist or invasive radiologist.

A decision tree for the evaluation and management of jaundice would list history, physical examination, and routine laboratory tests at the top. If the alkaline phosphatase or transaminases are normal, then the direction of investigation should be turned to evaluation for hemolysis and hereditary hyperbilirubinemias. On the other hand, if the alkaline phosphatase or transaminases are abnormal, and the clinical likelihood of biliary obstructive is low, one should proceed to biochemical studies for specific liver diseases. This might eventually require a liver biopsy for definitive diagnosis. If the clinical likelihood of biliary obstruction is high, one should consider having an ERCP or percutaneous transhepatic cholangiogram performed and therapeutic intervention accompany that procedure. If the clinical likelihood of biliary obstruction is low, then one should proceed with evaluation with a less invasive test such as abdominal ultrasound or CT scan. If at that time dilated bile ducts are found, then the patient should be evaluated for ERCP or percutaneous transhepatic cholangiogram. If the abdominal ultrasound or CT scan shows non-dilated bile ducts, further biochemical studies should be done looking for specific disease states.

Findings that are suggestive of obstructive jaundice include a history of abdominal pain, fever, prior biliary surgery or older age. Physical exam findings might include a high fever, abdominal tenderness, palpable abdominal mass or abdominal scar. Laboratory studies suggestive of obstructive jaundice include predominant elevation of serum bilirubin and alkaline phosphatase, elevated serum amylase, and a prothrombin time which is normal or normalizes with vitamin K administration.

On the other hand, findings more consistent with cholestatic liver disease include a history of anorexia, malaise, myalgias or possibly symptoms suggestive of a viral prodrome. Other history to consider in the evaluation of cholestatic liver disease includes known infectious exposure, receipt of blood products or use of intravenous drugs, exposure to known hepatotoxin, or family history of jaundice. Physical examination findings supporting of cholestatic liver disease include ascites, asterixis, encephalopathy and other stigmata of chronic liver disease (prominent abdominal veins, spider angiomata, gynecomastia and Kayser-Fleischer rings). Laboratory investigation might show a predominant elevation of the serum transaminases, prolonged prothrombin time which does not easily correct with vitamin K administration, or blood tests indicative of specific liver diseases.

Liver Disorders

Acute Hepatitis

Acute viral hepatitis is a syndrome of liver injury resulting from viral infection of the liver which by definition persists for less than 4 months. The clinical features of acute viral hepatitis are similar regardless of the etiology. Symptoms such as nausea, anorexia, abdominal pain, malaise, arthralgia, and fever, are common to all the etiologies of viral hepatitis. Findings on physical examination are also similar in the various forms of viral hepatitis. A detailed history may be suggestive, but is usually not conclusive for identifying the precise etiology. The viral etiologies of viral hepatitis can, therefore, only be distinguished by a series of sensitive and specific serological assays. Liver biopsy is usually not useful in acute hepatitis. In the majority of patients with acute viral hepatitis, the disease is asymptomatic and may only be detected in retrospect when antibodies are detected. In all cases, acute hepatitis is associated with elevation in serum aminotransferase activity; serum alkaline phosphatase, gamma glutamyl transferase and bilirubin levels may be elevated.

Hepatitis related to hepatic viruses A, B, C, D, and E is discussed in the following section (Table 45-3). Hepatitis may also be caused by other viruses such as Epstein-Barr virus (mononucleosis), cytomegalovirus, and herpes simplex virus.

Some etiologies of acute hepatitis, including viruses, can lead to chronic hepatitis, which is a term applied to liver disease that is protracted and necroinflammatory in nature. As a general rule, chronic hepatitis is defined as abnormal liver enzyme activity for at least a 6-month period. Such ongoing inflammation of the liver has the potential of culminating in cirrhosis. In addition to viruses, there are multiple other etiologies of chronic hepatitis including drugs, alcohol, Wilson's disease,

TABLE 45-3 Comparison of Features of the Three Common Forms of Acute Viral Hepatitis

	Hepatitis A	Hepatitis B	Hepatitis C
Virus	HAV	HBV	HCV
Source	Fecal-oral	Blood-borne	Blood-borne
Incubation	15–50 days	50–150 days	15–150 days
Chronicity	No, 0%	Yes, 10%	High, 50%
Antigens	HAV Ag	HB_s Ag HB_c Ag HB_e Ag	HCV Ag
Antibodies	Anti-HAV	Anti-HB_s Anti-HB_c Anti-HB_e	Anti-HCV

alpha$_1$ antitrypsin deficiency, hemochromatosis, autoimmunity, primary biliary cirrhosis, and primary sclerosing cholangitis. In some instances no specific etiology can be uncovered.

Hepatitis A (HAV) Hepatitis A, usually the least severe form of viral hepatitis, is caused by a small RNA virus. The epidemiology of hepatitis A is based on fecal-oral spread, and typically occurs as an outbreak. In the United States, epidemics are often traced to a common food source or to situations, such as institutional living or day-care, that facilitate this manner of spread. For those same reasons, hepatitis A is common among children in developing countries. It is generally an acute and self-limited illness, and although fulminant hepatic failure has been recorded, this is rare. There are no chronic carriers of hepatitis A. Virus appears in the blood stream at about the same time that symptoms commence, and can persist for up to 12 weeks. Virus does not persist thereafter; there is no chronic carrier state for hepatitis A. The detection of elevated titers of IgM anti-HAV indicates acute disease. A second antibody (IgG anti-HAV) appears approximately 3 months later and indicates immunity. Generally, no specific therapy is required other than supportive therapy. Corticosteroids may be useful if, as may occur rarely, there is a prolonged cholestatic phase. Gamma globulin provides short-term protection to close contacts.

Hepatitis B (HBV) This is a 42-μm DNA virus that consists of a central core which contains DNA, DNA polymerase, hepatitis B core antigen (HB$_c$ Ag), and hepatitis B$_e$ antigen (HB$_e$ Ag). This core is surrounded by an envelope of surface protein, hepatitis B surface antigen (HB$_s$ Ag). The interpretation of HBV serological tests is complex but clinically important. There are a few general guidelines for interpretation of these tests; complex cases often may need to be referred for interpretation. HB$_s$ Ag, the earliest marker, typically appears 4 to 12 weeks after infection. This is followed in sequence by the appearance of HB$_e$ Ag, IgM anti-HB$_c$, and subsequently, IgG anti-HB$_c$. HB$_s$ Ag indicates the presence of virus and that the patient is infected. Anti-HB$_s$ means the patient is immune. The detection of HB$_e$ Ag provides evidence of active viral replication. This replication stage can also be quantitated by an HBV DNA assay. The detection of IgM anti-HB$_c$ through an early antibody response does not indicate protection. IgM anti-HB$_c$ alone can be used to screen for acute hepatitis but this strategy could miss the very early stages of hepatitis B infection when HB$_s$ Ag alone will be detected. As the infection is resolving, there is seroconversion of HB$_e$ Ag to anti-HB$_e$ Ag, and seroconversion of HB$_s$ Ag to anti-HB$_s$ follows from a few weeks to several months later. IgM anti-HB$_c$ eventually disappears after the acute phase of the disease; however, IgG anti-HB$_c$ persists for years or perhaps for a lifetime.

Therapy for acute hepatitis B infection relies on supportive measures alone. The identification of chronic hepatitis B is based on the persistence of hepatitis B surface antigen for more than 6 months. Chronic disease can be treated with alpha-interferon (5 million units per day for 3 to 6 months), but only a small percentage of patients will be cured with interferon therapy.

A hepatitis B virus vaccine is now available that is safe, and the most effective means of preventing this disease.

Hepatitis C (HCV) Hepatitis C is a 55-μm RNA virus. There are several strains of this virus, some of which may differ in biological effects. This virus is transmitted parenterally and accounts for almost 95 percent of all cases of transfusion-related non-A, non-B hepatitis. The incubation period is 4 to 12 weeks but can be longer. Serum aminotransferase levels can be up to 10 to 20 times normal, but often demonstrate rather characteristic fluctuations in an individual patient. Approximately 50 percent of infected patients progress to develop chronic active hepatitis. Chronic infection can evolve to cirrhosis over a 10- to 20-year period, accompanied by a significant risk for the later development of hepatocellular carcinoma.

The hepatitis C antibody assay does not distinguish acute from chronic disease. Initial tests approved for the detection of hepatitis C detected antibody directed against a single epitope on HCV; second generation tests are now available which detect four antibodies with improved sensitivity.

Alpha interferon, 3 million units 3 times a week

for 24 weeks, is the current standard therapy for chronic HCV. However, recurrences and treatment failures are common. There is currently no vaccine available to prevent hepatitis C.

Hepatitis D (HDV) Hepatitis delta virus is a very small RNA virus that is a parasite of hepatitis B virus. The delta virus attaches itself to an HBV and requires its surface antigen coating to survive and multiply. This binding by delta virus may in turn prevent the detection of HB_s Ag. Hepatitis D virus should be suspected in patients with chronic hepatitis B who have negative HB_s Ag test results and persistent aminotransferase abnormality. Currently the only serologic marker for hepatitis delta virus is hepatitis delta virus antibody (HDV Ab).

Because hepatitis delta virus requires hepatitis B virus for replication, only populations at risk for B virus can be infected. HBV and HDV can be acquired simultaneously (coinfection) or sequentially (superinfection). Superinfection usually results in a chronic carrier state. Coinfection, in contrast, results in acute disease with resolution.

Alpha interferon is not active against this infection. The best strategy against this disorder is to prevent hepatitis B infection by vaccination.

Hepatitis E (HEV) This is another RNA virus that is spread by fecal-oral contamination. This virus has been responsible for water-borne epidemics, and for the most part, instances in the United States have been restricted to those who acquired infection in the course of overseas travel. This is usually an acute, self-limited disease which often has a prominent cholestatic phase. Pregnant women who acquire HEV have a high rate of fulminant hepatic failure. Serologic tests are not commercially available. There is no known therapy and no vaccine.

Chronic Liver Disease

Chronic Hepatitis Chronic hepatitis is a term applied to all liver disease that is protracted, generally greater than 6 months in duration, and necroinflammatory in nature. This disorder has the potential to develop into cirrhosis and possibly even to result in primary hepatocellular carcinoma. Chronic hepatitis is the consequence of numerous stimuli, differing mechanisms and sequelae, and responses to treatment that vary widely.

There are three main clinical circumstances that warrant consideration of the diagnosis of chronic hepatitis. 1. Persons with a previous history of acute viral hepatitis may continue to have elevated serum enzyme levels for longer than 6 months (see under Acute Hepatitis above for further details). 2. Patients may present with overt cirrhosis with portal hypertension or hepatic failure or with hepatocellular carcinoma. These individuals generally escape detection of the initial acute hepatitis because of the asymptomatic nature of the process. 3. The majority of patients with chronic hepatitis are identified when routine biochemical screening tests reveal abnormal aminotransferase activity.

A liver biopsy is required for a conclusive diagnosis of chronic hepatitis. There can be a wide variety of lesions of varying severity. Liver biopsy is important not only for diagnosis but for prognosis. The etiology of chronic hepatitis is heterogeneous in origin, consisting of viral, autoimmune, hepatotoxic, and metabolic disorders. It is imperative to distinguish the etiology of chronic hepatitis because prognosis and therapy vary accordingly.

The first step in any clinical evaluation involves obtaining a careful history. This should include family, social, travel, occupational, and medical history. Questions should address intravenous drug use; use of alcohol; sexual behavior; family history of liver, lung, neurologic, endocrine, or autoimmune diseases; travel; place of birth; workplace exposure to hepatotoxic chemicals; a complete medication summary including those medications used in the past; transfusions; needle sticks; acupuncture; tattooing; and previous history of jaundice or hepatitis. It is important to ask about current and past medications. The list of medications associated with chronic hepatitis is large and continues to grow. Some of the more common drugs implicated are listed in Table 45-4.

Physical examination should look for signs of chronic liver disease and of portal hypertension. Portal hypertension can manifest as ascites, esophageal varices, prominent hemorrhoids, caput medusa, and splenomegaly. Other stigmata of chronic liver

TABLE 45-4 Drugs Implicated as Causes for Chronic Hepatitis

Methyldopa
Sulfonamides
Nitrofurantoin
Dantrolene
Oxyphenisatin
Papaverine
Propylthiouracil
Isoniazid

disease include liver nails, palmar erythema, telangiectasias, and spider angioma.

Laboratory evaluation should include biochemical tests directed at defining the presence of liver disease such as total and direct serum bilirubin, AST, ALT, alkaline phosphatase, total serum proteins, serum albumin, protime, and hepatitis serologies as described in the section on acute viral hepatitis, above. Other specialized tests will be conducted once it has been concluded that chronic hepatitis probably exists. These tests will help identify the specific disease process inducing the chronic hepatitis. Examples would be: ordering a ceruloplasmin when evaluating for Wilson's disease or ordering a protein electrophoresis and Pi typing when looking for alpha$_1$ antitrypsin deficiency. Serum iron, transferrin saturation, and serum ferritin are used to further define hemochromatosis. Evaluation of chronic hepatitis is often best handled by a gastroenterologist. Liver biopsy may provide important pathologic clues for diagnosing the etiology of chronic hepatitis. Treatment will depend on the etiology of the chronic hepatitis.

Hemochromatosis Hemochromatosis is an autosomal recessive disorder of iron metabolism which leads to increased total body iron and excessive iron deposition in several organs. It can be either primary or secondary (e.g., due to excessive transfusion or excessive intake of iron, thalassemia, or other ineffective erythropoiesis/hemolysis syndromes). The classic tetrad of presentation is diabetes, cirrhosis, congestive heart failure, and bronze skin, all reflective of areas of iron deposition such as the pancreas, heart, liver, and skin. Hepatomegaly is almost invariably present. Hepatocellular carcinoma complicates the disease approximately 20 percent of the time. Iron studies show increased iron levels, transferrin saturation, and ferritin. Liver biopsy is still a standard of care for establishing the diagnosis and is useful for distinguishing primary from secondary forms. In hemochromatosis the total body iron is increased 5- to 10-fold and the standard of care is phlebotomy. One unit of blood will phlebotomize the equivalent of 250 mg of iron. Chelation therapy can be used for those patients who do not tolerate phlebotomy.

Wilson's Disease Wilson's disease is an autosomal recessive inherited disorder of copper metabolism that leads to accumulation of copper in tissues, including the liver, brain, eyes, skeleton, and kidneys. The clinical presentation is variable, but tends to be either hepatic or neurologic. Kayser-Fleischer rings are diagnostic. They may be absent when the patient presents with liver disease, but are always present when patients present with neurologic disease. Serum ceruloplasmin is typically low as is serum copper. Urine copper excretion is increased and liver copper is always elevated. Treatment is with copper chelation therapy, penicillamine.

Alpha$_1$ Antitrypsin Deficiency Alpha$_1$ antitrypsin deficiency is an inherited deficiency of serum protease inhibitor, variably associated with emphysema and liver disease. The protease inhibitor phenotype ZZ is the phenotype associated with clinical liver and lung disease. Orthotopic liver transplantation has been successful with patients with advanced liver disease.

Alcoholic Liver Disease Alcoholic liver disease has three major clinical pathologic settings: 1. alcoholic fatty liver, 2. alcoholic hepatitis, and 3. alcoholic fibrosis and cirrhosis. The clinical picture of cirrhosis is related to three separate entities: 1. portal hypertension, 2. loss of parenchymal function, and 3. extrahepatic injury produced by alcoholism. In advanced cirrhosis the chief manifestations result from portal hypertension, expressed as esophageal, gastric, or duodenal varices; splenomegaly; hypersplenism; and ascites. Hepatic encephalopathy is easily precipitated because of the distorted portal venous flow and inadequate parenchymal hepatic function. In patients with ascites, bacterial peritonitis is an easily overlooked and frequently fatal complication. The key to treatment is abstinence from alcohol and treatment of the complications of portal hypertension.

Primary Biliary Cirrhosis Primary biliary cirrhosis is a progressive, nonsuppurative, destructive intrahepatic cholangitis. It affects middle-aged women. Typically it presents as asymptomatic elevation in the alkaline phosphatase and it can present with pruritus, progressive jaundice, cirrhosis, or liver failure. Clinical manifestations more specific for primary biliary cirrhosis are xanthelasma and xanthomata and skin hyperpigmentation. Patients can have associated connective tissue diseases including Sjögren's syndrome and collagen vascular diseases. Diagnosis generally rests on the presence of an antimitochondrial antibody (AMA) and specific changes on liver biopsy.

Diarrhea: Differential Diagnosis and Treatment

Diarrhea can be defined as the "too frequent passage of too liquid stool." As a symptom, diarrhea can manifest as an increase in stool frequency, an increase in stool volume, or a decrease in stool consistency.

History and Differential Diagnosis

The frequency of bowel movements varies considerably in the general population, from three stools per week to three stools per day being normal, and it is considerably influenced by diet. In individuals on a typical American diet, diarrhea is defined as a stool weight in excess of 150 to 200 g per 24 h. In obtaining the history it is important to determine what is normal for each patient; recent changes often prove to be most significant. The clinical history is of paramount importance. If the duration of diarrhea is short, meaning less than 3 weeks, the diarrhea is most often infectious and the illness self-limiting. Chronic diarrheas, those of greater than 3 weeks duration, need complete investigation. Two major clinical distinctions need to be made when evaluating a patient complaining of diarrhea: 1. Is the diarrhea inflammatory or noninflammatory? 2. Is the diarrhea secretory or osmotic? Based on the answers to these questions four major clinical categories of diarrhea can be distinguished: 1. osmotic, 2. secretory, 3. inflammatory, and 4. functional (see also Inflammatory Bowel Disease, p. 494, and Irritable Bowel Syndrome, p. 514). This clinical categorization of diarrhea can be accomplished on the basis of clinical evaluation and two simple diagnostic tests.

On history, inflammatory diarrhea is characterized by frequent mucoid or bloody stools, at times accompanied by tenesmus, fever, and abdominal pain. Microscopic examination of a stool specimen typically reveals many fecal leukocytes and red blood cells. In contrast, in noninflammatory diarrhea, the diarrhea is watery, frequently of large volumes (over 1 liter per day) and blood and pus are absent. Abdominal pain and fever are also usually absent. The importance of examination of the stool smear for both the presence of fecal leukocytes and red blood cells is clear. White blood cells in the stool indicate the existence of an inflammatory process somewhere in the gastrointestinal tract.

There are several mechanisms involved in producing inflammation-induced diarrhea. The epithelium is stimulated to secrete by a variety of substances made by neutrophils, activated enteric nerves, and immune cells. Inflammatory reaction products may also lead to mucosal destruction, increased permeability, and nutrient malabsorption and maldigestion. Etiologies of inflammatory diarrhea include ulcerative colitis and Crohn's disease, antibiotic-associated colitis, radiation colitis, diverticulitis, and such infectious causes as shigella, campylobacter, salmonella, *E. coli,* and amoebiasis.

If diarrhea appears to be noninflammatory the next step in the evaluation is to determine whether the diarrhea is osmotic or secretory. The distinction is best made by measuring fecal sodium and potassium concentrations and osmolality, and then calculating the stool "anion gap." When requesting the stool osmolality assay, it is important to perform the test on a fresh stool sample. If the stool is allowed to sit for a period of time, bacteria will begin to act on the stool and this will change the osmolality. The sum of the measured sodium and potassium concentrations is multiplied by 2 to account for anions in the stool. If the stool osmolality exceeds that which can be accounted for by the measured electrolytes, then an osmolar gap exists and the diarrhea is defined as osmotic diarrhea. In secretory diarrheas, in contrast, stool osmolality is related almost entirely to the concentration of sodium and potassium and their related anions and an osmotic gap does not, therefore, exist. Secretory diarrhea tends to be of large volume, often greater than 1 liter per day, and continues during fasting, while osmotic diarrhea tends to be of smaller volume and ceases with fasting.

Osmotically induced diarrhea results when nonabsorbable ions or solutes are ingested or produced in the intestinal lumen. Since these solutes are not absorbed, they exert an osmotic force on the enterocytes resulting in water being drawn into the lumen and excreted. Causes of osmotic diarrhea include the ingestion of poorly absorbed solutes (prune juice, magnesium sulfate- and phosphate-containing laxatives, antacids, sorbitol, and sulfates), disaccharidase deficiency (e.g., lactase deficiency), maldigestion, pancreatic insufficiency, and any disorder of digestion or absorption that results in the intraluminal accumulation of unabsorbed carbohydrate.

Stimuli that drive the epithelium to actively secrete water and electrolytes result in secretory diarrhea. Infectious agents may cause secretory diarrheas by any one of four mechanisms: 1. the elaboration of an enterotoxin, such as occurs with cholera and *E. coli,* 2. the direct invasion of the intestinal epithelium, such as occurs with salmonella, shigella, and campylobacter, 3. the elaboration of cytotoxic substances, such as occurs with *Clostridium difficile,* some shigella species, and enterohemorrhagic *E. coli,* and 4. through an enteroadherent mechanism associated with a variety of *E. coli.* In addition to these bacterial agents, a number of protozoal agents and viruses may also be responsible. Examples include *Giardia, Cryptosporidia,* and *Microsporidia.* Peptides secreted by a variety of tumors can also cause secretory diarrhea. Examples include calcitonin from medullary carcinoma of the thyroid, serotonin from carcinoid tumors, gastrin in the Zollinger-Ellison syndrome, and vasoactive intestinal peptide (VIP) from ganglioneuromas. A number of luminal detergents also act as intestinal secretogogues, including bile acids, long-chain fatty acids, and certain laxatives. When the terminal ileum has been resected or severely damaged, such as in inflammatory bowel disease, unabsorbed bile salts and fatty acids are delivered into the colon, where they act as potent intestinal secretogogues, and result in the colonic secretion of electrolytes and water.

In the United States, the most common infectious causes of acute diarrhea are campylobacter, salmonella, shigella, enterohemorrhagic *E. coli, Giardia,* and a number of viruses. *Giardia* and bacteria should be sought initially by stool culture and three stool exams for ova and parasites. If this does not establish a diagnosis, a distal duodenal or jejunal biopsy and aspirate should then be obtained to further exclude *Giardia.* When an acute diarrhea develops in a hospitalized patient two specific etiologies must be considered: *Clostridium difficile* colitis (pseudomembranous colitis) or medication effects. Medication effects may be direct side effects (examples include methyl xanthines, beta blockers, antacids, antibiotics) or related to vehicles such as sorbitol and mannitol, which are common in various elixirs.

Treatment of Diarrhea

Treatment will, of course, depend on the etiology of the diarrhea, but should be mainly directed to preventing dehydration and restoring lost volume. This is frequently achieved with intravenous fluids; in many circumstances the same goal could be achieved with oral fluid and electrolyte therapy. The sodium substrate-coupled absorptive pathway is preserved in many diarrheal disorders and appropriate formulated solutions (such as Pedialyte) can take advantage of this intact absorptive pathway. Home remedies such as soda and fruit juices are suboptimal since they are generally deficient in electrolytes and poor replacements for diarrheal losses. Commercially available oral rehydration solutions are formulated to take advantage of the glucose sodium-coupled transport mechanism to stimulate sodium and thus water absorption. They are strongly recommended for use in adults as well as in children.

Constipation

Constipation is one of the most common gastrointestinal symptoms of patients seen in the general physican's office. A majority of patients will suffer from constipation at some point in their lives; however, it usually does not become a chronic, recurrent problem.

There is no one definition of constipation but one accepted definition of constipation is less than two or three bowel movements per week, or extreme straining with more than 25 percent of evacuation efforts. Simple measures such as dietary changes and fiber supplementation suffice in managing most patients.

A careful history is by far the most important method of delineating the problem. Important points in the patient's history include the onset of constipation and its duration. Severe constipation that has been lifelong often dating from early childhood suggests a congenital abnormality such as Hirschsprung's disease. Not infrequently, onset after an illness or traumatic event such as surgery will be noted. Diet and medications are also critical points to be examined. The use of medications, particularly laxatives, narcotics, and anticholinergics must be ascertained. The nature of the bowel movement must be outlined in some detail, including the frequency and timing of evacuation; time spent on the commode; alternate methods of evacuation (squatting, digital evacuation); color, consistency, and size of the stools; abdominal discomfort; and bleeding. Gynecologic disorders including urinary incontinence, cystocele, uterine prolapse, previous hysterectomy, endometriosis, and rectocele, and obstetric history are also factors to consider. Prior surgeries and anal-rectal complaints must be discussed. Child abuse or spouse abuse, sexual orientation, and anal receptive intercourse may all be significant factors.

On physical examination degree of abdominal distention and neurological examination, including sensation in the saddle area, must be assessed. The exam should also include a Valsalva maneuver as the physician checks for rectal prolapse. Especially in the parous woman, a large rectocele bulging into the vagina would be strongly suggestive of the etiology of constipation.

After a careful history and physical examination (including evaluation to make certain that the woman is not pregnant), a sigmoidoscopy and barium enema are usually done to rule out mechanical obstruction. Laboratory evaluation to rule out metabolic and endocrine disorders including hypercalcemia, hypothyroidism, and hypokalemia should be undertaken. If a history of infrequent defecation is noted, colonic transit may be measured by using radioopaque markers for assessment of transit time. No enemas or laxatives should be used during the transit study, and a written diary of bowel movements should be kept while markers are being evaluated by x-ray studies. A majority of patients assessed will show abnormal colonic transit. These patients with slow transit can further be subdivided into three groups. Most commonly colonic inertia is seen; transit seems to be delayed in the right colon or even throughout the entire colon. The left colon and rectosigmoid seem to be the areas of delay in hindgut dysfunction. In outlet dysfunction markers reach the rectum rapidly but stay there for long periods of time.

Anorectal manometry should be used to rule out short-segment Hirschsprung's disease in those patients in whom rectal retention seems to be the primary problem. Defecography (evacuation proctography) may also be used to assess relaxation and contractions or to identify rectoceles or intussusceptions that may interfere with evacuation. Defecography generally should be reserved for those patients whose symptoms indicate difficulty in evacuation of the rectum. In patients in whom colonic inertia is diagnosed by colonic transit studies, esophageal, gastric, and small intestinal motility should be evaluated to rule out one of the forms of chronic intestinal pseudoobstruction.

Most patients with constipation may be successfully treated with a conservative bowel management program consisting of a high-fiber diet, plenty of liquids, fiber supplementation (psyllium), and stool softener. A rigorous trial with this approach, and the occasional judicious use of laxatives such as milk of magnesia or enemas, is necessary for at least 3 to 6 months. Only a very small group of patients will not respond and will have no other identifiable etiology for their constipation. When anatomic abnormalities are found such as rectocele, these patients should be evaluated for surgical correction.

Colonic inertia rarely responds to cholinergic agents but cisapride, a relatively recently synthesized prokinetic agent, has been shown to be helpful in alleviation of constipation in some cases of colonic inertia. Surgery is quite useful in limited, clearly defined groups of patients, especially in those with short-segment Hirschsprung's disease.

Irritable Bowel Syndrome

This is a disease more commonly found in women. They are often middle aged or younger, and tend to be affluent. Affected patients have symptoms consisting primarily of abdominal discomfort and altered consistency of the stool, either recurrent diarrhea or recurrent constipation or most commonly, alternation between the two. This is a diagnosis of exclusion. The diagnosis requires that no anatomic or histologic explanations for the symptoms are found. Synonyms for irritable bowel syndrome include spastic colon, spastic colitis, and functional bowel disease. The term colitis actually should not be used since it implies inflammation and these patients do not have an inflammatory process.

The actual presentation varies from patient to patient, but usually includes abdominal distress which may vary from week to week in the same patient. These patients frequently complain of abdominal distention, flatulence, cramping, and belching. Their abdominal discomfort is most typically in the lower quadrants but is also seen in the left upper quadrant. It tends to be a diffuse type of discomfort and is not localized to one specific area. Patients with irritable bowel syndrome generally do not have pain that awakens them at night, and if diarrhea is one of their symptoms, the diarrhea is not nocturnal. Stool pattern and consistency are commonly diagnostic in their variability. Patients most frequently describe alternating constipation and diarrhea.

Typically patients will not have a bowel movement for several days followed by the frequent passage of hard stool, then passage of stools that the patient frequently describes as being wormlike, long, and accompanied by mucus. Bleeding is not a part of irritable bowel syndrome.

Physical exam is usually unremarkable except for perhaps lower quadrant tenderness to deep palpation. Since this syndrome is a diagnosis of exclusion, it is important to examine the colon with either a flexible sigmoidoscopy and barium enema or colonoscopy. Organic problems need to be excluded such as diverticular disease, inflammatory bowel disease, and microscopic or collagenous colitis.

This group of patients has documented abnormal motility tests in various parts of the gastrointestinal tract including the esophagus, small bowel, and colon. It is still debatable whether there is an underlying myoelectric abnormality in patients with irritable bowel syndrome. Studies suggest the volume of gas within the gastrointestinal tract in patients with irritable bowel syndrome is normal; however, the response to measured volumes of gas is abnormally perceived.

The mainstay of treatment of irritable bowel disease is a high fiber diet, and fiber supplementation such as bulking mucoloids (psyllium). The addition of antispasmodics is sometimes beneficial, whereas therapy with antispasmodics alone or with antidiarrheal agents is usually unsatisfactory. Reassurance is a key factor in the treatment process of patients with this disorder.

References and Selected Readings

1. McIntyre N, Benhomon JP, Bircher J, Rizzetto M, Rodes J (eds): *Oxford Textbook of Clinical Hepatology,* Oxford: Oxford University Press, 1991.
2. Sherlock S, Dooly J (eds): *Diseases of the Liver and Biliary System.* Oxford: Blackwell Scientific Publications, 1993.
3. Sleisenger MH, Fordtran JS (eds): *Gastrointestinal Disease.* 5th ed. Philadelphia: Saunders, 1993.
4. Wilson JD, Braunwald E, Isselbacher KJ, Petersdorf RG, Martin JB, Fauci ASi, Root RK (eds): *Harrison's Principles of Internal Medicine,* 12th ed. New York: McGraw-Hill, 1991.
5. Yamada T (ed): *Textbook of Gastroenterology.* Philadelphia: J.B. Lippincott, 1991.

46 The Acute Abdomen

Richard C. Pees
Rodrigue Mortel

The term acute abdomen is used when a patient presents with abdominal pain of sudden or gradual onset that increases in intensity over time. The pain may become diffuse or remain localized; frequently it is associated with nausea and emesis. Patients with an acute abdomen present a true diagnostic challenge. The underlying pathology may require either immediate surgical intervention or a period of close observation.

The perception and interpretation of pain are subjective and may be influenced by the patient's cultural, socioeconomic, and educational background. The level of anxiety and discomfort will be expressed differently in a stoic versus an hysterical individual. The physician's diagnostic task, however, can be made easier if there is a clear understanding of abdominal anatomy, neuroanatomy, and pathophysiology of disease.

There are several categories of abdominal pain. Visceral pain usually is poorly localized and is perceived as dull, burning, diffuse, waxing and waning, and/or crampy. Visceral pain fibers have their nerve endings in the parenchyma and walls of the various abdominal organs. They are sensitive to dilation/distention, stretch, and ischemia and are relatively insensitive to burning, cutting, compression, and crushing. Visceral pain frequently results in an autonomic response consisting of nausea, emesis, diaphoresis, hypotension, tachycardia, and diarrhea.[10]

Another category is somatic pain, which usually is perceived as sharper, knifelike, and well localized. These pain fibers are located in the mesentery and parietal peritoneum. The abdomen is a continuum, and pathology in one organ system frequently produces pain at distant locations.

The third category is referred pain. For example, subdiaphragmatic irritation secondary to a ruptured and/or bleeding ovarian cyst, intraabdominal bleeding or infection, or air under the diaphragm will be perceived by the patient as shoulder pain.

History

The evaluation of a patient with an acute abdomen requires answers to several questions. The ultimate goal is to characterize the nature, onset, location, severity, duration, quality, effect of activity, and radiation patterns of the abdominal pain. Answers to these questions coupled with knowledge of neuroanatomy and abdominal anatomy, will result in the development of an appropriate list of differential diagnoses.[3,13] A description of the sequence of events leading up to the onset of the pain is extremely helpful. It is also important to know whether the pain necessitated a change in the woman's lifestyle or activity. Particular attention should be paid to the pain patterns, which may provide important clues to the etiology.

It is essential to ascertain when the pain started and whether it was gradual or sudden in onset. The effect of meals, oral intake, changes in position, urination, and defecation should be assessed. Questions should be directed to determine where the pain is located; whether the pain is sharp, dull, knifelike, burning, tearing, crampy, ripping; how long the pain has been present; if there have been previous episodes of this pain; if there is any radiation pattern, and whether it is increasing or decreasing in intensity.

Pain that is sharp and sudden in onset tends to imply a potentially catastrophic event or disease process such as a ruptured viscus, ruptured ovarian cyst, or ruptured ectopic pregnancy. If the pain began suddenly and is severe, it is important to know if it began during intercourse or vigorous physical activity. Pain that is the result of inflammation usually is more gradual in onset, initially not as severe, and usually associated with a temperature elevation. If generalized peritonitis is present, the patient will be lying quite still and will tend to assume the fetal position, with legs drawn up toward the chest. Movement tends to exacerbate the pain when peritonitis is present.

A crampy type of pain is associated with muscular contractions, and is frequently seen in individuals with a partial small bowel obstruction, early complete bowel obstruction, ureteral calculi, enteritis/colitis, or biliary calculi. The location and radiation patterns of the pain will provide clues to the particular organ system involved. Epigastric and/or periumbilical pain is suggestive of small bowel origin; suprapubic pain implies large bowel, bladder, or reproductive organ origin; and flank/groin pain points to ureteral or kidney origin. Pancreatic pain usually is first perceived in the epigastric region and later radiates along the costal margins to the back.

The duration of the pain also is important. Pain that has been present for several hours and is intensifying implies a more severe process. The patient should be asked if there is any activity that exacerbates the pain. If the pain is relieved by simple measures such as antacids, and if there are no additional or associated symptoms, then the problem may be less important and may not require emergency therapy. If associated symptoms of diaphoresis, nausea, emesis, diarrhea, or chest discomfort are present, further evaluation is mandatory to rule out such catastrophic events as myocardial or pulmonary infarction, ruptured viscus, or severe peptic ulcer disease.

It is imperative that a complete menstrual history be obtained, including the date of the last menstrual period and whether it was normal in flow, duration, and timing. If the patient is sexually active, the method of birth control being used is very important, as well as whether birth control is being used regularly and correctly.

The patient also needs to be questioned about associated symptoms of nausea, emesis, diarrhea, constipation, last bowel movement, passage of flatus, chest pain or discomfort, shortness of breath, urinary tract symptoms (frequency, dysuria, burning, hematuria), hematemesis, hemoptysis, bloody or mucoid stools, loss of appetite, and anorexia. Emesis frequently occurs with small bowel obstruction, cholecystitis, appendicitis, and pancreatitis. It occurs within three to five hours following the onset of appendiceal pain, is present early and frequently in small bowel obstruction, and appears late or not at all in large bowel obstruction.[3] Anorexia is common with pancreatitis and appendicitis. Failure to pass flatus is common with complete bowel obstruction. Diarrhea, on the other hand, is common in individuals suffering from gastroenteritis, colitis, irritable bowel syndrome, and cyclically in those with endometriosis.

Additional inquiry should include a past history of abdominal surgery, drug allergies, prior similar episodes of this type of pain, current medications, any recent change in medications or ingestion of illegal substances, recent consumption of alcohol, and any history of abdominal trauma. A general review must address the following systems: cardiac, pulmonary, metabolic, and collagen. A myocardial infarction can present with upper epigastric pain and diaphoresis. Pneumonia and pulmonary emboli can cause diaphragmatic irritation and upper abdominal pain as well as shortness of breath, diaphoresis, fever, and tachycardia. Lupus and sickle cell crisis can precipitate an episode of acute abdominal pain.[3,10]

Persistent abdominal pain demands a thorough evaluation. A detailed history is critical in determining the cause of the acute abdomen. It should be remembered that a prior history of pelvic inflammatory disease (PID) does not rule out other etiologies for the pain.

Physical Examination

The examination of the patient with an acute abdomen begins by paying attention to how the patient is sitting or lying. Observe whether the patient is lying quietly, knees or hips flexed, pacing about, or agitated. Observe whether she appears pale, flushed, or diaphoretic. Examine the abdomen for surgical incisions, distention, erythema, and/or cutaneous lesions. Evaluate for tachycardia, hypotension, hypertension, tachypnea, and fever. Tachycardia implies a sympathetic reaction to severe pain via the release of catecholamines, hypovolemia, or severe dehydration. Hypotension is suggestive of sepsis or hypovolemia. Tachypnea may imply pneumonia, pulmonary emboli, or sepsis. Fever over 103°F suggests sepsis, pelvic abscess, pelvic inflammatory disease, pneumonia, early appendicitis, or pyelonephritis. Subnormal temperatures may occur in late sepsis, bowel gangrene, viscus perforation, pancreatitis, appendicitis, or pelvic inflammatory disease.[3,10,13]

Following visual inspection and review of the vital signs, direct examination of the abdomen is performed. The objective of this phase of the examination is to define the area of pathology and arrive at a diagnosis. Have the patient identify the area of most intense pain by asking her to outline that area with her finger. Then, auscultate the abdomen. Gently lay the stethoscope on the abdomen and listen to the quality of the bowel sounds. A silent abdomen or one with markedly decreased bowel sounds implies a complete bowel obstruction, severe peritonitis, or potentially a ruptured viscus. High-pitched and increased bowel sounds may imply an early bowel obstruction. The presence of a murmur may indicate the presence of arterial stenosis, aneurysm, or other vascular disease. A sense of the degree of tenderness can be gained by placing gentle pressure on the stethoscope while auscultating the abdomen.

Palpation of the abdomen should begin away from the point or area of maximum pain. Begin by applying light pressure and then gradually increasing this downward pressure. Evaluate for direct, rebound, and referred tenderness. Also evaluate for the presence or absence of guarding, rigidity, and masses. Rigidity may imply a ruptured viscus; rebound tenderness points toward an inflammatory process or peritonitis due to appendicitis, pancreatitis, cholecystitis, salpingooophoritis, or diverticulitis. Direct tenderness suggests an early inflammatory process, ruptured ovarian cyst or mass, or ectopic pregnancy—ruptured or unruptured. Percuss the abdomen to detect tympany, which may be due to a ruptured viscus or free air, dullness, and ascitic waves.

During the physical examination, the following maneuvers may be helpful in detecting an inflammatory process involving the peritoneum. If by flexing the thigh against the abdomen (iliopsoas sign), by rotating the flexed thigh internally (obturator sign), or by having the patient bounce on her heels (heel tap sign), severe pain is elicited, then the diagnosis of appendicitis, PID, diverticulitis, or peritonitis may be suspected. Likewise, push over the right costal margin while asking the patient to take a deep breath. If she stops the inspiration because of severe pain (Murphy's sign), then cholecystitis may be suspected.

Bimanual pelvic and rectal examination is essential. Is there discharge coming from the cervical os? Is the uterus enlarged, or are there unilateral or bilateral adnexal masses? Is there tenderness on cervical motion, or other pelvic tenderness? Is there a rectal tumor?

Examination of the heart, lungs, flanks, extremities, head, and neck is required to complete a thorough evaluation of a patient with an acute abdomen.

Laboratory Testing

The results of the following tests are often helpful in the evaluation of the patient:

CBC with differential
Urinalysis
Amylase
Liver function tests
Renal function tests
Electrolytes
Serum or urine pregnancy test
Abdominal/pelvic ultrasound

Additional testing that may be of some help includes:

Acute abdominal X-ray series to include the diaphragms
CT scan of abdomen and pelvis
Chest X-ray

Depending on the clinical level of suspicion regarding various potential etiologies in the differential diagnosis, a variety of other studies may also be appropriate.

Differential Diagnosis

At this point in the evaluation, a differential diagnosis should be possible (Table 46-1). This differential is developed through the knowledge of anatomy, pathophysiology, the history, and the physical examination.

The following discussion will be directed to the more common causes of an acute abdomen. Appendicitis and ectopic pregnancy will be discussed in some depth.

Generalized Peritonitis

These patients are lying quietly with their knees drawn up toward the chest. Movement makes the pain worse. The pain is relatively rapid in onset, usually localized at first, and then becoming diffuse. Tachycardia, hypotension, dehydration, hypoactive bowel sounds, and fever are present. Rebound tenderness is present to both percussion and palpation. WBC is elevated early, liver function tests are normal or mildly elevated, and amylase may be elevated. Treatment consists of identifying the cause, intravenous fluids, antibiotics, and on occasion a Foley catheter and nasogastric tube. Emergency surgery usually is required.

Perforated Ulcer

There is usually a history of prior ulcer disease. The pain is sudden in onset and sharp, usually starting in the epigastric area and then spreading over the entire abdomen. Shoulder pain may also be present. Nausea and emesis are common. The patient lies supine and avoids any undue motion. The abdomen is rigid and boardlike, with rebound in all quadrants. The bowel sounds are hypoactive to absent; tachycardia, tachypnea, hypotension, and shallow respirations are present. Serum amylase and WBC are elevated. Fever is usually present. The acute abdominal X-ray series is diagnostic, with free air under the diaphragm. Surgery is required.

Pancreatitis

This is a disease that is most common in patients 30 to 50 years old, and is usually associated with chronic alcoholism or biliary tract disease. Nausea, emesis, and anorexia are common. The pain usually begins over the epigastric area and rapidly increases in intensity. It radiates directly through to the back and around both costal margins. The patient appears acutely ill and lies quietly. There is severe tenderness to percussion and palpation, tachycardia, tachypnea, and fever. The amylase and WBC are elevated. Treatment includes hospitalization, intravenous fluids, nasogastric tube, and perhaps surgical drainage if a pseudocyst forms. Abdominal ultrasound and CT scan are very helpful in making the diagnosis.

TABLE 46-1 Differential Diagnosis of the Acute Abdomen

Right Upper Quadrant	Left Upper Quadrant
Pneumonia	Gastritis
Pulmonary emboli	Pulmonary emboli
Hepatic/subdiaphragmatic abscess	Pyelonephritis
Pyelonephritis	Renal calculi
Renal calculi	Diverticulitis
Peptic ulcer disease, perforation	Splenic flexure syndrome
Biliary disease	Splenic rupture
Myocardial infarction	Myocardial infarction
Pancreatitis	Mononucleosis
Appendicitis	Pneumonia
Congestive heart failure	Gastric ulcer disease
Fitz-Hugh Curtis syndrome	Perforation
Abdominal aortic aneurysm	Pancreatitis
Ischemic bowel	Abdominal aortic aneurysm
Intraperitoneal bleeding	Ischemic bowel
	Intraperitoneal bleeding
Right Lower Quadrant	**Left Lower Quadrant**
Appendicitis	Diverticulitis
Cholecystitis	Ureteral calculi
Diverticulitis	Colonic perforation
Cecal perforation	Volvulus
Ectopic pregnancy	PID with peritonitis
PID with peritonitis	Ectopic pregnancy
Ruptured ovarian mass/cyst	Ruptured ovarian mass/cyst
Tuboovarian abscess with peritonitis	Tuboovarian abscess with peritonitis
Mittelschmerz	Adnexal torsion
Ureteral calculi	Mittelschmerz
Mesenteric adenitis	Abdominal aortic aneurysm
Abdominal aortic aneurysm	Ischemic bowel
Ischemic bowel	Intraperitoneal bleeding
Intraperitoneal bleeding	
Regional enteritis	
Meckel's diverticulitis	

Diverticulitis

This problem is commonly seen in the fifth or sixth decade of life. The patient usually has a history of diverticulosis. Left lower quadrant tenderness and perhaps a mass are present. Nausea is common. WBC is elevated and the urinalysis contains many WBCs. Patients with diverticulitis occasionally are clinically misdiagnosed as having an ovarian cancer. CT scan is the most useful diagnostic test. Hospitalization usually is required.

Cholecystitis

This problem most commonly occurs in women in their 30s to 60s. The pain of cholecystitis commonly starts a few hours after a large meal. Fatty foods tend to make the episodes of pain worse. Nausea and emesis are common. Anorexia is not common. The pain begins in the RUQ and may radiate to the scapula or shoulder. Mild elevations of temperature (99 to 101°F), WBC, and the serum bilirubin are common. There may be mild abdominal distension.

Deep inspiration increases the pain, and a RUQ mass may be felt. Ultrasound is diagnostic. Hospitalization and intravenous antibiotics may be required. Surgical removal usually is required.

Small Bowel Obstruction

The pain usually begins suddenly, is sharp and colicky, and starts periumbilically. The patient usually is pain-free between attacks. There is usually a prior history of abdominal surgery. Nausea and emesis are common. Emesis is frequent in a high obstruction; early emesis is greenish in color and later becomes brownish with a fetid odor. Bowel sounds are high-pitched and come in rushes early; later the bowel sounds are hypoactive or absent. Lower abdominal cramping suggests a distal obstruction. Tachycardia, hypotension, increased hematocrit (from dehydration), elevated WBC, and fever (99 to 103°F) are present. Acute abdominal X-ray series is diagnostic and reveals dilated loops of bowel with air-fluid levels and no gas in the colon. Progression of crampy abdominal pain and hypoactive-to-absent bowel sounds with abdominal distention suggest bowel strangulation, perforation, and generalized peritonitis. Hospitalization, intestinal tube suction, intravenous hydration, antibiotics, and surgical exploration are required.[3] If nonsurgical management of small bowel obstruction does not succeed, it is essential that the physician be vigilant to insure that surgery is undertaken before bowel perforation occurs.

Large Bowel Obstruction

This disease process usually occurs in those over age 40. There is a gradual onset of pain, constipation, absence of flatulence, and abdominal distention. Nausea and emesis occur late, if at all. Tachycardia, tachypnea, and severe pain are absent unless perforation occurs. The hematocrit and WBC frequently are normal. The abdomen is distended and tympanitic. Common causes are carcinoma, diverticulitis, and volvulus. Acute abdominal X-ray series and/or CT scan are diagnostic. A left lower quadrant mass may be felt on abdominal and rectal examination. Hospitalization and surgical management are required.

Pelvic Inflammatory Disease

This category includes salpingitis, salpingooophoritis, and tuboovarian abscess. The initial episode may be mild and go unrecognized, or it may produce severe symptoms. There is usually a history of recent sexual activity or a new partner. The pain usually begins as mild and then intensifies over the course of 24 h. In severe cases, the pain is bilateral. Nausea and gradual loss of appetite are common. There may be a low-grade fever in mild cases or a fever of over 103°F in severe cases and in cases of tuboovarian abscesses. The patient usually lies still and shuffles when she walks. There will be bilateral (occasionally unilateral) lower quadrant direct and rebound tenderness. There may or may not be a mass present. WBC and ESR are generally elevated, and the pelvic examination elicits cervical motion tenderness and adnexal tenderness. The bowel sounds are hypoactive. A pelvic ultrasound is diagnostic in cases of tuboovarian abscess. Hospitalization and intravenous antibiotics are essential if tubal damage is to be minimized and fertility preserved. Recurrent episodes are common; if a tuboovarian complex forms, surgical removal is often required. Rupture of a tuboovarian abscess is a surgical emergency.

Adnexal Torsion

The history will reveal prior intermittent attacks of crampy pain. The onset of the pain usually coincides with an abrupt change in position or with vigorous activity and is sudden and unilateral. This pain will become constant and more severe over the course of a few hours. As the process progresses, nausea and emesis are common, and a low-grade fever and leukocytosis develop. This sequence of events should lead to the suspicion of tissue hypoxia and infarction. Physical examination will reveal unilateral tenderness and a mass. Treatment is often surgical removal of the affected adnexa, although if torsion has occurred but there is no tissue necrosis, sometimes the adnexa can be untwisted at surgery and salvaged. Common causes of adnexal torsion include large (>10 cm) ovarian masses/cysts, dermoid cysts, or a corpus luteum of pregnancy. Torsion of a pedunculated myoma results in the same symptoms and physical findings, and frequently requires removal of the pedunculated myoma.

Appendicitis

Appendicitis is a common disease and occurs over 250,000 times per year in the United States. It is slightly more common in males than in females, with a peak incidence in the teens and 20s. The incidence declines thereafter, and the disease is relatively uncommon in the 40s and 50s. The diagnosis of appendicitis is extremely difficult to make in the very young and very old. Under the best of circumstances, when the individual fulfills all the classic symptoms and signs of appendicitis, the diagnostic accuracy as confirmed by surgical and pathologic findings is only 70 to 90 percent.[5–7] The symptoms vary according to the location of the appendix, coexisting disease, age of the patient, and whether or not perforation has occurred.[3] For example, a retrocecal appendix may cause right upper quadrant pain; a pregnant uterus will cause rotation of the point of maximum tenderness upwards toward the right upper quadrant.[14]

Classic abdominal pain in appendicitis usually begins in the periumbilical area and migrates toward the right lower quadrant. Atypical location of the abdominal pain is quite common.[1] Nausea, emesis, and anorexia are frequently associated symptoms. Physical examination reveals RLQ direct and rebound tenderness. Bowel sounds may be hypoactive. A mild fever may be present and the WBC may be elevated or normal early in the course of the disease. The hematocrit usually is normal. The urinalysis is usually normal, or may reveal a few WBCs if the inflammatory process overlies the ureter. A rectal examination is essential in the evaluation of a patient with suspected appendicitis and may reveal a mass. Acute abdominal X-ray series usually are not very useful. Abdominal ultrasound and CT scanning may be more diagnostic. A barium enema also may be of value.

The differential diagnosis must include such other etiologies as: acute gastroenteritis, Meckel's diverticulum, mesenteric adenitis, salpingitis, ruptured ovarian cyst/endometrioma/mass, ectopic pregnancy, torsion of the adnexa, mittelschmerz, regional enteritis, and ureteral calculi.[1] Ovarian events often can be differentiated from appendicitis by taking a good menstrual and sexual history, performing a culdocentesis, and obtaining a pelvic ultrasound study. Ureteral calculi usually produce severe colicky pain, and urinalysis reveals multiple red and white cells. An acute abdominal series may reveal the calculi, or the CT scan will show a dilated ureter and the calculi.

Surgical exploration is needed. Laparoscopic evaluation results in earlier diagnosis, lower morbidity, and quicker return to full functional status. Early laparoscopic evaluation can yield a negative appendectomy rate of 2.2 percent.[5–7]

Ectopic Pregnancy

The incidence of ectopic pregnancy in the United States increased approximately fourfold between 1970 and 1989. Ectopic pregnancy occurs in 16.1/1000 pregnancies. Although the maternal mortality rate has decreased by 90 percent, mortality from ectopic pregnancies accounts for 10 percent of maternal deaths.[4] Extrauterine pregnancy is 50 times as likely to lead to maternal death as is a therapeutic first-trimester abortion and 10 times as likely to result in a maternal death as a full-term vaginal delivery. The usual causes of death in a woman with an ectopic pregnancy are related to hemorrhage, infection, delay in diagnosis, misdiagnosis, and anesthesia complications.[2] The substantial decrease in mortality is related to earlier detection, use of a more sensitive radioimmunoassay for beta HCG, development of sensitive vaginal ultrasound, and a higher index of suspicion.[8]

Certain risk factors are known to be associated with an increased incidence of ectopic pregnancy. The most significant is previous PID or salpingitis. Any infection that causes damage to the tubal epithelium increases the probability that a fertilized ovum will implant at a site other than the endometrial cavity.[8] Laparoscopically proven PID increases the risk of an ectopic pregnancy sixfold, and history of a prior ectopic pregnancy increases the risk by tenfold.[2] Other possible risk factors include endometriosis, prior or current IUD usage, advanced maternal age, progestin-only birth control pills, transmigration of the fertilized ovum, tubal reconstructive surgery, and assisted reproductive techniques.

The classic presentation is pelvic pain, an adnexal mass, and amenorrhea. Only about 14 percent of women present with this classic triad. Common presenting symptoms and signs are listed in Table 46-2.[9,11]

The history is suggestive of pregnancy, potentially including such factors as breast tenderness, nausea, urinary frequency, fatigue, unprotected intercourse, and an abnormal last menstrual period. If the patient is on oral contraceptives, there may be a history of missing a few pills. The last menses usually is late and shorter than usual. A spotty type of bleeding often is present. The examination may or may not reveal an adnexal mass or tenderness. Usually direct tenderness is present; if rupture has occurred, there will be rebound tenderness. The WBC will commonly be normal; the hematocrit will be normal unless significant hemorrhage has occurred. Use of a sensitive radioimmune assay for beta HCG is essential for early diagnosis. If the HCG titer is above 1500 mIU/ml, transvaginal ultrasound usually will detect an intrauterine gestational sac. More than 6500 mIU/ml is necessary to detect an intrauterine gestational sac when using an abdominal transducer.[8] The probability of an ectopic pregnancy with a positive culdocentesis and positive beta HCG is 86 to 99 percent. A positive culdocentesis is the return of nonclotting blood (hematocrit >35 percent) from the posterior cul-de-sac.[9] Positive culdocentesis also can be present with ruptured ovarian cysts, retrograde menstruation, endometriosis, adnexal torsion, and intraabdominal bleeding of unknown origin.

TABLE 46-2 Presentation of Ectopic Pregnancy

Symptoms	Percent
Abdominal pain	80–95
Abnormal bleeding	50–85
Amenorrhea	30–70
Symptoms of pregnancy	20–30
Syncope/faintness	6–40
Shoulder pain	5–22
Passage of tissue	6–10
Signs	**Percent**
Abdominal tenderness	85–98
Adnexal tenderness	85–95
Peritoneal signs	70–75
Adnexal mass	30–50
Enlarged uterus	6–30
Shock	2–20

Once the diagnosis of ectopic pregnancy is made, the two treatment options are medical and surgical.

Medical treatment of ectopic pregnancy is a much more recent development and is less commonly utilized. It consists of the use of methotrexate and citrovorum factor rescue. Contraindications for medical therapy include: an uncertain diagnosis, a gestational sac >3.5 cm, presence of fetal cardiac activity, poor patient compliance, active peptic ulcer disease, abnormal SGOT, active hepatic or renal disease, active bleeding, abdominal or pelvic pain, and hemodynamic instability.

Surgical options consist of laparoscopy or laparotomy. Laparoscopy is possible if the patient is hemodynamically stable, the size of the ectopic is <6 cm, hemoperitoneum is absent or small, an interstitial pregnancy is not present, and the surgeon has the necessary laparoscopic skills.[9] Linear salpingostomy, segmental resection, or salpingectomy are all accepted methods with either laparoscopy or laparotomy. Beta HCG titers must be followed until they are <10 mIU/ml.

Most ectopic pregnancies are located in the fallopian tube: ampullary, 78 percent; isthmic, 12 percent; interstitial, 2 to 3 percent; fimbrial, 5 percent; ovarian, <0.5 percent; cervical, <0.5 percent; and abdominal, 0.1 to 0.2 percent. Rupture usually occurs at 6 to 8 weeks in isthmic ectopic pregnancies, 8 to 10 weeks in ampullary ectopic pregnancies, and 8 to 16 weeks in interstitial ectopic pregnancies. If the patient is Rh negative, then RhoGam must be administered.

Systemic and Other Disorders

Other problems, including systemic diseases, may cause an acute abdomen. The following is a brief list of the more common causes: familial Mediterranean fever, lower lobe pneumonia, pseudomembranous colitis, pyelonephritis, sickle cell crisis, diabetic ketoacidosis, lead poisoning, and porphyria.[3,10]

References and Selected Readings

1. Coudon RE, et al: Appendicitis, in Sabiston DC Jr: *Textbook of Surgery.* Philadelphia: WB Saunders, 1991, pp 884–898.
2. DeCherney A, et al: Ectopic pregnancy, in Sciarra JJ (ed): *Gynecology and Obstetrics,* vol 2, chap 25. Philadelphia: JB Lippincott, 1991, pp 1–17.
3. Diethelm AG, Stanley RJ: The acute abdomen, in Sabiston DC Jr (ed): *Textbook of Surgery.* Philadelphia: WB Saunders, 1991, pp 736–755.
4. Centers for Disease Control: Ectopic pregnancy—United States. *MMWR* 41:591–595, 1992.
5. Graham A, et al: Laparoscopic evaluation of acute abdominal pain. *J Laparoscop Surg* 1(3):165–168, 1991.
6. MacFadyen BV, et al: Laparoscopic management of the acute abdomen, appendix, and small and large bowel. *Surg Clin North Am* 72(5):1169–1183, 1992.
7. Maxwell JM: Appendicitis. Improvements in diagnosis and treatment. *Am Surg* 57(5):282–285, 1991.
8. Montgomery-Rice V, et al: New options for the diagnosis and treatment of ectopic pregnancy. *Female Patient* 18:31–46, 1993.
9. Seigler A: Salpinotomy and salpingectomy: Indications and techniques for tubal pregnancy, in Sciarra JJ (ed): *Gynecology and Obstetrics,* vol 1, chap 68. Philadelphia: JB Lippincott, 1991, pp 1–8.
10. Shea DJ, et al: Abdominal pain, in Schwartz GR (ed): *Principles and Practice of Emergency Medicine.* Malvern, PA: Lea & Febiger, 1992, pp 374–388.
11. Stabile I, et al: Ectopic pregnancy: A review of incidence, etiology and diagnostic aspects. *Obstet Gynecol Surv* 45(6):335–347, 1990.
12. Stovall T, et al: Methotrexate treatment of unruptured ectopic pregnancy: A report of 100 cases. *Obstet Gynecol* 77(5):749–753, 1991.
13. Trott AT: Nontraumatic acute abdominal pain, in Rose P, et al: *Emergency Medicine,* St. Louis: CV Mosby, 1983, pp 1025–1035.
14. Varner M: General medical and surgical diseases in pregnancy, in Scott JR (ed): *Danforth's Obstetrics and Gynecology.* Philadelphia: JB Lippincott, 1990, pp 495–534.

47 Endocrine Disorders

Fred Benjamin

The physician responsible for the primary health care of women will frequently encounter disorders which are basically endocrine in origin. Many of these diseases occur in men as well, but the clinical presentation is often different in women and of particular importance to the female patient. For example, a large number of the endocrinopathies affect menstrual function so that the woman's chief complaint is frequently a menstrual disorder. Likewise, hormonal disorders associated with hyperandrogenism are often of much more concern to women because the manifestations will include the disturbing symptom of hirsutism.

This chapter will review the commonly occurring endocrine disorders that are encountered in women, how they present to the primary care physician, and the manner in which they can be recognized, diagnosed, and treated in the office setting. Thyroid disease, pituitary disorders, adrenal disorders, pheochromocytoma, carcinoid syndrome, hirsutism, metabolic bone disease, and parathyroid disorders will all be considered. However, some concerns which have a large endocrine component, such as the physiology of menstruation, menstrual disorders, normal and abnormal sexual development, the special needs of adolescents, infertility, and menopause are reviewed elsewhere in this book and will therefore not be dealt with in this chapter.

Thyroid Disease

Thyroid disease is of particular importance in the primary health care of women because practically all thyroid disorders, both benign and malignant, are much more common in women than in men. Hyperthyroidism is about 5 times, and hypothyroidism about 10 times more frequent in females than in males.

Thyroid disease usually presents itself to the clinician in one of three ways: 1. hypothyroidism, 2. hyperthyroidism, or 3. enlargement of the thyroid gland (thyromegaly or goiter). An understanding of these disorders presupposes a basic knowledge of the anatomy, physical examination, and physiology of the thyroid gland, as well as an understanding of the thyroid function tests.

Thyroid Anatomy and Physical Examination

Embryologically the thyroid gland is formed from the thyroglossal duct which migrates from the pharynx down into the neck. The gland consists of two lobes, one on either side of the trachea, each being 2 to 3 cm in length and 1 cm in width; the lobes are joined by a narrow isthmus which crosses the trachea just below the cricoid cartilage. Physical examination of the thyroid gland should begin by inspection both before and during swallowing. Palpation is best accomplished with the patient seated and the clinician standing behind. With the first three fingers on either side of the trachea at the level of the cricoid cartilage, the thyroid gland is readily identified by the fact that it moves up and down with swallowing. Normally it is readily palpated and may even be visible in thin patients.

Histologically the thyroid is composed of rounded follicles lined by cuboidal cells and filled with colloid, the storage form of thyroglobulin which is secreted by the thyroid cells. Iodide is incorporated into the amino acid tyrosine in thyroglobulin at one site to form monoiodotyrosine, or at two sites to form di-iodotyrosine. Monoiodotyrosine and di-iodotyrosine are then joined to form the active hormones tri-iodothyronine (T3) or tetraiodothyronine or thyroxine (T4); monoiodotyrosine plus di-iodotyrosine form tri-idothyronine, and di-iodotyrosine plus di-iodotyrosine form tetraiodothyronine.

The thyroid gland secretes 20 times more T4 than T3, but 30 percent of the T4 is converted in the periphery to T3, and 40 percent to inactive reverse T3. The action of thyroid in the body is mainly due to T3, because the thyroid hormone receptors have a 10-fold higher affinity for T3 than T4. However, the blood level of T3 is not a good reflection of thyroid function because: 1. T3 has a much shorter half-life than T4 (7 h versus 7 days), and 2. T3 is formed mainly in the periphery.

Thyroid Physiology

Thyroid hormone production within the thyroid gland is stimulated by thyroid stimulating hormone (TSH), secreted by the anterior pituitary gland. If the thyroid levels increase, TSH secretion is inhibited, a negative feed-back mechanism. Thyroid hormone has two major functions: 1. it increases protein synthesis in all body tissues (T3 and T4 enter cells, bind to nuclear receptors and influence the formation of RNA), and 2. it increases oxygen consumption.

Thyroid Function Tests

Total Serum T4 (Thyroxine) This is measured very accurately by radioimmunoassay (RIA), but this assay measures both the free (active) T4 and the bound T4. Thyroid binding globulin is increased by pregnancy, estrogen therapy, and hypothyroidism, and is decreased by androgen, hyperthyroidism, and obesity. The normal level is about 5 to 12 μg/dl.

Total Serum T3 This is measured by radioimmunoassay (RIA) and is normally about 80 to 200 ng/dl.

Free T4 and Free T3 Theoretically these determinations are the most valuable tests because they measure the active forms of thyroid hormone. However, these assays are difficult and expensive, and are therefore only really required in situations where changes in thyroid binding globulin are expected, e.g., pregnancy or birth control pills.

Thyroid Stimulating Hormone Thyroid stimulating hormone (TSH) used to be measured by RIA, but the drawback was insensitivity in the lower ranges. The development of monoclonal antibodies to TSH of high specificity has allowed the development of a sensitive TSH assay that is useful in testing for both hypo- and hyperthyroid states.[7] The normal values are 0.4 to 4.8 μU/ml.

TRH Stimulation Test When a bolus of 500 μg TRH is given to a normal person the serum TSH increases 2 to 5 times above baseline and by at least 6 μU/ml 30 min after the injection. In hyperthyroidism there is a blunted or absent response to TRH. This test was used to diagnose mild hyperthyroidism, but has now been replaced by the new sensitive monoclonal antibody TSH assay.

Thyroid Antibodies Two thyroid antibodies are used in studying patients with thyroid disease: thyroglobulin antibodies and microsomal antibodies. They are both positive in essentially all patients with Hashimoto's thyroiditis and in patients with Graves' disease.

Radioactive iodine (RAI) uptake A tracer dose of RAI is given and a count is taken over the thyroid gland 6 and 24 h later. Its main value is to determine whether a thyroid nodule is active or "hot" (i.e., benign) or inactive or "cold" (i.e., a tumor, potentially malignant).

Hypothyroidism

Etiology The most common type of hypothyroidism is "primary hypothyroidism" where the disorder is in the thyroid gland itself. "Secondary hypothyroidism" is rare and is due to lack of secretion of TSH by the pituitary or inadequate production of TSH-RH by the hypothalamus. The most common cause of primary hypothyroidism is Hashimoto's thyroiditis, an autoimmune disease which results in gradual destruction of the thyroid gland; it is 10 times more common in women than in men.[9] The second most common cause of primary hypothyroidism is posttherapeutic, following RAI therapy or surgery.

Symptoms Fatigue, lethargy, weakness, cold intolerance, weight gain, constipation, and menorrhagia are common symptoms; forgetfulness, intellectual impairment, and even frank psychosis (called "myxedema madness") may occur.

Signs Weight gain, bradycardia, cardiac enlargement and pericardial effusion, edema, slow relaxation of deep tendon reflexes, and hypercholesterolemia may occur. There may be loss of pubic, axillary, and scalp hair and hair of the lateral aspects of the eyebrows.

Diagnosis The thyroid gland may or may not be enlarged. The key to the diagnosis is an elevated TSH, and in the later stages, a low T4. In the most common type of hypothyroidism, Hashimoto's thyroiditis, there will always be thyroglobulin and microsomal antibodies present.

Treatment Thyroid replacement, usually for life, is required. Three forms of thyroid have been used: 1. Desiccated thyroid from animal sources (e.g., Thyrolar). This is not recommended because it is not standardized, and contains variable proportions of T3 and T4. The dose is 1 to 3 gr/day. 2. Synthetic T3, i.e., tri-iodothyronine (e.g., Cytomel). This is also not recommended because it has a short half-life of 7 h; accordingly, the serum concentrations are labile and are difficult to monitor, and at times there is hyper- and at other times hypothyroidism. 3. Synthetic thyroxine, i.e., T4 or tetraiodothyronine (e.g., Synthroid) is the best choice for therapy. It has a long half life of 7 days, and therefore the serum levels are stable and can be monitored at any time of the day. The average dose required is 0.1 to 0.15 mg/day (100 to 150 μg). Treatment should be started with 0.05 mg (i.e., 50 μg/day) and gradually increased by 25 μg every 4 weeks; rapid treatment may result in cardiac failure because of the cardiac effects of hypothyroidism. Response to treatment should be monitored by serum TSH levels; the aim is to achieve normal TSH levels (0.4 to 4.8 μU/ml) with normal or slightly elevated T4 values (5 to 12 μg/dl).

Hyperthyroidism

Etiology By far the most common cause of hyperthyroidism is Graves' disease (or toxic diffuse goiter), an autoimmune disease characterized by hyperthyroidism with goiter, exophthalmos, and pretibial myxedema. It is due to circulating thyroid stimulating immunoglobulins or thyroid stimulating antibodies which specifically stimulate the TSH receptors. The exophthalmos and pretibial myxedema are due to the autoimmune disease, the immunoglobulins causing inflammatory changes in these areas. Other less common causes of hyperthyroidism are: 1. Toxic solitary nodule or toxic multinodular goiter where one or more nodules function autonomously, producing thyroid hormones; they are treated surgically or with radioactive iodine. 2. Various forms of thyroiditis often begin with a hyperthyroid phase. 3. T3 thyrotoxicosis: here there are symptoms of hyperthyroidism, but the T4 is normal; this is difficult to diagnose, because the T3 is not ordinarily measured in patients presenting with hyperthyroidism. 4. Secondary hyperthyroidism due to overproduction of TSH by a tumor of the pituitary, embryonal carcinoma or choriocarcinoma (due to the TSH-like properties of chorionic gonadotropin), or to struma ovarii of the ovary producing thyroid hormones.

Symptoms The more frequent symptoms of hyperthyroidism are nervousness, increased sweating, heat intolerance, palpitations, fatigue, weight loss, and frequent bowel movements.

Signs The common signs are goiter, tremor, warm moist skin, and tachycardia. In addition, in Graves' disease there are exophthalmos and pretibial myxedema.

Diagnosis Diagnosis is made by the symptoms and signs, a high T4 and low TSH (and if the T4 is normal, an elevated T3).

Treatment a. *Propranolol (Inderal)* For the acute symptoms due to the adrenergic stimulation effects of hyperthyroidism (tremor, tachycardia, diaphoresis, and mental symptoms) the beta-adrenergic antagonist, propranolol, is very effective. It is used in thyroid storm and as an adjunctive therapy with antithyroid medications. The dose is 10 mg bid to 80 mg 4 times daily.

b. *Thiourea Drugs* Propylthiouracil and methimazole interfere with thyroid hormone synthesis (by blocking the organification of iodide).[3] A maintenance dose of 100 mg propylthiouracil daily, or methimazole 10 mg daily, is given for 1 to 2 years. There is a high recurrence rate of 50 to 80 percent on discontinuing the medication, but there is less posttherapy hypothyroidism than with RAI or surgery. Propylthiouracil is preferred during pregnancy because it crosses the placenta much less readily than methimazole.

c. *Radioactive Iodine* Radioactive iodine (^{131}I) is usually used in patients past their childbearing years, because of concerns about possible effects to any subsequent offspring, such as birth defects and neoplasia. However, extensive studies have failed to show such effects. Accordingly, there has been an increasing tendency to use RAI in younger patients, because it is easy to administer, can be given to outpatients, avoids surgery, is 100 percent effective if given in adequate dosage, and has no complications except hypothyroidism. This has an increasing incidence as time goes by, eventually reaching as high as 80 percent.

d. *Surgery* In experienced hands surgery is safe and effective and achieves euthyroidism rapidly. It is particularly indicated: 1. if the thyroid is very large; 2. if the patient is young and should not receive radioactive iodine; 3. if the patient has a toxic adenoma or toxic multinodular goiter; and 4. during pregnancy if the disease is not adequately controlled.

e. *Iodine* In pharmacologic doses iodide (3 drops of saturated potassium iodide tid or qid) rapidly inhibits the release of T4 and T3, inhibits the organification of iodine for a few days to a week, and decreases the vascularity of the thyroid gland. It is very helpful for situations in which a rapid response is required, e.g., thyroid storm or thyrotoxic patients undergoing emergency surgery.

f. *Thyroid Storm* This is a life-threatening emergency that can occur in patients with Graves' disease and is usually precipitated by infection, trauma, surgery, or toxemia of pregnancy. There is a sudden onset of acute thyrotoxicosis with fever, marked weakness, restlessness, confusion, and even coma, cardiovascular collapse, and shock. It is treated with iodine, propylthiouracil, propranolol, I.V. hydration and electrolytes, and if necessary cortisone.

Enlargement of the Thyroid Gland (Thyromegaly, Goiter)

Most pathologic states of the thyroid gland present as a diffuse or nodular enlargement of the gland. The various forms of hyperthyroidism and hypothyroidism discussed previously may have goiter. Other causes of thyroid enlargement are the following:

Euthyroid Goiter This is also known as simple, endemic, nontoxic, or colloid goiter. There is enlargement of the thyroid gland due to diminished thyroid hormone production, but there is no evidence of clinical hypothyroidism. It can be due to iodine deficiency, increased demand for thyroid (at puberty, during pregnancy or the menopause), or due to foods or medications that block the synthesis of thyroid hormone. Compensatory TSH elevations occur, preventing hypothyroidism, but causing enlargement of the thyroid gland in the process. An attempt should be made to identify the cause and to treat it, e.g., iodine deficiency. Levothyroxine may be necessary to suppress the TSH and decrease the goiter. Surgery may be necessary for very large goiters.

Silent Thyroiditis Mild transient enlargement of the thyroid may occur in the postpartum period, lasting from a few weeks to a few months. It may be associated with mild hyperthyroidism, but usually recovers spontaneously. The cause is undetermined but may be an autoimmune phenomenon.

Thyroid Cancer Thyroid cancer usually presents as a symptomless lump in the neck. There are four types of thyroid cancer: 1. papillary carcinoma is the most common (70 percent) and the least aggressive; 2. follicular, accounting for about 15 percent of cases; 3. medullary, about 5 percent; and 4. anaplastic, which is rare. Diagnosis is made by biopsy, and treatment is surgical. Suppressive doses of thyroid hormone may be given to prevent regrowth, and in some cases postoperative radioiodine may be advised.

Pituitary Disorders

Physiology

Some knowledge of the basic physiology of pituitary function is essential for an understanding of the causes, work-up, and management of pituitary disorders.

Seventy-five percent of the mass of the pituitary gland comprises the anterior pituitary, and 25 percent the posterior pituitary. The posterior pituitary is an extension of the hypothalamus, and consists of nerve tissue which serves as a storage site for two peptide hormones synthesized by the hypothalamus, namely, vasopressin and oxytocin. The anterior pituitary synthesizes and secretes six major polypeptide hormones: adrenocorticotropic hormone (ACTH), thyroid stimulating hormone (TSH), luteinizing hormone (LH), follicle stimulating hormone (FSH), prolactin (PRL), and growth hormone (GH). ACTH, TSH, LH, and FSH act by stimulating other endocrine glands, whereas GH and PRL act directly on target tissues. In the past, it was thought that the pituitary was the ''conductor'' of the whole ''endocrine orchestra'' or the ''master gland.'' It is now known that the pituitary is not the ''master'' but the ''slave''—it is completely subservient to the hypothalamus, which secretes small polypeptide hormones that are necessary to stimulate the pituitary to synthesize and secrete large polypeptide hormones. Practically all of the hypothalamic and pituitary hormones are secreted in a pulsatile fashion, one pulse occurring every 1 to 3 h; additionally, ACTH, GH, and PRL have a circadian rhythm with increased secretion between midnight and early morning.

Hypothalamic–Pituitary Diseases

Patients with hypothalamic-pituitary diseases present clinically in three ways: 1. hypofunction of one or more of the pituitary hormones; 2. hyperfunction of one or more of the hormones; and/or 3. symptoms such as headaches, visual disturbances, or neurologic signs due to a tumor or other hypothalamic pituitary lesions (e.g., inflammatory, granuloma, or lymphoma that is causing hypo- or hyperfunction).

Hypopituitarism

Etiology Anterior pituitary deficiency is due to a decrease of one or more of the hormones, and may be caused by lesions of the pituitary itself, the pituitary stalk, or the hypothalamus. Causative tumors include micro- or macroadenomas, craniopharyngiomas, pinealomas, and hamartomas. Other problems that may cause hypopituitarism are shock (especially postpartum, which can cause Sheehan's syndrome), inflammatory lesions, infiltrative disorders (such as hemochromatosis), and iatrogenic factors (e.g., radiation or surgery).

Symptoms and Signs The onset of the disease may be sudden, but is usually slow and insidious. The hormonal decrease often occurs in a definite order: gonadotropins are usually the first to decrease, resulting in amenorrhea (and impotence and oligospermia in men); growth hormone disappears next; the last hormones to be lost are usually TSH leading to hypothyroidism, and ACTH leading to hypoadrenalism, with resultant hypotension, fatigue, and intolerance to stress and infection.

Diagnosis When hypopituitarism is suspected or diagnosed, an underlying hypothalamic-pituitary lesion should be sought by visual fields and neurologic examinations, and by imaging techniques (sella x-ray, CT scan, and/or MRI). The specific hormone deficiencies must be diagnosed, with early emphasis on ACTH and TSH, which can be life-threatening. Assays required are serum FSH, LH, testosterone, estradiol, PRL, T4, TSH, and cortisol.[1] The most efficient method of evaluating pituitary function is by testing the pituitary reserve for several hormones simultaneously: 0.1 unit regular insulin/kg, TRH 200 μg and GnRH 100 μg are administered together I.V. over about 20 s. Glucose, cortisol, GH, TSH, PRL, LH, FSH, and ACTH are then measured at frequent intervals for 3 h.

Treatment Treatment consists of replacing the specific hormone(s) that is/are deficient. The target gland hormone(s) rather than the pituitary hormone is used (i.e., thyroid hormone, cortisone, estrogen, or testosterone). However in the case of GnRH deficiency, if infertility is the problem and ovulation induction is required, pituitary FSH and LH (or the LH surrogate HCG) are used. GH deficiency does not require replacement in adults. Isolated deficiencies of GnRH, ACTH, TSH, or HGH may occur, but more than one, or all of the hormone deficiencies may coexist and must be sought.

Hyperpituitarism

Excessive secretion of any of the pituitary hormones may occur, resulting in hyperpituitarism. Excess secretion of growth hormone results in gigantism or acromegaly, excess ACTH secretion causes Cushing's disease, and excess secretion of PRL causes hyperprolactinemia. In most of these situations the hormone is overproduced by a pituitary tumor. For many years, three types of pituitary tumors have been recognized, depending on the type of staining of the granules in the cells of the tumor as seen by ordinary light microscopy. Tumors with basophilic staining granules produce excessive amounts of ACTH resulting in Cushing's disease; tumors with acidophilic staining granules produce excessive amounts of growth hormone; the third type of pituitary tumor, and by far the most common type, is the chromophobe adenoma, so-called because neither basophilic nor acidophilic granules are seen in the cells. As a result of the development of the radioimmunoassay for prolactin, it is now known that these tumors produce excessive amounts of prolactin. In fact, the rate of prolactin turnover is so great and so rapid that the small granules containing prolactin do not have time to coalesce into larger granules which are necessary for basophilic or eosinophilic staining. These tumors, previously called chromophobe adenomas, are now called prolactinomas.

Acromegaly and Gigantism Excess of GH before closure of the epiphyses results in gigantism; much more commonly the hypersecretion occurs later in life, resulting in acromegaly.

Acromegaly is characterized by coarsening of the facial features, thickening of the skin, enlargement of the hands and feet, and protrusion of the jaw called prognathism. Diagnosis is made by the characteristic appearance, and by elevation of serum GH which is not suppressed by glucose administration.

Treatment methods include transsphenoidal resection of the causative adenoma, radiotherapy, and/or bromocriptine.

Cushing's Disease Hypercortisolism due to excess pituitary ACTH secretion is called Cushing's disease; all other types of hypercortisolism are referred to as Cushing's syndrome. Treatment modalities for Cushing's disease are transsphenoidal removal of the basophil adenoma, radiotherapy, and/or bromocriptine.

Pituitary Hyperthyroidism Occasionally, hyperthyroidism is due to a pituitary adenoma that secretes TSH. The management again consists of surgical removal of the tumor, irradiation, or bromocriptine.

Hyperprolactinemia By far the most common type of hyperpituitarism is excess secretion of prolactin. As previously indicated this is due to prolactin secreted by the most common pituitary tumor, the prolactinoma. Most of these tumors are less than 1 cm in diameter and are termed microadenomas; those that are 1 cm or larger are called macroadenomas.

Although the most important cause of hyperprolactinemia and/or galactorrhea is a pituitary tumor or other lesion of the hypothalamus (generically called the Forbes-Albright syndrome), there are several other causes, namely, tranquilizers, narcotics, antihypertensive drugs, birth control pills, stimulation of the nipples or breasts, hypothalamic-pituitary dysfunction, hypothyroidism, chest lesions, chronic renal disease, and certain nonpituitary prolactin-producing tumors (e.g., of the lung or kidney).

Symptoms Since there are receptors for prolactin in many tissues of the body, hyperprolactinemia can cause one or more of several symptoms: galactorrhea, oligomenorrhea, infertility, hirsutism, or osteoporosis.

Diagnosis Diagnosis is made by finding an elevated serum prolactin level, above the upper limit of normal (20 ng/ml in most laboratories). A serum prolactin assay should be carried out in all cases of galactorrhea and a screening prolactin assay should be done in all patients complaining of infertility, oligomenorrhea, hirsutism, infertility, or osteoporosis.

If the prolactin is elevated, the patient is not on any medications, and the TSH and chest findings are normal, the pituitary and hypothalamic area should be imaged by conventional radiology, or by CT scan or MRI.

Treatment In most cases the nonsurgical treatment of hyperprolactinemia is very satisfactory.[13] If a nonpituitary cause is found, it should be treated, e.g., discontinuation of the causative drug, treatment of hypothyroidism that may be present, or therapy for any underlying treatable chest or renal disease. In most other situations the mainstay of treatment is bromocriptine, i.e., 2-bromo-alpha-ergocriptine (Parlodel); it is a long-acting dopamine agonist, directly inhibiting the pituitary lactotropes from secreting prolactin. It is effective in functional hyperprolactinemia as well as in cases with micro- or macroadenoma. In cases of microadenoma the medication should be discontinued every 1 to 2 years, with measurement of the prolactin levels 6 weeks later, because there is a permanent remission in 10 percent of cases after 1 year and 20 percent after 2 years of bromocriptine treatment. In addition, in half of those patients in whom the prolactin level rises again after discontinuing the bromocriptine, the levels are much lower than they were before treatment, and it may not be necessary to restart the bromocriptine. There is a high incidence of side effects with bromocriptine: gastrointestinal (nausea, vomiting, and abdominal cramps), as well as symptoms due to hypotension caused by inhibition of sympathetic nerve activity with resultant relaxation of the splanchnic and renal vascular beds, dizziness, and syncope. Bromocriptine should therefore be started in a small dosage (half of a 2.5-mg tablet) at night and then gradually increased to twice daily administration until the prolactin levels are in the normal range. Vaginal administration obviates the gastrointestinal symptoms and, because of the slower absorption from the gut and slower metabolism by the liver, necessitates only once daily administration.

Surgery for macroadenomas has a high morbidity and mortality rate and an 80 percent recurrence rate. There is a 40 percent recurrence with microadenomas. Accordingly, surgery is reserved for patients who cannot tolerate the side effects or expense of prolonged bromocriptine treatment. Radiotherapy requires considerable expertise and may be associated with several complications, so it has assumed only a minor role in the treatment of prolactinomas.

Women with infertility due to hyperprolactinemia can achieve a pregnancy in most cases by normalizing the prolactin levels with bromocriptine. The therapy is usually discontinued during pregnancy, but studies have shown that it causes no teratogenic or other side effects. Only 5 percent of microadenomas and 20 percent of macroadenomas enlarge during pregnancy and, if this occurs, treatment with bromocriptine is very satisfactory.

Posterior Pituitary Disorders

The posterior pituitary is a direct extension of the hypothalamus, and serves as a storehouse and site of release of two hormones synthesized by the supraoptic and paraventricular nuclei of the hypothalamus, namely oxytocin and arginine-vasopressin. Oxytocin has two physiologic effects, ejection of milk and stimulation of uterine contractions; however, there are no significant clinical disease states associated with excess endogenous oxytocin secretion. The major function of arginine-vasopressin is the regulation of osmolality and blood volume. It does this by being a powerful vasoconstrictor and an antidiuretic hormone, and is therefore called the antidiuretic hormone or ADH. When plasma osmolality rises ADH release increases; conversely, water-loading inhibits ADH thereby increasing diuresis.

The only significant posterior pituitary disease seen clinically is deficiency of ADH, resulting in excretion of excessive quantities of very dilute urine, the disease being known as diabetes insipidus (DI).

Diabetes Insipidus *Etiology* The major cause of diabetes insipidus is a hypothalamic-pituitary disorder resulting in deficient secretion of ADH, known as central or ADH-sensitive DI. Occasionally ADH secretion is normal, but the kidney is ADH-resistant, a condition known as nephrogenic diabetes insipidus (NDI). This review is limited to the major type of DI, central DI. A variety of hypothalamic and posterior pituitary diseases can cause central DI: primary or idiopathic, hypophysectomy, cranial lesions, granulomatous disease, infections, and vascular lesions.[10]

Symptoms The only symptoms of DI are polydipsia and polyuria. The patient may consume enormous quantities of fluid, and large volumes (up to 30 liters) of very dilute urine may be excreted daily.

Diagnosis Diabetes insipidus must be distinguished from other causes of polyuria, including chronic renal disease, diabetes mellitus, and compulsive water drinking. Measurement of circulating levels of ADH by radioimmunoassay would appear to be the most specific method of making a diagnosis. However, this assay is difficult and not generally available, and the water deprivation test is simple and reliable and makes the RIA ADH assay unnecessary. The water deprivation test should be performed with the patient under close supervision. A normal response is one in which the maximum urine osmolality after dehydration exceeds the plasma osmolality and does not increase more than an additional 5 percent after injection of vasopressin.

Treatment If an underlying cause is found, it should be treated. Aqueous vasopressin can be administered by injection (subcutaneously or intramuscularly) 5 to 10 units, but this is not very practical because it has to be given every 6 h. Synthetic vasopressin (Pitressin) may be given bid or qid as a nasal spray. Vasopressin tannate in oil IM (0.3 to 1 ml) may control symptoms for up to 96 h. In partial or mild DI, various diuretics (especially thiazide) may be helpful as may be ADH-releasing drugs such as chlorpropamide or carbamazepine.

Adrenal Diseases

Anatomy and Physiology of the Adrenal Glands

The adrenal gland consists of an outer cortex which synthesizes and secretes steroid hormones and an inner medulla which is part of the sympathetic autonomic nervous system, the cells of which synthesize the catecholamines, dopamine, norepinephrine, and epinephrine, all derived from tyrosine. Unlike other sympathetic neurons that secrete mostly norepinephrine, the adrenal medulla secretes mostly epinephrine, which is about 5 to 10 times more potent than norepinephrine.

The adrenal cortex consists of three zones:

1. An outer zone, the zona glomerulosa, secretes the mineralocorticoids, the most potent of which is aldosterone. Mineralocorticoids cause retention of sodium and excretion of potassium. Aldosterone secretion is not under the control of ACTH, but is stimulated mainly by renin (via angiotensin II) and to some extent by hyperkalemia.
2. A middle zone, the zona fasciculata, which secretes mainly the glucocorticoid cortisol, is under the control of ACTH. During stress (including trauma, infection, and exercise) cortisol is secreted and is life-saving; it makes increased amounts of glucose and fatty acids available for energy, and attenuates defense mechanisms, thereby protecting against their potentially dangerous overactivity. The increased cortisol levels during stress cause vasodilation to protect against possible dangerous vasoconstriction.

3. An inner zone, the zona reticularis, synthesizes mainly the sex steroids, androgens and estrogens. The zona reticularis is also under the control of ACTH.

The main diseases of the adrenal gland are those that involve either hypofunction or hyperfunction of the adrenal cortex.

Adrenal Cortical Hypofunction

Adrenal cortical hypofunction is usually due to disease of the adrenal cortex itself, when it is known as primary adrenocortical insufficiency or Addison's disease. Occasionally the adrenal cortex is normal, but due to a deficiency of ACTH a secondary adrenal cortical insufficiency occurs; this is known as secondary adrenal insufficiency.

Addison's Disease (Primary Adrenocortical Insufficiency) *Etiology* In about 75 percent of cases of Addison's disease there is atrophy of the adrenal cortex without any obvious local disease. This has been called ''idiopathic'' Addison's disease, but it is probably due to an autoimmune process in most cases because it is often associated with other autoimmune diseases such as hypo- or hyperthyroidism, hypoparathyroidism, primary ovarian failure, diabetes mellitus, or pernicious anemia. In the remaining 25 percent of cases there is destruction of the adrenal cortex by tuberculosis, amyloidosis, or neoplasm.[14]

Symptoms Weakness, fatigue, anorexia, nausea, vomiting, diarrhea, and abdominal pain occur, with weight loss. Dizziness and syncopal attacks may occur.

Signs Inability to concentrate the urine, together with changes in electrolyte balance, result in severe dehydration, hypotension, and collapse. Reduced cortisol levels cause increased ACTH and beta-lipoprotein which stimulates the melanocytes and produces hyperpigmentation of the skin and mucous membranes. Pigmentation is therefore not present in secondary adrenocortical insufficiency.

Diagnosis The disease can be suspected from the symptoms and signs. In primary failure there is a high plasma ACTH level, and in secondary adrenal failure, a low level. The specific diagnosis can be made by performance of an ACTH stimulation test: plasma cortisol levels normally range from 5 to 25 mcg/dl; following an IV injection of 0.25 mcg of ACTH the plasma cortisol level doubles in 30 to 60 min, whereas in Addison's Disease, the levels are low and do not rise following IV ACTH.

Treatment With appropriate cortisol replacement therapy the prognosis is very good and patients can lead normal lives. Patients may also need mineralocorticoids.

For acute adrenocortical insufficiency, dehydration and hyponatremia are treated with IV fluids and electrolytes, and IV hydrocortisone is given. For chronic insufficiency hydrocortisone 20 mg is given in the morning and 10 mg in the afternoon with adjustment of the dose as necessary.

Secondary Adrenal Insufficiency This is due to Sheehan's syndrome, or to pituitary or hypothalamic tumors, infections, or trauma. The treatment is the same as for Addison's disease.

Hyperfunction of the Adrenal Cortex

Hyperfunction of the adrenal cortex may involve any of the three zones: hyperfunction of the zona fasciculata causes production of excess cortisone resulting in Cushing's syndrome; hyperfunction of the zona reticularis is associated with excess androgen production resulting in adrenal virilism called the adrenogenital syndrome; and hyperfunction of the outer zone, the glomerulosa, causes excess aldosterone production with resultant aldosteronism. However, there may be some overlapping of these three areas of hyperfunction.

Cushing's Syndrome Cushing's syndrome is the generic term used to include all the clinical syndromes resulting from chronic excess cortisol stimulation.

Etiology Excess cortisol activity or Cushing's syndrome in its broad sense can be due to several causes:

1. Hypersecretion of ACTH by the anterior pituitary. This is usually referred to as Cushing's disease. In many of these cases a basophil adenoma or chromophobe adenoma is the source of the excess ACTH and the tumor can be visualized by CT scan or MRI. How-

ever, a microadenoma may be difficult to see, and sometimes despite the finding of excess ACTH, no histologic abnormality can be identified;

2. Occasionally excess ACTH or cortisone may be administered exogenously or may be produced by a nonpituitary tumor such as carcinoma of the lung;
3. Cushing's syndrome may also result from cortisol production by an adenoma or carcinoma of the zona fasciculata of the adrenal cortex.

Symptoms The patient may complain of weakness and fatigue due to muscle wasting, and may have obesity, or acne and hirsutism, or bruising. Women often have oligomenorrhea.

Signs The patient may show truncal obesity with moon face, buffalo hump, and supraclavicular fat pads, with thin extremities due to muscle wasting. The skin may show acne, hirsutism, bruising, and purple striae. The patient may have hypertension, diabetes, or osteoporosis.

Diagnosis Normally there is a circadian rhythm of cortisol secretion, the plasma level being about 15 μg/dl in the morning (6 to 8 A.M.) and 5 μg/dl in the evening (6 P.M.). The presence of such diurnal variation rules out Cushing's syndrome and its absence is diagnostic of the disease. Likewise, the administration of 1 mg of dexamethasone at bedtime yields a 7 to 8 A.M. serum cortisol of less than 5 μg/dl; lack of such suppression is diagnostic for Cushing's syndrome in most cases.

Treatment If the pituitary gland is the source of the excess ACTH secretion (i.e., it is a case of Cushing's disease), transsphenoidal exploration of the pituitary should be carried out, and if a tumor is found it should be excised. If it is a microadenoma there is about an 80 percent success rate, but macroademonas frequently recur. If no tumor is found then treatment choices are total hypophysectomy, irradiation of the pituitary, or adrenalectomy.

Adenomas and carcinomas of the adrenal gland have to be removed surgically. Since the remainder of the adrenal cortex will have been suppressed and therefore become atrophic, supplementary cortisol must be given during surgery and the postoperative period.

Hyperaldosteronism Aldosterone, a potent mineralocorticoid, is produced by the zona glomerulosa, the outer zone of the adrenal cortex. It causes retention of sodium and water, and excretion of potassium. When secreted in response to stimuli such as hypertension or edematous disorders (such as cardiac failure or the nephrotic syndrome) it is called secondary aldosteronism.

When excess aldosterone is produced by a lesion of the adrenal itself (usually an adenoma, but occasionally a carcinoma or hyperplasia) it is called primary aldosteronism or Conn's syndrome.[6] In many cases the only manifestation is a mild to moderate hypertension, but the patient may have hypernatremia, hypervolemia, and hypokalemic alkalosis resulting in weakness, paresthesias, and tetany. A CT scan of the adrenal often reveals a small adenoma.

If the diagnosis of primary aldosteronism is made both adrenals should be explored for possible multiple adenomas. The prognosis is good when an adenoma is identified and removed. With adrenal hyperplasia a large number of patients remain hypertensive, but the hyperaldosteronism can usually be controlled by spironolactone.

Adrenogenital Syndrome (Adrenal Virilism) When there is excess secretion of androgens by the inner reticularis zone of the adrenal cortex, the condition is called the adrenogenital syndrome or adrenal virilism. Very occasionally this is due to an adrenal adenoma or carcinoma. In most cases it is caused by an enzyme block in the synthesis of hydrocortisone, in which case it is known as congenital adrenal hyperplasia (CAH).

Congenital Adrenal Hyperplasia Congenital adrenal hyperplasia (CAH) is an important disease for several reasons: it is one of the most frequent autosomal genetic disorders in humans, being transmitted via an autosomal recessive inheritance pattern; it is the most common of all the intersexual states—of all infants born with ambiguous genitalia 40 to 50 percent have CAH; it is the most common cause of heterosexual precocious pseudopuberty in girls; it is the main disorder that must be excluded before a diagnosis of polycystic ovarian disease (PCOD) can be made; and lastly, it is the next most common cause of hirsutism and acne after PCOD and constitutional hirsutism.

Etiology and Pathogenesis The basic defect in this syndrome is a failure in the production of hydrocortisone due to an enzyme block in its biosynthetic pathway. In most cases (about 90 percent) the block is at the stage of 17-alphahydroxyprogesterone (17-OHP), because the enzyme 21-hydroxylase, which is essential for the conversion of 17-OHP into desoxycorticosterone, and hence to hydrocortisone, is defective. The deficiency of hydrocortisone results in absence of inhibition of the output of ACTH by the pituitary, and the excess ACTH stimulates the adrenal to secrete increased amounts of androgens, because the adrenal pathways to androgens [the delta-5 pathway through dehydroepiandrosterone-sulfate (DHEA-S) and the delta-4 pathway through progesterone] are not blocked. The blood contains not only increased amounts of DHEA-S but also increased amounts of 17-alphahydroxyprogesterone, and the urine contains not only increased amounts of 17-ketosteroids which are the excretion product of DHEA-S, but also large amounts of pregnanetriol which is the excretion product of 17-OHP.

There are also two other possible enzyme blocks. In one type, a hypertensive form, the 21-hydroxylase is competent but the deficiency is at the next step, 11-hydroxylase, which is necessary for the conversion of desoxycorticosterone to hydrocortisone. This results in the production of excessive amounts of desoxycorticosterone which is a potent hypertensive agent. The third block is very rare. Here the block is very early in the biosynthetic pathway. Pregnenolone cannot be converted into progesterone because of a deficiency of 3-beta-ol-dehydrogenase. This results in profound adrenocortical insufficiency and early death, so that unless this deficiency is very mild these cases are not seen clinically.

Clinical Presentations There are three different clinical presentations of CAH, depending on the severity of the block; the more severe the block the earlier in life the condition manifests itself clinically. The three clinical presentations are: 1. a severe form which presents at birth as a child with ambiguous genitalia, a female pseudohermaphrodite; 2. a moderately severe form which presents in late childhood as heterosexual precocious pseudopuberty; and, 3. a mild or attenuated form (also called "cryptic" or "late onset" or "adult onset" or "acquired form") where the child appears normal at birth and throughout infancy and childhood, but presents in her late teens or early twenties simulating a case of PCOD.

The severe form presents at birth. There is greatly increased production of androgens even in fetal life, so that the development of the genital organs is disturbed in utero. The ovaries, tubes, uterus, and upper part of the vagina are basically unaffected because adrenal function is not present at their formative stage, and particularly because androgens have no influence on their development. However, the external genitalia, the development of which is completed later and which are influenced by androgens, become malformed. The clitoris is enlarged, and there may be a single urogenital sinus. The child is born with ambiguous genitalia and as a female pseudohermaphrodite.

In addition, about a third of these patients have a salt-losing state, as in Addison's Disease, and they present with neonatal vomiting, diarrhea, and collapse due to loss of sodium and water, and a resultant profound electrolyte imbalance. This is due to deficiency of 21-hydroxylase in both the zona glomerulosa and the zona fasciculata. It is very important to recognize this condition in the neonate because it can be treated and the whole clinical picture can be altered.

The second clinical presentation is a moderately severe form which presents in late childhood as a heterosexual precocious pseudopuberty. The child is normal at birth but in late childhood develops a precocious puberty along male lines. As a result of the excess androgens there is a preliminary stimulation of growth so that at first the patient is taller than her peers, but ends up being short in stature due to premature closure of the epiphyses due to the androgens. So, the patient presents not only with precocious pubic and axillary hair, but also with hirsutism all over the body and acne. She also has all the other signs of a precocious puberty along male lines—a muscular body and deep voice, together with primary amenorrhea and absent breast development.

The third clinical presentation is the mild, attenuated, late-onset form, which is the most common type. The child appears normal at birth and throughout childhood. However, in her late teens or early twenties she presents with acne, hirsutism, oligomenorrhea, and possibly an enlarged clitoris, a clinical picture very similar to that seen in cases of PCOD.

Diagnosis The diagnostic approach must be directed to the type of clinical presentation. In the severe form that presents at birth with an enlarged clitoris, the main differential diagnosis is from a male pseudohermaphrodite of the developmental type (i.e., a male with a small penis, hypospadias, a bifid scrotum, and undescended testes); a Swyer's syndrome; or, very rarely, a true hermaphrodite. The differential diagnosis also includes a female pseudohermaphrodite due to exogenous male hormone taken by the mother in pregnancy or endogenous masculinizing hormone during fetal life other than CAH, i.e., an androgen-producing ovarian or adrenal tumor. The main diagnostic measures required to make a diagnosis are karyotyping and endocrine assays. However, the most important initial laboratory test is the measurement of the serum electrolytes, because one third of these patients have a deficiency of aldosterone, and this is a life-threatening disease which can easily be corrected.

In the moderately severe and the late onset mild forms that occur in childhood and in the late teens, respectively, the diagnosis is made by the finding of an elevated DHEA-S and particularly by an elevation of the 17-OHP level which is specific for CAH. In severe cases, the 17-OHP will be markedly elevated, and will be elevated all the time. However, in the moderately severe and mild cases it may only be slightly elevated or it may only be elevated in the early morning when the circadian rhythm of the adrenal hormones is at its peak, or it may not be elevated at all and may require an ACTH stimulation test to uncover it.

Accordingly, the procedure that should be adopted to make a diagnosis of CAH is as follows: a basal follicular morning serum 17-OHP and progesterone (P) should be obtained. If this 17-OHP is above 8 ng/ml, the diagnosis of CAH is established; if it is below 2 ng/ml, CAH is very unlikely. If it is above 2 but less than 8 ng/ml, an ACTH stimulation test should be done. A level above 20 ng/ml one half to 1 h after an intravenous injection of 0.25 mg ACTH (Cortrosyn, Organon) is diagnostic for CAH.

Treatment The logical and specific treatment is cortisone. This replaces the cortisone that is lacking, suppresses the excess ACTH secretion by the anterior pituitary, and prevents the oversecretion of androgens by the adrenal cortex. With this treatment the patient with severe CAH can be prevented from developing a heterosexual precocious pseudopuberty, and the patient with a heterosexual precocious pseudopuberty can be restored to normal femininity; the breasts develop, the uterus grows, ovulation and menstruation occur, and fertility is present. The usual daily dose of oral cortisone required is 25 mg cortisone acetate, or 5 mg prednisone or their equivalents. The dose should be sufficient to suppress the 17-OHP to below 2 ng/ml; however, if the dose suppresses the morning blood cortisol to below 2 μg/dl the dose should be reduced to avoid an inability to react to stress. Patients with a salt-losing syndrome should additionally be given fludrocortisone (e.g., Florinef 0.1 to 0.2 mg p.o. daily) and serum electrolyte levels and blood pressures should be monitored closely. Fluids and sodium must be given as necessary.

Pheochromocytoma Pheochromocytoma is a tumor of chromaffin cells, which are cells of the sympathetic nervous system which secrete catecholamines, i.e., dopamine, norepinephrine, and epinephrine.[5]

Etiology In 80 percent of cases the tumors are in the adrenal medulla, but they may be found in any other chromaffin tissues such as the ganglia of the sympathetic chain. They are usually about five centimeters in diameter, and 95 percent are benign.

Symptoms and Signs The clinical manifestations are variable and depend mainly on the relative amounts and patterns of norepinephrine and epinephrine secretion. About 90 percent of patients have hypertension, which may be paroxysmal or continuous, and they may have headaches, palpitations, tremors, and hot flushes.

Diagnosis Diagnosis is suspected from the symptoms and signs. It is made by imaging techniques including CT scan and MRI. It is also made by measuring the main urinary excretion product of the catecholamines, namely, vanil-mandelic acid (VMA); normally there is less than 10 mg VMA per 24-h urine.

Treatment Phenoxybenzamine, an alpha blocker, with the subsequent addition of propanolol, a beta blocker, may be used to reduce the symptoms and in preparation for surgery. However, surgery is the treatment of choice for most patients with pheochromocytoma, after adequate preoperative preparation.[12]

Carcinoid Syndrome

Carcinoid syndrome is a syndrome in which the patient experiences recurrent bouts of flushing of the skin, and abdominal cramps with diarrhea. It is usually due to secretion of vasoactive substances by carcinoid tumors of the intestine.

Etiology and Pathology The usual etiology of the carcinoid syndrome is tumor formation that arises from enteroendocrine cells in the ileum, pancreas, thyroid, gonads, or bronchi. These cells produce vasoactive substances including serotonin, histamine, prostaglandins, and polypeptide hormones. Histamine causes vasodilation and hence results in flushing. Serotonin stimulates smooth muscle and hence causes diarrhea and abdominal cramps.

Symptoms The most prominent symptoms are flushing of the skin, (especially the head and neck), abdominal cramps, and recurrent diarrhea. Some patients develop bronchial spasm leading to asthmatic-like wheezing.

Diagnosis The condition should be suspected from the aforementioned symptoms. The diagnosis is confirmed by testing for increased urinary excretion of the serotonin metabolite, 5 hydroxyindoleacetic acid (5-HIAA). Liver scan and imaging techniques may be used to demonstrate the causative tumor, and laparotomy is usually required.

Treatment Treatment is difficult and often unsatisfactory. Resection of some carcinoid tumors may be feasible. Radiation therapy is unsuccessful and no effective chemotherapy is available currently. However, even with metastatic carcinoid tumors, long term survival up to 15 years is fairly common. Numerous palliative medications have been tried for the symptoms of flushing and diarrhea, including phenothiazine, prednisone, and peripheral serotonin antagonists such as cyproheptadine. Success with these drugs is variable.

Hirsutism

Hirsutism, the presence of excessive facial or body hair in women, is a common condition, and often an unpleasant symptom. It is always due to excess androgen activity. However, although the most common, it is only one of the clinical manifestations of hyperandrogenism, the others being acne, oligomenorrhea, enlargement of the clitoris, hoarseness of the voice, temporal recession of scalp hair, and increased masculinity. Except for acne and hirsutism, the other symptoms are uncommon, and usually signify markedly increased androgen production.

Causes of Hirsutism Although there are a large number of causes of hirsutism, the problem as encountered by the clinician is a fairly simple one, because, in practice, 95 percent of cases of hirsutism are due to one of only four causes:[4] 1. polycystic ovarian disease (PCOD) is by far the most common cause of hirsutism, being responsible for about 80 percent of the cases; 2. CAH is the cause in 5.5 percent; 3. hyperprolactinemia is the cause in 3.5 percent; and 4. end-organ hyperresponsiveness is the cause in 6.8 percent. There are numerous other rare causes of hirsutism (such as ovarian and adrenal tumors, Cushing's syndrome, acromegaly, the taking of dilantin, and hermaphroditism), but all of these together are responsible for a total of only 5 percent of all cases of hirsutism.

PCOD: The basic defect in this syndrome revolves around an increase in LH. LH normally acts on the theca interna of the follicle to induce the synthesis of androstenedione, which diffuses into the follicular fluid where it is aromatized to estrogen. The increased LH in PCOD stimulates the theca interna to produce increased amounts of the androgen androstenedione, which results in hirsutism.

CAH: The basic defect in CAH is an enzyme deficiency resulting in decreased production of cortisol. The ACTH therefore rises and stimulates the zona reticularis of the adrenal cortex to produce increased amounts of androgens, resulting in hirsutism.

Hyperprolactinemia: Numerous studies have shown that in as many as 40 percent of cases of hyperprolactinemia there are increased levels of DHEA-S and free testosterone, and in about 20 percent there are clinical manifestations of these excess androgens such as acne and hirsutism. These increased androgens may be due to a direct action of prolactin on the adrenals and ovaries, or due to anovulation and PCOD caused by the hyperprolactinemia.

End-organ hyperresponsiveness: In this cause of hirsutism the plasma levels of all the androgens are normal, and therefore this used to be called "idiopathic," "familial," or "constitutional" hirsutism. It is now known, however, that this is due either to increased androgen receptors, or more commonly, to increased activity of 5-alpha-reductase, resulting in increased peripheral production of dihydrotestosterone, the most potent of all of the androgens. There are increased serum and urinary levels of 3-alpha-androstanediol glucuronide, a metabolite of dihydrotestosterone, which is directly related to the rate of conversion of testosterone to dihydrotestosterone; the upper limit of normal of this metabolite in serum is approximately 200 ng/dl; in end-organ hyperresponsiveness it is above 400 ng/dl.

Diagnosis The clinician needs to obtain the laboratory tests for only four diseases in order to diagnose the etiology of 95 percent of cases of hirsutism. 1. To diagnose PCOD, an FSH, LH, and androstenedione are required. In PCOD, there is an inverse FSH/LH ratio and/or an increased LH, and the androstenedione is elevated. 2. To diagnose CAH, assays of DHEA-S and 17-OHP should be done, and they are both elevated. 3. For hyperprolactinemia only a prolactin level is needed. 4. End-organ hyperresponsiveness is diagnosed by finding that all tests are normal, and confirmation can be achieved by a serum 3-alpha-androstenediol glucuronide determination.

If the serum testosterone is above 200 ng/dl or the DHEA-S is above 7000 ng/ml, an ovarian or adrenal tumor should be suspected.

Treatment The hirsutism due to PCOD can be treated specifically by suppressing the elevated LH with the combination birth control pill, or by treatment with medroxyprogesterone acetate (Provera). CAH and hyperprolactinemia are treated specifically with cortisone or bromocriptine respectively. For end-organ hyperresponsiveness one of the antiandrogens can be used: spironolactone or cimetidine which are available in the United States (FDA approved but not specifically for hirsutism); or cyproterone acetate (CPA) which is not approved for use in the United States but has been used successfully in Europe. Although all of these modalities will prevent further hair growth, the hair already present will not fall out, and will have to be removed by shaving, waxing, tweezing, or electrolysis (i.e., electrocoagulation of the dermal papillae).

Parathyroid Disorders and Bone Metabolism

The homeostatic regulation of calcium metabolism involves calcium fluxes in and out of bone, changes in calcium absorption from the intestine, and calcium excretion in the urine. All of this is controlled primarily by parathyroid hormone (PTH), an 84-amino acid single-chain polypeptide secreted by the parathyroid glands. Secretion of PTH from the parathyroid glands is regulated by serum calcium levels through a classic negative feedback mechanism—a low serum calcium stimulates PTH secretion while a high level suppresses it. PTH stimulates the renal tubules to reabsorb calcium and also stimulates the kidneys to produce 1-25-dihydroxyvitamin D which enhances the absorption of calcium from the gut. By these mechanisms normal serum calcium levels between 8.8 and 10.4 mg/dl are constantly maintained.

Hypercalcemia/Hyperparathyroidism

Etiology Hypercalcemia, i.e., a serum calcium of greater than 10.5 mg/dl, is most often due to primary hyperparathyroidism, but may be due to malignancy (especially breast), medications (thiazides, lithium, vitamin A and D preparations, calcium, and antacids), immobilization (especially with Paget's disease), thyrotoxicosis, adrenal insufficiency, and acute renal failure (especially in the diuretic phase). Primary hyperparathyroidism is usually due to a single parathyroid adenoma (which is found in more than 80 percent of cases); in the remaining cases hyperplasia, multiple adenomas, and occasionally carcinoma may be found.

Symptoms Many patients are asymptomatic, the disorder being discovered on routine serum chemistry screening. When symptoms do occur they may be gastrointestinal or renal; ureteric colic due to a stone; or bone pain, especially when osteitis fibrosa cystica, the bone disease of severe hyperparathyroidism, occurs.

Diagnosis The hallmark of the diagnosis of primary hyperparathyroidism is hypercalcemia without appropriate suppression of PTH levels. Because of the technical difficulty in locating the source of the excess PTH at surgery, several imaging techniques have been used and proven effective: ultrasound, CT scan, MRI, and thallium scan of the neck.[15]

Treatment Medical management of primary hyperparathyroidism using measures such as increased fluid intake, additional sodium chloride and oral phosphate have been tried, but with little success. Ultimately, surgery is required for most cases of primary hyperparathyroidism and may be totally curative if there is a well-defined single adenoma. However, when there is hyperplasia or supernumery or ectopic glands, there may be persistent disease despite multiple operations.[11]

Hypocalcemia/Hypoparathyroidism

Hypocalcemia is defined as a total serum calcium level of less than 8.8 mg/dl in the presence of normal serum albumin.

Etiology The major cause of hypocalcemia is hypoparathyroidism which can be primary, i.e., due to deficient PTH secretion, or secondary, where the end-organs are insensitive to circulating PTH.[2] There are many other causes which must be ruled out, but if hypocalcemia is accompanied by hyperphosphatemia the diagnosis is almost certainly hypoparathyroidism. Among the other etiologies are hypo- or hypermagnesemia, chronic renal failure (with accompanying hyperphosphatemia), metastatic carcinoma (which may cause hypo- or hypercalcemia), and acute pancreatitis. Primary hypoparathyroidism is often due to surgical damage or removal of the parathyroid glands during thyroidectomy or radical neck dissection, or removal of the glands for hyperparathyroidism. Infection, metastatic tumor, or infiltration by granuloma may also occasionally be the cause of damage to the parathyroid glands. Secondary hypoparathyroidism, also known as pseudohypoparathyroidism (PHP), is an uncommon inherited disorder.

Symptoms The hypocalcemia may cause carpopedal spasm, paresthesias, and muscle cramps, and occasionally tetany and convulsions.

Signs Most signs are due to the hypocalcemia. Chvostek's sign consists of contraction of the facial muscles when the facial nerve is gently tapped. The occurrence of carpopedal spasm within 3 min of impeding the return of blood from the forearm with a blood pressure cuff is known as Trousseau's sign. Hyperreflexia may be seen, and the teeth may reveal enamel hypoplasia and caries.

Diagnosis The serum calcium will be low. The PTH will be low in primary hypoparathyroidism and high in pseudohypoparathyroidism. Renal function must always be evaluated, because hypocalcemia may be due to renal disease.

Treatment In severe, acutely symptomatic hypocalcemia, intravenous calcium chloride or calcium gluconate should be given. The mainstay of the treatment of chronic hypocalcemia is oral calcium. Calcium carbonate is the preferred form because it contains more calcium than most other calcium salts. Up to 2 g of elemental calcium may be required daily. Serum calcium levels should be monitored and maintained at or near 8 mg/dl.

References and Selected Readings

1. Abboud CF: Laboratory diagnosis of hypopituitarism. *Mayo Clin Proc* 61:35, 1986.
2. Ahn TG, et al: Familial isolated hypoparathyroidism: A molecular genetic analysis of eight families with 23 affected persons. *Medicine* 65:73, 1986.
3. Allanic H, et al: Antithyroid drugs and Graves' disease: A prospective randomized evaluation of the efficacy of treatment duration. *J Clin Endocrinol Metab* 70:675, 1990.
4. Benjamin F, Deutsch S, Sapertein H, Seltzer VL: Prevalence of and markers for the attenuated form of congenital adrenal hyperplasia and hyperprolactinemia masquerading as polycystic ovarian disease. *Fertil Steril* 46:215, 1986.
5. Benowitz NL: Phenochromocytoma. *Adv Intern Med* 35:195, 1990.

6. Bravo EL: Primary aldosteronism. *Urol Clin North Am* 16:481, 1989.
7. Caldwell G, et al: A new strategy for thyroid function testing. *Lancet* 1:1117, 1985.
8. Gesundheit N, et al: Thyrotropin-secreting pituitary adenomas: Clinical and biochemical heterogeneity—Case reports and follow-up of nine patients. *Ann Intern Med* 111:827, 1989.
9. Kidd A, et al: Immunologic aspects of Graves' and Hashimoto's Diseases. *Metabolism* 29:80, 1980.
10. Maesaka JK, et al: Hyponatremia and hypouricemia: Differentiation from SIADH. *Clin Nephrol* 33:174, 1990.
11. Potts JT Jr: Management of asymptomatic hyperparathyroidism. *J Clin Endocrinol Metab* 70:1489, 1990.
12. Sheps SG, et al: Recent developments in the diagnosis and treatment of pheochromocytoma. *Mayo Clin Proc* 65:88, 1990.
13. Vance ML, et al: Treatment of hyperprolactinemia. *J Clin Endocrinol Metab* 68:336, 1989.
14. Vita JA, et al: Clinical clues to the cause of Addison's disease. *Am J Med* 78:461, 1985.
15. Winzelberg GG: Parathyroid imaging. *Ann Intern Med* 237:893, 1989.

48 Diabetes Mellitus

Abbas E. Kitabchi

Diabetes mellitus (DM) is a clinical disorder characterized by abnormal metabolism of carbohydrate, fat, and protein, resulting in inappropriate hyperglycemia. It may be due either to a deficiency in secretion of or ineffectiveness of insulin, or both. According to the latest statistics in the United States, 14 million Americans have diabetes, of whom about 50 percent are unaware of their disorder.[9]

Table 48-1 shows the latest classification of diabetes and hyperglycemia. It depicts not only the two major types of spontaneous diabetes [i.e., *type 1,* or *insulin-dependent, diabetes* (IDDM), formerly called "juvenile-onset diabetes," and *type 2,* or *non-insulin-dependent diabetes* (NIDDM), formerly called "adult-onset diabetes"], but also gestational diabetes as well as other types associated with endocrinopathies. This table provides a new terminology for the formerly named "chemical diabetes," which is now known as *impaired glucose tolerance* (IGT). Of all of these forms of diabetes, by far the most frequent in the United States is type 2, which constitutes more than 90 percent of all diabetic cases. Table 48-2 provides the clinical characteristics of the two major forms of diabetes.

TABLE 48-1 **Types of Diabetes Mellitus and Other Categories of Hyperglycemia**

Disease Classifications
Clinical Classes
Diabetes mellitus (DM)
Type 1: Insulin-dependent diabetes mellitus (IDDM)
Type 2: Non-insulin-dependent diabetes mellitus (NIDDM) (obese or nonobese)
Maturity onset diabetes of the young (MODY)
Other types of diabetes:
Pancreatic disease
Endocrinopathies (Cushing's syndrome, acromegaly, pheochromocytoma, hyperaldosteronism)
Drug-induced
Gestational diabetes mellitus (GDM)
Impaired glucose tolerance (IGT) (obese or nonobese)

SOURCE: (Adapted from National Diabetes Data Group: Classification and diagnosis of diabetes mellitus and other categories of glucose intolerance. *Diabetes* 28:1039–1057, 1979.

TABLE 48-2 Major Characteristics of Types 1 and 2 Diabetes Mellitus

Features	Type 1 (IDDM)	Type 2 (NIDDM)
Age at onset	Usually < 20	Usually > 40
Proportion of all diabetes	About 10%	About 90%
Seasonal trend	Fall and Winter	None
Appearance of symptoms	Acute or subacute	Slow
Metabolic ketoacidosis	Frequent	Rare
Obesity at onset	Uncommon	Common
Beta Cells	Decreased	Variable
Insulin	Decreased	Variable
Inflammatory cells in islets	Present initially	Absent
Family history of diabetes	Uncommon	Common
Concordance in identical twins	25–50%	90–95%
HLA association	Yes	No
Antibody to islet cells (ICA)	Yes	No
Insulin autoantibodies (IAA)	Yes (in younger age)	No
"64K" antibodies	Yes	No
Treatment	Diet and insulin	Diet, OHA's, insulin

*OHAs = oral hypoglycemic agents.

SOURCE: (Adapted from Kitabchi AE, Fisher JN: Diabetes mellitus, in Conn R (ed): *Current Diagnosis*. Philadelphia: Saunders, 1992, pp 766–774.

Non-insulin-dependent diabetes (NIDDM) is ethnic group–related. The prevalence of the disease is in Pima Indians (35 percent), in native Americans (17 percent), in Hispanics (12 percent), and African Americans (5 percent) as compared to 2.5 percent for the general population. The incidence of NIDDM increases with age, the number of family members with a history of diabetes, and other risk factors, which are summarized in Table 48-3. A 60-year-old Pima Indian, for instance, has an approximately 60 percent chance of being diabetic.

TABLE 48-3 Population at Risk for Development of Type 2 Diabetes Mellitus

1. Persons with classic signs and symptoms of diabetes (i.e., polyuria, polydipsia, polyphagia, and loss of weight).
2. Obesity (particularly upper body adiposity).
3. Strong family history of diabetes.
4. Ethnic groups (i.e., African Americans, Hispanics, and Native Americans).
5. History of Gestational Diabetes Mellitus (GDM).
6. History of delivering infant weighing greater than 9 lb.
7. History of recurring skin, genital, or urinary tract infections.
8. History of impaired glucose tolerance.
9. History of coronary artery disease (CAD).

SOURCE: (Adapted from Kitabchi AE, Fisher JN: Diabetes mellitus, in Glenn RH, Peters SP (eds): *Clinical Studies in Medical Biochemistry*. New York: Oxford University Press, Chap 12, 1987, pp 102–117.

Table 48-4 summarizes some statistics on the microvascular complications of diabetes, and Table 48-5 depicts its macrovascular complications. NIDDM is more often associated with macrovascular, and IDDM more often with microvascular, effects. According to the latest statistics from the American Diabetes Association (ADA), more than $90 billion in direct and indirect costs were spent on diabetes and its complications in 1992.[3] This included the costs of management and therapy as well as loss of wages associated with the disease. NIDDM in certain ethnic groups has reached epidemic proportions in the United States. Since NIDDM—along with cancer and cardiovascular diseases—accounts for three-quarters of the deaths in this country and is related to lifestyle, an effort to modify lifestyle in order to reduce the incidence of these disorders is important.

Both type 1 and type 2 diabetes are heterogeneous. IDDM, however, is more often associated with ketosis and is characterized by insulinopenia. It is believed to be an autoimmune-related disease that may be initiated as a result of viral infection or a toxic component in the environment. It is strongly

TABLE 48-4 Microvascular Complications of Diabetes Mellitus

Eye (retinopathy)	Leading cause of new cases of blindness in adults (increased risk: 20×). Relative risk for cataracts and glaucoma increased 2–3×.
Kidney (nephropathy)	Occurs in 35% of type 1 and 20% of type 2 patients. Accounts for 30% of new cases of end-stage renal disease (ESRD) each year (increased risk: 25×).
Nerve (neuropathy)	Common in both type 1 and type 2 patients. Important cause of morbidity.

SOURCE: Adapted from Harris MI: Undiagnosed NIDDM: Clinical and public health issues. *Diabetes Care* 16:642–652, 1993.

TABLE 48-5 Macrovascular Complications of Diabetes Mellitus

Coronary heart disease	Increased 4× in women.
Cerebrovascular disease	Risk for stroke increased 4×.
Peripheral vascular disease	Present in 8% at diagnosis, 45% at 20 y. Foot or ankle ulcers occur in 15%. Occurs in 40–50% of nontraumatic amputations. 50% 3-year survival after amputation.

SOURCE: Adapted from Harris MI: Undiagnosed NIDDM: Clinical and public health issues. *Diabetes Care* 16:642–652, 1993.

associated with the human leukocyte antigen (HLA), particularly with DR_3 and DR_4 genes. More specifically, the DQ locus (DQW32) has been identified as a susceptibility gene for IDDM. The deficiency of insulin and excess counterregulatory hormones (such as cortisol, catecholamines, and glucagon) in an uncontrolled diabetic brings about a series of metabolic decompensations resulting in (1) a breakdown of protein in muscle (*proteolysis*), which brings about an excess of amino acids; (2) a breakdown of triglycerides in fat tissue, leading to increased free fatty acids (*lipolysis*); and (3) a breakdown of glycogen to glucose and increased gluconeogenesis (glucose production from noncarbohydrate precursors), both of which lead to hyperglycemia. Decreased insulin availability in the presence of increased glucagon and increased free fatty acids lead to excessive ketone production, which can eventually cause severe metabolic ketoacidosis and, if not treated, coma and death. Table 48-6 correlates these clinical conditions with various metabolic defects.

NIDDM, or type 2 diabetes, which is also heterogeneous, is not an autoimmune disease but is characterized by the presence of insulin resistance. The disease may be insidious at the start, with normal fasting blood glucose but postprandial hyperglycemia, which at the outset is characterized by hyperinsulinemia and impaired glucose tolerance (IGT). In certain cases, IGT may lead to frank NIDDM, and finally insulinopenia, a stage during which patients become insulin-requiring (as opposed to insulin-dependent) diabetics. The hyperinsulinemic stage may be variable, from a short period to a long duration, before the appearance of clinical diabetes. The hyperinsulinemia is an effort on the part of the pancreas to maintain fasting euglycemia by excess secretion of insulin, and, therefore, the ratio of insulin to glucose at this stage remains elevated, denoting endogenous insulin resistance. Although the pathogenesis of NIDDM has not been fully elucidated, insulin resistance is the hallmark of the disease, and obesity is a strong contributing factor, as 85 percent of NIDDM patients are also obese.[17]

A subclassification of NIDDM is MODY (Matu-

TABLE 48-6 Correlation of Uncontrolled Diabetic Syndromes with Various Metabolic Defects

Metabolic Defects	Chemical Abnormalities	Clinical Symptoms
	Carbohydrate Metabolism	
1. Diminished uptake of glucose by muscle, adipose, and liver cells	Hyperglycemia	Polyuria, polydipsia, polyphagia, fatigue, muscle weakness, pruritus
2. Overproduction of glucose (via glycogenolysis and gluconeogenesis) by the liver	Hyperglycemia	Blurred vision Diminished mental alertness
	Protein Metabolism	
1. Diminished uptake of amino acids and diminished synthesis of protein	Negative nitrogen balance Elevated levels of branched-chain amino acids and blood urea nitrogen	Loss of muscle mass and weakness
2. Increased proteolysis	Elevated serum potassium	
	Fat Metabolism	
1. Increased lipolysis	Elevated plasma fatty acids and glycerol	Loss of adipose tissue Nausea and vomiting
2. Decreased lipogenesis		Loss of adipose tissue
3. Increased production of triglycerides	Hypertriglyceridemia	Exudative xanthoma (skin lesions) Lipemia retinalis Pancreatitis (abdominal pain)
4. Decreased removal of ketones and increased ketone production	Elevated plasma and urine ketones	Hyperventilation, metabolic acidosis, abdominal pain, acetone on breath

SOURCE: Adapted from Kitabchi AE, Fisher JN: Diabetes mellitus, in Conn R (ed): *Current Diagnosis.* Philadelphia: Saunders, 1991, pp 766–774.

rity Onset Diabetes of the Young) or NIDDY (Non-Insulin-Dependent Diabetes of the Young), which occurs in a young age group and is transmitted via autosomal dominant inheritance with possible alteration of a glucokinase gene in the pancreas.

Diagnosis of Diabetes Mellitus

Based on the latest consensus report, there are now three accepted methods by which DM is diagnosed in nonpregnant adults.[16] Two of them consist of the use of a single blood glucose determination, and the third method involves the use of a 2-h oral glucose tolerance test (OGTT) with 75 g glucose. The first two methods consist of having either (1) a fasting blood glucose level equal to or greater than 140 mg/dl on two separate occasions or (2) a random blood glucose level that is unequivocally elevated (greater than 200 mg/dl) in a subject who has the classical signs and symptoms of diabetes (i.e., polydipsia, polyuria, polyphagia, and possibly weight loss). Table 48-7 summarizes the criteria for these three methods of diagnosis.

Indications and Criteria for Screening Tests for NIDDM

In general, as IDDM patients present themselves with a decompensated metabolic condition, the early

TABLE 48-7 Diagnostic Criteria for Diabetes Mellitus (DM), Impaired Glucose Tolerance (IGT), and Gestational Diabetes Mellitus (GDM)

Nonpregnant Adults

DM criteria: at least one of the following:

1. Random plasma glucose level of ≥ 200 mg/dl plus classic DM signs and symptoms, including polydipsia, polyuria, polyphagia, and weight loss.
2. Fasting plasma glucose level of ≥ 140 mg/dl on at least two occasions.
3. Fasting plasma glucose level of < 140 mg/dl but sustained elevated plasma glucose levels during an oral glucose tolerance test. The 2-h sample and at least one other between 0 and 2 h after 75 g glucose dose should be ≥ 200 mg/dl. Oral glucose tolerance testing is not necessary if criteria 1 or 2 have been met.

IGT criteria: all the following:

1. Fasting plasma glucose < 140 mg/dl.
2. Plasma glucose in 2nd h of OGTT should be between 140 and 199 mg/dl.
3. During oral glucose tolerance test, at least one other plasma glucose value at 30, 60, or 90 min should be ≥ 200 mg/dl.

Gestational Diabetes Mellitus (GDM) criteria:

Following an oral glucose load of 100 g, two plasma glucose values equal or exceed the following: fasting, 105 mg/dl; 1 h, 190 mg/dl; 2 h, 165 mg/dl; 3 h, 145 mg/dl.

Children

DM criteria: one of the following:

1. Random plasma glucose level of ≥ 200 mg/dl plus classic DM signs and symptoms, including polyuria, polydipsia, ketonuria, and rapid weight loss.
2. Fasting plasma glucose level of ≥ 140 mg/dl on at least two occasions and sustained plasma glucose levels during an oral glucose tolerance test. Both the 2-h plasma glucose and at least one other between 0 and 2 h after the glucose dose (1.75 g/kg/IBW up to 75 g) should be ≥ 200 mg/dl.

SOURCE: Adapted from National Diabetes Data Group: Classification and diagnosis of diabetes mellitus and other categories of glucose intolerance. *Diabetes* 28:1039–1059, 1979.

screening is not recommended at this time. Such screening, however, is under consideration for first-degree relatives of IDDM patients because of investigational purposes. On the other hand, with recent reports on the results of the Diabetes Control and Complications Trial (DCCT), indicating that control of blood glucose can significantly reduce complications of diabetes in IDDM patients,[18] one may deduce that such control may also benefit NIDDM patients. Therefore, any method to detect early NIDDM in those people with a high risk of NIDDM (Table 48-3) is highly desirable, if not imperative, in order to take preventive steps to curtail development of NIDDM. It is recommended that persons with a high risk be screened for NIDDM.

Performance of OGTT

As stated under the methods of diagnosis of DM, the screening tests used to detect DM consist of fasting blood glucose, random blood glucose, or OGTT.

Table 48-8 summarizes the conditions under which an OGTT should be performed. Meticulous attention should be given to the adequate intake of carbohydrates (CHO) by the patient (>150 CHO/day × 3 days), use of no drugs, and no prolonged bed confinement or stress.[5] It should be emphasized that OGTT is not recommended for those individu-

TABLE 48-8 Standardized Conditions for the Performance of an Oral Glucose Tolerance Test (OGTT)

1. Administer only to otherwise healthy ambulatory subjects in whom diabetes mellitus is strongly suspected, or are otherwise at risk, and a fasting or random glucose is not diagnostic.
2. At least 3 days of unrestricted diet (greater than 150 g of carbohydrates) and physical activity should precede this test.
3. Subject should have fasted for 10 to 14 h.
4. Test should be performed in the morning.
5. 75 g of oral glucose for adults, 100 g for pregnant adults, and 1.75 g per kilogram of body weight for children up to a maximum of 75 g.
6. Subject should remain seated and nonsmoking during the test and should use no caffeine.
7. Venous plasma glucose determination for 2 h at 30-min intervals (3 h for pregnant women with samples every hour).

SOURCE: Adapted from Harris MI: Undiagnosed NIDDM: Clinical and public health issues. *Diabetes Care* 16:642–652, 1993.

als who have had a diagnosis of DM by either fasting blood glucose or random blood glucose since the ingestion of the glucose load may precipitate DKA or a hyperglycemic hyperosmolar nonketotic state (HHNS).

Assessment of Glycemic Control

For many years it was assumed that urine glucose testing was a good indicator of glycemic control, but recent studies suggest a poor relationship between blood glucose and urine glucose by numerous dip stick/test tapes, including the glucose oxidase–containing dip stick/test tape.[14] The only acceptable method for assessment of glycemic control is determination of blood glucose with the use of direct enzymatic methods (i.e., glucose oxidase). In addition to the standard laboratory method, many meters are now available that use strips containing glucose oxidase enzyme for direct measurement of glucose in the whole blood. The accuracy of such machines has been well documented. Those with an easier method of analysis (no wiping of blood from the strip) and memory have become more acceptable by patients and health care providers. Urine tests for "ketone bodies" still remain a useful and quick way to assess ketosis. We advise patients to check their urine for ketones when their blood glucose continues to remain above 250 mg/dl, and, if moderate ketones are present, to seek immediate medical advice. Self glucose monitoring (SGM) systems are now an accepted method of monitoring for those patients who must adjust their medication and activities based on their blood glucose.

Glycohemoglobin

Glycohemoglobin is a product of a ketoamine reaction between glucose in the blood and N-terminal amino acids of the beta (β) chains of hemoglobin; it consists of hemoglobin A_{1a}, A_{1b}, and A_{1c}. Since the half-life of red blood cells is about 120 days, the glycohemoglobin level generally reflects the glycemic state over the last 12 weeks.[2] A more specific form of glycohemoglobin (Hb A_{1c}), although more difficult to assay, is more specific for the stable form of glycohemoglobin and is preferred by most diabetologists for assessment of chronic glycemic control. The normal level of this compound is between 4 to 6 percent (depending on the laboratory method used), and, therefore, values up to 7 percent are considered good for patients with diabetes while values above 10 percent are considered poor control. A falsely decreased level of glycosylated hemoglobin can be found in patients with severe anemia or shortened red blood cell half-life, as in patients with hemolytic anemias or hemoglobinopathies. Inversely, falsely elevated levels of glycosylated hemoglobin can be found in patients with uremia and hemoglobin F elevation.

Although SGM is a useful method of monitoring day-to-day glucose variations, Hb A_{1c} provides an accurate reflection of an average level of blood glucose in the past few weeks. Hb A_{1c}, however, cannot demonstrate the severe fluctuations that a brittle diabetic may experience during such a period. In that situation, daily SGM is the most useful method of monitoring. Obtaining Hb A_{1c} levels several times a year is clinically beneficial in most patients, but some insurance companies restrict payment if done more frequently, particularly in the elderly.

Treatment Regimens of Patients with Diabetes

It is incumbent on those who manage patients with diabetes to provide appropriate education for the patients. This should either be done in the physician's office or the patient referred to a facility or organization with enough expertise that its program has been approved by the American Diabetes Association (ADA) and certified by the American Association of Diabetes Educators (AADE).

Table 48-9 summarizes the goals and methods of therapy for patients with diabetes. Table 48-10 provides general guidelines for management of patients with diabetes. Since education is by far the most important aspect of management, the author has summarized in Table 48-11 the pertinent points of an educational program that every patient and family member need to know. It cannot be overstated that a well-informed patient (regardless of level of education) is essential for good care. Therefore, any physi-

TABLE 48-9 Goals and Methods of Therapy of Patients with Diabetes Mellitus

A. GOALS OF THERAPY
   1. Normalize metabolism
   2. Normalize physical well-being
   3. Normalize psychological well-being
   4. Avoid complications
      a. Acute complications
      b. Long-term complications

B. METHODS OF THERAPY
   1. Education
   2. Diet/meal planning
   3. Exercise
   4. Hypoglycemic agents
      a. Sulfonylurea (only in NIDDM)
      b. Insulin

TABLE 48-10 General Guidelines for Diabetes Management[a]

1. Establish diagnosis of diabetes mellitus (DM).
   A. FBG ≥ 140 mg/dl × 2 *or*
   B. Classical signs and symptoms of DM and random BG ≥ 200 mg/dl *or*
   C. By OGTT (BG at 120 min ≥ 200 mg/dl and one other BG from zero to 120 min ≥ 200 mg/dl). *Do not perform OGTT if the diagnosis of DM is already established.*
   D. Classify DM as to type 1, type 2, etc.
2. Inform patient of diagnosis of diabetes and refer to diabetes education classes (to learn about signs and symptoms, complication, blood glucose monitoring, diabetes medications, sick days, etc.)
3. Place patient on ADA diet with appropriate caloric, sodium, and lipid restrictions.
4. Identify cardiac risk factors.
5. Determine status of kidney function (serum creatinine, 24-h urine albumin).
6. Evaluate for presence of neuropathy (refer to neurologist prn).
7. Establish extent of fundoscopic lesion (refer to ophthalmologist prn).
8. Check feet pulses, and skin, and toenails at each visit.
9. Use finger stick blood glucose for daily diabetic control and urine check only for ketones.
10. Follow chronic glycemic control by Hb A_{1c} approximately every 3 months

[a]In addition to the above specific management procedures, it is understood that all patients who are seen for diabetes evaluation and have not been seen by other physicians for general health evaluation should have a complete history and physical examination and the following laboratory tests: CBC with differential, chemisty profile, lipid profile, urinalysis, thyroid function tests, and ECG (if indicated).

cian attempting to manage a diabetic should ideally have access to a team of health care professionals, including a nutritionist, a diabetes educator, and a mental health professional, in addition to the physician. In some locales the patient may not have access to such individuals, in which case the physician will need to fill these roles. In the DCCT studies, the team approach has proven to contribute enormously to the successful management of IDDM. Complications of neuropathy, retinopathy, and nephropathy were reduced by 40 to 70 percent in patients who received intensive therapy (accomplished by a team approach) as compared to the standard therapy group.[18]

Diet Therapy

Probably the most important step to take after the diagnosis and education of a diabetic is a discussion of diet. Although many patients have traditionally been frightened by the thought that as a result of their diabetes they are ''sentenced'' to a miserable and unpalatable diet, adherence to such old beliefs is no longer justified.

With the availability of a large number of innovative recipes it is imperative that the health care team uses a common sense approach to the diet and impress on the patient that the ADA diet is similar to every other common sense diet.

The most important aspects of the diet regimen are (1) moderation, (2) avoidance of large amounts of refined sugar, and (3) a decrease in the size of food portions. In my practice, I emphasize that my patients follow a diet consistent with both the ADA and American Heart Association (AHA) diets, i.e., 50 to 55 percent carbohydrates (mostly complex carbohydrates and less refined sugar), 15 to 20 percent protein, and 30 percent fat, of which no more than 10 percent should be saturated fat, plus an adequate

TABLE 48-11 Educational Components Which Need to Be Discussed with Patients (and Their Relatives) with Diabetes

1. Types, incidence, and definition of diabetes.
2. Signs and symptoms of diabetes.
3. Acute and chronic complications of diabetes.
4. Importance of diet.
5. Technique of insulin injection and frequency of medication.
6. Influence of exercise on diet and treatment.
7. Testing and keeping of records of blood glucose and blood glucose target range.
8. Testing of urine ketones if blood glucose levels are greater than 250 mg/dl or patient is nauseated or vomiting.
9. Emergencies and needed action.
10. Sick days.
11. Importance of foot and skin care.
12. Identification card (Medic Alert).
13. Follow-up care [Hb A_{1c}, self glucose monitoring (SGM)].
14. Importance of glucose control and its relationship to diabetic complications (DCCT studies).
15. Continuing education in conjunction with the ADA program.

TABLE 48-12 Simple Formula to Calculate Ideal Body Weight (IBW) and Caloric Requirements

Build	Women
Medium	Allow 100 lb for first 5 ft of height plus 5 lb for each additional inch.
Small	Subtract 10%
Large	Add 10%

Caloric need for maintenance of IBW for adults can be estimated by using a food nomogram or by adding basal calories and calories needed for activity, using the following:

Basal calories:	IBW (lb) × 10
Sedentary:	IBW (lb) × 10 + 30%
Moderate:	IBW (lb) × 10 + 50%
Strenuous:	IBW (lb) × 10 + 100%

SOURCE: Adapted from Bittle J, Kitabchi AE: Obesity: An overview, in Givens JR (ed): *The Hypothalamus.* Chicago: Year Book, 1984, pp 73–96.

amount of fiber (20–30 g/day). Probably the most important aspects of a diet to emphasize are (1) timeliness of food intake in relation to medication, (2) moderation in consumption of any food group, and (3) food servings of smaller portions.

The author's team proposes that calorie requirements be based on ideal body weight (IBW) as derived from the Modified Metropolitan Insurance Company table. This is summarized in Table 48-12.[1]

Treatment of NIDDM

Table 48-13 provides more specific guidelines for the management of patients with NIDDM. As stated above, diet is the backbone of DM treatment. Our approach to overweight diabetic individuals would consist of three major strategies: weight loss, a low-fat diet (≤30 percent Kcal from fat with low-saturated fat), and physical exercise. Obese patients should be advised to reduce their weight to the ideal body weight as detailed in Table 48-12.

Weight reduction in overweight individuals is associated with improved triglyceride levels, insulin sensitivity, total cholesterol and low-density lipoprotein (LDL) cholesterol, increased high-density lipoprotein (HDL), improved glucose, and decreased insulin resistance. Although the greater the weight loss the greater the improvement, even with a weight loss of < 5 kg an improvement in lipid disorders has been observed.

Physical exercise helps not only with weight reduction, but also significant weight loss, and regular exercise has been shown to improve insulin sensitivity and dyslipidemia in those people who are in high-risk groups for cardiovascular and microvascular diseases.

Oral Hypoglycemic Agents (OHAs): Sulfonylureas

As stated in Table 48-13, the use of oral hypoglycemic agents (OHAs) is recommended for all NIDDM patients who (1) fail diet therapy, (2) have had diabetes less than 10 years, (3) require less than 30

TABLE 48-13 General Guidelines for Management of Type 2 (NIDDM) Diabetes

1. Place patient on ADA reducing diet (50 % CHO, 30 % fat, 20 % protein, high fiber) with 3 meals per day to achieve and maintain ideal body weight or reduce weight by 5–15 % in 3 mo (if ≥ 130 % above ideal body weight).
2. Encourage risk-factor interventions (smoking, exercise, lipids, etc.).
3. While on diet, check fasting blood glucose by finger stick daily for 2 mo. If diet is effective, FBG will gradually decline during this period. If FBG does not decline or increases, consider use of oral hypoglycemic agents (OHAs) if:
   a. Patient has had diabetes for less than 10 y.
   b. Patient does not have severe hepatic or renal disease.
   c. Patient is not pregnant.
   d. Patient is not allergic to sulfonylurea.
4. Patients with FBG (on diet) ≥ 250 mg/dl (after adequate dietary restriction) are not suitable candidates for oral hypoglycemic agents.
5. While on OHA check patient for FBG and 2 HPPBG every 2 mo (with daily FBG and 2 HPPBG monitoring at home. If 2 HPPBG < 200 mg/dl, omit OHA and place on diet alone and follow every 1–2 mo. If FBG > 200 mg/dl consistently while on OHA, place patient on insulin.
6. Insulin dosage should be calculated on actual body weight (0.5–1.0 U/kg body wt).
7. If total insulin requirement is less than 30 U/day, may try to give the entire dose as NPH or Lente before a major meal and check for glycemic control (*Goal:* FBG < 140, 2 HPP < 200, and no BG < 60 mg/dl).
8. If the goal is not achieved by a single insulin injection, insulin may be given as a mixture of Regular: NPH (50:50) bid, 1/2 h before breakfast and 1/2 h before supper.
9. Very obese NIDDM may require more insulin/kg body wt and greater percentage of total insulin as regular insulin than less-obese NIDDM.
10. If above regimen fails to control blood glucose, consider multiple regular insulin injections before each meal with bedtime NPH or Lente insulin.

NOTE: Refer insulin-resistant patients (requiring > 200 U insulin/day) to a Diabetologist.

units of insulin, and (4) do not have contraindications to the use of OHAs (sensitivity to OHAs, pregnancy, and severe liver and kidney damage).

Table 48-14 lists first- and second-generation sulfonylureas as the only OHAs available and approved by the FDA in the United States.[7] The effect of sulfonylureas may be twofold, one enhancing insulin secretion from the pancreas and the other providing an extrapancreatic benefit. However, it is very rare that OHAs can provide any beneficiary effect in a patient whose insulin secretion (as measured by C-peptide) is nil (less than 0.2 pmole/ml) and whose fasting blood glucose on an adequate diabetic diet is greater than 250 mg/dl.

It is also important to remember that OHAs have an annual failure rate of 3 to 5 percent. Therefore, patients must be evaluated frequently, and when OHAs fail to control blood glucose (2-h postprandial > 200 mg/dl), insulin therapy may be needed.

TABLE 48-14 FDA-Approved Sulfonylureas (OHA)

OHA	Trade Name	Daily Dose	Duration of Action (h)
Tolbutamide*	Orinase	1.5–3.0 g in divided dose	6–12
Tolazamide*	Tolinase	200–1000 mg in divided dose	12–24
Acetohexamide*	Dymelor	250–1500 mg as single dose	12–24
Chlorpropamide*	Diabinese	100–500 mg as single dose	Up to 60
Glyburide†	Glibenclamide, Glynase, Micronase, DiaBeta	2.5–20 mg	10–24
Glipizide†	Glucotrol, glydiazinamide	2.5–20 mg	3–8

*First generation

†Second generation

SOURCE: Adapted and modified from Karam JH, Salber PR, Forsham PW: Pancreatic hormones and diabetes mellitus, in Greenspan FS (ed): *Basic and Clinical Endocrinology,* 3rd ed. Norwalk, CT: Appleton and Lange, 1991.

Insulin Therapy

Table 48-15 lists various preparations of insulin and their bioavailability. Table 48-13 provides a general guideline for the use of insulin in NIDDM patients.

Although not completely documented, studies at certain centers suggest that the combination of an evening dose of insulin (NPH or combined NPH + regular) at supper or bedtime followed by a morning dose of OHA may be effective in the control of hyperglycemia in NIDDM. Although this method of therapy is not uniformly accepted, in difficult situations where patients are reluctant to use multiple insulin injections, it may be worth a trial.

The newly available preparations of combined intermediate (NPH) and regular insulin (70/30; 50/50) may be important adjuncts to the therapy of IDDM patients who are too young or unable to mix regular and NPH insulin or in certain NIDDM patients who may use these preparations alone or in conjunction with OHAs.

Implications of DCCT Studies in the Management of NIDDM Patients

It is important to point out that although the DCCT studies showed an impressive reduction in complications of IDDM patients with intensive therapy, these studies cannot be summarily extrapolated to NIDDM patients. Some of the reasons for this caveat have been discussed recently,[13] but it must be emphasized that whereas control of hyperglycemia in IDDM patients is of paramount importance, in NIDDM patients prevention of the disease may be the most crucial factor in management. The two most important components of such management are diet and exercise, but as NIDDM is more prevalent in minority groups, such measures must be culturally and ethnically acceptable to the patients.

Treatment of IDDM

Table 48-16 recommends several steps in the management of patients with IDDM. It is important to note, however, that all modes of treatment must be individualized, and a general approach needs to be tailored to the needs of the individual, taking into consideration activity, dietary preference, work place, and family support.

Various studies suggest that the pancreas in adults secretes basal insulin and C-peptide in equimolar concentrations.[10] It is estimated that the basal rate of insulin secretion is 1 unit/h daily for a total of about 24 units/day. In addition, the pancreas, through a multiple mechanism of cephalic and gastric phases, secretes postprandially approximately 25 units per day. We have shown this graphically in Fig. 48-1 for the three meals (realizing that this is an approximation and that the secreted amounts are influenced by multifactorial events). The total estimated daily secretion of insulin is therefore 49 units in a 70-kg person, which calculates to about 0.7 units of insulin/kg. As can be seen from the figure, about half of this insulin has a low steady level (resembling

TABLE 48-15 Summary of Bioavailability Characteristics of the Insulins

	Insulin Type	Onset	Peak Action	Duration
Short-acting	Regular, Actrapid, Velosulin	15–30 min	1–3 h	5–7 h
	Semilente, Semitard	30–60 min	4–6 h	12–16 h
Intermediate-acting	Lente, Lentard, Monotard, NPH, Insulatard, Protaphane	2–4 h	8–10 h	18–24 h
Long-acting	Ultralente, Ultratard, PZI	4–5 h	8–14 h	25–36 h
	Beef*			
	Human stated to be shorter in duration of action.*			

*Author's comments.

SOURCE: Adapted from Karam JH, Salber PR, Forsham PH: Pancreatic hormones and diabetes mellitus, in Greenspan FS (ed): *Basic and Clinical Endocrinology,* 3d ed. Norfolk, CT: Appleton and Lange, 1991, pp 592–650.

Figure 48-1 A simplified representation of baseline and postprandial insulin secretion in a 70-kg subject (total of 49 U/day).

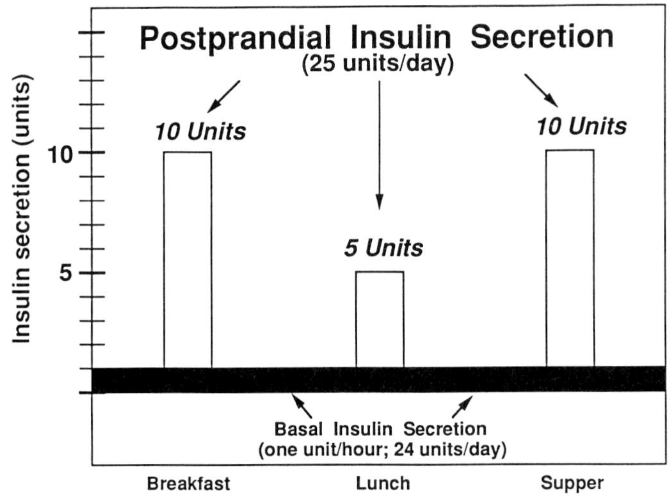

intermediate-NPH or long-acting ultralente insulin), while the remaining 25 units are secreted on demand as a fast-acting insulin (resembling a regular insulin preparation).

Based on this assumption, we have suggested in Table 48-16 a dosage of insulin in IDDM that simulates the pancreas (i.e., 50 percent intermediate or long-acting and 50 percent regular insulin), of which two-thirds of the dose (combined NPH and regular insulin) is given before breakfast and the remaining one-third (combined NPH and regular insulin) before supper. As stated, however, there are tremendous individual variabilities for combined insulin therapy. As an example, we have depicted in Fig. 48-2 various proposed schedules for insulin injections that one may use in adult IDDM patients.

In general, human insulin is preferred to other animal sources of insulin since animal insulins are more immunogenic than the human form of insulin. Also, in general, regular insulin produces less insulin antibodies than intermediate or long-acting preparations (even human preparations). It should also be noted that in a patient who is allergic to insulin, the allergic response can occur even with human insulin.

With the advent of intensive therapy, it is essential to note that no IDDM patient can achieve euglycemic control—even with excellent dietary compliance—with one insulin injection per day. Almost all such patients will require two injections (i.e., before

TABLE 48-16 General Guidelines for the Management of Type 1 (IDDM) Diabetes

1. Place patient on ADA diet (50 % CHO, 30 % fat, 20 % protein) suitable for growth, development, and maintenance of ideal body weight. Give at least 3 meals a day plus bedtime snack (see below).
2. Do not give oral hypoglycemic agents for type 1 DM.
3. All patients must receive at least bid insulin (with short- and intermediate-acting insulins).
4. Give insulin based on actual body weight (0.5–0.8 U/kg b.wt.), 40–60 % of total as intermediate-acting and 60–40 % as regular insulin.
5. Goal of therapy: FBG 70–120 mg/dl and 2 hpp ≤ 180 mg/dl with no blood glucose below 60 mg/dl.
6. Split dosage of intermediate-acting insulin to give about half of it in the morning and remainder at supper or HS.
7. If bid insulin does not achieve the therapeutic goal, consider injection of regular insulin before each meal with intermediate- or long-acting insulin at bedtime.
8. Regular insulin must be given half hour before each meal or snack. Adjust regular insulin based on AC blood glucose and/or grams of CHO intake.
9. If regular insulin is prescribed at HS, be sure to give snack (if BG ≤ 200 mg/dl).
10. See patient for follow-up initially every 2 weeks, then every 1–3 mo for glycemic control, dietary compliance, and chronic complications.

NOTE: Refer brittle diabetic (i.e., wide swing of hypo- and hyperglycemia) to a diabetologist.

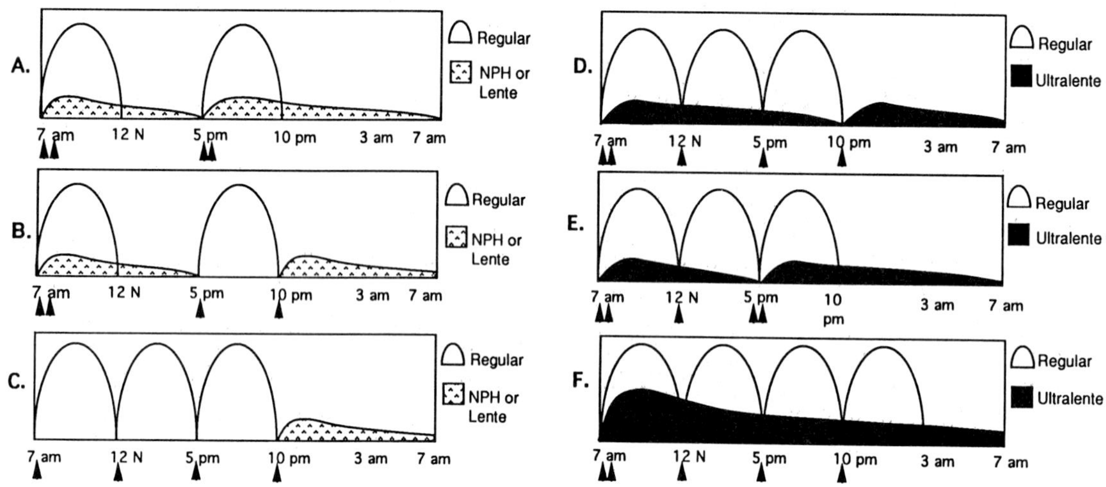

Figure 48-2 Proposed methods of insulin injection schedule in IDDM patients. The Ultralente insulin dose in *F* is twice as much as in *D* or *E*.

breakfast and before supper), and the majority will require three injections of insulin (morning, supper, and bedtime). Some patients may need small doses of regular insulin at lunch (Fig. 48-2).

Hypoglycemia is one of the most serious side effects of intensive therapy. As a result, such therapy in young children (<13 years) or older IDDM patients with multiple complications of hypoglycemic unawareness is not recommended.[18]

Outpatient Management of Patients with Diabetes

Until 1993, there were no clear studies to correlate hyperglycemia with the complications of diabetes in IDDM,[15] but the recent report of the DCCT studies[18] clearly demonstrates the benefit of glycemic control. All physicians who manage patients with diabetes should have clear in their minds a numerical goal for glycemic control and emphasize these target ranges to the patient, in addition to the other factors mentioned in Tables 48-9 through 48-13. The desired level of Hb A_{1c} should also be discussed. Although 7.2 percent was the approximate average of the Hb A_{1c} of DCCT patients on intensive therapy, it is important to note that the studies showed *any* reduction in Hb A_{1c} was beneficial in reducing complications.[18]

Since admission of patients to the hospital for diabetes control is difficult to obtain from health insurance carriers in the absence of acute metabolic decompensation (i.e., DKA, HHNS, or hypoglycemia), outpatient care is the prevailing method of management. The author recommends that IDDM patients be seen at least every 2 months and that patients do a minimum of two blood glucoses per day (SGM), but, more importantly, communicate with the health care team when repeated levels of hypoglycemia or hyperglycemia are experienced.

We particularly encourage patients to fax their glucose data to us so we can advise them on proper adjustment of their insulin. In such cases, a quarterly visit may be adequate for a more stable patient. A similar schedule should also be followed for NIDDM patients, as these patients may need just as much behavioral modification and support for their control of diet and weight as the IDDM patients require for their insulin, particularly in coordination with the nutritionist and mental health professionals (who know about diabetes). It is important to realize that no therapy can substitute for a highly motivated patient assured by a compassionate and knowledgeable health care provider team that help is available; the major responsibility for care, will, however, rest on the shoulders of the patient herself.

Complications of Intensive Insulin Therapy—Hypoglycemia

This chapter has dealt with the day-to-day ambulatory management of patients with diabetes. The author has not discussed management of the acute complications of diabetes, such as DKA and HHNS, but readers are referred to some comprehensive reviews on this subject in others articles.[8,11]

Since hypoglycemia is becoming more frequent with the use of intensive insulin therapy, it should be emphasized that patients prone to hypoglycemia must carry on their person not only a Medic Alert identification, but also a glucagon injection kit as well as glucose tablets (or a tube of Write-A-Cake icing, which requires no refrigeration). The preferred method of therapy for hypoglycemia in an alert patient is a glass of milk, which will provide a longer-lasting euglycemia than a glass of orange juice or sugar cubes. Obviously an unconscious patient at home needs either parenteral administration of glucagon (subcutaneous or IM) or sugar paste on the gum (but not in the mouth) by another person prior to taking the patient to the emergency room, where IV glucose may be administered.

References and Suggested Reading

1. Bittle J, Kitabchi AE: Obesity: An Overview. In Givens JR. (ed): *The Hypothalamus.* Chicago, Year Book, 1984, pp 73–96.
2. Bunn HF: Evaluation of glycosylated hemoglobin in diabetic patients. *Diabetes* 30:613–617, 1981.
3. Ray NF, Wills S, Thamer M: Direct and Indirect Costs of Diabetes in the United States in 1992. The American Diabetes Association Report. Medical Technology and Practice Pattern Institute, Washington, D.C., December 1993.
4. Gavin JR, Davidson JA: Type II diabetes in minorities. *Current Concepts.* Kalamazoo: Upjohn, 1992.
5. Harris MI: Undiagnosed NIDDM: Clinical and public health issues. *Diabetes Care* 16:642–652, 1993.
6. Harris MI, Hadden WC, Knowler WC, Bennett PH: Prevalence of diabetes and impaired glucose tolerance and plasma glucose levels in U.S. population, aged 20–74 yr. *Diabetes* 36:523–534, 1987.
7. Karam JH, Salber PR, Forsham PH: Pancreatic hormones and diabetes mellitus, in Greenspan FS (ed): *Basic and Clinical Endocrinology,* 3d ed. Norwalk: Appleton and Lange, 1991, pp 592–650.
8. Kitabchi AE, Fisher JN, Murphy MB, Rumbak MJ: Diabetes ketoacidosis and hyperglycemic hyperosmolar nonketotic state, in Kahn CR, Weir G (eds): *Joslin's Diabetes Mellitus Textbook,* 13th ed. Philadelphia: Lea and Febiger, 1993, pp 738–770.
9. Kitabchi AE, Fisher JN: Diabetes mellitus, in Conn R (ed): *Current Diagnosis.* Philadelphia: Saunders, 1991, pp 766–774.
10. Kitabchi AE, Duckworth WC, Stentz FB: Insulin synthesis, proinsulin and C-peptide, in Rifkin H, Porte D (eds): *Diabetes Mellitus,* 4th ed. New York: Elsevier, 1990, pp 71–88.
11. Kitabchi AE, Rumbak MJ: Management of diabetic emergencies. *Hosp Pract* 24:129–160, 1989.
12. Kitabchi AE, Fisher JN: Diabetes mellitus, in Glew RH, Peters SP (eds): *Clinical Studies in Medical Biochemistry.* New York: Oxford University Press, 1987.
13. Lebovitz HE: The DCCT and its implications for NIDDM. *Clin Diabetes* 12:3–4, 1994.
14. Morris LR, McGee JA, Kitabchi AE: Correlation between plasma and urine glucose in diabetes. *Ann Intern Med* 94:469–471, 1981.
15. Nathan DM: Long-term complications of diabetes mellitus. *N Engl J Med* 328:1676–1685, 1993.
16. National Diabetes Data Group: Classification and diagnosis of diabetes mellitus and other categories of glucose intolerance. *Diabetes* 28:1039–1057, 1979.
17. Reaven GM: Banting lecture 1988: Role of insulin resistance in human disease. *Diabetes* 37:1595–1607, 1988.
18. The DCCT Research Group: The effect of intensive treatment of diabetes on the development and progression of long-term complications in insulin-dependent diabetes mellitus. *N Engl J Med* 329:977–986, 1993.
19. *The Physician's Guide to Type II Diabetes (NIDDM): Diagnosis and Treatment,* 2d ed. New York: American Diabetes Association, 1988.

49 HIV Infection

Howard Minkoff

By the end of the decade approximately 40 million people around the world will be infected with human immunodeficiency virus (HIV). An increasing percentage of them will be women. AIDS is the fourth leading cause of death of reproductive age women in the United States and is *the* leading cause in many large cities. Children who acquire the virus do so in the overwhelming majority of cases perinatally. In the face of this epidemic, providers of health care to women will be called on to perform several vital functions: educate their patients about prevention, diagnose and treat HIV infection, and provide obstetric and gynecologic care focused on the unique needs of HIV-infected women. This chapter is intended to prepare the primary care physician for the performance of these tasks.

Education and Prevention

Approximately 13 million Americans will acquire a sexually transmitted disease (STD) next year. The consequences of their doing so will range from infertility to death from AIDS. Primary care physicians have an obligation to be involved on a routine basis in emphasizing the prevention message. The core of this message depends on an understanding of HIV's modes of transmission. Intravenous drug use and heterosexual contact continue to be the predominant routes of infection, and health care providers must focus on these two issues.

Absolutely safe sex would involve abstinence or mutual monogamy with an uninfected partner. Partners who are bisexual or intravenous drug users would, of course, be considered at high risk. Realistically, however, it is unlikely that many women will know the HIV status of sexual partners, and, particularly in high prevalence communities, any casually known partner poses a risk. Therefore women will have to rely on other safety techniques. Although noninsertive sex is also very safe, it is not widely accepted. As a result, most safer sex strategies will—to a greater or lesser extent—have to rely on condoms. The use of condoms in the prevention of STDs, particularly HIV, has been widely heralded. The evidence for their efficacy comes from studies of prostitutes, discordant couple studies, and in vitro experiments. The latter have even demonstrated efficacy in the prevention of transmission of hepatitis B, which is a smaller particle than HIV. Most evidence of efficacy is limited to latex condoms, however, since natural skin condoms have much wider variation in pore size. A controversial area is the role of viricidal agents such as nonoxynol-9. Although they have the potential to inactivate the virus should a condom break, there is concern that chronic frequent usage might result in vaginal ulcerations.

Diagnosis of HIV Infection

Testing for antibody to HIV became a practical clinical tool in 1985. Given the limited treatment options available for the care of HIV-infected women and children in the early 1980s, the driving force behind testing at that time was to allow women to make informed reproductive choices. Shortly thereafter, however, researchers[54] demonstrated that serostatus did not substantively alter reproductive choice. Despite that fact, it was clearly important that each woman have the right to all information germane to her individual decision and that HIV tests be made available.

The strategy used to provide access at that time was to offer the test selectively. Women who volunteered a history of "risk" behavior had the advantages and disadvantages of the test discussed at their prenatal visit. The failure of that approach to engage many women in the process of learning their serostatus soon became apparent. Several researchers compared HIV serosurveys with anonymously collected patient histories and found that a large percentage of infected individuals had not acknowledged any risk behaviors.[34] Apparently, since a history of intravenous drug use or sex with bisexual men was perceived to be stigmatizing, many women chose not to acknowledge these behaviors when the sole advantage was perceived to be access to a test.[38]

In response to these reports, many clinicians, particularly those in high prevalence communities, started to offer the test universally. As expected, it was then found that many women who at the time of pretest counseling acknowledged no risk but whose test result confirmed an HIV infection, did indeed know their risk factor but had chosen not to discuss it until their serostatus had been established.[39]

As therapeutic interventions for both the mother and child were developed in the late 1980s, many clinicians came to believe that a nondirectional offering of the test was too passive a process and that the imprimatur of the physician should be given to the test through the substitution of "recommending" for "offering."[1]

Currently many obstetrical services in high-prevalence communities are recommending that all prenatal patients take an HIV test. There are clinicians who feel, however, that the time has come to go even further in testing. Some, who advocate either mandatory or "right of refusal" approaches to testing, do so based on their belief that substantive medical advantage is available to children whose serostatus is known and that children cannot speak out for themselves and attain those advantages by opting to have an HIV test. Consequently, there is a debate at the moment between those who prioritize fetal-neonatal beneficence and those who champion maternal autonomy.

The posttest counseling session for a seropositive women should be planned before the woman arrives for her result. This planning includes a review of the woman's support network and the development of a follow-up plan for ongoing psychosocial support and medical evaluation.

When women learn they are HIV-seropositive, their reactions range from despair and anger to total denial and withdrawal.[26] In general it can be anticipated that women will react to learning this diagnosis in much the same way they have reacted to other stressful events in their lives. It is important to allow them sufficient time during the session to work through some of these initial reactions. Such beginning counseling sessions often last between 45 and 75 mins.

The content of the counseling that a seropositive woman receives must be sufficient to assure an informed decision regarding reproductive choice. Information about the perinatal transmission of the virus, the consequence of pregnancy on the natural history of HIV disease, the natural history of pediatric HIV disease, and the therapeutic options for the women should be described in lay language. If abortion is still an option, depending on the woman's due date and the state's legal limit for abortion, it should be discussed. The woman's decision—whether or not she chooses abortion—should be supported, and a liaison with psychosocial supports should be established.

Primary Care of HIV Infection

Once a woman has been identified as HIV-infected and received appropriate counseling and emotional and social support, the physician must turn his or her attention to a baseline medical evaluation of the patient.[2] A complete history and physical examination that includes but is not limited to mental status, fundoscopic, pelvic, genital, and rectal examination should be performed in order to ascertain the presence of any HIV-related stigmata.

Baseline laboratory studies should also allow the clinician to assess both the patient's susceptibility to infection (immune status) and any evidence of prevalent infections (e.g., syphilis). Therefore, the patient needs a complete blood count and CD4 lymphocyte studies that include the absolute numbers and percentages of CD4 and CD8 cells and a T4/T8 ratio. Additionally serologic tests for syphilis, hepatitis, and toxoplasma should be obtained. The patient needs a tuberculin skin test (PPD), and an anergy panel using two or more antigens (*Candida,* mumps, tetanus toxoid) should be given. Finally an SMA12, urinalysis, chest x-ray, and Pap smear are required.

This initial assessment can be used to classify the status of the woman's disease based on the revised CDC definitions.[11] Basically, individuals have their disease status subcategorized depending on whether they (A) are asymptomatic or have generalized lymphadenopathy only, (B) have symptoms that are not AIDS-defining, or (C) have AIDS. They are further stratified based on whether their CD4 count is (1) 500 or over, (2) 200 to 499, or (3) under 200.

The laboratory results will also guide decisions regarding preventive strategies such as tuberculosis prophylaxis and pneumocystis prophylaxis (CD4 < 200). Appropriate vaccinations with hepatitis vaccine, pneumonia vaccine, and influenza vaccine can be given as necessary. Any sexually transmitted diseases that are diagnosed should also be treated.

It is at this point that considerations of antiretrovirals should also occur. Two drugs, zidovudine (AZT) and didanosine (ddI), are currently approved for the treatment of HIV infection. A third drug, zalcitabine (ddC), has been approved for combination chemotherapy with zidovudine. The timing of initiation of therapy is linked to CD4 counts.

The New York State AIDS Institute[2] recommends that CD4 counts be measured every 6 months until they approach 500/mm^3. At that point they should be obtained on an every 3 months basis. Consideration of antiretroviral therapy begins at a count under 500/mm^3, though recommendations are in a state of flux pending more data on the benefits of early therapy. When the count falls below 200/mm^3, pneumocystis carinii pneumonia (PCP) prophylaxis should be instituted.

When a patient is placed on AZT (500 mg/day), the provider should be aware of the potential adverse effects. The most common complications are anemia, thrombocytopenia, and granulocytopenia—all of which are generally reversible. Nausea, headache, myalgias, and myopathy are often reported but may be transient. Patients should be followed with CBCs and serum chemistries. Patients with advanced HIV disease who are intolerant or failing AZT may be placed on ddI. The major toxicities are pancreatitis and neuropathy. The dosage is 200 mg bid for adults who weigh over 60 kg and 125 mg bid if they weigh less.

Although the management of the protean infectious diseases that occur in the setting of HIV infection is well beyond the scope of this chapter and falls more appropriately within the purview of a specialist in infectious diseases, the primary care physician should be familiar with the manifestations of disease that are clinically significant and require consultation and/or referral. These complications can be broadly categorized into infectious, neoplastic, and neurologic.

Infectious complications range from local fungal infections (thrush, esophageal candidiasis) through a wide array of pulmonary, gastrointestinal, and other infections caused by parasites (*Pneumocystis carinii* pneumonia, *Toxoplasma gondii, Cryptosporidium* spp.), fungal organisms (*Candida albicans, Cryptococcus neoformans, Histoplasma capsulatum*), bacterial organisms (mycobacterial infections, *Salmonella, Treponema pallidum*), and viruses (herpes simplex virus, cytomegalovirus, varicella zoster). These infections frequently present as pneumonia, watery diarrhea, or as neurologic impairment.

AIDs-defining neoplastic complications include Kaposi's sarcoma, B-cell lymphomas, and primary central nervous system (CNS) lymphomas. In some other neoplasias, such as oral and anal squamous cell carcinoma and Hodgkin's disease, a link with AIDS has been suspected. Treatment of AIDS-associated neoplasia should be instituted under the guidance of a hematologist-oncologist and be appropriate for the specific neoplasm.

Management of neurologic complications is extremely complex. Neurologic dysfunction in patients with AIDS may result from HIV infection of the CNS (AIDS dementia) or toxic metabolic disorders. It may also be a consequence of infectious or neoplastic complications of AIDS.

Pregnancy and the HIV-Positive Woman

The "golden rule" in the care of a pregnant woman with any medical complication is to provide optimal care in a fashion that is unmodified by gender or childbearing considerations unless there is compelling evidence that such care poses an unacceptable risk to the fetus. If fetal risks are substantial, then the counsel of the mother is sought in order to best balance the maternal-fetal risks and benefits associated with an alternative approach. The same principle holds in the case of the HIV-infected woman.

In reality there are very few examples of HIV therapies that need to be modified because of pregnancy. Thus the clinician's first responsibility is to ensure that the standard interventions are in place. Pneumovax, influenza, and hepatitis vaccines should be administered as necessary. Testing should be performed to detect any sexually transmitted diseases such as syphilis, gonorrhea, and chlamydia. Tuberculosis should be ruled out, and baseline toxoplasmosis titers should be obtained.

During the antepartum period the clinician must be wary of nonspecific symptoms that may, in other circumstances, be attributed to pregnancy per se. Fatigue and weight loss are common in the first trimester but may also be early manifestations of HIV disease. Upper respiratory tract symptoms (e.g., fever and tachypnea), in particular, warrant aggressive investigation. Patients should be encouraged to report all symptoms immediately. Nutritional counseling should be instituted if difficulty is encountered in maintaining appropriate weight gain. Although no cofactors have proved to adversely affect the rate of disease progression, it seems prudent to advise patients to avoid factors shown to alter T4/T8 ratios (sleep deprivation, stress) or enhance viral replication in vitro (e.g., antigenic stimulus from unprotected intercourse with an infected male, infections). Alcohol and illicit drugs should be prohibited.

The timing of initiation of many of the therapeutic agents used in the management of HIV infection is determined by an individual's CD4 count. These counts, therefore, must be followed closely during pregnancy. Since pregnancy itself may lead to changes in the CD4 count, more frequent monitoring may be warranted.[1] Although some component of the decline of CD4 counts during pregnancy may be attributable to pregnancy alone (as opposed to a viral effect), it should not be assumed that the prognostic significance of a low count is less reliable than in nonpregnant populations.

Standard approaches to prophylaxis against *Pneumocystis carinii* pneumonia should be maintained during pregnancy. Women whose CD4 counts drop below 200/mm^3 should receive either pentamidine or bactrim therapy. Although pentamidine has the advantage of less frequent side effects and extremely low blood levels, access to the aerosol form may not be readily available to all women, and its use can be associated with breakthrough. Bactrim is readily available and highly effective. Adverse maternal reactions are common (most often, rash), but neonatal consequences have not been serious, and kernicterus has not been reported in settings in which sulfa derivatives were not also used during the neonatal period. The specific agent that is employed is probably less important than the fact that some therapy is prescribed during gestation.

It is currently recommended that nonpregnant individuals whose CD4 counts drop below 500/mm^3 receive antiretroviral therapy. There is some question, however, regarding the degree of advantage to starting therapy at that level as opposed to an even lower count (e.g., 200/mm^3).

The benefit related to the perinatal use of ZDV has been demonstrated. A double-blinded study known as ACTG 076 (AIDS Clinical Trials Group 076), which was designed to evaluate the efficacy, safety, and tolerance of ZDV in preventing maternal transmission of HIV to the fetus, was halted in February 1994 when preliminary results did in fact indicate a substantial reduction in HIV infection among infants born to women treated with zidovudine. There are clearly many issues which remain to be resolved, but the U.S. Public Health Service has recommended that pregnant women be informed of these results. Data on 364 births indicated a 67 percent relative reduction in risk of HIV infection in those infants whose mothers had taken ZDV. The rate of perinatal infection was 25.5 percent in the placebo group and only 8.3 percent in the treated group. The long-term risks of ZDV therapy to the fetus are not presently known. The current recommendation of the U.S. Public Health Service is that until the risk for teratogenicity and other complications from ZDV therapy given in the first trimester can be assessed, it is recommended that when ZDV is being used only for the purposes of reducing the risk for perinatal transmission it should not be instituted earlier than the 14th week of gestation. On AIDS Clinical Trial Protocol 076, zidovudine is administered orally during the pregnancy, intravenously during labor and delivery, and then orally to the newborn for the first six weeks of life.

Other than the use of intravenous ZDV during labor as per protocol 076, the intrapartum management of the HIV-infected mother is not substantively altered by serostatus, though to some extent the care of all mothers and neonates in the labor and delivery suite has been influenced by the HIV epidemic. The introduction of universal precautions into the labor and delivery area, for example, has changed some of the standards in that setting. Delee suctioning is no longer performed with suction generated by a clinician. The mucous trap is now attached to wall suction. With this new approach caution must be exercised lest excessive pressure be utilized, which could theoretically damage the neonate's gut. It has been recommended that less than 140 mmHg be used.

The possibility that fetal scalp electrodes and scalp clips can act as potential vectors of viral transmission continues to be raised. This concern is based on the presence of virus that has been documented in the vaginal secretions and the prolonged contact that the fetus might have in the hours before birth, after the membranes have ruptured, with those viral particles. Some component of the fetal protection at that point could be intact skin. Thus, piercing that skin to obtain a scalp blood sample or placing an electrode into the skin could pose a theoretical risk of inoculating the fetus with virus. There are, however, scant empiric data to address this concern. Some investigators have reported that infants who underwent the types of invasive procedures described above were not more likely to become infected than infants not so exposed, but the sizes of those cohorts were too small to have the requisite statistical power to rule out the level of risk generally associated with needle-stick injuries. Thus clinicians must continue to balance the theoretical risk of these procedures with the clinical benefit to be derived from their performance. In any event, "routine" use should be avoided.

In the postpartum period universal precautions should be extended to the neonate. Additionally there is an ever-increasing body of evidence that breastfeeding can be associated with viral transmission and should therefore be proscribed (in developed countries). Since new protocols for management of pediatric and adult HIV are constantly under development, appropriate referral of mother and child to physicians with expertise in the management of HIV disease should be made before their discharge from the hospital.

Gynecologic Care of the HIV-Positive Woman

Candidiasis

Clinicians were aware of an association between vaginal candidiasis and depressed immune function long before the HIV epidemic began. A woman's immunologic defense against *Candida albicans* is primarily cell-mediated.[59] Since an increased frequency of vaginal candidiasis is found to accompany even the mild cell-mediated immunocompromise associated with pregnancy, it is not surprising that candidal infections have also been described in association with HIV infection. In fact, the association between candidial infections at a variety of anatomical sites and both the stage and prognosis of HIV disease was noted in some of the earliest reports on HIV infections.[50]

The relationship between HIV and candida, among women in particular, has been the subject of a small but growing body of research. In 1982, in one of the first reports on AIDS in women, Masur et al reported oral or esophageal candidiasis in four of five patients with the syndrome.[37] In a widely cited study, Rhoads and colleagues (1987) reported on chronic vaginal candidiasis in women with relatively advanced immunocompromise.[47] Among 29 women with HIV, 7 (24 percent) were found to have chronic recurrent vulvovaginal candidiasis. The severity of the infection in these women (symptoms and discharge for at least 1 year and requiring almost constant use of intravaginal antifungal agents for suppression) was more remarkable than the percentage infected. Of the 7 women with chronic vaginal candidiasis, 6 had severe depletion of the CD4 cells, with counts below 100/mm^3, and were diagnosed with AIDS. None of the HIV-positive women without mucocutaneous candidiasis developed AIDS over the study period.

More recently a clinical continuum of candidiasis that is linked to progressive immunocompromise has been described.[28] Mean CD4 counts among women with vaginal candidiasis only were generally still in the normal range while among women with thrush but not esophageal candidiasis average CD4 counts were 230/mm^3. CD4 counts among women with esophageal candidiasis averaged 30/mm^3. In another study of 97 HIV-infected women, vaginal candidiasis was present more commonly in the women with CD4 counts of $<$ 100/mm^3.[24] It is important to be aware, therefore, that the rate of vulvovaginal candidiasis seen in HIV-infected women prior to immune compromise may not exceed the background level among HIV-negative women.

There have been increasing reports of nonalbicans species that may be refractory to the azole therapeutics; these have been suggested as etiologic factors in recurrent candidiasis.[31] There is little information available about the prevalence of such yeast species among HIV-infected women or whether they are linked to refractory disease.

Current management of vaginal candidiasis for HIV-infected women includes an initial attempt at topical therapy for the symptomatic individual. It is reasonable to assume that among relatively immunocompetent women cure rates should not be markedly lower than those seen in seronegative women. When a woman has recurrent or refractory disease, ketoconazole can be utilized (400 mg per day for 14 days, followed by 400 mg per day for 6 days each month for 6 months; liver function should be monitored). Recently the use of fluconazole for treatment of severe or recurrent vulvovaginitis has been proposed as an alternative therapy.[33]

Sexually Transmitted Diseases

Sexually transmitted diseases (STDs) have been clearly implicated in the transmission of HIV. Genital ulcer disease in particular is thought to increase the risk of both HIV acquisition and transmission.

Somewhat less is known about the impact of HIV infection on the natural history and response to therapy of STDs. It has been reported that the natural history of many STDs may be modified by HIV infection. Disseminated or chronic, severe herpes infections, for example, have been reported in association with advanced HIV disease when immunosuppression is more marked.[53] Quinnan et al. summarized several studies that noted increased prevalence and severity of herpes simplex and zoster in other immunosuppressed populations such as those receiving bone marrow transplants.[45] Among 200 HIV-positive women followed in Rhode Island,

20 had chronic recurrent genital or generalized mucocutaneous herpes simplex. "Recurrent" was defined as at least eight discrete clinical episodes in a year or recurrences occurring at least twice as often as the patient's past outbreak pattern. Severe genital herpes was more common in this group of women than observed in groups of men.[10]

Another study of cell-mediated immunity and HSV reported on the prevalence of herpes simplex virus (HSV) ulcerations in relation to CD4 counts among HIV-infected patients. Patients with CD4 counts of $< 50/mm^3$ had a significantly higher risk of HSV ulceration. Despite their observation, the authors did not recommend anti-HSV prophylaxis for patients with low CD4 counts but did suggest appropriate empirical therapy when individuals presented with ulcers.[4] Other authors have also recommended that indications for the use of suppressive acyclovir be the same for HIV-seropositive patients as they are for HIV-seronegative patients.[45] An example of an indication for therapy would be for individuals whose recurrences are very frequent (more than six per year). Restricting the use of suppressive acyclovir to such individuals might help to limit acyclovir-resistant strains of HSV. Self-treatment with acyclovir is a common practice among patients with recurrent herpes. Whether such a practice can contribute to the development of HSV resistance in HIV infected patients has not been the subject of controlled trials.

An association between syphilis and HIV has also been reported. In Baltimore STD Clinics for example, 24.3 percent of patients with a reactive syphilis serology were HIV-infected compared with 3.5 percent of patients with a nonreactive test for syphilis. In heterosexual women without a history of intravenous drug use (IVDU), the risk of HIV was 6.8 times greater among those with a positive syphilis serology.[44] Additionally, syphilis may follow a more fulminant course among HIV-infected individuals, and laboratory diagnosis may be more complicated with increased rates of false-negative and false-positive reactions. Syphilitic infection of the CNS, which usually occurs after years of infection, has been documented with primary syphilis in HIV-infected individuals. Johns et al (1987) reported four cases of neurosyphilis in HIV-infected patients. They warned of an increased propensity of the disease to progress to neurosyphilis and a shortened latency before the onset of symptomatic neurosyphilis.[29]

The occurrence of documented CNS involvement in early syphilis in patients with HIV has led some to recommend increasing the standard dose of benzathine penicillin to three doses over 3 consecutive weeks.[41] Treatment failures documented by rising treponemal titers and recurrence of symptoms have been reported in latent syphilis. It has been recommended that a lumbar puncture be performed as part of an evaluation for neurosyphilis in HIV-infected patients with a history of syphilis.[41] There have been no studies to date clearly evaluating the benefits of this, as opposed to alternative, management.

Current CDC guidelines call for three injections of benzathine penicillin (PCN) for secondary or early latent syphilis. Treatment failures have been reported for penicillin and ceftriaxone in HIV-positive patients with latent or asymptomatic neurosyphilis.[31] Treatment failure is difficult to document; CNS involvement may be present even with negative tests for *Treponema pallidum*. Other measures of CSF abnormality (alterations in glucose, protein, and cell counts) should lead to suspicion of neurologic involvement.

Interpretation of serologic tests for nontreponemal and treponemal antibodies must be made with caution. Biologic false positives [positive rapid plasma reagin (RPR) with negative fluorescent treponemal antibody absorption (FTA-ABS) tests] have been noted to be more common in those with HIV, although the phenomenon is relatively rare.

Another concern is that specific serologic tests for syphilis may become falsely negative in individuals with HIV infection.[34] Negative specific serology does not exclude a past history of syphilis infection in patients with AIDS. Ten percent of AIDS patients in one study showed negative FTA-ABS and *T. pallidum* hemagglutination (TPHA) within 3 years after known syphilis infection. In the same study, a significantly greater proportion of HIV-infected patients showed decreasing titers of specific antibody compared to HIV-negative controls.[30]

Serologic testing may miss patients with persistent syphilis infection. Conversely, even with adequate treatment, RPR titers may not fall as expected.[41] Careful history taking about exposure to and treatment of STDs and complete medical and sexual histories may reveal past infection in HIV-positive patients undetected by standard screening tests.

Very little data have been published on the course and response to therapy of gonorrhea and chlamydia. A gender-specific consequence of such infections is pelvic inflammatory disease (PID). The course of PID among HIV-infected women has been the subject of only a few preliminary reports. Given the similar etiology (sexual transmission) of HIV and PID it is not surprising that the reported prevalance of HIV in a population of women with PID is higher that that among other women in the same community. In Brooklyn, the prevalance of HIV among women hospitalized with PID was 13 percent compared to 2 percent among women giving birth in the same hospital. In this population, in contrast to the two previous studies, there was a trend toward a higher rate of syphilis among HIV-positive women, though HIV seropositivity was not associated with a higher frequency of other STDs.[25]

It is less clear whether women coinfected with HIV have a different course of PID than seronegative women. Studies to date have been limited to inpatients and cannot address issues such as the relative likelihood of need for hospital admission based on serostatus. Hoegsberg et al. (1993) reported in a small study that women admitted with PID were significantly less likely to have a leukocytosis if they were HIV-seropositive. On admission, 40 percent of the HIV-positive patients and 89 percent of the HIV-seronegative women had a white blood cell count of $\geq 10{,}000/\text{mm}^3$ ($p < .001$). HIV-infected women were twice as likely to have a tuboovarian abscess and three times as likely to fail antibiotic therapy, although these differences did not reach statistical significance. Currently the CDC recommends that HIV-infected women who develop PID should be followed closely with early hospitalization and IV antibiotic therapy.[38]

Cervical Diseases

Human papilloma virus (HPV)–associated cervical intraepithelial lesions have been reported to occur with increased frequency and severity among women who are immunocompromised. Renal transplant recipients are an example of that phenomenon. More recently it has been reported that cervical dysplasia is also found with increased frequency among women with HIV infection. The prevalence and severity of cervical dysplasia are linked to the degree of immune compromise.[32,36]

The possibility of more rapid progression of cervical disease in HIV-infected women has been raised. A preliminary report on the follow-up of women with untreated lesions found higher rates of progression and lower rates of regression in association with HIV-infected women.[3]

Whether response to therapy is altered among HIV-infected women remains unclear. Maiman (1993) reported CIN recurrence rates of 39 percent and 9 percent ($p < .01$) in HIV-positive and HIV-negative women, respectively. While other groups have also found that persistent or recurrent disease is more common among HIV-infected women,[58] still others have failed to detect increased rates of recurrence or progression after standard treatment[18] or find higher recurrence rates for vulvar and vaginal condylona only.[32] These discrepancies may arise because of differences in degree of immunosuppression in the groups of HIV-infected women who were followed or to differences in stage of cervical disease at time of treatment.

The adequacy of Pap smear screening in HIV-infected women remains controversial. An early report by Maiman indicated that a high proportion of cervical pathology among 32 HIV-infected women was not detected on Pap smear.[43] In a similar study of 68 HIV-infected women, all of whom received Pap smears, colposcopy, and biopsy, the sensitivity of Pap smears relative to biopsy was 38 percent.[52] In an unpublished study of 300 HIV-infected women followed with Pap smears, colposcopy, and biopsy (as indicated by colposcopy) the sensitivity of Pap smears (with respect to biopsy) was 76 percent and the specificity was 95 percent,[46] which is consistent with literature values for uninfected women cited by the author.[60] The reasons for these disparities are unclear; nonstandardized methodology and noncomparability of control groups may account for some of the differences seen. At present, neither the CDC nor

ACOG advocate routine colposcopy for HIV-infected women[13,48]; Pap smear screening at least once yearly is recommended.

Contraceptive Options for Seropositive Women

The fertility of HIV-infected women appears to be unaffected by their serostatus. Decisions regarding contraception need to be made on the basis of safety and efficacy of the contraceptive method and whether the health effects of the method may be influenced by HIV infection. The impact of the method on HIV infection, if such information becomes available, is another important consideration.

Condoms As indicated previously, condom use is very important in helping to prevent further HIV transmission. When avoidance of pregnancy is of primary concern, barrier methods alone may not confer optimal protection. Supplemental methods may be indicated to ensure effective contraception.

Although Goedert et al. found no evidence of accelerated progression to AIDS among seropositive patients who practiced unprotected intercourse,[20] the possibility that such behavior may introduce more virulent viral strains or, through antigenic stimulation, activate viral replication cannot be ruled out. The use of condoms can also reduce the risk of secondary infections with other STDs.

Hormonal Contraceptives Variations in humoral and cell-mediated immune activity related to gender have been reported. Although the natural history of HIV disease has not been demonstrated to vary with gender, any medication that affects immune status could theoretically contribute to a difference between women and men in disease progression. Gonadal steroids, adrenal glucocorticoids, pituitary hormones including growth hormone and prolactin, thymic hormones, and factors elaborated by activated lymphocytes all influence immune function, with ovarian production of estrogen playing a central role.[21] Sex steroid–mediated immunodepression is also postulated to explain the immune system down regulation noted to occur during pregnancy, which may act to prevent rejection of developing fetal tissue.

At present the potentially multiple biological effects of steroid hormone–containing oral contraceptives (OCs) remain incompletely understood. Possible mechanisms by which OC use might affect progression of HIV disease in seropositive women include inhibition of cell-mediated immunity, with possible simultaneous enhancement of susceptibility to opportunistic infections and suppression of stimulation of CD4 cells, which may lead to decreased viral expression. The estrogen component of OCs may also be associated with a variety of perturbations of the immune system including decreased natural killer cell activity and neutrophil function, potentiation of the production of systemic antibody, and decreased local antibody responses.

Pending confirmed evidence of risk, there is at present no justification for modifying standard recommendations for the use of hormonal contraception in the setting of HIV infection.

IUDs Because of concerns about the possible increased risk of upper genital tract infections among IUD users, IUDs are not recommended for women at risk for STDs, including HIV. Multiple concerns have been raised over their use among HIV-infected women. A theoretical risk of decreased efficacy due to reduced local inflammatory response among women with advanced immunosuppression has been raised. Anemia may be exacerbated by the increased menstrual blood flow associated with IUD use, and concern has been expressed that tailed IUDs may provide a route for ascending infection leading to PID, which may be more severe in immunocompromised patients.

Tubal Ligation Tubal ligation offers a very effective means of contraception but may not be an option for all women because of its irreversible nature.

Conclusion

Unfortunately, the clinician who provides primary care to reproductive age women will be spending increasing time dealing with HIV infection. The care of HIV-infected women requires compassion, energy, and expertise. Providers must work to maintain their patients' health by attempting to slow the intractable progression of immune compromise and by confronting the myriad complications carried in the wake of declining CD4 counts. Additionally clinicians must recognize that these women are in the reproductive age range and will have many gynecologic and obstetric needs. Those needs will be made infinitely more complex by HIV. Despite the daunting nature of these challenges, no other aspect of medicine can, by requiring a total commitment of knowledge and concern, so thoroughly fulfill a physician's social, ethical, and medical obligation to the patient and the community.

References and Selected Readings

1. American College of Obstetricians and Gynecologists (ACOG): Human Immunodeficiency Virus Infection. *Tech Bull (Rev),* 162:1–11, 1992. [Also published by ACOG, Washington D.C.]
2. AIDS Institute, New York State Dept. of Health: *Criteria for the medical care of adults with HIV infection.* 1:109–111, 1993.
3. Anastos K, Dememberg R, Solomon L, Rein S: Relationship of CD4 cell counts to cervical cytologic abnormalities and gynecologic infections in 150 HIV-infected women (abstract no. TuB0532). Amsterdam: Eighth International Conference on AIDS. 1992.
4. Bagdades EK, Pillay D, Squire SB, et al: Relationship between herpes simplex virus ulceration and CD4 cell counts in patients with HIV infection. *AIDS* 6:1317–1320, 1992.
5. Baker DA, Hameed C, Tejani N, et al: Lymphocyte subsets in women on low-dose oral contraceptives. *Contraception* 32:377–382, 1985.
6. Baker DA, Salvatore W, Milch PO: Effect of low-dose oral contraceptives on natural killer cell activity. *Contraception* 39:119–124, 1989.
7. Barnes EW, Loudon NB, MacCuish AC: Phytohaemagglutinin-induced lymphocyte transformation and circulating autoantibodies in women taking oral contraceptives. *Lancet* (suppl 1)898–900, 1974.
8. Ben-Nathan D, Lachmi B, Lustig S, Feuerstein G: Protection by dehydroepiandrosterone in mice infected with viral encephalitis. *Arch Virol* 120:263–271, 1991.
9. Bisset LR, Griffin JFT: Humoral immunity in oral contraceptive users: I. Plasma immunoglobulin levels. *Contraception* 38:567–572, 1988.
10. Carpenter CCJ, Mayer KH, Stein MD, et al: Human immunodeficiency virus infection in North American women: Experiences with 200 cases and a review of the literature. 70:307–325, 1991.
11. Centers for Disease Control: 1993 Revised classification system for HIV infection. 41:1–144, MMWR 1992.
12. Centers for Disease Control: Pelvic inflammatory disease: Guidelines for prevention and management. 40:1–24, MMWR 1991.
13. Conti M, Agaopssi A, Muggiasca M, et al: High progression rate of HPV and CIN in HIV infected women (abstract no. PoB3050). Amsterdam: Eighth International Conference on AIDS, 1992,
14. Delhart DJ: HIV testing in women with vaginal candidiasis (letter). *Am J Med* 90:536, 1991.
15. Dowell ME, Ross PG, Mucher DM, et al: Response of latent syphilis or neurosyphilis to ceftriaxone therapy in persons infected with human immunodeficiency virus. *Am J Med* 93:481–487, 1992.
16. Farizo KM, Buehler JW, Chamberland ME, et al: Spectrum of disease in persons with human immunodeficiency virus infection in the United States. *JAMA* 267:1798–1805, 1992.
17. Farizo KM, Kelly JJ, Buehler JW, et al: Provision of gynecologic care at outpatient medical facilities serving HIV infected persons. *J Wom Hlth* 1:193–196, 1992.
18. Feingold AR, Vermund SH, Burk RD, et al: Cervical cytologic abnormalities and papillomavirus in women infected with human immunodeficiency virus. AIDS 3:896–903, 1990.
19. Glatt AE, Stoffer HR, Forlenza S, Alierie RH: High titer positive nontreponemal tests with negative specific treponemal serology in patients with HIV infection and/or intravenous substance use. *AIDS* 4:861–864, 1991.
20. Goedert JJ, Eyster ME, Biggar RJ, Blattner WA: Heterosexual transmission of human immunodeficiency virus: association with severe depletion of T-helper lymphocytes in men with hemophilia. *AIDS Res Hum Retrovir* 3:355–361, 1987.
21. Grossman C: Possible underlying mechanisms of sexual dimorphism in the immune response, fact and hypothesis. *J Steroid Biochem Mol Biol* 34:241–251, 1989.
22. Grossman CJ: Interactions between the gonadal steroids and the immune system. *Science* 227:257–261, 1985.
23. Haas JS, Bolan G, Larsen SA, et al: Sensitivity of treponemal tests for detecting prior treated syphilis during human immunodeficiency virus infection. *J Infec Dis* 162:862–866, 1990.
24. Hawley P, Clayton D, Clayton A: Correlation of CD4 counts in HIV seropositive women with and without vaginal candidiasis (abstract no. PoB3052). Amsterdam: Eighth International Conference on AIDS, July 19–24, 1992.
25. Hoegsberg B, Abulafia O, Sedlis A, et al: Sexually transmitted diseases and human immunodeficiency virus infection among women with pelvic inflammatory disease. *Am J Obstet Gynecol* 163:1135–1139, 1990.
26. Holman S, Sunderland A, Brethard M: Counseling of the HIV infected pregnant woman. *Clini Obstet Gynecol* 32:486–491, 1989.
27. Hurley R, deLouvois J: Candida vaginitis. *Postgrad Med J* 55:645–647, 1979.
28. Imam N, Carpenter CC, Mayer KH, et al: Hierarchical pattern of mucosal candida infections in HIV seropositive women. *Am J Med* 89:142–146, 1990.
29. Johns DR, Tierney M, Felsenstein D: Alteration in the natural history of neurosyphilis by concurrent infection with the human immunodeficiency virus. *N Engl J Med* 316:1569–1572, 1987.
30. Johnson PD, Graves SR, Stewart L, et al: Specific syphilis

serologic tests may become negative in HIV infection. *AIDS* 5:419–423, 1991.
31. Just G, Streinheimer D, Schenellbach M, et al: Change of causative organisms under antifungal treatment in immunosuppressed patients with HIV infections. *Mycoses* 32(suppl 2):47–51, 1989.
32. Kreiss JK, Kiviat NB, Plummer FA, et al: Human immunodeficiency virus, human papillomavirus, and cervical intraepithelial neoplasia in Nairobi prostitutes. *Sex Transm Dis* 19:54–59, 1992.
33. Kutzer E, Oittner R, Leodolter S, Brammer KW: A comparison of fluconazole and ketoconazole in the oral treatment of vaginal candidiasis; report of a double-blind multicenter trial. *Eur J Obstet Gynecol Reprod Biol* 29:305–313, 1088.
34. Landesman S, Minkoff HL, Holman S, et al: Sero survey of human immunodeficiency virus infection in parturient. *JAMA* 258:2701–2703, 1987.
35. Maiman M, Fructer R, Serur E, et al: Recurrent cervical intraepithelial neoplasia in HIV seropositive women. *Obstet Gynecol* 82:170–174, 1993.
36. Mandelblatt JS, Fahs M, Garibaldi K, et al: Association between HIV infection and cervical neoplasia: implications for clinical care of women at risk for both conditions. *AIDS* 6:173–178, 1992.
37. Masur H, Michelis MA, Wormser GP, et al: Opportunistic infections in previously healthy women: initial manifestations of a community acquired cellular immunodeficiency. *Ann Intern Med* 97:533–537, 1982.
38. Minkoff H, Duerr A: HIV infection and pregnancy, in Pizzo P, Wilfert CM (eds): *Pediatric Aids.* Baltimore: Williams and Wilkins, 1994.
39. Minkoff HL, Landesman SH, Delke I, et al: Routinely offered prenatal HIV testing (letter). *N Engl J Med* 319:1018, 1988.
40. Mulder JW, Jos Frissen PH, Krijnen P, et al: Dehydroepiandrosterone as predictor for progression to AIDS in asymptomatic human immunodeficiency virus infected men. *J Infect Dis* 165:413–418, 1992.
41. Musher DM, Jammil RJ, Baugh RE: Effect of human immunodeficiency virus infection on the course of syphilis and on the response to treatment. *Ann Intern Med* 113(11):872–881, 1990.
42. Notenboom R, MacFadden DK: Reliability of syphilis tests in patients with HIV (abstract no. PoB3044). Amsterdam: Eighth International Conference on AIDS, 1992.
43. Palefsky J, Holly EA, Ahn DK: Progression of anal cytologic changes in men with group IV HIV disease (abstract no. WSB176). Berlin: IX International Conference on AIDS, 1993.
44. Quinn TC, Cannon RO, Glasser D, et al: The association of syphilis with risk of human immunodeficiency virus infection in patients attending sexually transmitted disease clinics. *Arch Intern Med* June 150:1297–1302, 1990.
45. Quinnan GV, Masur H, Rook AH, et al: Herpes virus infections in the acquired immune deficiency syndrome. *JAMA* 252:72–77, 1984.
46. Relliham MA, Dooley DP, Burke TW, et al: Rapidly progressing cervical cancer in a patient with human immunodeficiency virus infection. *Gynecol Oncol* 36:435–443, 1990.
47. Rhoads JL, Wright C, Redfield RR, Burke DS: Chronic vaginal candidiasis in women with human immunodeficiency virus infection. *JAMA* 257:3105–3107, 1987.
48. Rogo KO, Kavoo-Linge: Human immunodeficiency virus prevalence among cervical cancer patients. *Gynecol Oncol* 37:87–92, 1990.
49. Rompalo AM, Cannon RO, Quinn TC, Hook EW 3d: Association of biologic false-positive reactions for syphilis with human immunodeficiency virus infection. *J Infect Dis* 165:1124–1126, 1992.
50. Roy S: Nonbarrier contraceptives and vaginitis and vaginosis. *Am J Obstet Gynecol* 165:1240–1244, 1991.
51. Schafer A, Friedmann W, Mielke M, et al: The increased frequency of cervical dysplasia-neoplasia in women infected with the human immunodeficiency virus is related to the degree of immunosuppression. *Am J Obstet Gynecol* 164:593–599, 1991.
52. Schwartz LB, Carcangiu ML, Bradham L, Schwartz PE: Rapidly progressive squamous cell carcinoma of the cervix coexisting with human immunodeficiency virus infection (Clinical opinion) *Gynecol Oncol* 41:255–258, 1991.
53. Seigal FP, Lopez C, Hammer GS, et al: Severe acquired immunodeficiency in male homosexuals manifested by chronic herpes simplex lesions. *N Engl J Med* 305:1439–1444, 1981.
54. Selwyn PA, Carter RJ, Schoenbaum EE, et al: Knowledge of HIV antibody status and decisions to continue or terminate pregnancy among intravenous drug users. *JAMA* 261:3567–3571, 1989.
55. Sobel JD: Pathophysiology of vulvovaginal candidiasis. *J Reprod Med* 34:572–579, 1989.
56. Sperling RS, Stratton P, and members of the Obstetric-Gynecologic Working Group of the AIDS Clinical Trials Group of the National Institute of Allergy and Infectious Disease et al: Treatment options for HIV virus infected pregnancy women. *Obstet Gynecol* 79:443–447, 1992.
57. Vermund ST, Kelly KF, Klein RS, et al: High risk of human papillomavirus infection and cervical squamous intraepithelial lesions among women with symptomatic human immunodeficiency virus infection. *Am J Obstet Gynecol* 165:392–400, 1991.
58. Williams A, Darragh T, Osmond D, et al: Anal/cervical HPV infection and risk of anal/cervical dysplasia associated with HIV-1 (abstract no. WSB175). Berlin: IX International Conference on AIDS, 1993.
59. Witkin SS: Immunologic factors influencing susceptibility to recurrent candidal vaginitis. *Clin Obstet Gyn* 34:662–627, 1991.
60. Wright T, Chaisson MA, Ellerbrock T: Cervical intraepithelial neoplasia in women infected with HIV: Prevalence, Pap smear validity and the role of immunosuppression. Presented at the VIIIth International Conference on AIDS, Amsterdam, 1992.

50 Other Infectious Diseases

Eileen Hilton
Leonard J. Rossoff

Approach to the Febrile Patient

The approach to the febrile patient involves a full history and physical examination with a focus on specific issues. These include an assessment of how long the fever has been present, the maximum daily temperature spike and its timing, the presence of chills and rigors, and possible precipitating factors. The patient should be questioned regarding possible exposure to illness in others, foreign travel, and unexplained weight loss. Is there diarrhea? If so, what is the quality? Is it bloody, mucousy, or watery? Has the patient taken antibiotics or an antipyretic? Did these have any effect on the fever or the symptoms? Is there a cough and, if so, is it productive? Does the patient report dysuria, hematuria, foul-smelling urine, frequency, or urgency? Does the patient's household include pets? If so, are they healthy?

On physical examination, skin rashes must be carefully evaluated. Palpation of the ethmoid, maxillary, and frontal sinuses should be done to determine if there is any tenderness or warmth. A pharyngeal examination will note the presence of exudates or vesicular lesions. Bulging of the tympanic membrane and redness of the canal should be noted on examination of the ear. The neck should also be evaluated for stiffness, especially when headache is a complaint. A careful lymph node examination should be performed. It is helpful to have the patient raise and slowly lower her arms while the examiner palpates for axillary nodes. On lung examination, the apices should be auscultated anteriorly and above the clavicles. The right middle lobe is often overlooked on physical examination; one should auscultate anteriorly and to the right of the breast.

Auscultation of murmurs, especially those with a diastolic component, may suggest a diagnosis of endocarditis. Palpation of the spleen is accomplished with the patient lying on her right side while the examiner's hand is placed below the edge of the rib cage. The patient is asked to inhale deeply while the examiner feels for the spleen tip. The abdomen should be evaluated for peritoneal signs indicative of infection. A pelvic examination should be performed to seek a gynecologic etiology for the fever. Is there discharge coming from the cervical os, tenderness on cervical motion, or a tender uterus or adnexa? Splinter hemorrhages under the fingernails are viewed using a flashlight transilluminating the tips of the fingers. This will enable the examiner to differentiate superficial nail markings from embolic phenomena. Unequal peripheral pulses are also suggestive of embolic episodes. The skin should be evaluated for evidence of cellulitis, the joints for evidence of inflammation, and the extremities for evidence of phlebitis.

Differential Diagnosis and Evaluation of the Febrile Patient (Table 50-1)

Acute Fever

The differential diagnosis of the febrile patient includes infectious and noninfectious inflammatory disease such as rheumatological and granulomatous disorders (e.g., sarcoid and inflammatory bowel disease). It also includes malignancy, especially lymphomas and leukemias.

Infectious causes of fever fall into two categories: *prolonged* or *acute*. Acute fever is only 2 to 3 weeks in duration and in many cases does not require an extensive workup since self-limited infection is often the culprit. If the cause is viral, myalgias and sore throat are prominent, as is a recent exposure to another individual with a "viral syndrome." In evaluating an acute bacterial infection, common etiologies include sinusitis, pharyngitis, cellulitis, lower respiratory tract infections, salpingo-oophoritis and urinary tract infections (UTIs).

Chronic Fever

If a fever persists longer than 3 weeks with no obvious source, it falls under the category of fever of unknown origin (FUO). In the past, infection accounted for about one third of all FUOs. With the increased empiric use of antibiotics, this percentage appears to be decreasing. The most common infectious causes of FUO include abscesses and infections of the kidney, bone, and heart valves. Since the recent increase in infection with human immunodeficiency virus (HIV), there has been a resurgence of tuberculosis as a cause of FUO. Some viruses such as Epstein-Barr and cytomegalovirus may cause prolonged fever.

Laboratory Studies

Initial blood tests should include complete blood count (CBC), platelet count, and a manual differential. An atypical lymphocytosis suggests a viral illness and a left shift a bacterial infection. Anemia may be associated with more chronic infections.

The erythrocyte sedimentation rate (ESR) can be useful in the evaluation of a fever of unknown origin. A viral illness is more likely to present with a normal ESR and a bacterial infection with an elevated ESR. A sedimentation rate over 100 suggests a long-standing infection (e.g., endocarditis, occult abscess, osteomyelitis).

Abnormalities in blood chemistries and liver function tests may provide clues to the site of infection. If liver tests are abnormal and there is no other obvious etiology of the fever, imaging studies [computerized tomography (CT) scan, magnetic resonance imaging (MRI), sonography, and HIDA] may reveal the source. Rheumatological disorders are initially evaluated with an antinuclear antibody (ANA) and a rheumatoid factor.

Blood cultures are necessary in a patient with prolonged fever. No more than six should be performed. All blood cultures need to be obtained with sterile skin preparation and from different venipuncture sites.

Any site that is oozing pus, appears inflamed, or seems to be infected should be cultured. If the pa-

TABLE 50-1 Some Causes of Persistent Fever

Etiology	Diagnostic Aid
Infectious-inflammatory	
Abdominal	
Cholecystitis Cholangitis	HIDA, ultrasound
Abscess Diverticulitis Appendicitis	CT scan, MRI, Gallium scan, In-labeled WBC scan
Genitourinary	
Pelvic inflammatory disease (PID)	Culture, ultrasound, CT, MRI
Urinary tract infection (UTI)	Laparoscopy
Intravascular	
Endocarditis Indwelling catheter	Blood cultures, echocardiogram
Other	
Sinusitis	Sinus films, CT scan
Osteomyelitis	Bone scan
Granulomatous	
Mycobacteria (typical/atypical)	Culture
Fungal	Biopsy
Nonbacterial	
Viral (Hepatitis, CMV) Rickettsial Chlamydial Parasitic (amebiasis) Spirochetal (Lyme, Syphilis)	Serology, culture, smear
Miscellaneous	
Sarcoidosis	ACE, biopsy
Inflammatory Bowel Disease	Endoscopy, biopsy
Drug Reaction	
Radiation	
Thyroiditis	Thyroid function tests, scan
Hemolysis	Blood smear, serum haptoglobin/hemoglobin
Neoplasm	
Lymphoma	
Solid tumor (Renal cell, Hepatoma)	
Disorder of thermoregulation	
Brain Tumor	
Stroke	
Encephalitis	
Seizure	
Heatstroke	
Malignant Hyperthermia	

tient complains of a chronic cough, sputum cultures for pathogens should be obtained. Sputum may be induced with a bronchodilator or nebulized 0.45% saline. If there is any history of tuberculosis exposure, early morning sputum for mycobacterial culture should be procured on 3 consecutive days. An initial Gram stain is important to evaluate the presence of inflammatory cells and the predominant organism. All patients with an FUO need a urine analysis and culture. Cultures of other areas should be based on symptoms.

Serological testing Serology is largely used for the evaluation of illnesses such as Epstein-Barr virus, cytomegalovirus, hepatitis, and toxoplasmosis. Occasionally, it may be useful for diagnosis of fungal illnesses such as coccidiomycosis.

Skin Testing

It is important to test for a positive reaction to a tuberculin skin test in patients with prolonged fever. It should be noted that patients may be anergic in the face of overwhelming tuberculosis, malnutrition, and immunocompromising states. Therefore, an anergy panel using several immunoantigens such as *Candida,* streptokinase-streptodornase, and tetanus toxoid should be placed to assess cell-mediated immunity. There are commercially produced multitest panels available for this purpose. An intradermal purified protein derivative (PPD) is preferred to a tine test as it has been better standardized. It is only the widest diameter of induration that should be measured and recorded in ''millimeters of induration.'' The interpretation of a positive PPD has been recently modified (Table 50-2), and the influence of a previous Bacillus Calmette-Guérin (BCG) inoculation should be discounted.

TABLE 50-2 Interpretation of a "Positive PPD"

5 mm is considered positive in a patient under the following circumstances.
- Recent contact with infectious case
- CXR consistent with "old TB"
- Known or suspected HIV

10 mm is considered positive in a patient under the following circumstances.
- Risk factor for TB
- Foreign-born in high-prevalence area
- High-risk population (African American, hispanic, Native American)
- Intravenous drug abuser
- High prevalence locality

15 mm is considered positive in a patient under the following circumstances.
- Anybody

Other Diagnostic Studies

All patients who have a fever of unknown origin need a chest x-ray. Sinus and panorex dental films may be useful as well if sinus or dental infection is suspected. Sonography is valuable for confirming a suspicion of renal, biliary, retroperitoneal, and pelvic infection. In the evaluation for endocarditis, a transesophageal echocardiogram has shown promise in revealing valvular lesions. CT scans are also frequently helpful, especially in defining the retroperitoneum. MRI is most beneficial for evaluating soft tissue, brain, bones, and joints. Nuclear scans are occasionally worthwhile, and technetium bone scans may uncover areas of osteomyelitis. Gallium scans are frequently nonspecific but may be helpful in AIDS patients with *Pneumocystis* pneumonia who present with a normal chest x-ray, cough, or hypoxemia. Gallium will also concentrate in the lung in interstitial pneumonitis. Currently, In-111 labeled leukocyte scanning has been found to be helpful in the diagnosis of abscesses.

Biopsies

Biopsies are recommended when less-invasive testing has not revealed the diagnosis. If liver abnormalities are present, a biopsy of the liver might be indicated. An enlarged lymph node should be biopsied if all other workup is negative. Bone marrow biopsy may clarify the causes of anemia or show the presence of granulomatous disease. A needle biopsy aspiration of any suspicious area or collection guided by sonography, CT scan, or fluoroscopy may also be indicated. In patients unable or unwilling to undergo surgery, drainage may be effected by a guided percutaneously placed catheter. All biopsies should be sent for culture in addition to histology.

Empiric Therapy

In the absence of a clear source of infection, empiric trials of broad-spectrum antibiotics may be introduced. This can lead to confusion; i.e., if the patient defervesces, how long should treatment be continued? Additionally, toxicities may be associated with antibiotics. If antibiotics fail, a course of antituberculous therapy may be instituted while awaiting results of cultures. Empiric corticosteroid therapy for presumed collagen vascular disease should be withheld unless the index of suspicion is very high and supported by suggestive serology and histological findings.

Common Infections

Urinary Tract Infections (UTIs)

One of the most common afflictions of the female patient is the urinary tract infection (UTI). Some women appear clearly predisposed to them, and an increasing number of host and bacterial factors are being identified. This discussion will focus on the practical aspects of diagnosis and treatment of lower and upper UTIs.

Lower UTI Lower UTIs involve the urethra and bladder. Symptoms of infection include frequency, burning, foul smell, and hematuria. The most common causative organisms are *Escherichia coli* and *Enterococcus.* Clearly other organisms can also be involved. In chronically infected patients or with the use of indwelling catheters, almost any organism may be implicated.

Optimally the workup should include microscopy of the urinary sediment, Gram stain, and urine culture and sensitivity. In this age of cost containment, a more practical approach can be utilized provided the patient does not appear to be significantly ill, has no findings suggestive of pyelonephritis, and is not immunocompromised or at high risk for progression of infection. If on dipstick analysis of the urine the leukocyte esterase is positive and the pH is high, infection may be presumed.

Empiric treatment may be initiated with an antibiotic likely to cover the most common pathogens. Good choices include trimethoprim-sulamethoxizole or ampicillin. These may be given in a single dose or for 3 days. The latter course is preferred by many clinicians as that is the usual time to symptomatic improvement, and there is a higher failure rate with single dose therapy. At the end of therapy a urine culture should assure bacterial eradication. Persistence of infection may represent either a resistant organism or an upper tract infection. Resistant organisms should be treated on the basis of their established antibiotic sensitivity.

Upper Tract Infection (Pyelonephritis) As stated above, failure of short-course therapy often suggests an upper tract infection. Other signs and symptoms of upper tract infection include fever, rigors, flank pain, nausea, and vomiting. Some patients may present with acute sepsis and hypotension. A toxic presentation or inability to tolerate oral antibiotics mandates hospitalization.

The organisms implicated in upper tract infections are similar to those found in the lower tract. Again, a chronically infected patient may have any causative pathogen. The workup of an upper tract infection should include a urinalysis with microscopy as well as culture and sensitivity. Initial antibiotics should be based on urine Gram stain results and subsequently modified when the organism and its sensitivity have been identified. If gram-negative rods are seen on Gram stain, therapy can be started with sulfa agents or one of the quinolones. Gram-positive cocci require coverage for enterococcus with ampicillin. Initial empiric parenteral antibiotic choices include ampicillin-sulbactam or pipercillin-tazobactam (pseudomonas suspected). A traditional, less-expensive approach is ampicillin and an aminogylcoside, pending final identification of the organism. Therapy should be continued for 2 weeks for an acute pyelonephritis and 4 to 6 weeks for chronic infection.

Prevention of UTIs Some patients with frequent infections may benefit from long-term low-dose (once daily trimethoprim-sulfamethoxazole) antibiotic administration. Success has also been reported with thrice weekly dosing regimens. For the woman who notes frequent infection after sexual intercourse, a single prophylactic postcoital dose may prove helpful. All pregnant women should be screened for bacteriuria in the first trimester and treated even if asymptomatic.

Respiratory Infections

Upper Respiratory Tract Infections A frequent problem seen in office practice is the upper respiratory tract infection. It usually begins with a vague malaise, sore throat, and, if viremia is present, myalgias. Cough may ensue, and the quality of the cough should be elucidated. By far the most common cause of the upper respiratory tract infection is viral. The time of year and epidemiologic information regarding community outbreaks may aid in the diagnosis. Occasionally, even after initial improvement, a bacterial superinfection may intervene with high fever and purulent nasal discharge or sputum. If a viral infection is probable, symptomatic therapy with decongestants and antipyretics should be given with instructions to call for additional investigation should bacterial superinfection be suspected.

The therapy for superinfection of an upper respiratory tract infection may include erythromycin or a newer macrolide (e.g., clarithromycin) which has *Haemophilus influenzae (H. influenzae)* activity in addition to providing coverage against streptococcus and atypicals *(Mycoplasma* and *Legionella).* The optimal initial approach, albeit somewhat impractical and expensive, includes a Gram stain and culture of any purulent fluids with treatment tailored to the pathogens recovered. In general, the macrolides will adequately cover most infections of the upper respiratory tract including sinusitis, otitis, and pharyngitis. Alternative choices include oral cephalosporins, some of which have additional *H. influenzae* coverage (cefaclor), ampicillin, and ampicillin–clavulinic acid. A failure to respond to empiric therapy should result in a determined effort to culture for specific pathogens.

Lower Respiratory Tract Infections (Table 50-3) A frequent outpatient complaint is cough. Symptoms of a lower respiratory tract infection with clinical or radiographic evidence of consolidation is labelled "pneumonia." If these findings are absent, particularly in a smoker, they are referred to as a "bronchitis."

Any complaint of cough or pleurisy should prompt a detailed physical examination. There may be dullness on percussion (pneumonia or effusion), and tactile or auditory fremitus may be increased (pneumonia) or decreased (pleurisy). Fremitus should be tested with a resonant phrase such as "99" or "toy boat." The finding of crackles (rales, crepitations), tubular ("bronchial") breath sounds, egophony, or whispered pectoriloquy strongly support pneumonia. Egophony represents the change in sound harmonics with transmission through consolidation, i.e., an "EEE" to bleating "AAA" sound. Whispered pectoriloquy refers to the clear transmission to the stethoscope of a whispered phrase such as "1-2-3."

Unfortunately, the presentation of pneumococcal pneumonia in the elderly can frequently be misleading. The symptoms may be nonspecific findings of sepsis without cough or other pulmonary complaint. Thus, if pneumonia is at all suspected, a screening chest x-ray should always be performed. If no evidence of a definite lower respiratory tract infection is found and the cough persists, other causes should be entertained. These include a postnasal drip, "cough-equivalent" mild asthma, chronic bronchitis, gastroesophageal reflux, or even an occult lung malignancy.

There are no clear-cut guidelines regarding admission to the hospital for a patient with pneumonia. If the patient is elderly; immunocompromised; diabetic; noncompliant; unable to tolerate fluid, food, or medication by mouth; living alone; unable to travel; or in respiratory distress, hospitalization is prudent. If on chest x-ray more than two lobes are involved or there is a diffuse bilateral reticular (interstitial) infiltration suggesting an atypical (e.g., *Mycoplasma, Legionella*) or opportunistic (e.g., *Pneumocystis*) infection, the patient should be hospitalized.

The outpatient treatment of lower respiratory tract infections is similar to that of upper respiratory tract

TABLE 50-3 Community-Acquired Typical and Atypical Pneumonia

	Typical	Atypical
Organism	Bacterial	Nonbacterial (viral, *Mycoplasma, Chlamydia, Legionella*)
Onset	Abrupt	Insidious
Cough	Productive	Nonproductive
Sputum	Purulent	Scant, mucoid
Tachycardia	Frequent	Occasional
Gram stain	Polys and Bacteria	Polys
Chest x-ray	Focal infiltrate Pleural effusion common	Diffuse infiltrate Pleural effusion uncommon
Treatment: po	Penicillin, erythromycin, cefaclor	Erythromycin, doxycycline, clarithromycin
Treatment: IV	Cefuroxime, penicillin, ampicillin-sulbactam, trimethaprim-sulfa	Erthromycin, doxycycline

infections. If available, Gram stain and culture of the sputum are used to guide appropriate therapy. The most common pathogen is *Pneumococcus.* Other pathogens include gram-negative organisms, most commonly *H. influenzae,* and the atypicals *(Mycoplasma* and *Legionella).* If Gram stain is unrevealing, initial empiric therapy may be started with a macrolide (erythromycin or clarithromycin). If *Pneumococcus* is the most likely pathogen, penicillin is the drug of choice. Other alternatives include cephalosporins (cefaclor) and sulfa agents (sulfamethoxizole-trimethaprim).

The treatment of community-acquired pneumonia in the inpatient setting is also aimed at the *Pneumococcus* and the most frequently found atypicals and gram-negatives. The choice of antibiotics should be based on Gram stain and culture results. Parenteral antibiotics that may be used include cefuroxime, ampicillin-sulbactam, sulfas, and if there is a clinical suspicion of atypicals, intravenous erythromycin or doxycycline may be added. It should be noted that there are many other choices of treatment for both in- and outpatient therapy.

Patients at risk for lower respiratory tract infection should receive pneumococcal and seasonal influenza vaccines.

Tuberculosis (TB) Tuberculosis (TB) is once again a major health problem. Patients with chronic cough, unexplained fever, weight loss, anemia, or other signs of chronic illness should be investigated for the possibility of primary or reactivation tuberculosis. This organism, the "great masquerader," may infect one or multiple body sites. The lung is most frequently involved in reactivation, usually in the upper lobes, and frequently with a background of chronic changes (calcifications, scarring), suggesting the old infection.

New, or primary, TB is difficult to distinguish from any other lower respiratory tract infection. The diagnosis rests on clinical suspicion and a positive stain for acid-fast organisms in the sputum. The ability to culture and type tuberculous organisms is rapidly improving. Sputum collections for this purpose should be obtained in the morning on 3 separate days.

TB prophylaxis. The healthy purified protein derivative (PPD) converter should be viewed as infected with the tuberculosis bacillus. The risk of active TB developing in household contacts and new converters is 3.0 percent during the first year and 0.5 percent each year thereafter. If there are children in the household, immediate chemoprophylaxis should be instituted despite the results of the skin test. The test should be repeated in 3 months. If the skin test is negative, therapy may be discontinued.

When evaluating the patient with a positive PPD (Table 50-2), the following should be done: a careful exposure history, physical examination, chest x-ray [posteroanterior (PA) and lateral], urine analysis, and serum and liver chemistries. If the urinalysis is abnormal, three specimens of urine for TB culture should be obtained. If there are no signs of active infection and conversion is suspected within the last 3 or so years, therapy with isoniazid (INH) for 6 to 9 months is advised. HIV-infected patients should be treated for a minimum of 1 year (Table 50-4).

Patients should be followed monthly for evaluation of INH toxicity. At these visits, symptoms of abdominal discomfort, nausea, change in the color of the stool or urine, fevers, rashes, and signs of jaundice or liver tenderness should be elicited. The utility of routine liver function testing is controversial. Mild elevations in liver function tests should not discourage therapy, and most experts would not discontinue INH until liver enzymes rise to three times baseline. The risk of INH hepatitis increases with age, and some choose not to provide prophylaxis to patients over 35 years old if the timing of PPD conversion is unclear. However, if conversion occurred within the last year, INH prophylaxis should be instituted at any age.

If a patient has a known exposure to a multiresistant strain of TB, there is no consensus as to the best form of prophylaxis, and consultation with a local expert should be sought.

Therapy for patients with active TB. Shorter course antituberculous regimens have proven effective. The routine short-course treatment of a sensitive strain includes INH, rifampin, and pyrazinamide. The pyrazinamide is given for the first 2 months then discontinued, and the INH and rifampin are continued for a total of 6 to 9 months. Some clinicians continue with pyrazinamide until sputum is AFB–smear negative. All patients with active TB should be offered HIV testing.

The recommended therapy for extrapulmonary tuberculosis varies depending on the site and severity of the infection, but most physicians will treat it for a minimum of 1 year. Follow-up should be monthly with focus on the symptoms and signs of toxicity of the agents in use. Additionally, sputum samples should be obtained to document smear and culture conversion.

Infection with a resistant strain should prompt consultation with a specialist as multiple second-line drugs of higher toxicity will likely be used for a prolonged duration of therapy.

Isolation and communicability. Tuberculosis is communicable when the patient has pulmonary or laryngeal disease. The most contagious forms of tuberculosis occur when cavitary lesions are present. These cavities may teem with mycobacteria. Transmission usually occurs by droplets emitted during coughing, sneezing, or vocalizing. About 2 weeks after institution of therapy, the patient is considered noninfectious even if a few acid-fast organisms are

TABLE 50-4 Therapy for Tuberculosis

Condition	Drug	Duration	Potential Toxicity	Follow-Up
PPD converter (HIV-negative)	INH	6–9 mo	Hepatitis, neuropathy	Monthly
PPD converter (HIV-positive)	INH	12 mo	Hepatitis, neuropathy	Monthly
Pulmonary TB	INH	9 mo	Hepatitis, neuropathy	
	RIF	9 mo	Hepatitis, flulike syndrome	Monthly
	PZA	2 mo	Rash, arthralgias, ↑ uric acid	
Extrapulmonary TB	INH	12 mo	Hepatitis, neuropathy	
	RIF	12 mo	Hepatitis, flulike syndrome	Monthly
	PZA	2 mo	Rash, arthralgias, ↑ uric acid	

INH = isoniazid, 300 mg/day
RIF = rifampin, 600 mg/day
PZA = pyrazinamide, 25 mg/kg/day

seen. Household and close contacts should have screening tuberculin (5tu-PPD) skin testing, and only if the skin test is positive should a chest x-ray be done.

Endocarditis

In most instances, endocarditis is treated in the inpatient setting. This discussion will focus on the outpatient diagnosis, follow-up, and prophylaxis of endocarditis.

The patient with endocarditis will usually present with fever. Occasionally fever may not be present, and nonspecific symptoms such as fatigue and weight loss may be the only clues. Recent dental manipulations or intravenous abuse of drugs raise a red flag.

The physical examination may reveal microembolic phenomena, i.e., splinter hemorrhages and subconjunctival petechiae. Findings such as Roth spots and Osler's nodes are rare and usually associated with long-standing infection. Of paramount importance is a careful evaluation of the heart sounds. A new murmur, especially one with any diastolic component, should alert the physician to the possibility of endocarditis.

Laboratory findings in endocarditis include an elevation in the white blood cell (WBC) count and ESR as well as microscopic hematuria and a positive rheumatoid factor. Sonography of the heart valves, especially with transesophageal echocardiography, may reveal valvular vegetations.

If the diagnosis of endocarditis is suspected, blood cultures should be done. Optimally two to four cultures should be taken from different sites with at least 15 min between samples. This approach is aimed at decreasing contamination and the confusion that arises when two blood cultures from the same venipuncture are positive with an organism of low pathogenicity. If prior antibiotics were given, the microbiology laboratory should be alerted to hold the cultures for a minimum of 14 days to maximize the possibility of isolation of an organism.

Treatment of endocarditis is based on the organism isolated. Once sensitivities are obtained, an antibiotic with a minimum of side effects and ease of administration should be selected. The latter is important as many patients are now discharged home on long courses of intravenous antibiotics. The microbiology laboratory will most likely provide two different sets of sensitivity tests, one an inhibition zone test using discs impregnated with the antibiotic and the other a measurement of the minimum inhibitory concentration (MIC) of each drug required to inhibit growth of the pathogen. The latter method is considered more accurate in predicting which antibiotic will be effective.

Rarely, blood cultures will be negative despite a strong suspicion of endocarditis. This may be due to previous antibiotic therapy or infection with a more fastidious organism such as *H. parainfluenzae*. Empiric therapy in these cases should address such possibilities. Possible therapeutic regiments include ampicillin and aminoglycoside or ampicillin-sulbactam and an aminoglycoside.

The duration of therapy for endocarditis is 4 to 6 weeks of parenteral antibiotics. As previously stated, outpatient therapy, usually after 2 weeks of hospitalization, is now common practice. Weekly follow-up in the office should include observation for signs of clinical deterioration such as a changing murmur, heart failure, embolic phenomena, and antibiotic toxicity. Electrocardiograms (ECGs) should be done to monitor new bundle branch blocks as this may indicate myocardial abscess formation. Any serious clinical decompensation should prompt readmission to the hospital for further evaluation.

Patients with a history of previous endocarditis, mitral valve prolapse with regurgitation, aortic or mitral stenosis, or artificial heart valves should be given antimicrobial prophylaxis before dental, genitourinary (GU), or gastrointestinal (GI) manipulations. Endocarditis prophylaxis is reviewed in Chaps. 41 and 59.

Central Nervous System Infections

Bacterial Meningitis Bacterial infection of the central nervous system (CNS) is a medical emergency. If unrecognized, patients can succumb to a bacterial meningitis in less than 24 h. The onset of a headache associated with a stiff neck and fever comprise the classic triad of bacterial meningitis. Unfortunately, not all of these symptoms and signs may be present. The best approach is to maintain a high degree of clinical suspicion.

Bacterial meningitis may be caused by pneumococcus, meningococcus, and, less frequently, other organisms, depending on the clinical setting. Group B streptococcus and *H. influenzae* in the very young, and pneumococcus and *H. influenzae* in the elderly should be suspected. Immunocompromised patients and alcoholics may be infected by *Listeria.* AIDS patients should have *Cryptococcus* and toxoplasmosis included in the differential diagnosis. Thus, the clinical setting is critical in the determination of the possible pathogen in bacterial meningitis.

The diagnosis of meningitis relies on an examination of the cerebrospinal fluid (CSF). If there is any question of CNS infection, a lumbar puncture should be performed immediately. If there is any evidence of papilledema or focal neurological findings, a CT scan or MRI of the brain should be done to rule out a space-occupying lesion prior to doing a lumbar puncture if possible. This should be done in an emergency room with access to a microscope for evaluation of spinal fluid. In bacterial meningitis, white blood cells are found in the CSF. Early on in the course, there may be only a few cells. If the cells are predominantly polymorphonuclear cells, bacterial meningitis is likely. Additionally, chemistries of the fluid may reveal a glucose less than half that of a simultaneous peripheral glucose. Gram stain of the fluid should be examined immediately for the presence of microbiota.

Treatment should be tailored to results of the Gram stain. If gram-negative or gram-positive cocci are seen, treatment with penicillin should be started immediately. Gram-negative coccobacillary forms may be *H. influenzae,* and a later generation cephalosporin (ceftriaxone) should be effective. Unfortunately, the Gram stain may be unrevealing, either because of the skill of the technician, a paucity of organisms, or previous therapy with antibiotics. In these cases, the clinical setting should help in choosing effective therapy. Unless there are unusual circumstances, therapy with a third-generation cephalosporin will be sufficient to cover most of the usual pathogens. Once the organism is isolated, therapy can be simplified. Treatment should be continued for 10 days in the hospital.

Aseptic Meningitis Aseptic meningitis is more common than the bacterial form. There are multiple causes of a sterile spinal fluid culture. The infectious causes in order of likelihood include viral, partially treated bacterial, mycobacterial, syphilitic, borrelial, fungal, leptospiral, or a parameningeal focus. It should be noted that many of these entities require antimicrobial therapy; therefore, a vigorous attempt at diagnosis should be made.

Some patients can be observed while withholding antibiotics. If the patient is less than 45 years old, has had a recent viral illness (in summer or fall), does not appear toxic, and the CSF shows a predominance of lymphocytes, a normal glucose, and a negative Gram stain, a viral process is likely. If there is any question of a partially treated meningitis, the clinician should err on the side of treatment.

Patients with meningococcal and *H. influenzae* meningitis should be isolated for the first 24 h of therapy. The physician should notify appropriate health authorities. Prophylaxis is indicated for close contacts, not coworkers or schoolmates. However, all contacts should be offered chemoprophylaxis if they report close exposure. Chemoprophylaxis is with rifampin (*H. influenzae:* 20 mg/kg/day for 4 days; meningococcus: 10 mg/kg twice a day for 2 days).

Infections Requiring Surgical Intervention

There are a number of instances where surgery should be considered as an essential part of management. These will be discussed by organ system.

Head and Neck Infections of the sinuses usually do not require surgery. However, if there is pansinusitis, surgical drainage may prevent retrograde spread into the cavernous sinus or the cranium. The diagnosis of pansinusitis is suspected when erythema, warmth, and tenderness are noted over the frontal, maxillary, and ethmoid sinuses. It is usually associated with a fever and significant toxicity, and is confirmed by sinus x-rays. In addition to drainage, parenteral antibiotics are given to cover pathogens including the pneumococcus and *H. influenzae.* Ampicillin-sulbactam or second- to third-generation cephalosporins are possible agents.

Ludwig's Angina or Infection of the Submandibular Spaces Deep fascial space infections are an emergency and require immediate surgery. These infections are usually secondary to dental manipulations. Danger signs are bilateral involvement of the submandibular and sublingual spaces with rapid spread of cellulitis. Eating, swallowing, and eventually breathing may be impaired. In addition to surgical drainage, high doses of parenteral antibiotics are required. These should cover the usual mouth organisms and, hence, anaerobes. Appropriate agents might include imipenem, clindamycin, cefoxitin, ticarcillin-clavulinate and ampicillin-sulbactam. If the patient is immunocompromised, an aminoglycoside should be added. Treatment should be continued until there is complete resolution of the cellulitis.

Abdominal Infections Infections in the abdominal cavity frequently require surgical intervention. In general, abscesses complicating diverticulitis, appendicitis, or microperforations of the bowel should be drained. Drainage may be attempted percutaneously by an "interventional" radiologist (if the abscess is walled off) or surgically if more definitive therapy is required. The presence of free pus in the abdomen is a surgical emergency and requires prompt surgical intervention.

Antibiotic treatment should be aimed at gastrointestinal organisms, including aerobic gram-negatives, gram-positives, and anaerobes. In the majority of cases, enterococcal coverage is not necessary for initial therapy. Enterococcal coverage should be added if the organism has been isolated or if the patient is not responding to the initial coverage. Appropriate antibiotics include cefoxitin, cefotetan, clindamycin, or metronidazole plus an aminoglycoside. If enterococcal coverage is indicated, appropriate drugs might be ampicillin-sulbactam, ticarcillin-calvulanate, imipenem, or piperacillin. Duration of therapy varies, and a decrease in the abscess size should be determined by sonography or CT scanning.

Salpingo-oophoritis and other gynecologic infections will be discussed in other chapters.

Acute Cholecystitis Acute cholecystitis usually follows obstruction of the cystic duct by a stone and is frequently accompanied by bacterial infection. The diagnosis is suspected when the patient has a combination of right upper quadrant pain, tenderness (Murphy's sign), fever, and leukocytosis. The bilirubin is elevated in about half and transaminase in about one quarter of patients. Diagnostic imaging includes a radionuclide (HIDA) scan, which may visualize the biliary tree but not the obstructed gallbladder. Ultrasonography may reveal a stone (9 out of 10 cases). Although three-quarters of patients with acute cholecystitis may initially be successfully treated medically, the recurrence rate is so high (60 percent in 6 years) that early surgery is usually indicated. Complications of acute cholecystitis (empyema, perforation) occur in one quarter of cases and require urgent surgical intervention. Endoscopic surgery is gaining widespread acceptance. Antibiotics should cover the most common pathogens; *E. coli, Enterococcus,* and *Klebsiella.* Ampicillin-sulbactam or ampicillin and aminoglycoside represent good initial choices.

Diverticulitis The etiology of diverticulitis is felt to be inflammation induced by fecal material and bacteria (fecalith) entrapped in a diverticulum. Acute colonic diverticulitis is suggested by fever, left lower quadrant pain, tenderness, and leukocytosis. Appropriate antibiotics include those that cover bowel flora as listed above. A patient with diverticulitis will commonly require surgical intervention. If a patient with diverticulitis has a perforation of the lesion, this may result in peritonitis, septic shock, or, if walled off, in a diverticular abscess.

Soft Tissue and Bone Infections Soft tissue infections may, under certain circumstances, require surgical debridement. A rapidly ascending infection of the fascia is a medical emergency, especially when it occurs in a closed space—for example, the hand. An infection in a diabetic in the perineum or around the vulva (Fournier's gangrene) may be a synergistic mixed aerobic and anaerobic infection and requires immediate extensive debridement with aggressive use of antibiotics. Choices might include ampicillin-sulbactam, imipenem, or "triple antibiotics" (ampicillin in addition to metronidazole and an aminoglycoside).

Osteomyelitis is another infection that may require debridement. It can present with fever, an elevated sedimentation rate, and pain over the affected area. A bone scan or indium-labeled WBC study should help to define the problem. Bone biopsy with culture is essential to diagnosis as cultures of the overlying area may not reflect the causative bacteria. In cases of chronic osteomyelitis, debridement may be indicated.

Therapy of osteomyelitis should be based on the results of biopsy or debridement cultures. *Staphylococcus* is a frequent pathogen and excellent coverage is provided by nafcillin, oxacillin, cefazolin, and vancomycin. However, another gram-positive or gram-negative organism may be present. Duration of parenteral antibiotic therapy for osteomyelitis is 4 to 6 weeks. Many clinicians opt for home antibiotic therapy after the initial evaluation in the hospital. Office follow-up of the ambulatory osteomyelitis patient should include weekly monitoring for efficacy as well as drug toxicity. A normal bone scan and ESR several months after the initial diagnosis support eradication of infections.

Hepatitis

Hepatitis, or inflammation of the liver parenchyma, may have multiple causes. Only viral hepatitis will be discussed. In the past, hepatitis A (infectious hepatitis) and hepatitis B (serum hepatitis) assays were the only agents to be identified serologically. Newly defined agents of hepatitis include hepatitis C (previously non-A, non-B hepatitis) and hepatitis E (enterically transmitted non-A, non-B hepatitis). There is also the potential for a superinfection with Delta agent, which requires previous infection with hepatitis B in order to produce disease.

Hepatitis A Hepatitis A in the United States is most frequently found in food-borne outbreaks. It is, however, endemic in other parts of the world and should therefore be a consideration in evaluating a returning traveler with illness. Spread is via the fecal-oral route and the incubation period is 2 to 6 weeks. The case fatality rate is less than 0.5 percent and it is not associated with chronic hepatitis. The diagnosis is made based on a history of possible exposure, an acute influenza-like illness with headache, myalgia, fever, and malaise. At the end of the prodromal phase, the stool will appear clay-colored, and the urine darkens. At this point the patient becomes clinically jaundiced with pruritis developing if there is substantial bilirubin deposition in the skin. The liver may be enlarged and tender. Serological testing will reveal elevated IgM antihepatitis A virus antibody. After approximately 1 month, an elevation of IgG antibody to the hepatitis A virus will appear.

The management of hepatitis consists of supportive care. Hospitalization is indicated for patients with evidence of hepatic failure such as a prolonged prothrombin time. Bed rest with bathroom privileges is recommended, but once symptoms have abated, patients may resume normal activities. Alcohol and medications that are metabolized in the liver should be avoided. No specific treatment is recommended, and corticosteroids should be deferred unless there is fulminant hepatic failure and cholestatic hepatitis. Even in these circumstances, their use is controversial.

Hepatitis A is extremely contagious and is a reportable disease. Unfortunately, there is often a delay between the time of exposure and the diagnosis. Prophylaxis of intimate contacts should be postponed until the identity of the agent is confirmed. Once confirmed, all family members and close contacts should quickly receive immune serum globulin. It is probably only effective within 7 to 14 days of exposure; however, it can be given up to 4 weeks later. Hospitalized patients should be in a private room with separate toilet facilities. At home, the patient should use a private toilet if possible and should be instructed to avoid food preparation.

Hepatitis B In the United States, acute hepatitis B infection is most commonly seen in intravenous drug abusers, sexual contacts of carriers, and health care workers. In a significant number of patients, there is no obvious route of transmission. The incubation period is 2 to 6 months, with a mean of 12 weeks. The fatality rate is 1 to 3 percent and, unfortunately, infection may become chronic in as many as 85 percent of neonates, 25 percent of children, and 10 percent of young adults.

The onset of hepatitis B is more insidious than that of hepatitis A, but it cannot be differentiated on clinical grounds alone. A polyarthritis has been associated with the preicteric phase. Diagnostic serology reveals the hepatitis B surface antigen, which is found in almost all patients during the icteric phase. Occasionally, the patient may be in a "window" phase that occurs before antihepatitis B surface antibody appears. During this period antibody to core antigen is found. The surface antigen usually disappears with convalescence; however, 5 to 10 percent of patients do not clear their surface antigen. These patients may remain asymptomatic but can transmit their infection to others. This chronic state should be suspected if antigen titers do not disappear after 5 months of infection.

Patients who have past infection with hepatitis B may become infected with Delta virus with a mortality as high as 20 percent. This should be suspected in surface antigen–positive patients who present with a severe infection. Serological testing can confirm the diagnosis with the detection of antihepatitis Delta agent antibody in the serum.

Hepatitis B is less contagious than hepatitis A. Prophylaxis is recommended for regular sexual contacts. Specific hepatitis B immune globulin (HBIG) should be administered as soon as possible and repeated in 1 month. Additionally, hepatitis B vaccine should be given simultaneously and repeated 1 and 6 months later.

Current ACOG guidelines for hepatitis B are the following: (1) Women who have risk factors for hepatitis B should be vaccinated; pregnancy is not a contraindication to vaccination. (2) Individuals who have been exposed to hepatitis B virus before they are vaccinated should initially receive passive immunization with HBIG and then undergo a vaccination series. Of note, the combination of passive and active immunization is particularly effective in reducing the perinatal transmission of hepatitis B virus. (3) All pregnant women should have hepatitis B virus screening, and women in high-risk groups who initially test negative for the virus should be targeted for vaccination if they have not been vaccinated previously. (4) Universal vaccination of all neonates with hepatitis B vaccine is now recommended both by ACOG and by the CDC. Infants born to seropositive or untested mothers at risk should also receive HBIG.

Hepatitis C Hepatitis C is the cause of most cases of transfusion-associated hepatitis. Unlike hepatitis B, the risk of transplacental transmission is low. Mothers who are carriers have about a 10 percent risk of transmitting the infection to the fetus. There is also some evidence of sexual transmission. The propensity to become a carrier is quite high—about 50 percent more likely than in hepatitis B. The incubation period is 6 to 12 weeks with a mean of 8 weeks. Diagnosis is made serologically with a positive antibody to hepatitis C detected in the serum. Currently, there is no available vaccine, and immunoglobulin has not been proven effective in its prevention.

Hepatitis E Hepatitis E is referred to as enterically transmitted non-A, non-B hepatitis. It was first described in a 1955 Egyptian epidemic. In the 1980s, electron microscopy demonstrated the virus-like particle thought to be the cause of this disease. This type of hepatitis is a risk for foreign travelers. Outbreaks have occurred in India, Pakistan, Nepal, the former Soviet Union, North Africa, subSaharan Africa, and Somalia.

Epstein-Barr Virus (Mononucleosis)

Epstein-Barr Virus (EBV) is a member of the herpesvirus family, which also includes cytomegalovirus and herpes simplex types 1 and 2. Most U.S. residents have been infected with this virus in their teens and twenties with seroprevalence above that age approaching 90 percent. The symptoms of acute EBV include severe sore throat, fever, and lymphadenopathy. Other symptoms may be retroorbital headaches, myalgias, and the sensation of abdominal fullness. Fever may take 10 to 14 days to resolve. A rash may be seen after administration of ampicillin in over 90 percent of the cases. A majority of the cases resolve spontaneously, but an unfortunate few are complicated by autoimmune hemolytic anemia, splenic rupture, or encephalitis.

In recent years, chronic fatigue syndrome has been linked with EBV because of elevations of the early antigens of EBV. These serological abnormalities may represent a nonspecific activation of the immune system that may be secondary to many other infectious and inflammatory conditions. The link with EBV has been inconclusive. There are, however, rare patients who suffer from what appears to be reactivation of latent EBV. Their EBV serologies are markedly abnormal as compared to the previously mentioned group. There is no proven efficacious treatment of this syndrome or of EBV infections in general.

Varicella Zoster Virus

Varicella-zoster virus (VZV), one of the herpesvirus family, is the causative agent of chickenpox and, when reactivated, shingles. Most adults have had chickenpox and are considered immune. However, there are some women who will not remember ever having had the disease. It is worthwhile to assess antibody status in these patients, especially if they are of childbearing age. This relatively benign disease of childhood may be life-threatening in adults and dangerous to a fetus.

Chickenpox presents with vesicular, pustular, pruritic lesions on an erythematous base. They are typically found at the hairline at the base of the scalp and spread to other parts of the body. High fevers may precede the appearance of the lesions. The incubation period after exposure is from 10 to 21 days. In children, the disease causes irritability but little toxicity; in adults, however, severe complications involving the respiratory tract may ensure. It is recommended that all adults with chickenpox be carefully observed for any respiratory symptoms. Any sign of respiratory involvement should prompt an immediate chest x-ray and an arterial blood gas, with hospitalization if any abnormalities are found. High-dose acyclovir has been used for therapy in VZV pulmonary infections. Some have advocated the use of acyclovir in all adults with chickenpox, but this is controversial.

Varicella immune globulin may be used in an attempt to prevent the disease in patients with a compromised immune system and in the newborn whose mother developed chickenpox within 5 days before or 2 days after delivery.

Chickenpox is highly contagious by the respiratory route. Spread may occur before the appearance of skin lesions and may continue until all lesions have crusted over.

Like other herpesviruses, VZV may persist in a latent state. This virus prefers neural tissue and when reactivated presents as a painful vesicular rash in a dermatomal distribution. Although reactivation is more common in the elderly, it may occur at any age. Shingles, or VZV reactivation, has been associated with decreases in cell-mediated immunity (malignancy, chemotherapy) but may also be seen in healthy patients.

VZV may reactivate in any dermatome but is commonly seen on the thorax. Spread outside a dermatome suggests immunocompromise, and further workup may be indicated. Facial herpes may be very debilitating, especially if there is involvement of the eye. Involvement of the tip of the nose should prompt aggressive examination of the cornea, as both areas are supplied by branches of the nasociliary nerve. In fact, all patients with facial herpes zoster near the eye should be examined by an ophthalmologist to exclude corneal involvement.

The treatment of VZV is symptomatic. Acyclovir in doses as high as 15 mg per kilogram of body weight may be given to the immune-compromised patient to prevent dissemination. Topical acyclovir has not been shown to be effective. The use of steroids to decrease postherpetic neuralgia is controversial and not recommended. VZV is also spread by contact with the infected lesion but is only of concern in a person who has never had chickenpox. Contacts may contract chickenpox but not shingles.

Measles

Measles, or rubeola, a common childhood disease, may prove a serious illness in adults. Most adults are immune, but those born after 1956 have vaccine-induced immunity, which may not be lifelong. This is suggested by recent reports of epidemics in colleges.

Measles is a highly contagious virus with transmission by droplets from nasopharyngeal secretions occurring from 5 days after exposure until 5 days after the initial appearance of skin lesions.

Manifestations of the measles include fever, malaise, cough, coryza, and conjunctivitis. The maculopapular rash occurs about 2 weeks after exposure, beginning on the forehead and spreading downward to the feet by the third day. In adults, fever and rash may be more severe. Additionally, as with chickenpox, respiratory complications may be life-threatening. Any progression of respiratory complaints should be taken very seriously. Measles may be prevented or the course attenuated by the administration of gamma globulin within 6 days of exposure. There is no treatment for the measles virus. Bacterial superinfection should be treated based on the causative pathogen (usually pneumonia due to streptococcus, staphylococcus, or *H. influenza*).

For recommendations regarding immunization, refer to the chapter on immunization (see Chap. 11). In addition to those general recommendations, all adults born after 1956 should have a booster vaccination for prevention of measles if foreign travel to areas of risk is planned.

Rubella

Rubella, or German measles, is usually a benign infection but is a serious problem in pregnancy, when it may lead to fetal malformations. The infection, less contagious than chickenpox or measles, is spread via nasopharyngeal secretions with an incubation period from 14 to 21 days. After a prodrome of malaise, fever, headache, and conjunctivitis, a maculopapular rash begins on the forehead and spreads downward.

Lymphadenopathy occurs with postauricular and suboccipital involvement being most characteristic. In young women, arthralgias and slight joint swelling may occur. The diagnosis of rubella is confirmed by virus isolation or more easily with detected changes in antibody titers.

The prevention of congenital rubella is the aim of vaccination programs as the disease itself is relatively benign. Gamma globulin can abort the clinical manifestations of the disease, but fetal transmission may still occur. Therefore, active immunization has been practiced since 1969. Women contemplating pregnancy should be screened for rubella antibodies if there is any doubt of immune status and should be vaccinated if they are not immune. Rubella vaccine is a live attenuated virus and thus should be avoided during, and for 3 months prior to, a planned pregnancy as there is a theoretical risk of fetal damage.

Mumps

Mumps, an acute viral disease, is transmitted via the respiratory route and has an incubation period of 12 to 25 days. It typically manifests with acute parotitis and a prodrome of malaise, anorexia, feverishness, and sore throat. There are few complications in adult females. (Up to 35 percent of adult males develop orchitis.) Treatment is symptomatic. Prevention is with vaccination of a live attentuated virus and should be avoided in pregnancy. Recommendations for MMR vaccination are further discussed in the chapter on immunization.

Lyme Disease

Lyme disease is caused by the spirochete *Borrelia burgdorferi* and is the most common tick-borne infection in this country. The disease is prevalent in the Northeast, the Great Lakes region, and the far West. Transmission is greatest during the warm weather months when people are more likely to be outdoors. About 10 days after the bite of an infected tick, a flulike illness usually begins. About half of patients develop a rash, characteristically a bulls-eye pattern, the hallmark of which is rapid enlargement. Left untreated, Lyme disease may progress to involve the heart (heart block, myocarditis), joints (arthritis), nervous system (aseptic meningitis, encephalopathy, neuropathy), and the eyes (uveitis, conjunctivitis). The disease, like syphilis, is protean in its manifestations. This is unfortunate, as diagnosis rests heavily on clinical judgment. Laboratory confirmation may be difficult since many of the commonly used serological assays are unreliable. Thus, Lyme disease has become a popular catchall diagnosis for patients with nonspecific complaints.

The treatment of Lyme disease is based on its stage of progression. Duration of treatment is controversial, but in general the following recommendations apply. Early Lyme disease (flulike symptoms and rash) is treated with amoxicillin (500 mg, tid) and probenecid (500 mg, tid) or doxycycline (100 mg, bid) for 10 to 21 days. Later Lyme disease may be treated with oral medication in the above doses or with parenteral ceftriaxone (2 g, od) for 4 weeks. If neurological involvement is suspected, a lumbar puncture and referral to a Lyme disease specialist should be considered. The Lyme spirochete may be transmitted transplacentally and has resulted in fetal infections and death. Therefore, treatment in pregnancy should be aggressive if Lyme is suspected. Prevention of this disease involves avoidance of tick-infested areas and the wearing of protective attire. Tick repellents can be used on clothing but not directly on skin. Currently, empiric treatment of a tick bite with antibiotics is not recommended. Instead, a baseline Lyme titer repeated in 6 weeks to assess for seroconversion is advised. Vaccines may be available in 2 or 3 more years.

International Travelers

The woman traveling to an underdeveloped country should be counselled about avoidance of the local water. In general, water is safe to drink if it has been boiled for longer than 10 min. If this is not possible, bottled water may be purchased preferably with carbonation to avoid bottles illicitly filled with tap water and sold to tourists. Foods to be avoided include salads, fruits, and uncooked vegetables that have been peeled or prepared by someone else. The risk of water-borne infections includes the previously discussed hepatitis A and E, typhoid, cholera, traveller's diarrhea (enterotoxigenic *E. coli, Clostridium perfringens, Campylobacter,* and viruses).

Pregnant women should be advised to postpone travel to high-risk areas until after delivery. Many of the antimalarials and treatments of tropical diseases are problematic during pregnancy. Hepatitis E may be prevalent in some regions and can be fatal in pregnancy. If travel to high-risk areas during pregnancy is unavoidable, a consultation with a travel medicine specialist is advised.

Preparation for foreign travel includes vaccination, especially for diseases particular to the area being visited. In general, patients should be up to date on their polio and tetanus vaccinations. Tetanus toxoid should be given every 10 years and polio vaccination within the last 5 years for international travel. Other recommendations depend on the area visited (e.g., Africa: yellow fever, meningococcus, and typhoid; Asia: Japanese encephalitis and typhoid; South America: yellow fever and typhoid). Yellow fever injections are only obtainable at licensed centers.

The patient traveling or camping out in rural areas must be treated somewhat differently. Many underdeveloped areas have a high incidence of rabies, and vaccination for this disease may be indicated. If there is any question regarding current recommendations for vaccination, the physician (or the patient) can contact the Centers for Disease Control (CDC) vaccination division in Atlanta [(404)332-4559].

Malaria is one of the leading causes of death in the world. International travelers visiting endemic areas should be given appropriate chemoprophylaxis. In the past, chloroquine was the preferred agent. Currently, there are many areas with chloroquine-resistant malaria (Africa, South America, and Asia). For these regions, mefloquine is now the drug of choice. Antimalarials are given for 1 to 2 weeks prior to international travel and continued once weekly until 4 weeks after the patient leaves the region. Recommended dosages are 500 mg of chloroquine weekly if visiting areas with chloroquine-sensitive organisms or 250 mg of mefloquine weekly for other regions. Side effects, including nightmares and worsening of depressive states, have been reported with mefloquine. Additionally, there is a question of drug interaction with calcium channel and beta blockers. Alternative antimalarials such as doxycycline should be chosen for these patients. There are some areas in southeast Asia which now have mefloquine-resistant organisms. For patients traveling to rural Thailand or along the Burmese (Myanmar) borders, doxycycline (100 mg daily) should be given. The traveler should take stringent precautions to avoid mosquito bites, especially during the evening hours, the feeding time for the vector of malaria.

If a patient reports ten or more mosquito bites after travel, she should be instructed to contact her physician. One of the forms of malaria *(P. vivax)* has an autoinfectious cycle and a course of primaquine is indicated to eradicate the liver cycle. A G6PD deficiency should be assessed prior to giving primaquine.

Patients should be cautioned to avoid sexual contact with residents of developing countries. Hepatitis B is endemic in many parts of Asia, and HIV infection is becoming more prevalent. Some countries require a traveler to have a certificate of HIV negativity prior to entry into the country for extended periods of time.

Illness in the Returning Traveler

Fever in the returning traveler is usually self-limited and rarely related to the foreign travel. However, in view of the potential for life-threatening illnesses, it should be treated as a medical emergency. Along with the usual causes of fever, the clinician should evaluate the patient for malaria, enteric fever, hepatitis, and amebiasis. Screening procedures should include a history and physical examination; complete blood count; blood chemistries; G6PD; urinalysis; hepatitis B surface antigen; syphilis screen; HIV testing; stool for ova, parasites, and enteric pathogens; malaria smear; and schistosomiasis serology (if returning from endemic areas).

Even if the traveler has taken adequate antimalarial prophylaxis, malaria is still a possibility. The typical presentation of malaria includes fever, chills, headache, and myalgia. Diagnosis is made by blood smear examination, noting that a single negative smear does not exclude malaria. The incubation period for *falciparum* malaria is 5 to 42 days. An evaluation should be performed to detect the presence of thrombocytopenia. If platelets are normal, it is unlikely that the patient has malaria. A patient with a high degree of parasitemia, anemia, or any signs of cerebral malaria should be admitted to the hospital for specialist consultation and treatment.

Enteric Infections

Diarrhea in the returning traveler may have numerous causes, including bacterial *(Salmonella, Shigella, Campylobacter, E. coli,* and *Yersinia enterocolitica),* protozoal *(Giardia lamblia, Entamoeba histolytica, Blastocystis hominis, Cryptosporidium,* and *Isospora belli), Stronglyoides,* and schistosomiasis.

Traveler's diarrhea is usually an acute illness caused by enterotoxigenic *E. coli.* Stool cultures should be done to determine if any other of the above-listed diarrheal pathogens are present. Another consideration is the possibility that the patient has *Clostridium difficile* overgrowth complicating previous treatment with antimalarials or antibiotics. If suspected, a *C. difficile* titer should be obtained.

Empiric treatment of diarrhea should cover the usual bacterial pathogens. The quinolones (e.g., ciprofloxacin, ofloxacin, norfloxacin) afford excellent coverage for many of the possible causes. Once culture and sensitivity results are known, the agent can be changed if indicated. If *C. difficile* toxin is discovered, either oral metronidazole or vancomycin are used for therapy. Treatment should continue until the diarrhea resolves. For diarrhea caused by parasites, metronidazole covers amebiasis, giardiasis, and numerous other pathogens.

Complications of Antibiotics

The most frequently occurring adverse effects of antibiotics are mild and include gastrointestinal distress (occurring to some extent with all antibiotics but more commonly the erythromycins and tetracyclines), rashes, candidal vaginitis, and antibiotic-associated diarrhea. Many of these problems may be treated symptomatically or by switching to another agent. Diarrhea associated with antibiotics may be caused by an overgrowth of a toxin-elaborating bacterium, *C. difficile.* When this is suspected, a stool for *C. difficile* toxin should be collected. The treatment of this diarrhea is with oral metronidazole or oral vancomycin. Additionally, the causative antibiotic should be discontinued. If this is not possible, then oral metronidazole or vancomycin should be continued until the other antibiotics have been stopped, even if the diarrhea appears to have resolved.

Life-threatening reactions to antibiotics include anaphylaxis and severe dermatological problems, i.e., Stevens-Johnson syndrome.

Patients who report antibiotic sensitivities should be questioned carefully regarding the nature of the reaction. A history of a rash is alarming if urticaria, desquamation, or mucosal involvement is reported.

Any history of bronchospasm related to the use of an antibiotic should be heeded very seriously. If the antibiotic in question must be used, then an allergist should be consulted for skin testing and possible desensitization.

References and Selected Readings

1. American College of Obstetricians and Gynecologists (ACOG) Technical Bulletin: Hepatitis in pregnancy. 174:1–9, 1992.
2. American Heart Association: Prevention of bacterial endocarditis: Recommendations by the American Heart Association. *JAMA* 164:2919–2922, 1990.
3. Bia FJ (ed): *Travel Medical Advisor: The Physician's Update on International Health.* Atlanta: American Health Consultants, 1993.
4. Braunwald E, Isselbacher KJ, Petersdorf RG, Wilson JD, Martin JB, Fauci AS (eds): *Harrison's Principles of Internal Medicine,* 11th ed. New York, McGraw-Hill, 1987.
5. Centers for Disease Control: Health Information for International Travel [HHS Publication No. (CDC) 92-8280]. Washington: U.S. Department of Health and Human Services, 1992.
6. Mandell GL, Douglas RG, Bennet JE (eds): *Principles and Practice of Infectious Diseases,* 3d ed. New York, Churchill-Livingston, 1990.
7. New York City Department of Health: City health information, Bureau of TB Control. *New York City Department of Health,* 2(5), 1992.

51 Hematologic Disorders

Kanti R. Rai
Henny Billett

History and Physical Examination

Physicians who provide primary health care to women should be knowledgeable about hematologic disorders which affect women of all ages—the elderly as well as the young, and among the latter, the nonpregnant as well as the pregnant. Special considerations in history taking and physical examination of patients with hematologic disorders are discussed below.

Symptoms

Thorough history taking is a requisite in the management of all medical problems. The following symptoms, however, deserve special emphasis when a hematologic disorder is suspected. Many of these may be the presenting symptoms, while others may only be elicited on direct questioning of the patient or a family member.

1. A sense of malaise, general weakness, easy fatigability. These symptoms may be present in a myriad of nonhematologic conditions, but they have a special significance in patients with anemia, leukemias, and bleeding disorders.
2. Bleeding history: Is the patient an easy bruiser (platelet disorder, congenital or acquired disorders of coagulation factors)? Does she recall having bled excessively following a minor (dental procedure) or major surgery? The extent and duration of bleeding during the menstrual cycle is a critical part of the history to determine whether the estimated iron loss far exceeds dietary and supplemental iron intake.
3. Does the patient have an increased frequency of infections (neutropenia)?
4. Does the patient complain of dyspnea and/or palpitations on minor exertion (e.g., walking a flight of stairs)? This may be suggestive of anemia of a relatively abrupt onset.

Other salient aspects of the history include:

1. Dietary and nutritional habits
2. Past history of hemorrhoids, venous or arterial occlusions; of any hematologic complications of pregnancy or childbirth

3. Current and past medications, birth control pills, antibiotics, psychiatric drugs
4. History of previous transfusions
5. Occupational history: Exposure to radiation and organic chemicals

Physical Examination

During physical examination of a patient with a known or suspected hematologic disorder, special emphasis should be placed on the following: 1. skin: pallor and texture; 2. hair; 3. fingernails and evidence of clubbing; 4. conjunctiva, tongue, and oral mucosa; 5. fundi; 6. lymphadenopathy; 7. thyroid; 8. spleen; 9. liver; 10. bone tenderness.

Evidence of pallor of the skin and conjunctivae is a tell-tale sign of anemia. The presence of petechiae and ecchymoses indicates an abnormality of platelets or other bleeding disorders. Skin turgor is an indication of the state of hydration, as well as of overall nutritional status. Clubbing of the fingers may indicate an underlying chronic disease such as sickle cell anemia or thalassemia. Fundi may reveal hemorrhages or sludging of vessels as seen with hyperviscosity syndromes of polycythemia, multiple myeloma, or Waldenstrom's macroglobulinemia. Enlargement of lymph nodes, spleen, and liver may suggest a wide range of disorders from infectious mononucleosis to leukemia and lymphomas, and bone tenderness may be indicative of hyperactivity in the bone marrow as is sometimes seen in leukemias or sickle cell crises, as well as in multiple myeloma.

In a majority of cases of hematologic disorders, the primary care physician can develop a very short list of differential diagnoses after a thorough history and physical examination. The next step, then, is to formulate the plans for the most appropriate laboratory and radiologic tests to speedily establish the final diagnosis.

Hematologic disorders can be broadly classified in the following categories, although it should be borne in mind that some diseases may affect more than one of them:

Diseases Primarily Affecting the Red Cells

Anemias
Polycythemia

Diseases Primarily Affecting the Leukocytes

Leukopenia
Leukocytosis

Diseases Primarily Affecting Hemostasis

Von Willebrand disease
Factor XI deficiency (Hemophilia C)
Presence of an inhibitor to the coagulation cascade or of a circulating anticoagulant
Hypercoagulable state
Disseminated Intravascular Coagulopathy (DIC)
Thrombocytopenias and platelet abnormalities
Thrombocytosis

Disorders of Erythrocytes

Anemia

After the age of 12, hemoglobin levels in women remain relatively stable. This contrasts with males in whom the hemoglobin rises until age 17 due to testosterone-induced hematopoiesis. The normal hemoglobin level for females is approximately 12 to 14g/dl and the range of normal mean red cell volume for women is 80 to 98 fl.

In general, the routine care of the nonpregnant female need not include a complete blood count and/or chemistries but when a patient is first seen and examined, baseline values may be obtained as a basis for future comparison.

For the pregnant woman, an expansion in total blood volume occurs as early as the first trimester. This increase can be detected as early as 6 weeks of gestation and continues until 26 to 30 weeks. Erythropoietin levels are increased during pregnancy by about 30 percent. Both red cell mass and plasma volume increase. The increase in plasma volume occurs earlier and tapers off at about 35 weeks. Red cell mass increases less than plasma volume but continues to increase until delivery. This increase in red cell mass is greater in those women receiving iron

TABLE 51-1 Differential Diagnosis of Anemia

Low or Normal Reticulocyte Count
Iron deficiency
Folate/B_{12} deficiency
Myelodysplasia
Myeloproliferative disease
Drugs
Chemotherapy
Immunosuppressives
Marrow infiltration
Tumor
Infection
HIV
Chronic disease
Renal disease
Collagen vascular disease
Diabetes and other endocrinopathies
Aplastic anemia
Increased Reticulocyte Count
Congential red cell disorders
Hemoglobin abnormalities
• Thalassemias
β°, β^{+}, α, Hb H
• Hemoglobinopathies
SS, SC, Sβ°Thal,
Hb E and C syndromes
Membrane abnormalities: Spherocytosis
Enzyme abnormalities: G-6-PD, PK
Acquired red cell disorders
Autoimmune hemolytic anemia
Drug-induced hemolysis
Microvascular
Preeclampsia
TTP, HUS
DIC

supplementation than in those who are not. Most women reach their hemoglobin nadir at 26 to 30 weeks of gestation, and from 30 weeks on, hemoglobin levels rise until delivery. Delivery often entails the loss of approximately one unit of blood. Within 1 month after delivery, total blood volumes should return to normal.

A healthy young woman who is not at high risk for anemia probably does not need to have her hemoglobin levels checked. Therefore, the initial hemoglobin determination for many women is often performed at the first prenatal visit. This serves to screen patients for anemias that may have been previously unrecognized, such as thalassemia trait or an insidious iron deficiency.

Hemoglobin levels below 11.5 g/dl in the nonpregnant female and hemoglobin levels below 10 g/dl at any time during pregnancy signal a nonphysiologic anemia. The most common cause of anemia in women is iron deficiency. The majority of menstruating women have decreased or absent iron stores and many of these women will develop an iron deficiency anemia during their lifetime and especially during pregnancy. Typically, the iron deficiency occurs as a result of further depletion of initially meager stores. Whereas men require an investigation as to the source of bleeding causing an iron deficiency anemia, women who are still menstruating or only a few years postmenopausal are assumed to be iron deficient secondary to menstruation and pregnancies and often do not require further evaluation other than inquiring about the amount of menstrual flow. In women whose anemia is either normocytic or microcytic, a diagnosis of iron deficiency anemia should be considered first, especially if this is an anemia *newly* arisen during pregnancy. Although the iron deficient blood smear usually demonstrates microcytic hypochromic cells, automated analyses may miss this population, especially during pregnancy when there is a mild increase in mean corpuscular volume (MCV) (approximately 5 percent). The white cell (WBC) count is normal and the platelet count may be normal, low, or high. The reticulocyte count will be inadequate for the anemia. Serum ferritin will be diagnostic if it is low. Falsely normal levels of ferritin may be seen secondary to a general increase in phase-reactive proteins in some patients with acute and/or chronic disease and during pregnancy. In iron deficiency, serum iron will be decreased and the total iron binding capacity (TIBC) levels will usually increase, resulting in a decreased percent saturation. Typically a bone marrow examination is not required to make the diagnosis in a healthy female, pregnant or nonpregnant. If there is still a question of etiology, a trial of iron therapy

(60 to 180 mg/day) may be started and the patient's response should be observed. An anemia that does not respond to iron with a reticulocytosis within 1 week and a demonstrable rise in hemoglobin within 2 to 3 weeks should prompt further investigation *and* the discontinuation of iron therapy until a diagnosis has been firmly established.

Both iron and folate are required by an active hemopoietic system, but folate cannot be reutilized by the body. Consequently, folate requirements are increased during periods of rapid growth and during pregnancy. Folate deficiency most often occurs in hemolytic anemias, in hemoglobinopathies, and during late pregnancy when folate requirements are almost double that of the nonpregnant state. Folate requirements may be further increased in multiple gestations. Although normal pregnant women may increase their MCV during pregnancy, folate deficiency must be considered when the MCV rises excessively.

Folate deficiency typically manifests itself as a macrocytic anemia *with* hypersegmentation of the neutrophils. There may be an accompanying leukopenia or thrombocytopenia. Folic acid deficiency may be silent, however, or it may yield a mixed peripheral blood picture due to an accompanying iron deficiency. Serum folate levels will often be diagnostic. During pregnancy folate levels may decrease secondary to the increased plasma volume of pregnancy and red cell folate levels may be more helpful. However, even red cell folate levels may miss a relatively new folate deficiency since these levels reflect the folate incorporated into the cell at inception and therefore represent, on average, the level of folate in cells about 6 to 8 weeks old. Folate therapy for the deficient state should be given at levels of 1 to 2 mg/day. A reticulocytosis should be seen in 1 week and a rise in hemoglobin levels should be seen within 2 to 3 weeks.

Megaloblastic anemia secondary to folic acid deficiency is not uncommon; megaloblastic anemia secondary to vitamin B_{12} deficiency is. Vitamin B_{12} deficiency typically occurs in the elderly, particularly in Nordic populations, but there is a subgroup of younger women with pernicious anemia. The hematologic manifestations are similar in both B_{12} and folate deficiencies. Central nervous system (CNS) sequelae, from peripheral neuropathy to a flagrant organic mental syndrome, occur only in vitamin B_{12} deficiency. Treating a vitamin B_{12}–deficient patient with folate will ameliorate the anemia but will leave unchanged or possibly worsen the neurologic complications. Therefore, the diagnosis of pernicious anemia must be considered before ascribing all macrocytic anemias to folate deficiency. Measuring B_{12} and folate levels is the easiest way to diagnose these deficiencies. In the younger female population with B_{12} deficiency, an anti-intrinsic factor antibody will often be positive. When the anti-intrinsic factor is positive, a Schilling test need not be done. If negative, a Schilling test will help diagnose pernicious anemia and differentiate it from malabsorption. A Schilling test is contraindicated in pregnancy since it involves radioactivity. In severe megaloblastic anemia, the peripheral blood smear may be mistaken for a myelodysplastic syndrome. Treatment of pernicious anemia is simple, with daily injections of B_{12} for 1 to 2 weeks and then monthly injections thereafter.

Anemia accompanies myelodysplasia, myeloproliferative diseases, and many tumors. This anemia can be secondary to marrow replacement by nonerythropoietic precursors, as well as a suppression of cytokine production and response. Many of the so-called chronic anemias which result from diabetes, chronic infections, HIV, or collagen vascular diseases are multifactorial in etiology. Typically these states do not require therapy as the hemoglobin levels are usually not very low. If a severe anemia does result, however, many of these respond to pharmacologic doses of erythropoietin. The prototype of an erythropoietin-responsive anemia is, of course, chronic renal disease, and all patients with anemia secondary to chronic renal failure should be treated with erythropoietin and iron. Even patients on chronic chemo- or immunotherapy often are able to mount an erythropoietin-induced red cell response.

Aplastic anemia, manifested by a decrease in all hemopoietic elements, is generally a rare disease, but it does have an increased propensity to occur in females and during pregnancy, and to recur with each successive pregnancy. Depending on the degree of leukopenia and thrombocytopenia, therapy may be merely supportive. However, in the event that the degree of suppression is severe, therapy may involve antithymocyte globulin and/or bone marrow transplantation. The advisability of continuing a pregnancy in which severe aplastic anemia has occurred is questionable, although there are reports of infants surviving both therapies.

Although less than 10 g/dl of hemoglobin signals an anemia that requires investigation, most pregnant women can tolerate hemoglobin levels of 8 g/dl or higher. There is some evidence, however, that this moderate anemia in the pregnant woman may predispose to increased fetal morbidity.

Very low hemoglobin levels may require acute therapy. This therapy can be vastly different depending on the etiology of the anemia. A patient with an autoimmune hemolytic anemia should avoid transfusions for as long as possible since the antibody is likely to destroy transfused cells as well and not yield any lasting benefit. A patient with a hemoglobinopathy may also tolerate a somewhat lower hemoglobin level since tissue oxygenation may be adequate. In contrast, a patient with a refractory hypoplastic anemia may need to be transfused earlier. If a deficiency such as iron or folate is the cause of the anemia, supplementation alone is typically sufficient.

In caring for the woman with thalassemia, therapy is directed on two fronts. Most patients with β°thalassemia (thalassemia major) are on a transfusion regimen aimed at hemopoietic suppression, so the level of hemoglobin will be acceptable if transfusions are maintained. Pregnancy is not advisable if the patient is symptomatic from iron overload and has evidence of impaired cardiac, pulmonary, or liver function. Patients with well-controlled thalassemia, however, have delivered normal, healthy infants successfully. A more difficult issue regards iron chelation. All patients on chronic transfusion regimens should be on chelation therapy in order to delay the consequences of hemosiderosis. A question exists regarding whether or not to continue iron chelation therapy during pregnancy. There are no data concerning the safety of desferoxamine therapy either during pregnancy or during breast feeding. Consensus is to stop chelation therapy during pregnancy and to restart after delivery of the infant and after breast feeding has been discontinued.

Patients with β^{+}thalassemia (thalassemia intermedia) or HbH disease (only one of the four α genes present) are not as symptomatic. They should therefore not routinely be placed on chronic transfusion regimens. These patients can be followed on a regular basis. Care must be taken during viral illness since the normal hematosuppression that may occur during mild viral illnesses may render these patients quite anemic. When pregnant, close observation in a high-risk clinic, folic acid supplementation, and transfusion as necessary is our standard protocol. Hemoglobin electrophoresis of the partner is advisable for genetic counseling and to predict potential obstetric problems for the mother and the fetus.

Usually, the patient with thalassemia major or intermedia has been diagnosed in childhood and is under a regular schedule of care. For many patients, the first time they learn that they have thalassemia trait is on a routine blood screening when a mild anemia is seen with microcytic, hypochromic red cell indices accompanied by a relatively normal red cell count. Differentiating this group from patients with iron deficiency is usually not difficult *if* the diagnosis is considered. Patients with βthalassemia trait will often have a mild degree of splenomegaly and the reticulocyte count may be increased. On hemoglobin electrophoresis, an increase in Hb A_2 is present. Hb F is usually normal. If the diagnosis of βthalassemia trait is made during pregnancy, care should be taken to ensure that patients receive the necessary folate. If the hemoglobin is low and/or the patient is symptomatic, transfusion may be indicated, but this is usually not necessary. Hemoglobin testing of the partner is advisable. If there is a hemoglobin abnormality in a potential father (thalassemia trait, β^{s} or other abnormal hemoglobins) genetic counseling is important.

In Asian populations, a higher proportion of patients are seen with microcytosis secondary to HbE or HbE trait. Patients with HbEE may have a mild anemia, but typically whether homo- or heterozygous, these patients do not have ill effects. The same is not true for HbE-β° which behaves more like a thalassemia major.

Other causes of congenital hemolytic anemia are uncommon. Glucose-6-phosphate dehydrogenase deficiency is rare in women. Hereditary spherocytosis when first seen in adulthood is typically mild. The anemia seen in this syndrome, if requiring therapy, can be mitigated by splenectomy. Most patients with hemolysis will have an increase in bilirubin gallstones. Typically these are soft stones and do not cause the same symptomatology as cholesterol-based cholelithiasis.

The adverse effects of sickle cell anemia are well recognized. Patients with sickle cell disease may have episodes of painful crises with severe bone pain which may require hospitalization for analgesic therapy and which may recur with frequencies ranging from less than once a year to almost continual hospitalization. In addition, they may suffer from stroke, leg ulcers, kidney failure, aseptic necrosis, and frequent infections, especially pneumonia. Acute pulmonary vasoocclusion, known as acute chest syndrome, can be a life-threatening emergency and requires immediate transfusion. Aplastic anemia, typically secondary to parvovirus B19, can cause a precipitous hemoglobin drop within one day as can splenic and/or hepatic sequestration crisis.

There is no evidence that routine transfusion of patients with sickle cell disease is necessary or even desirable. Patients should be transfused if their level of hemoglobin is too low (usually less than 8 to 9g/dl) or if they experience acute chest syndrome or *refractory* painful crises unresponsive to therapy. It is, at present, unclear whether patients with sickle cell disease require preoperative exchange transfusion or whether attaining a satisfactory hemoglobin level (above 10g/dl) by simple transfusion is sufficient. Nonpregnant and pregnant patients with sickle cell trait do not have any significant increased morbidity. Genetic counseling and hemoglobin electrophoresis of the father is desirable.

Pregnancy in women with sickle cell disease is associated with increased risk. There is an increase in morbidity, typically in the form of increased infections (notably urinary tract and pulmonary) and vasoocclusive and/or thromboembolic complications. Infants are often small for gestational age, of low birth weight, and/or premature; an increase in miscarriages also occurs. Patients with Hb SC have less difficulty with pregnancy and painful crises, but may have more aseptic necrosis and CNS events. Care should be taken in all these groups to make certain that, when pregnant, they are placed in a high-risk category and seen frequently. All patients should receive folate therapy. All pregnant patients with sickle cell disease should have their blood screened for the presence of alloantibodies, the frequency of which is higher in this population than in other equivalently transfused groups. If possible, the father's blood type (ABO, Rh, Kell, and probably Duffy and Jka) and hemoglobin type should be ascertained in order to be prepared for potential problems should they arise.

Autoimmune hemolytic anemia is more common in women than in men, and is often associated with collagen vascular diseases, the use of certain medications [especially methyldopa (Aldomet), penicillin, quinidine, and cephalosporins] or some proliferative disorders. These patients may present with a profound anemia for which compatible blood is unavailable secondary to a panagglutinin. Although many of these women will respond initially to steroids and/or intravenous gammaglobulin, more than two thirds will eventually have a recurrence and approximately one-third will ultimately require splenectomy as a means of controlling their hemolysis.

Erythrocytosis

Patients with increased hemoglobin levels have erythrocytosis. Care should be directed to determining whether this is secondary (due to chronic lung disease or to aberrant erythropoietin production) or primary (polycythemia vera). An erythrocytosis may sometimes occur in association with renal cysts, hemangiomas, and liver tumors. Patients who have secondary polycythemia are typically comfortable if their hematocrit levels are less than 60 percent; patients with polycythemia vera should maintain their hematocrit levels at less than 45 percent. Phlebotomy is a simple means of lowering hemoglobin levels; for patients with p. vera who are not contemplating pregnancy, therapy with hydroxyurea may be more appropriate.

Disorders of Leukocytes

The total leukocyte count in the nonpregnant woman commonly ranges between 4.5 and 10.0×10^9/L. It has been observed that these counts are generally somewhat lower in the normal African-American population. Approximately 60 percent of leukocytes are neutrophils. The most commonly encountered abnormalities are leukopenia and leukocytosis.

Leukopenia

A leukocyte count below 3500/μl on repeated examination is defined as leukopenia. Although all types of white cells may be decreased (granulocytes, lymphocytes, monocytes), the most frequent clinically important abnormality is neutropenia where the absolute neutrophil count is less than 1500/μl. It has been observed that some African-Americans and Yemenite Jews normally have a low neutrophil count. On occasion, a viral infection can cause a significant leukopenia. However, these events are transitory and blood counts tend to normalize on recovery from the acute infection. Patients with AIDS may also have leukopenia as a result of neutropenia as well as a markedly reduced absolute lymphocyte count.

When a woman presents with a fever and sore throat, and is found to have a profound neutropenia, the physician should be immediately alerted to the possibility of drug-induced neutropenia or agranulocytosis. In agranulocytosis, the absolute neutrophil count is at a dangerously low level ($\leq$500/μl). Such a patient should be hospitalized and consultation with infectious disease and hematology specialists should be obtained to institute appropriate antibiotic therapy and to determine the cause of the problem. The infection in such a case can rapidly spread, resulting in substantial risk to the patient's life.

There are numerous drugs which can cause agranulocytosis or neutropenia. Generally, these drugs belong to one of the following broad classes: 1. nonsteroidal anti-inflammatory; 2. anticonvulsants; 3. antipsychotics; 4. antidepressants; 5. anxiolytics; 6. antimicrobials; 7. antiarrhythmics; 8. diuretics; and 9. antineoplastic agents. Some of the examples of drugs prescribed in the office-practice settings associated with agranulocytosis or neutropenia are imipramine, indomethacin, carbamazepine (Tegretol), clozapine, methimazole (Tapazol), and aminopyrine. The physician must formulate a complete list of all the medications a patient with neutropenia is currently taking or has taken in the recent past, and then thoroughly check to determine whether any of those drugs have neutropenia included in their toxicity profiles. The first important step is to promptly discontinue those drugs. In certain cases, it may be necessary to substitute another drug which is free of such toxicity if an abrupt discontinuance of the medication suspected to cause agranulocytosis puts the patient at some other risk (especially patients with seizure disorders or schizophrenia). In nonsevere situations, when absolute neutrophil counts are between 1000 and 1500/μl, it may not be necessary to hospitalize the patient, but efforts to find out which is the suspected drug should be the same as in cases of agranulocytosis.

The mechanism of toxicity of various groups of drugs that cause neutropenia or agranulocytosis is not known in all cases. In some cases it may be an abrupt idiosyncratic reaction, and it may be immunologic or direct suppression of bone marrow in others. Once the causative agent of neutropenia has been discovered and eliminated, the blood leukocyte count generally starts to return toward normal in about 1 week, taking up to 3 or 4 weeks for its complete normalization. For severe neutropenia (especially associated with fever or overt infection), the use of filgrastim (Neupogen) administered under the care of a hematologist is indicated. These patients should be monitored with blood counts at 3- to 6-month intervals for about 1 year to ensure that no other hematologic abnormality is being missed.

In addition to the above, a primary care physician should also keep in mind that occasionally conditions such as systemic lupus erythematosus, Hodgkin's disease, and leukemias may be associated with leukopenia. If a leukopenic picture persists after a suspected causative drug has been discontinued, consultation with a hematologist should be sought.

Leukocytosis

A leukocytosis (total leukocyte count in excess of 12,000/μl) with neutrophilia in a nonpregnant woman generally indicates an acute infection or inflammation. Sometimes, with an acute infection, the blood neutrophil concentration may be as high as 20,000 to 40,000/μl. There may be an associated increase in the band-forms, and metamyelocytes may be seen on the peripheral blood smear. Neutrophils may contain coarse cytoplasmic granules (toxic granules). This pattern is called a leukemoid reaction. With successful treatment of the underlying infection or inflammation the blood count returns to normal.

Hematologic Malignancies

If the blood leukocytosis is persistent or there is no evidence of any obvious acute infection or inflammation, a hematology consultation should be obtained. Leukemias, lymphomas, and other bone marrow diseases manifest themselves with leukocytosis as well as other abnormalities in the blood counts. If the report of the blood count reveals the presence of blast forms (lymphoblasts or myeloblasts) accounting for more than 20 percent of all leukocytes, acute leukemia should be suspected. If, however, the differential count report shows a preponderance of mature cells, a diagnosis of chronic leukemia is very likely [morphologically mature–appearing lymphocytes in chronic lymphocytic leukemia-CLL; myelocytes, metamyelocytes, bands and polymorphonuclear neutrophils in chronic myelocytic leukemia (CML)]. A thorough physical examination may reveal the presence of palpable lymphadenopathy, hepatomegaly, or splenomegaly. Although leukemias and lymphomas may occur at all ages, CLL is generally a disease of the elderly, and CML generally has a bimodal age incidence—teenage and young adults and again in the fourth and fifth decades. Hodgkin's disease and non-Hodgkin's lymphomas can occur at all ages, although the former is seen less frequently among the elderly. Palpably enlarged lymph nodes that are nontender, discrete, and nonadherent to the adjacent tissue, with splenomegaly, are the usual abnormal findings on physical examination in cases of lymphoma. A brief overview of malignancies involving the hemopoietic system is provided in the following section.

Acute myelocytic leukemia [syn. acute myeloblastic leukemia (AML), acute non-lymphocytic leukemia, (ANLL)] is the most common form of acute leukemia affecting adults, and accounts for 80 percent of all cases of acute leukemia. Patients with congenital chromosomal abnormalities such as Down's syndrome and Fanconi anemia have a higher risk of developing AML. Although all the associated high-risk factors for AML are not known, there is an association with exposure to benzene, radiation, and chemotherapy. Based on morphologic and histochemical features of the leukemic blasts, AML has been classified by the FAB (French, American, British) system into acute myeloblastic, promyelocytic, myelomonocytic, monoblastic, erythro- and megakaryoctic leukemias. The following are recognized as poor prognostic markers in AML: older age (especially older than 60), AML developing after a period of preleukemic syndrome, the presence of certain chromosomal abnormalities, and the inability to achieve a complete remission after one cycle of remission induction therapy. Disseminated intravascular coagulaopathy may complicate the clinical picture of patients at the time of initial diagnosis of AML, but today with improved chemotherapy agents and judicious use of clotting factors, heparin, and transfusions, the overall survival of such patients has markedly improved. Chemotherapy to induce remission requires hospitalization of the patients because bone marrow ablation (rendering it hypocellular or acellular) is a requisite before one can expect regeneration of normal cells in the marrow. Therefore, during the chemotherapy and for a few weeks thereafter, the patients are pancytopenic, requiring frequent transfusions of red cells and platelets and intravenous antibiotics for presumed or overt sepsis. The major components of remission induction chemotherapy are cytosine arabinoside by continuous intravenous infusion and an anthracycline drug (such as daunorubicin) given intravenously. Virtually all patients require central venous access (either a subcutaneously placed infusaport or Hickman catheter) to protect from extravasation of vesicant drugs. There is a significant morbidity associated with chemotherapy, including hair loss, mucositis, neutropenic fevers, sepsis, and bleeding. In general, AML patients need to remain hospitalized for 4 to 6 weeks for the remission induction therapy. A regular visit to the hospital by the primary care physician is helpful both for continuity of care and for general reassurance and psychological purposes, to protect the patients from a sense of abandonment at the time when they are emotionally most vulnerable. Following an achievement of complete remission (CR), AML patients need continued chemotherapy as consolidation or maintenance regimens at intervals of 1 to 2 months. The overall median survival with AML has shown slow but clear improvement over the past 15 years, and today is about 3 years from diagnosis. Nearly 30 percent of those who achieve a CR are living beyond 5 years.

Acute lymphocytic leukemia [syn. acute lymphoblastic leukemia (ALL)] is the most common form of leukemia in children but accounts for only 20 percent of acute leukemias in the adult population. The FAB classification of ALL is based on the degree of maturity of lymphoblasts on morphologic grounds. The most primitive appearing undifferentiated lymphoblastic ALL and those with Burkitt morphological features are associated with poor prognosis. Other poor prognostic features include leukocyte counts higher than 50,000/μl, myeloid surface markers, older age, extensive hepatosplenomegaly or adenopathy, CNS involvement, presence of Philadelphia chromosome, and failure to achieve a CR after the first 4 weeks of remission induction therapy. Women, in general, tend to have a better prognosis with ALL than men.

The major components of remission induction therapy are vincristine, prednisone, L-asparaginase, cytosine arabinoside, and CNS prophylaxis with intrathecal methotrexate. Maintenance therapy is given for about 2 years. Patients with ALL generally are hospitalized during the first 4 weeks of chemotherapy, and the subsequent therapy is provided on an outpatient basis. Adults with ALL have an overall median survival of only approximately 2 years. Therefore, today there is an increasing trend towards encouraging patients less than 60 years of age with an available HLA-compatible sibling to undergo bone marrow transplant therapy, especially in those patients presenting with bad prognostic features.

Chronic myelocytic leukemia [syn. chronic myelogenous leukemia (CML)] accounts for nearly 20 percent of all leukemias in the adult. Most patients have splenomegaly at the time of initial presentation. An increased blood leukocyte count with a preponderance of myelocytes, metamyelocytes, and polymorphonuclear cells with an increase in eosinophils and basophils, and the presence in the bone marrow (or peripheral blood) of an abnormality in the Philadelphia chromosome (a translocation between chromosomes 9 and 22) are the diagnostic criteria for CML. Many patients present because of a feeling of excessive fatigue. There are three recognizable phases of CML: chronic, aggressive, and blastic. Therapy is directed towards control of the leukocyte count and splenomegaly during the chronic phase, with the use of hydroxyurea or busulfan (Myleran) and alpha-interferon. Overall survival seems to be improved if the disease control features include elimination or marked decrease in the abnormal Philadelphia chromosome. There is no satisfactory therapy for the aggressive and blastic phases, although treatment strategies generally used for AML are applied. Long-term (more than 10 years) survival has been reported in 30 to 40 percent of patients who are less than 50 years of age following bone marrow transplantation with HLA-compatible sibling marrow during the chronic phase of CML. The overall median survival with CML is 4 to 5 years.

Chronic lymphocytic leukemia (CLL) is generally considered to be a disease of the elderly, but is now being diagnosed in increasing numbers in younger (40- to 50-year-old) patients. CLL is the most common form of leukemia in the adult. It occurs in women somewhat less frequently than in men. The diagnosis of CLL is suspected when a blood count reveals a high total leukocyte level with a preponderance of lymphocytes. In order to establish a diagnosis of CLL, the following three criteria must be met: 1. a sustained and absolute lymphocytosis in the blood (>5000/μl) with mature appearing lymphocytes; 2. lymphocytosis in the bone marrow which is hypercellular or normocellular; and 3. phenotypic features of blood lymphocytes showing monoclonal B-cell proliferation. Presenting symptoms and abnormal findings on physical examination may vary; some patients have no symptoms at all and there may be no abnormalities on physical exam, while others may have significant weakness, fever without sepsis, night sweats, and weight loss with generalized enlargement of lymph nodes and splenomegaly. A majority of patients present with features in between these two extremes. The survival of CLL patients also varies over a wide spectrum. Some patients die within 2 years after diagnosis while others remain alive and well for 10 to 15 years and may die of causes unrelated to CLL.

A clinical staging system identifies patients according to their survival outlook: low-risk group patients have no abnormalities except for the minimum diagnostic features and have a long median survival time (>11 years); intermediate-risk patients have adenopathy or hepatosplenomegaly and have a median survival time of about 6 to 7 years; and high-risk patients have significant anemia (hemoglobin ≤11g%) and/or thrombocytopenia (platelets <100,000/μl) and have a median life-expectancy of about 2 years. CLL patients are not started on cytotoxic therapy until they develop symptoms from their disease or the palpable organomegaly starts to become problematic. Treatment is based on the use of chemotherapy—chlorambucil (Leukeran), cyclophosphamide, and fludarabine. Prednisone is used when autoimmune complications are present. Radiation therapy to an enlarged spleen or to large, bulky lymphoid masses is of benefit in selected cases. Splenectomy has also been useful for control of hypersplenism. Patients with CLL are at increased risk of bacterial infections and sometimes intravenous immunoglobulin therapy can be very helpful in affording protection from such infections.

Hodgkin's disease is a lymphoid malignancy which can affect all age groups. Often there is a painless enlargement of lymph nodes with no associated symptoms, but some patients present with what are known as "B" symptoms of lymphoma: night sweats, fever without infections, and weight loss of 10 percent or more of the baseline weight without trying. There may be palpably enlarged lymph nodes with or without enlargement of the spleen. Diagnosis is made by pathologic examination of a lymph node, spleen, or bone marrow which shows the characteristic Reed-Sternberg cell. The pathologic subtype of nodular sclerosing Hodgkin's is the most common (40 to 75 percent of cases), followed by mixed cellularity (20 to 40 percent), while lymphocyte predominance and lymphocyte depletion subtypes each account for 5 to 10 percent of all cases of Hodgkin's disease. The latter type of Hodgkin's disease is associated with a poor prognosis. To establish the extent of disease, a staging work-up is necessary and consists of a chest x-ray; CT scans of chest, abdomen, and pelvis; bone marrow examination; and, in selected cases, lymphangiogram and gallium scan. Splenectomy and exploratory laparotomy for biopsies of the liver and lymph nodes are done in selected cases of Hodgkin's disease. The Ann Arbor classification of extent of disease classifies Stage I as involvement of a single lymph node region, Stage II as involvement of two or more lymph node regions on the same side of the diaphragm, Stage III as involvement of lymph node regions on both sides of the diaphragm, and Stage IV as involvement of extralymphatic sites (i.e., bone marrow, liver, lungs). Each stage is further classified as either B (presence of classical symptoms of lymphoma) or A (absence of symptoms). Treatment strategies are governed by the staging; radiation therapy is appropriate for Stages I and II A. Some cases of Stage III A are also treated with radiation therapy. Chemotherapy is used for all Stage II B, III B, and IV patients. For bulky mediastinal masses with Stages II, III, and IV, both radiation therapy and chemotherapy are necessary to achieve a complete response. Chemotherapeutic drugs are used in combinations known by the acronyms MOPP [nitrogen mustard, vincristine (Oncovin), procarbazine, prednisone] and ABVD [doxorubicin (Adriamycin), bleomycin, vinblastine, and dacarbazine]. By the combination of newer antiemetic drugs (ondansetron, granisetron) with older ones (prochlorperazine, lorazepam, diphenhydramine), chemotherapy-induced severe nausea and vomiting has been reduced to a significant degree. Similarly, the use of filgrastim (Neupogen) has significantly reduced the incidence of chemotherapy-induced severe neutropenia. With these modern approaches to the therapy of Hodgkin's disease, an increasing proportion of patients are living 5, 10, and 15 years without evidence of disease. Once the patients have completed their chemotherapy or radiation therapy, they can resume their follow-up with their primary care physician. Primary care physicians must remain alert to the fact that long-term survivors of Hodgkin's disease may develop a second malignancy, including AML and myelodysplastic syndrome.

Non-Hodgkin's lymphoma (NHL) is a diagnosis given for a heterogeneous group of lymphoid malignancies with either B-cell or T-cell monoclonal origin. Although all the etiologic factors for NHL are not known, there is a higher than expected rate of occurrence in immunosuppressed patients (renal transplantation, AIDS) or those exposed to radiation or various viruses (Burkitt's lymphoma and Epstein Barr virus). Presenting symptoms and physical findings bear some resemblance to those seen in Hodgkin's disease. Diagnosis is established by pathologic examination of a biopsied enlarged lymph node or other involved tissue including the bone marrow. Pathologic subtyping was formerly done by the Rappaport criteria, but now the International Working Formulation (IWF) is used widely. IWF divides NHL into low-grade (small lymphocytic, follicular cleaved or mixed cell types); intermediate-grade (follicular large cell, diffuse small-, mixed-, or large-cell types); and high-grade (large cell, immunoblastic, lymphoblastic small noncleaved, or Burkitt or non-Burkitt cell types). The classification for extent of disease is similar to the Ann Arbor method described under Hodgkin's disease. However, NHLs present with extranodal involvement more often than Hodgkin's and NHL tends to be more disseminated than Hodgkin's. The treatment and prognosis of NHL depends on a combination of both pathologic IWF subtype and Ann Arbor clinical stage. Generally speaking, chemotherapy is the mainstay of treatment in most cases of NHL. The choice of drugs varies from single agent cyclophosphamide to combinations known by acronyms, e.g., COP (cyclophosphamide, vincristine, prednisone), CHOP (COP + doxorubicin). Some patients with NHL have a relatively indolent course and may be followed without instituting any cytotoxic therapy until "B" symptoms develop. Selected patients have benefited from radiation therapy to the involved lymphoid masses. Autologous bone marrow transplantation can be curative in selected cases of NHL as well as of Hodgkin's disease. With the improvement in chemo–radiation therapy methods and in supportive therapies (antiemetic and protection from severe neutropenia) the overall survival in patients with NHL is improving continuously, but cures remain at relatively low frequencies.

Multiple myeloma (syn. myeloma) and other malignancies involving plasma cells (Waldenstrom's macroglobulinemia, solitary plasmacytoma) are relatively rare B-cell neoplasms. The presenting features may vary from an accidental discovery of abnormally high total protein in the serum in an otherwise asymptomatic patient to symptoms of profound weakness, bone pain, and the discovery of pathological fractures. The main diagnostic criteria are the presence of paraproteinemia, consisting of monoclonal immunoglobulin (IgG, IgA, and free light chains in myeloma and IgM in Waldenstrom's macroglobulinemia), with bone marrow infiltration by plasma cells (myeloma) or lymphoplasmacytic cells (Waldenstrom's). These patients usually have anemia and an elevated sedimentation rate. They may have an increased vulnerability to infections and a bleeding diathesis. A hyperviscosity syndrome may result from severe paraproteinemia. The presence of renal insufficiency (elevated serum BUN and creatinine), hypercalcemia, and lytic lesions in the skeleton (with pathological fractures) portend a bad prognosis. The mainstay of treatment is chemotherapy (melphalan, prednisone). Radiation of painful skeletal lesions offers relief from symptoms. Therapeutic plasmapheresis is necessary prior to initiating chemotherapy when the serum viscosity is very high. The overall median survival of patients is about 3.5 to 5 years.

Disorders of the Coagulation System

Congenital and Acquired Disorders

The most common congenital coagulation disorders in females are Von Willebrand's disease (VWD) and Factor XI deficiency (Hemophilia C). Factor VIII (Hemophilia A) and IX (Hemophilia B) deficiencies are sex-linked and although they can occur in females, this is rare. Patients with von Willebrand's disease will present with easy bruisability and menorrhagia; patients with Factor· XI deficiency will more often present with a posttraumatic hemorrhage. Both of these deficiencies can manifest widely disparate symptomatology and the best indicator for the patient's future prognosis is the prior surgical history of the family or the patient. If the patient and/or the patient's family has no history of bleeding during previous surgical procedures, the patient is unlikely to bleed and should require no blood product. Thus a patient with 5 percent factor XI who has bled from a previous operation will require plasma coverage in the next one; a similar patient with 5 percent factor XI who has not bled should merely have plasma reserved for her in the blood bank. Similarly many patients with VWD may be treated with desmopressin alone or desmopressin and epsilon aminocaproic acid (Amicar); others will require treatment with either Humate P (the only Factor VIII product shown to contain functional VWF) or cryoprecipitate.

TABLE 51-2 Coagulation Disorders

Congenital
von Willebrand's disease Factor XI deficiency Factor VIII deficiency (rarely)
Acquired
Antiphospholipid syndrome DIC

Probably the most common prothrombotic disorder seen in the female population is a prolonged prothrombin time (PT) and/or partial thromboplastin time (PTT) with no prior history of bleeding. The patient may have a history of previous miscarriages, deep venous thrombosis, stroke, or myocardial ischemia. These patients often have positive mixing studies which demonstrate the presence of an inhibitor to the coagulation cascade. Usually, these are antiphospholipid antibodies (APA). Patients may also have anticardiolipin antibodies (ACL) present, and the patient is said to have the "antiphospholipid syndrome," also known as "the lupus anticoagulant." Therapy for this group is uncertain. There is general agreement that no therapy is needed when the patient is asymptomatic, but when thrombosis occurs, anticoagulation at higher than normal levels may be necessary.

Disseminated Intravascular Coagulopathy

DIC in women is most often associated with amniotic fluid embolism, fetal demise, abruptio placenta, incomplete abortion, intraamniotic saline injection, eclampsia, drugs, HIV and sepsis. The laboratory features of schistocytes on smear, an increased PT, PTT, decreased platelet count, relatively low fibrinogen and positive D-Dimers are usually characteristic.

Thrombocytopenia

Thrombocytopenia most commonly occurs as a side effect of medication (especially alcohol, chemotherapeutic agents and antibiotics) or as a result of infection (especially viral). Occasionally, low platelet counts may be secondary to a nutritional deficiency (B_{12} or folate) or myelo- or lymphoproliferative disease with a packed bone marrow. A most troublesome, and not uncommon, thrombocytopenia is immune thrombocytopenia purpura (ITP). In its adult chronic form, it is recurrent and sometimes

TABLE 51-3 Thrombocytopenia

Nonpregnant
ITP
Drugs
Chemotherapy
Antibiotics
Marrow invasion and/or infiltration
Infection
Viral
Sepsis
HIV
B_{12}/folate deficiency
TTP, HUS
Pregnant (All of the Above Plus)
Incidental thrombocytopenia
Preeclampsia
HELLP

associated with collagen vascular disorders. Like autoimmune hemolytic anemia, it often responds to steroids or intravenous gamma-globulin (IVGG) initially, only to recur or recrudesce. Because the platelets are often quite large, the platelet counts tolerated by this group are much lower than those of patients with hypoproliferative thrombocytopenias. Still, when platelet counts are less than 10,000, these patients have increased morbidity and an increase in CNS bleeds.

The therapeutic options for pregnant women with ITP are similar to those for the non-pregnant patient. However, many of these options may benefit the mother without increasing the fetus's platelet counts. Mothers with ITP may have their platelet counts increased by steroids or IVGG but the evidence that this affects fetal platelet counts significantly is slim. Therefore the current recommendations are to treat with steroids if the platelet count is low enough to be dangerous for the mother. IVGG will typically give only a transient rise and should probably be reserved for those whose delivery dates are planned.

Thrombotic thrombocytopenia purpura (TTP) or hemolytic uremic syndrome (HUS) also have an increased incidence in women. Both TTP and HUS occur in young women and manifest as fever, a microangiopathic hemolytic anemia, and a thrombocytopenia. Renal vasoocclusion is more prevalent in HUS, while CNS events are more common in TTP. There may be a recurrent form for both these illnesses.

Therapy for patients with TTP is similar whether the patient is pregnant or not: plasma exchange and infusion with fresh frozen plasma. Plasma infusion, with or without exchange, aspirin, and/or steroids ameliorates the problem in most patients and mortality is less than 20 percent as compared to 60 to 80 percent without therapy. In contrast, HUS with its more prominent renal component, has a different prognosis in pregnant as compared to nonpregnant women. HUS in pregnancy, however, typically occurs within the first month postpartum, is often associated with a premorbid gastroenteritis, and carries with it a 60 percent mortality even with therapy. An examination for retained products of conception may prove fruitful. This postpartum type of HUS often requires dialysis.

Platelet Release Defects

Ingestion of aspirin and other nonsteroidal anti-inflammatory drugs can have an adverse effect on platelet release and aggregation resulting in a prolonged bleeding time. There are no good predictors, bleeding time included, of who will bleed on aspirin.

Thrombocytosis

Thrombocytosis is uncommon. Typically it is associated with bleeding, tumors, chronic inflammation, and postsplenectomy. It may also be secondary to a myeloproliferative syndrome, either essential thrombocytosis (ET) itself or associated with polycythemia vera (PV) or Chronic Myelogenous Leukemia (CML). Although the myeloproliferative diseases tend to occur in the middle aged (PV or CML) or the elderly (ET), there is a subgroup of ET that occurs in younger women and is associated with acrocyanosis, digital thrombosis, and ischemia. Although typically thrombocytosis itself is not dangerous and requires no therapy, thrombocytosis secondary to myeloproliferative disease requires treatment with chemotherapeutic agents and/or aspirin, and requires close observation.

Splenomegaly

A physical examination should normally include palpation of the liver and the spleen. The technique of splenic palpation differs from that of the liver in that it requires merely light laying of hands just under the lateral lower left or midaxillary part of the rib cage. The hard palpation used for liver assessment often results in propelling the spleen away rather than its capture. Since lung sizes may be quite disparate, spleens may be enlarged but remain under the costal margin or may be normal in size but palpable below the costal margin. True splenomegaly occurs in 2 to 5 percent of the United States population but at much higher rates in the tropical population. When the spleen enlarges, "hypersplenism" may occur resulting in an increased level of hematopoietic destruction within the spleen. Hypersplenism may cause anemia, leukopenia, and/or thrombocytopenia. Typically the bone marrow response is active but inadequate to meet the demand.

Overall, a large spleen does not require attention unless the cytopenia demands action or there is a potential for rupture. The ctiology of the splenomegaly will often help determine whether therapy is or will be necessary. Splenomegaly may be due to simple cysts and hemangiomas or increased portal or splenic vein pressure from cirrhosis, idiopathic or thrombotic causes. Infection typically causing both hepatomegaly and splenomegaly results from hepatitis (mononucleosis, malaria, CMV, Hepatitis A, B, or C) or a chronic granulomatous infiltrative process (TB, histoplasma, echinococcus). Noninfectious infiltrative etiologies such as amyloid, Gaucher's disease and glycogen storage diseases typically have been present for long periods of time. Occasionally diabetes may cause an enlarged spleen. Neoplasms may cause enlargement of the spleen either through infiltrative processes such as leukemias, diffuse lymphomas or via invasion by metastatic tumors.

Connective tissue disorders such as systemic lupus erythematosus, sarcoid, or rheumatoid arthritis often have an accompanying splenomegaly without liver enlargement. Acquired splenomegaly is associated with autoimmune syndromes such as autoimmune hemolytic anemias, chronic idiopathic thrombocytopenia purpura and Felty's syndrome (neutropenia and splenomegaly).

Hematologic causes of splenomegaly may be congenital or acquired. Congenital etiologies of splenomegaly are usually due to increased hematopoietic demand secondary to hemoglobinopathies and thalassemias. In these diseases, the increased demand has been present since birth and has inhibited the natural repression of fetal splenic hematopoiesis. In the acquired disorders, the spleen may be enlarged in myelodysplastic ("preleukemic") syndromes and in acute or chronic myeloid and lymphoid leukemias. Polycythemia vera may be differentiated from other causes of erythrocytosis by the almost univer-

TABLE 51-4 Differential Diagnosis of Splenomegaly

- Hepatitis
  - CMV
  - Hepatitis A, B, C
  - Infectious mononucleosis
  - Malaria
- Infiltrative
  - Infectious
    - TB
    - Histoplasma
  - Noninfectious
    - Amyloid
    - Gaucher's
  - Neoplastic
- Hematologic
  - Acute leukemias
  - Chronic leukemias
  - Myelodysplasia
  - Polycythemia
  - Myelofibrosis
  - Hemoglobinopathies
  - Thalassemia

sal splenic enlargement while some of the largest myeloproliferative spleens are seen in agnogenic myeloid metaplasia with myelofibrosis.

Surgical therapy is indicated only in cases of severe discomfort, potential rupture, or hypersplenism that outstrips hematopoietic capability. Although there is some question of an increased incidence of sepsis in splenectomized children, there is no data that splenectomy is harmful in the adult population. The peripheral smear in the splenectomized adult will typically show Howell-Jolly bodies (fragments of chromatin left within the red cells that would normally have been removed), target cells, and there may be a thrombocytosis either acutely and/or chronically.

References and Selected Readings

1. Jandl JH: *Textbook of Hematology,* Boston, Little Brown, 1987.
2. Hoffbrand AV, Pettit JE: *Essential Hematology,* 3rd ed. Cambridge, MA, Blackwell Scientific Publications, 1993.
3. Spivak JL, Eichner ER (eds): *The Fundamentals of Clinical Hematology,* 3d ed. Baltimore, The Johns Hopkins University Press, 1993.
4. Williams MD, Wheby MS: Anemia in pregnancy. *Med Clin North Am* 76:631–647, 1992.

52 Clinical Neurology

Ronald Kanner

Neurologic diseases are frightening and often devastating, affecting the very functions that make us human. The problem is further compounded by the commonly held belief that there are few therapeutic options for most neurologic disorders. While this latter statement may currently be true of the "interesting" inherited/degenerative diseases of the nervous system, most neurologic problems seen in office practice can be addressed quickly and effectively.

Accurate diagnosis and treatment depend on a well-directed history, a careful neurologic examination, and the judicious selection of ancillary tests. This chapter covers the neurologic history and physical examination and discusses the ancillary tests with each of the presenting problems. The orientation is by symptoms, rather than diseases, because that is the way patients present in the office.

Neurologic History

The neurologic history is more focused than a general medical history. After hearing the current complaint, the physician considers three major issues: location, onset, and progression. Location is the easiest point to obtain. The patient complains of a specific deficit (pain, weakness, sensory loss) and can simply point to the area involved. The "geographic" pattern of impairment provides insight into the syndrome diagnosis (e.g., proximal weakness in myopathies, distal weakness in neuropathies, hemiparesis in cerebral disorders, radicular sensory loss in herniated discs). The temporal pattern (onset and progression) provides etiologic insight (sudden and stable or improving in vascular disease; gradual and progressive in tumor or degeneration). These issues are addressed more fully in the sections describing the individual syndromes.

Neurologic Examination

In most cases, an adequate neurologic examination can be performed in 5 min. Following a set pattern of examination with emphasis on the area of complaint can expedite the process. One possible approach is a "top-to-bottom" orientation, starting with mental status, then progressing to cranial nerves, motor, sensory, reflex, coordination, and gait examinations.

Mental Status

The two main components of the mental status examination are the *level* of consciousness and the *content* of consciousness. Level of consciousness is purely descriptive. ''Fully awake, alert and oriented'' and ''comatose and unresponsive to all stimuli'' represent ends of the spectrum that are easily understood. The problems lie in between. Vague terms, such as ''lethargic,'' ''stuporous,'' and ''semicomatose'' are not useful unless they are accompanied by an accurate description of the patient at rest, the stimuli that are required to arouse the patient, and the patient's best level of function when aroused.

The two most important parts of the content of consciousness are language function and memory. Language function usually can be assessed during simple conversation and history-taking. If there is any doubt, the patient should be asked to follow some simple commands, repeat simple phrases, and name common objects. On the basis of these tests, the most common aphasias can be classified (Table 52-1).

Memory function can be tested only after it is ascertained that the patient has adequate language function and attention. The level of education and sophistication should be known, so that the patient's current level of memory function can be assessed in the context of her usual baseline function. The patient is asked to spell a five-letter word (e.g., world) and then spell it backward (testing attention). Recent recall is then tested by asking the patient to recall three objects after 5 min of distraction with other tasks (e.g., arithmetic function, reasoning). Remote recall should be tested using facts that can be verified (e.g., political events or family names when other family members are present).

TABLE 52-1 Common Aphasias[a]

	Broca	Wernicke
Location	Anterior Inferior frontal	Posterior Temporal
Type	Motor Expressive	Sensory Receptive
Output	Nonfluent	Fluent
Hemiparesis	Yes	No

[a]Most commonly, aphasias are mixed, showing characteristics of both anterior and posterior types. In a ''global'' aphasia, both components are fully represented and the patient has neither comprehension nor significant output.

Cranial Nerves

I: *Olfactory* function is not always checked, but is important in cases of trauma and dementia. It should be checked in each nostril, individually, using a familiar substance, such as coffee. Do not use alcohol; it produces a noxious stimulus.

II: *Optic nerve* function involves visual acuity, visual fields, and direct inspection of the nerve (funduscopic exam). It is the afferent part of the pupillary reflex.

III, IV, VI: *Oculomotor, trochlear,* and *abducens nerve* functions are tested together, first by observing the eye position on primary gaze, then by having the patient track an object in all directions. When there is paresis of a muscle or nerve, diplopia is the resulting complaint. The false image is cast further out in the direction of movement of the paretic muscle. The oculomotor nerve also serves the efferent part of the pupillary reflex.

V: The *trigeminal nerve* has a motor component that supplies the muscles of mastication [masseters, temporalis, and pterygoids (lateral movement of the jaw)], and three sensory divisions. V1 covers the area from the coronal suture to the upper lids and part of the cornea. Note that V1 does not stop at the hairline, which is where hysterical or factitious sensory loss often stops. V2 covers the area of the zygomatic arches and cheeks. V3 covers the mandible, except for the angle of the jaw.

VII: The *facial nerve* supplies motor function to the muscles of expression and, through the chorda tympanae, supplies taste to the anterior two-thirds of the tongue. A branch to the stapedius dampens noise; the greater superficial petrosal supplies the lacrimal glands.

VIII: The *statoacoustic nerve* subserves hearing and balance. Hearing can be tested either with a high frequency tuning fork or by whispering a number in the patient's ear while rubbing the fingers near the other ear (to test the ear individually). Balance is tested by having the patient stand with her feet together and arms outstretched. This testing is described further in the section on gait disorders.

IX and X: *Glossopharyngeal and vagal* functions are usually tested together, with the gag reflex. The glossopharyngeal nerve supplies sensation to the oropharynx. Voluntary and reflex (gag) elevation of the palate should be tested.

XI: The *spinal accessory nerve* supplies the trapezii (shoulder shrug) and the sternocleidomastoid muscles (contralateral head turning). Weakness is clinically manifest by shoulder droop.

XII: The *hypoglossal nerve* protrudes the tongue. When there is dysfunction, the tongue deviates toward the side of the weakness.

Motor Examination

The issues to be addressed are bulk, tone, and strength. Muscles are checked visually for atrophy and fasciculations. This should be done in a warm room, because fasciculations may appear in otherwise normal muscles in a cold environment. Tone is defined as involuntary resistance to passive stretch. It is generally increased in upper motor neuron lesions (spasticity) and decreased in lower. Specific types of increased tone may be diagnostic of certain disease states (e.g., cogwheel rigidity in parkinsonism).

Strength is graded on a 0 to 5 scale. Zero is no flicker of movement; 1 = isometric contraction, without movement of the extremity; 2 = movement, but only parallel to the ground (not against gravity); 3 = movement against gravity; 4 = ability to overcome some resistance; 5 = full strength. In manual motor testing, the examiner should be positioned in such a way that the muscle being tested is put against an appropriate amount of force. That is, finger extensors should be tested against muscles of similar strength. Plantar flexion of the feet should be tested functionally by having the patient try to stand on tiptoe, because manual testing cannot exert enough power to test the gastrocnemius muscles.

Sensory Examination

The sensory exam should be tailored to the individual complaint. Testing every sensory function in patients without sensory complaints is time-consuming and confusing. Light touch, pin, vibratory, and position sense testing usually suffice. Light touch and pin are self-explanatory. Vibration should be tested with a low frequency tuning fork held against a toe or finger, with the examiner's finger beneath the patient's, using the examiner's sensation as normal. Position sense is tested by holding a distal phalanx on the side and displacing the digit a few millimeters.

Reflexes

Deep tendon reflexes are examined by tapping a muscle tendon where it crosses a joint, and looking for contraction of the muscle. Greater sensitivity can be obtained by holding the joint in the hand, with a finger over the tendon, and tapping the finger. Reflexes are generally increased in upper motor neuron lesions and decreased in lower.

The Babinski response, present in upper motor neuron lesions, is elicited by scratching the lateral aspect of the plantar surface of the foot and looking for extension of the great toe, with fanning of the others.

Coordination and Gait Examinations

The most important cerebellar functions can be tested by watching the patient walk and perform simple tasks. Appendicular dysfunction can be brought out by having the patient put her heel on her knee and run it down her shin, and by having her touch alternately her nose and the examiner's finger. Appendicular ataxia or dysmetria is caused by lesions in the cerebellar hemispheres or their connections in the brain stem. Truncal dysfunction can be brought out by having the patient tandem walk. Truncal ataxia is caused by lesions in the cerebellar vermis or its connections.

Common Classes of Neurologic Disease Seen in Office Practice

Episodic Loss of Consciousness

The two most common causes of episodic loss of consciousness are seizures and syncope. Syncope usually is preceded by a sense of "graying out," light-headedness, and diaphoresis. Recovery from syncope usually is rapid and complete, while seizures may be followed by post-ictal confusion, lethargy, and, rarely, paralysis (Todd's). Occasionally, a patient may have some clonic movements during a syncopal event if they are maintained in an upright position. These jerks are due to transient global ischemia and are not truly epileptic. The movements are generally less prolonged and less violent than those seen in generalized seizures.

Seizures The most clinically useful classification of seizure divides them into generalized and focal (partial). Generalized seizures involve the entire brain from their onset and are associated with alterations of consciousness. The most commonly recognized type is the generalized major motor seizure, or "grand mal." There usually is a phase of tonic muscular contraction, lasting 10 to 20 s, followed by clonic movements of the extremities, gradually decreasing in frequency over 30 to 60 s. The seizures often are accompanied by tongue biting and incontinence. Absence seizures, another type of generalized epilepsy, involve loss of contact with the environment, but no convulsive activity. When these seizures appear in childhood and are accompanied by a specific EEG pattern (three per second spike and wave), they are referred to as petit mal.

Partial seizures have a focal onset. The focal clinical symptoms depend on the area of the brain affected. If a seizure is preceded by an aura, it is partial (focal). There may be focal motor or sensory signs. If there is no alteration of consciousness, these are called simple seizures; if there is clouding of consciousness, they are complex seizures. Partial complex seizures with psychomotor symptoms usually originate in the temporal lobe (fewer than 10 percent may originate in the frontal lobe). These were previously referred to as temporal lobe or psychomotor seizures. Partial seizures can spread and evolve into generalized major motor seizures (secondary generalization).

When a patient comes to the office with a history of having had a first seizure, the decisions are how far to go in the clinical investigation and whether or not to treat. Decisions are guided by the type of seizure, the clinical circumstances in which it occurred, and the neurologic examination. Partial (focal) seizures and/or focality on the neurologic exam necessitate imaging (MRI or contrast CT), EEG, and lumbar puncture (if there is no large mass) to rule out local pathology as the cause. In the case of generalized major motor seizures with a clear cause (e.g., head trauma, alcohol withdrawal), imaging and EEG probably are sufficient.

The decision regarding whether or not to treat a first seizure is more difficult. If there is a structural cause for the seizure, or if there is an epileptic EEG, most clinicians would opt for treatment. Even in relatively benign seizures, the psychosocial impact of repeated seizures must be considered. In New York State, for example, epilepsy patients must be seizure-free for one year before being allowed to drive. Furthermore, in women taking oral contraceptives, phenytoin may alter the efficacy of the contraceptive.

The most commonly used drugs for the various seizure types are listed in Table 52-2, along with side-effects. Only adult doses are listed. If phenytoin is given without a loading dose, it will take nearly one week to reach therapeutic levels. An oral loading dose of approximately 15 mg per kilogram body weight will achieve therapeutic levels within hours.

The issue of epilepsy in pregnancy is particularly thorny. The balance to be struck is between the risk of seizures to the mother and the fetus, and the risk to the fetus of medication. The effect of pregnancy on epilepsy is unpredictable in any given patient, but about half of all patients may have an increase in their seizure frequency. The ones most at risk for worsening are those with difficult seizures prior to pregnancy. Some increase in seizure activity may be related to an alteration in antiepileptic drug pharmacokinetics. These changes may be due to changes in protein binding, drug clearance, and volume expansion, requiring more careful monitoring of serum anticonvulsant levels.

The teratogenic effects of anticonvulsants certainly exist, but in my opinion are probably overstated. Antiepileptic drugs do have teratogenic potential, especially carbamazepine and valproic acid, but the effects are most pronounced during the first three or four months of pregnancy. Carbamazepine

TABLE 52-2 Commonly Used Antiepileptic Drugs

Drug (Generic)	Indication (S)	Side Effects	Dosing Schedule
Dilantin (phenytoin)	Tonic-clonic Partial	Nystagmus, hirsutism elevated LFTs[b] gingival hyperplasia	300–500 mg/day[a]
Luminal (phenobarbital)	Same	Somnolence	30–60 mg tid[a]
Tegretol (carbamazepine)	Tonic-clonic	Dizziness Agranulocytosis[c]	200 mg 3–6/day[a]
Klonopin (clonazepam)[d]	Absence	Somnolence	0.5–5 mg tid[a]

[a]Dosing ranges vary considerably with the individual and, when there are problems obtaining seizure control or questions of toxicity, serum levels should be checked. The average therapeutic ranges are 10–20 μg/ml for Dilantin, 10–40 μg/ml for Luminal, 4–10 μg/ml for Tegretol, and 0.01–0.07 μg/ml for Klonopin. These are mean effective ranges and should not be considered firm boundaries.

[b]These side effects appear even at therapeutic levels. A mild elevation of alkaline phosphatase does not necessarily represent toxicity. Gingival hyperplasia can be lessened with good oral hygiene.

[c]Agranulocytosis is a rare and idiosyncratic reaction to Tegretol, not a true side effect. Blood counts should be checked weekly for the first month of therapy, and then monthly for two or three months.

[d]Klonopin is a benzodiazepine anticonvulsant that also has anxiolytic properties.

and Depakote cause neural tube defects, and patients on these drugs should consider plasma and amniotic fluid alpha-fetoprotein assessment as well as other evaluation. A fetal hydantoin syndrome is clearly recognized, characterized by craniofacial and limb malformations accompanied by mental deficiency. However, the benefits of phenytoin to the mother and fetus versus the incidence of fetal hydantoin syndrome must be evaluated in context for each woman.

The issue of whether to change drugs in a pregnant epileptic woman whose seizures are well controlled is very difficult and involves choices outside the field of epilepsy. These include whether or not the patient would consider abortion if a neural tube defect were found, the patient's understanding of and decisions regarding the risk/benefit ratio of changing, and the relative risks of increased seizures. Prolonged maternal seizures with hypoxia have a deleterious effect on the fetus, and many mothers and fetuses do not survive status epilepticus.

Approximately 5 to 10 percent of pregnant mothers who are taking antiepileptic drugs may develop vitamin K deficiencies. This can lead to hemorrhagic complications in the newborn. It is suggested that women on antiepileptic drugs take oral vitamin K daily for the last two to four weeks of pregnancy.

Syncope Syncope is defined as loss of consciousness due to lack of blood flow to the brain. It usually is preceded by a feeling of faintness. The possible causes are legion, but the three most common broad categories are loss of peripheral vascular resistance (vasovagal), loss of cardiac output (arrhythmias), and loss of blood volume (e.g., dehydration, blood loss). The neurologic examination is normal, and treatment is directed at the underlying cause.

Dizziness Dizziness is one of the most common neurologic complaints. The most important step in diagnosis is to determine what the patient really means by the term. Most often, it is lightheadedness or a sense of giddiness. True vertigo, on the other hand, is the sensation that the patient or the environment is moving abnormally. If the patient cannot give a clear description, it may be helpful to have her hyperventilate for three minutes. This will produce mild lightheadedness and swaying in most people. If that matches the patient's symptoms, a search for brain stem or peripheral causes of vertigo is unnecessary.

In cases of true vertigo, the issue is to differentiate between potentially lethal brain stem disease and relatively benign disorders of the peripheral vestibular system. Vestibular lesions produce vertigo that is sensitive to changes in position. There is a brief latency between the time the patient changes position and when she develops dizziness and nystagmus. The nystagmus tends to diminish with repeated exercises. A lengthy discussion of the evaluation and treatment of dizziness can be found in Chap. 57.

Loss of Intellect, Memory, or Language Function

Dementia Dementia is defined as a progressive decline in intellectual and cognitive function. Early signs may be so subtle that they go unnoticed. Commonly, patients progressively restrict their spheres of activity so that they continue to function well, but in a progressively more limited range. The dementia may not become apparent until the patient tries to function in a broader context, and gets lost or shows very significant confusion. The history should be directed at ascertaining what specific losses of cognitive function have occurred. Further clinical investigation is directed toward finding potentially curable causes of dementia. In broad terms, the causes of dementia can be lumped into three groups: cases in which the brain is the target of a systemic illness (metabolic and nutritional disorders, infections, vascular, and inflammatory diseases); primary structural causes (tumors, other space-occupying lesions, and hydrocephalus); and primary degenerative diseases of the nervous system (senile dementia of the Alzheimer type, Pick's disease, and other syndromes). To clarify these issues, the initial work-up for a presumed dementing illness should include a detailed neurologic history and clinical examination, an imaging procedure of the brain (noncontrast CT scan usually is sufficient), B_{12} and folate levels, thyroid function tests, and a serologic test for syphilis. In subtle cases, neuropsychometric testing may be needed.

Metabolic causes of dementia: B_{12} deficiency may produce a gradually progressive dementia that is accompanied by signs of combined systems degeneration (corticospinal tract and posterior column dysfunction) with some degree of spasticity and marked position sense loss. The cbc usually shows a macrocytic anemia. A Schilling test confirms the diagnosis.

Hypothyroidism rarely causes dementia without significant systemic signs of hypothyroidism, including weight gain, cold intolerance, sparse hair and rough skin. Patients appear generally slowed, without any clear focal neurologic deficit or specific area of intellectual dysfunction. With thyroid replacement in these cases, care must be taken not to precipitate an addisonian crisis.

CNS complications of syphilis were becoming very rare; however, with the AIDS epidemic, the frequency is on the rise and, what used to be considered late stages of syphilis are appearing within one to two years. Patients may demonstrate confabulatory states and severe memory deficit. In suspected cases, lumbar puncture should be performed along with a serum VDRL and FTA-ABS. CSF characteristically shows an elevated protein (50–200 mg/dl) and a lymphocytic pleocytosis. CSF VDRL is almost always positive, but it may require a number of lumbar punctures to demonstrate positivity. Serum FTA-ABS is invariably positive in neurosyphilis.

Recommended treatment is aqueous crystalline penicillin G, 2 to 4 million units IV every 4 h for 10 to 14 days. An approved alternative is procaine penicillin G, 2.4 million units IM daily for 10 to 14 days, along with oral probenecid, 500 mg four times a day.

In immunocompromised hosts, *opportunistic infections,* such as cryptococcosis, must be considered. Again, diagnosis is made by lumbar puncture.

Thiamine deficiency, when prolonged, can produce the Korsakoff syndrome, which is primarily an amnesic syndrome. Patients have severe impairment of recent recall and are confabulatory. At this stage, thiamine replacement may stop progression of the disease, but usually does not reverse it fully.

Structural lesions of the central nervous system as a cause of dementia: Brain tumors and subdural hematomas may produce progressive dementia, with surprisingly little in the way of focal neurologic signs. Usually, there is a subtle hemiparesis associated with the dementia, which tends to be more rapidly progressive than that seen in Alzheimer's disease, usually occurring over a matter of weeks to months. CT scan reveals the underlying lesion. In hydrocephalus, patients may show more slowness of response than true dementia. There is often an associated gait disturbance, and urinary incontinence may be part of the clinical presentation. Again, this is rapidly diagnosed on brain imaging. When vascular disease causes dementia, a stepwise progression of impairment usually can be elicited, and there are signs of focal cerebral dysfunction.

Senile dementia of the Alzheimer's type (SDAT), previously called Alzheimer's disease, is the most common form of dementia. Incidence increases exponentially with advancing age. While some areas of cognition may be affected more than others early in the disease (recent recall more than distant), there is a gradual decline in all cognitive functions. In early cases, tacrine (an ergot derivative) may produce some benefit. There is no known cure, and the disease is progressive.

Memory Loss Pure memory loss, without decline in other cognitive functions (amnesic syndrome), is unusual. In transient global amnesia, there is brief (minutes to hours) loss of memory. The patient is fully awake and alert, but does not recognize her surroundings nor have any recall of how she arrived at the current place. It clears spontaneously, and usually there are no sequelae. It is believed to be due to bilateral mesial temporal lobe transient ischemia, but this has not been firmly established, and usually there are no further events. Korsakoff's psychosis is a pure amnesic syndrome caused by prolonged thiamine deficiency. It is most commonly seen in alcoholic patients and is accompanied by confabulation and peripheral signs of thiamine deficiency (peripheral neuropathy). Occasionally, elderly patients will have minor lapses of memory, such as forgetting names or where they put objects, but no further deterioration. This is called benign senile forgetfulness and is not a harbinger of future senile dementia of the Alzheimer type. Most commonly, however, memory loss in the elderly is only the start of the syndrome, and they then progress to other fields of cognitive impairment.

Aphasias Language function is predominantly in the left hemisphere in all right-handed patients and in more than half of left-handed patients. Thus, the left hemisphere is dominant for language in well over 95 percent of the population. Patients with language disorders (aphasias), have difficulty with all types of communication, not just the spoken word. Aphasias are broadly divided into two groups, anterior and posterior. The nomenclature and characteristics of the major aphasic syndromes are shown in Table 52-1. Broca's area is in the inferior frontal gyrus of the left hemisphere. It is intimately related with the motor strip. Lesions in this area produce an expressive aphasia. Patients have trouble expressing themselves, they are nonfluent and often have accompanying motor signs. Wernicke's area is in the posterior part of the left superior temporal gyrus. Lesions in this area produce difficulty in understanding language. Patients may be fluent, but their speech output makes no sense. Pure receptive aphasias may be associated with a field cut, but usually are not associated with a hemiparesis. The easiest way to remember the difference is that the motor strip is anterior to the sensory strip, so anterior aphasias are motor, expressive, nonfluent, and associated with motor paresis. Most commonly, aphasias are mixed, showing elements of both expressive and receptive aphasias.

Weakness

The approach to the patient with a complaint of weakness is anchored in three concepts: localization (pattern), onset, and progression. The pattern of weakness can give an initial indication of what part of the nervous system is affected. Upper motor neuron lesions (brain or spinal cord) characteristically present with a hemiparesis or paraparesis. Rarely, a cerebral lesion may lead to a monoparesis. Muscle disease tends to be proximal, while peripheral neuropathy tends to be distal. Diseases of the neuromuscular junction, such as myasthenia, tend to be patchy and multifocal, often involving the ocular muscles. Weakness can occur with lesions virtually anywhere in the nervous system. It is useful to differentiate between upper motor neuron (central) and lower motor neuron (peripheral) lesions. The upper motor neuron is anywhere from the cortex to the synapse on the anterior horn cell in the spinal cord. From the anterior horn cell to the neuromuscular junction is the lower motor neuron. Lower motor weakness can occur anywhere in the path of the lower motor neuron. The course, from proximal to distal, is anterior horn, root, plexus, nerve, neuromuscular junction, muscle. Upper motor neuron lesions are characterized by increased tone, hyperreflexia, and Babinski signs. Lower motor neuron lesions are characterized by decreased tone, decreased reflexes, atrophy, and fasciculations. Using the approach just summarized, some of the common neurologic disorders that present with weakness are discussed below.

Central Lesions Affecting the Brain *Cerebrovascular disease:* The discussion of cerebrovascular disease is limited here to thrombotic and embolic cerebrovascular accidents (CVAs) because these account for the vast majority of strokes, and it would be unusual to manage hemorrhagic CVAs in the office. Clinically, strokes are characterized by the sudden onset of neurologic dysfunction, limited to an area of the brain supplied by a specific artery. Deficits tend to resolve slowly, over weeks to months. If the deficits clear within 24 h, the event is technically considered a transient ischemic attack (TIA), although deficits lasting more than one hour usually reflect an actual stroke. Even in completed strokes, the CT scan is often normal in the first 24 h and in small infarctions. If the patient's condition rapidly deteriorates, it is imperative to rule out superimposed hemorrhage, edema, or an incorrect diagnosis (tumor presenting as stroke). The greatest risk for postischemic brain swelling is 48 to 72 h after the stroke. Since there is no proven prevention, observation and supportive care are necessary.

Listing all the possible stroke syndromes is beyond the scope of this book. Table 52-3 shows some of the common syndromes and the arterial supplies responsible for them. When weakness occurs, it is usually in the form of a hemiparesis, with the extensors of the arms and the flexors of the legs being weaker than their antagonist muscles. Weakness is usually accompanied by hyperreflexia and a Babinski sign. The involvement of cranial nerves on one side and the body on the other is indicative of brain stem disease. For office practice, a much more common issue than either stroke recognition or care is stroke prevention.

Stroke prevention can be viewed in three ways: stroke prevention in the population with specific risk factors, stroke prevention in patients who have had transient ischemia, and prevention of recurrent stroke.

Hypertension is the most clearly recognized and easily treated risk factor for stroke. Good blood pressure control can greatly reduce the likelihood of stroke. While diabetes is a risk factor, it is less clear that tight control of blood sugar will alter the incidence of stroke. Atrial fibrillation is a clear risk factor for embolic CVA, and low-dose anticoagulation can reduce the risk. While smoking has not been defined clearly as a risk factor on its own, the vascular effects of smoking behoove all health care providers to advise the elderly (and all patients) to stop smoking. Young women who smoke and take oral contraceptives increase their stroke risk and should be cautioned that if they wish to take oral contraceptives they should not smoke.

Transient ischemic attacks are a harbinger of stroke. Transient monocular blindness (amaurosis fugax) may be considered in the same category as a TIA and usually is due to platelet emboli from the

TABLE 52-3 Common Stroke Syndromes

Artery	Area Supplied	Clinical Syndrome
Anterior cerebral	Interhemispheric	Paresis of leg > arm Contralateral
Middle cerebral	Lateral hemisphere	Face > arm > leg Motor + sensory Aphasia, if dominant
Posterior cerebral	Occipital poles +/− temporoparietal	Hemianopsia +/− sensory
Vertebrobasilar	Brain stem	Crossed syndromes, with cranial nerves on one side and body findings on the other

carotid artery. Patients who have a TIA have approximately a 10 percent chance of suffering a CVA in the coming year. Aspirin can reduce this risk to about 5 percent. Other antiplatelet drugs, such as ticlopidine, are slightly more effective, but the side effect profile (e.g., reversible neutropenia) requires regular blood monitoring for the first three months of therapy. The data on anticoagulation are inconclusive. If a tight carotid stenosis (greater than 70 percent) can be demonstrated, there is clear benefit from carotid endarterectomy.

Patients who have had a stroke are more likely to have a second stroke than the general population is to have a first stroke. Prevention of that second stroke depends mainly on identifying the causes of the first. There are experimental studies currently in progress to determine whether or not aspirin, anticoagulation, or other drugs can prevent stroke recurrence.

Brain tumors: Headache is the most common presenting complaint in patients found to have brain tumors. The "classic" brain tumor headache is described as worse in the early morning and improving with aspirin or as the day progresses. More commonly, the headache is more of a tension-type (see Chap. 63), and the indications of a brain tumor are that the headache is progressive over weeks to a few months and there may be focality on the neurologic examination.

Weakness, when present, is most commonly in the form of a progressive hemiparesis. As in other upper motor neuron lesions, the extensors of the arm and the flexors of the leg are most affected. Severe, bilateral, progressive headaches are indicative of increased intracranial pressure and require emergency management. Other signs of decompensation requiring rapid attention include obtundation, nausea and vomiting, papilledema, and rapidly progressive neurologic deficits.

MRI scan with gadolinium demonstrates virtually all clinically significant brain tumors. If MRI is unavailable, contrast-enhanced CT is sufficient in most cases. EEG and lumbar puncture add little or nothing to the diagnosis.

Treatment of metastatic brain tumors is directed at controlling intracranial pressure, reducing focal deficits, and lessening the tumor burden. Steroids (the equivalent of about 16 mg of dexamethasone/day) provide initial relief of most tumor symptoms, because the edema surrounding the lesions is vasogenic. For metastatic lesions, most commonly arising from lung, breast, melanoma, or colon primaries, surgical removal may be indicated for solitary lesions or those that are causing rapidly progressive deficits and are accessible. Radiation therapy is generally considered palliative and is rarely curative. Steroid therapy should be continued throughout the course of radiation and tapered as tolerated. About 20 percent of patients with metastatic lesions will remain steroid-dependent until death.

Seizures occur in about 25 percent of patients with brain tumors, usually early in the course, and may be the presenting symptom. There is some disagreement about the need for prophylactic anticonvulsant therapy in patients with brain tumors who have not had seizures. Given the fact that seizures tend to be an early occurrence and that anticonvulsive therapy carries certain risks, many practitioners opt for treating only patients who have had seizures or have undergone surgery.

Multiple sclerosis is a demyelinating disease that affects the central nervous system. While there are scattered reports of peripheral nervous system involvement, the brain and spinal cord are the two primary targets. The disease is defined clinically as "two lesions separated in space and time and not attributable to any other cause." This means that two different parts of the central nervous system are affected at two different times. It most commonly presents with gait difficulties that may be due to weakness, spasticity, or incoordination. While eye movement disorders, optic neuritis, and multifocal cerebral disorders are common, about one-third of cases are strictly spinal. It is the most common cause of asymmetrical paraparesis in young adults. Onset is most commonly in the third or fourth decade of life, and it is more common in women than in men. It usually takes an exacerbating-remitting course, but there are chronic progressive forms. Even with remissions, deficits usually tend to increase. High doses of steroids or ACTH may shorten individual exacerbations, but nothing has been definitely shown to alter the overall course. About 25 percent of patients with multiple sclerosis are still working after 20 years. Poor prognostic factors include male sex, early age of onset, and presentation with primarily motor signs.

Compressive myelopathies. Cervical spondylosis: In severe cases of degenerative disease of the spine, mainly in elderly patients, there can be encroachment by disc material and overgrown bone on the cervical spinal cord. This generally has a very slow progression, associated with mild spasticity of the lower extremities. In cases in which the progression is rapid, or there is loss of bowel or bladder function, surgery is indicated to correct the compressive lesion. Many cases, however, can be followed conservatively.

Malignant epidural spinal cord compression: Five to 10 percent of patients with systemic cancer develop epidural spinal cord compression from a metastasis to the spinal column. Rarely, this can be the presenting symptom of the malignancy. The syndrome is characterized by severe back pain with a radicular radiation, followed by progressive paraparesis. Any patient with cancer and back pain should be suspected of having epidural cord compression. If there is a vertebral collapse on plain radiographs, there is better than a 50–50 chance that the compression will be at that level. These patients must be treated emergently, with high-dose steroids and radiation therapy.

B_{12} deficiency also can present with myelopathic features and is recognized by the marked position and vibratory sense loss in the toes, added peripheral neuropathy, and megalocytic anemia.

Peripheral Lesions Anything affecting the nervous system from the anterior horn cell in the spinal cord, to the muscle fiber, produces a "lower motor neuron" pattern of weakness.

Guillain-Barré syndrome (GBS) is an acute, demyelinating, polyradiculoneuropathy. Demyelination occurs from the nerve roots out to the nerves. The characteristic pattern is the development of a mild, distal paresthesia, following an upper respiratory tract infection. This is superseded by a rapidly progressive weakness and areflexia, reaching a maximum in a few days to a week. In fulminant cases, patients can go from normal to quadriplegic and respirator-dependent in a matter of hours. The syndrome should be suspected in anyone with progressive weakness and hyporeflexia. Sensory findings, when present, are minimal. Diagnosis can be confirmed early by showing markedly slowed nerve conduction velocities. The characteristic CSF picture of increased protein, but no cells, does not develop until seven to ten days into the disease. If GBS is suspected, the patient should be hospitalized immediately, in an intensive care unit, with careful monitoring of vital capacity (VC). If VC drops below 1250 ml, or if there is a marked deterioration in a few hours, the patient should be intubated and placed on a respirator.

Treatment is both supportive and etiologic. The most common cause of death is respiratory failure, and patients may be respirator-dependent for weeks. With adequate care, 80 to 90 percent of patients make a full functional recovery.

Etiologic treatment is aimed at the presumed immune mechanism of demyelination, and includes plasma exchange (plasmaphoresis) and infusions of human immune globulin, both of which appear to shorten the time that the patient requires a respirator. The data on the use of steroids are less convincing.

The natural history of the disease is seven to ten days of progression, two to four weeks of stabilization, and many months of recovery. During the paralytic phase, passive range of motion of the joints must be performed to avoid contractures.

Other polyradiculopathies: Nerve roots are formed by the motor and sensory fibers that leave or enter the spinal cord. The spinal cord itself ends at about the L1-L2 spinal column level. Below that, there are only lumbar and sacral roots. Roots can be affected by demyelination, compression, or inflammation. Single roots are most commonly affected (monoradiculopathy) by compressive lesions, such as herniated disks. The syndrome is marked by the sudden onset of pain after lifting or other strenuous movement. Pain radiates down the affected extremity in a dermatomal distribution, with the pattern and reflex changes depending on the root affected (Table 52-4). In most cases of lumbar radiculopathy, a few days of bed rest will bring about resolution. If there

TABLE 52-4 **Common Radicular Syndrome**

Root	Dermatome	Muscles[a]	Reflexes
C5	Cap of shoulder	Deltoids, biceps, brachioradialis	Biceps
C6	Upper arm and thumb	+/− biceps	Biceps
C7	Arm to middle finger	Triceps	Triceps
C8	Inner arm to fifth finger	Hand intrinsics	None
L2	Upper, inner thigh	Iliopsoas, quads, adductors[b]	Quadriceps
L3	Anterior to medial thigh	Same	Same
L4	Lateral thigh to medial knee	Same +/− anterior tib	Same
L5	Lateral hip to medial shin and foot	Anterior tibial	None[c]
S1	Posterior thigh to lateral foot	Plantar flexors, hamstrings	Achilles

[a]Only the major muscles are listed, not every one innervated.

[b]The adductors are innervated by the anterior divisions of these roots, while the quadriceps are by the posterior. If only one of the muscles is weak, the lesion is likely in the nerve, rather than the root.

[c]Some neurologists test a posterior tibial reflex, but it is difficult to elicit.

is significant motor impairment or sphincter involvement, surgical correction is indicated. With cervical disks, there is the added problem of cord compression. If signs of cord compression (paraparesis, hyperreflexia, Babinski) appear, decompression should be considered. Further discussion of back pain and radiculopathy can be found in Chap. 63.

When systemic tumors metastasize to the meninges, they can affect multiple roots. The characteristic syndrome includes headache, along with involvement of cranial and/or spinal nerves. Diagnosis is made on lumbar puncture, which demonstrates increased protein and cells, with a cytology positive for malignant cells. Inflammatory processes, such as systemic lupus erythematosus, also can affect multiple roots in a similar fashion.

Plexopathies: Brachial plexopathy is characterized by pain and weakness in the upper extremity. More than one root or nerve is involved. The course of the disease depends on its underlying cause. There are benign idiopathic cases, in which pain precedes the weakness and then diminishes as weakness progresses. These are self-limited disorders and resolve in weeks, and probably are a form of localized demyelination. More ominous is a progressive, painful plexopathy involving the lower roots (C8-T1) and accompanied by a Horner's syndrome (ptosis, myosis, and anhydrosis). This distribution is indicative of tumor in the apex of the lung, invading the brachial plexus (Pancoast's syndrome). Therapy must be directed quickly at the underlying tumor. Pain in the upper, inner aspect of the arm, radiating to the elbow, is rarely due to benign disease and should raise the suspicion of tumor.

Lumbar plexopathy: The lumbar plexus is most often affected by processes in the retroperitoneal space. Tumors, such as renal cell cancer, lymphoma, and ovarian cancers commonly spread to this area and cause a progressive, painful plexopathy. In patients who are anticoagulated, the sudden onset of leg pain should raise the suspicion of retroperitoneal hematoma with lumbar plexus involvement. Clinically, both present as pain with weakness and patchy sensory and reflex loss in the leg. Retroperitoneal hematoma may resolve spontaneously; however, if weakness progresses, exploratory laparotomy is indicated. Tumor involvement of the lumbar plexus requires direct therapy, either by surgery or radiation therapy.

Peripheral neuropathies: As with all other neurologic diseases, peripheral neuropathies can be defined by their onset, distribution, and progression. The main objective is to differentiate between mononeuropathies (in which individual nerves are affected) and diffuse polyneuropathies (in which peripheral nerves in general are affected). Mononeuropathies usually are compressive or inflammatory lesions, confined to one or a few nerves. The weakness, sensory loss, and reflex changes are confined to just that nerve distribution. In a polyneuropathy, however, there is more often symmetrical sensory loss and weakness, with a progression from distal to proximal. There are exceptions to these rules, particularly the demyelinating neuropathies, but they are beyond the scope of this book.

The mononeuropathies commonly seen in obstetric practices are postpartum femoral neuropathy, sciatic neuropathy, and intercostal neuropathy. After a woman has had her delivery in the dorsal lithotomy position, on rare occasions she may subsequently have trouble extending her leg at the knee (quadriceps weakness). The knee jerk is absent, and there may be sensory loss over the anterior thigh. These problems are secondary to stretching of the femoral nerve. Other muscles are intact, unless the obturator nerve is stretched at the same time, causing weakness of the adductors of the thigh. Isolated obturator injury is uncommon. Both of these nerve injuries usually resolve spontaneously, but may take many months, depending on the severity of the injury. Sciatic neuropathy may occur from pressure from the fetal head. It is invariably on the side of repose of the head.

Intercostal neuropathy produces numbness and burning pain along the inferior part of the rib cage late in pregnancy. It is believed to be due to stretching of the intercostal nerves at the junction with the spine.

The neuropathies seen most often in clinical practice are those due to diabetes. They commonly present as a distal, symmetric sensory motor loss that starts in the toes and ascends. Later in the disease, the fingers and hands may be affected. There is a shading of sensory loss from distal to proximal. In some cases, this neuropathy is quite painful, with burning dysesthesia. Low doses of tricyclic antidepressants may be effective for the burning pains. If they are shooting, stabbing pains, anticonvulsants may be useful. This subject is covered in greater depth in the section on pain.

Occasionally, diabetes may present as a mononeuropathy, or as mononeuropathy multiplex (multiple single nerves involved). The most common is femoral neuropathy, in which there is pain in the anterior thigh and weakness in the quadriceps. This resolves spontaneously within months. The third and sixth cranial nerves also are involved occasionally. These are believed to be ischemic neuropathies. There is some debate about diabetic neuropathy in general, but it is believed that tight control of diabetes can forestall the appearance of neuropathic complications.

Nutritional neuropathies seen in clinical practice include B_{12} deficiency, which is characterized by peripheral neuropathy along with "combined systems disease" that includes signs of spinal cord dysfunction such as hyperreflexia and severe position sense loss. Thiamine deficiency produces a typical neuropathy but, in a florid picture, may be combined with a Wernicke's encephalopathy. It is seen most commonly in alcoholics, but can present in anyone with severe nutritional deprivation over many months. Thiamine replacement will resolve the problem.

Pyridoxine, vitamin B_6, in very high doses can produce a peripheral neuropathy. This has been seen in a number of women taking high doses of B_6 for premenstrual syndrome.

Myasthenia gravis is a disease of the neuromuscular junction characterized by weakness of many muscles (commonly starting with the extraocular and pharyngeal muscles) and fatigue. The most frequent initial complaints are double vision, lid ptosis, weakness, and fatigue. Muscles become weaker on repetitive testing.

The disease is most common in young women and elderly men and is believed to be autoimmune in origin. The postsynaptic membrane of the neuromuscular junction is blocked by an autoantibody, so acctylcholine released from the presynaptic membrane does not bind adequately. The diagnosis is made when the clinical syndrome is drastically improved by the administration of edrophonium (Tensilon). Tensilon is a very short-acting cholinesterase inhibitor that makes more acetylcholine available at the neuromuscular junction, thus partially overcoming the blockade. The "Tensilon test" should not be undertaken in the office unless there is ECG monitoring and resuscitation equipment is available.

Treatment of myasthenia gravis is directed at increasing acetylcholine availability with the use of cholinesterase inhibitors (Mestinon) or at modulating the immune system with plasmapheresis, steroids, thymectomy, or immunosuppressants. Decompensation can be precipitated by intercurrent illnesses or by incorrect medication dosing. When Mestinon doses are too high, patients become cholinergic and have abdominal cramps and hypersecretion. The major cause of death in myasthenia is respiratory failure.

Patients with myopathies present with proximal weakness. They complain of difficulty climbing stairs or combing their hair, as a result of weakness of proximal muscles of the legs or arms. The reflex and sensory examinations are normal. The most common myopathies seen in office practice are inflammatory, such as polymyositis, which can present with aching pain, and metabolic, such as those associated with thyroid disease (hypo- and hyper-) or electrolyte imbalance (most commonly hypo- or hyperkalemia). Therefore, the initial approach to a patient who presents with proximal weakness and shows the appropriate signs, is to check a serum CPK, thyroid function tests, and serum electrolytes. EMGs and muscle biopsy, if necessary, can confirm the diagnosis, and treatment is based on the underlying cause.

Disorders of Gait and Movement

Disorders of gait may be due to disorders of pyramidal function (weakness and spasticity), extrapyramidal function (increased tone and postural instability), sensory function (position sense loss), and cerebellar function (uncoordination). Weakness and spasticity are fairly obvious, but the other changes may be more subtle.

Spastic gait is characterized by ''scissoring'' of the legs, in which there is circumduction and crossing. It can be due to spinal or cerebral disease. Cerebral lesions that can cause spastic gait without arm weakness are usually midline (parasagittal tumors, hydrocephalus, etc.). Both intrinsic and extrinsic lesions of the spinal cord also can cause spastic gait. Structural lesions must be addressed first. If there are localizing signs (a sensory level, back pain, reflex changes), imaging should be directed at the area in question. Work-up for demyelinating disease or metabolic problems is guided by the history and associated findings.

In Parkinson's disease, the most representative of the extrapyramidal disorders, the constellation of symptoms includes masked facies, bradykinesia, increased muscle tone with cogwheel rigidity, a characteristic ''pill-rolling tremor,'' postural instability, stooped posture, and a shuffling gait. Any one of the features may predominate in a given patient. Approximately one-fourth to one-half of patients develop dementia late in the disease. In many cases, it turns out to be senile dementia of the Alzheimer type. Depression is also very common.

The tremor of parkinsonism is a resting tremor and attenuates briefly with volitional actions. The oscillations are slower than those seen in a nervous (adrenergic) tremor and are differentiated from benign essential tremor because the latter occurs more with action.

Brain imaging should be performed to rule out the rare cases of structural lesions masquerading as parkinsonism (subdural hematomas, multiple CVAs, basal ganglia tumors).

The underlying pathophysiology of parkinsonism is a paucity of dopamine. Therapy is directed at replacing the deficit. Sinemet, a combination of levodopa and carbidopa, is the first-line drug in most cases. L-Dopa is converted to dopamine within the central nervous system. Carbidopa prevents that conversion from taking place in the periphery, thus allowing more to be presented to the CNS. Dosing should be started low and titrated up gradually, as the patient needs and tolerates. The most common side effects are nausea and dizziness. Anticholinergic agents and direct-acting dopamine agents also can be used, but probably should be managed by a neurologist.

Gait disorders due to sensory impairment usually are the result of position sense loss. This can be tested by having the patient stand with her eyes open, and then close them. If the patient has severe sensory loss, she may be able to keep her balance by using visual cues, but will lose it with the eyes closed (positive Romberg). Cerebellar gait disorders, on the other hand, present with a broad-based gait and inability to tandem. These patients may lose their balance with their eyes open.

One of the most common abnormal movements seen in office practice is tremor. The defining points of tremor are its frequency, amplitude, and time of appearance (i.e., at rest or with movement).

Physiologic tremor can be seen in everyone. It may be irregular in frequency and amplitude, but usually is fine and fast. It is enhanced by anxiety and by maintaining an outstretched posture of the arms. A similar tremor can be caused by anticholinergic and adrenergic drugs, including caffeine, as well as by lithium and thyroid disease.

Familial or benign essential tremor is a coarse tremor that occurs during movement. It is seen mainly in the upper extremities, but the voice and head (titubation) may be affected. It can impair function and occasionally responds to benzodiazepines or beta-blockers.

Intention tremor is not present at rest or during the first part of a movement. It is most pronounced during the terminal phase of a movement and may be interpreted as "end-point dysmetria." It is most characteristic of hemispheric cerebellar dysfunction.

References and Selected Readings

1. Donaldson JO: *Neurology of Pregnancy,* 2d ed. London: WB Saunders, 1989.
2. Porter RJ: *Epilepsy: 100 Elementary Principles.* London: WB Saunders, 1984.
3. Adams RD, Victor M: Motor paralysis, in *Principles of Neurology,* 5th ed. New York: McGraw-Hill, 1993.
4. Adams RD, Victor M: Derangements of intellect, behavior and language due to diffuse and focal cerebral disease, in *Principles of Neurology,* 5th ed. New York: McGraw-Hill, 1993.
5. Adams RD, Victor M: Diseases of the spinal cord, peripheral nerve, and muscle, in *Principles of Neurology,* 5th ed. New York: McGraw-Hill, 1993.
6. Adams RD, Victor M: Multiple sclerosis and allied demyelinative diseases, in *Principles of Neurology,* 5th ed. New York: McGraw-Hill, 1993.
7. Cerebral ischemia: treatment and prevention, in: Barnett HJM, Hachinski VC (eds): *Neurologic Clinics.* WB Saunders, Philadelphia, vol 10, 1992.

53 Rheumatic and Musculoskeletal Disorders

Elise Belilos
Steven Carsons

Approach to the Patient with Arthritis

There are several key factors that help the clinician decide what type of arthritis a patient has. The first is the distribution of the joints involved. For example, rheumatoid arthritis (RA) tends to involve the wrists and the metacarpal phalangeal (MCP) and proximal interphalangeal (PIP) joints of the hands, while osteoarthritis (OA) tends to involve primarily the PIP and distal interphalangeal (DIP) joints of the hands and weight-bearing joints such as the hips and knees. The seronegative spondyloarthropathies tend to involve the low back or sacroiliac joints with an asymmetric oligoarthritis peripherally. The second factor is whether the arthritis is inflammatory or noninflammatory. In addition to objective inflammation in the joints, factors that suggest an inflammatory arthritis include morning stiffness (generally greater than 1 h) and gelling (stiffness after sitting for a prolonged period). The third factor is duration of symptoms. For example, gouty arthritis tends to be episodic, with acute attacks generally resolving within 1 to 2 weeks, while RA and OA have more prolonged symptoms.

Physical examination reveals the presence or absence of objective synovitis in addition to assessing possible loss of range of motion of joints. The general medical evaluation is of extreme importance in discovering extraarticular features that may suggest a particular form of arthritis, such as nodules in RA or psoriasis or nail pitting in psoriatic arthritis.

Radiographs may be helpful in revealing characteristic changes of a particular form of arthritis such as marginal erosions at the MCPs, PIPs, or ulnar styloid processes in RA or sacroiliitis in the spondyloarthropathies. Laboratory data are often supportive of the clinical diagnosis, but generally are not diagnostic. For example, older patients with clinical evidence of OA are often misdiagnosed as having RA simply on the basis of a positive rheumatoid factor. Examination of synovial fluid, if present, is helpful in differentiating inflammatory from noninflammatory effusions, to look for crystals, and to rule out infection.

Osteoarthritis

Osteoarthritis is the most common rheumatic condition; the prevalence currently is thought to exceed 60 million people in the United States.[1] The incidence increases dramatically with advancing age, being less common before the age of 50 and estimated to exceed 50 percent by the age of 60.[1] Osteoarthritis of the hip is equally common in females and males, but OA of the knees and hands is more common in older females than in males of the same age.[1] Much OA is idiopathic, but in some cases predisposing factors may be elicited. Factors that may predispose patients to OA include genetic background, obesity or mechanical factors, previous trauma to the joint, or prior damage from other joint diseases.

Osteoarthritis is a degenerative arthritis with fissuring and wearing down of the cartilage, primarily of the weight-bearing surfaces. This leads to asymmetric joint space narrowing with secondary osteophyte or spur formation. As it is a disease of weight-bearing joints, it involves the hips, knees, feet, lumbosacral spine, lower cervical spine, and the PIP and DIP joints of the hands (from excessive use). It is generally a noninflammatory arthritis, but patients may at times have inflammation of one or more joints secondary to other causes, such as superimposed crystalline disease. The natural history of OA is one of gradual progression of symptoms over time.

The chief complaint of a patient with OA usually is joint pain. The patient's pain generally is worse after physical activity or at the end of the day. Patients often will report that they have difficulty going up or down stairs. Morning stiffness, if present at all, generally lasts only a few minutes. In addition, patients may complain of a gradual and progressive loss of joint function.

On physical examination, there often is evidence of bony swelling secondary to osteophyte formation. In the hands, this swelling is referred to as Heberden's nodes at the DIP joints and Bouchard's nodes at the PIP joints. The CMC joint (at the base of the thumb) is often involved in osteoarthritis and may be tender on examination. While not commonly appreciated, the carpometacarpal (CMC) is one of the most common sites of OA in persons who use their hands excessively. There may be hallux valgus (bunion) at the first MTP joint of the foot. The joints are generally cool without evidence of synovitis. There may be decreased range of motion in involved joints, and crepitus may be palpated.

Laboratory data generally are not helpful except in the sense that they are usually normal, including normal ESR and negative rheumatoid factor. If joint effusion is present, it generally will be "noninflammatory" with WBC counts of less than 2000 WBC/μl. Radiographs show asymmetric joint space narrowing of the weight-bearing surfaces (for example, the medial compartment of the knee is more commonly involved), and osteophyte formation. In addition, there may be evidence of subchondral sclerosis and cyst formation.

Treatment of osteoarthritis, like all diseases, begins with patient education. Physical therapy helps strengthen the structures around the affected joint(s) to relieve stress on the joint. Nonsteroidal anti-inflammatory drugs (NSAIDs) generally are the mainstay of medical management of symptomatic and/or inflammatory osteoarthritis. Examples of these are given in the Table 53-1.

The most common and worrisome side effects of NSAIDs include gastrointestinal (GI) intolerance or GI bleeding and renal toxicity. The risk of GI bleeding may be reduced by the coadministration of misoprostil (Cytotec), 100 to 200 μg qid pc, in selected patients. Varying degrees of hepatotoxicity may be seen with different NSAIDs (Voltaren being the most frequent). Thus, a CBC and renal and hepatic profiles should be checked at baseline and

TABLE 53-1 Examples of NSAIDS

Medication	Usual Starting Dose	Comments
Choline magnesium trisalicylate (Trilisate) or Salicyl salicylate (Disalcid)	750–1000 mg po bid pc	Nonacetylated; less renal and GI toxicity; useful in the elderly when only a mild NSAID is needed; may cause tinnitus
Ibuprofen (Motrin)	400, 600, or 800 mg po tid–qid pc (max dose = 3200 mg/day)	Inexpensive
Naproxen (Naprosyn)	375–500 mg po bid pc	
Diclofenac (Voltaren)	50–75 mg po bid pc	May have higher incidence of increased LFTs
Etodolac (Lodine)	200–300 mg po tid–qid pc	May have less GI toxicity
Nabumatone (Relafen)	500–750 mg (2 tabs po qd pc)	May have less GI toxicity
Sulindac (Clinoril)	150–200 mg po bid pc	May have less renal toxicity; may have CNS side effects
Indomethacin (Indocin)	25–50 mg po tid–qid pc	Very potent NSAID with frequent GI intolerance (best if used for short intervals such as acute gout attack); CNS side effects common, especially in the elderly
Piroxicam (Feldene)	10–20 mg po qd pc	Good in the younger patient for improved compliance (once a day) but should be used with caution in the elderly because of long half-life

every three to four months while the patient is on an NSAID. Table 53-2 summarizes instructions that should be given to all patients using NSAIDs. In addition, patients on these medications may develop fluid retention or hypertension, so that blood pressure also should be carefully monitored. NSAIDs have an anticoagulant effect and should be avoided in patients on anticoagulant therapy. In general, NSAIDs should be withheld approximately one week prior to surgery in order to avoid enhanced bleeding due to their antiplatelet effects. In patients who cannot take NSAIDs, such analgesics as acetaminophen may be a useful alternative. Muscle relaxants such as cyclobenzaprine (Flexeril) or chlorzoxazone (Parafon Forte) may be helpful, especially in osteoarthritis of the cervical or lumbosacral spine where paraspinal muscle spasm may be contributing significantly to the patient's symptoms. In advanced OA, joint replacement should be considered, the timing of which should be determined by the degree of damage evident radiographically, together with the patient's pain or limitation of daily activities, with the latter being the more important determinant.

Additional therapeutic considerations for degenerative joint disease of specific anatomical regions are discussed in the section below.

Osteoarthritis of the Hand Heberden's and Bouchard's nodes are often quite painful when they first appear, sometimes accompanied by significant erythema and swelling. However, these nodes generally will become much less painful over time. Reassurance that symptoms will improve and that their arthritis will not cause severe deformities is very helpful for patients. In addition to analgesics or anti-inflammatory medications, local heat with hot soaks

TABLE 53-2 Instructions for Patients Using NSAIDs

- Always take with food
- Notify physician of any abdominal pain or change in bowel movement
- Have your blood checked regularly while on the medication (every 3–4 months)
- Avoid aspirin or other over-the-counter anti-inflammatory medications

or paraffin baths may provide symptomatic relief during the initial painful phase.

Osteoarthritis at the base of the thumb (in the first CMC joint) is very common and deserves special attention. In addition to the above measures, use of a hand splint that immobilizes this joint may be helpful. With severe pain in this joint, intra-articular steroid injection should be considered.

Osteoarthritis of the Hip In addition to the medical management of OA of the hip (see above), common sense measures to reduce stress on the joint should be employed. Obese patients should be encouraged to lose weight. Use of a walking aid such as a cane or walker is often helpful; a cane should be used on the contralateral side. The use of higher chairs and avoidance of activities such as climbing stairs, kneeling, squatting, or standing for prolonged periods also will help to reduce stress on the hip joint.[2] Non-weight-bearing exercises (such as swimming) are ideal for strengthening the structures around the joint. In advanced cases, total hip replacement should be considered and generally has excellent results, with relief of pain and restoration of hip motion.

It is important to note that some patients who complain of ''hip'' pain actually have a trochanteric bursitis rather than a true hip problem. These patients will have marked point tenderness of the upper lateral thigh (over the greater trochanter) and minimal symptoms on rotation of the hip. Trochanteric bursitis generally responds well to injection of steroid into the bursa.

Osteoarthritis of the Knee Similar to the treatment principles applied to OA of the hip, treatment of OA of the knee includes: 1. avoidance of excessive stress on the joint; 2. strengthening of the structures around the joint with specific exercises; 3. medical management (see above); and 4. surgical management. Again, weight loss is essential in obese patients. Elastic supports or knee braces may help to stabilize the knee and relieve stress on the joint. Exercises to strengthen the quadriceps (such as leg lifts) are an essential part of the treatment plan.

Patients with OA of the knee commonly develop acute flares with joint effusion (sometimes secondary to superimposed calcium pyrophosphate dihydrate crystalline disease). Joint aspiration with intra-articular steroid injection is especially helpful in this setting. Not uncommonly, a patient may develop an associated anserine bursitis (with point tenderness over the anserine bursa, which is located superficially at the inferomedial aspect of the knee); this also generally responds well to local steroid injection.

In advanced cases of OA of the knee, arthroscopic debridement may provide relief and allow the patient to postpone total knee replacement.

Osteoarthritis of the Foot The most common cause of pain at the first metatarsal phalangeal (MTP) joint (at the base of the big toe) is osteoarthritis. The use of metatarsal pads, metatarsal bars, or stiffening the sole of the shoe to minimize dorsiflexion during walking may be a useful adjunct.[2] In severe cases where conservative measures and medical management are ineffective, surgery may be required. Inflammation of the bursa medial to the first MTP joint may be helped by local steroid injection.

Evaluation of Low Back Pain

Low back pain is extremely common and accounts for up to one-third of all rheumatic complaints.[3] Heavy physical labor, anxiety, depression, cigarette smoking, and pregnancy are considered to be associated risk factors.[3] Degenerative disease is a common cause of low back pain in older patients, but there are numerous causes of low back pain. Both degenerative and nondegenerative causes will be discussed in this section. In most cases, a careful history and physical examination together with appropriate imaging techniques can elucidate the etiology of low back pain.

The character of a patient's pain, together with aggravating or alleviating factors, can be an important clue to the source of the pain. Spinal pain is felt locally, may be sharp or dull, and typically is aggravated by motion. Spinal pain secondary to degenerative disease typically is worse after exercise or at the end of the day, whereas patients with inflammatory spondyloarthropathies usually describe their pain as a stiffness that is worse in the morning or after periods of prolonged inactivity (see Spondyloarthropathy section). Pain secondary to disc disease is worse with activities that increase intradiscal pressure such as lifting, bending, sitting, coughing, or the Valsalva maneuver. Nerve root pain is typically radicular and often is accompanied by numbness and paresthesias and occasionally by motor weakness. It usually is exacerbated by maneuvers that stretch the nerve root (such as bending) and relieved by rest. Sciatic pain (pain running from the buttock down the back of the leg) may arise from the lumbar spine (with impingement of nerve roots) or anywhere along the course of the sciatic nerve. Spinal stenosis, which may be congenital or caused by degenerative disease and/or disc herniation, is suggested by claudication-like symptoms. Patients with spinal stenosis will report that their symptoms are worse with walking and relieved upon resting or sitting. Low back pain may also be referred from abdominal or pelvic viscera, and usually is a deep, aching pain felt in a dermatomal distribution. Referred pain generally is not affected by activity or rest. Gynecologic causes of referred back pain include endometriosis, fibroids, pelvic infection, and invasive carcinoma of the uterus, cervix, or bladder.[3] Malignant invasion of the lumbosacral plexus may give rise to radicular symptoms. Sacral pain can occur with menstruation, and sacral pain on standing may be secondary to prolapse of the uterus.[3] Assessment of bowel, bladder, and sexual function should always be included in evaluating the patient with low back pain as these may be abnormal in patients with central disc herniations, conus tumors, and occasionally spinal stenosis.[3] A history of fever or other constitutional symptoms may suggest infection of the vertebral body or disc space or malignancy. Pyogenic vertebral osteomyelitis occurs via hematogenous spread. *Staphylococcus aureus* is the organism most commonly implicated, but gram-negative bacilli are increasingly involved, especially in the setting of genitourinary manipulations.[3] In patients with more indolent back pain and constitutional symptoms, tuberculosis (especially with involvement of L1) and other nontubercular granulomatous infections of the spine should be considered.

On physical examination, simple observation will reveal normal lumbar lordosis and dorsal kyphosis; the presence of scoliosis or straightening of the spine (which may be present with paraspinal muscle spasm) should be noted. Abnormalities in gait or posture may signify a low back problem; for example, the patient may flex her lower extremities to relieve root tension. Local tenderness or paraspinal muscle spasm may be palpable. Palpation also may reveal malalignment of the spinous processes secondary to spondylolisthesis (forward slippage of one vertebra on another). Range of motion of the lumbar spine should be tested with normal anterior flexion to 90 degrees, extension to 30 degrees, and lateral flexion to 30 degrees. Hyperextension may elicit pain from inflamed facet joints; asymmetric lateral bending may be a clue to unilateral root entrapment.[3] The neurologic exam is extremely important in evaluating patients with low back pain. L5–S1 and L4–L5 are the most common levels involved in disc herniations, followed by L3–L4.[3] Findings referable to the L4 root (L3–L4 disc) include absent or diminished patellar reflex, weakness of the quadriceps or tibialis anterior (inversion and dorsiflexion of the foot) muscles, or sensory findings including the medial aspect of the lower leg and foot. Involvement of the L5 root (L4–L5 disc) may lead to weakness of the extensor hallucis longus (raising big toe) or sensory findings including the lateral leg and dorsum of the foot. S1 foot involvement may lead to a diminished Achilles tendon reflex, weakness of the peroneus longus and brevis (eversion and plantar flexion of the foot), or sensory findings including the lateral aspect of the foot. Certain maneuvers may be helpful in further evaluating the patient with low back pain. For example, the straight leg raise stretches the sciatic nerve and reveals problems originating at the nerve roots or along the sciatic nerve.

Laboratory data generally are not helpful in evaluating the patient with low back pain, with the exception of an abnormal CBC or elevated ESR, which may signal an underlying infection or malignancy.

Imaging studies, on the other hand, often are quite useful. Plain radiographs of the lumbosacral spine are often the first step in evaluating low back pain of almost any etiology and are particularly useful in evaluating patients for tumor, infection, or osteoarthritis. In degenerative disease, radiographs typically show loss of disc space, sclerosis, and osteophyte formation. Technetium-99 bone scanning is useful in detecting bony infection or malignancy and in detecting early sacroiliac disease in patients with spondyloarthropathies. Gallium or indium-labeled leukocyte scans are useful for early diagnosis of infection. To evaluate patients with suspected disc herniations or spinal stenosis, imaging with CT or MRI is necessary. In patients with spinal stenosis, these techniques can reveal impingement on the cord or nerve root by bulging of the disc, thickening of the ligamentum flavum, osteophytic entrapment of the facets, and obliteration of the epidural fat.[3] CT scanning appears to be more than 95 percent reliable in detecting herniated discs.[3] MRI has the advantages of excellent soft tissue contrast, multiplanar images, and the ability to view the vertebrae, discs, and spinal canal of an entire anatomical region without contrast.[3] Myelography is not used as a diagnostic technique, but rather as a preoperative tool to help define the anatomy of a surgical lesion.

Treatment of low back pain obviously will depend on the etiology. In cases of suspected vertebral body or disc space infection, culture of the site either by CT-guided needle aspiration or open biopsy is essential. For vertebral osteomyelitis, treatment with appropriate antibiotics for 6 weeks is recommended.[3] For disc herniation, most cases can initially be treated conservatively with a combination of bed rest, anti-inflammatory medications, analgesics, and muscle relaxants. Once the patient improves, a program of back protection and exercises should be started. Patients who do not respond to this regimen or have severe, recurrent symptoms may be candidates for surgery. Marked muscular weakness and progressive neurologic deficit in spite of conservative measures probably require surgery.[3] One absolute and emergent indication for surgery in patients with disc herniation is the cauda equina syndrome, where a midline herniation causes paralysis of the sacral roots with bowel and bladder dysfunction and inability to walk.[3] For patients with degenerative disease of the low back, a combination of anti-inflammatory medication or analgesics and an exercise program to strengthen the low back is the mainstay of treatment (see above). In patients with accompanying paraspinal muscle spasm, muscle relaxants may be a useful adjunct. For patients with spinal stenosis, similar measures may be helpful. If conservative measures are not helpful or symptoms are severe, surgical decompression generally provides good symptomatic relief in patients with spinal stenosis. Epidural steroid injections have also been used in the treatment of spinal stenosis.

Rheumatoid Arthritis

It is estimated that 1 percent of the adult population in the United States has rheumatoid arthritis (RA).[4] It is two to three times more common in women than in men. The cause of rheumatoid arthritis remains unknown. There is, however, a genetic predisposition, with a strong association of RA with the immunogenetic marker HLA-DR4. Rheumatoid arthritis is a symmetrical polyarthritis involving the wrists and the MCP and PIP joints of the hands in addition to multiple other joints, including the MTP joints of the feet, ankles, knees, elbows, and upper cervical spine. The disease is inflammatory in nature, with prominent morning stiffness and gelling. Swelling of the joints usually is present for weeks to months, and, in fact, should be present for at least six weeks before a diagnosis of RA can be made (see Table 53-3). It should be noted that there may be multiple patterns of onset, including an insidious onset (most common) over weeks to months, an acute onset, or an intermediate onset. Occasionally, the arthritis may begin in a more asymmetric fashion, but will generally become more symmetric later on. Patients with RA can go on to develop erosions and multiple joint deformities. Unlike osteoarthritis, RA is a sys-

TABLE 53-3 Key Signs of Rheumatoid Arthritis

- Symmetric polyarthritis, especially small joints of hands and wrists
- Prominent morning stiffness (>1 h)
- Duration of symptoms > 6 weeks
- Nodules overlying elbows and other extensor surfaces
- Positive rheumatoid factor (~80%)
- Marginal erosions on x-ray

temic illness, and patients may have constitutional symptoms as well as extraarticular manifestations of their disease. Extraarticular manifestations include: rheumatoid nodules; ocular involvement (scleritis, scleromalacia perforans); peripheral neuropathy or nerve compression syndromes such as carpal tunnel syndrome; pericarditis and other cardiac manifestations; vasculitis (which may be cutaneous or visceral); and pulmonary nodules (note: a single pulmonary nodule in a patient with RA should still be biopsied to rule out malignancy). Patients with RA may develop dry eyes, dry mouth, and salivary gland swelling consistent with secondary Sjögren's syndrome (see below). A small percentage of patients with RA (usually severe, erosive disease) may develop neutropenia and splenomegaly (Felty's syndrome).

The chief complaint of patients with RA usually is pain, swelling, and stiffness of multiple joints in a symmetric pattern as described above. It is uncommon for RA to occur without wrist or hand (MCP/PIP) involvement. In addition to swelling, patients may note warmth or erythema of their joints. Patients report marked morning stiffness, usually lasting more than an hour and often lasting several hours or even all day. Patients will also describe gelling after sitting for prolonged periods of time. Their stiffness typically improves as they move around during the course of the day.

Examination of the joints reveals synovitis in multiple symmetric joint areas, including the MCPs, PIPs, and wrists. These joints will be warm, swollen, tender, and painful on motion. Joint effusions are common and there may be decreased range of motion of the involved joints. Characteristic deformities such as ulnar deviation, swan-neck deformity (flexion at the MCP, hyperextension at the PIP, and flexion at the DIP), and boutonniere deformity (flexion at the PIP and hyperextension at the DIP) may be found. A careful search for rheumatoid nodules over extensor surfaces (most commonly over the olecranon processes, at the occiput or over extensor tendons) should be performed. A thorough general medical examination always should be done to look for evidence of the extraarticular manifestations described above.

Laboratory studies may reveal a mild normochromic normocytic anemia, slight leukocytosis (with normal differential) or slight thrombocytosis, elevated ESR, and positive rheumatoid factor (positive in approximately 80 percent of cases). It should be noted that there are many possible causes for a "false-positive" rheumatoid factor and that 15 to 20 percent of cases of RA are seronegative. Thus, the rheumatoid factor should be used to support the clinical diagnosis of RA but is not diagnostic. The presence of rheumatoid factor may have some prognostic significance in definite cases of RA, as patients with high titer rheumatoid factor and nodules tend to have more severe erosive disease.

Analysis of rheumatoid synovial fluid reveals that it is inflammatory with WBC counts ranging from 5000 to 25,000 WBC/μl, usually with greater than 85 percent PMNs.[4] Crystal analysis and culture are negative.

Radiographs of the hands, wrists, and feet are often helpful in both establishing the diagnosis and evaluating patients for the presence or absence of erosive disease. Early on, there may be evidence of soft tissue swelling and periarticular osteopenia. Marginal erosions may be seen at the MCP, PIP, or MTP joints. Erosions also are commonly seen at the ulnar styloid, but may be seen in any joint involved in RA. With severe, long standing disease, radiographs may show loss of joint space. Radiographs of the cervical spine should be part of the preoperative evaluation of the patient with RA, as possible C1-2 subluxation is an important consideration in any patient undergoing general anesthesia.

Treatment of RA begins with patient education. As this is generally a chronic disease, it is critical that patients understand the disease and what they can do to minimize their disability. Physical therapy is important in maintaining range of motion of the joints; patients with RA must achieve a balance between rest and exercise. The first line of medical management is generally NSAID therapy (see Table 53-1). Often patients will require treatment with "second-line agents" or "disease-modifying antirheumatic drugs" (DMARDS), such as hydroxychloroquine, gold, methotrexate, or azathioprine. While not yet FDA-approved for use in RA, sulfasalazine has been used extensively. If a diagnosis of RA is suspected, the patient should be referred to a rheumatologist for evaluation and early intervention with these second-line agents in appropriate cases. In general, these medications require weeks to months before maximal effect is seen. Arthrocentesis and local injection with corticosteroids may be a helpful adjunct with large or particularly symptomatic joint effusions (one should always be careful to rule out coexisting infection if a single joint appears inflamed out of proportion to the rest of the joints). Systemic corticosteroids should be used very sparingly in the smallest possible dose for the shortest possible time. The side effects of systemic steroids (especially long-term use) are numerous and include edema and weight gain, hypertension, hyperglycemia, osteoporosis (and subsequent risk of fracture), irregular menses, cataracts, glaucoma, aseptic necrosis of bone, GI bleeding, increased susceptibility to infections, and pituitary axis suppression. Patients who have been receiving corticosteroids chronically require stress-dose steroids for surgery, trauma, or other major stresses. In severely damaged joints with markedly restricted range of motion, joint replacement should be considered; the timing of surgery should be determined mostly by the patient's ability to function.

Rheumatoid Arthritis and Pregnancy Marked improvement of RA during pregnancy has been well described. Approximately 70 percent of patients with RA improve significantly during pregnancy, with improvement most commonly occurring in the first trimester and generally being sustained throughout pregnancy.[5] This improvement probably is even greater, considering that second-line agents are generally discontinued during pregnancy and first-line anti-inflammatory medications often are reduced.[5] Unfortunately, more than 90 percent of these patients will have a relapse of their RA within 6 to 8 months after delivery.[5] Women who experience significant improvement in their arthritis during pregnancy are likely to have similar improvement during subsequent pregnancies.[5] Increased risk to the fetus during gestation in RA has not been conclusively demonstrated; most fetal complications in pregnant women with RA have been limited to cases of severe active systemic disease or related to pharmacologic therapy.[5] In managing the pregnant patient with RA, all medications with known major toxicities should be discontinued as soon as pregnancy is known. Most authors recommend stopping all second-line agents. Methotrexate, chlorambucil, and cyclophosphamide all cause congenital malformations and ideally should be stopped at least 4 months prior to conception.[5] The smallest possible dose of aspirin or prednisone may be the safest alternatives to control symptoms during pregnancy.[5] Complications of aspirin use during pregnancy include an increased incidence of the postmaturity syndrome, prolonged labor, increased peripartum hemorrhage, cephalohematoma, and intracranial hemorrhage in premature infants; for these reasons, it is generally recommended that salicylates be discontinued in the final weeks of pregnancy.[5] Intra-articular corticosteroid injections offer the advantage of minimal systemic effects and no significant exposure to the fetus.[5]

The Spondyloarthropathies

The spondyloarthropathies are a group of related disorders including ankylosing spondylitis (AS), psoriatic arthritis (PSA), Reiter's syndrome (RS), enteropathic arthritis [the arthritis associated with inflammatory bowel disease (IBD)], and reactive arthritis (following enteric infection). The spondyloarthropathies as a group are more common in men, but the incidence in women has probably been underestimated. In psoriatic arthritis, arthritis associated with IBD, and reactive arthritis, for example, the female-to-male ratio is approximately 1:1.[6] In all the spondyloarthropathies, there is a familial occurrence and a strong association with HLA-B27. Clinically, the spondyloarthropathies are inflammatory in nature and are characterized by spinal and sacroiliac involvement, an asymmetric oligoarthritis peripherally, enthesopathy (inflammation at the site of tendon or ligamentous insertion onto bone), and the absence of serum rheumatoid factor. Extraarticular manifestations are common and vary in each syndrome. In ankylosing spondylitis, for example, aortic insufficiency, apical pulmonary fibrosis, or uveitis may be seen. As in IBD alone, a variety of cutaneous, mucosal, and ocular manifestations may occur in patients with arthritis associated with Crohn's disease or ulcerative colitis. In addition to skin lesions, nail pitting and onycholysis often are found in patients with psoriatic arthritis. Of note, some patients with psoriatic arthritis will have had psoriasis prior to the onset of the arthritis, some patients will have simultaneous psoriasis and arthritis, and still others will not develop psoriasis until months to years after their presentation with arthritis. Reiter's syndrome typically follows infection with *Chlamydia trachomatis* of the GU tract or enteric pathogens in the GI tract. It is characterized by urethritis, conjunctivitis or other ocular involvement, painless oral or urogenital ulcerations, and occasionally skin lesions such as keratoderma blennorrhagica (a hyperkeratotic skin lesion usually present on the soles of the feet in approximately 10 percent of patients with RS). Women with RS may have asymptomatic cervicitis as their only genitourinary manifestation. Thus, gynecologic examination with genital cultures or serologic testing for Chlamydia may help establish the diagnosis. Salpingitis, vulvovaginitis, and asymptomatic cystitis also have been reported in RS.[7]

The history often reveals chronic low back symptoms and swelling and warmth of one or more peripheral joints in an asymmetric fashion, with prominent morning stiffness and gelling. In addition to the musculoskeletal symptoms, a careful history should be taken to elicit any symptoms of rashes or psoriasis, recurrent eye inflammation, oral or genital ulcers, urethritis, or history of IBD. A family history of spondyloarthropathy or psoriasis should be sought.

Examination may reveal decreased range of motion of the spine (in both anterior and lateral directions), decreased chest expansion, or tenderness over one or both sacroiliac joints. There may be straightening of the spine with loss of the lumbar lordosis or an exaggerated stooped posture in more severe cases (especially in ankylosing spondylitis). Inflammation in one or more peripheral joints in an asymmetric distribution often is found. In psoriatic arthritis and Reiter's syndrome, diffuse swelling of an entire digit may be seen ("sausage digits"). The general medical examination should be comprehensive to search for extraarticular manifestations (see above), including a careful look at the nails and skin for evidence of psoriasis on the scalp, behind the ears, over the elbows and knees, and in the umbilicus and anal crease.

Laboratory tests generally are not helpful except to document the absence of rheumatoid factor. Although HLA-B27 is positive in a fairly high percentage of patients with spondyloarthropathy, it is not a useful screening tool because it is expensive and is present in 6 to 8 percent of normal individuals. Radiographs of the sacroiliac joints are much more helpful, as the presence of sacroiliitis on x-ray is highly suggestive of a spondyloarthropathy. Bone scan may be helpful in detecting early sacroiliac disease not yet apparent on plain radiographs. Radiographs of the lumbar spine may reveal nonmarginal bridging syndesmophytes or a "bamboo spine" appearance, especially in classic ankylosing spondylitis. Radiographs of involved peripheral joints may be helpful in evaluating for the presence of erosive disease (especially in psoriatic arthritis). Aspiration of joint fluid, if present, will reveal nonspecific inflammatory effusions.

Treatment of the spondyloarthropathies begins with patient education and an exercise program. For patients with spine disease primarily (as in ankylosing spondylitis), maintaining good posture is an important goal. For those with peripheral inflammatory arthritis, medical management usually starts with NSAID therapy (see Table 53-1). Patients with erosive disease (as in psoriatic arthritis) are candidates for second-line agents (see treatment of rheumatoid arthritis) and should be evaluated by a rheumatologist early in their course for possible initiation of these medications. Local aspiration and injection with corticosteroids may be a helpful adjunct for peripheral joint disease.

Crystalline Arthropathies: Gout and Pseudogout

Gout is primarily a disease of men. However, the male:female ratio approaches 1:1 at menopause.

The disease is fairly common, with a prevalence of approximately 275/100,000.[8] The risk of developing gout increases with age and serum uric acid levels.[8] Other risk factors for the development of gout include obesity, hypertension, and alcohol abuse. An acute attack may be precipitated by alcohol intake or abrupt shifts in fluid status, such as dehydration (or diuresis) or hydration in a hospitalized patient on intravenous fluids. Gout is caused by the precipitation of uric acid crystals within the joint, which subsequently causes an inflammatory response. A total body overload of urate may lead to extraarticular deposits of uric acid in tophi (most commonly in the olecranon bursae, over the extensor surfaces of the forearms, on the pinnae of the ears, or overlying joints) or to the development of urate nephrolithiasis. Acute gouty arthritis is episodic in nature, with attacks lasting for 1 to 2 weeks with symptom-free intercritical periods. It often begins as an inflammatory monoarthritis, commonly in the first MTP joint (large toe), ankle, or knee. Although podagra (gout of the first MTP joint) is a common presentation, the most common cause of first MTP pain is osteoarthritis. Later, the attacks may become polyarticular, with more frequent attacks or shorter intercritical periods. In more advanced cases, patients may develop chronic tophaceous gout with erosions and deforming arthritis that may mimic rheumatoid arthritis (although gout tends to be less symmetric).

On physical exam, a patient with an acute gout attack may have one or more swollen, warm, erythematous joints that are markedly tender (gout is one of the most painful forms of inflammatory arthritis). Often there is marked warmth, erythema, and swelling of the surrounding soft tissue, which may be confused with an infectious cellulitis and, in fact, has sometimes been referred to as "gouty cellulitis." In addition, patients with an acute attack of gout may also have fever. A careful search for tophi should be done; their presence will influence the long-term treatment plan.

Radiographs generally are not helpful in the initial attack, but, in longstanding disease, may suggest the diagnosis of gout as tophaceous deposits around the joint that may cause oval-shaped erosions with characteristic "over-hanging edges."

Laboratory studies usually, but not always, reveal hyperuricemia; one can have an acute gout attack with a normal serum uric acid level. Additionally, there are patients who have hyperuricemia and arthritis but do not have gout. The only way to establish a definitive diagnosis of gout is to demonstrate the presence of intracellular monosodium urate (MSU) crystals in synovial fluid using a compensated polarized light microscope. MSU crystals are needle-shaped crystals slightly longer than the diameter of a WBC and strongly negatively birefringent (they are bright yellow when parallel to the plane of compensated polarized light and bright blue in the direction perpendicular to this). Joint effusions are usually highly inflammatory, with WBC counts ranging from 2000 to 100,000 WBC/μl.[8] A synovial fluid culture always should be ordered to rule out coexisting infection.

There are many possible therapeutic approaches to an acute gout attack. Which is chosen depends on the patient's concomitant medical problems and the duration of symptoms. For example, intravenous or oral colchicine will be effective for an acute attack only if used within the first 24 to 48 h of the attack. NSAIDs are useful for an acute attack of gout (see Table 53-1) if the patient has no contraindications to their use. If only one joint is involved, aspiration and local injection of corticosteroids is often the simplest and safest alternative. If multiple joints are involved and the patient is not a candidate for NSAID or colchicine therapy, a short tapering course of moderate dose systemic corticosteroids should be considered (less than 30 mg prednisone/day or its equivalent tapered over 1 to 2 weeks). Alternatively, ACTH gel may be given IM in dosages of 40 to 80 units IM every 12 hours for 1 to 3 days. The major drawback of using either ACTH or systemic corticosteroids is that patients may have rebound flares when these medications are withdrawn; this may be minimized by giving low-dose prophylactic colchicine (0.6 mg/day) during and after therapy. The use of allopurinol during an acute gout attack is absolutely contraindicated; it may abruptly shift the uric acid levels and worsen an attack. Patients with chronic tophaceous gout, a history of urate nephrolithiasis, or frequent gouty attacks unresponsive to prophylactic NSAIDs or colchicine and who are hyperuricemic are candidates for urate-lowering agents such as allopurinol (once the acute attack resolves). Dosage of allopurinol should be adjusted for body weight and creatinine clearance.

Calcium pyrophosphate dihydrate deposition disease (CPPD), or pseudogout, is another crystalline arthropathy. The female-to-male ratio in this disorder is about equal, and the incidence increases with age. CPPD disease often occurs in the setting of preexisting damage to a joint, as in osteoarthritis. CPPD disease sometimes is associated with an underlying metabolic disorder such as hyperparathyroidism, hemochromatosis, hypomagnesemia, hypothyroidism, hypocalciuric hypercalcemia, hypophosphatasia, gout, diabetes, and amyloidosis.[9] There is also a hereditary form of this disorder that shows an autosomal dominant pattern (with variable penetrance) of inheritance.[9] CPPD crystals set up an inflammatory response within the joint analogous to what happens in gout. Joints most commonly affected are the knee and the wrist. Attacks may be acute, subacute, or chronic, and may be monoarticular or polyarticular. CPPD disease may mimic gout (except for the noted absence of podagra) or, when polyarticular, rheumatoid arthritis. The history and physical generally will suggest an inflammatory arthritis, commonly in the knee or the wrist. Radiographs show evidence of chondrocalcinosis (linear stippled calcification seen within the joint space). Like gout, the definitive diagnosis of CPPD disease is made by demonstration of the appropriate crystals in synovial fluid. CPPD crystals are rhomboidal in shape and are weakly positively birefringent (pale blue when parallel to the plane of compensated polarized light and pale yellow in the direction perpendicular to this). Laboratory tests are most helpful in screening for a possible associated metabolic disorder; all patients in whom a diagnosis of CPPD is made should have measurement of serum calcium, phosphorus, magnesium, alkaline phosphatase, iron studies, thyroid function tests, glucose, and uric acid. Treatment of CPPD disease is symptomatic, with the use of NSAID therapy (see Table 53-1), local aspiration and injection with corticosteroids, or a short tapering course of low-dose systemic corticosteroids. Low-dose colchicine occasionally may be useful for prophylaxis in refractory recurrent cases, but usually this is not necessary as the attacks generally are spaced farther apart than those of recurrent gout.

Septic Arthritis

Septic arthritis should always be considered in an acutely swollen and warm joint, especially when associated with fever and chills. Prompt diagnosis and treatment of septic arthritis is of extreme importance; infection with *S. aureus,* for example, can rapidly destroy a joint. Spread to the joint is usually via a hematogenous route; septic arthritis is most commonly a monoarthritis and the joint most commonly affected is the knee. Diagnosis is made by aspiration of synovial fluid with Gram stain and culture. Synovial fluid leukocyte counts are very high, generally above 50,000 WBC/μl, and synovial fluid glucose often is much lower than a simultaneous serum glucose. (These findings are not specific, however, and can be seen in rheumatoid arthritis, for example; the ultimate diagnosis rests on the results of the culture). The most common organism in septic arthritis is *S. aureus,* followed by streptococci and gram-negative bacilli. In young patients with one more probable septic joints associated with tenosynovitis or skin lesions, gonococcal arthritis should be suspected. Gonococci are fastidious organisms and difficult to grow from synovial fluid cultures. In suspected cases of gonococcal arthritis, cultures of the pharynx and genitourinary sites have a much higher yield and always should be performed. All cases of suspected septic arthritis should be treated in a hospital setting with appropriate intravenous antibiotics and thorough drainage of involved joints. Repeated arthrocentesis may be necessary to achieve adequate drainage.

Lyme Disease

Lyme disease is a multisystem illness caused by the spirochete *Borrelia burgdorferi,* which is carried by Ixodes ticks. Because of the small size of these ticks, many patients do not recall a tick bite. The initial manifestations of Lyme disease may include the characteristic rash, erythema chronicum migrans (ECM), which, when present, usually appears within a month of the tick bite. Lyme disease is discussed in Chap. 50. Early musculoskeletal manifestations generally consist of transient or migratory arthralgias. Later in the course (with a mean of about 6 months after onset), approximately 60 percent of patients will develop frank arthritis.[10,11] The arthritis is most commonly a monoarthritis or an asymmetric oligoarthritis, often involving the knee.

Common Conditions That Mimic Arthritis

Polymyalgia Rheumatica (PMR) and Temporal Arteritis

PMR is a fairly common clinical syndrome in patients over 50, most commonly in caucasians. It is more common in women, with a ratio of 2:1.[12] It is an inflammatory disorder characterized by pain and stiffness in the shoulder and hip girdle muscles, with prominent morning stiffness and gelling. Patients often will complain of difficulty raising their arms to comb their hair or of difficulty arising from a chair. Physical examination reveals that the joints are normal. Weakness is absent. Laboratory data reveal an elevated ESR of >40 to 50 mm/h (often >100 mm/h). Elevated alpha-2 globulins are often seen on serum protein electrophoresis. A mild normochromic, normocytic anemia may be noted. In addition, abnormalities of liver function tests may be seen, especially alkaline phosphatase. Treatment is with low doses of prednisone (10–15 mg/day) and the response of PMR to steroids often is dramatic. The response usually is so dramatic that, if a patient suspected of having PMR does not respond to 15 mg/day of prednisone within 2 weeks, another diagnosis should be considered. In patients where steroids are problematic (for example, in diabetes), NSAIDS may also be tried (see Table 53-1). The natural history of PMR is that it is generally self-limited within several months to years. Steroids should be tapered to the lowest dose that will control the patient's symptoms.

The major concern in PMR is that approximately 15 percent of cases will develop an associated Temporal arteritis (giant cell arteritis), a serious vasculitis that can lead to blindness. Patients with PMR should always be warned about this association and told about symptoms to watch for. Temporal arteritis is discussed in Chap. 63.

Fibromyalgia

Fibromyalgia or fibrositis is a common disorder, mostly affecting young and middle-aged females. Its prevalence was found to be 2.1 and 5.7 percent in a family practice and a general internal medicine clinic, respectively.[13] The female predominance is striking; it has been reported that 80 to 90 percent of patients with fibromyalgia are women.[13] The disease is characterized by reproducible paired tender points or trigger points in the absence of arthritis. These tender points generally are accompanied by disturbed sleep or ''nonrestorative'' sleep. Fatigue often is a prominent symptom of fibromyalgia. In fact, fibromyalgia and chronic fatigue syndrome are overlapping disorders.[13] Patients also may complain of morning stiffness that can mimic that seen in rheumatoid arthritis. Often patients will have a history of irritable bowel syndrome or dysmenorrhea. Approximately 12 percent of patients with fibromyalgia will have a ''female urethral syndrome,'' defined as urinary frequency, dysuria, and suprapubic discomfort with negative urine cultures.[13] Although patients often complain of subjective swelling (especially in the hands), there is no objective evidence of swelling or inflammation on examination. Except for the characteristic tender points, the physical examination is normal. Patients have some or all of the following eight paired symmetrical tender points: 1. insertion of the nuchal muscles into the occiput; 2. upper trapezius (midportion); 3. pectoralis muscle just lateral to the second costochondral junction; 4. 2 cm below the lateral epicondyle; 5. upper gluteal area; 6. 2 cm posterior to the greater trochanter; 7. medial knee in area of anserine bursa; and 8. gastrocnemius-Achilles tendon junction.[14] Patients with fibromyalgia may present with costochondritis or an anterior chest wall syndrome. Laboratory tests (including CBC, chemistries, ESR, RF, ANA, TFTs, and CPK) and radiographs should all be normal. Treatment of fibromyalgia is often difficult. Patient education and a program to improve physical fitness are extremely important. Medications that restore sleep [such as amitriptyline (Elavil) 10–25 mg po hs or cyclobenzaprine (Flexeril) 10–20 mg po hs] are helpful.

Regional Disorders: Tendinitis and Bursitis

Tendinitis often occurs in the setting of overuse, which may be a sports-related injury or may be occupational. Areas commonly affected include the supraspinatus and bicipital tendons of the shoulder and the lateral epicondyle (tennis elbow). Supraspinatus tendinitis is suggested by a painful arc from about 70 to 100 degrees of active abduction. Bicipital tendinitis is suggested by localized tenderness over the bicipital groove and by a positive Yergason's test (pain on resisted supination). Epicondylitis is suggested by point tenderness at or near the lateral epicondyle. Treatment of these disorders is by cessation of the offending repetitive motion; local injection of corticosteroids is often effective.

Bursitis may be caused by local irritation or trauma. Septic bursitis may occur when organisms are introduced by puncture wounds or overlying cellulitis. There are numerous bursae throughout the body, but common sites for bursitis include subacromial bursitis, trochanteric bursitis, olecranon bursitis, prepatellar bursitis, and anserine bursitis (inferomedial aspect of the knee). Treatment of bursitis (in the absence of infection) is by local injection of corticosteroids. Because it is an area susceptible to trauma and introduction of infection, the olecranon bursa is a common site for septic bursitis. Septic bursitis should be treated with aspiration (repeated drainage often required) and appropriate antibiotics.

Systemic Rheumatic Diseases

Systemic Lupus Erythematosus

Systemic lupus erythematosus (SLE) is a complex disease that can involve multiple organ systems and is associated with the production of autoantibodies. The cause of SLE remains unknown; genetic, hormonal, and environmental factors have all been implicated. Estimates of prevalence of SLE have varied widely, from 4 to 250 cases per 100,000 population.[15] In the United States, the prevalence is higher among Asians and blacks than among whites or hispanics.[15] SLE is much more common in women, with a female: male ratio ranging from 8:1 to 13:1.[15]

Major clinical manifestations (Table 53-4) of SLE include rash (including malar or "butterfly" rash, photosensitivity, or discoid lesions), oral ulcers (typically painless), arthritis (often associated with morning stiffness but typically nonerosive), serositis (including pericarditis or pleurisy), renal disease, CNS disease, Raynauds phenomenon, or alopecia. Patients may also present with fatigue, fever, weight loss or other constitutional symptoms, and may have hepatosplenomegaly or lymphadenopathy. Patients with renal or CNS disease have a worse prognosis. Renal disease is generally manifested by proteinuria (often nephrotic range), active urinary sediment, and later by renal insufficiency. A variety of renal lesions may be seen (with diffuse proliferative glomerulonephritis having the worst prognosis and requiring aggressive intervention), and renal biopsy may be helpful in selected cases. Countless manifestations of CNS lupus have been described, but the most common are seizures, psychosis, and migraine-type headaches. MRI may be helpful in evaluating patients for possible CNS lupus, but the findings are nonspecific. A subset of patients may give a history

TABLE 53-4 Important Features of SLE

- Rash
    - Malar rash
    - Discoid lesions
    - Photosensitivity
- Oral ulcers
- Alopecia
- Arthritis
- Raynaud's phenomenon
- Pleuritis/pericarditis
- Renal disease
- CNS involvement

of previous thrombotic events (such as DVT, PE, or stroke) or multiple spontaneous abortions and may have an associated "lupus anticoagulant" or anticardiolipin antibody (see below).

Physical examination often will give clues to the diagnosis. Alopecia may be noted that may be diffuse or that may manifest as short broken hairs along the frontal hairline ("lupus hairs"). Discoid skin lesions generally will appear as rounded, slightly scaling lesions with a region of central atrophy; these lesions tend to scar. When discoid lesions involve the scalp, scarring can lead to permanent alopecia (other forms of alopecia are temporary and tend to fluctuate with disease activity). The malar rash typically appears on the cheeks and across the bridge of the nose, but characteristically spares the nasolabial folds. A livedo reticularis rash (a fine lacy rash) may be noted, particularly in patients with an associated anticardiolipin antibody. Peripheral edema or hypertension may signify the presence of renal disease. Oral or nasal mucosal ulceration may be found; the patient may be unaware of these lesions, which tend to be painless. Examination of the chest may reveal evidence of pericardial or pleural involvement. The arthritis of SLE generally will have less pronounced synovitis than that of rheumatoid arthritis; deformities (such as Jaccoud arthropathy), if present, generally are completely reducible. In cases of severe Raynaud's phenomenon, the hands or feet may appear dusky and cool.

Laboratory data are extremely helpful in diagnosing and managing SLE (Table 53-5). The ANA will be positive in more than 95 percent of cases of SLE, and thus is a useful screening test. The major limitation of the ANA is its lack of specificity. More specific but much less sensitive tests for SLE include anti-double stranded DNA and anti-Smith antibodies. Some patients with SLE have hypocomplementemia, with decreased C3 and/or C4 levels. The presence of hypocomplementemia and high titers of anti-ds DNA antibodies may predict the onset of renal disease and often fluctuates with disease activity; it is useful to follow serial measurements in patients with these abnormalities in order to assess disease activity and to help gauge therapy. Routine urinalysis should always be obtained at baseline and periodically in patients with SLE.

TABLE 53-5 Laboratory Findings in SLE

- Anemia
- Leukopenia
- Thrombocytopenia
- Abnormal urinalysis
- Serologies
  - ANA (>95%)
  - Anti-native (ds) DNA
  - Anti-Smith (Sm)
  - BFP VDRL

Hematologic involvement in SLE is common, and patients may have evidence of a hemolytic anemia, leukopenia (especially lymphopenia), or thrombocytopenia. Patients may also have a "false-positive" VDRL (positive VDRL with negative FTA). Patients with an associated "lupus anticoagulant" may have an elevated PTT, a positive dilute Russel viper venom time (DRVVT), a false-positive VDRL, or IgG or IgM anti-cardiolipin antibodies.

Treatment of SLE is complex and depends on the specific manifestations of the disease. Avoidance of the sun and use of sunscreens should be advised. The arthritis of SLE often is managed initially with NSAIDs (see Table 53-1). Patients who have cutaneous disease, arthritis, and serositis as their major manifestations are candidates for treatment with the antimalarial, hydroxychloroquine (Plaquenil) in dosages of 200 to 400 mg/day. Patients should be evaluated by an ophthalmologist at baseline and every 4 to 6 months while on this medication, as they may (rarely) develop retinal changes. Screening for G6PD deficiency also should be performed prior to starting hydroxychloroquine; patients with G6PD deficiency may develop hemolysis on this drug. Topical steroid preparations may be a useful adjunct in patients with severe skin disease. Systemic corticosteroids are generally used in two types of clinical settings in SLE. The first is in low doses (less than 10 mg prednisone/day) for patients with mild disease such as arthritis or mild serositis not controlled with NSAIDs or hydroxychloroquine alone. The second is in high dosages (prednisone 1 to 2 mg/kg/ per day) in patients who are severely ill with major organ involvement such as lupus cerebritis, lupus nephritis, severe autoimmune hemolytic anemia, or thrombocytopenia or systemic vasculitis.[16] In patients in whom there is any question of absorption, intravenous steroids should be used in equivalent doses. Immunosuppressive agents such as azathioprine (Imuran) and cyclophosphamide (Cytoxan) may be necessary in patients with major organ involvement who fail to respond to corticosteroids. The use of intravenous cyclophosphamide has been shown to be of significant benefit in lupus nephritis, particularly class IV or diffuse proliferative glomerulonephritis. This drug is an alkylating agent with significant toxicity, including risk of subsequent malignancy, bone marrow suppression, leukopenia and risk of serious infection, hemorrhagic cystitis, premature ovarian failure and infertility.[17] As SLE is mainly a disease of women of child-bearing age, the significant risk of infertility with Cytoxan is a serious consideration. Loss of ovarian function may also contribute to osteopenia and accelerated atherosclerotic disease; the latter especially in women on long-term corticosteroid therapy. In addition, cyclophosphamide is teratogenic; pregnancy should be ruled out before the drug is given, and adequate birth control is mandatory during its use. Azathioprine is used frequently as a steroid-sparing agent or for manifestations of SLE unresponsive to NSAIDS, hydroxychloroquine, or steroids alone. Azathioprine, although less toxic than cyclophosphamide, shares many of the same potential serious adverse effects, including bone marrow suppression, risk of serious infection, risk of subsequent malignancy, premature menopause, and infertility (much less frequent than with cyclophosphamide). In addition, patients on azathioprine may develop hepatitis.

SLE and Pregnancy

Exacerbation of SLE occurs in 30 to 50 percent of pregnancies in women with this disorder, and there is an increased risk of fetal loss in SLE patients compared with normal populations.[18] Subsequently, pregnancy in women with SLE is considered high-risk, but many women with SLE have successful pregnancies. Exacerbations of SLE during pregnancy occur in all three trimesters (in approximately equal frequency) and in the immediate postpartum period, although the rate of exacerbation during and after pregnancy has been decreasing progressively over the past 30 years, possibly due to increased use of corticosteroids or improved care.[15] Mothers with active disease at the time of pregnancy have worse pregnancy outcomes, with an increased risk of prematurity. The risk of fetal death is increased in lupus patients with renal disease.[15] A flare of lupus nephritis may be difficult to distinguish from preeclampsia in lupus patients; lupus nephritis is more likely to be associated with hypocomplementemia and/or elevated titers of anti-dsDNA antibodies.[15] Thus, patients with SLE who are contemplating pregnancy should be advised that the optimal time for pregnancy is when their disease is quiescent or well controlled (especially renal disease). In addition, screening for an associated antiphospholipid syndrome (see below) and anti-RO (SSA) antibodies should be done because of an associated risk of recurrent miscarriages[19–22] and congenital heart block, respectively. Ideally, second line or cytotoxic medications should be discontinued at least 4 months prior to conception; the lowest possible dose of corticosteroids alone should be used to control their disease prior to and during pregnancy.

SLE and Menstrual Abnormalities

A small number of patients with SLE report a monthly flare in their symptoms around the time of their menses, most commonly manifested by increased joint pain, transient facial rash, or pleuritic chest pain.[23] Some women may have menorrhagia, possibly secondary to the use of NSAIDs, thrombocytopenia, or an inhibitor of one of the clotting factors.[23] In addition, women with SLE may have irregular menses secondary to their underlying disease or to the use of corticosteroids. Premature menopause may occur in patients treated with medications such as cyclophosphamide or azathioprine.

Antiphospholipid Syndrome

The antiphospholipid syndrome (or anticardiolipin antibody syndrome) may occur in association with other rheumatic diseases (most commonly with SLE, as discussed above) or may occur in the absence of any rheumatic disease (primary antiphos-

TABLE 53-6 Features of the APL Syndrome

- Arterial or venous thrombotic events
- Recurrent fetal loss
- Livedo reticularis
- Migraine headache
- Thrombocytopenia
- Laboratory evidence of circulating anticoagulant
  ↑ PTT
  DRVVT
- BFP VDRL
- Antiphospholipid antibody

pholipid syndrome). It is characterized (Table 53-6) by recurrent venous and arterial thrombotic events (including DVT, PE, and stroke), recurrent spontaneous abortions (especially in the second trimester), and thrombocytopenia. Migraine-type headaches and a livedo reticularis rash are common. Patients may have abnormalities of phospholipid-dependent tests of coagulation, such as prolongation of the PTT or dilute Russel viper venom time (DRVVT). Sometimes this may be referred to as a ''lupus anticoagulant,'' although this is a misnomer for two reasons. First, patients don't necessarily have lupus; second, patients are paradoxically hypercoagulable *in vivo.* Patients may also have a biological false-positive test for syphilis or IgG or IgM anticardiolipin antibodies (ACL). Patients may have abnormalities in any one or any combination of these tests; it is thus useful to screen with all these tests (PTT, DRVVT, VDRL, and ACL) when this syndrome is suspected clinically. In nonpregnant patients with this syndrome and recurrent thrombotic events, life-long anticoagulation with coumadin is warranted. During pregnancy, a combination of subcutaneous heparin and low-dose aspirin may be used.

Drug-Induced Lupus

Patients taking certain medications may develop a syndrome similar to SLE. The medications most commonly implicated in drug-induced lupus include procainamide, hydralazine, INH, methyldopa, and chlorpromazine.[15] While drug-induced lupus may resemble SLE, there are several important differences. Patients with drug-induced lupus generally have arthralgias or arthritis, symptoms of pleuropericarditis, and constitutional symptoms; renal and CNS disease are distinctly uncommon. Unlike SLE, drug-induced lupus occurs with equal frequency in males and females and is rare in African Americans.[15] As in SLE, ANAs are seen in approximately 95 percent of cases of drug-induced lupus, but patients with drug-induced lupus generally do not have anti-dsDNA or anti-Smith antibodies, and serum complement levels are generally normal. Approximately 90 percent of patients with drug-induced lupus will have antihistone antibodies (but these antibodies will also be present in approximately 25 percent of cases of native SLE).[15] The treatment for drug-induced lupus is to discontinue the offending drug. Some patients will develop a positive ANA while on medication but will not have any signs of symptoms of drug-induced lupus; in these patients, it is not necessary to discontinue that medication.

Scleroderma and Crest Syndrome

Systemic sclerosis (or scleroderma) is a generalized disorder of connective tissue in which there is thickening and fibrosis of the skin associated with internal organ involvement. The etiology is unknown. It is three to four times more common in women than in men, and most commonly presents between the ages of 30 and 60.[24] Familial cases of scleroderma are rare, but it is not uncommon for patients with scleroderma to have first-degree relatives with other rheumatic disorders.[24] In addition, patients may have an ''overlap syndrome'' with features of other rheumatic diseases (especially SLE and dermatomyositis/polymyositis) in addition to features of scleroderma.

Scleroderma may be rapidly progressive, with extensive skin and internal organ involvement (diffuse form), or may be more limited, with a more indolent course. Limited scleroderma has been termed the CREST variant (prominent features are *C*alcinosis, *R*aynaud's phenomenon, *E*sophageal dysmotility, *S*clerodactyly, and *T*elangiectasias).

Patients with CREST may have stable disease for many years and tend to have involvement of the skin only of the distal extremities (up to MCPs or proximal forearms) and face. They generally do not have other major organ involvement, with the notable exception of pulmonary hypertension. There is a cooccurrence of primary biliary cirrhosis in some patients. In contrast, patients with diffuse scleroderma have widespread involvement of the skin, including the skin of the proximal as well as distal extremities, the face, and the trunk (especially the anterior chest and abdomen). Early internal organ involvement is frequent, including involvement of the GI tract, lungs, heart, and kidneys.

The first symptoms are often in the hands, with either Raynaud's phenomenon, puffiness of the hands, and/or polyarthralgias.[24] Generally, thickening of the skin of the hands will follow several weeks or months later. In limited scleroderma, Raynaud's phenomenon (episodic digital ischemia with cold exposure and reactive hyperemia with rewarming) is almost always present, and often precedes other symptoms of scleroderma by many years. In diffuse scleroderma, Raynaud's is present in only 75 percent of cases, and its absence is associated with an increased risk of renal disease.[24] Joints and tendons may be involved, and coarse, leathery friction rubs may be palpated over the flexor and extensor tendons of the fingers, distal forearms, knees, and ankles; these are found almost exclusively in patients with diffuse scleroderma.[24] Patients may have either a bland, noninflammatory myopathy characterized by fibrotic replacement of muscle or an inflammatory myositis (one of the few indications for steroids in scleroderma). Involvement of the GI tract most commonly takes the form of esophageal dysmotility, but other complications such as malabsorption, pneumatosis intestinalis (air in the wall of the intestine), or wide-mouth diverticulae can occur. Patients with scleroderma may develop bibasilar pulmonary fibrosis, which may be evident on chest radiography. Pulmonary function tests may show decreased diffusing capacity or evidence of restrictive lung disease. Pulmonary hypertension occurs more commonly in patients with limited scleroderma. Clinical evidence of cardiac involvement occurs uncommonly and may be manifested by arrhythmias or severe congestive heart failure. "Scleroderma renal crisis" is a major cause of death in patients with scleroderma and generally presents with malignant hypertension (which may be associated with hypertensive encephalopathy) associated with proteinuria, microscopic hematuria, or worsening renal function. Therapy with angiotensin converting enzyme inhibitors (such as captopril) has dramatically improved survival in these patients.

In early cases, physical examination may reveal edematous or puffy hands; discoloration characteristic of Raynaud's phenomenon may be noted in some patients. Soon after this, the skin may appear shiny and taut (generally starting on the fingers), and there is loss of the normal skin creases. Taut skin on the face may lead to decreased ability to open the mouth fully and a characteristic "pursed lip" appearance. Taut skin over the joints may lead to flexion contractures in severe cases. Telangiectasias may be noted (especially in the CREST variant), and there may be areas of hypo- or hyperpigmentation. Leathery friction rubs may be palpated over tendons as discussed above. Nailfold capillary microscopy is helpful in establishing the diagnosis, and may reveal dilated, tortuous vessels or capillary drop-out. There may be pitting or loss of digital pulp of the fingertips. Examination of the chest may reveal bibasilar crackles suggestive of pulmonary fibrosis.

More than 90 percent of patients with scleroderma will have positive ANAs.[25] Twenty to 50 percent with diffuse scleroderma will have antibodies to topoisomerase I (Scl-70), although this antibody may also be found in up to 15 percent of patients with the limited form.[24,25] More than 50 percent of patients with limited scleroderma will have anticentromere antibodies; this antibody is helpful in identifying patients with limited disease as it rarely occurs in those with diffuse scleroderma (<5 percent).[25]

Prognosis in patients with diffuse disease and early internal organ involvement is poor, but the disease course in scleroderma is extremely variable. Factors that may be associated with a worse outcome include male sex, older age, diffuse cutaneous disease, and renal, cardiac, or lung involvement.[25] Unfortunately, there is no drug or combination of drugs of proven value in treating patients with scleroderma.[25] Some success has been reported with the use of D-penicillamine, especially in patients with early diffuse disease or interstitial lung disease.[25] However, this agent is associated with significant toxicity, including bone marrow suppression, nephrotic syndrome and glomerulonephritis, pemphigus, and myasthenia gravis.[25] Treatment with corticosteroids is generally of no benefit, except in associated inflammatory conditions such as inflammatory myositis or serositis. In fact, the use of high-dose steroids has been associated with the development of renal failure and other vasoocclusive complications of the disease.[26] In scleroderma renal crisis, prompt recognition and treatment with angiotensin converting enzyme inhibitors may be lifesaving. Supportive measures are important in the overall management of patients with scleroderma. Patients with Raynaud's phenomenon should be instructed about common sense preventive measures such as keeping their hands and feet warm and smoking cessation. Calcium channel blockers such as nifedipine often are helpful in managing Raynaud's. Meticulous skin care, especially in those who develop digital ulceration or other areas of breakdown, is of extreme importance. In patients with esophageal involvement, metoclopramide may improve esophageal motility. Simple measures such as avoiding eating before bedtime and elevation of the head of the bed may minimize symptoms of esophageal reflux.

Polymyositis and Dermatomyositis

Polymyositis and dermatomyositis are inflammatory myopathies of unknown etiology. They are relatively uncommon, with an annual incidence of five cases per 1 million.[27] These disorders are more common in women than in men. Both are characterized clinically by symmetric proximal muscle weakness; dermatomyositis has the additional feature of characteristic skin lesions. The heart, lungs, and GI tract also may be involved. An increased risk of malignancy has been reported in patients with polymyositis and dermatomyositis; all patients with these diagnoses should have a comprehensive history and careful physical examination as well as routine screening procedures.

Initially, patients usually complain of symptoms referable to hip girdle weakness, such as progressive difficulty arising from a chair or climbing stairs. Subsequently, patients develop weakness of shoulder girdle muscles and complain of difficulty with activities that require raising their arms, such as combing their hair or putting heavy objects onto a high shelf. Patients with involvement of the anterior neck flexors may complain of difficulty raising the head from the pillow. Fewer than half of patients with polymyositis or dermatomyositis will complain of pain in the hip or shoulder girdle muscles;[27] weakness is generally the predominant symptom.

On physical exam, almost all patients will have symmetric proximal muscle weakness. Tenderness of these muscles may be noted in some patients. In dermatomyositis, a variety of skin lesions may be seen, including diffuse erythema or duskiness of the face and upper chest in a ''shawl'' distribution. Patients may have the classic ''heliotrope'' rash (purplish discoloration over the eyelids) and/or periorbital edema. Gottron's papules (violaceous flat papules over the dorsal surface of the interphalangeal joints of the fingers) and Gottron's sign (erythematous smooth or scaling lesions over the dorsal IP or MCP joints, elbows, knees, and medial malleoli) are the only skin findings pathognomonic of dermatomyositis.[27]

Laboratory data reveal elevated muscle enzymes, with CPK and/or aldolase being elevated in the majority of patients at some point during the course of their disease. Serum transaminases and LDH may also be abnormal. Other routine laboratory tests generally are normal. A variety of autoantibodies have been described in patients with polymyositis and dermatomyositis, including antibody to Jo-1 (antihistidyl t-RNA synthetase), which is present in 20 to 30 percent of patients with polymyositis. The presence of Jo-1 antibody has been associated with an increased incidence of interstitial lung disease.

EMG studies show characteristic findings in patients with myositis and are often helpful in establishing the diagnosis. Demonstration of inflammation on muscle biopsy confirms the diagnosis and should be performed in almost all patients with suspected myositis before starting long-term and potentially toxic therapy.

Treatment of polymyositis and dermatomyositis usually is with high-dose daily oral corticosteroids (1 to 2 mg/kg per day prednisone). High-dose steroids generally are continued until normalization of muscle enzymes, which may require several months; steroids should then be gradually tapered to the lowest dose that controls the disease. Patients who fail to respond to high-dose steroids or have unacceptable complications require the addition of an immunosuppressive agent.

Mixed Connective Tissue Disease

Mixed connective tissue disease (MCTD) occurs with a frequency similar to that of scleroderma and is a disease mostly of women, with a mean age of onset of 37 years.[28] It is characterized clinically by puffy hands, polyarthritis, Raynaud's phenomenon, and myositis. Patients often have pulmonary involvement, including pulmonary hypertension. In addition, patients often have features of other rheumatic disorders, especially SLE or systemic sclerosis (see above), and, indeed, may eventually experience transition into these disorders. Patients with MCTD generally have high-titer positive ANAs with a speckled pattern. MCTD is characterized by the presence of antibody to the extractable nuclear antigen, ribonucleoprotein, (anti-RNP) in the absence of other autoantibodies. Treatment of this syndrome depends on the specific manifestations (see treatment of SLE, systemic sclerosis, and polymyositis). In general, inflammatory manifestations such as myositis respond to treatment with corticosteroids, while scleroderma-like disease and pulmonary hypertension do not. Raynaud's phenomenon should be treated with conservative measures (such as prevention of cold exposure) and calcium channel blockers (such as nifedipine), if needed. The prognosis for patients with MCTD is generally fairly good, with the exception of patients with scleroderma-like features or pulmonary hypertension.

Sjögren's Syndrome

Sjögren's syndrome has been estimated to affect 2 to 3 million people in the United States.[29] The majority of patients with this disorder are women (>90%), with an average age of onset of 50 years.[29] Sjögren's syndrome may be primary or may be associated with other rheumatic conditions, most commonly RA, SLE, and systemic sclerosis. It is a disorder of unknown etiology in which there is lymphocytic infiltration of lacrimal and salivary glands. This leads to the clinical manifestations of keratoconjunctivitis sicca (dry eyes), xerostomia (dry mouth), and salivary gland swelling. Patients with primary Sjögren's syndrome may have extraglandular manifestations, including involvement of the lungs, kidneys, nervous system, and skin. Of importance, patients with primary Sjögren's syndrome have a significantly increased risk of developing lymphoma (approximately 40-fold) or other lymphoproliferative disorders.[30]

Patients with dry eyes often complain of a sandy or "gritty" feeling in their eyes or a "foreign body sensation." Patients may also complain of dry, red, or painful eyes. It is important to ask the patient about use of medications that may cause dry eyes, such as cold remedies, antidepressants, and some antihypertensives. In addition, the normal production of tears and saliva decreases with age, and this decrease appears to be more common in women and to intensify after menopause.[30] Patients with dry mouth may complain of frequent thirst or inability to eat dry foods (such as a saltine cracker) without a drink. There may also be a sudden increase in dental caries secondary to decreased saliva. Patients with Sjögren's syndrome also may notice parotid gland swelling, which usually is bilateral. Women with Sjögren's syndrome may also complain of vaginal dryness, sometimes associated with a burning sensation or dyspareunia. Arthralgias, myalgias, and fatigue also may be reported; hypothyroidism should always be ruled out in these cases, as it is relatively common in patients with Sjögren's syndrome.

On physical exam, dry or injected eyes may be noted. There may be decreased sublingual salivary pooling or evidence of poor dentition with accelerated dental caries. Fissuring of the tongue or corners of the mouth may be noted. Patients may also have evidence of oral candidiasis. Enlargement of the parotid glands may be apparent on palpation. A careful search for lymphadenopathy should be done in addition to a comprehensive general medical examination.

Laboratory data often reveal evidence of autoimmunity, including a positive ANA and/or RF. More specifically, patients with Sjögren's syndrome often have anti-Ro (SSA) and/or anti-La (SSB) antibodies, although these antibodies also may be seen in other rheumatic disorders, such as SLE. A mild normocytic normochromic anemia, leukopenia, or eosinophilia (about 6 percent eosinophils) may be seen in some patients, and an elevated sedimentation rate is common.[29] Serum electrolytes and urinalysis may reveal evidence of renal tubular acidosis. In addition to routine laboratory screening, serum protein electrophoresis and immunoelectrophoresis should be performed to look for evidence of a monoclonal protein. Quantitative immunoglobulins should be performed at baseline and periodically; a sudden change in immunoglobulin levels may indicate a transformation to lymphoma.

A Schirmer's test should be performed to provide more objective evidence of dry eyes. In this simple test the examiner places the end of a small standardized sterile strip of filter paper under the patient's lower eyelids. The patient is asked to close her eyes, and the Schirmer's paper is left in place for 5 min. The amount of moisture on the paper after this time is recorded; the patient is considered to have dry eyes if less than 8 mm of the paper is wet in 5 min. Additionally, patients should have a slit lamp exam by an ophthalmologist with staining with rose bengal dye to demonstrate keratoconjunctivitis sicca.

Objective evidence of dry mouth can be obtained by salivary flow studies or salivary scintigraphy. In addition, minor salivary gland biopsy (lip biopsy) will demonstrate lymphocytic infiltration and help establish the diagnosis.

Treatment of Sjögren's syndrome is mostly symptomatic. Artificial tears (such as Tearisol, Liquifilm, or 0.5% methylcellulose) are helpful in patients with dry eyes.[29] Patients should be counseled on the need for fastidious dental care. Special toothpastes and oral preparations are available, although xerostomia is more difficult to treat. Oral candidiasis should be treated with topical preparations such as clotrimazole or nystatin.[30] Hydroxychloroquine (Plaquenil) has been used to treat the arthralgias, myalgias, and fatigue that may be associated with Sjögren's syndrome. Steroids generally are not used in the management of Sjögren's syndrome, except in life-threatening vasculitis, hemolytic anemia, and pleuropericarditis resistant to nonsteroid anti-inflammatory drugs.[30]

Vasculitic Syndromes

The vasculitic syndromes, a group of disorders whose main pathologic feature is inflammation of the blood vessels, are generally classified by their dominant clinical and pathologic features, including the size of the vessels involved. Recent clinical use of the ANCA (antineutrophil cytoplasmic antibody) has improved our ability to identify and classify patients with these syndromes. Unlike most other rheumatic diseases, most of the vasculitic syndromes are more common in men. The cause of vasculitis is not known in most cases, but some cases have been associated with such infections as hepatitis B and HIV. Many clinical entities can mimic systemic vasculitis, including atrial myxoma, septicemia (especially gonococcemia, meningococcemia, and Rocky Mountain spotted fever), endocarditis, Lyme disease, and the multiple cholesterol emboli syndrome.[31] Hypersensitivity vasculitis is a fairly common disorder and will be discussed in some detail. Other vasculitic syndromes are summarized in Table 53-7.

Small Vessel Leukocytoclastic Vasculitis

Leukocytoclastic vasculitis is a pathologic diagnosis that describes infiltration of small vessel walls (especially postcapillary venules) with PMNs and subsequent fragmentation of the PMNs and destruction of the vessel wall.[31] It is found on biopsy of involved tissue in syndromes such as hypersensitivity vasculitis, Henoch-Schönlein purpura (primarily in children), mixed cryoglobulinemia, and urticarial vasculitis.[31] In all these disorders, the skin manifes-

TABLE 53-7 Vasculitic Syndromes

Syndrome	Key Clinical Findings	Laboratory Findings
Large and medium vessel		
Temporal arteritis	Age > 50 Association with PMR Headache, visual changes, fever, jaw claudication Tender TA with ↓ pulsation	↑↑ ESR ↑ globulin ↑ Alk phos. Anemia
Takayasu arteritis	Young Asian women Claudication; UE > LE Absent / unequal pulses or BP	↑ ESR Anemia Leukocytosis
Small-medium vessel		
Polyarteritis (PAN)	Multisystem including skin, joints, GI tract, kidney, nervous system	Hypocomplementemia Hepatitis B SAg p-ANCA (not specific)
Wegener's granulomatosis	Upper airway inflammation Pulmonary involvement Renal involvement	c-ANCA (specific)
Churg-Strauss angiitis	Multisystem including lung, skin, joints History of asthma and atopy	Eosinophilia ↑ IgE p-ANCA (not specific)

tations (palpable purpura) usually are the most prominent clinical feature.

Hypersensitivity Vasculitis Hypersensitivity vasculitis is a fairly common condition that may develop after exposure to various drugs or infectious agents. It may occur following exposure to a number of bacterial, parasitic, or viral agents. Although drug-induced hypersensitivity vasculitis most commonly occurs within the first few days of treatment, it may occur at any time after the start of a medication and is not time- or dose-dependent.[31] The most commonly implicated medications are penicillin or its derivatives and sulfa drugs.[31] The key clinical finding in this disorder is "palpable purpura." These slightly raised purpuric lesions do not blanch with pressure and are not related to thrombocytopenia. The lesions occur most commonly on the lower extremities or on dependent areas in bedridden patients. Individual lesions usually are fairly small, but may appear larger in areas where multiple lesions coalesce. They generally resolve in 1 to 4 weeks (sometimes leaving hyperpigmented areas or atrophic scars), but recurrent crops of skin lesions often occur.[31] Biopsy of these lesions will show leukocytoclastic vasculitis (see above). In addition to the skin manifestations, patients with hypersensitivity vasculitis commonly develop fever and other constitutional symptoms and arthralgias or, occasionally, arthritis. Patients may also develop renal involvement (proteinuria, hematuria), GI involvement (abdominal pain, GI bleeding), pulmonary involvement (nodular or diffuse infiltrates, pleural effusion), or neurologic involvement [headache, diplopia, organic brain syndrome (OBS) rarely].[31] Treatment of hypersensitivity vasculitis should start with a search for a possible inciting agent or medication. All suspect or nonessential medications should be discontinued. In mild cases, no further treatment is necessary. In more severe cases or in patients with internal organ involvement, systemic corticosteroids usually are needed. Steroid dosage should be individualized depending on the severity and extent of involvement (prednisone, 20 to 60 mg/day or equivalent) and should be tapered to the lowest effective dose once symptoms are controlled.

Behçet's Disease

Behçet's disease occurs primarily in young adults (age 25 to 35) and is slightly more common in women.[32] The disease is more prevalent and more severe in Japan and the eastern Mediterranean countries.[31] The cardinal manifestations of Behçet's disease include recurrent oral and genital ulcerations, ocular lesions, and cutaneous lesions. Oral aphthous ulcers usually are the initial manifestations and are present in almost all patients. They are most common on the lips, tongue, buccal mucosa, palate, and pharynx.[31] They are typically painful and appear as rounded or oval ulcerations with whitish or yellowish pseudomembranes and well-demarcated erythematous borders.[32] The lesions may be multiple and generally heal without scarring in 1 to 3 weeks.[31] Genital ulcers are similar in appearance and also painful, but tend to recur less frequently. Women with Behçet's disease may have involvement of the vulva, perianal area, cervix, or vaginal mucosa. Recurrent anterior and posterior uveitis or retinal vasculitis may lead to blindness. The skin manifestations include erythema nodosum-like lesions, papules, pustules, folliculitis, ulcers, and cutaneous pathergy (formation of a pustule at the site of a sterile needle puncture 24 to 48 h later).[31] In addition to these features, patients may also have arthritis, GI lesions (ulcerations), vascular lesions (major vessel occlusion or aneurysm, thrombophlebitis), and CNS lesions (cerebral vasculitis, aseptic meningitis).[31] Laboratory tests in this disorder are nonspecific; acute phase reactants may be elevated in active disease, but may be normal in uveal disease.[31] Biopsy of lesions may reveal vasculitis (especially skin or vulva ulcerations). In patients with active CNS disease, CSF may show elevated protein and a mononuclear pleocytosis; MRI of the brain may show areas of increased signal in the periventricular white matter, brain stem, and cerebellum.[31] Treatment of Behçet's disease with systemic corticosteroid may help some of the skin and joint inflammation but is ineffective in controlling ocular or CNS manifestations. Cytotoxic agents, particularly chlorambucil and cyclophosphamide, are more effective.[31]

References and Selected Readings

1. Mankin HJ: Clinical features of osteoarthritis, in Kelly WN, Harris ED Jr, Ruddy S, Sledge CB (eds): *Textbook of Rheumatology,* 4th ed. Philadelphia: WB Saunders, pp 1374–1384, 1993.
2. Brandt K: Management of osteoarthritis, in Kelly WN, Harris ED Jr, Ruddy S, Sledge CB (eds): *Textbook of Rheumatology,* 4th ed. Philadelphia: WB Saunders, pp 1385–1399, 1993.
3. Lipson SJ: Low back pain, in Kelly WN, Harris ED Jr, Ruddy S, Sledge CB (eds): *Textbook of Rheumatology,* 4th ed. Philadelphia: WB Saunders, pp 441–458, 1993.
4. Harris ED Jr: Clinical features of rheumatoid arthritis, in Kelly WN, Harris ED Jr, Ruddy S, Sledge CB (eds): *Textbook of Rheumatology,* 4th ed. Philadelphia: WB Saunders, pp 874–911, 1993.
5. Klipple GL, Cecere FA: Rheumatoid arthritis and pregnancy. *Rheum Dis Clin North Am* 15 (No. 2):213–239, 1989.
6. Calin A: Ankylosing spondylitis and the spondyloarthropathies, in Schumacher HR Jr (ed): *Primer on the Rheumatic Diseases,* 9th ed. Atlanta: Arthritis Foundation, pp 142–147, 1988.
7. Fan PT, Yu DTY: Reiter's syndrome, in Schumacher HR Jr (ed): *Primer on the Rheumatic Diseases,* 10th ed. Atlanta: Arthritis Foundation, pp 158–161, 1993.
8. Tate G, Schumacher HR Jr: Gout: Clinical features, in Schumacher HR Jr (ed): *Primer on the Rheumatic Diseases,* 9th ed. Atlanta: Arthritis Foundation, pp 198–202, 1988.
9. Moskowitz RW: Diseases associated with the deposition of calcium pyrophosphate or hydroxyapatite, in Kelly WN, Harris ED Jr, Ruddy S, Sledge CB (eds): *Textbook of Rheumatology,* 4th ed. Philadelphia: WB Saunders, pp. 1337–1354, 1993.
10. Steere AC: Lyme disease, in Kelly WN, Harris ED Jr, Ruddy S, Sledge CB (eds): *Textbook of Rheumatology,* 4th ed. Philadelphia: WB Saunders, pp 1484–1493, 1993.
11. Steere AC: Lyme disease, in Schumacher HR Jr (ed): *Primer on the Rheumatic Diseases,* 9th ed. Atlanta: Arthritis Foundation, pp 188–190, 1988.
12. Hunder GG: Polymyalgia rheumatica and temporal (giant cell) arteritis, in Schumacher HR Jr (ed): *Primer on the Rheumatic Diseases,* 9th ed. Atlanta: Arthritis Foundation, pp 134–135, 1988.
13. Yunus MB, Masi AT: Fibromyalgia, restless legs syndrome, periodic limb movement disorder, and psychogenic pain, in McCarty DJ, Koopman WJ (eds): *Arthritis and Allied Conditions,* 12th ed. Philadelphia: Lea & Febiger, pp 1383–1405, 1993.
14. Bennett RM: The fibrositis-fibromyalgia syndrome, in Schumacher HR Jr (ed): *Primer on the Rheumatic Diseases,* 9th ed. Atlanta: Arthritis Foundation, pp 227–230, 1988.
15. Schur PH: Clinical features of SLE, in Kelly WN, Harris ED Jr, Ruddy S, Sledge CB (eds): *Textbook of Rheumatology,* 4th ed. Philadelphia: WB Saunders, pp 1017–1042, 1993.
16. Quismorio FP Jr: Systemic corticosteroid therapy in systemic lupus erythematosus, in Wallace DJ, Hahn BH (eds): *Dubois' Lupus Erythematosus,* 4th ed. Philadelphia: Lea & Febiger, pp 574–587, 1993.
17. Wallace DJ: Cytotoxic drugs, in Wallace DJ, Hahn BH

(eds): *Dubois' Lupus Erythematosus,* 4th ed. Philadelphia: Lea & Febiger, pp 588–599, 1993.

18. Mintz G, Rodriguez-Alvarez E: Systemic lupus erythematosus. *Rheum Dis Clin North Am* 15 (No. 2):pp 255–274, 1989.
19. Pattison NS, McKay, EJ, Liggins, GC, Lubbe WF: Anticardiolipin antibodies: Their presence as a marker for lupus anticoagulant in pregnancy. *NZ Med J* 100:61, 1987.
20. Hahn BH: Management of systemic lupus erythematosus, in Kelly WN, Harris ED Jr, Ruddy S, Sledge CB (eds): *Textbook of Rheumatology,* 4th ed. Philadelphia: WB Saunders, pp 1043–1056, 1993.
21. Dudley DJ, Branch DW: Antiphospholipid syndrome—a model for autoimmune pregnancy loss. *Infertil Reprod Med Clin North Am* 2 (No. 1):158, 149–164, 1991.
22. Asherson RA, Cervera R: Anticardiolipin antibodies, chronic biologic false-positive tests for syphilis and other antiphospholipid antibodies, in Wallace DJ and Hahn BH (eds): *Dubois' Lupus Erythematosus,* 4th ed. Philadelphia: Lea & Febiger, pp 233–245, 1993.
23. Rothfield NF: Systemic lupus erythematosus: Clinical aspects and treatment, in McCarty DJ, Koopman WJ (eds): *Arthritis and Allied Conditions,* 12th ed. Philadelphia: Lea & Febiger, pp 1155–1177, 1993.
24. Medsger TA Jr: Systemic sclerosis and localized scleroderma, in Schumacher HR Jr (ed): *Primer on the Rheumatic Diseases,* 9th ed. Atlanta: Arthritis Foundation, pp 111–116, 1988.
25. Medsger TA Jr: Systemic sclerosis (scleroderma), localized forms of scleroderma, and calcinosis, in McCarty DJ, Koopman WJ (eds): *Arthritis and Allied Conditions,* 12th ed. Philadelphia: Lea & Febiger, pp 1253–1292, 1993.
26. Seibold JR: Scleroderma, in Kelly WN, Harris ED Jr, Ruddy S, Sledge CB (eds): *Textbook of Rheumatology,* 4th ed. Philadelphia: WB Saunders, pp 1113–1143, 1993.
27. Cronin ME, Miller FW, Plotz PH: Polymyositis and dermatomyositis, in Schumacher HR Jr (ed): *Primer on the Rheumatic Diseases,* 9th ed. Atlanta: Arthritis Foundation, pp 120–123, 1988.
28. Sharp GC, Singsen BH: Mixed connective tissue disease, in McCarty DJ, Koopman WJ (eds): *Arthritis and Allied Conditions,* 12th ed. Philadelphia: Lea & Febiger, pp 1213–1224, 1993.
29. Talal N: Sjögren's syndrome and connective tissue diseases associated with other immunologic disorders, in McCarty DJ, Koopman WJ (eds): *Arthritis and Allied Conditions,* 12th ed. Philadelphia: Lea & Febiger, pp 1343–1356, 1993.
30. Fox RI, Kang HI: Sjögren's syndrome, in Kelly, WN, Harris ED Jr, Ruddy S, Sledge CB (eds): *Textbook of Rheumatology,* 4th ed. Philadelphia: WB Saunders, pp 931–942, 1993.
31. Conn DL, Hunder GG, O'Duffy JD: Vasculitis and related disorders, in Kelly WN, Harris ED Jr, Ruddy S, Sledge CB (eds): *Textbook of Rheumatology,* 4th ed. Philadelphia: WB Saunders, pp 1077–1102, 1993.
32. Choi SJ: Behçet's syndrome, in Schumacher HR Jr (ed): *Primer on the Rheumatic Diseases,* 9th ed. Atlanta: Arthritis Foundation, pp 192–193, 1993.

54 Allergy and Immunology

John E. Rooney
Eric S. Applebaum
Vincent R. Bonagura

Allergic Rhinoconjunctivitis

History

Symptoms characteristic of allergic rhinoconjunctivitis are listed in Table 54-1. Ocular and nasal symptoms may be present simultaneously or in isolation. The disease exists in two forms: perennial, which is due to indoor substances such as house dust, mites, and animal dander; and seasonal (''hay fever'') due to pollens. Ascertaining the time course of symptom exacerbations is therefore essential (Table 54-2). A history of fever, myalgia, or green nasal discharge (as opposed to clear) suggests infection. A complete list of over-the-counter, prescription, and illicit drug use should be obtained. Frequently, patients with allergic rhinoconjunctivitis have concomitant eczema or asthma and a family history of allergies.

Physical Exam

The nasal mucosa is pale or cyanotic in up to 60 percent of patients with allergic rhinitis. Nasal polyps, which are white and firm, should be distinguished from swollen turbinates, which are pink and boggy. Examination of the eyes may reveal injection of the conjunctivae and chemosis (swelling of the conjunctival tissue around the cornea).

Differential Diagnosis

Symptoms of perennial allergic rhinoconjunctivitis are present for more than nine months per year,

TABLE 54-1 Allergic Rhinoconjunctivitis: History

Symptoms
Sneezing
Rhinorrhea or ocular discharge
Nasal or ocular pruritus or burning
Nasal congestion
Postnasal drip: nocturnal cough, throat-clearing

Time Course of Symptoms (season, diurnal pattern)

Symptom Triggers
Irritants: e.g., smoke, perfume, pollution, cleaning fluids
Emotion
Exercise
Food
Specific allergens

Environmental Aeroallergens
Pollens: e.g., seasonal symptoms, cut grass, raking leaves
House dust mites: e.g., curtains, carpet, bedding
Feathers: e.g., pillows, comforters
Pets: e.g., cat, dog, birds
Molds: e.g., basements, bathrooms, humidifiers, plants

Current Medications

Family History

TABLE 54-2 Allergy Seasons

Perennial
House dust mites
Indoor molds
Pets
Cockroaches
Pyrethrum (insecticide)
Feathers (pillows, comforters)

Seasonal
Weeds
- Mid-August through first frost (northeastern and northwestern U.S.)
- August through October (southern U.S.)
- July through October (Central Plains, California)

Trees
- March through June (eastern U.S.)
- January through June (southern and northwestern U.S.)
- December through May (Central Plains, southwestern U.S.)
- January through May (California)

Grasses
- Mid-May through mid-July (northeastern U.S.)
- March through September (southern U.S.)
- March through November (California)
- May through August (northwestern U.S.)

Molds
- Autumn, spring, summer (warm and temperate climates)

whereas symptoms of seasonal rhinoconjunctivitis follow the allergy seasons outlined in Table 54-2. There are, in addition, several forms of nonallergic rhinitis.

Rhinitis medicamentosa is caused by prolonged use of α-adrenergic nasal decongestants (e.g., oxymetazoline or phenylephrine). After as little as five days of regular use, rebound nasal congestion can occur upon withdrawal of the medication, and tachyphylaxis to the medication may develop. The nasal mucosa appears dark red and dry with small areas of bleeding. It is treated by weaning the patient from the medication over one week and administering topical steroids to reduce inflammation. Regular intranasal administration of cocaine also produces this syndrome.

Various prescription medications may cause rhinitis. Aspirin, nonsteroidal anti-inflammatory drugs, and a variety of antihypertensives are most commonly responsible. Hydralazine, prazosin, hydrochlorothiazide, nadolol, labetalol, clonidine, guanabenz, and reserpine have been associated with rhinitis.

Patients with nonallergic rhinitis with eosinophilia syndrome (NARES) have perennial symptoms and eosinophilia in the nasal secretions, but do not have specific allergic triggers. NARES is associated with chronic sinusitis and nasal polyps in up to two-thirds of patients.

Although food allergy per se is rarely a cause of rhinitis, gustatory rhinitis is manifested as copious clear nasal discharge during eating, particularly spicy foods. It is due to a vagal reflex rather than an allergic mechanism and may be treated with topical anticholinergics (e.g., ipratropium bromide, two sprays per nostril, qid prn).

Rhinitis of pregnancy is a common syndrome usually beginning after the first trimester and resolving spontaneously after delivery. Hormonal changes are responsible for producing nasal congestion and hypersecretion. Medical treatment is generally of limited benefit.

Sinusitis is suggested by fever, green nasal discharge, headache, nocturnal cough, maxillary teeth pain when chewing, persistent halitosis, postnasal drip, and tenderness on exam. Not all symptoms need be present at one time. Three weeks of an appropriate antibiotic (e.g., trimethoprim-sulfamethoxazole, amoxicillin-clavulanate, clarlthromycin), decongestants, and topical anti-inflammatory agents are indicated. A sinus CT scan, including coronal views, is indicated for recurrent or persistent sinusitis or when nasal polyps are suspected.

Laboratory Evaluation

A smear of nasal secretions should be obtained and examined for eosinophils under light microscopy with Wright's stain. Eosinophils are often present in abundance in allergic rhinoconjunctivitis and NARES. Total serum IgE elevation supports the diagnosis of allergic rhinoconjunctivitis. Although in vitro assessment of IgE antibody to specific allergens is readily available through the radioallergosorbent test (RAST), this method is less sensitive than allergic skin testing.

Treatment

Environmental control is an essential component of the treatment of allergic rhinoconjunctivitis. Pollens may be avoided by remaining indoors in an air-conditioned building and by driving in an air-conditioned automobile with the windows closed. Outdoor activities should be limited during the patient's allergy season. House-dust mite exposure is reduced by replacing curtains with window shades and by either removing carpeting from the home or vacuuming weekly with the patient out of the room. Vinyl dust covers may be used to cover pillows and mattresses. Such encasement of bedding permits regular cleaning and traps dust mites within the mattress. Washing bedding in hot water (130°F) for one hour also kills dust mites. Pets, especially cats, should be removed from the home. Mold may be reduced by thorough cleaning of warm, humid areas such as bathrooms and by reducing humidity in the home.

The mainstay of medical treatment for allergic rhinoconjunctivitis is H_1-receptor antagonists (antihistamines). They relieve sneezing, itching, and rhinorrhea, but not nasal congestion. Three nonsedating antihistamines are currently available in the United States; loratadine (Claritin, 10 mg po qd); terfenadine (Seldane, 60 mg po bid); and astemizole (Hismanal, 10 mg po qd). Astemizole has a longer onset of action (days) and a longer half-life, making it less suitable as a "prn" medication.

Cases refractory to environmental control and as-needed antihistamines may be treated with topical anti-inflammatory drugs. Cromolyn sodium (e.g., Nasalcrom) is safe and relieves symptoms of sneezing, itching, and rhinorrhea, but must be used every 3 to 4 h. Topical steroids may be used once or twice daily; these include beclomethasone (Beconase), flunisolide (Nasalide), or triamcinolone (Nasacort). Onset of action for both cromolyn and intranasal steroids is within several days, with peak effect obtained only after weeks of regular use. Thus, these medications must be used regularly rather than as needed.

Decongestants are α-adrenergic agonists and are available as oral and topical preparations. Oral forms include pseudoephedrine (Sudafed), phenylpropanolamine (Entex, Naldecon, Triaminic), and phenylephrine (Rynatan). They may be contraindicated in patients with hypertension or glaucoma, or in those taking monoamine oxidase inhibitors. Topical decongestants such as phenylephrine (Neo-Synephrine) and oxymetazoline (Afrin) should be used cautiously and for no longer than 3 days to prevent rhinitis medicamentosa. Intranasal saline sprays (e.g., Ocean, NaSal), by keeping the mucosa moist, may provide safe symptomatic relief.

Immunotherapy is the administration of specific allergens to individuals with documented sensitivity in whom medical therapy is inadequate or intolerable. While not a cure for allergic rhinitis, it provides significant relief in over 85 percent of patients. Patients with a history suggestive of allergic triggers and symptoms refractory to simple treatment should be referred to an allergist for further evaluation.

Follow-up should be obtained within one month after the onset of new medication to assess efficacy of treatment and side effects.

Asthma

History

Classic symptoms of asthma include wheezing, coughing, and shortness of breath. Exacerbations may be triggered by the allergens shown in Tables 54-1 and 54-2, by cold air, or by exercise. Symptoms may be seasonal or perennial. The patient may have coexisting allergic rhinoconjunctivitis or eczema or a family history of allergic disease.

Physical Exam

Wheezing, prolonged expiration time, and diminished air movement are characteristic of acute asthma but may be absent in chronic stable disease. Intercostal or supraclavicular retractions with tachypnea suggest an acute exacerbation requiring emergency treatment. Signs of allergic rhinitis or conjunctivitis may coexist.

Differential Diagnosis

Extrinsic asthma is worsened by a specific, IgE-producing allergen, whereas intrinsic asthma is not. In reality, these two entities most often overlap. A brief differential diagnosis of wheezing is presented in Table 54-3.

TABLE 54-3 Brief Differential Diagnosis of Wheezing

α-1 Antitrypsin deficiency
Allergic bronchopulmonary aspergillosis (ABPA)
Asthma
Chronic obstructive pulmonary disease (COPD)
Bronchiectasis
Chronic bronchitis
Emphysema
Chronic sinusitis
Congestive heart failure
Cystic fibrosis
Gastroesophageal reflux
Interstitial lung disease
Primary ciliary dyskinesia
Pulmonary embolism
Respiratory infections
Bronchiolitis
Bronchitis
Pneumonia
Upper airway obstruction
Foreign body
Laryngeal edema

Laboratory Evaluation

Pulmonary function testing reveals obstructive disease [normal to low forced vital capacity (FVC), low forced expiratory volume (FEV_1)] and diminished FEF_{25-75} indicating air trapping and small airway obstruction. These abnormalities may be elicited by cold air provocation or by exercise. Improvement usually is seen after administration of a bronchodilator.

Asthmatic patients should be given a peak flow meter, which records peak expiratory flow rate. A patient's expected peak flow may be extrapolated based on sex, age, and height. A "personal best" peak flow should also be recorded during a symptom-free interval. The patient's peak flow during an exacerbation can therefore be used to gauge the severity of that exacerbation. A value of 80 percent or greater of the personal best indicates that emergency treatment is not required; 60 to 80 percent of personal best indicates a moderate exacerbation requiring immediate home treatment; below 60 percent personal best warrants immediate emergency room evaluation if not rapidly improved with home or office treatment.

Severe asthmatics should be screened for cystic fibrosis with a sweat test. RAST or skin testing for specific allergens implicated by the patient's history may be useful in identifying allergic triggers. Markedly elevated serum IgE and peripheral eosinophilia may suggest allergic bronchopulmonary aspergillosis (ABPA). These patients should be referred to an allergist for further evaluation.

Treatment

Treatment of asthma begins with an inhaled $\beta 2$-agonist bronchodilator (e.g., albuterol) used as needed. Aerosolized bronchodilators are far more effective and have fewer side effects than the same medication given orally. Using a spacer device, such as the Aerochamber or InspirEase, may aid in drug delivery. β2-agonists are best used as needed rather than as part of a set regimen.

If symptoms are not controlled adequately with a bronchodilator as needed, an anti-inflammatory agent such as inhaled cromolyn or an inhaled corticosteroid is added. Either of these medications must be used regularly, as a therapeutic effect may not be observed until the second to fourth week of treatment. Cromolyn (Intal) has fewer side effects than steroids and is deliverable via a home nebulizer for those unable to use a metered dose inhaler. Nedocromil (Tilade) is a new anti-inflammatory drug with efficacy similar to cromolyn; it is delivered by metered dose inhaler. Unlike cromolyn, nedocromil given together with aerosolized steroids may have an additive effect. Aerosolized steroids in common use include triamcinolone (Azmacort) flunisolide (Aerobid), and beclomethasone (Beclovent). Any inhaled steroid should be used with a spacing device to reduce oral deposition and susceptibility to thrush.

Theophylline may be added to control symptoms in moderate asthma. While its efficacy in the in-hospital treatment of acute asthma exacerbations is controversial, it is clearly effective in suppressing the symptoms of chronic disease. Sustained release theophylline preparations (e.g., Slo-bid, Theo-Dur) may be useful in controlling nocturnal and early morning symptoms when given at bedtime. Once-daily preparations (e.g., Uniphyl) are available, but generally have not been shown to be effective in once-daily dosing. Average initial adult dosage is 300 mg bid of a long-acting preparation such as Theo-Dur. Serum theophylline level must be monitored initially until a therapeutic dose is established (generally serum concentration 10 to 20 μg/ml) and then checked every six months. Many patients, however, achieve therapeutic benefits with serum concentrations below 10 μg/ml. Theophylline clearance may be decreased and dosage reduction required in patients with heart failure or liver disease or in those taking certain medications (e.g., cimetidine, erythromycin, ciprofloxacin). Since different theophylline preparations differ widely in their bioavailability and rate of release into serum, generic substitution should not be given without the knowledge of the physician. Signs and symptoms of theophylline toxicity include nausea, vomiting, agitation, tachycardia, seizures, and arrhythmias.

Severe asthmatics may require treatment with oral corticosteroids; for example, prednisone or methylprednisolone (Medrol). Side effects can be minimized by giving steroids every other day. A one-week course of prednisone or methylprednisolone (40 mg per day) during an asthma exacerbation may lead to rapid symptom improvement. Such a brief course of therapy causes few side effects and little adrenal suppression. Methylprednisolone has fewer mineralocorticoid side effects than does prednisone. Any patient requiring more than six courses per year of oral steroids should be considered for chronic steroid therapy.

Acute asthma exacerbations may be treated with a nebulized β2-agonist (e.g., albuterol, 2.5 mg in 3 ml normal saline) or epinephrine (0.3 mg or 0.3 ml of a 1:1000 solution subcutaneously). Patients requiring treatments more frequently than every four hours should be referred to an emergency department. Although steroids are frequently prescribed during an acute exacerbation, onset of action takes several hours.

Immunotherapy also is effective in limiting the symptoms of extrinsic asthma. Patients with moderate or severe asthma and those having suspected allergic triggers should be referred to an allergist for further evaluation.

Routine follow-up of asthmatic patients should occur every three to four months—more frequently for those with severe disease. Ideally, an office visit should be scheduled at the beginning of a patient's "bad season" to assess the need for further therapy.

Treatment in Pregnancy

During pregnancy, one-third of asthmatic patients worsen, one-third improve, and one-third remain unchanged. Peak asthma severity occurs between 29 and 36 weeks' gestation. Patients experience a similar pattern of change in their asthma with each pregnancy.

Effective asthma management is essential to prevent fetal hypoxia. Albuterol, pirbuterol (Maxair), theophylline, inhaled and oral steroids are pregnancy category C; cromolyn and nedocromil are category B. Mild asthmatics are best treated with inhaled β-agonists used as needed. Terbutaline (Brethaire) is the inhaled β-agonist of choice in pregnancy. If the patient requires daily treatment or has poor response to treatment, cromolyn or an inhaled steroid is added. Beclomethasone (Beclovent) is the inhaled steroid of choice in pregnancy. More severe asthmatics and those with acute exacerbations may be treated with oral prednisone. Systemic corticosteroids have not been associated with fetal malformation; however, long-term use may cause decreased birth weight and increased incidence of premature delivery. Theophylline may be used safely if serum concentrations are monitored carefully to remain in therapeutic range; however, inhaled agents are preferred. α-Adrenergic agents may be administered during an acute exacerbation; however, other agents should be used first because of the possibility of uterine vasoconstriction. Terbutaline (0.25 mg sc) is preferred over epinephrine. Nonpharmacologic intervention such as environmental control (especially smoke avoidance) and allergen avoidance is crucial. Immunotherapy may be safely continued, but is not initiated during pregnancy.

Drug Allergy

History

Drug allergies may be divided into three reactions: immediate (occurring in <1 h after drug administration); accelerated (1 to 72 h); and delayed (>72 h). Examples are anaphylaxis (immediate), rashes (accelerated), and serum sickness (delayed). Table 54-4 outlines a brief directed history. In general, drug allergies are not manifested within a week of the patient's first exposure to a drug. Furthermore, while drug allergy may develop after months of asymptomatic chronic use of a drug, this is unlikely. Allergy to shellfish does not predispose one to allergy to radiographic contrast material; this is a common misconception. Allergy to multiple antibiotics can be familial.

TABLE 54-4 Drug Allergy: History

Symptoms
Rash
Wheezing
Arthralgia
Respiratory distress
Pruritus
Face/tongue swelling
Trouble swallowing
Lip/mouth pruritus
Cough
Fever
Hives
Time course of symptom onset and resolution
Location of eruption
Medication history
All medication taken in past month
Temporal relation between medication and reaction
New medications
Topical agents
Over the counter medications
Latex exposure
Past history of allergy
Type of allergic reaction
Known allergies
Past medical history
Thyroid disease
Collagen vascular disease
Malignancy
Contact dermatitis
Family history of
Drug allergy
Food allergy
Allergic rhinoconjunctivitis
Asthma or autoimmune disease

Physical Exam

Urticaria, anaphylaxis, or angioedema may occur acutely. Urticaria is raised, erythematous, and pruritic; it may have areas of central clearing. Bronchospasm and hypotension may be seen in anaphylaxis. Angioedema is characterized by swelling, usually involving the perioral and periorbital regions, tongue, extremities, or genitalia. It generally is not pruritic, although patients may report a burning sensation. Rashes occur in an accelerated reaction, and usually are hives or a pruritic maculopapular exanthem. Classic signs of serum sickness, a delayed reaction, include pruritic rash, fever, polyarticular arthritis, and lymphadenopathy.

Differential Diagnosis

Angioedema and urticaria also may be associated with occult malignancy, collagen vascular disease, hypothyroidism, hyperthyroidism, infection, physical stimulation (e.g., cold, sunlight, pressure), or food allergy. Certain medications, such as vancomycin and opiate analgesics, cause a nonspecific histamine release that can mimic an allergic reaction.

Patients demonstrating allergic reactions during surgery in the hospital, or during physician contacts may have allergy to latex. They may have similar reactions when exposed to balloons, condoms, latex gloves, or certain foods (e.g., avocado, bananas, chestnuts, figs).

Laboratory Evaluation

Skin testing will detect only immediate IgE medicated hypersensitivity reactions and is not useful for predicting reactions such as fever or serum sickness. Testing is practical and reliable for penicillin, insulin, streptokinase, latex, and other large-protein antigens.

A screen for nonallergic causes of urticaria and angioedema includes erythrocyte sedimentation rate, thyroid function tests, C4 level (the fourth component of complement), and complete chemistry profile.

Treatment

Most drug reactions resolve within one week after discontinuation of the drug. Symptoms may be relieved with an antihistamine, and in severe cases, systemic steroids. Treatment of anaphylaxis is discussed separately. Concomitant use of β-blockers increases the severity of systemic allergic reactions and makes patients more refractory to treatment. β-blockers should be discontinued and another agent substituted in any patient having a systemic allergic reaction.

A protocol has been established to pretreat patients with anaphylactoid reactions to radiographic contrast who must undergo contrast studies. It involves administration of prednisone (50 mg po given 13, 7, and 1 h prior), diphenhydramine (50 mg IV or po 1 h prior), and ephedrine (25 mg if not contraindicated). Nonionic contrast should be used.

In cases where a life-threatening disease exists, treatable only by a medication to which the patient is allergic, desensitization may be possible. This is performed by an allergist in the hospital setting.

Food Allergy

History

Manifestations of food allergy include eczema, urticaria, angioedema, and anaphylaxis. Less commonly, there may be gastrointestinal manifestations, such as abdominal pain, nausea, vomiting and diarrhea, or respiratory manifestations such as bronchospasm. A reaction generally occurs within two hours of ingestion. Symptoms occurring more than 48 h after ingestion are unlikely to be due to food allergy. The most common food allergens in adults are peanuts, tree nuts, fish, and shellfish. The type of allergic reaction to a particular food is usually consistent; the same food elicits the same kind of reaction with each exposure.

The history should include the type and severity of symptoms, the timing of symptoms in relation to food ingestion, the quantity of food ingested, and the relationship of symptoms to exercise. The patient should complete a food diary for the 24 h prior to the reaction. Ascertain any prior history of food allergy or effort to eliminate certain foods from the diet.

Physical Exam

The primary role of the physical exam is to rule out other disorders, such as inflammatory bowel disease, that may be causing gastrointestinal symptoms. Any atopic features, such as rash or angioedema, are assessed. Note whether food intolerance or avoidance has affected the patient's nutritional status.

Differential Diagnosis

Oral allergy syndrome is swelling and itching of the mouth in response to food allergens. The syndrome tends to coexist with certain pollen allergies. For example, patients with ragweed allergy react to melon and bananas. Patients with birch tree allergy react to apples, carrots, potatoes, or hazelnuts.

Exercise-induced anaphylaxis occurs during or after exercise and in some cases depends on prior food ingestion. It may be associated with specific foods, particularly celery, shrimp, oysters, peaches, wheat, and chicken.

Nonallergic *food intolerance* must be differentiated from true food allergy. *Lactose intolerance* causes diarrhea and cramps with milk ingestion due to lactase deficiency. *Chinese restaurant syndrome* is an adverse effect of the food additive monosodium glutamate (MSG). MSG can cause headache, burning dysesthesias, and facial and chest pain. Headache may be caused by the pharmacologic action of tyramine (in cheese and chocolate), histamine (in red wine), and nitrites (in smoked foods and cold cuts). Caffeine overdose or withdrawal also may cause headache.

Laboratory Evaluation

RAST or skin testing should be based on information gained from a food diary and thorough history. A negative test has a high negative predictive value. However, even when correlated with a good history, a positive test has a positive predictive value of only 40 to 50 percent. Therefore, these tests are commonly confirmed with a double-blind placebo controlled food challenge.

Treatment

The best treatment is avoidance of foods to which the patient is allergic. Patients with anaphylaxis should carry an EpiPen for self-administration of epinephrine at the beginning of a reaction.

Any patient with a severe systemic reaction, frequent symptoms, or poor response to simple food avoidance should be referred to an allergist for further evaluation. Immunotherapy is not effective.

Anaphylaxis

History and Physical Exam

Symptoms and signs of anaphylaxis may be cutaneous (urticaria, angioedema, flushing), respiratory (wheezing, chest tightness), gastrointestinal (nausea, vomiting, diarrhea), or cardiovascular (hypotension, shock). Most anaphylactic reactions occur within 2 h of allergen exposure, although a late reaction may occur hours after the initial event.

Differential Diagnosis

Medications, food, vaccines, blood products, latex, and insect stings are among the more common agents associated with anaphylactic reactions. Stings from Hymenoptera (wasps, hornets, yellow jackets, and bees) are particularly implicated and may be life-threatening. Patients with IgA deficiency are predisposed to anaphylactic reactions from blood products. Exercise-induced anaphylaxis may occur in isolation or in relation to food. The syndrome of idiopathic anaphylaxis is well described.

Laboratory Evaluation

Patients experiencing anaphylactic reactions should be referred to an allergist for complete evaluation. Obviously, in the acute situation emergency care must be rendered immediately.

Treatment

The mainstay of treatment for anaphylaxis is epinephrine (0.3 mg subcutaneously). Epinephrine may be given in the office or self-administered with an EpiPen. Antihistamines (e.g., diphenhydramine 25 to 50 mg qid) and prednisone (40 mg po qd) also may be given until symptoms resolve completely. A 1- to 2-week course is generally advisable. β-blockers should be discontinued in patients at risk for anaphylaxis. They can increase the severity of the allergic reaction and hamper pharmacologic response to epinephrine.

Treatment for an acute reaction should be initiated immediately and the patient should be transferred to an emergency department and observed for 24 h.

Immunotherapy is recommended for those with insect sting anaphylaxis. A large local reaction to a sting—even swelling of an entire extremity contiguous with the sting site—does not warrant immunotherapy. Desensitization to a medication may be attempted in the hospital in the case of a life-threatening illness where no other treatment options are available.

Immunodeficiency Diseases

History and Physical Exam

The hallmark of immunodeficiency is recurrent, persistent, or unusual infections (e.g., *Pneumocystis carinii* pneumonia). Excluding AIDS, which is discussed elsewhere (Chap. 49), the diseases seen most often in adults are defects in humoral immunity. They generally predispose to bacterial sinopulmonary infections. Encapsulated organisms, such as *Streptococcus pneumoniae* and *Hemophilus influenza* may predominate. Recurrent skin infections, meningitis, osteomyelitis, gastroenteritis, colitis, and bacteremia also are seen.

Differential Diagnosis

IgA deficiency is common, occurring in about one person in 400 in the general population. Its clinical significance is uncertain. Patients with IgA deficiency are at risk for anaphylactic reactions from blood products.

Patients with common variable immunodeficiency (CVID) may present in young adulthood. Levels of IgG, IgA, and IgM are low, but not absent. B lymphocyte count is normal. CVID is associated with increased incidence of autoimmune diseases such as rheumatoid arthritis. It is also associated with lymphoid malignancies, particularly non-Hodgkin's lymphoma.

Bruton's X-linked agammaglobulinemia is characterized by absent B lymphocytes and markedly reduced immunoglobulins of all classes.

Immunodeficiency with thymoma affects adults in their fourth decade or older. The thymoma usually is a benign spindle cell tumor. All immunoglobulins are decreased, as is the absolute B lymphocyte count.

Less common immune deficiencies may involve abnormalities of T lymphocyte or neutrophil function or complement deficiency.

Recurrent infections also may be caused by nonimmunologic mechanisms. For example, anatomical abnormalities hampering sinus drainage may predispose to recurrent sinusitis.

Laboratory Evaluation

An appropriate initial screen evaluates many components of the immune system. Serum immunoglobulins (IgG, IgA, IgM, IgE), total T and B lymphocytes, and T cell subsets should be quantitated. Delayed hypersensitivity skin testing to PPD, mumps, and Candida, if positive, is evidence of functional cellular immunity. Specific antibody response to immunization should be demonstrated. Measuring antitetanus antibody evaluates response to a protein antigen, while measuring anti-pneumococcal antibodies in a patient who has received the pneumococcal vaccine evaluates response to carbohydrate antigens.

Treatment

A patient suspected of having an immune deficiency should be referred to an allergist-immunologist for complete evaluation. Deficiencies of humoral immunity may be treated with infusions of gamma globulin. In some cases, prophylactic antibiotics may be warranted.

References and Selected Readings

1. Bochner BS, Lichtenstein LM: Anaphylaxis. *N Engl J Med* 324:1785–1790, 1991.
2. Buckley RH: Immunodeficiency diseases. *JAMA* 268:2797–3807, 1992.
3. Eghrari-Sabet JS, Slater JE: Latex allergy: A potentially serious respiratory disorder. *J Respir Dis* 14:473–482, 1993.
4. Lieberman P: Anaphylactoid reactions to radiocontrast material. *Ann Allerg* 67:91–100, 1991.
5. Naglerio RM: Allergic rhinitis. *N Engl J Med* 325:860–869, 1991.
6. National Asthma Education Program. Expert Panel Report: Guidelines for the Diagnosis and Management of Asthma. Bethesda MD: National Heart, Lung and Blood Institute, National Institutes of Health, Publication No. 91-3042, 1991.
7. Patterson R, DeSwarte RD, Greenberger PA, Grammar LC: Drug allergy and protocols for management of drug allergies. *NER Allerg Proc* 7:325–342, 1986.
8. Sampson HA, Metcalfe DD: Food allergies. *JAMA* 268:2840–2844, 1992.
9. Sneller MC, Strober W, Eisenstein E, et al: New insights into common variable immunodeficiency. *Ann Intern Med* 118:720–730, 1993.

55 Evaluation of Chronic Fatigue

Roy M. Pitkin

Complaints of protracted and disabling fatigue are encountered quite commonly in ambulatory practice. The sensation of tiredness may be either persistent or recurrent, but it is severe enough that it comes to dominate the lives of those affected. Although it may be tempting to regard such individuals as casualties of the stresses of modern life, there is evidence that the problem is of much earlier origin. Indeed, Hippocrates seems clearly to have recognized the various forms of muscular fatigue, observing that "fatigue pains" can occur in those out of training after the slightest exercise, but also in "trained bodies" after unusual exercises and even after usual exercises "if they be excessive."

In the 19th century the term "neurasthenia" was coined to relate chronic fatigue to a dissipation of energy in the nervous system. The term and the concept of nervous energy persisted until well into the 20th century. Names used in more modern times include effort syndrome, fibrositis, fibromyalgia, myalgic encephalomyelitis, and postviral fatigue syndrome. Current thinking seems to favor the terminology "chronic fatigue syndrome," even though the nature—and indeed the existence—of a "syndrome" remain a contentious and emotional issue.

Regardless of whether or not a chronic fatigue syndrome exists as a specific and definable entity, conditions and diseases that may present primarily with complaints of abnormally persistent to severe fatigue are both numerous and varied. For this reason, it is appropriate to consider first the differential diagnosis of chronic fatigue as a symptom.

Differential Diagnosis

When a patient presents with a complaint of fatigue, several general medical conditions should be considered, of which the first to come to mind is usually anemia. Because of the decreased oxygen-carrying capacity of the blood, an individual anemic for any reason will, especially if her anemia has developed fairly quickly, complain of tiredness with less than ordinary exertion. Malignancies, especially lymphomas and leukemias, occasionally will be seen in patients whose primary complaint is feeling excessively tired.

Many endocrine-metabolic disorders can cause fatigue. Fairly often, fatigue heralds the onset of diabetes mellitus. Thyroid disease, more often hypothyroidism but occasionally hyperthyroidism, and hyperparathyroidism sometimes are characterized by malaise and weakness. Addison's disease and hypopituitarism also can present with chronic fatigue.

Lassitude accompanies many different infections and sometimes can dominate the clinical picture. Chronic infections such as tuberculosis and brucellosis are classic cases in point. On a more modern note, weakness and inability to carry out ordinary activities probably are the most common early symptoms of the acquired immunodeficiency syndrome. Infectious mononucleosis and chronic pyelonephritis are notorious for presenting as fatigue.

The most difficult problems to differentiate are usually neurologic and psychiatric conditions. Fatigue is a prominent and at times early symptom of multiple sclerosis. Psychiatrically, the relevant disorder is depression; the distinction can be especially difficult because, as will be seen later, the chronic fatigue syndrome can include depression as well as forgetfulness, confusion, difficulty thinking, and inability to concentrate.

Chronic Fatigue Syndrome

Over the last 60 years, there have occurred throughout the world a number of apparent epidemics characterized by intense fatigue, myalgia, irritability and depression, and difficulty with memory and concentration. The clinical picture of what has come to be known as the chronic fatigue syndrome, though somewhat variable from epidemic to epidemic and in nonepidemic or sporadic cases, has enough consistency to merit designation as a syndrome.

There are three types of ''normal'' fatigue—that resulting from physical exertion unaccustomed in type or amount, that following sustained mental stress or effort, and that due to inadequate sleep—and the patient with chronic fatigue syndrome typically complains of perniciously exaggerated forms of all three. This is the primary and dominating symptom, and the affected individual complains of it bitterly and with a wide variety of descriptive illustrations. For research purposes, a duration of at least six months is required, a criterion also useful clinically to distinguish chronic fatigue syndrome from postviral syndromes such as those following influenza and infectious mononucleosis.

Muscle pain and tenderness is a common, though not invariable, accompaniment. The myalgia is generalized but seems to involve particularly the long muscles of the extremities. Patients complain of pain both with and without physical activities. Much of the time there is also arthralgia, but joint stiffness is somewhat less common. Examination may reveal tenderness at specific and consistent sites.

Nearly all patients with chronic fatigue syndrome experience an inexplicable decline in their ability to cope with the events and circumstances of everyday life. There may be an apparent personality change, inability to concentrate, and memory deficits. Depression, if present at all, is clearly secondary to concern about medical status. The presence of these mental and emotional symptoms raises the possibility of a primary psychological disorder, such as neurosis or hypochondriasis, but most authorities regard the weight of the evidence as favoring a specific physical basis.

Definition and quantification are essential for research, and a group of American investigators has proposed criteria to define chronic fatigue syndrome (Table 55-1). For a case to be acceptable for research purposes, it must exhibit both major criteria (severe fatigue for at least six months and exclusion of other chronic medical and psychiatric conditions) plus either six symptomatic criteria plus two physical criteria, or eight symptomatic criteria. Although intended to provide the kind of rigor in definition and quantification needed in research, these criteria also can be useful in clinical assessment.

The etiology of the chronic fatigue syndrome is particularly controversial and, not surprisingly, theories of causation are both numerous and varied. They may be grouped conveniently under infectious, immunologic, and psychological headings.

The most popular theories involve infections, usually viral. An infectious cause is suggested strongly by the well-described epidemics occurring periodically over the last 50 to 60 years in various parts of the world. Much interest over the last decade has centered on the Epstein-Barr virus. However, most studies have failed to find a difference in antibody titers between patients who meet the criteria for chronic fatigue syndrome and those who do not. Enteroviruses and Coxsackie viruses also have been

TABLE 55-1 Criteria for Chronic Fatigue Syndrome[a]

Major criteria

- Persistent or relapsing fatigue for at least 6 months that does not respond to rest and reduces activity by at least half
- Other clinical conditions, including psychiatric disease, excluded

Minor criteria—Symptomatic or historical

- Mild fever or chills
- Sore throat
- Lymph node pain in cervical or axillary chains
- Generalized muscle weakness
- Myalgia
- Fatigue for longer than 24 h after levels of exercise that previously were well tolerated
- Generalized headache
- Migratory noninflammatory arthralgia
- Neuropsychiatric symptoms
- Sleep disturbance
- Onset of symptoms acute or subacute

Minor criteria—Physical (on two occasions, at least 1 month apart)

- Low grade fever
- Nonexudative pharyingitis
- Cervical or axillary lymph nodes

[a]Definition of a research case requires both major criteria plus either at least 6 historical criteria and 2 physical criteria, or 8 historical criteria.

SOURCE: Modified with permission from Holmes GP, Kaplan JR, Gantz NM, et al: Chronic fatigue syndrome: A working case definition. *Ann Intern Med* 108:387–389, 1988.

considered carefully. They are clearly capable of causing epidemic acute illnesses, and the enteroviruses probably were responsible for most of the "nonparalytic poliomyelitis" of former times. However, the issue of their causing a chronic and persisting form, especially involving the central nervous system, remains controversial. As with Epstein-Barr virus, antibody studies have not been rewarding. The highest level of interest currently is centered on retroviruses, which unquestionably can cause a chronic smoldering infection. About viruses generally, current thinking tends to assign them a triggering role, rather than one of chronic infection.

Some sort of immunologic basis is suggested by a common history of allergy or atopy. Moreover, several laboratory test abnormalities have been reported in individual studies, although not often confirmed in independent studies. The abnormalities described include diminished natural killer cell function, impaired T-cell response to mitogenic or antigenic stimuli, and activated T-cell subsets. Both hyper- and hypogammaglobulinemia have been reported.

The concept of a primary psychological basis has been particularly persistent. To be sure, most patients complaining of chronic fatigue will have primary depressive illnesses or anxiety rather than chronic fatigue syndrome. Moreover, unraveling the temporal sequence in a patient who presents with complaints of "feeling tired all the time" but with obvious depression and anxiety can be a chicken-egg problem. Most patients with chronic fatigue syndrome *become* depressed and anxious within a month or two from the onset of this condition; for some, the depression is the most debilitating aspect of their condition. The question of whether there was evidence of a psychiatric disorder *before* the onset of chronic fatigue can be difficult to resolve by even the most careful history. Nevertheless, most authorities are persuaded by the sometimes epidemic nature and the laboratory abnormalities (even though not reported consistently) that a primary psychological cause is unlikely.

Under the circumstances in which the etiology is so unclear, it is not surprising that the number and variety of treatments are both huge. The list of drugs tried and, at least in noncomparative reports or research involving open comparisons, found to offer some benefit is a long one. Among the pharmacologic agents studied the most and in a controlled manner are: acyclovir; liver extract, folic acid, and vitamin B_{12}; intravenous immunoglobulin; magnesium sulfate; essential fatty acids; tricyclic antidepressants; and nonsteroidal anti-inflammatory drugs. Although promising results have been reported in the case of each of these agents, subsequent independent studies generally have failed to confirm the initial positive outcome.

Clinical Assessment and Management

History

In a patient presenting with complaints of chronic fatigue, a careful and detailed history is the first and most important step. The nature of the onset is often the most critical piece of information. It is usually abrupt in chronic fatigue syndrome, often accompanying or following a flulike illness, whereas if the patient says she "has always been tired," the likelihood of an underlying psychiatric disorder is high. The duration of the illness should be sufficient to rule out recognized postviral conditions, and the research case definition of six months (Table 55-1) is probably useful clinically as well. Similarly, an effort to quantitate the disability, such as the 50 percent level suggested for research purposes, can be valuable.

Perhaps the most important, and at the same time the most difficult, distinction involves primary depressive disorders. Fatigability is a common complaint with depression and, as noted earlier, most chronic fatigue patients experience some secondary depression. A careful history is critical in determining whether depression preceded or followed the onset of the illness. Other features that point more to depression than to chronic fatigue syndrome include diurnal rhythm, terminal sleep disturbance, weight loss, and pervasive feelings of unworthiness and self-blame.

There may be a variety of other symptoms, of which unexplained generalized muscle pain is probably the most common. Weakness and arthralgias also may be present, as may sore throat, cervical adenopathy, and headache. Psychological complaints (difficulty concentrating, confusion, irritability, anxiety, and depression) are encountered commonly. As with the primary complaint of debilitating fatigue or easy fatigability, these other symptoms should be of new onset and should not have existed to any significant degree before the beginning of the present illness.

A complete listing of current and past medications is essential, since more than 250 drugs listed in the *Physician's Desk Reference* include fatigue as a side effect. There should be specific inquiry about various forms of substance abuse. Alcoholism per se may often lead to fatigue complaints but alcoholics may invoke fatigue to try to cover up inadequate performance.

The history is not generally remarkable in a patient with chronic fatigue syndrome, except possibly for an unusually frequent incidence of atopy or other allergies.

Physical Examination

A complete physical examination should be performed. Its major goal is to rule out other illnesses in the differential diagnosis. Particularly important is the neurologic examination.

Positive physical findings are infrequent in the chronic fatigue syndrome. Perhaps the most common, present in one-third or so, are enlarged and/or tender lymph nodes in the cervical or axillary areas. Even when lymphadenopathy is present, the degree of nodal enlargement is modest, and nodes larger than two centimeters in diameter should suggest other causes.

The physical examination also offers an opportunity for assessment of intellectual capacity by, for example, evaluating the patient's orientation and ability to perform serial sevens. Individuals with chronic fatigue syndrome may have some degree of cognitive impairment, but severe forms are more consistent with primary psychiatric illness.

Laboratory Studies

There are no specific diagnostic laboratory tests in chronic fatigue syndrome, but some abnormalities

TABLE 55-2 Laboratory Tests in Chronic Fatigue Syndrome

Hematology	Complete blood count Erythrocyte sedimentation rate
Urine	Complete urinalysis Test for infection
Chemistry	Electrolytes Liver function tests BUN and creatinine
Thyroid	Thyroxine Thyroid stimulating hormone
Immunologic	Antinuclear antibodies Circulating immune complexes Immunoglobulins (IgG, IgA, IgM)

are seen to occur with increased frequency in the condition. Moreover, carefully selected laboratory tests may be helpful in excluding other diseases. Table 55-2 lists those that might be included in routine assessment.

A complete blood count is essential to rule out anemia and the more overt forms of infection. The erythrocyte sedimentation rate can help in excluding infection and other inflammatory states. About 20 percent of patients with chronic fatigue syndrome will have either leukocytosis or leukopenia, and a similar proportion will exhibit minor elevation of the sedimentation rate.

Serum electrolytes, including calcium and phosphorus, should be measured, and liver function tests (transaminases, alkaline phosphatase, and bilirubin) included as well. Urea nitrogen and creatinine are important to evaluate renal status. All of these blood chemistry tests usually can be performed by an automated technique as part of a panel.

Routine urinalysis should be included, as well as some chemical or microbiologic test for urinary tract infection. Thyroid evaluation should include measurement of serum thyroxine and thyroid-stimulating hormone. If either is abnormal, antithyroid microsomal antibodies should be tested.

Although the number of immunologic tests found to be positive in individual studies is large, few have been observed consistently in different investigations. Antinuclear antibody tests have been positive (usually weakly) and circulating immune complexes have been low, each in as many as one-half of patients with chronic fatigue. A similar proportion has been observed to have modest elevations in levels of one or another class of immunoglobulin (IgG, IgA, IgM).

Management

In a patient diagnosed as having chronic fatigue syndrome, with other causes of the complaint ruled out, the important guiding principles of management are to provide compassionate emotional support and to avoid unproved and exotic remedies. The patient needs understanding and reassurance as she seeks to modify her life-style to come to terms with her chronic condition. She should eat a balanced diet and get sufficient rest, although she needs to understand that there is no evidence that prolonged rest is curative.

Chronic fatigue syndrome patients typically find that any physical activity leads to exacerbation of their symptoms, leading to a vicious cycle of progressive physical deconditioning. This sequence can be broken by a specific program of very gradual graded exercise therapy, preferably under the direct supervision of an exercise therapist. Some success has been reported with cognitive behavior therapy, an approach that attempts to modify the individual's attitudes and perceptions regarding the symptoms.

Pharmacologic treatment has a limited role, chiefly in treating specific symptoms. If depression is prominent, antidepressant medication, with an agent that seems appropriate for the clinical picture and that the patient can tolerate, may be given. Some antidepressants have sedative side effects, and these generally should be avoided, except perhaps at bedtime. If anxiety or panic disorders occur, a drug such as alprazolam can be useful. For those in whom myalgias and arthralgias are troublesome, a nonsteroidal anti-inflammatory drug like ibuprofen may give relief.

Referral is sometimes indicated for either diagnosis or management. Usually the proper consultant will be a neurologist, although, depending on the individual clinical picture, a rheumatologist, psychiatrist, or other specialist may be appropriate. If the need is more therapeutic than diagnostic, referral to a psychologist or other counsellor may be appropriate.

References and Selected Readings

1. Bock GR, Whelan J (eds): *Chronic Fatigue Syndrome.* Chichester: John Wiley (Ciba Foundation Symposium 173), 1993.
2. Buchwald D, Kornacoff AL: Review of laboratory findings for patients with chronic fatigue syndrome. *Rev Infect Dis* 13(suppl 1):S12–18, 1991.
3. Dawson DM, Sabin TD (eds): *Chronic Fatigue Syndrome.* Boston: Little, Brown, 1993.
4. Holmes GP, Kaplan JR, Gantz NM, et al: Chronic fatigue syndrome: A working case definition. *Ann Intern Med* 108:387–389, 1988.
5. Thomas PK: The chronic fatigue syndrome: What do we know? *BMJ* 306:1557–1558, 1993.

Color Plates

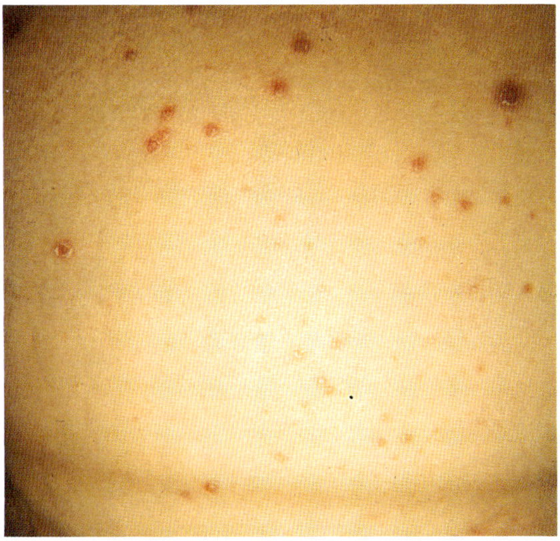

Color Plate 1 Folliculitis in a diabetic patient.

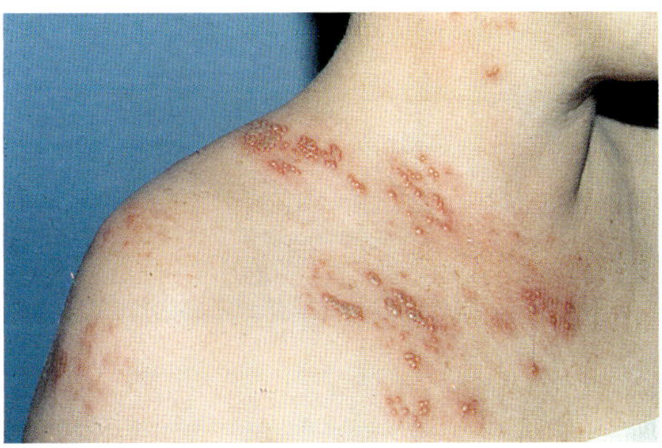

Color Plate 2 Herpes zoster.

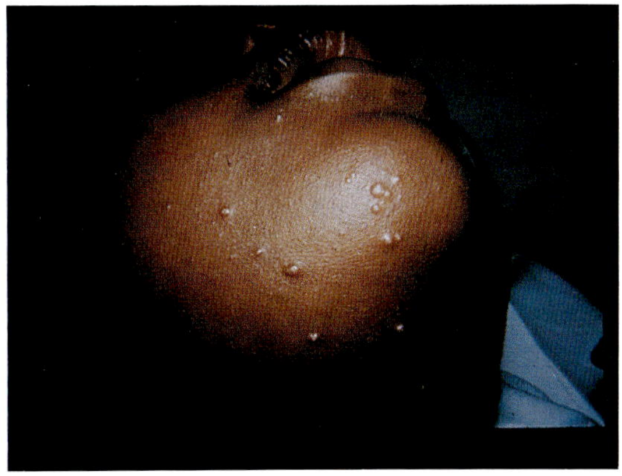

Color Plate 3 Molluscum contagiosum.

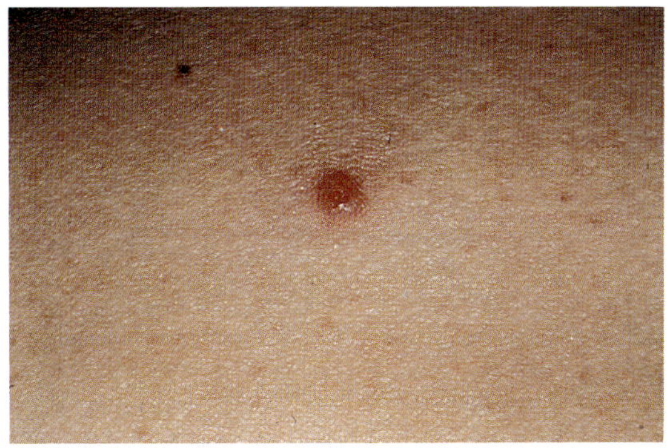

Color Plate 4 Insect bite.

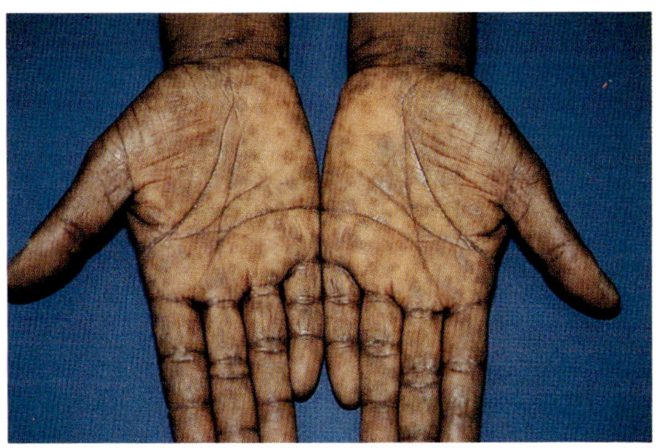

Color Plate 5 Secondary syphilis.

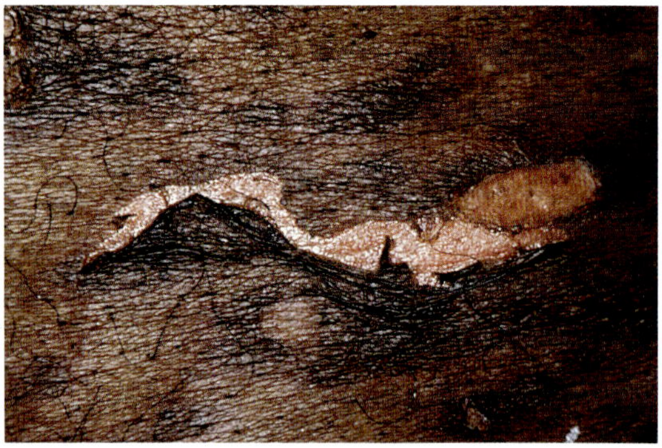

Color Plate 6 Toxic epidermal erythema multiforme.

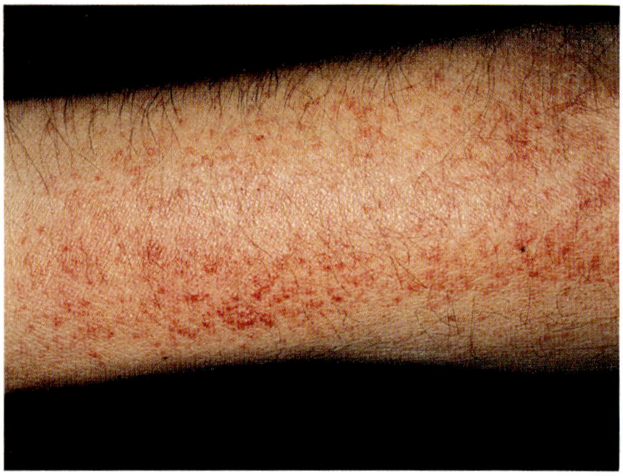

Color Plate 7 Polymorphic light eruption.

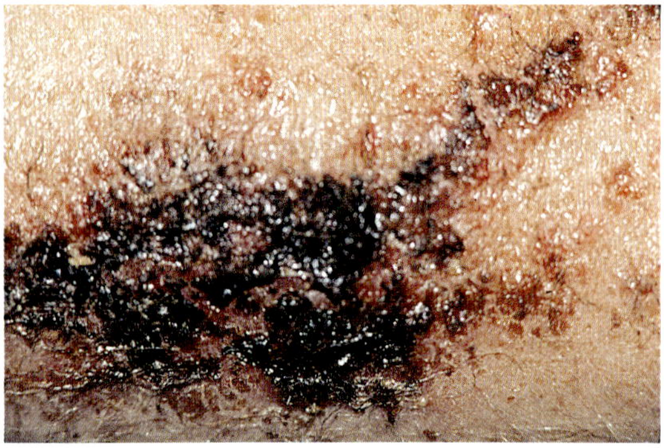

Color Plate 8 Contact dermatitis from poison ivy.

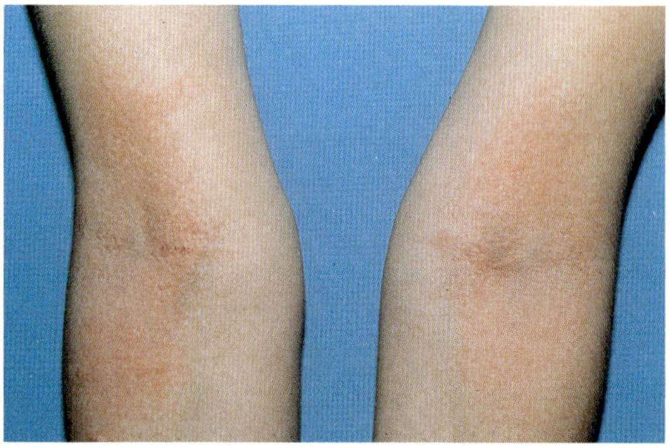

Color Plate 9 Atopic dermatitis.

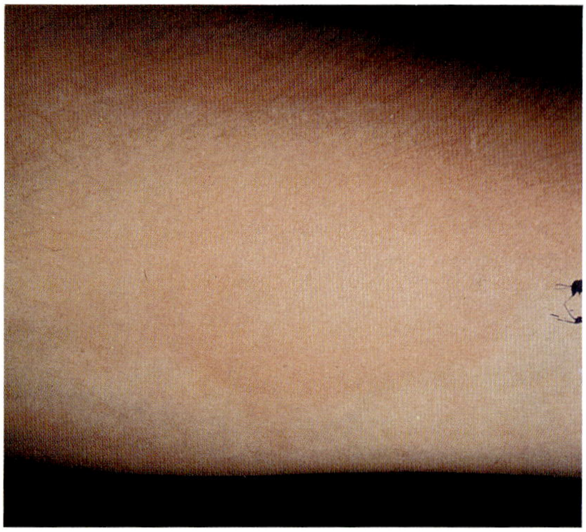

Color Plate 10 Urticaria.

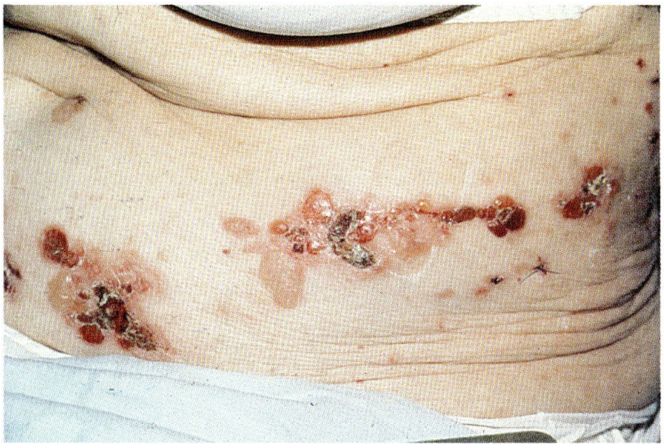

Color Plate 11 Bullous pemphigoid, flared by herpes zoster.

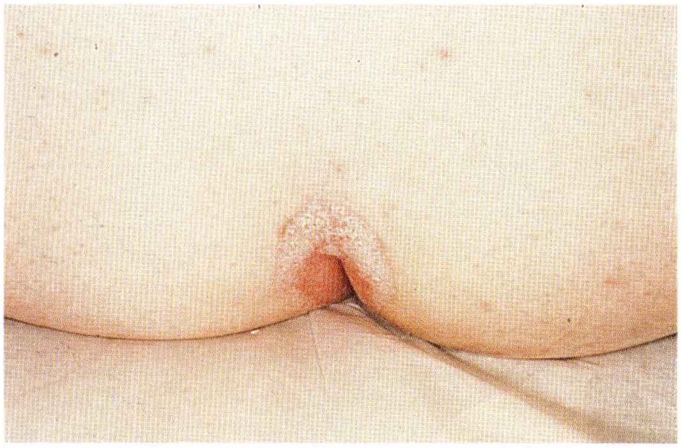

Color Plate 12 Psoriasis.

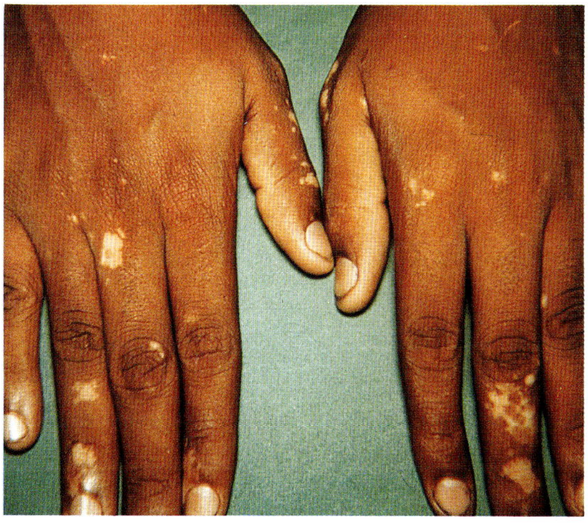

Color Plate 13 Vitiligo.

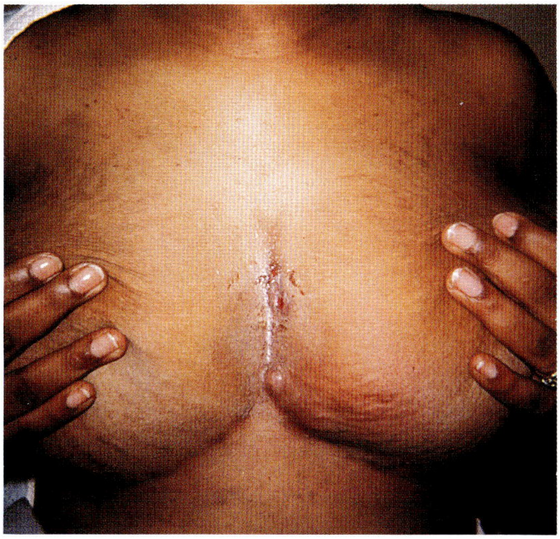

Color Plate 14 Hidradenitis suppurativa.

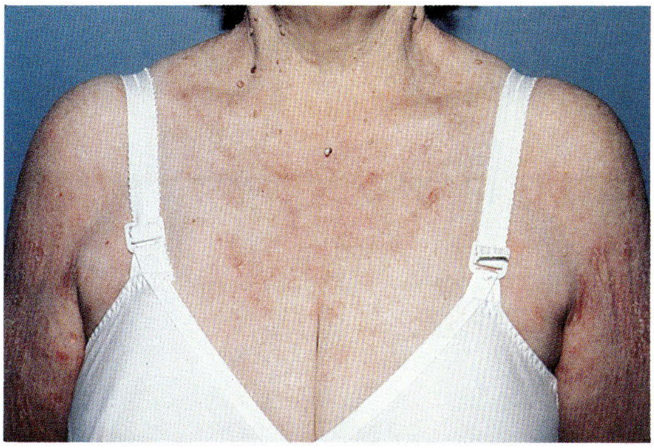

Color Plate 15 Subacute cutaneous lupus erythematosus (drug-induced).

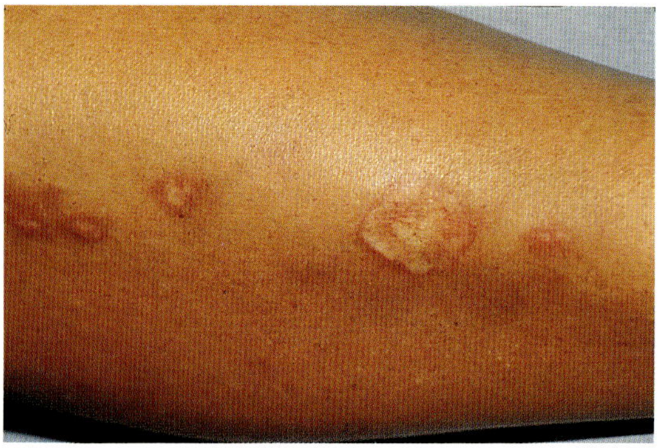

Color Plate 16 Necrobiosis lipoidica diabetecorum.

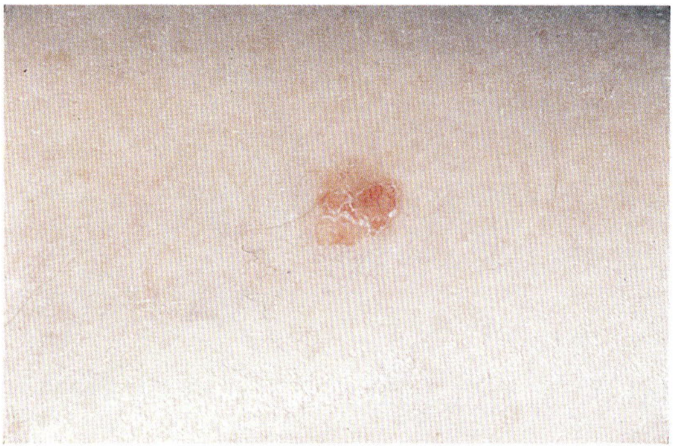

Color Plate 17 Superficial squamous cell carcinoma.

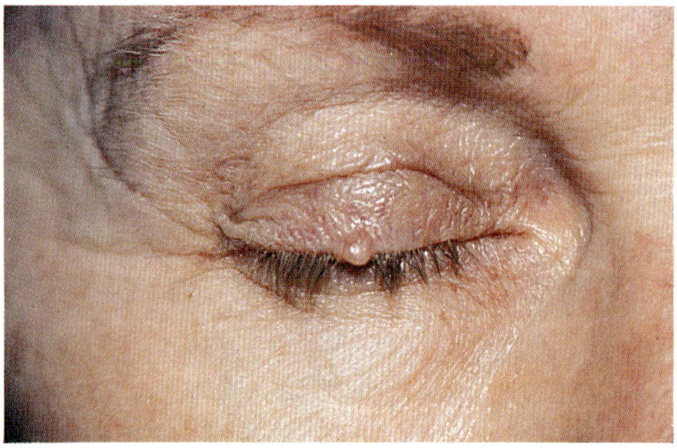

Color Plate 18 Basal cell carcinoma.

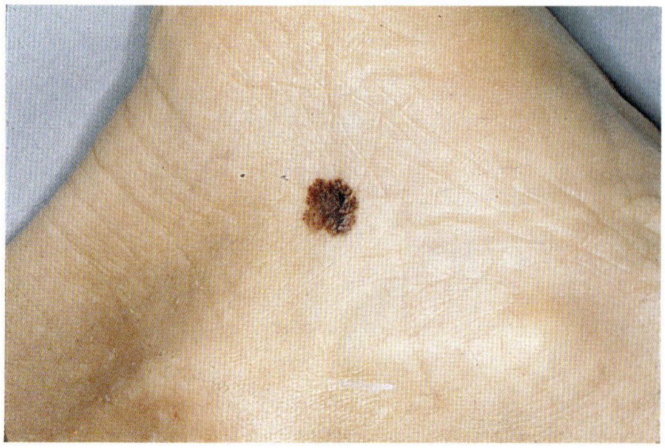

Color Plate 19 Superficial malignant melanoma.

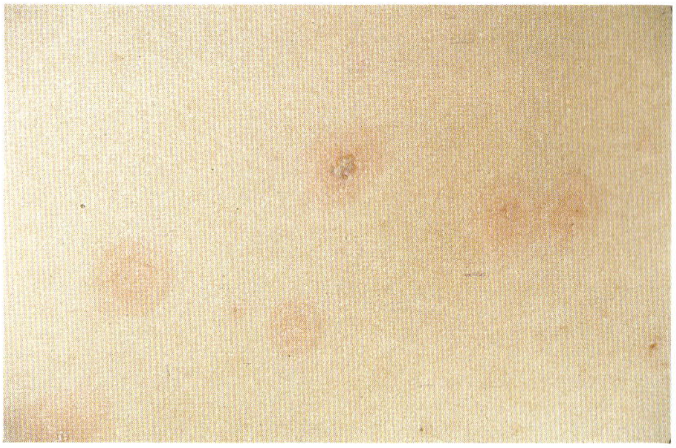

Color Plate 20 Pemphigus gestationis–herpes gestationis.

56 Dermatologic Disorders

W. Kenneth Blaylock

The History and Physical Examination in Dermatologic Diagnosis

The clinical approach to a patient with a skin complaint should begin with a good history and a thorough physical examination. Access to the skin by visual inspection, i.e., seeing the gross pathology, is an advantage to the clinician. Special diagnostic procedures should be available, and are listed below (see Table 56-1).

The history of the skin eruption should include a description of the presentation of the first primary lesion and its location and configuration, as well as the type and duration of symptoms. The sequence of events in the progression of the eruption is important, and the relationship to drugs or other possible environmental flare factors can be very helpful in the evaluation process.

Cutaneous lesions are either primary or secondary. Primary lesions may present with fluid or may be free of fluid (see Table 56-2). The solid lesions are the macule, papule, nodule, tumor, and wheal. The fluid-filled lesions are vesicles, bullae, pustules, and cysts. Secondary lesions usually follow trauma to the primary lesions, or they may occur as a manifestation of the healing skin. These secondary lesions include crusts, flakes, erosions, and ulcers (see Table 56-3).

TABLE 56-1 Cutaneous Diagnostic Procedures

Procedure Type	Procedure, Supplies, and Equipment	Clinical Condition Where Helpful
Hand lens or head magnification	Magnification 5–10×	Scabies, melanoma and other tumors
Potassium hydroxide (KOH)	KOH, glass slide, microscope	Tinea versicolor; tinea pedis; tinea corporis
Wood's light	360–400 nm wavelength light	Tinea versicolor; erythrasma
Skin biopsy	3- or 4-mm punch; formalin	Tumors; bullous diseases (adjacent skin or edge of lesion); nodules
Tzanck prep	Scalpel blade, skin scraping, glass slide, Wright stain	Herpes zoster; herpes simplex
Scabies	Scalpel blade (#15), oil	Papules or burrows; scabies or suspected scabies

TABLE 56-2 Primary Skin Lesions

Type	Description	Examples
Macule	Flat, 1–30 mm	Freckle, viral eruption, purpura
Papule	Solid, elevated, 5 mm or less	Drug or viral eruption, psoriasis, purpura
Nodule	Solid, elevated, 5–20 mm	Panniculitis (subcutaneous), sarcoid—sarcoidosis (dermal), keloid (dermal)
Tumor	Solid, elevated, large nodule	Basal cell cancer carcinoma, melanoma, dermatofibroma
Wheal	Elevated, fluid in dermis	Urticaria
Vesicle	Elevated, clear fluid, less than 5 mm	Eczema, herpes zoster, contact dermatitis
Bullae	Elevated, clear fluid, greater than 5 mm	Herpes zoster, erythema multiforme
Pustules	Round, elevated, white or yellow, fluid	Impetigo, pustular psoriasis

Skin Infections: Bacteria

Impetigo

Impetigo (contagiosa) is the most common bacterial infection of the skin. It is caused by gram-positive bacteria, i.e., coagulase-positive *Staphylococcus aureus* or β-hemolytic *Streptococcus* spp., or both. These lesions are thin-walled subcorneal vesicles or pustules on erythematous bases; they break easily and are seen most commonly on exposed areas of skin. When the lesions rupture, they exude serum. There is usually peripheral extension, often develop-

TABLE 56-3 Secondary Skin Lesions

Type	Description	Clinical Example
Crust	Dried serum or exudate on surface	Healing wound or excoriation
Flake	Scales, stratum corneum	Seborrheic dermatitis
Plaque	Coalescing papules	Psoriasis, granuloma annulare
Fissure	Break or crack in epidermis	Ichthyosis or chronic eczema
Erosion or excoriation	Epidermis missing	Impetigo or scratching
Ulcer	Loss of epidermis and dermis	Venous stasis ulcer
Scar	Healing with dermal fibrosis	Acne
Atrophy	Loss of epidermis and dermis	Topical steroid abuse, sun damage

ing a connected round pattern. Mixed infections are common.

Some strains of streptococci associated with impetigo and scabies with secondary impetigo can produce glomerulonephritis. Culture and Gram stain of exudate from a lesion are helpful in confirming the diagnosis of this bacterial infection. Treatment requires both local care and systemic antibiotics (see Table 56-4).

Ecthyma

This is a deeper infection of the skin produced by beta-hemolytic Streptococcus organisms. The lesions initially may resemble impetigo, but later deeper ulcers occur in the skin. Impetigo is common on the face and hands, while ecthyma is usually on the lower legs and follows dry fissures or insect bites. The diagnosis is established by the clinical picture, Gram-stained smear, and culture. Treatment is the same as for impetigo, although antibacterial therapy may need to be continued for as long as 2 to 4 weeks.

TABLE 56-4 Skin Infections: Therapy

Infection	Organisms	Therapy
Impetigo	Group A beta-hemolytic streptococcus or *S. aureus*	Penicillinase-resistant penicillins, 250–500 mg po qid, or Erythromycin, 250–500 mg., po qid
Ecthyma	Group A beta-hemolytic streptococcus	Same as impetigo, antibiotic for 2–4 wks
Erysipelas	Group A beta-hemolytic streptococcus	Systemic IV penicillin, such as nafcillin Hospitalization
Cellulitis	Group A, C, G streptococcus	Same as erysipelas (for severe cases) For mild cases: 500 mg erythromycin, or dicloxacillin, qid × 10 days and bed rest
Folliculitis	*S. aureus*	Moist heat and antiseptic cleansers In severe cases: erythromycin, 250–500 mg. po qid × 10 days
	Pseudomonas	Stop exposure to contaminated water; local therapy and antibiotics as indicated
Furuncle	*S. aureus*	Erythromycin or dicloxacillin, a semisynthetic penicillin, 250–500 mg po qid × 10 days Moist heat, incision and drainage Bacitracin or mupirocin, bid × 7 days in nose
Toxic shock syndrome	*S. aureus* toxic shock syndrome toxin-1	Managed in hospital

Erysipelas

This form of infection is produced by group A, β-hemolytic streptococci. The clinical manifestations are fever; malaise; and skin erythema, with distinct sharp borders, induration, and tenderness. This eruption usually occurs on the face, arms, or legs.

Erysipelas is seen frequently in the elderly. Hospitalization is often indicated. Early intravenous antibiotic therapy may be replaced by oral therapy in two to three days, as disappearance of the redness occurs. Recurrences are common in the same site, particularly on the lower legs, where fissures between the toes may provide the site at which pathologic organisms enter the skin. Antibiotic therapy in this setting should be followed by careful attention to any fungal infection of the feet.

Cellulitis

This infection closely resembles erysipelas. It usually is caused by beta-hemolytic streptococci; however, the *Staphylococcus aureus* occasionally can produce cellulitis. Recurrent cellulitis in the lower leg is treated with the same antibiotics used for erysipelas. Recurrent cellulitis requires the prevention of tinea pedis between the toes.

Folliculitis

Folliculitis develops in traumatized skin as a primary infection. Bacterial folliculitis is characterized by inflammatory papules surrounding a central hair. *Staphylococcus aureus*-induced folliculitis has perifollicular erythema and pustule formation. A Gram stain of the pustular contents usually shows the gram-positive organism. Folliculitis caused by *Pseudomonas aeruginosa* is associated with contaminated water in hot tubs or whirlpools. Folliculitis without infection may also occur in traumatized skin from rubbing or scratching (Fig. 56-1).

Furunculosis

Furuncles and carbuncles are painful, hot erythematous nodules ("boils") containing pus, usually caused by *S. aureus.* All fluctuant lesions should receive incision and drainage and systemic antibiotics. The use of topically applied antibiotics in the nose may be indicated to prevent nasopharyngeal colonization and recurrence. Family members may need to be treated to reduce colonization of *S. aureus* in the nasopharyngeal and flexural skinfolds.

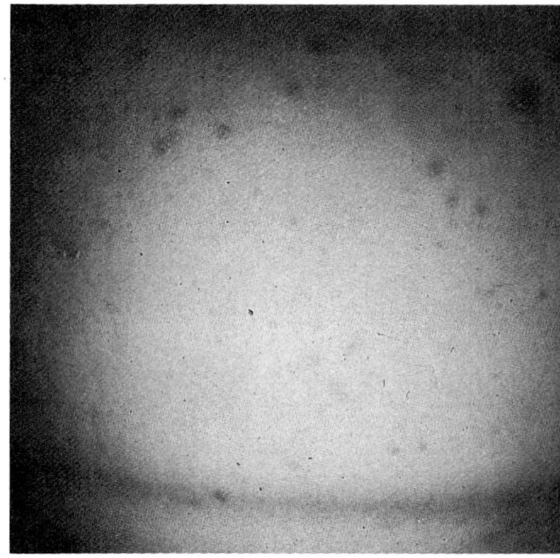

Figure 56-1 Folliculitis in a diabetic patient. (See Color Plate 1.)

Erythrasma

This eruption is produced by a short, gram-positive rod, *Corynebacterium minutissimum.* The clinical eruption is a scaly, reddish or brownish, slightly thickened macule, seen in intertriginous areas such as the axillae, groin, and toe web spaces, especially between the fourth and fifth toes. The Wood's light examination reveals a coral-pink fluorescence. Therapy includes topical antifungal creams, e.g., miconazole and/or oral erythromycin 250 mg po, qid for 2 weeks (see Table 56-5).

Toxic Shock Syndrome

Although this is not a bacterial skin infection, there is a close relationship between toxic shock syndrome and infection with *Staphylococcus aureus.* Prolonged tampon use may support bacterial growth and precipitate this syndrome and skin eruption. A proportion of Staphylococcus isolates produce an antigen referred to as toxic shock syndrome toxin-1. This toxin can act as a super antigen.

Toxic shock syndrome evolves in a few days. Although it occurs in healthy menstruating women, it also may occur in nonmenstruating women and in

TABLE 56-5 Cutaneous Fungal and Yeast Infections

Infection	Therapy
Tinea corporis, Tinea cruris, Tinea faciale	Imidazole creams, Chlotrimazole, or Miconazole cream bid × 2 weeks or until eruption is clear and then additional 1–2 weeks
Tinea manum and Tinea pedis	Chlotrimazole or miconazole cream bid × 3–4 weeks, until clear, then an additional 2 weeks If refractory and chronic, ultramicronized griseofulvin, 250 mg po bid for 1–2 months
Tinea unguium finger nails	Ultramicronized griseofulvin, 250 mg po bid × 6 months
Tinea versicolor	Zinc pyrithione shampoos, Imidazole creams, bid × 2–4 weeks
Candidiasis	Imidazole creams, bid until clearing and then one additional week Keep the affected area dry

men. The syndrome begins with a sudden onset of high fever, with headache, myalgia, vomiting, diarrhea, and hypotension. The clinical criteria for the syndrome include temperature more than 38.9°C, hypotension, and an erythroderma of the palms and soles, with subsequent desquamation. The mucous membranes may be inflamed. If organ failure occurs in three or more systems such as the hepatic, renal, cardiovascular, or neurologic systems, with the skin signs and no evidence for other causes of sepsis, the syndrome is established.

Treatment includes hospitalization, volume expanders, and appropriate antimicrobial drugs. Death can occur with sepsis and multiorgan failure.

Skin Infections: Fungal and Yeast

Dermatophyte infections, tinea versicolor, candidiasis, and erythrasma are common skin infections in this category.

Dermatophyte

The dermatophytic infections are the most common cutaneous fungal infections. These superficial infections occur in skin, hair, and nails, and usually are produced by Microsporum or Trichophyton organisms. Occasionally *Candida albicans* may produce this infection. All scaling eruptions should have a KOH examination performed to exclude a fungus or yeast infection. Hyphae or pseudo-Hyphae on the slide are diagnostic for dermatophyte or Candida infection.

Tinea corporis is a dermatophyte infection involving glabrous skin areas other than the hands, feet, and groin. This infection produces a red, scaly patch with sharp advancing borders and central clearing.

Tinea cruris is usually symmetrical, and develops on the upper, inner surfaces of the thighs. This infection spreads peripherally with central clearing. The disorder flares in hot weather or with occlusion. Itching is common and severe. Organisms that may produce this eruption are *T. rubrum, T. mentagrophytes,* or *Candida albicans.* When the eruption is produced by *C. albicans,* small pustules may be observed at the border of the lesions.

Tinea manum is usually a dry, scaly, erythematous eruption that involves the palms and may extend to the dorsal surface of the hands. *Trichophyton rubrum* usually produces this eruption. *T. rubrum* can cause a dry infection on both feet as well in a moccasin distribution. *T. mentagrophytes* infections generally produce an inflammatory, blistering eruption of hands and feet, and these lesions may become hemorrhagic.

Tinea faciale presents on the face with scaling red patches with a scaling border. It must be differentiated from sunlight eruptions, seborrheic eczema, and actinic skin damage.

Tinea pedis, or athlete's foot, is prevalent in warm weather and is recurrent and commonly undertreated. Fissures between the toes with maceration is a common presentation. An erythematous, scaling eruption that covers the soles is an additional type of infection. A third form presents with cutaneous blisters that occasionally are hemorrhagic.

Tinea unguium, i.e., onychomycosis, an infection of the nails, is usually caused by a *T. rubrum, T. mentagrophytes,* or *E. floccosum* infection or by *C. albicans. Trichophyton mentagrophytes* produces an invasion of the surface of the nail plate, resulting in white patches. Other organisms such as *Trichophyton rubrum* and *C. albicans* produce a thick yellow-brown discoloration of the nails, with nail brittleness.

Tinea Versicolor

This exceedingly common superficial fungal infection is caused by a lipophilic yeast, *Pityrosporum orbiculare,* which resides on the scalp and on the skin of the chest and back. Lesions appear as macules with slight scales. The infected areas do not pigment in a normal manner; as a result, this infection is quite apparent in summer, producing a white or semitanned appearance in tanned persons. The lesions of tinea versicolor produce a gold fluorescence with the Wood's light examination. Diagnostic confirmation is easily made with a KOH preparation, following scraping with a scalpel blade or glass microscopic slide.

Candidiasis

Candidiasis (*C. albicans*) is a more common cutaneous infection today owing to the prevalence of immunosuppression. This organism, which resides in the intestinal tract and on mucosal surfaces, thrives on damaged skin and in a moist, alkaline environment. Candidiasis is commonly flared by antibiotic therapy, especially in persons with immune defects (e.g., leukemia, lymphoma, AIDS), or in persons on chemotherapy for inflammatory diseases. Severe atopic diseases, e.g., hay fever, asthma, and atopic dermatitis enhance this eruption. Iron deficiency anemia and mild diabetes also promote candidiasis.

Viral Infections of the Skin

Vesicular Disorders

Herpes Simplex The cutaneous lesions of herpes simplex infections are produced by: HSV-1 (most commonly oral-facial), and HSV-2 (commonly associated with genital infection). Each of these viral types can infect any skin area. Recurrence in the genital area from type 1 infection is less common than from type 2 infection.

Recurrent herpetic infection is the most common clinical presentation of HSV-1, since primary HSV-1 infections are frequently subclinical. This reactivation of the latent herpes virus HSV-1 may be flared by sunlight, trauma, or immunosuppression. The first symptom of recurrence is skin fullness and burning. This is followed by small blisters in 12 to 24 h. The eruption usually occurs in the same area and resolves in 7 to 14 days.

A systemic complication of recurrent herpes simplex infection is erythema multiforme, a serious bullous disorder. In individuals with atopic dermatitis, superimposed herpes simplex viral infection can occur as eczema herpeticum.

Recurrent herpes simplex infection is best treated with acyclovir (Zovirax), a purine nucleoside analog. Intravenous acyclovir is the treatment of choice in recurrent mucocutaneous herpes simplex infection in immunocompromised adults, and in severe primary genital herpes in nonimmunocompromised patients. Acyclovir taken orally is helpful in controlling the reactivation of the virus in the genital area. Recurrent herpes labialis should be managed with acyclovir in selected patients, especially in those patients developing erythema multiforme following this infection. Acyclovir should not be used during pregnancy unless the potential benefit justifies the potential risk to the fetus.

Herpes zoster, which is becoming more common, especially in immunosuppressed patients, is believed to develop with the reactivation of latent varicella virus. Following varicella (either overt or subclinical infection), the virus remains in a dormant state within sensory ganglia. This eruption may occur with normal immunity in middle-age or later. When the eruption occurs in individuals less than 40 years of age, immunosuppression with AIDS or other diseases should be suspected. Herpes zoster is best treated with oral acyclovir. Adequate hydration and pain relief are important as well as compresses for active blisters (Fig. 56-2).

Solid or Wart Lesions

Molluscum Contagiosum In this viral infection, papules erupt anywhere on the skin surface, but particularly in areas that are scratched, i.e., face, hands,

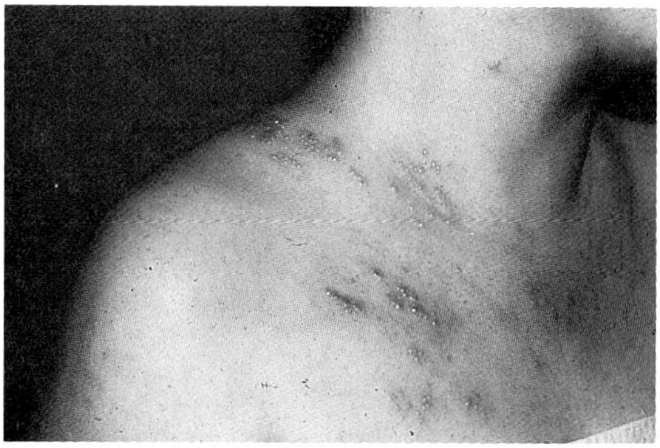

Figure 56-2 Herpes zoster. (See Color Plate 2.)

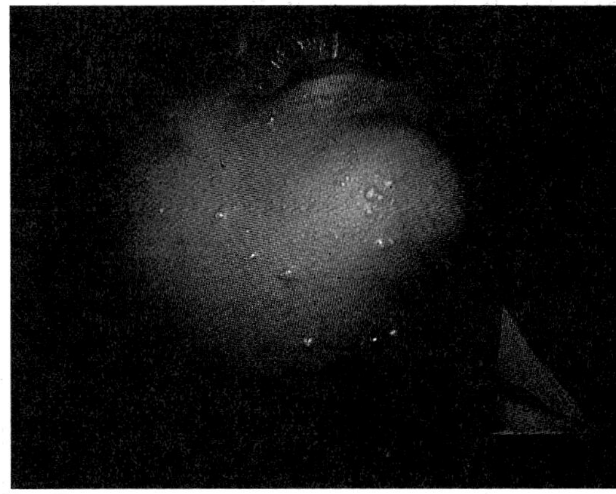

Figure 56-3 Molluscum contagiosum. (See Color Plate 3.)

and genital region. Molluscum contagiosum frequently is transmitted by sexual contact, and it may be quite extensive in the immunosuppressed patient and in patients with the atopic diseases. The lesions erupt as papules after an incubation period of 2 to 7 weeks. These tiny papules grow to a final diameter of 2 to 5 mm. Occasionally, large lesions are seen. A curetted lesion can be examined with the microscope after a Wright stain has been utilized. A positive preparation has a characteristic inclusion body, which establishes the diagnosis. The best therapy is local curettage or cryosurgery. Gentle evacuation of the lesion with an 18 gauge needle and/or a chalazion curette also can be helpful (Fig. 56-3).

Warts Caused by Human Papilloma Viruses The classic "warts" occur with the highest incidence in childhood or the teenage years, but are not uncommon among young adults. The clinical course is unpredictable, with the duration usually less than 3 years. Immunosuppressed patients, especially those who have undergone transplantation, are particularly susceptible to this eruption. Local trauma allows viral implantation, particularly on the fingers, the plantar surfaces of the feet, and the genitalia.

The causative agent, human papillomavirus (HPV), is a spherical DNA virus 50 mm in diameter. The human papillomavirus is host- and tissue-specific. There are more than 30 different types of HPV. Certain HPV infections have malignant potential. Spontaneous remission is immunologic in nature.

The phenotypical appearance of warts depends on the location as well as secondary lesions, such as hyperpigmentation and scarring. The common verruca vulgaris presents as an elevated papule or nodule with a hyperkeratotic verrucous surface. Plane or linear lesions may occur in areas of trauma, especially on the face and on lower extremities in women who shave their legs.

Wart destruction is the usual therapy. Liquid nitrogen freezing is the most useful technique in wart therapy. The lesion is frozen until the wart and a surrounding thin rim of normal-appearing skin turn white. A blister usually occurs in 24 to 48 h, followed by healing within 3 weeks. Cryotherapy may produce cutaneous nerve damage, scarring, and/or pigment loss or gain. Patients should be informed of this possibility. Freezing warts on the lower legs is not recommended because of the scarring potential.

Mild electrodesiccation and curettage can be useful in removing small warts from the skin surface. Caution again is important since these physical modalities may produce scarring and other side effects as listed above. It is important that the physician does not overtreat a lesion that usually will resolve without treatment in most patients.

Arthropod Bite Eruptions

Arthropod bites and stings by insects are common and produce many types of skin lesions. These lesions are papular, urticarial, or nodular in type (Fig. 56-4). The immediate effect of a sting is pain. In some patients, symptoms from bites and stings are related to scratching the area of the bite with the release of toxins. Later effects are usually allergic. Insects can transmit a variety of infections, including Rocky Mountain spotted fever, Lyme disease, and Ehrlichiosis.

Most patients recognize the stinging or burning pain of an insect bite, including erythema and the edema that results. Most bites occur on exposed areas, especially the face and extremities. The lesions usually are red papules or nodules with a central opening in the epidermis. The best treatment includes eliminating the insect exposure and a low strength topical steroid cream, plus a topical antibiotic if infection is suspected. Oral antihistamines can be very helpful in reducing itch.

Pediculosis

Pediculosis is caused by sucking lice. These include: *Pediculus humanus* var. capitis (head louse); *P. humanus* var. corporis (body louse); and *Phthirius pubis* (pubic or crab louse). Each of these can produce an infestation.

Body lice are most common in adults while head lice occur more often in children. Pubic and crab louse infestations usually occur in adults and are sexually transmitted. Patients with pubic lice should have other venereal diseases excluded. The adult louse attaches to the hair, and nits are distributed on these hairs. The pubic crab lice may also involve the eyebrows and eyelashes. Pruritus is extreme. The diagnosis of this infestation is frequently made by the patient. Topical therapy with lindane or permethrin is indicated.

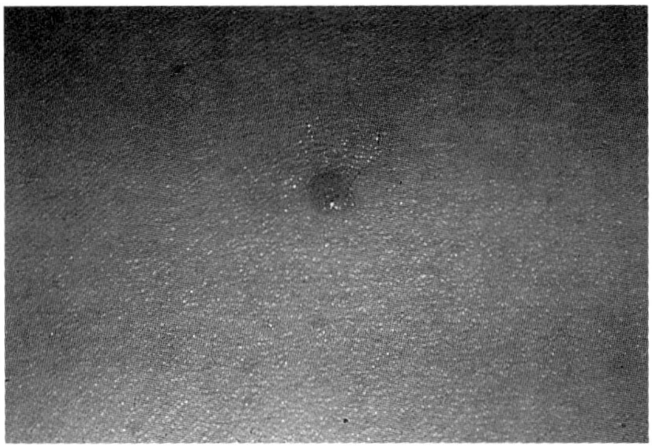

Figure 56-4 Insect bite. (See Color Plate 4.)

Scabies

This disorder is caused by a small mite, *Sarcoptes scabiei.* Scabies occurs in individuals in all socioeconomic groups. The disease is spread by physical contact.

The female mite, after burrowing into the stratum corneum, deposits eggs in these burrows. The larvae emerge in three to five days and mature in about two weeks. With continued propagation of the organism, the infestation can persist indefinitely. The skin lesions are papules, excoriations, and burrows. The marked pruritus usually occurs at night.

The diagnosis is established by a mineral oil preparation from fresh skin scrapings. The papules and excoriations can mimic other skin conditions associated with pruritus, e.g., atopic dermatitis, contact dermatitis, or other arthropod bites. The best therapies are 1% lindane (Kwell) lotion and 5% permethrin (Elimite) cream. A single application is applied from neck to toe, and it is washed off the next morning. One application is recommended. Multiple applications of lindane may produce neurotoxicity.

Sexually Transmitted Diseases: Genital Ulcers

An extensive discussion of sexually transmitted diseases can be found in Chap. 25. The dermatologic manifestations of sexually transmitted diseases are discussed below.

Syphilis

Genital ulcers suggest venereal disease (i.e., syphilis, herpes, chancroid, or granuloma inguinale).

Syphilis is caused by the spirochete *Treponema pallidum.* It can be detected in most of the primary and secondary skin lesions by darkfield examination. The most common mode of transmission is sexual contact. HIV infection must be excluded with any ulcerative sexually transmitted disease since, in addition to the fact that individuals with one sexually transmitted disease are at greater risk to have another, ulcer formation enhances the chance for this infection.

Syphilis is divided into three stages. Primary syphilis, a chancre with small ulcers, develops in one to four weeks after contact with an infected source. Regional lymphadenopathy is present.

The secondary lesion, a papulosquamous lesion without ulcer, begins 2 to 12 weeks after onset of the chancre. Secondary lesions involve the body and the feet and hands, especially the ventral surface (Fig. 56-5). Ulcers may be present on mucous membranes of the labial or buccal mucosa with secondary syphilis. The patient with these cutaneous features may have toxic symptoms, i.e., fever and malaise, as well as nontender lymphadenopathy. Secondary syphilis can produce alopecia. Condylomata lata, with papules and nodules found in intertriginous areas in the perineum, are very contagious. Tertiary syphilis, occurring two years after the primary infection, is rare today because of the initial use of antibiotic agents.

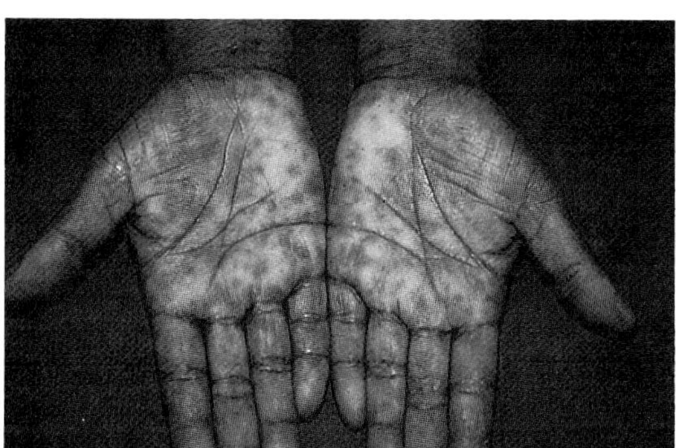

Figure 56-5 Secondary syphilis. (See Color Plate 5.)

Herpes Progenitalis

Primary genital herpes occurs following an incubation period of three to seven days. Localized burning or paresthesia is followed by a typical eruption of grouped vesicles on the genitalia, followed by ulcer formation. Constitutional symptoms and lymphadenopathy occur with the primary infection. Healing occurs over a two- to three-week period. Secondary lesions are common, and heal within two weeks. Recurrent attacks become less frequent and less severe as times passes. Sexual contact should not occur while lesions are present on the skin or mucous membranes. Viral shedding occurs in some individuals after the resolution of all active lesions.

Chancroid

Chancroid is an infectious disease of the genitalia caused by a gram-negative bacillus, *Hemophilus ducreyi.* It is characterized by painful, nonindurated ulcers that develop after an incubation period of three to five days. Multiple lesions are common. A positive diagnosis requires the demonstration of the organism by means of smears or culture. Smears are taken after cleansing a lesion with normal saline, and securing material from the ulcer border. The sample is applied to a glass slide, heat-fixed, and then Gram stained. Clusters of gram-negative bacilli establish and confirm the diagnosis. It is difficult to culture the organism. Lymphadenopathy is present. The simultaneous presence of syphilis and/or HIV should always be excluded in these patients.

Lymphogranuloma Venereum

This sexually transmitted disease is caused by *Chlamydia trachomatis,* an intracellular parasite. The primary lesion is a small papule that rapidly ulcerates. Lymphadenopathy is present and prominent.

Granuloma Inguinale

Granuloma inguinale is a slowly progressive ulcerative disease caused by a gram-negative bacillus with features similar to Klebsiella. The disease begins as a papule or ulcer. Ulcers enlarge and spread from the labia minora to the inguinal region or perineum (Table 56-6).

Condyloma Acuminatum

Condyloma acuminatum, a wart variant, occurs as a fleshy, papillomatous growth on genital skin and mucous membranes.

Common Drug Reactions

For an in-depth discussion of this issue, the reader is referred to Chap. 66. The discussion of drug reactions in this chapter focuses on dermatologic manifestations.

Eruptions may occur in the skin and on mucous membranes following systemically administered drugs used either for establishing a diagnosis or for therapy. The eruption usually is not related to a therapeutic effect of the drug. The clinician must decide how the patient was exposed to the drug and which of many possible drugs is producing the eruption. The clinical presentation and proposed mechanism for each drug reaction will be helpful in deciding whether the drug should be discontinued.

TABLE 56-6 Sexually Transmitted Diseases: Genital Ulcers

Diagnosis	Organism	Diagnostic Methods
Genital herpes	*Herpes simplex*	Culture or Tzanck prep
Primary and secondary syphilis	*Treponema pallidum*	Dark field or immunofluorescence
Chancroid	*H. ducreyi*	Gram stain and culture from lesion; no aspiration
Granuloma inguinale	*Granulomatis donovani*	Donovan bodies: material from lesion edge Wright or Giemsa stain
Lymphogranuloma venereum	*C. trachomatis*	Culture from urethra, cervix, node, or rectum

The morphology of a drug eruption may resemble many other skin diseases. A drug may produce one or several different primary lesions. A drug can produce a localized urticarial response in one patient, while in another person a blistering eruption may occur.

Topical or intradermal skin testing is not reliable except in the cases where penicillin allergy is suspected.

Anaphylaxis, a type I immunologic reaction, as a clinical syndrome can include urticaria, angioedema, laryngeal edema with hoarseness and stridor and advancement to cardiovascular collapse. Severe bronchospasm may occur. This eruption can occur within a few minutes after a drug is administered.

Serum sickness typically develops 8 to 12 days after exposure to a drug, and is characterized by fever, urticaria or vasculitis, lymphadenopathy, splenomegaly, arthritis or arthralgias, and nephritis.

Delayed hypersensitivity, a type IV immunoresponse, may produce a maculopapular eruption that can evolve into an exfoliative dermatitis. These reactions may result from systemic administration of a drug to which a patient has been sensitized by previous topical administration; thus, this type of reaction has the characteristics of systemic allergic contact dermatitis.

Among the most severe drug reactions are toxic epidermal necrolysis (TEN) and/or erythema multiforme (Fig. 56-6). This usually begins as a macular erythema and progresses to bulla formation and desquamation of skin, leaving a raw, denuded surface.

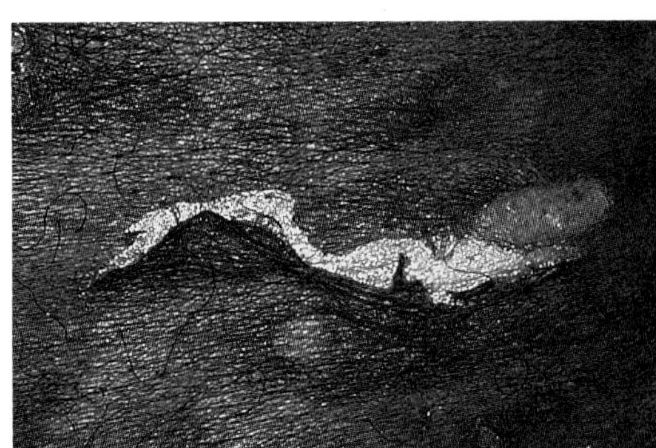

Figure 56-6 Toxic epidermal erythema multiforme. (See Color Plate 6.)

Mucosal erosions and conjunctivitis also may be present. Loss of fluid and electrolytes is a significant problem. Other evidence for systemic toxicity includes fever, lethargy, vomiting, and diarrhea. Death occurs in a high percentage of patients (25 to 30 percent), unless early intervention with grafting occurs. Toxic epidermal necrolysis must be distinguished from staphylococcal scalded skin syndrome (SSSS). A skin biopsy can be very helpful.

Fixed drug eruptions, lichenoid eruptions, and vasculitis are less common manifestations of drug hypersensitivity (see Table 56-7).

Photosensitivity (Phototoxicity and Photoallergy)

Many chemicals and drugs can combine with components of skin and allow the skin to respond excessively to ultraviolet light. This can result in a photosensitivity response—either phototoxicity or photoallergy. The usual wavelengths of light responsible for these reactions are between 290 to 400 nm. The 290 to 320 nm range is UVB, the spectrum producing sunburn and skin cancers and some photoallergic reactions; the 320 to 400 nm range UVA light

TABLE 56-7 Drug Eruptions

Signs and Symptoms	Common Causes or Stimulus	Therapy
Urticaria angioedema	Many drugs	Discontinue suspected drugs Hospitalization if anaphylaxis occurs Subcutaneous epinephrine Systemic steroids Antihistamines
Maculopapular	Many drugs	Discontinue offending drugs Cool or tepid baths Antihistamines for pruritus Topical steroids for severe eruptions
Exfoliative erythroderma	Many drugs	Stop suspected drug Topical corticosteroids Systemic steroids in severe cases
Fixed drug eruption	Barbiturates Tetracyclines Sulfonamides Anovulatory drugs	Discontinue suspected drug Topical steroid creams
Erythema multiforme	Sulfonamides Penicillins Many other drugs	Stop suspected drug or drugs Systemic steroids for severe cases Hospitalization
Toxic epidermal necrolysis	Allopurinol Sulfonamides Phenytoin	Do not use systemic steroids Stop suspected drug Hospitalization; skilled nursing care Skin grafting
Lichenoid eruption	Gold, thiazides, Beta-blockers	Antihistamines Topical corticosteroids Systemic steroids for severe cases
Lupus erythematosus	Related to manifestation of photosensitivity or immunologic disorders	Protection from ultraviolet light Local steroids for cutaneous manifestations
Vasculitis	Allopurinol Penicillins Sulfonamides	Discontinue offending drug

is responsible for most phototoxic and photoallergy drug eruptions.

Phototoxicity

This drug eruption is dose-related. The erythema is similar to an exaggerated sunburn reaction, occurring 6 to 8 h after exposure to sunlight. Tetracycline and many other drugs can produce phototoxicity in some patients.

Photoallergy

This drug reaction, which is secondary to a drug or chemical plus ultraviolet light, is due to an immune mechanism. Only small quantities of the drug are necessary to elicit a response. Photoallergic reactions can occur after topical as well as systemic administration of certain drugs. Photoallergic drug reactions have resulted from exposures to sulfonamides, chlorpromazine, sulfonylureas, and many other drugs.

Polymorphic light eruption is a photosensitivity skin eruption occurring with sun exposure; it is immunologically mediated (Fig. 56-7). It can be produced by ultraviolet light of any wavelength. The skin lesions appear within a few hours after sun exposure, and the eruption is not related to the length of exposure to the sun. Pruritus is common, and the eruption usually occurs with first sun exposure in the spring. Edema, red papules, vesicles, or eczematous lesions are the usual skin manifestations (see Table 56-8).

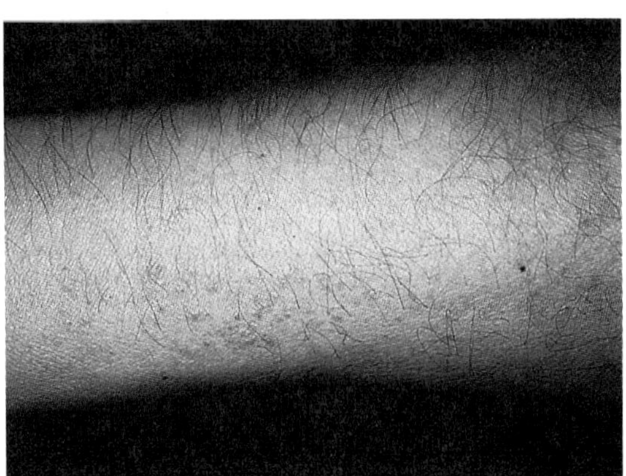

Figure 56-7 Polymorphic light eruption. (See Color Plate 7.)

Eczematous Dermatoses

"Dermatitis" or "inflammation of the skin" is synonymous with the term "eczema," which refers to boiling. Eczema is characterized by a red papulovesicular eruption, with oozing and crusting, followed by scaling and thick skin (lichenification), with or without pigment loss. This eruption is markedly pruritic. The common forms of eczema are contact dermatitis, seborrheic dermatitis, atopic dermatitis, and stasis dermatitis.

Contact Dermatitis

Contact dermatitis is induced by a contact with an antigenic substance or irritant. Irritants, if applied in

TABLE 56-8 Photosensitivity Diseases

Type	Disease	Flare Factor	Therapy
Genetic	Erythropoietic photoporphyria	Sun	Sun screens Beta carotene
Metabolic	Pellagra, sporadic porphyria, cutanea tarda	Alcohol/sun Drugs Hepatitis C	Niacin Phlebotomy and sun protection
Photoaggravated	Lupus erythematosus	UVB	Sun screens Topical steroids
Dermatoses	Atopic dermatitis or lichen planus	UVB	Sun screens and topical steroids
Immunologic	Polymorphic light eruption	UVA UVB	Sun protection Topical steroids PUVA for hyposensitization

sufficient concentrations, will produce a dermatitis in any individual. Irritant dermatitis can be a dermatitis or a minimal burn. Allergic contact dermatitis is a T-cell mediated immune response to an allergen following a previous sensitizing contact with the chemical. Many chemicals and drugs can be both irritants and allergic sensitizers. The eczematous response in allergic contact dermatitis is vesicles or bullae at sites of exposure to the allergen.

Rhus dermatitis is usually produced by poison ivy, oak, or sumac, and is the most common form of contact dermatitis (Fig. 56-8). The pattern of vesiculation is produced as the oleoresin from the plant strokes the skin. This resin attaches directly to the skin; at that point, oil can be spread by the fingers. The antigen is similar in poison ivy, poison oak, and poison sumac. After the appearance of the dermatitis, the blister fluid from the lesion is not antigenic to other skin areas in the patient, and is not transferrable to other sensitive individuals.

Patients must be questioned at length about the history of any form of dermatitis. Other common causes of allergic contact dermatitis include nickel, potassium dichromate, paraphenylenediamine, rubber compounds, and formalin. To establish the cause when the history is nondiagnostic, careful skin testing should be done after the acute eruption has subsided. This should be accomplished when the disease has cleared and when the patient has discontinued corticosteroids. Distinguishing irritant from allergic contact dermatitis is difficult. This problem frequently requires the help of an expert in dermatology. Skin biopsy generally is not helpful, except where psoriasis is to be excluded.

Figure 56-8 Contact dermatitis from poison ivy. (See Color Plate 8.)

Therapy should begin with removal of the offending allergen. Topical soaks with cool water, or Burow's 1/40 solution, and shake lotions are helpful. Prednisone, 1.0 mg/kg of body weight, for 4 to 5 days, with tapering over a 5- to 10-day period can also be very helpful. Antihistamines, can be used to provide relief from itching, and antibiotics may be necessary for secondary infections.

Hand Eczema

This eruption occurs anywhere on the hands or feet, and is usually a localized form of either atopic or contact eczematous dermatitis. A history of atopy in the patient or her family may be helpful in determining the type of hand eczema—i.e., atopic or contact. The hands and feet may become sensitive to excess water, detergents, or other chemicals. The relationship to emotions is not clear. Allergic contact dermatitis may produce the eruption or flare underlying atopic dermatitis. Bacterial and yeast infections should be excluded in evaluating the condition. Chronically inflamed skin, especially when exposed to excess moisture and irritants, becomes dry and produces painful fissures.

The acute eruption is treated similarly to contact dermatitis. A chronic eczematous eruption that has not cleared with conservative topical therapy is best handled by a specialist in dermatology.

Seborrheic Dermatitis

Seborrheic dermatitis or eczema involves the regions of skin where many sebaceous glands are present. It is a common condition and may produce regional scaling and mild exfoliation. It is often flared during a severe illness. Although seborrhea is associated with hypersecretion of sebum and growth of *Pityrosporum orbiculase* in most patients, there are individuals with a high output of sebum and no dermatitis. The therapy for this condition depends on the location of the eczema (see Table 56-9).

TABLE 56-9 Seborrheic Dermatitis

Location	Treatment
Scalp	Increase frequency of shampooing with shampoo containing selenium sulfide or zinc pyrithione Shampoo 2–3 times per week Low strength topical steroid solution once daily for a few days, then 2–3 days per week
Face	1% Hydrocortisone cream, 2 × day for one week, then once daily × 1 week, then discontinue Avoid applying around the eyes
Ears, neck, chest, and back	Hydrocortisone cream, bid for 1 week, then daily × 1 week, then discontinue
Skin folds	1% Hydrocortisone cream, plus miconazole, or clotrimazole cream if *C. albicans* infection exists

Stasis Dermatitis

Stasis dermatitis is secondary to venous hypertension. Edema and infection are flare factors for the eruption. Diseases that produce edema and venous stasis, i.e., congestive heart failure, renal disease, and cirrhosis, flare the eruption in the susceptible individual. The medial surface of the lower leg is the most common site for the eruption. Fungal infection must be excluded by a KOH preparation and culture. Contact dermatitis to medications is common. Treatment should be directed toward reducing the edema and inflammation. Low-strength topical steroids, applied twice daily for 2 weeks, are helpful. Systemic prednisone may be required for the severe form of this dermatitis. Once treatment has been completed the prednisone should be tapered gradually over a 2-week period and discontinued. Support hose, limiting the standing position, and weight reduction are usually necessary for managing the chronic form of this eruption.

Atopic Dermatitis

Atopic dermatitis is a form of eczema that can occur in all age groups. It is characterized by severe itching and a cutaneous papulovesicular eruption flared by scratching. The scratching can induce the physical findings; the excoriations and bleeding promote bacterial infections, followed by oozing and weeping and more infection. The eruption occurs as a local or generalized dermatitis. The flexural folds of skin and the hands and feet are typical locations for the eruption.

This eczema usually occurs in persons with a personal or family history of asthma, hay fever, eczema, or urticaria. Patients with atopic dermatitis have increased sweating on the face, hands, and feet. There is increased itching, often followed by excessive scratching. The eruption often occurs from exposure to heat, sun, simple trauma or stress. Severe skin infections may complicate this dermatitis.

The diagnosis of atopic dermatitis is established by the recognition of the cutaneous features (Fig. 56-9) as well as by establishing an association with other components of the atopic state (asthma, hay fever, sinusitis) in the patient or the family members.

Most patients do not require hospitalization except during a severe flare of the dermatosis, which is usually followed by a severe secondary bacterial infection or exfoliative dermatitis. These patients often are carriers of *Staphylococcus aureus* in the nasopharynx and on the skin; they also are at high risk for developing a generalized viral infection when exposed to the herpes simplex virus.

The management of this disorder should include reducing or eliminating all flare factors, especially dry skin and infection. The elimination of some foods, inhalant antigens, and other environmental

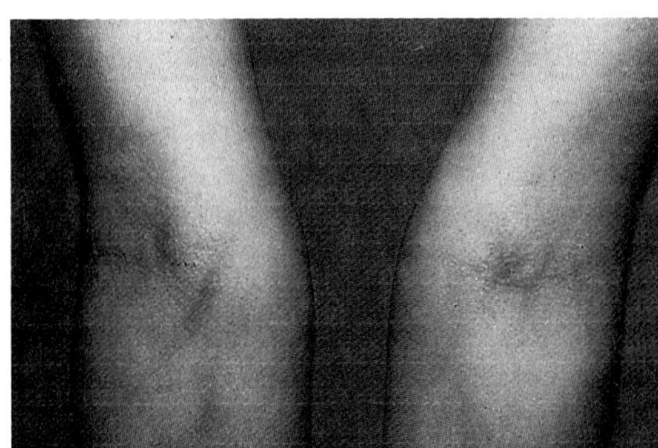

Figure 56-9 Atopic dermatitis. (See Color Plate 9.)

antigens can be helpful. House dust can aggravate the condition in some individuals with atopic dermatitis, and some patients will clear the eruption with a change in their home environment.

Specific therapy for the dermatitis includes topical as well as systemic medication. Good topical therapy is most important because local therapy may prevent the need for systemic therapy, particularly systemic steroids.

Halogenated corticosteroid preparations are the most effective form of topical therapy. The delivery system in which the steroid is placed is quite important. A moisturizing agent, such as a hydrophilic or emollient cream to prevent dryness, is helpful. Emollients should be applied after each bath or water exposure. Soaps should be avoided if possible; particularly, they should not be placed on red inflamed or fissured skin. The topical application of emollients containing a low concentration of coal tar can be helpful in the management of chronic, noninflamed atopic dermatitis.

If topical therapy is inadequate, light therapy or systemic therapy should be considered. The chronic unstable form of the eruption should be managed by a specialist in this disorder when light therapy or systemic therapy is required. Immunotherapy with inhalant extracts is not helpful.

Urticaria

Urticaria is a common and troublesome pruritic eruption with wheals or generalized swellings in the skin or mucous membranes. It is generally a transient eruption, but it can be quite severe and very symptomatic and chronic (Fig. 56-10).

Some agents can produce urticaria through a direct release of histamine or other mast cell mediators; examples include foods such as shellfish, tomatoes, strawberries and chocolate, and drugs, such as aspirin. Allergic urticaria is a type I, immunoglobulin E-mediated reaction.

The primary lesion in urticaria is a wheal, or red swelling, which may be annular (ring-shaped) or flat. Urticaria due to pressure may produce large and deep lesions with erythema. Itching or stinging or slight burning pain are the main symptoms, and each

Figure 56-10 Urticaria. (See Color Plate 10.)

lesion may last as long as 24 h. New wheals come in crops as old lesions disappear. The eruption will frequently occur where there is pressure from clothing. The waistline is a common site.

Acute urticaria is 6 weeks or less in duration; urticaria that lasts longer than 6 weeks is considered chronic. There are several different forms of urticaria (see Table 56-10).

Skin Diseases with Blisters

Bullous Pemphigoid

Bullous pemphigoid usually occurs in persons over age 60. This is a bullous eruption produced by an immune reaction involving the basement membranes. Bullous pemphigoid typically presents with large (2 to 5 cm diameter), firm bullae on a red base on the trunk and extremities (Fig. 56-11). They also may arise on otherwise normal-appearing skin. Mucous membrane lesions rarely occur. They are frequently seen in patients with pemphigus vulgaris.

A related disorder that occurs in elderly patients is benign mucous membrane or cicatricial pemphigoid. In this disease, bullae occur with frequency on the oral mucosa and on the eyelids. Skin involvement is less common. This disease causes scarring, which may occur on other mucous membrane surfaces, such as the vagina, larynx, or esophagus.

TABLE 56-10 Urticaria: Therapy

Type	Cause	Therapy
Urticaria (acute and chronic)	Drugs NSAIDs Food and food additives Insect bites Infection Emotions Physical trauma Systemic diseases	Nonsedating antihistamine therapy
Cold urticaria	Produced by cold environment	Cyproheptadine
Cholinergic urticaria	Induced by exercise challenges	Reduce hot showers Cool compresses Nonsedating antihistamine therapy
Solar urticaria	Exposure to defined wavelengths of sunlight	Nonsedating antihistamine therapy
Aquagenic urticaria	Tap water	Avoid water UVA light Nonsedating antihistamine therapy
Angioedema	Drugs or hereditary deficiency Cholinesterase inhibitor deficiency	Stop drugs for hereditary[a] Angioedema Avoid trauma

[a]Should be managed by rheumatologist or dermatologist

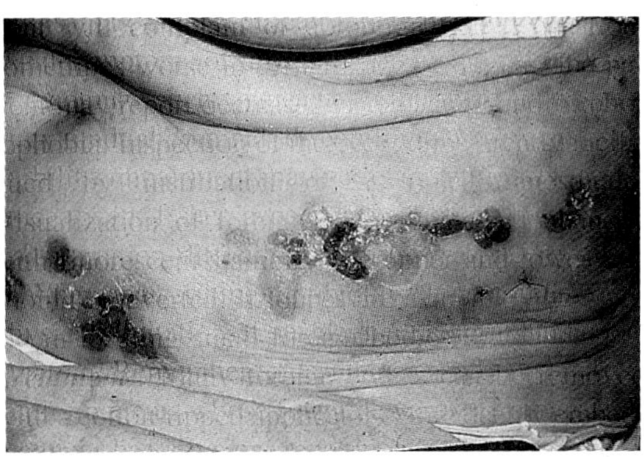

Figure 56-11 Bullous pemphigoid, flared by herpes zoster. (See Color Plate 11.)

The lesions in bullous pemphigoid and benign mucous membrane pemphigoid differ from pemphigus vulgaris because the blisters are tense and not easily broken. The patients usually are healthy. The cutaneous blisters in bullous pemphigoid are similar to the lesions seen in erythema multiforme, although erythema multiforme is not chronic as is bullous pemphigoid.

Bullous pemphigoid is treated with systemic corticosteroids. The usual dose is to 60 to 80 mg of prednisone by mouth each day. This dose is reduced to 5 to 10 mg over a 30-day period. In some patients, a low dose of oral prednisone is required for several months. If possible, a dermatologist should evaluate all patients with chronic bullous eruptions and should supervise their management.

Erythema Multiforme

In erythema multiforme, the blisters are tense and the skin is inflamed. This inflammatory reaction can be induced by several antigens. The severe forms of erythema multiforme are accompanied by constitutional symptoms, e.g., fever, malaise, and, frequently, upper respiratory symptoms. The initial lesion is a red macule, wheal, or an edematous papule. These lesions usually evolve to form an iris or target lesion.

Erythema multiforme is symmetrical and usually erupts on the palms and soles, on the dorsal area of the hands and feet, and on the arms and legs. The trunk is involved when the disease is generalized. Involvement of mucous membranes usually is present. The eyes, nose, mouth, rectum, and genitalia may be involved.

Lesions erupt in crops over a 2- to 4-week period. Eye involvement with blisters on the conjunctivae may occur, and corneal ulceration may be a problem. Toxic epidermal necrolysis, a variant of erythema multiforme, may evolve from erythema multiforme.

Many antigens trigger erythema multiforme. They include bacterial, viral, and fungal infections, drugs, the collagen vascular diseases, inflammatory bowel disease and malignancy. The diagnosis depends upon the clinical recognition of the lesions. A drug history, chest film, and bacterial and viral cultures are a part of the evaluation process.

The best therapy is to eliminate the underlying cause and correct any abnormality produced by the disease. Any infection should be treated, and suspected drugs should be discontinued. Mild cases require only local treatment, such as compresses for blisters (1:20 Burow's solution, applied for 15 to 30 min qid). With a severe eruption, fluid and electrolyte balance must be maintained. Viscous xylocaine, applied locally, may help the patient to eat. This medication should be rinsed over the mucous membranes for about five minutes and then removed from the mouth. Systemic steroids should be reserved for those patients who are extremely toxic, and should be given early in the disease process. If toxic epidermal necrolysis follows (Fig. 56-6), the systemic steroids should be withdrawn.

Papulosquamous Disease and Ichthyosis

Psoriasis

Psoriasis is a papulosquamous eruption with a papule as the primary lesion. These papules are thickened and red, with silver scales that bleed when the scales are physically removed. The degree of thickness of the scale is greatest when the disease is chronic but minimal when the disease is active and inflammatory. The following help establish the diagnosis: 1. a positive family history; 2. a history of severe scalp eruption as an infant, with or without a severe diaper dermatitis; 3. prominent dandruff in the adolescent and adult; 4. nail changes including pinhead-size pits, brown spots or oil drops, and subungal keratin deposition beneath a loose nail edge; 5. genital and intergluteal eruption; and, 6. symmetrical disease. A history of a flare of the disease with an infection, such as streptococcal pharyngitis or a *C. albicans* infection in the mouth, suggests psoriasis. Several drugs flare psoriasis, including lithium and beta-blocking agents (Fig. 56-12). Psoriasis must be differentiated from chronic eczema when the eruption involves the hands and feet. Psoriasis is frequently associated with arthritis.

In summary, a clinical diagnosis is not difficult to establish if the patient has: 1. symmetrical papulosquamous lesions, elbows and knees; 2. scalp and nail involvement; and 3. intergluteal and genital involvement. A biopsy of the skin may be helpful in some individuals when the hands are involved or where disease is minimal.

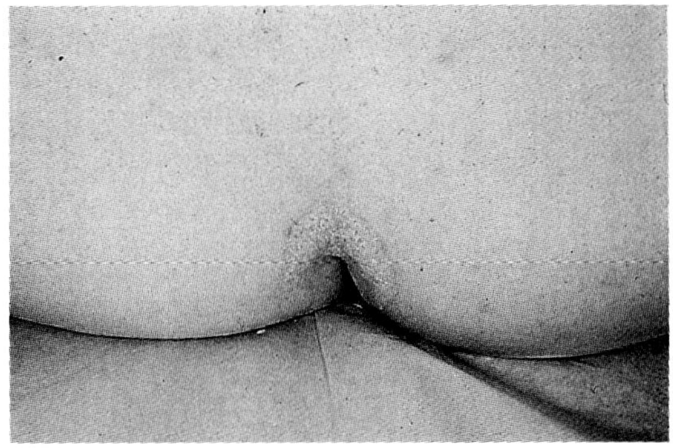

Figure 56-12 Psoriasis. (See Color Plate 12.)

Treatment sometimes is difficult. The early management of this chronic eruption should include a discussion with the patient regarding the diagnosis and the morbidity of the disease. This should include: a discussion of the relationship of anxiety in aggravating the illness, the noncontagious nature of the eruption, and the possible impact on the family. Psoriasis is a dynamic disease process with fluctuations of the eruption throughout the patient's life (see Table 56-11).

The therapy of psoriasis can be enhanced if special attention is given to the control of infections of the tracheobronchial tree, sinuses, throat, and vagina. The eradication of any *C. albicans* infection frequently is more helpful than topical therapy in controlling psoriasis lesions.

The use of any therapy for psoriasis and other generalized chronic skin disease requires an understanding of the dynamic aspects of the inflammatory process, training with the disease, and experience with the therapeutic modalities. This can ensure the correct use and enhance the safety of the therapy. Any unstable inflammatory skin process will usually require the consultative expertise of a dermatologist, especially when therapies require UV light, retinoids, systemic steroids, and other chemotherapeutic agents.

TABLE 56-11 Psoriasis: Therapy

Type	Location	Management
Localized plaque psoriasis	Elbows, knees, scalp	Potent topical steroids used intermittently[a] 3% Salicylic acid ointment UVB light with dermatologist supervision Vitamin D_3 preparations (recently released)
Guttate generalized	Abdomen, back, arms, legs	Oral antibiotics when indicated for infection Topical steroids (as above) UV light (with dermatologist supervision)
Erythroderma exfoliative dermatitis	All skin areas	Etretinate[b], Methotrexate (MTX)[c] or systemic steroids Consultation and supervision by a dermatologist
Pustular psoriasis, localized	Hands, feet	Etretinate[b] (retinoid) Topical steroids Consultation with dermatologist
Pustular psoriasis, generalized	Entire body	MTX[c] Etretinate[b] Consultation with dermatologist

[a]Intermittent use for 2 weeks with a rest period of 7–14 days (use less potent steroids in rest period).

[b]A teratogen with a long half-life; it should not be used in women with childbearing capability or future capability.

[c]Hepatotoxic. Should be monitored by a physician with expertise in MTX use.

Pityriasis Rosea

This is an acute, self-limited disease characterized by papulosquamous lesions on the body and extremities. The cause of pityriasis rosea is unknown, although a viral etiology has been suspected because of a preceding fever or upper respiratory symptoms.

The eruption occurs in males and females, usually between the ages of 20 and 40. Fever, cough, or malaise may occur, but most patients are asymptomatic. The initial eruption is a round or oval scaly lesion, the herald patch. A generalized eruption occurs with smaller lesions on the trunk. The lesions generally disappear in six to eight weeks. Postinflammatory hyperpigmentation may occur. Recurrences are rare. The treatment of pityriasis rosea is symptomatic. A severe eruption with intense itch will respond to nonsedating antihistamine therapy.

Dry Skin and Ichthyosis

Patients with ichthyosis have very dry skin. Disorders in this category are associated with a retention of stratum corneum. There are four major types of inherited ichthyosis. The most common inherited form of the eruption is dominant ichthyosis vulgaris. Acquired, noninherited ichthyosis is seen as a manifestation of nutritional deficiency, sarcoidosis, AIDS, or an underlying malignancy.

In ichthyosis vulgaris, fine scaling occurs on the trunk and extremities, usually on the lower legs. Follicular hyperkeratosis is present over the lateral surface of the extremities, with increased palmar markings noted. The eruption is worse in dry winter weather. Many of these patients have an atopic disorder, e.g., hay fever or atopic dermatitis.

Many patients are helped by symptomatic therapy with emollients and bath oils. Emollient creams and lotions, free of allergic sensitizers, should be applied after a bath or shower while the skin is moist. Lotions, creams, or emollients containing alpha-hydroxy acids reduce dryness and improve skin texture and appearance.

Disorders of Pigmentation

Melasma

Melasma is a patchy form of overproduction of pigmentation occurring on the face. It occurs commonly in women who are pregnant or are taking oral contraceptives. Melasma is flared by sunlight.

Melasma can involve the forehead, face, upper lip, and chin. The pigmentation varies in intensity and shade related to the location of the pigment in the skin, i.e., epidermal-brown and dermal-gray. A Wood's light exam demonstrates superficial epidermal pigmentation. This eruption is difficult to manage. Experience with depigmenting agents is desirable. A 2% concentration of hydroquinone is frequently helpful. Sensitization can occur. Good sunscreens are absolutely necessary (15 to 30 SPF).

Vitiligo

Vitiligo is a hypopigmenting disorder that can produce severe cosmetic defect. This patchy eruption is characterized by smooth, complete depigmentation. Although the cause is unknown, there is evidence of an immune dysfunction. There is a familial tendency.

The pigment loss results in white macules, which involve extensor surfaces and are bilateral and symmetrical (Fig. 56-13). Depigmentation of the hair can occur. Depigmentation is noted in areas subjected to trauma including surgical trauma.

In persons with a dark complexion, vitiligo is especially noticeable, and results in a severe cosmetic problem. In persons with a fair complexion, vitiligo often is not as noticeable. The lesions will sunburn more easily than normal skin, and they never tan because of the loss of melanocytes. A Wood's light examination will demonstrate the difference between these lesions and postinflammatory hypopigmentation.

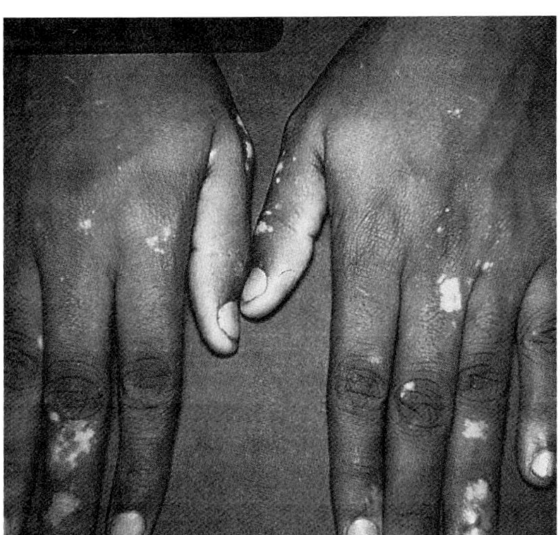

Figure 56-13 Vitiligo. (See Color Plate 13.)

The treatment of vitiligo is difficult, and the results are not entirely satisfactory. Depigmentation therapy for small areas of hyperpigmentation and PUVA therapy to stimulate new pigment production should be monitored by an expert in dermatology and light therapy.

Oral Mucous Membrane Lesions

Aphthous Stomatitis

Aphthous stomatitis (canker sores) are common recurrent painful erosions of the oral mucosa. Although the cause is unknown, trauma is a definite flare factor. Herpes simplex must be excluded as a cause of any recurrent group of small mouth ulcers, but most aphthous ulcers are not due to herpes simplex infections.

The typical lesion occurring on the tongue and buccal mucosa begins as a tender spot that evolves into a round, shallow ulcer, surrounded by erythema. Multiple lesions also can occur. The lesion generally is less than 1 cm in diameter. The pain in the lesion is quite severe, and new lesions are flared by rough foods and trauma from the teeth. A single ulcer will clear in ten to 14 days in most patients. Lesions similar to aphthous stomatitis occur with ulcerative colitis and Behçet's syndrome.

Topical steroid therapy, e.g., Kenalog in Orabase, is generally helpful in reducing pain with eating. Topical anesthetics can reduce the local pain. Mouth lesions produced by *C. albicans* infections are white patches with crusting; when the crust is removed, a red eroded area is noticed. Nystatin mouthwash four times per day is good therapy for oral Candida infections. Any indurated white patch, plaque, or nodule in the mouth requires a biopsy to exclude cancer.

Cheilitis

Cheilitis is an inflammatory dermatitis of the lips with mild exfoliation. The inflammation may be secondary to such skin diseases as psoriasis or atopic dermatitis, or it may be allergy or irritation. An allergic contact reaction to food, metals, or cosmetics such as lipsticks may be present. Angular cheilitis results from accumulation of moisture at the mouth angle with fissuring. Topical allergens must be identified. Low strength topical steroid preparations in an emolient base are helpful in managing an allergic cheilitis.

Acne

Acne Vulgaris

Acne vulgaris is not a diagnostic problem. A broad experience with the many topical and systemic preparations is helpful in managing this eruption. Adult sebaceous glands and follicles have wide openings on the skin surface, and the sebaceous lobules are large. Obstruction due to hyperkeratinization occurs in the follicular neck of the pilosebaceous unit. Sebum is continually being generated. In addition, the anaerobic bacteria *Propionibacterium acnes* in sebaceous follicles reproduce in large numbers. Good therapy is aimed at these changes.

Acne occurs in families. Testosterone is implicated in the flare of acne at puberty. Although the level of the hormone in the serum is not elevated, follicular hypersensitivity is present. Acne begins with closed comedones (usually white), and then proceeds to form pustules, nodules, or cysts over the face, neck, shoulders, chest, and back. Some patients have only nodulocystic acne from the beginning of the eruption; others have only open and closed comedones. Cystic disease is the most severe form; inflammatory nodules and deep cystic lesions scar.

Although most acne occurs in the adolescent, many cases begin in patients over 20. When papular acne develops in women during their late 20s and early 30s with no prior history of the disease, cosmetics, hormones, and stress should be suspected as flare factors. Acne often flares premenstrually. Drugs such as corticosteroids, phenytoin, and lithium can flare acne.

The therapeutic objective is to control the process until the condition enters a natural state of remission. The prognosis is good. An important management goal is patient education. She should recognize the chronicity of her condition, the flare factors, and should be motivated to manage the condition properly.

Retin-A cream is helpful in reducing hyperkeratinization in comedonal and papulopustular acne, as is benzoyl peroxide, 2.5 or 5% solution. Gentle washing with a gentle skin cleanser should be done only twice daily.

Topical antibiotics are also helpful agents. Antibiotics work by reducing numbers of *P. acnes*. Benzoyl peroxide, tetracycline, minocycline, erythromycin, and clindamycin, as topical preparations, are useful in the management of papulopustular acne.

Oral antibiotics are the most helpful systemic form of acne therapy. Tetracycline and erythromycin are commonly used. The dose depends on disease activity. The usual dose is 250 mg administered three or four times a day for 2 weeks, followed by 500 mg per day for 6 months. 1.5 to 2 g therapy, per day, may be necessary for the drug to be effective in the more severe nodulocystic forms of the disease.

Minocycline, a semisynthetic tetracycline derivative, can be given when resistance to tetracycline develops. The usual dose is 50 to 100 mg per day. Photosensitivity is less with minocycline therapy. Common side effects of minocycline include dizziness and pigmentation of the skin and mucous membranes. Pseudomembranous colitis can occur following any orally administered antibiotic.

The oral retinoid, Accutane, isotretinoin, is recommended only in managing severe nodulocystic acne resistant to other therapies. Pregnancy precautions are mandatory because of the teratogenic potential for this drug.

Rosacea (Acne Rosacea)

Rosacea is an inflammatory disease that affects adults. It commonly occurs in women over the age of 40. Although its cause is unknown, the eruption of rosacea is flared by many factors. Alcohol, coffee, tea, chocolate, and other foods and beverages are possible flare factors. Heat, rather than caffeine or beverage constituents, is responsible for the flushing associated with drinking hot liquids. Fluorinated corticosteroids applied to the face over several weeks may produce a rosacea-like eruption. The clinical presentation includes facial erythema, telangiectasia, and pustules. The most severe form of the eruption is associated with red nodules and cysts. The best therapy is to avoid all flare factors, especially heat. Topical antibiotics, erythromycin or metronidizole, are important treatments for rosacea. Oral tetracycline, 250 mg three or four times a day, is required in some patients to control this eruption, although the usual dose for this problem is 250 to 500 mg of tetracycline a day.

Hidradenitis Suppurativa

Hidradenitis suppurativa is a chronic, inflammatory eruption occurring in the axillae, groin, and buttocks. The clinical eruption appears as red nodules that become painful. The nodules are elongated, and may or may not form an abscess. Draining fistulous tracts may develop. Initial cultures are sterile, but secondary infection may occur due to *S. aureus*. Proteus and Pseudomonas organisms can be grown from many of these lesions. The disease is persistent. The medical treatment includes oral antibiotics—tetracycline, erythromycin, or the cephalosporins. The only cure is surgical excision of the lesions (Fig. 56-14).

Hair Loss

Alopecia Areata

Alopecia areata is a form of acute hair loss. It presents with patches of apparently complete hair loss, occurs without signs of inflammation, and without scarring. Hairs at the periphery of new patches can be easily plucked, and a clubbed hair root is noted with thinning of the hair shaft. There is usually spontaneous regrowth of hair after an interval of 2 to 6 months, and 90 percent of the hair is regrown in one year in most patients. Some clinical features indicate a poor prognosis for hair regrowth. These are extensive generalized and/or persistent hair loss, and a pattern of interlocking patches of alopecia involving the posterior scalp.

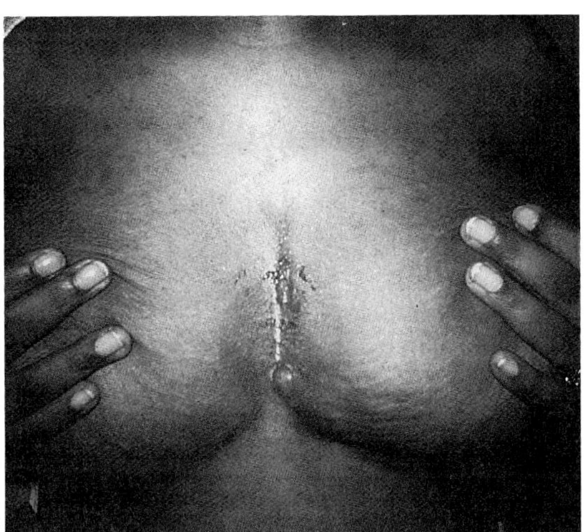

Figure 56-14 Hidradenitis suppurativa. (See Color Plate 14.)

The evaluation of treatment for alopecia areata is difficult because spontaneous remission is common. Oral corticosteroids for a short term may be considered in some cases of generalized hair loss, but their side effects should be discussed with the patient before using them. Topical corticosteroid therapy generally is not effective. Intralesional corticosteroid therapy can be helpful for a small patch of alopecia, but skin atrophy can occur. Reassurance is the best therapy for a single lesion.

Androgenic Alopecia

This form of alopecia occurs in both males and females. This condition is genetic, with the onset occurring in patients usually between 20 and 30 years of age. Androgenic alopecia is associated with a short anagen (growth phase) in the hair cycle, and hairs plucked from involved regions show a high proportion of telogen (resting) hairs. A biopsy may be useful in separating this condition from other forms of alopecia. Topical 2% minoxidil (Rogaine), applied bid, can be helpful in some patients. Long-term treatment is required, and the hair falls out when therapy is discontinued. Hair transplantation usually is not necessary.

Telogen Effluvium—Loss of Resting Hairs; Stress Alopecia

Telogen effluvium, loss of resting hairs, occurs after pregnancy. Other stressful events may cause this form of hair loss. There is an excellent prognosis for hair regrowth. Telogen effluvium occurs when a higher than normal proportion of scalp hairs enter the telogen or resting phase. Several months of shedding may occur before there is hair regrowth. In addition to pregnancy, this form of hair loss may occur following a high fever, a severe illness, or sudden physical or emotional trauma. If the stress is resolved, the hairs return with 6 months.

Endocrine abnormalities can cause alopecia, and must be excluded when considering telogen effluvium. These include hyper- and hypothyroidism. Hyperthyroidism is associated with dry, fine, thin hair; in hypothyroidism, the hair is coarse and brittle.

Traumatic Alopecia

Any injury to the hair and scalp can cause traumatic alopecia. Excessive handling, combing, and brushing or frequent waving can damage the hair.

Cutaneous Lesions with Systemic Disease

Lupus Erythematosus

There are three major forms of lupus erythematosus: discoid lupus erythematosus (DLE); subacute cutaneous lupus erythematosus (Fig. 56-15); and systemic lupus erythematosus (SLE).

Discoid lupus erythematosus is generally limited to the skin. These patients may develop systemic manifestations. Patients with established SLE, especially when the eruption occurs early in life, may develop discoid skin lesions as part of their generalized disease. DLE begins as an erythematous papule that enlarges to form a plaque. Follicular plugging may be observed. The majority of these patients do not have a positive ANA. They usually can be managed with topical therapy with sunscreens and medium strength topical steroids. The more severe forms may require systemic anti-inflammatory drugs.

Systemic lupus erythematosus is a multisystem disease that may be mild to life-threatening. Women are affected more frequently than men. Cutaneous findings helpful in establishing the diagnosis of SLE include: 1. mucosal ulcers; 2. a malar erythematosus eruption; 3. photosensitivity; and 4. cold sensitivity in the hands and feet. The commonly affected organs include the joints, kidneys, and central nervous system. Renal disease is the most common cause of

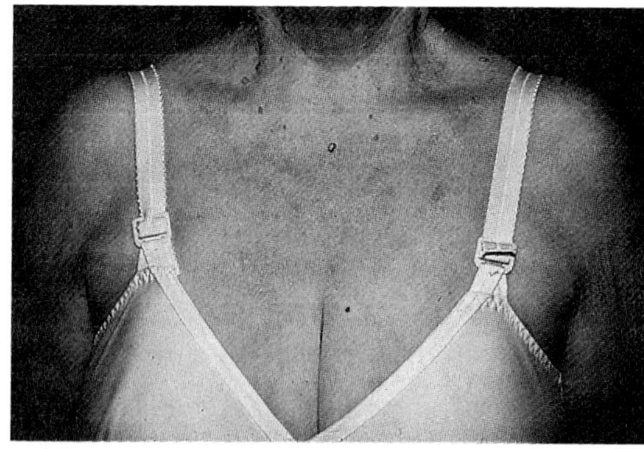

Figure 56-15 Subacute cutaneous lupus erythematosus (drug-induced). (See Color Plate 15.)

death in SLE. Systemic lupus erythematosus and subacute cutaneous lupus erythematosus can be caused by many drugs, including procainamide and hydralazine.

The diagnosis of SLE depends on clinical assessment and laboratory findings. A skin biopsy is important in the diagnostic process in most patients with possible lupus erythematosus. Light microscopy and immunofluorescent studies help to establish the diagnosis in the skin.

Dermatomyositis

Dermatomyositis is an inflammatory disorder affecting muscle and skin. It includes polymyositis (without cutaneous changes), myositis as a feature of other connective tissue disorders, and a dermatitis without myositis. Dermatomyositis may be acute, with fever and toxicity, or may present with progressive muscle weakness accompanied by myalgia.

The cutaneous findings usually are noted before the development of polymyositis. A red macular eruption, which is photosensitive, often appears over the face, neck and upper trunk, and over the joints. Edema and scales may be present. Atrophy, telangiectasis, and pigmentation may be noted. Internal malignancy must be excluded.

Morphea

Morphea is a localized sclerosis of the skin of unknown cause. Although systemic scleroderma is rare in this condition, a generalized or linear form may be present. Morphea begins as a red macule that becomes a yellow-brown, indurated plaque with pigment loss. The surface skin is not elevated. Some lesions have a characteristic violaceous border, while old lesions may have postinflammatory hyperpigmentation. Topical steroids are helpful in the management of this condition. The linear form of the disease may have systemic manifestations that may require evaluation by a rheumatologist, an orthopaedic surgeon, or both.

Scleroderma

Hardening of the skin is a feature of systemic scleroderma, and the internal involvement may include the vascular system, the lungs, esophagus, and other organs.

In progressive systemic sclerosis, the cutaneous changes are regularly associated with systemic manifestations. Raynaud's phenomenon usually is present, and digital ulcers with gangrene may occur on fingers or toes followed by loss of digits.

Erythema Nodosum

Erythema nodosum presents with tender erythematous nodules, 1 to 5 cm in diameter, on the anterior tibial area of the leg. Fever and arthralgias may be present. The skin lesions are short-lived, lasting a few weeks to several months. A chronic form of the disease may occur and persist. Erythema nodosum is a hypersensitivity phenomenon. The common precipitating factors include a streptococcal infection and/or drug sensitivity. Other causes include infectious diseases, such as deep fungi, sarcoidosis, and inflammatory bowel diseases, e.g., ulcerative colitis or Crohn's disease. The best treatment is short term bed rest, aspirin for pain reduction, support hose, and management of any underlying disease.

Sarcoidosis

Sarcoidosis is a systemic disorder characterized by granulomas in many organ systems. Sarcoidosis occurs in both sexes and in all races. One-third of patients with sarcoidosis develop skin lesions. In the acute form of the disease, patients may have erythema nodosum, fever, bilateral hilar adenopathy, and polyarthralgia. In addition to erythematous nodules, other skin lesions may include papular eruptions of the face and extremities, cutaneous plaque formation, nodules, ichthyosis, and ulcers. These skin lesions will resolve in a satisfactory manner only when systemic therapy is given for the sarcoidosis.

Rheumatoid Arthritis (Rheumatoid Nodules)

Rheumatoid nodules occur on the skin in patients with rheumatoid arthritis and they represent vasculitis. They are seen in patients with high positive serum levels of rheumatoid factor. These nodules usually occur around the elbows but may arise anywhere. Systemic therapy for the rheumatoid arthritis is the treatment of choice.

Cutaneous Manifestations of Diabetes Mellitus

A variety of skin eruptions may occur in patients with diabetes (see Table 56-12).

Tumors of the Skin (see Tables 56-13, 56-14, and 56-15)

Benign Tumors and Cysts of the Epidermis

Epidermal tumors are common. When carefully examined, all persons will be found to have one or more of these tumors. Although the growths occasionally may resemble premalignant and malignant lesions, their recognition enables the experienced clinician to reassure the patient about their benign nature. Excision for cosmetic reasons is optional.

Common Epithelial Cysts There are three types of epithelial cysts: the epidermal pilar cyst in the scalp; the milium, which may occur anywhere on the face; and the epidermal inclusion cyst. Heat, erythema, and tenderness may be pronounced if a cyst has recently leaked or ruptured. The most effective treatment for epithelial and pilar cysts is surgical drainage or removal. Often it is possible to make a small

TABLE 56-12 Diabetes Mellitus

Cutaneous Eruptions	Morphology	Therapy
Diabetic dermopathy	1.0–2.0 cm patches, red-brown on legs	None
Diabetic bullae	Tense blisters, small or large, hands and feet	None, except avoid trauma
Thick skin scleroderma	Thick skin dorsal hands; marked increase in skin thickness, back and neck	No proven therapy; emollients for dryness of skin
Perforating disorders	Hyperkeratotic papules; elimination of dermal collagen elastin	Therapy for renal disease; emollients and peeling agents
Necrobiosis lipoidica diabeticorum[a]	Cutaneous marker for diabetes; annular plaque with elevated border; telangiectasia	Potent topical steroids applied at the periphery of the lesion

[a]See Fig. 56-16.

TABLE 56-13 Epithelial Tumors

Tumor	Location	Therapy	Prevention
Seborrheic keratosis	Face, body, leg	Cryosurgery, shave excision, or mild electrodesiccation	None
Sebaceous gland hyperplasia	Face	Electrodesiccation with epilating current and curettage	Sunscreens, protective clothing, hat
Actinic keratosis	Face	Cryosurgery or topical 5-fluorouracil	Sunscreens, hat
Keratoacanthoma	Any location	Surgical excision with adequate margin	Sunscreens, hat
Cutaneous horn	Any location	Surgical excision	Sunscreens, hat
Bowen's disease	Any location	Surgical excision	Sunscreens, hat
Squamous cell carcinoma	Any location	Surgical excision	Sunscreens, hat
Basal cell carcinoma	Face, body	Surgical excision	Sunscreens, hat

linear incision and remove the well encapsulated cyst, or the cyst may be removed through a 3-mm biopsy site. Incision and drainage usually provide only temporary therapy and may be followed by a recurrence. Residual fragments may produce a foreign body granuloma or serve as the nidus for a new cyst formation.

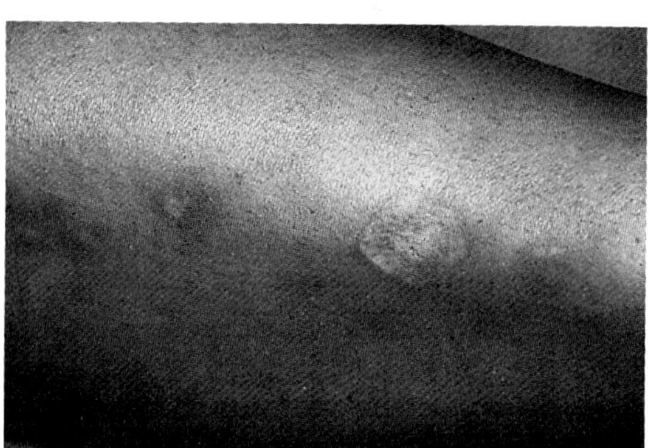

Figure 56-16 Necrobiosis lipoidica diabeticorum. (See Color Plate 16.)

Milia are small (1- to 2-mm diameter), superficial, white cystic lesions that may arise spontaneously or secondary to trauma. They are frequently found around the eye, and must be distinguished from sebaceous hyperplasia and syringomas. Milia may be successfully removed in a variety of ways. One method is to make a small nick in the overlying skin and then apply pressure to evacuate the contents with a comedone extractor.

Epidermal Nevi Epidermal nevi are wartlike lesions that arise on the skin early in life. They may, however, begin in the adult. They are frequently

TABLE 56-14 **Nonepithelial Skin Tumors**

Type	Location	Therapy
Skin tags	Neck, axilla, groins	Cryosurgery or complete excision
Granuloma pyogenicum	Any skin area	Shave excision, followed by electrodesiccation of lesion base
Dermatofibroma	Any skin area	Cryosurgery
Lipoma	Any skin area	Simple excision or excision through a 4-mm punch biopsy of skin with pressure to the area to push the lipoma through the opening

noted on the face or behind the ear and on the neck. These lesions are usually brownish, hyperkeratotic papules that form a linear or sometimes swirling configuration. Localized epidermal nevi can be treated by local excision or dermabrasion, but a large lesion presents a distinct management problem and should be managed with a good cosmetic result as the primary goal. Plastic surgery usually is required when the lesion is large. Local recurrence after surgery is not uncommon.

Seborrheic Keratosis This common benign epithelial tumor arises in the skin in adult life. Many of these lesions are present in older adults, and they may occur on any area of skin on the body except the palms and soles. They may occasionally itch. The lesions vary in color from a normal flesh-color to tan-brown or black, and they vary in size from a tiny papule (2 mm), to a large plaque or nodule, several centimeters in diameter. They usually have a warty surface and appear to be sitting on top of the skin. They can resemble a malignant lesion, such as Bowen's disease (squamous cell carcinoma in situ), pigmented basal cell carcinoma or malignant melanoma. There is no medical reason for removing most of these seborrheic keratoses. Pigmented seborrheic keratosis may require a biopsy to exclude malignant melanoma. Cosmetic removal may be accomplished with cryosurgery or mild electrodesiccation and curettage. If there is a question about the nature of a pigmented seborrheic keratosis, a biopsy should be performed.

TABLE 56-15 **Cutaneous Characteristics of Pigmented Lesions**

Type	Feature
Benign nevi	Small, uniform color, distinct border
Atypical nevi	Large, irregular border, several colors
Seborrheic keratosis	Flesh colored, brown, or black, with keratin
Pigmented basal cell carcinoma	Uniform color, distinct border, no keratin
Blue nevus	Small, blue, stable
Junctional nevus	Flat, distinct border
Malignant melanoma	Multiple colors, indistinct borders, rapid growth

Adnexal Tumors These tumors may resemble, to a degree, portions of cutaneous adnexal structures—hair follicles, sebaceous glands, apocrine glands, and eccrine sweat glands. It is important to be knowledgeable about the more common adnexal tumors since they can resemble basal cell carcinoma. Sebaceous gland hyperplasia is a condition seen in fair-skinned adults who have a history of excessive exposure to ultraviolet light. The lesion is a yellow papule or a small nodule on the face. Telangiectasia and a central punctum can be similar to findings with a basal cell carcinoma. A biopsy distinguishes this lesion from a basal cell carcinoma. A second adnexal tumor, the trichoepithelioma, is a solitary nodule that presents on the face. A third adnexal tumor is the syringoma, which is a flesh-colored papule frequently found in the skin just below the lower lid margin. A biopsy confirms the diagnosis in each case. The lesions may be removed surgically to produce a good cosmetic appearance by simple excision or electrodesiccation and mild curettage.

Common Nonepithelial Skin Tumors (see Table 56-14)

Skin Tags Skin tags, or squamous papillomas or skin polyps, are elevated, flesh-colored or tanned papular or filiform lesions commonly occurring in adults in flexural areas, e.g., neck, axillae, and groin. Obesity and local factors such as sweating and friction are flare factors. Patients are usually most concerned about the cosmetic appearance of these lesions as well as bleeding from trauma.

Hypertrophic Scars and Keloids Injury to the skin below the epidermal basement membrane results in scarring. The size and appearance of a scar is dependent on the injury, location on the body surface, and genetic factors. Scars may be tan to red-brown to black. Excess proliferation of fibrous tissue occurs in genetically susceptible individuals. Keloids are often difficult to manage (see Chap. 60).

Dermatofibroma The dermatofibroma is a common tumor of fibrohistiocytic origin. It occurs after trauma or infection. The tumor is a firm papule or nodule. Although it may occur anywhere, it frequently appears on the lower extremities.

Lipoma Lipomas are common and asymptomatic unless they have an angiomatous component. They present in a subcutaneous location, and must be distinguished from epithelial cysts and neurofibromas. Small lipomas are of no cosmetic importance and are best left untreated. Large lesions may be removed surgically.

Vascular Tumors

Hemangiomas The most common blood vessel tumors are varieties of hemangioma. They may be present at birth as a macular congenital form, i.e., nevus flammeus, or papular (strawberry) or cavernous. The acquired adult form of capillary hemangioma, the cherry angioma, is regularly seen on covered skin areas. This lesion is cosmetically unacceptable to many patients, but it is always benign.

Granuloma Pyogenicum This common tumor represents an exuberant growth of vascular tissue. The precise cause is unknown, but the lesions may be initiated by trauma or hormonal stimulation such as during pregnancy. Granuloma pyogenicum is red and usually presents as a solitary, polypoid lesion. The finger is a common location for this lesion; however, it may occur anywhere following skin trauma.

Premalignant and Malignant Epithelial Tumors

The most common premalignant lesion occurring on the skin is actinic keratosis. Other lesions occurring in sun-damaged skin include cutaneous horns (keratoacanthoma), Bowen's disease, and basal cell and squamous cell carcinoma.

Actinic Keratosis Actinic or solar keratoses are the most common precancerous skin lesions. They usually appear in the third or fourth decade of life in people who have a light complexion. Actinic keratoses range in color from pink or red to brown. The lesion size and the degree of accumulation of melanin pigment determines the color. They usually have a slight surface scale, and range in size from 0.2 to 1.5 cm in diameter. The lateral borders may be indistinct. The malignant potential for these lesions is low; however, a firm hypertrophic lesion or a lesion with a small ulcer formation, or both, suggests malignancy. A biopsy should be obtained when malignancy is suspected or when a lesion previously treated with cryosurgery returns on the skin surface.

All persons who develop an actinic keratosis have sun damaged skin and are likely to have many similar lesions in the future. Sun protection is mandatory, and topical therapy is often indicated.

Keratoacanthoma This tumor is generally considered to be benign, although it may be hard to differentiate the lesion, clinically and pathologically, from squamous cell carcinoma. It is a lesion that likely is produced by excessive ultraviolet light exposure. Tar exposure and viral infection are possible flare factors. The usual history is a papule occurring on sun-exposed skin that evolves rapidly (in a matter of weeks) to form a nodule with a central crater filled with keratin. The lesion remains stationary for a 6- to 8-week period and then regresses. The major consideration in the differential diagnosis is squamous cell carcinoma.

Cutaneous horns are produced as a reaction to chronic sunlight exposure. The lesion is an elevated horny papule. These lesions have a malignant potential at the base and should be excised and evaluated histologically to exclude malignancy.

Bowen's Disease (Squamous Cell Carcinoma in

Situ of the Skin) Bowen's disease is squamous cell carcinoma in situ of the skin. The epidermal malignancy is confined to the epidermis and has not invaded the dermis. It may occur anywhere on the skin surface, and the occurrence is not always related to the skin complexion, type or sun exposure. Bowen's disease can resemble psoriasis or nummular eczema. A biopsy should be done to establish the diagnosis.

Squamous Cell Carcinoma Squamous cell carcinoma, a malignant epithelial tumor with a potential for invasion and metastasis, is commonly noted on the scalp, face or lip. It should be considered a potentially dangerous skin malignancy, especially when it occurs in the T zone on the face, which includes the skin on the forehead, around the eyes, and over the nose. The ears, the oral mucosa, and any burn site are dangerous locations for metastases from these lesions.

Squamous cell carcinoma usually is related to chronic sun exposure. Arsenic or radiation exposure also may be factors in causing squamous cell cancer. Squamous cell carcinomas are highly variable in appearance. Some are hyperkeratotic, some are verrucous nodules, and others form papules or plaques. Ulcer formation may occur. The treatment of choice is adequate surgical excision. (Fig. 56-17).

Basal Cell Carcinoma Basal cell carcinoma is the most prevalent cutaneous malignancy. It is an epithelial tumor which arises as a consequence of an intrinsic defect in basal cells that prevents these cells from maturing and forming normal keratin. Although local skin destruction and invasion can occur, this lesion rarely extends beyond the skin (Fig. 56-18).

Figure 56-17 Superficial squamous cell carcinoma. (See Color Plate 17.)

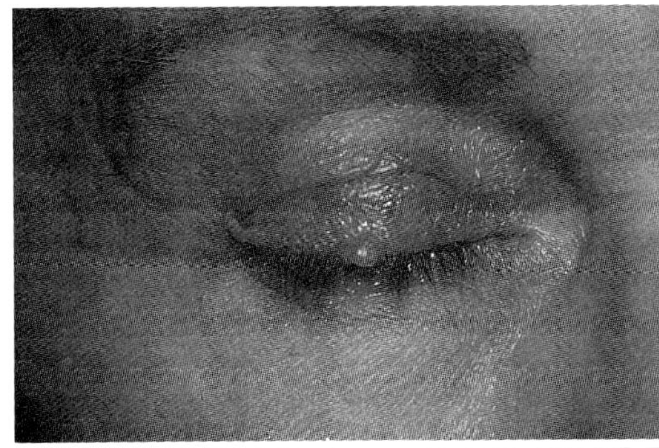

Figure 56-18 Basal cell carcinoma. (See Color Plate 18.)

Lymphoma and Leukemia Lymphoma of the skin presents with violaceous papules and nodules. Lymphomas of T-cell origin commonly begin in the skin.

Mycosis fungoides is an indolent T-cell lymphoma that originates in the skin and has an early course resembling a persistent eczematous dermatitis or psoriasis. Erythematous, atrophic patches frequently are seen in the early or ''patch'' stage of the disease. As progression occurs, violaceous plaques and tumors develop in the skin. The diagnosis is made by frequent biopsies in several skin sites. Early therapies include topical nitrogen mustard and ultraviolet A or B light.

Melanocytic Tumors (Table 56-15)

Melanocytic Lesions Melanocyte cell growth occurs within the epidermis or dermis. The nevus cell is a form of melanocyte and involves the epidermis, dermis, or both. Benign epidermal melanocytic tumors include ephelis and lentigo. Nevus cell tumors are numerous and may be benign or malignant.

Ephelis (Freckle) Freckles are especially numerous in many Caucasians. The freckles occur in sun-exposed areas. The melanocytes in freckles are normal, but appear larger than normal. No therapy is indicated.

Lentigo Lentigines (pigmented macules) occur in young adults, with or without sun exposure. When they occur in older adults, the sun-exposed area is involved. In adults, lentigines occur on the face, neck, dorsa of the hands, shoulders, and back. Lentigos and seborrheic keratoses are the usual examples of "liver" spots. Lentigines, although benign, are a cosmetic problem and they can mimic malignant melanoma when the pigment is irregular. Suspicious lesions should be biopsied. Cosmetic therapy for benign lentigos can be accomplished with light cryosurgery.

Lesions Composed of Nevus Cells Nevus cell nevi ("moles") occur in all human beings and are the most common tumors of the skin. Nevus cells are of melanocyte origin. Very few are clinically present at birth. Adults may have 60 or more nevi. As the patient advances in age, many of these lesions regress.

Nevus cell nevi begin as nests of cells at the dermoepidermal junction (junctional nevi). When nevus cells are found solely in the dermis, the lesions are intradermal nevi. Nevi may be seen anywhere on the body, including the palms, soles, and genitalia. Most nevi do not require excision. A nevus that has changed in color, shape, or size, or is symptomatic—or is merely suspicious to the patient or physician—should be biopsied to exclude malignant melanoma.

Malignant Melanoma Malignant melanoma arises from melanocytes in the skin as well as from melanocytes in other locations, such as the eye and the vagina. 1.5 to 3 percent of all skin cancers are melanomas. Melanoma occurs in any location on the skin surface, but is especially common on the head and neck, upper back, and lower extremities. Sunlight plays a role in the development of malignant melanoma and is a risk factor, especially when an acute sunburn occurs early in the life of the patient.

The majority of malignant melanomas arise spontaneously. Melanomas can arise in pre-existing nevi—especially in giant congenital nevi. The major risk factors for melanoma are a family history of melanoma, a personal history of melanoma, and an atypical mole in a patient with immunosuppression or who has a light complexion with a previous history of excess sun exposure.

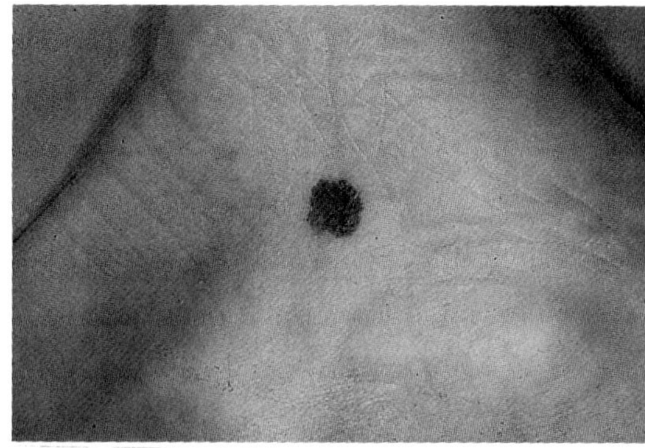

Figure 56-19 Superficial malignant melanoma. (See Color Plate 19.)

Malignant melanomas are divided into four major clinical types. The superficial spreading malignant melanoma (Fig. 56-19) is a slightly elevated lesion with an irregular, indistinct margin and irregular dis-

TABLE 56-16 Cutaneous Disorders in Pregnancy

Eruption	Type	Therapy	Prognosis
Hyperpigmentation	Physiologic	None	Good
Spider angioma and Palmer erythema	Physiologic	None required	May recur
Pruritic papules and plaques of pregnancy (PUPPP)	Related to pregnancy	Should be minimal and should be prescribed by dermatologist and obstetrician	Resolves postpartum; does not recur
Pemphigus or herpes gestationis (Fig. 56-20)	Related to pregnancy	Systemic steroids	Prognosis for mother good; prognosis for baby is variable; may recur

Figure 56-20 Pemphigus gestationis—herpes gestationis. (See Color Plate 20.)

tribution of colors, including black, brown, red, and occasionally blue. The nodular melanoma usually is uniform in color, i.e., black. Lentigo maligna melanoma occurs in a sun-exposed area, usually beginning as a lentigo with gradual enlargement. A fourth variety of malignant melanoma is acral lentiginous melanoma. This form presents as an irregular, pigmented, macular, or slightly elevated lesion on the palms, soles, or digits.

Early diagnosis and surgery offer the only chance for cure in any malignant melanoma.

Cutaneous Disorders in Pregnancy

Many skin changes can occur in pregnancy, many of which are physiologic. Cutaneous eruptions also occur in pregnancy, and skin diseases can be altered by pregnancy (see Table 56-16).

References and Suggested Reading

1. Arnold HL, Odom RB, James WD: *Andrew's Disease of the Skin, Clinical Dermatology.* Philadelphia: WB Saunders, 1990.
2. Beutner KR: Human papillomavirus infection. *J Am Acad Dermatol* 20:114–123, 1989.
3. Bigby M, Jick A, Jick H, Arndt K: Drug-induced cutaneous reactions: A report from the Boston Collaborative Surveillance Program on 15,438 consecutive inpatients, 1975–1982. *JAMA* 256:3358–3363, 1986.
4. Borelli D, Jacobs PH, Nall L: Tinea versicolor: Epidemiologic, clinical, and therapeutic aspects. *J Am Acad Dermatol* 25:300–305, 1991.
5. Coskey RJ, Coskey LA: Diagnosis and treatment of impetigo. *J Am Acad Dermatol* 17:62–63, 1987.
6. Chuang TY: Condylomata acuminata (genital warts): An epidemiologic view. *J Am Acad Dermato* 16:376–384, 1987.
7. Drake LA, Ceilley RI, Cornelison RL, et al: Guidelines of care for atopic dermatitis. *J Am Acad Dermatol* 26:485–488, 1992.
8. Drake LA, Ceilley RI, Cornelison RL, et al: American Academy of Dermatology: Guidelines of care for basal cell carcinoma. *J Am Acad Dermatol* 26:117–120, 1992.
9. Farber EM, Abel EA, Charuworn A: Recent advances in the treatment of psoriasis. *J Am Acad Dermatol* 8:311–321, 1983.
10. Glass AG, Hoover RN: The emerging epidemic of melanoma and squamous cell skin cancer. *JAMA* 262:2097–2100, 1989.
11. Hanifin JM: Atopic dermatitis: New therapeutic considerations. *J Am Acad Dermatol* 24:1097–1101, 1991.
12. Hook EW, Hooton TM, Horton CA, et al: Microbiologic evaluation of cutaneous cellulitis in adults. *Arch Intern Med* 146:295–297, 1986.
13. Howland WW, Golitz LE, Weston WL, Huff JC: Erythema multiforme: Clinical, histopathologic, and immunologic study. *J Am Acad Dermatol* 10:438–446, 1984.
14. Hughes BR, Murphy CE, Barnett J, Cunliffe WJ: Strategy of acne therapy with long-term antibiotics. *Br J Dermatol* 121:623–628, 1989.
15. Isselbacher KJ, Braunwald E, Wilson JD, Martin JB, Fauci AS, Kasper DL (eds): *Harrison's Principles of Internal Medicine,* 13th ed. New York: Mcgraw-Hill, 1994.
16. Kaye FJ, Bunn PA, Steinberg SM, et al: A randomized trial comparing combination electron-beam radiation and chemotherapy with topical therapy in the initial treatment of mycosis fungoides. *N Engl J Med* 321:1784–1790, 1989.
17. Koh HK: Cutaneous melanoma. *N Engl J Med* 325:171–182, 1991.
18. Kwa RE, Campana K, Moy RD: Biology of cutaneous squamous cell carcinoma, *J Am Acad Dermatol* 26:1, 1992.
19. Lesher JL, Smith JG: Antifungal agents in dermatology. *J Am Acad Dermatol* 17:383–384, 1987.
20. Marks R: The role of treatment of actinic keratoses in the prevention of morbidity and mortality due to squamous cell carcinoma. *Arch Dermatol* 127:1031–1033, 1991.
21. Parsons JM: Pityriasis rosea update: 1986. *J Am Acad Dermatol* 15:159–167, 1986.
22. Patterson JW, Blaylock WK: *Dermatology, A Concise Textbook.* New York: Medical Examination Publishing, 1987.
23. Sacks MK: Cutaneous cellulitis. *Arch Dermatol* 127:493–496, 1991.
24. Schultz MW, Gomez M, Hanson RC, et al: Comparative study of 5% permethrin cream and 1% lindane lotion for the treatment of scabies. *Arch Dermatol* 126:167–170, 1990.

25. Soter NA; Urticaria: Current therapy. *J Allergy Clin Immunol* 86:1009–1014, 1990.
26. Stern RS, Boudreaux C, Arndt KA: Diagnostic accuracy and appropriateness of care for seborrheic keratoses. *JAMA* 265:74–77, 1991.
27. Stern RS, Pass TM, Komaroff AL: Topical v. systemic agent treatment for papulopustular acne: A cost effective analysis. *Arch Dermatol* 120:1571–1578, 1984.
28. Stern RS, Wintroub BU, Arndt KA: Drug reactions. *J Am Acad Dermatol* 15:1282–1288, 1986.
29. Stevens DL, Tanner MH, Winship J, et al: Severe group A streptococcal infections associated with a toxic shock-like syndrome and scarlet fever toxin A. *N Engl J Med* 321:1–7, 1989.

57 Otolaryngology

Gerald D. Zahtz
David Myssiorek

The field of otolaryngology deals with disease processes involving the head and neck region. This chapter will provide a broad overview of the diagnosis and office treatment of common otolaryngologic problems. Within the head and neck, very few disease processes are specific for women, except for hormonally related rhinitis, the increased incidence of cancer of the hypopharynx, otosclerosis, and Meniere's disease.

As in all fields of medicine, accurate history taking is essential for proper diagnosis and must be followed by a thorough physical examination.

Physical Examination

Ears

Initially, the external ear and postauricular areas should be inspected for swelling, erythema, cysts, and congenital malformations. After this inspection, the pinna is grasped and gently pulled superoposteriorly to straighten the ear canal as the otoscope is inserted. If the patient complains of pain during this maneuver, one must consider a diagnosis of otitis externa involving the external auditory canal. The normal ear canal should have no erythema or exudate. Cerumen should be removed gently by curettage or irrigation to allow proper evaluation, unless there are signs of infection or tympanic membrane perforation. The tympanic membrane (TM) is then visualized and should appear as an intact, pearly white translucent membrane. Mobility of the tympanic membrane should be ascertained by pneumatic otoscopy. This is done using the insufflator bulb attachment of the otoscope. By blowing air through the head of the otoscope and into the ear canal, the mobility of the tympanic membrane can be evaluated.

Nose

Initial evaluation should begin with the examination of the external nose, with documentation of external deformities, as well as erythema or edema. Intranasal examination can be performed with an otoscope, but is best performed with a headlight and nasal speculum. The largest speculum should be placed into the patient's nostril carefully. Abnormalities in the position of the midline septum, the presence of masses, and the color and size of the turbinates should be noted, as well as the character of any intranasal secretions.

The intranasal examination should be performed twice, before and after the use of vasoconstrictors, such as oxymetazoline or phenylephrine. The postvasoconstrictor examination allows septal deformities, nasal masses, and purulent secretions to be easily diagnosed.

Pharynx

The entire oral cavity must be examined for mucosal and dental lesions. All bridgework and dentures must be removed. Optimal examination requires both a bright light and a tongue depressor to allow proper visualization of the oral mucosa and the posterior pharynx. The presence or absence of tonsils should be noted, as well as any asymmetric finding in the oral cavity. Careful attention should be given to the lateral borders of the tongue to examine for any suspicious lesions.

Larynx

The laryngeal examination is very important for the evaluation of hoarseness. This area is not easily accessible except by use of headlight and mirror or a fiberoptic nasopharyngoscope. This procedure is usually performed by the otolaryngologist.

Neck

The entire neck should be inspected for any masses, bruits, scars, or deformities, and should then be palpated. If any masses are found, their size, position, fluctuancc, and mobility should be recorded. The contour (irregularity, lobularity) should also be noted. A careful evaluation of the thyroid gland is also essential as part of this examination.

Nasal Obstruction/Sinusitis

Nasal obstruction/sinusitis are common complaints in a general practice. Their evaluation requires an accurate history, physical exam, and occasionally diagnostic tests. Most nasal mucosal abnormalities cause bilateral disease with varying degrees of severity that can fluctuate over hours, days, or seasonally. Structural abnormalities are usually unilateral, fixed, and unchanging; however, their severity can vary.

The time of onset and duration of symptoms should be ascertained. Antecedent trauma, symptom laterality, and whether symptoms are intermittent or constant, seasonal or perennial, should be determined. If any factors seem to trigger the symptoms or relieve them, these should be recorded. The patient's hormonal status must be determined, as rhinitis of pregnancy, menopause, hypothyroidism, and hormonal therapy (replacement therapy or birth control pills) can also cause nasal obstruction.

The examination of the nose has been previously discussed. Extra effort in the visualization of the nasal cavity will reward the practitioner with a proper diagnosis. Nasal obstruction usually can be divided into the following categories: mucosal disease, structural abnormalities, nasal masses. The differential diagnosis of mucosal disease includes acute rhinitis, allergic rhinitis, vasomotor rhinitis, atrophic rhinitis, rhinitis medicamentosa, hormonally related rhinitis, and sinusitis.

Acute rhinitis, also known as the "common cold," is the most common cause of nasal obstruction. It has no "cure," but is treated symptomatically with various drying agents, such as antihistamines, decongestants, antihistamine/decongestants, and topical decongestants. It can also be the first stage of an acute sinus infection. As the nasal mucosa becomes edematous, the sinus opening (ostium) becomes blocked and the oxygen saturation in the affected sinus decreases; bacteria begin to proliferate inside the sinus, causing an acute infectious process. The diagnosis of acute sinusitis is made as the patient's "cold" does not resolve over the normal 24 to 48 h; instead, the patient begins to develop purulent rhinorrhea. Swelling of the face, toothache and facial pain may be associated with acute sinusitis. The patient suspected of having sinusitis should be sent for paranasal sinus x-rays to confirm the diagnosis. CT scans are necessary when an underlying etiology such as tumor or polyp is being sought. The CT also can distinguish fluid from solid tissue in the sinus. Culture of the nasal drainage may identify the infecting organism; however, approximately half the time, these cultures do not adequately represent the sinus pathogen. The most common organisms in adults are Streptococci (including Pneumococci) and Haemophilus strains.

Treatment of sinusitis is similar for all the sinuses. Systemic nasal decongestants and short-term topical nasal decongestants (neosynephrine or oxymetazoline) should be started unless the patient is taking medications that preclude their use or has certain cardiac conditions. Humidification and warm compresses over the affected sinus help. If orbital complications are present referral to an otolaryngologist and an ophthalmologist usually is necessary.

Acute bacterial sinusitis should be treated aggressively with antibiotic therapy, as well as decongestant therapy to maintain drainage. The mainstay of antibiotic therapy is amoxicillin; however, in view of the increasing resistance of bacteria to this medication, one must consider change of therapy to amoxicillin/clavulanic acid, cephalosporins, clarithromycin, or trimethoprim-sulfamethoxazole (for patients allergic to penicillin) if improvement is not seen. Patients who present with increasing pain, headache, or facial cellulitis should immediately be referred to an otolaryngologist for further therapy unless the primary care physician has substantial expertise with this problem.

Diagnosis of allergic rhinitis is based on the history of seasonal symptoms, nasal itching, paroxysmal sneezing and rhinorrhea. It can be exacerbated by exposure to antigens that will trigger an allergic response. Nasal examination reveals clear, watery discharge with pale blue nasal turbinates. Further discussion of this problem can be found in Chap. 54.

Vasomotor rhinitis is a problem in which there is excessive swelling and congestion of the nasal mucosa in the absence of allergic disease. The findings on physical examination are the same as seen in allergic rhinitis except for the absence of response to skin tests and the lack of eosinophils on nasal smear. Factors causing symptoms include stress, changes in weather and humidity, and irritating fumes. The treatment is symptomatic, using the previously mentioned medications. Medical management is less successful in this disease, and patients may require surgical therapy of the turbinates for effective treatment of this problem.

Atrophic rhinitis is a rare disease caused by atrophy of mucosa and bone in the nasal cavity characterized by excessive crusting, foul-smelling rhinorrhea, epistaxis, and anosmia. Treatment is aimed at local therapy, with frequent cleaning of nasal crusts and debris, and moisturization of the nasal cavity.

Rhinitis medicamentosa is caused by the chronic use of topical nasal decongestants. This condition is discussed in Chap. 54.

Other medications that can cause nasal obstruction include alcohol, antithyroid medications, aspirin, cocaine, estrogens and birth control pills, ephedrine, epinephrine, iodides, marijuana, reserpine, and tobacco.

The diagnosis of hormonally related rhinorrhea requires a good history. Each of the following endocrine factors can play a role in nasal obstruction: 1. pregnancy—especially the second and third trimester; 2. menstruation—congestion can fluctuate with the woman's cycle; 3. diabetes mellitus; 4. hypothyroidism—causes increased nasal congestion. In the latter two instances, control of the endocrine disease may be necessary to help control the congestion. These problems occasionally will respond to topical intranasal steroids.

Structural abnormalities include extranasal deformities, deviated septum, nasal valve collapse, and choanal atresia. The most common nasal masses seen are nasal polyps, which usually are found in patients with severe allergies and asthma. Other neoplastic processes can be found in the nasal cavity. Both the structural abnormalities and the nasal masses are disease processes that usually will require referral to the otolaryngologist.

Dizziness

The proper evaluation of the "dizzy" patient is one of the most difficult problems for the physician. Vertigo with its sensation of motion must be distinguished from disequilibrium, a sensation of imbalance not related to motion. Care must be taken when obtaining the history to decipher and define the patient's symptoms. Symptoms of visual disturbances, weakness in the legs, near-syncope, mild nausea, and spatial disorientation are not caused by inner ear disease.

Vertigo can be described by the patient as "things spinning around me" or "I am spinning around." It can also, on occasion, present with a tilting sensation. The association of symptoms with loss of hearing, ringing in the ears, and pressure in the ears will shift the diagnosis to a peripheral disorder; headaches, seizures, loss of consciousness, visual change, and lightheadedness will shift the diagnosis away from peripheral disease. Other important questions concern the duration and frequency of the symptoms and the circumstances under which they occur (e.g., after meals or related to position), and response to medications. It must be remembered that the "balance mechanism" requires normal vestibular function, an intact optical system, as well as proprioception, which is then interpreted by the central nervous system as "balance." A breakdown in any one of these factors can cause "dizziness." Physical examination requires a brief neurologic examination of the cranial nerves, gait, and balance. Observation of the extraocular movement of the eyes for nystagmus is also important. Vertigo that can be elicited by change of position needs to be documented and distinguished from orthostatic changes.

With the above information, the physician should be able to differentiate dizziness caused by labyrinthine disease and that which is nonlabyrinthine in origin. Nonlabyrinthine disease will require further medical and neurologic evaluation.

The differential diagnosis of vestibular disease is divided into two types: peripheral disease and nonperipheral disease. Nonperipheral disease includes cerebellar or cerebellopontine angle tumors, multiple sclerosis, and temporal lobe epilepsy. These processes usually are diagnosed by eliminating peripheral causes and by direct imaging techniques of the brain using MRI. Vascular lesions causing brainstem ischemia usually have additional neurologic symptoms such as slurred speech, visual problems, and difficulty swallowing. A whiplash injury to the neck also can cause cervical vertigo, which is confirmed only by excluding all other forms of vertigo. Metabolic disorders such as hypoglycemia, hypothyroidism, and syphilis have all been associated with vertigo. These diseases are diagnosed by obtaining appropriate blood tests. Symptoms usually will resolve with treatment of the underlying disease process.

Peripheral lesions of the labyrinth present with "true" vertigo. This differential diagnosis includes Meniere's disease, benign positional vertigo, vestibular neuronitis, labyrinthitis, ototoxicity, motion sickness, and multiple sclerosis (MS). Meniere's disease classically presents with episodes of vertigo, aural fullness, ringing, and fluctuating hearing loss. It is felt to be caused by endolymphatic hydrops, an increase of endolymphatic fluid in the inner ear due to an abnormality in the sodium-potassium pump of the inner ear. The classic episode lasts for hours, not days; however, unsteadiness may persist for some time after the episode. These attacks are episodic and may be separated in time by months or even years. An accurate history is very important in helping to make the diagnosis. Its treatment comprises a salt-restricted diet, diuretics, and the use of vestibular suppressants (meclizine, promethazine, diazepam). If symptoms continue, surgical therapy may be necessary.

Benign paroxysmal positional vertigo usually is described as a sudden onset of vertigo while in a certain position (e.g., turning one's head, turning to one side in bed). The labyrinth usually responds to this disease process by accommodation (i.e., the body learns to compensate for the fact that the labyrinthine impulses on the two sides are different). This causes a resolution of symptoms over time. Relief can be obtained by the use of vestibular suppressants; however, these must be used sparingly as they may delay the accommodation process. Labyrinthine exercises can help enhance this accommodation process. In these exercises, the head and the body are placed in prescribed positions to allow both labyrinths to re-equilibrate.

Vestibular neuronitis presents with a sudden onset of vertigo lasting for hours, which slowly abates. It has been related to antecedent viral diseases, but can occur at any time. The acute symptoms usually abate within 24 h; however, prolonged unsteadiness can persist for months. This disease has no aural symptoms and should not be confused with Meniere's disease or labyrinthitis. Vestibular suppressants and labyrinthine exercises also can be used for treatment of this problem.

Labyrinthitis presents with the same symptoms as noted above, except for the addition of hearing loss. This disease process must be monitored carefully, because it can be caused by bacterial infection and can lead to meningitis.

Perilymphatic fistula is a controversial area in otolaryngology. It is caused by a leak of "inner ear fluid" in the region of the round or oval windows. It presents with sudden vertigo, occasional hearing loss, and a history or antecedent barotrauma (e.g., scuba diving or airplane flight). It should be treated with bedrest and, if the symptoms do not improve, surgical therapy may be necessary.

Ototoxicity and vestibular toxicity can be caused by numerous medications that affect the vestibular and auditory system. These include aspirin, aminoglycosides, loop diuretics, and antineoplastic agents. These problems can present at any time during therapy and have been reported to develop even months after discontinuing medication.

Motion sickness should be mentioned, and it is distinguished by its direct causal effects, secondary to repetitive motions, such as experienced in ships, airplanes, and automobiles. Scopolamine patches have been shown to have a good effect in the prevention and control of this problem.

Multiple sclerosis (MS) can present with vertigo in 10 percent of cases. Its diagnosis is based upon multiple presentations of various neurologic symptoms and signs. Approximately 30 percent of all MS patients will have vertigo during the course of the disease.

Hearing Loss

Hearing loss is divided into two categories, conductive and sensorineural. Conductive loss is caused by abnormalities of the external ear, tympanic membrane and cavity, and the ossicles. It is this type of loss that is theoretically correctable either through medications or surgery. A sensorineural hearing loss implies damage to the auditory nerve caused by abnormalities in the cochlea or along its neural pathways to the brain.

A simple tuning-fork test can help one distinguish between these two types of hearing loss. A 512-Hz tuning-fork is used to perform the Weber and Rinne test. Lower frequency tuning-forks do not test hearing; rather, they test vibrotactile sensation. In the Weber test, the examiner places a vibrating tuning fork on the midline of the forehead, bridge of the nose, or the midline on the teeth. Normally, the patient will perceive the sound equally in both ears or will be unable to localize the sound. In patients who have conductive hearing loss, the sound will be louder in the ear with the conductive defect. In sensorineural hearing losses, the sound would be greater in the opposite ear. Thus, if a patient notices the sound to be lateralized into one ear, it suggests either a conductive hearing loss in that ear or a sensorineural hearing loss in the opposite ear.

The Rinne test is then used to distinguish between a conductive hearing loss and sensorineural hearing loss. The vibrating tuning fork is placed along the ear and on the mastoid. In normal situations and in sensorineural hearing loss, the patient will perceive a louder noise when the tuning fork is placed alongside the ear (air conduction) versus placing it on the mastoid region. If the sound is louder when the tuning fork is placed on the mastoid, the patient has a conductive hearing loss. Thus, once a patient has been shown to have an abnormal Weber test, each ear is then examined by the Rinne test, which will then distinguish conductive from sensorineural hearing loss.

These tests can be used as a rough gauge to determine the type of loss, but this must be confirmed on audiometric evaluation. A physical examination of the ear, with removal of impacted cerumen for visualization of the tympanic membrane, to rule out perforations or fluid behind the ear should be performed, as these are the most common causes of conductive hearing loss and are easily diagnosed. Treatment should be directed to the specific disease, and usually will warrant referral to an otolaryngologist.

Some specific etiologies of hearing loss primarily affect women. Otosclerosis is an abnormality of the stapes, which becomes fixed, thus impeding the normal conduction mechanism of sound to the inner ear. It is frequently bilateral, has a genetic predisposition, and seems to present between the ages of 15 and 45, with a 2:1 predominance in women. It is seen most frequently in white patients and is known to cause a rapid progression of hearing loss in younger women, during pregnancy, and in women taking estrogens. The diagnosis is made by a normal examination which has ruled out external and middle ear pathology, and tuning-fork tests, which show a conductive hearing loss. Audiometry is then used for confirmation. These patients should be referred to the otolaryngologist for definitive surgical therapy.

There are many other causes of hearing loss, including trauma, ototoxicity due to drugs, and presbycusis.

Otalgia

Otalgia (pain in the ear) may be due primarily to ear pathology, from local tissue inflammation or tumor (e.g., parotitis), temporomandibular joint syndrome, or referred from the throat. Approximately one-half of ear pain is nonotologic in origin. Sensory innervation to the ear is derived from the trigeminal, facial, glossopharyngeal and vagal nerves. The greater auricular nerve (derived from C_3) provides sensation to the lower half of the auricle and its anterior canal wall. Consequently, if the patient has otalgia, it is not enough to examine only the ear.

In general, laboratory tests for otalgia are not necessary unless constitutional symptoms and signs are present. Appropriate cultures, complete blood count, and sedimentation rate may assist in determining treatment of infectious causes. Serologic tests in cases of Wegener's granulomatosis or relapsing polychondritis are needed to direct diagnostic investigation.

The most common source of ear pain over all age groups is infection. The patient should be questioned about recent trauma, upper respiratory tract infections, water exposure, travel, and instrumentation (cotton swabs, match sticks). Deeper trauma or spread of infection can lead to damage to the middle ear and/or inner ear. Symptoms to elicit include hearing loss, vertigo, tinnitus, and autophony (hearing one's self). During warm months, swimming quite often causes otitis externa. The physical examination of the external auditory canal will reveal swelling, erythema, and tenderness of the canal. The tympanic membrane (TM) may also be injected. If discharge or cerumen is noted in the canal, local care in the form of curettage or suctioning should be performed to allow the ear's pH to lower and humidity to decrease. If significant edema of the ear canal or TM exists, a Rinne test may show a bone conduction greater than air conduction. Nonototoxic, pH-buffered eardrops should be started and the ear kept dry. If the canal is very swollen, a wick should be placed to allow eardrops to enter the ear and prevent complete collapse of the canal. Attention should be turned to the periauricular lymph nodes. Enlargement of these nodes implies that the infection has spread beyond the local tissues and probably requires systemic antibiotics.

The middle ear and mastoid, when inflamed, also can cause otalgia. Acute otitis media may occur at any age. In adults, the common predisposing factors include allergies, barotrauma, and upper respiratory infections. Symptoms include hearing loss, severe pain, and fullness. Some patients will complain of tinnitus and/or dizziness. The patient should be asked if she has flown or scuba-dived recently. Previous ear surgery or trauma is significant, since these patients are more prone to the complications of otitis media. Unilateral otitis media should prompt an investigation of the nasopharynx since nasopharyngeal masses can obstruct the Eustachian tube orifices, resulting in otitis media. Unchecked, otitis media can result in TM perforation, sigmoid thrombophlebitis, meningitis, epidural/subdural abscess, and brain abscess.

The TM in otitis media appears thickened and red. The light reflex is absent and the drum will not move on pneumotoscopy. If the external ear is projecting from the head at a greater than usual angle ($\tilde{}30°$), acute mastoiditis may be present. Obtaining cultures from draining ears may not necessarily reveal the infecting organism since the external auditory canal is usually colonized by *Pseudomonas aeruginosa.* Treatment for acute otitis media includes oral systemic antibiotics such as amoxicillin and decongestants. Recalcitrant otitis or suspected mastoid disease usually requires referral to a specialist.

If the ear exam is normal, pain may originate from facial structures such as the skin, teeth, or parotid gland. The skin should be examined for red, swollen tender areas consistent with infection (abscess or acne). Gentle tapping of the dentition with an instrument handle may reveal a sensitive tooth, requiring evaluation by a dentist. The parotid gland should be palpated for irregularity, tenderness, and masses. Stensen's duct, which usually is opposite the second molar, is examined for stones, pus, and lack of saliva. Pus is indicative of a gland infection. Lack of saliva, particularly in an older, dehydrated patient, is suggestive of obstruction or Sjogren's syndrome. These patients need intravenous hydration, antibiotics for Staphylococcus species, and sialagogues.

If uncertainty persists, the pharynx and hypopharynx should be examined. Otalgia may be based on referred sensation via the glossopharyngeal nerve in patients with tonsillitis/pharyngitis or secondary to eustachian tube dysfunction caused by inflammation. If infected, the tonsils may appear red and cryptic with exudate. In mononucleosis, the exudate is thick and the tonsils are markedly red and enlarged. A peritonsillar abscess will deviate the uvula to the opposite side, cause trismus from pterygoid muscle involvement, and result in drooling from inability to swallow. Following tonsillectomy and/or adenoidectomy, pain in the ear is common.

Cancers in this region become painful when nerves or muscles are invaded or if the tumor becomes infected. One of the earliest symptoms of hypopharyngeal cancer is otalgia. Similarly, patients with laryngeal cancer or chondritis may experience otalgia. Again, the neck should be examined because a mass in the neck is also an "early" sign of hypopharyngeal carcinoma. Referral to an otolaryngologist is mandatory if a cancer is suspected or cannot be ruled out.

When no tumor or infection can be detected and a dental examination is normal, the temporomandibular joint (TMJ) should be suspected as the source of the pain. These patients may clench their teeth, grind them during sleep (bruxism), or have had recent dental manipulations resulting in spasm of the pterygoid musculature. The pain usually is described as dull, radiating to the scalp, neck, TMJ, face, or temple. It often is exacerbated by biting or chewing. The patient should be asked about gum-chewing or holding her chin in her palm while sitting. During the examination, the joint should be palpated during opening and closing of the jaw. The mandible should be observed for unusual or unequal excursions as well. An intraoral digital examination may reveal tenderness over the pterygoid musculature. Disorders specific to joints should also be suspected, e.g., the patient with rheumatoid arthritis may have TMJ arthritis. If the diagnosis of TMJ syndrome is entertained, initial treatment with warm, moist heat, soft diet, and nonsteroidal antiinflammatory drugs is indicated. If this fails, the patient should be evaluated by an oral surgeon who treats this entity, since an appliance may be necessary.

Hoarseness

Although hoarseness may have many etiologies, the most common site of pathology is the larynx. Occasionally the patient with poor pulmonary reserve or psychological difficulty develops hoarseness without laryngeal pathology. Speech is produced when a column of air passes through the vocal folds causing them to vibrate. This requires the coordination of the muscles of respiration, phonation, an intact laryngeal lining, and an intact cerebrum and brainstem. Hoarseness includes subjective complaints of breathiness, harshness, diplophonia (speaking in two pitches at the same time), change in pitch, or change in loudness.

The history should include the patient's age and sex, occupation, and the season. Certain professionals, e.g., teachers, singers, and preachers subject their voices to excessive daily use. Associated illness (sinusitis, neoplasms, pneumonia) may change the voice. Trauma resulting in hoarseness may result in permanent voice loss if not attended to early. Allergy, substance abuse (tobacco, alcohol), and medication use (anticholinergic medications) can lead to hoarseness from drying of the mucous membranes of the larynx or tumor formation. Reflux esophagitis may cause hoarseness by creating a chemical burn at the level of the arytenoid mounds of the larynx. Specifically, the onset and duration of the voice change should be noted. Any previous treatment(s) should be noted. Hemoptysis may be noted in supraglottic tumors or laryngeal tuberculosis. Constitutional symptoms of weight loss, shortness of breath, and fatigue should be sought.

Hoarseness usually represents a vocal fold irregularity that does not allow this structure to vibrate correctly. If a patient has inspiratory stridor, this suggests that a mass at or above the level of the vocal cords is present. Expiratory stridor may represent a subglottic or extrathoracic tracheal lesion.

All patients with unexplained hoarseness of greater than two weeks' duration should be evaluated. Following a thorough head and neck examination, the external larynx should be palpated. Tenderness over the prominence (Adam's apple) in the face of laryngeal trauma is indicative of cartilaginous fractures.

The larynx should elevate during swallowing. Grasping the larynx and rocking it side to side should produce crepitus in the normal patient; however, it will glide smoothly in a patient with a cancer in the postcricoid region.

The larynx cannot be visualized in a routine examination without the proper equipment. For this reason, most physicians refer patients for evaluation of suspected laryngeal lesions. If a suspicious lesion is detected on physical examination, particularly in a patient who smokes, a biopsy performed in the operating room is indicated. A paralyzed vocal fold in the absence of trauma, thyroid surgery, or CVA requires systematic evaluation of the chest and skull base for lesions affecting the vagus nerve along its course. MRI or contrast CT scans of these structures and the neck should be performed to rule out lesions of the lung, esophagus, larynx, and thyroid gland.

When no lesion can be detected, or if adequate equipment is lacking, the patient should be referred to an otolaryngologist for further workup. The cause of hoarseness in the patient with no paralysis and no obvious lesion may be minor edema of the mucous membrane of the vocal cord itself, reflux, or misuse of the vocal organ. Voice rest is indicated (avoidance of screaming, singing, excessive speaking, whispering, grunting, and heavy weight lifting). An antireflux regimen (no late meals, antacids, no acidic foods, head-of-bed elevation, nonrestrictive clothing), and hydration will help.

References and Selected Readings

1. English GM (ed): *Otolaryngology.* Philadelphia: JB Lippincott, 1992.
2. Goodhill V (ed): *Ear Diseases, Deafness and Dizziness.* Hagerstown MD: Harper & Row, 1979.
3. Josephson JS, Mattox DE (eds): Update in otolaryngology I. *Med Clin North Am* 75, No. 6: 1991.
4. Kimmelman CP (ed): Otolaryngologic office evaluation and management. *Otolaryngol Clin North Am* 25, No. 4: 1992.
5. Lee KJ (ed): *Essential Otolaryngology, Head and Neck Surgery,* 5th ed. Medical Examination Publishing, 1991.
6. Paparella MM, Shumrick DA, Gluckman JL, Meyerhoff (eds): *Otolaryngology.* Philadelphia: WB Saunders, 1991.

58 Eye Disorders

J. Stephen Hudgins

When faced with what they believe to be a medical problem with their eyes, many patients will turn to their primary care physician for evaluation and treatment. This provider must therefore be comfortable in the assessment of ocular signs and symptoms and in determining what conditions may be treated in his or her office and what conditions need to be stabilized and referred.

Although the source of the patient's ocular problem may be obvious, eliciting a chief ocular complaint, a history of present illness, and a personal and family ocular history is usually time well spent. Likewise, a thorough ocular examination will help the clinician avoid missing unsuspected ancillary problems when the primary problem is known.

Diagnostic Equipment

The equipment needed for a screening ocular examination in the primary care setting includes:

- A visual acuity chart (Snellen)
- An occluder with pinhole
- A penlight or flashlight with a cobalt-blue filter
- A pair of loupes (optional, but useful)
- An ophthalmoscope
- A Schiotz tonometer
- Sterile saline irrigating solution
- Fluorescein strips
- Short-acting mydriatic agent (Tropicamide 1%)
- Topical anesthetic (proparacaine, 0.5%, or tetracaine, 0.5%)

Ocular Symptoms

Decreased Visual Acuity

A rapid or significant decrease in visual acuity may be associated with a serious ocular condition and should be referred for ophthalmologic evaluation. More gradual reductions in vision, especially when visual acuity remains unchanged at some distances usually is indicative of a change in refractive error. If visual acuity significantly improves when the patient is looking through a pinhole, this suggests either an error in focusing or a problem with the clarity of some part of the ocular media (e.g., cornea or lens).

Diplopia

When examining patients with double vision, the first priority is to determine if the diplopia is monocular or binocular. In binocular diplopia, the patient's double vision goes away when either eye is covered. The etiology of this double vision is that the two eyes are aimed in different directions and therefore two different images are sent to the visual cortex. The images may be offset vertically, horizontally, or both, or even tilted. Ocular misalignment can arise from problems with the orbit, the extraocular muscles, the cranial nerves that innervate these muscles, or the brain. Ophthalmologic and sometimes neurologic evaluation is mandatory for adults complaining of binocular diplopia.

In monocular diplopia, the double vision will persist in at least one of the eyes when the other eye is covered. This usually is the result of a problem with the clarity of the ocular media (often the lens, frequently due to cataract formation).

Floaters

New-onset floaters, especially when accompanied by flashes of light seen in the periphery of vision at night, warrant prompt evaluation by an ophthalmologist. While these symptoms usually are attributable to a shifting of the vitreous jelly that fills the back of the eye, they may indicate the onset of a tear or detachment of the retina. Other serious causes of new-onset floaters include vitreous hemorrhage (often seen in diabetics) and inflammatory conditions involving the retina and vitreous.

Scotomas

A blind or blurry spot in the vision of one eye may be due to problems with the retina (e.g., macular hole, retinal hemorrhage, or aging macular degeneration) or optic nerve (e.g., glaucoma). Congruent scotomas in both eyes are presumed to be due to problems in the visual pathways or visual cortex. Migrainous auras, with or without the headache, may cause transient bilateral scotomas.

Photophobia

New-onset photophobia may be due to corneal abrasions or infections, or to intraocular inflammations such as uveitis. Increased glare caused by cataracts or other disturbances in ocular media clarity, or by problems associated with transition from dark to light (as seen with aging macular degeneration) may be confused with photophobia. When a patient complains that she has always been slightly sensitive to bright light, this usually does not suggest a significant problem.

Pain

Assessing the character, location, duration and severity of ocular pain symptoms can be quite helpful in determining the etiology of the pain. Foreign body sensation described as a "sharp, scratchy" pain may be associated with a foreign body or may be seen with corneal abrasions in the absence of a foreign body. A "dull, achy" pain that may be referred to the brow and may be associated with nausea is the hallmark of glaucomatous pain. Headaches often cause pain around or behind the eye and on occasion may be attributed to the eye. Sinus pain also can be referred to the eye. Pain noted with movement of the eye is a serious symptom and may indicate involvement of the retrobulbar region by infectious or other processes.

Orbit

Orbital Cellulitis

Diagnosis Patients usually give a history of trauma to the lids or orbit or sinus disease, or they may have a history of an infection elsewhere in the body. Symptoms may include orbital pain, pain with movement of the eyes, diplopia, decreased vision, fever, and malaise. Examination usually will reveal swelling and rubor of the lids, hyperemia, and chemosis of the conjunctiva. Exophthalmos and restricted ocular motility may be seen.

Treatment Because of the risk of optic nerve injury and the risk of spread of the infection to the cavernous sinus or to the brain, treatment must be aggressive, with hospitalization, culturing of the infection if possible, appropriate IV antibiotics, urgent ophthalmologic and sometimes ENT evaluation, and often imaging of the orbit to look for suppuration.

Exophthalmos

Diagnosis If a patient reports onset of proptosis over a short period of time (not attributable to trauma), retrobulbar hemorrhage, or inflammation or extension of an adjacent sinus infection should be suspected. Proptosis developing over a few weeks is more consistent with orbital pseudotumor or other more chronic inflammatory conditions. Proptosis developing over months is more consistent with thyroid orbitopathy or with an orbital neoplasm. An arteriovenous aneurysm of the cavernous sinus may cause proptosis and may have an associated bruit. Onset can be rapid or more gradual.

Because of the various etiologies of proptosis, imaging of the orbit usually is diagnostic. The urgency of ophthalmologic evaluation is related to the rapidity of onset of the proptosis.

Treatment After the etiology of the proptosis has been determined, treatment objectives are twofold: to treat the underlying cause of the proptosis and to protect the eye from the deleterious side effects of proptosis. The most common side effect is corneal and conjunctival exposure, and this should be treated aggressively with lubricating drops and ointments. Mild misalignments of the eyes sometimes can be treated with prism glasses. Optic nerve impingement can be serious and may require systemic corticosteroids or even orbital surgical decompression.

Eyelids

Blepharitis

Diagnosis Patients with blepharitis complain of ocular irritation (often described as burning or gritty), redness, and increased tearing. They also may report red, scaly lids that may be gummy or matted on awakening. Ocular examination reveals a red, sometimes scarred lid margin with telangiectatic vessels, lid margin debris, and conjunctival hyperemia.

Treatment Blepharitis may represent a chronic low-grade bacterial (usually staphylococcal or streptococcal) infection of the meibomian glands and lash follicles. In other patients, the etiology may be more akin to skin conditions such as seborrhea. In either case, the bulwark of the treatment is lid hygiene using warm compresses and some mild scrubbing action twice a day. When an infectious component is suspected, erythromycin or bacitracin ointment twice daily to the lid margin after the warm soaks is useful. Lubricant eye drops during the day may be of symptomatic benefit.

Hordeolum (Stye)

Diagnosis Styes represent a localized infection of a lash follicle or meibomian gland at the lid margin.

Examination reveals a localized area of redness, swelling, and tenderness at the lid margin. If the lesion has started to point, a whitish or yellowish area of induration may occupy the center of the lesion.

Treatment Drainage of the lesion is encouraged by application of warm compresses for 5 to 10 min, three to four times a day. Because the infecting organism is usually staph or strep, an antibiotic ointment with good gram-positive coverage such as erythromycin or bacitracin may be applied twice daily. Occasionally the lesions will not drain or clear and will require surgical incision and drainage.

Chalazion

Diagnosis Meibomian glands located in the tarsal plates of the upper and lower lids produce oil that exits at the lid margin. When the gland's orifice is blocked, oil production is backed up; the gland is dilated; and a small, round, smooth, nontender mass may be noted in the lid. This stagnant collection of oily/waxy material is easily infected. When infected it becomes hot, red, irritated, and tender. Eversion of the lid may aid in diagnosis, especially if the lesion has started to point.

Treatment Treatment is similar to that of the stye, with warm compresses and topical antibiotics. Rarely, systemic antibiotics are required if a large region of the lid appears to be involved.

Preseptal Cellulitis

Diagnosis This condition simulates some of the signs and symptoms of orbital cellulitis with lid redness and swelling. Because this represents infection anterior to the orbital septum, proptosis, motility disorder, visual reduction, pain on ocular movement, and inflammation of the bulbar conjunctiva should never be seen.

Treatment If orbital cellulitis has been completely ruled out, the condition can be treated in compliant adult patients with systemic antibiotics on an ambulatory basis. Patients should be alerted to signs and symptoms that might indicate progression to orbital cellulitis and instructed to seek follow-up immediately if they occur.

Structural Lid Problem

Diagnosis Trauma, burns, chronic blepharitis, and aging can lead to lid abnormalities such as entropion, ectropion or lid margin irregularity or scarring. This, in turn, can lead to irritation of the globe either directly or due to poor distribution of tears and/or exposure.

Treatment Lubricating drops or ointments may be sufficient to prevent significant discomfort or damage. Epilation of inturned lashes and, in some cases, surgical correction are required.

Skin Cancers of the Lid

Diagnosis Skin cancers are not uncommon around the eyes. Basal cell carcinomas are the most common, but squamous cell carcinomas, melanomas, and even metastatic lesions are seen. Sun exposure and skin type are risk factors; the lower lid is most often involved.

Treatment Treatment of skin cancers of the lids must satisfy two objectives: complete removal of the lesion and maximum preservation of lid tissue and function.

Lacrimal Apparatus

Overflow Tearing

Diagnosis Epiphora may arise from excessive tear production, usually secondary to ocular irritation, structural abnormalities of the eyelid or lid margin, or from poor drainage of tears through the tear ducts. Poor drainage may be due to blockage or stenosis of the duct passages or by a functional abnormality of its pumping action. Epiphora in adults is more often due to functional abnormalities or lid problems.

Treatment Congenital overflow tearing in children often spontaneously resolves with or without treatment. Treatment consists of lacrimal sac massage performed twice a day and antibiotic drops. When the symptoms persist, probing or placement of tubes in the tear ducts usually is effective. In adults, evaluation and treatment can be combined in irrigation and probing of the tear ducts. Occasionally, in children and adults, more definitive surgical treatment is needed.

Dacryocystitis

Diagnosis Ocular examination usually reveals pain, redness, swelling and tenderness overlying the lacrimal sac. Massage of the lacrimal sac may express purulent material through the puncta (the opening of the lacrimal duct). Because the tear ducts are partly or totally obstructed, the patients may complain of epiphora.

Treatment Hot compresses over the lacrimal sac and systemic antibiotics are indicated. Culturing of the expressed purulent material during the initial evaluation often is useful. Unfortunately, these infections may be difficult to eradicate; even when stabilized, they may leave residual scarring and stenosis in the tear ducts.

Conjunctiva

Subconjunctival Hemorrhage

Diagnosis The cause of subconjunctival hemorrhage is the breakage of a small blood vessel in or under the conjunctiva. Patients often first notice the condition when they look in the mirror or when a friend or co-worker asks what happened to their eye. Vision is usually unaffected; there is no discharge, and at most there is mild ocular awareness; there is never any pain. The history may reveal recent use of nonsteroidal anti-inflammatory medications. Onset is sometimes associated with coughing or sneezing, emesis, rubbing the eye or straining while having a bowel movement. Ocular examination reveals that all or part of the conjunctiva is bright red. The redness stops at the corneal limbus and there is never blood in the eye.

Treatment The patient should be instructed not to rub her eye. Acetaminophen should be substituted for the nonsteroidal anti-inflammatory medication if possible. Cool compresses may help if the patient complains of ocular awareness.

Conjunctivitis

Conjunctivitis may have an allergic or infectious origin. Less frequently it may be due to a toxic reaction or have a systemic cause.

Allergic Conjunctivitis

Diagnosis Patients with allergic conjunctivitis invariably complain of itch. Without significant itching, the physician should not diagnose an allergic etiology. Patients also may complain of burning, increased tearing with a mucus discharge, and may report conjunctival redness and eyelid swelling. They usually give a history of allergies, and the symptoms often are seasonal. If the offending allergen is airborne or ingested, the condition usually will be bilateral, though it may be asymmetric in intensity. However, if the causative allergen was touched with the finger before touching the eye, the condition may be unilateral.

Treatment There are two goals of treatment: 1. alleviating the signs and symptoms of past and present exposure; 2. preventing future exposure. Ice-cold ocular compresses are quite effective in reducing redness, swelling, and itch. Topical vasoconstrictor/antihistamine drops are useful when not overused. Mast cell inhibitors which are now once again available in drop form are effective agents for chronic treatment. The use of steroid eye drops should be restricted to ophthalmologists.

Infectious Conjunctivitis

Diagnosis Infectious conjunctivitis can be bacterial, viral or chlamydial in origin. Viral conjunctivitis probably is the most common. Patients with adenoviral conjunctivitis complain of a red, scratchy eye and increased tearing. Patients often have a simultaneous URI, and a preauricular node may be palpable. The condition eventually is bilateral in 80 percent, but usually starts in one eye. Herpes conjunctivitis may present in a similar fashion; however, lid vesicles may be seen and the condition is more typically unilateral. Preauricular adenopathy may be seen with chlamydial conjunctivitis but usually not with bacterial conjunctivitis. A history of sexually transmitted Chlamydia may be elicited with chlamydial conjunctivitis.

Treatment If chlamydial conjunctivitis is suspected, appropriate cultures should be obtained. Though topical antibiotics may provide symptomatic relief in chlamydial conjunctivitis, oral antibiotics usually are needed to effect a cure. As with other sexually transmitted chlamydial diseases, sexual partners may need to be treated. If bacterial conjunctivitis cannot be ruled out by history or exam, treatment with a broad-spectrum antibiotic such as topical ciprofloxacin or trimethoprim/polymyxin B should be initiated. Because these infections are usually due to gram-positive organisms, gentamycin (Garamycin) or tobramycin are not good first choices. Many organisms are now resistant to topical sulfonamides, so these also should be avoided. The high rates of allergic reaction to preparations containing neomycin should discourage their use.

Cornea

Pterygium

Diagnosis Patients with pterygia may be asymptomatic or may report mild chronic ocular irritation and sensitivity to dust and wind. Many patients will ask what is growing into their cornea. Ocular examination reveals a winglike, whitish growth extending from the conjunctiva onto the cornea at 3 or 9 o'clock along the corneal limbus. The lesion may or may not appear inflamed. A small, yellow-whitish bump on the conjunctiva called a pinqueculum is usually the progenitive lesion.

Treatment Minimizing sun and wind exposure by sunglasses, wearing a hat or restricting time spent unprotected out of doors may slow the lesion's growth. Artificial tear supplements may decrease inflammation and increase comfort. When the lesions become large, they should be surgically removed, although they may grow back.

Keratoconjunctivitis Sicca (KCS)

Diagnosis Patients with KCS complain of dry, gritty eyes. In most patients the symptoms are less on awakening and increase during the day, or with exposure to wind. Symptoms tend to be worse in the winter owing to lower humidity levels in the air. The eyes may be red, and vision may be normal or reduced. Paradoxically, some patients with dry eyes complain of episodic teariness, probably caused by chronic irritation triggering a short period of excess lacrimal secretion. Ocular examination may appear normal. Rose bengal staining by an ophthalmologist often will prove diagnostic by revealing mild to moderate exposure in the interpalpebral region.

Treatment Tear supplements are useful. When needed more than four times a day, preservative-free drops should be used. In more severe cases, closure of the tear ducts may be useful.

Infectious Keratitis

Diagnosis Patients with corneal infections complain of pain, photophobia, increased tearing, and often of decreased vision in the affected eye. When the infection is due to bacteria, the patients may have had prior corneal trauma or foreign bodies, or they may use contact lenses. Patients with fungal infections of the cornea often report trauma with vegetable material, such as being struck in the eye with a branch. Patients with herpes simplex infection may give a history of cold sores, blistering around the eye, or a past similar infection in the same or other eye. Ocular examination reveals conjunctival hyperemia and a corneal lesion that stains with fluorescein. Mucoid material may be adherent to the lesion. A hypopyon (accumulation of white blood cells in the anterior chamber of the eye) may be present.

Treatment Because of the risk of permanent visual loss or even loss of the eye, infectious keratitis should be treated only by an ophthalmologist. Antibiotics should not be started by the primary care physician because the lesion may need to be cultured. Ophthalmologic evaluation should be performed within a few hours if possible.

Glaucoma

Chronic Open Angle Glaucoma (COAG)

Diagnosis The great majority of patients with COAG never have any symptoms attributable to their glaucoma. Because of this, it is thought that up to half of the patients with COAG are unaware of their condition. COAG is thought to represent a mild to moderate elevation in intraocular pressure brought on by a chronic gradual reduction in outflow facility (at the iridocorneal angle). In other words, fluid flows into the eye, but outflow becomes more difficult over time and the fluid pressure then rises. The elevated pressure damages the optic nerve, with the fibers subserving peripheral vision being the most vulnerable and therefore the first destroyed. As the nerve is damaged, its appearance slowly changes, with the nerve head's anatomical cup becoming larger and larger over time. Asymmetric optic cups, large optic cups, and optic nerve head hemorrhages are all signs of possible glaucoma. The measurement of intraocular pressure, usually by Schiotz tonometer, is another way to detect glaucoma. Because intraocular pressure demonstrates significant fluctuation over time, a normal reading does not rule out glaucoma. Likewise, a high reading, especially if only mildly elevated, does not prove glaucoma, but is sufficient basis for ophthalmologic evaluation. The few patients who have symptoms prior to diagnosis may experience eye ache or headache, may see halos around lights, or may note decreased peripheral vision. Because these symptoms are associated with higher pressure levels or more advanced disease, more urgent evaluation and referral is indicated.

Treatment Most but not all patients with glaucoma can achieve complete control of their disease with daily topical and/or oral medication. A few patients require laser treatments to reach good control and a very few require surgery. Regular ophthalmologic follow-up with periodic visual field testing is usually required for the rest of the patient's life.

Angle-Closure Glaucoma

Diagnosis Unlike chronic open angle glaucoma, patients with angle closure glaucoma are almost always symptomatic. Patients often complain of a severe achy pain in the eye or brow and ocular tenderness. Visual symptoms include halos around lights due to corneal edema and/or sudden loss of vision. The patients may have nausea and vomiting. Ocular examination reveals a red eye with limbal injection, corneal cloudiness, and a significant elevation in intraocular pressure. Other findings may include a shallow anterior chamber and/or a fixed mid-dilated pupil.

Treatment Because the decrease in outflow facility, and therefore the pressure elevation, often is due to the peripheral iris tissue blocking the angle, constriction of the pupil with pilocarpine 2% is indicated. In patients for whom beta-blockers are not contraindicated, Betoptic 0.5% may be instilled. Carbonic anhydrase inhibitors [e.g., acetazolamide (Diamox) 500 mg] given orally in patients for whom they are not contraindicated aid in reducing pressure. Oral glycerin (or isosorbide for diabetics) also will usually result in the reduction of pressure. Ophthalmologic referral during the initial treatment or after the patient's condition is stabilized is recommended. Laser surgery is usually recommended and has been generally effective in preventing recurrences of the angle closure attack.

Secondary Glaucoma

Diagnosis Glaucoma can arise secondary to trauma, prolonged systemic or topical corticosteroid treatment, vascular disturbances in the eye or in the blood flow to the eye, or following cataract or other intraocular eye surgery. Uveitis, intraocular tumors, or even advanced cataracts can cause glaucoma.

Treatment Treatment involves simultaneous control of pressure and correction, if possible, of the underlying cause of the glaucoma.

Uveitis

Diagnosis Uveitis refers to inflammation of the uveal tissues which include the iris, ciliary body and choroid. When the inflammation primarily affects the anterior uveal structures, patients complain of pain, photophobia, and possibly reduced vision; they report ocular redness. Ocular examination reveals circumcorneal injection. Adhesions from the iris to the lens may distort the pupillary opening. Intraocular pressure may be high, low, or normal. When the inflammation is more posterior in the eye, patients complain primarily of reduced vision and floaters. The external eye usually is quiet, and pain and photophobia may be minimal or absent.

Treatment Along with the treatment of the acute manifestations of the condition comes the search for and treatment of the underlying cause of the problem. Some causes, such as syphilis, tuberculosis, and Lyme disease, can be cured with antibiotics. Others, such as herpes zoster, herpes simplex, and toxoplasmosis have specific palliative treatments, but no cure. Still others, such as sarcoidosis and juvenile rheumatoid arthritis (JRA), while not curable, alert the practitioner to search for and treat systemic manifestations of the conditions. Because uveitis may present in many subtly different forms and because these different forms suggest different etiologies, early ophthalmic evaluation is mandatory. Likewise, because of the potentially serious nature of the condition and the risk of permanent eye damage, vision loss, and glaucoma, treatment should be initiated and followed by an ophthalmologist.

Lens

Cataract

Diagnosis Adult patients with cataracts report painless progressive loss of vision. Patients may also report loss of contrast and increased glare. Cataracts usually can be seen with the direct ophthalmoscope, viewing the eye from a distance of approximately one foot. Dilation of the pupil will aid diagnosis, but usually is not required.

Treatment Mild cataracts may be followed. Visually significant cataracts (best corrected visual acuities of 20/50 or worse attributable to the cataract) may be surgically removed. Surgical intervention also may be indicated with acuities greater than 20/50 when glare is significant or the patient's driving or work is affected. Rarely, cataracts grow and cause glaucoma, in which case prompt removal is indicated. If, as rarely happens, the cataract causes intraocular inflammation, rapid removal is indicated.

Retina

Aging Macular Degeneration (AMD)

Diagnosis AMD is a leading cause of blindness in elderly white patients. The condition is painless and affects only the central vision; the peripheral vision is spared. Patients may notice blurring, distortion, or both in the center of their vision. The condition usually is bilateral, although the presentation and severity may be quite asymmetric. In mild cases, ocular examination may reveal the loss of the foveal reflex or mild heterogeneity in the macular retinal pigment epithelium. Macular hemorrhage or scarring may be seen in more severe cases.

Treatment In the great majority of patients with AMD, the changes are gradual and untreatable. In 15 percent of patients however, an acute worsening of the condition will be noted, usually secondary to subretinal hemorrhage and scar formation. In some of these patients, laser treatments may be of limited benefit in halting or reversing the acute exacerbation. Referral to an ophthalmologist is indicated.

Retinal Detachment

Diagnosis Unfortunately, there are no signs nor symptoms pathognomonic for retinal detachment. The most reliable is the loss of part of the peripheral vision in one eye. The patient may report this as a shadow in the periphery of the vision. Floaters or flashes may be associated with retinal detachment but usually are indicative of a posterior vitreous detachment without retinal detachment. Detachment of the macula will result in significant unilateral vision loss. Confrontation visual field testing may be useful. Ophthalmoscopy through a dilated pupil may reveal vitreous hemorrhage or pigment, or the detachment itself may be seen. However, because much of the fundus cannot be visualized with the direct ophthalmoscope, nothing abnormal may be seen.

Treatment If retinal detachment is seen or suspected, the patient needs prompt referral for ophthalmologic evaluation. Trauma, recent cataract or other intraocular surgery, or diabetes are risk factors and should raise the level of suspicion. Some small detachments can be treated with laser surgery. Larger detachments usually require placement of plastic devices called buckles on the outside of the eye. Some detachments also require intraocular surgery to repair.

Diabetic Retinopathy

Diagnosis Diabetes often leads to vascular changes in the retina. In mild or early diabetes, the retina may look normal. The first changes typically seen are microaneurysms and hemorrhage; this is designated "background retinopathy." Hard exudates and macular edema may result from the vascular changes, and these may mildly or markedly reduce vision. When vascular changes become more pronounced, areas of local retinal infarction called cotton-wool spots may develop. More severe changes produce abnormal new blood vessel formation called neovascularization. These vessels bleed easily and may contract, causing traction to—and sometimes detachment of—the retina. For patients with adult-onset diabetes, ophthalmologic evaluation should be done at least once yearly, and more frequently as the severity of the condition increases. Pregnant diabetics should be seen at a minimum of every three months during pregnancy. Patients with juvenile-onset diabetes almost never develop problems during the first five years of their disease, but require yearly examinations from then on.

Treatment The great majority of diabetic patients never require treatment for their diabetic retinopathy. However, most patients with neovascular changes eventually require a laser treatment called panretinal photocoagulation. Some patients with macular swelling and exudates can benefit from a different laser treatment called focal or grid treatment. Rarely, surgery is required. Good diabetic control has been shown to slow the onset of significant retinopathy and should be encouraged.

Retinal Vascular Occlusions

Diagnosis Patients with central retinal artery occlusion complain of painless unilateral blindness. If the patient is awake when the occlusion occurs, onset will be described as sudden; otherwise, it will be noticed on awakening. If one of the major retinal arterial branches is occluded, blindness in a part of the visual field is reported. If a smaller branch is occluded, the patient may be asymptomatic. Examination reveals retinal pallor in the area affected. Occasionally the obstructing plaque or emboli may be visualized. The affected retinal arteries may appear attenuated, and stagnant, discontinuous segments of blood may be seen in the vessels. An afferent pupillary defect may be noted in the affected eye. Patients with venous obstructions report more gradual onset of less severe unilateral vision loss. Hemorrhages and edema will be seen in the affected area of the retina, and the affected veins may appear distended.

Treatment Unless corrected within approximately one hour, retinal artery occlusion will result in permanent damage to the affected areas of the retina; therefore, this is a true ophthalmic emergency. No treatment works all the time, but intermittent massage of the eye and/or inhalations of 5% CO_2 have been recommended. An ophthalmologist may attempt an anterior chamber paracentesis to reduce intraocular pressure, and thereby may dislodge or move the obstruction. Evaluation to identify embolic sources or temporal arteritis is of utmost importance to prevent stroke and/or damage to the other eye. Because venous obstruction is usually seen in patients with hypertension, heart disease, diabetes, or peripheral vascular disease, a thorough history and physical examination usually will be indicated. Although venous obstructions usually clear over a period of months, neovascular changes of the retina and iris and severe glaucoma can result. Therefore, the patient should receive periodic ophthalmic evaluations until the condition clears, and laser treatments if problems appear.

Optic Nerve

Optic Neuritis

Diagnosis Patients complain of decreased vision in one eye and may report problems with color vision or decreased color saturation. Occasionally there is pain with movement of the eye. Ocular examination may reveal visual acuity from 20/20 to the complete absence of light perception. An afferent pupillary defect is present in the affected eye, although it may be subtle when vision is only minimally affected. The eye appears quiet, and ophthalmoscopic exam may reveal blurring of the disk margin, nerve head hyperemia, peripapillary swelling, and hemorrhages and venous congestion.

Treatment Prompt referral to an ophthalmologist or neurologist is indicated.

Papilledema

Diagnosis Patients may complain of headache, blurring of vision, and brief obscurations of vision. Other neurologic signs or symptoms related to increased intracranial pressure may be present. Ophthalmoscopic examination of the optic nerves will show disk head elevation bilaterally.

Treatment Prompt neurologic evaluation is indicated.

Injuries

Ocular injuries can range from the trivial to the blinding. The extent of the injuries may not be immediately apparent; a careful examination and a complete history with detailed documentation almost always are indicated. If the history of injury includes possible chemical burns, irrigation should be initiated promptly (see ocular burns). In most other circumstances, a more detailed history may be obtained before initiating treatment. If the history suggests possible penetrating or perforating injuries to the eye, examination and manipulation of the eye should be minimized. A determination of visual acuity, pupillary response, extraocular motility, the location and extent of orbit and lid injuries, and the location(s) of any foreign bodies should be made. The presence or absence of conjunctival hemorrhage, laceration, corneal abrasion or laceration, and hyphema should be noted. If possible, direct ophthalmoscopy should be performed and the ease or difficulty of visualization recorded.

Superficial Foreign Bodies

Diagnosis Usually, but not always, the patient will give a history of "something in the eye." The patient will complain of a foreign body sensation, sometimes worse in certain gaze positions. The patient may report decreased visual acuity and/or photophobia. Inspection of the eye will be greatly facilitated by instillation of a topical anesthetic. Visualization of foreign bodies may be enhanced with fluorescein staining. The upper and lower lids should be everted. If loupes are available, they will aid in locating small foreign bodies.

Treatment Many foreign bodies can be removed with a cotton-tipped applicator. More deeply embedded foreign bodies can be removed with the edge of a large gauge hypodermic needle or foreign body spud, although this should be done by a physician skilled in this procedure. Deeper foreign bodies or metallic foreign bodies that have rusted require removal by an ophthalmologist. If the eye is thought to be infected, prompt referral to an ophthalmologist is indicated. Otherwise, a topical antibiotic ointment such as erythromycin or bacitracin may be instilled, and, if the cornea is abraded, an eye-patch applied to keep the eyelid closed overnight.

Intraocular Foreign Bodies

When an intraocular foreign body is suspected, manipulation and examination should be minimized and the patient promptly referred to and seen by an ophthalmologist. A rigid shield should be placed over the eye. No ointment should be placed in the eye. In consultation with the ophthalmologist, broad-spectrum antibiotic therapy may be initiated.

Orbital Trauma

Trauma to the orbit from such injuries as falls, motor vehicle accidents, assaults, and industrial accidents often result in bruising and extravasation of blood in the adnexal region, leading to what is commonly known as a "black" eye. If this is the extent of the injury, treatment consists of cold compresses for 24 to 36 h and elevation to minimize swelling. Significant hemorrhage behind the eye as evidenced by exophthalmos, subconjunctival hemorrhage, extraocular motility disorder, and/or decreased vision is potentially quite serious, and urgent ophthalmologic evaluation is indicated. Orbital trauma may result in fracture of the orbital rim or a blow-out fracture involving one or more of the bones that make up the orbit. Signs and symptoms may include enophthalmos, periorbital crepitance, diplopia, and numbness of the cheek. Work-up usually involves radiologic imaging of the orbit. When a blow-out fracture is suspected, prompt evaluation by an ophthalmologist or ENT specialist is indicated.

Lid Trauma

Lacerations of the eyelids are common. Repair of these lacerations, when indicated, must be done by an ophthalmologist under the following circumstances:

- When there is significant tissue loss
- When the lid margin is involved
- When the lacrimal apparatus is potentially damaged
- When the laceration is deep or when eyelid structures other than the skin may be involved.

Conjunctival Trauma

Subconjunctival hemorrhages are quite common and usually resolve without complication. However, subconjunctival hemorrhage may obscure deeper, more serious injuries. If this is a possibility, ophthalmologic evaluation is indicated. Because some conjunctival lacerations need to be repaired, ophthalmologic follow-up is indicated when these are diagnosed.

Corneal Trauma

Diagnosis Patients usually report pain and/or a foreign body sensation, and may report photophobia or reduced vision. Corneal trauma often is associated with a foreign body that may or may not be in the eye when the patient is seen. Damage to the corneal surface (e.g., corneal abrasion) may be demarcated after the instillation of fluorescein. Application of a topical anesthetic drop such as proparacaine will improve patient comfort dramatically and will facilitate evaluation.

Treatment If foreign bodies are seen, they should be removed as previously described. If there are signs of deeper corneal injury such as a corneal laceration or some indication or suspicion of corneal infection, the patient needs prompt ophthalmologic evaluation. Otherwise, instillation of an antibiotic ointment such as erythromycin or bacitracin followed by application of an eye-patch to keep the lid shut is indicated. In extreme abrasions, one drop of homatropine, 2% may be instilled prior to patching to ease ciliary spasm. Next day follow-up with an ophthalmologist is indicated.

Intraocular Trauma

Intraocular trauma usually, but not invariably, causes decreased vision and often pain. Sometimes there are externally visible signs of inflammation, such as conjunctival hyperemia. Hyphemia, or blood in the anterior chamber, usually indicates trauma to the uveal structures. Because of the risk of elevated intraocular pressure, emergent ophthalmologic evaluation is indicated. A shallow anterior chamber, distortion of the pupil, and/or decreased clarity of the internal ocular media are all signs of potential intraocular injury and need ophthalmologic evaluation. Patient visual symptoms such as new floaters, flashes, scotomas, or other new visual field defects strongly suggest intraocular damage and should be specifically asked about when ocular trauma has occurred.

Ocular Burns

Chemical Burns

Diagnosis Significant ocular chemical burns will produce mild to marked lid swelling, conjunctival hyperemia and chemosis, and corneal haze. This may be generalized or may be greater in the interpalpebral region. Because tearing tends to wash chemicals inferiorly, the inferior conjunctiva may be more affected. Sometimes lid swelling is so pronounced as to make examination and treatment quite difficult.

Treatment After instillation of several drops of a topical anesthetic agent, initiate irrigation of the eye with isotonic sterile saline. The present recommendation for chemical injuries due to caustic agents is to irrigate for one-half hour or more. The eyelids should be everted to facilitate irrigation under the lids and to allow for visualization and removal of material that may be lodged in the cul-de-sac. Except for the most trivial of chemical injuries, prompt ophthalmologic evaluation is indicated.

Thermal Burns

Diagnosis Thermal burns to the eyes are seldom seen in isolation; usually, facial or other burns are present. The skin of the eyelids may have suffered first-, second-, or third-degree burns. Lashes are often singed or absent. The conjunctiva usually is hyperemic and/or chemotic. Corneal haze and edema often are present.

Treatment Significant thermal lid or eye burns require prompt ophthalmologic evaluation.

Ultraviolet Burns

Diagnosis The patient usually will give a history of exposure to the light from arc welding, exposure to a tanning booth or bed, or sun exposure usually associated with reflection from snow or water. The light exposure usually precedes the typical symptoms of pain, increased tearing, decreased vision, and photophobia by 6 to 12 h. Examination reveals conjunctival hyperemia, corneal haze, and fluorescein uptake in a diffuse, often interpalpebral, pattern.

Treatment After instillation of a topical anesthetic agent, a mild antibiotic agent such as erythromycin or bacitracin may be instilled, followed by patching to keep the lids shut. The patient should be informed that the pain usually recurs when the topical anesthetic wears off and that she may need oral analgesics until her eyes heal in a day or so. Because topical anesthetic agents may slow or prevent healing, their use after diagnosis should be minimized.

Contact Lenses

For many millions of women, contact lenses are a safe, effective, and in some cases superior alternative to spectacle glasses for the correction of refractive errors. Unfortunately, however, the use and misuse of contact lenses represents a risk factor for a wide variety of ocular conditions. Poorly fitted, damaged, or contaminated contact lenses may injure the surface of the eye. Improper insertion or removal, over-wearing, or sleeping in contact lenses not meant to be slept in may lead to a red, irritated eye. The risk of corneal infection is greatly increased in contact lens wearers. In the presence of ocular irritation, redness, or decreased vision, the patient needs to know that the first step in treatment and sometimes the only step needed is to stop wearing the lenses. However, if the patient's symptoms do not quickly and completely resolve, ophthalmologic evaluation is needed.

Physiologic Changes and Problems During Pregnancy

Physiologic ocular changes due to pregnancy include chloasma of the eyelids, decrease in intraocular pressure, transient loss of accommodation, changes in corneal thickness and sensitivity, and changes in the tear film. These latter changes may interface with previous successful contact lens wear. Pre-existing conditions potentially exacerbated by pregnancy include diabetic retinopathy, Graves disease and pituitary adenomas. Sarcoidosis may improve during pregnancy. Pathologic conditions that may develop during pregnancy include central serous retinopathy and ptosis. Toxemia of pregnancy can induce ocular changes, including retinal hemorrhages and ischemia, ischemic optic neuropathy, papilledema, and retinal detachment. Transient cortical blindness with eclampsia has been reported.

References and Suggested Readings

1. American Academy of Ophthalmology: Basic and Clinical Science Course 1992–1993, Sections 1–11. San Francisco, 1992.
2. Kanski JJ: *Clinical Ophthalmology, A Systematic Approach,* 2d ed. London: Butterworths, 1989.
3. Mills J: *Current Emergency Diagnosis and Treatment,* 3d ed. Los Altos, CA: Lange Medical Publications.
4. Tremain S, Abbot R: *The Diagnosis and Treatment of Red Eye.* Kansas City, MO: American Academy of Family Physicians, 1991.
5. Tasman W (ed): *Duane's Clinical Ophthalmology,* Philadelphia: JB Lippincott, 1993.
6. Berkow R: The Merck Manual, 16th ed. Rahway, NJ: Merck Research Laboratories, 1992.
7. Behrmann RE: *Nelson's Textbook of Pediatrics,* 14th ed. Philadelphia: WB Saunders, 1992.
8. Sumress JS: *The Pregnant Woman's Eye.* Survey of Ophthalmology vol. 32, No. 4, Jan–Feb 1988.

59 Dental and Medical Interrelationships

Peter A. Mychajliw
James J. Sciubba

As advances in diagnostic technologies, research, and treatment modalities continue, the identification of patients with acute and/or chronic dental problems will increase. It is imperative that dentists and physicians manage these patients jointly and comprehensively based on their medical, dental, physical, and psychological findings. Although many women receiving medical care may seem to have adequate oral health, one must continually be aware of the intimate interrelationships between medicine and dental medicine. Appropriate referrals must be made for a wide array of conditions (Table 59-1).

After referral for dental evaluation, the physician should receive a comprehensive report detailing the patient's chief complaint, positive findings of the history, (limited) physical, laboratory, radiology, and clinical examinations. An overview of the proposed treatment plan, including any preventive/interceptive or emergent care, and an overall diagnosis also should be included. If the patient has or subsequently develops a medically related problem, the dentist and physician must agree on any modifications or contraindications to the proposed dental treatment based on those variables. The patient should then be counseled accordingly before beginning comprehensive dental treatment. Should the request for consultation originate from the dentist, the same scenario would apply.

Dental Care during Pregnancy

A classic example of the importance of coordinated care by the dentist and the physician is in the case of the pregnant patient. Therapeutic dental care must

TABLE 59-1 Conditions Likely to Benefit from Dental Medicine Consultation

Systemic diseases that may have oral manifestations/complications, e.g., AIDS, Sjögren's syndrome
Before cancer chemotherapy
Before head and neck cancer radiation therapy or extirpative oncologic surgery
Before organ transplant
Before cardiac valve surgery
Oral complications of pregnancy
Eating disorders
Xerostomia
Infection suspected of soft/hard tissues in the head and neck region
Developmental or acquired physical or mental disabilities
Dentofacial deformities

be rendered to the patient without endangering the fetus. The physician must provide an evaluation of the patient's current medical condition, a plan for prenatal management, a history of any previous pregnancies, and information regarding any complicating factors. A comprehensive treatment plan is formulated that stresses maintenance of optimal oral hygiene throughout the pregnancy, and tailors the treatment sequence to minimize or avoid exposure to such potentially harmful procedures as radiation, drugs, supine hypotension in late pregnancy, and breast milk transmission of drugs to the infant.

Radiographs crucial to an accurate dental diagnosis are best obtained in the second or early third trimester. Radiography is to be avoided, if possible, during the first trimester, as the fetus is particularly susceptible to damage from radiation at this time. Radiographic procedure precautions that must be in place include lead apron, high-speed film, collimation, filtration, long cone, and high voltage.

In some human and animal studies, exposures as high as 5 to 10 cGy total dose have shown no associated increase in gross congenital malformations, intrauterine growth retardation, or abortion. A chest radiograph delivers an approximate fetal dose of 0.08 cGy. A complete diagnostic series of dental radiographs with a lead apron in place yields 0.0001 cGy fetal dose. A single dental radiograph taken with the precautions outlined, does not pose a substantial radiation risk to the fetus.[3,10]

Ideally, no drug should be administered during pregnancy. Unfortunately, that is not always possible. Many of the drugs commonly used in dentistry may be used with relative safety. The current issues of the Food and Drug Administration Drug Bulletin and *Physician's Desk Reference* (PDR) may need to be consulted, and the dentist should speak with the obstetrician prior to prescribing. The major concerns are fetal toxicity or teratogenicity and maternal problems that could result in fetal hypoxia. Local anesthetics such as lidocaine and mepivicaine and antibiotics such as penicillin and the cephalosporins may be utilized with relative safety during all trimesters. Tetracyclines are contraindicated owing to the potential for tooth discoloration and tooth enamel hypoplasia in the developing dentition. Aminoglycosides, streptomycin in particular, also are contraindicated. Several medications should be avoided when a woman is breastfeeding; the dentist should check with the PDR and with the patient's physician before prescribing if there is any question regarding safety.

Oral complications of pregnancy commonly include gingival changes, exacerbation of existing gingivitis and periodontal disease, and a generalized increase in tooth mobility. An exaggerated inflammatory response to local irritants, especially bacterial plaque secondary to hormonal influences and vascular changes, becomes readily apparent at the second month, progressing to a maximal effect at the eighth month, with resolution postpartum. The marginal gingiva and interdental papillae are most affected; these areas often become enlarged, painful, edematous, and bleed readily upon minimal provocation. Periodontal pseudopocketing also may occur secondary to interdental papillae hypertrophy. Pyogenic granulomas or pregnancy tumors occur in approximately 5 percent of pregnant women, usually appearing during the second trimester. The most common site is the labial gingiva of the anterior maxilla. They can be pedunculated or sessile, are usually painless, and bleed readily. These generally disappear after delivery, but may need surgical removal earlier if indicated. This would best be accomplished during the second trimester.

Tooth mobility is believed to be associated with the degree of gingival disease and attachment apparatus disturbance. It generally resolves postpartum. The ''soft teeth'' myth in pregnancy is predicated on the old belief that maternal teeth satisfy fetal calcium requirements. This is not the case, as the calcium in teeth is a crystalline type unavailable to the systemic circulation.[9,10,20]

The timing of dental treatment during pregnancy is relatively straightforward. During the first trimester, only plaque control therapy, including nonsurgical periodontal management, oral hygiene instruction, and emergency care should be rendered. Elective care should be deferred to the second and early third trimesters. As previously mentioned, the second trimester is the safest time to provide most elective dental care; however, anything that can be safely postponed until after childbirth should be. Plaque control and nonsurgical periodontal therapy may continue through the second and third trimesters.[10]

The dentist should also seize these opportunities to educate the patient and her spouse, if possible, about the baby's dental development, dental disease and prevention, the importance of a good plaque control program, and fluoride supplementation, if warranted. The American Academy of Pediatric Dentistry recommends an oral examination and preventive health education within six months of eruption of the first primary tooth and no later than at one year of age.

Dentistry in Relation to Other Common Health Care Issues

Oral Contraceptives

As with pregnant patients, it is of paramount importance that the dentist who is prescribing certain medications be knowledgeable about drug administration to women taking oral contraceptives. Currently, there may be more than 10 million American women taking these agents. Numerous reports have implicated a wide variety of drugs that may cause reduction of contraceptive efficacy. These include ampicillin, penicillin, tetracyclines, clotrimazole, griseofulvin, phenytoin, phenobarbital, phenylephrine, phenylbutazone, phenacetin, diazepam, and cyclophosphamide, among others. The prescriber must advise the patient of potential reduction of effectiveness of the oral contraceptive owing to drug interaction.[22]

Endocarditis

Various forms of congenital heart disease, coarctation of the aorta, cardiac valve abnormalities, artificial cardiac valves, rheumatic heart disease, hypertrophic aortic stenosis, indwelling vascular catheter (right heart), hypertrophic cardiomyopathy, ventriculoatrial shunts for hydrocephalus, mitral valve prolapse with regurgitation, and mitral valve surgery may place patients at risk for infective endocarditis and/or endarteritis subsequent to bacteremia. Such exposure can be traced to many invasive procedures, including those of the upper respiratory, genitourinary, and gastrointestinal tracts, and to invasive dental treatment involving mucosal surfaces or contaminated tissues.[6,13] Prophylactic use of antibiotics is recommended for patients at risk for endocarditis when undergoing dental procedures likely to cause bacteremia with organisms commonly associated with endocarditis. Table 59-2 outlines the American Heart Association's most recent recommendations for the antibiotic prophylactic regimens for dental, oral, or upper respiratory tract procedures in patients who are at risk for infective endocarditis.[6]

Well-coordinated medical-dental consultation is essential in establishing an appropriate comprehensive dental treatment plan for the patient at risk for endocarditis. The goal here is to eliminate existing pathology, reduce gingival inflammation, and establish an effective prevention program. These patients must have a preoperative dental evaluation and treatment prior to cardiac surgery, medical circumstances permitting.

Oral Cancer

Emphasis on a team approach to management is also critically important for oral cancer patients undergoing surgery, radiation, or chemotherapy. The goal here is the same as for the cardiac patient. The dentist may also be called upon to help treat some of the acute and short- and long-term complications associated with cancer treatment. These include mucositis, opportunistic fungal infections, trismus, xerostomia, and surgical site prosthetic repair. These patients invariably require frequent follow-up visits and usually have continued dental needs. The benefit of early detection of the cancer by clinical and/or radiographic examination, with biopsy as necessary, cannot be overemphasized.

Smoking and Alcohol Abuse

Studies report an increased incidence of smoking among women. Alcohol abuse appears to be a growing problem as well.[12] These have been linked to an

TABLE 59-2 Prophylactic Antibiotic Regimens

Drug	Adult Dosing Regimen[a]
Standard Regimen (oral)	
Amoxicillin	3.0 g 1 h before procedure; then 1.5 g 6 h after initial dose
Amoxicillin/penicillin-allergic patients (oral regimen)	
Erythromycin	Erythromycin ethylsuccinate, 800 mg, or erythromycin stearate, 1.0 g 2 h before procedure; then 1/2 dose 6 h after initial dose
OR	
Clindamcyin	300 mg 1 h before procedure; then 150 mg 6 h after initial dose
Patients unable to take oral medications	
Ampicillin	IV or IM administration of 2.0 g 30 min before procedure; then 1.0 g IV or IM or 1.5 g oral amoxicillin 6 h after initial dose
Ampicillin/amoxicillin/penicillin-allergic patients unable to take oral medications	
Clindamycin	300 mg IV 30 min before procedure; then 150 mg IV or oral 6 h after initial dose
Patients considered high risk (i.e., not considered candidates for standard regimen)	
Ampicillin, gentamycin, and amoxicillin	IV or IM administration 2 g ampicillin plus 1.5 mg/kg gentamycin 30 min before procedure, followed by 1.5 mg oral amoxicillin 6 h after or repeated parenteral regimen 8 h after initial dose
Amoxicillin/ampicillin/penicillin-allergic patients considered at high risk	
Vancomycin	IV administration of 1.0 g vancomycin over 1 h starting 1 h before procedure; no repeat dose necessary

[a]Dose of gentamycin not to exceed 80 mg

increased incidence of oral cancer. Smoking and smokeless tobacco also have been linked to many premalignant and benign oral and perioral conditions and diseases.[5] This is another area in which medical-dental intervention is important.

Trauma

The physician may be the first consulted on trauma involving tooth avulsion. It is imperative to determine whether the tooth is a primary (baby) tooth or a permanent tooth, as reinsertion of primary teeth is contraindicated owing to inherent poor prognosis. The root surface should not be manipulated; it should be cleansed by irrigation only, preferably with saliva, saline, or milk. Tap water is least desirable. The tooth should be reinserted as soon as possible. Teeth reinserted more than two hours out of their socket generally have an extremely poor maintenance prognosis. The patient's tetanus immunization status should be evaluated, and systemic antibiotic and topical antimicrobial therapies are recommended. If reinsertion was achieved, the tooth should be held in place with finger or gauze pressure. If the tooth could not be reinserted by the physician, it should be placed in the buccal vestibule of the mouth or in milk for transport. An immediate dental consultation is required, as the dentist will need to stabilize the tooth with a nonrigid splint and perform further treatment.[19] Recently, a tooth-preserving transport system (Emergency Tooth Preserving System)[8] consisting of Hank's balanced salt solution, a cushioning device, and an outer hard impermeable container has become available.[8]

AIDS

The AIDS patient presents a complex challenge for the health care profession. As the patient becomes increasingly immunosuppressed, susceptibility to opportunistic infections, thrombocytopenia, and benign and malignant processes dramatically increases. The most common oral manifestations of AIDS include hairy leukoplakia, candidiasis, Kaposi's sarcoma, squamous cell carcinoma, lymphoma, periodontal disease, and xerostomia.[18] The AIDS patient does not need a referral to a hospital for dental treatment unless her health status is such that she requires the medical support of a hospital setting. The patient's dental treatment plan may need to be modified due to changes in her physical well being, degree of immunosuppression, and evidence of thrombocytopenia. The goal of treatment is to prevent or eliminate infection and pain, and to deliver comprehensive dental care commensurate with the patient's ability to undergo the planned procedure. An aggressive oral home care protocol should be instituted with frequent office follow-up visits. Frequent medical or dental reconsultations as the disease progresses often are necessary.

There are many other instances in which the physician may wish to initiate a dental consultation, or the converse may apply. The patient can only benefit from this input.

Acknowledgment

We wish to thank Dr. Paul Crespi for his input.

References and Suggested Reading

1. American Academy of Pediatric Dentistry: *Reference Manual,* 1991–1992.
2. Berlin CM: Pharmacologic considerations of drug use in the lactating mother. *Obstet Gynecol* 58(suppl):1755–2355, 1981.
3. Brent RL: The effects of embryonic and fetal exposure to x-ray, microwaves, and ultrasound. *Clin Obstet Gynecol* 26:484–510, 1983.
4. Briggs GG, Freeman RK, Yaffe SJ: *Drugs in Pregnancy and Lactation,* Charles W. Mitchell, eds. Baltimore: Williams & Wilkins, 1994.
5. Christen AG, McDonald JL, Christen JA: *The impact of tobacco use and cessation on nonmalignant and precancerous oral and dental diseases and conditions.* June 1991; An Indiana University School of Dentistry Teaching Monograph, Department of Preventive and Community Dentistry, Indiana University School of Dentistry, Indianapolis, Indiana.
6. Dajani AS, Bisno AL, Chung KY, et al: Prevention of bacterial endocarditis: Recommendations by the American Heart Association. *JAMA* 164:2919–2922, 1990.
7. Donahus AH: Women's health: A national plan for action. *J Dent Ed* 57(10):738–741, 1993.
8. Krasner P, Person P: Preserving avulsed teeth for replantation. *JADA* 123:80–88, 1992.
9. Lamley PJ, Lewis MAO: Oral medicine in practice: The compromised patient. *Br Dent J* 168(10):389–394, 1990.
10. Litle JW, Falace DA: *Dental Management of the Medically Compromised Patient,* 3d ed. St. Louis: CV Mosby, 1988.
11. Mason JO: A national agenda for women's health. *JAMA* 267(4):482, 1992.
12. Nicotine transdermal system. *Physicians' Desk Reference,* 48th ed. Montvale, NJ: Medical Economics Data Production Co., pp 1759–1762, 1994.
13. Pallasch TJ: A critical appraisal of antibiotic prophylaxis. *Int Dent J* 39:183–196, 1989.
14. Pinkham J, et al: *Pediatric Dentistry: Infancy Through Adolescence,* Philadelphia: WB Saunders, pp 160–162, 1988.
15. Public Health Service: *Health United States 1991 and Prevention Profile.* Washington, DC: U.S. Department of

Health and Human Services, Public Health Service, Centers for Disease Control and Prevention. NCHS 1992; DHHS Publication No. (PHS)92–1232.

16. Public Health Service: *Women's Health Issues: A Presentation at the 159th Meeting of the National Heart, Lung and Blood Advisory Council.* Bethesda MD: U.S. Department of Health and Human Services, National Institutes of Health. NHLBI, 1990.
17. Redford M: Beyond pregnancy gingivitis: Bringing a new focus to women's oral health. *J Dent Ed* 57(10):742–748, 1993.
18. Regezi JA, Sciubba JJ: *Oral Pathology: Clinical-Pathologic Correlations.* Philadelphia: WB Saunders, 1993.
19. Surace L, Crespi P: Acute management of dental avulsions, *Children's Hosp Quart* 1(3):273–277, 1989.
20. Tarsitano BF, Rollings RE: The pregnant dental patient: Evaluation and management. *Gen Dent* 41(3):226–231, 1993.
21. Zachariasen RD: Effect of antibiotics on oral contraceptive efficacy. *J Dent Hyg* 65(7):334–338, 1991.

60 Plastic Surgery

Frederick Neil Lukash

Women often request information from their primary care physicians regarding plastic or reconstructive surgery. In addition, there are situations in which it will be clear to physicians that their patients would benefit from such information (e.g., a patient who is to have a mastectomy or one who has sustained severe facial trauma in an auto accident). Cosmetic surgery also may be beneficial to a patient's psychological well-being. It is therefore important for primary care physicians to be well informed about what is potentially available to their patients and the relative benefits and risks of the various procedures. This chapter will discuss the most common types of cosmetic and reconstructive surgery procedures that primary care physicians will likely discuss with their female patients.

Breast Surgery

Some women are quite concerned because they perceive their breasts to be different from the "societal" norms, and they may inquire about breast surgery. In addition, women who are facing possible mastectomy (or those who have had one) should be advised regarding the potential for breast reconstruction.

Breast Reduction

Overly large breasts can be problematic both physically and psychologically. Excessive weight of the breasts can result in back pain and poor posture. Pressure from brassiere straps can cause deep grooves in the shoulders and skin discoloration. Rashes often develop under large breasts from sweating and rubbing against the skin of the abdomen. Some women with pendulous breasts also may suffer psychological discomfort. Young women may be more likely to be stared at and commented on as sexual objects. Self-consciousness may lead to attempts at concealment, and they may shy away from sports or social events.

The ideal candidate for "reduction mammoplasty" is a person who has achieved a body weight appropriate for her size and has maintained it. Large weight swings up or down after surgery will influence breast size and alter the result. Age is not a barrier to reduction. Girls in their teens and older women many years beyond the menopause have successfully undergone this surgery. With younger patients an endocrine evaluation may be needed, and it is important to be certain that teenage breast development is essentially complete and that further breast growth after surgery is unlikely. Women contemplating pregnancy are encouraged to defer this procedure until their family is complete, because child bearing can markedly influence breast size and shape and the ability to breast-feed may be impaired.

Reduction mammoplasty usually takes between three and four hours and is performed under general anesthesia. Hospital stay is usually 24 to 48 h. Since this is an elective operation that can result in blood loss, patients should be encouraged to donate their own blood for autotransfusion if needed.

Two basic types of techniques are used to reduce the size of a breast. In women with moderate hypertrophy, the breasts can be reduced and recontoured while leaving the nipple-areolar complex attached to the remaining breast tissue. This preserves nipple viability and sensitivity. When dealing with very pendulous breasts, the nipple-areolar complex is detached from the breast and repositioned as a graft on the newly reshaped breast. This technique is the safest with overly large breasts, but results in temporary anesthesia to the nipples, which slowly regain sensation over a one-year period.

Breast Uplifts

Time, pregnancy, weight changes, and gravity can lead to sagging of the breasts. This condition is called "mammary ptosis." It can occur with both small and large breasts and represents a combination of decreased breast volume and increased skin stretching.

The diagnosis of breast ptosis is made by looking at the position of the nipple-areolar complex with respect to the inframammary fold. When the nipple is below the fold, ptosis is present.

In many patients, although there is significant sagging there is adequate breast volume, and an uplift alone will provide rejuvenation. In others, however, there is not enough breast tissue; here, an augmentation in combination with an uplift will be needed. The procedure to correct mammary ptosis is called mastopexy. Although it can be performed under local anesthesia, most patients elect general anesthesia. The procedure can easily be done on an ambulatory basis; it takes about 2 to 3 h and is strictly a cosmetic operation.

Breast Augmentation

Each year over 100,000 women in the United States seek out cosmetic surgery for breast enlargement. Size-enhancement surgery has been performed since the 16th century; however, the modern age of breast augmentation began in 1960 with the creation of silicone sheeting. This allowed the creation of a bag that contained either silicone gel or saline. Since that time, many variations of the prototype have appeared, but the basic design has remained. There has been recent controversy over the safety and efficacy of silicone implants; however, the number of problems in relation to the total number of implants appears to be very small. At present ongoing studies under FDA auspices are attempting to bring this issue to a conclusion and to allow patients to know the scientific status of silicone implants. At present, most surgeons are utilizing the silicone bag that is filled with physiologic normal saline.

Before undergoing breast augmentation, a woman should have a complete physical examination. Any history of collagen diseases such as scleroderma and rheumatoid arthritis should be specifically ascertained. (This would be a contraindication to implant surgery since it is believed that certain individuals may experience symptoms akin to these diseases many years following implantation.) Likewise, a mammogram should be performed to rule out occult malignancy and to establish a normal baseline. Obviously any problems with breast disease should eliminate surgical augmentation as an option and should be appropriately treated.

Augmentation mammoplasty is performed on an ambulatory basis under either local or general anesthesia. The incisions are small (2 to 3 cm). They are made either under the breast, around the lower portion of the areola, or in the axilla. Through these incisions a pocket is made either beneath the breast itself or beneath the pectoralis muscle. The implant is then placed in the pocket.

Complications from breast implant and augmentation surgery can be divided into early, late, and very late categories. The early problems are very clear-cut and rectifiable. These include bleeding and infection. Implant removal usually is warranted in the presence of infection around the prosthesis. Late problems usually relate to what is called "capsular contracture." This hardening of the tissues around the implant is not really a complication but, rather, an exaggeration of the normal process of the body walling off foreign material. In 85 percent of patients this encapsulation process is minimal and the implants remain soft. In 15 percent, capsular contracture alters the esthetics of the breast. Current thinking is that if the contractures are a problem to the patient, the implants should be removed. Capsular contracture is not physically harmful, but can be frustrating to both patient and doctor. Finally, there is the issue of whether a woman who has had silicone breast implants is at higher risk for collagen vascular disease. This is currently under investigation. One theory has been proposed that suggests there may be a subset of women who are prone to collagen disease and in whom breast implants may act as a catalyst.

Women who have had breast augmentation should have screening mammography, physician-performed breast examination, and breast self-examination utilizing the same schedule as patients who have not had this surgery. Mammography is somewhat more difficult to perform in these women, but innovative techniques have been described.

Breast Reconstruction Following Mastectomy

Breast reconstruction following mastectomy is one of the most rewarding procedures that a plastic surgeon can perform. Reconstruction is quality-of-life surgery and has no influence on the outcome of the disease. The decision for reconstruction should rest with the affected individual.

There are many methods and timing sequences for reconstruction. Surgery can be immediate at mastectomy, or it can be delayed to any time convenient for the patient. Reconstruction also can utilize the silicone implant or can involve transfer of the patient's own tissue from other areas, such as the abdomen. Most breast reconstruction surgery is staged. Whereas the mound can be part of the immediate surgical process, such refinements as fabrication of the nipple and areola and potential modification of the other breast (to match the reconstructed breast) are staged to allow for artistic precision. Most plastic surgeons who deal extensively with breast reconstruction like to see the patient as soon as the diagnosis of breast cancer is made. That way, assurances can be offered to allay her anxiety. It also provides the best opportunity to plan for the appropriate type and timing of the reconstruction, and to establish the plan with the oncologic surgeon. Breast reconstruction is not a purely "cosmetic" operation, but rather one that restores to normal tissues altered by disease and surgery.

The Aging Face

As people age, the elasticity in their skin decreases and the strong collagen fibers weaken. The firm fatty tissue beneath the skin shrinks. The skin "fits" more loosely, and lines appear where the facial muscles attach to the skin's undersurface. These are most apparent under the chin and around the mouth and eyes. Many factors play a role in the rate and degree of the aging process. First and foremost is genetics. People with thin, dry, fair skin will realize the signs earlier. Overexposure to sunlight and excessive use of tobacco and alcohol accelerate the aging process. The aging of skin involves wrinkling and sagging; therefore, rejuvenation procedures are aimed at these two processes.

Wrinkles

Facial wrinkling is the end-result of constant muscle action on the skin. As the skin and underlying fat thin, the lines of facial expression become accentuated. These lines are predictable and are referred to as "crow's feet" (around the eyes), "frown lines," and "laugh lines" (around the nose and mouth). The treatment of wrinkling is directed to the crease itself, and has no effect on sagging skin. Isolated wrinkles are currently managed by filling the creases with biocompatible materials. Most often this is accomplished with either collagen or fat. Collagen, a purified animal protein, is capable of incorporating with one's own collagen to elevate the depressed skin of a wrinkle. Any patient choosing this treatment requires a skin test to insure that there is no allergy to the "foreign protein." If there is an allergy, this option is eliminated. The other option is fat, which is taken from one's own body and therefore is totally compatible. The fat is harvested by liposuction techniques and then reinjected into the wrinkles. Both of these techniques render good short-term results, varying from 6 months to 2 years. By that time, the material has absorbed, and repeat procedures are needed.

Generalized wrinkling is managed by various types of chemical treatments to the surface of the skin. The most superficial type of chemical "peel" utilizes the alpha hydroxy acids. These compounds are derived from fruits and have been nicknamed "fruit peels." They act on the upper levels of the skin and work to improve the complexion and reverse the effects of sun damage. When used in combination with Retin-A, there is a noticeable improvement in superficial wrinkling (fine lines around the eyes). To maintain the benefits of alpha hydroxy acid treatments, a home maintenance program is essential. Cessation of treatment results in a return to the pretreatment state.

Another group of chemicals are the trichloroacetic acids. These compounds attack the middle levels of the skin and can have a significant effect on improving wrinkling. The peel is performed in the doctor's office and requires no anesthesia. It takes about 4 days for the process to be completed. Strict compliance with protocol is necessary to avoid complications. The final group of compounds are in the phenol family. These attack the deeper layers of the skin and have the most profound effect on wrinkles. A side effect of phenol peels is a lightening of the skin. Therefore they are reserved for fair-complected people. As with the trichloroacetic acids, strict attention to protocol is mandatory, or disastrous complications such as scarring can occur.

Sagging Skin

Loose sagging skin cannot be improved by chemical peels. Lifting procedures such as face lifts and brow lifts are necessary. The most dramatic results are seen with the loose skin of the neck, jowls, and the sagging eyebrows. Surgery of the face and brows can be performed on an ambulatory basis. Anesthesia can be either local or general, according to the patient's preference.

Lifting and peeling procedures produce significant improvement in the aging face. Many people have combination problems that require both techniques. Treatment, however, does not stop the aging process. Over time, the forces of elastic collagen degeneration and gravity work to cause further sags and wrinkles. At that time many people seek out re-do surgery.

Surgery of the Eyelids and Eyebrows

Cosmetic plastic surgery of the eyelids is called a blepharoplasty. The procedure takes between 60 and 90 min, and most often is done under local anesthesia on an outpatient basis.

Prior to any surgery on the eyelids, careful medical and ophthalmologic examinations are essential. Conditions such as dry eye syndrome, glaucoma, thyroid disease, hypertension, and bleeding disorders are absolute contraindications. Most plastic surgeons will practice conservatism when operating on the eyelids. A removal of too much skin can risk exposure and possible ulceration of the cornea.

Resuspension of the eyebrows is commonly referred to as a brow lift. This surgery is performed when there is an overhanging of skin on the outside corners of the eye (hooding), and crowding of tissue at the nasal root and inner aspects of the eyes. Many patients who think they need a blepharoplasty are really in need of a brow lift.

The brow lift procedure, like a blepharoplasty, can be performed on an ambulatory basis and under local anesthesia. Blepharoplasty and brow lift often are performed together and may also be a part of additional facial rejuvenation procedures such as face lift and chemical peel.

Blepharoplasty and brow lift procedures are among the most frequently performed cosmetic surgery operations. Complications are unusual, but can occur. These include bleeding and infection. The most feared complication with a blepharoplasty is blindness. This is extremely rare, but has happened. Brow lift complications also include nerve injury and alopecia (spotty baldness).

Nasal Surgery

More than 70,000 people in the United States seek out cosmetic nasal surgery each year. Nasal plastic surgery is called rhinoplasty and can be performed any time from the mid-teen years, when midfacial growth is complete. Surgery can be either under local or general anesthesia, and usually is performed on an ambulatory basis.

Chin Surgery

In some patients facial balance involves more than the nose itself. Not only may a nose be too large, but the chin can be too small and thus offset facial symmetry. An astute surgeon viewing the entire face will realize that more than refining the nose may be necessary, and in some situations may recommend chin augmentation as well.

Body Contouring

Perceptions of appropriate body image have changed drastically in recent times. Although diet and exercise remain the most important cornerstones for maintaining a healthy and fit body, there are indications for surgical assistance. When dealing with youthful elastic skin, liposuction is the ideal method to remold by removing isolated fat deposits. When the skin tone is poor from age, large weight losses, or from pregnancy, when stretching has destroyed the skin's elastic fibers, only redraping procedures will restore the desired contour.

Liposuction

This operation was endorsed by the American Society of Plastic and Reconstructive Surgery in 1982. The premise of liposuction is that once fat tissue is physically removed it will not return. Current medical theories agree that people are born with a certain number of fat cells. The number does not change, but rather the cells themselves increase and decrease in size. For many people this means a constant struggle with diet and exercise to overcome genetic predispositions. In spite of their best efforts, certain areas will not respond. These are commonly found under the chin, around the waist and hips, and on the upper, outer thighs. It is for these localized areas of fat that fail to respond to diet and exercise that liposuction deserves consideration. Liposuction is not a substitute for general weight control and is not a panacea to treat obesity.

The ideal candidates for liposuction are younger people with good skin tone. The elastic recoil of the skin is what allows for shrinkage and recontouring in the areas where fat has been removed. Liposuction in people with poor skin tone results in wrinkling and drooping of tissues, which may require additional surgical correction.

Depending on the size of the area to be recontoured, the operation can be performed in the office operatory, an ambulatory facility, or may require overnight hospitalization. Likewise, anesthesia may be either a local to the involved area, a regional such as an epidural, or general anesthesia. Liposuction, as with any surgical procedure, is not without the risks and complications of bleeding and infection.

Body Contouring Surgery

As stated previously, when skin tone is poor, redraping surgery is the appropriate treatment for dysmorphias. The most common of these procedures is the abdominoplasty, or 'tummy tuck.'' Thigh and buttock lifts are less frequent requests, but still remain an important aspect to body contouring.

Abdominoplasty is a major plastic surgical procedure designed to remove excess skin and fat between the umbilicus and the pubic hair line. The procedure takes between two and four hours, and is always done under general anesthesia in a hospital setting. As with most large surgical procedures, complications are possible. The most frequent is bleeding at the time of surgery. For this reason, patients should donate their own blood in advance for autotransfusion if needed.

Scars

The paramount role of a plastic surgeon regarding scars is the understanding of the biology of tissue injury and wound repair. This enables a plastic surgeon to sometimes revise and improve an unslightly scar, to tell patients what their scars might be like following various types of procedures—and periodically to give the unwelcome news that their existing scars are permanent and will remain as is.

All wounds, whether from accident or surgery, heal by the same basic mechanism—that of fibrous scar tissue. This applies to bones and internal organs as well as to skin. The main ingredient in wound repair is collagen. Following injury there are three phases of healing. The first lasts only a few days and involves the body's "signaling system" to manufacture collagen to "glue" the wound together. The next phase lasts about three weeks and is an intense period of wound healing in which collagen is manufactured and deposited into the wound. Scars during this period usually appear red and thick. The final phase of wound healing is called the "maturation" phase. This period starts at approximately the fourth week following injury and lasts more than a year. During this time the body attempts to remodel the scar to make it as close to the original tissue as possible. It is during this final period that scars begin to soften and fade, but never totally disappear.

Many factors influence a scar's outcome. Foremost is location. There are areas of the body such as the eyelids where the skin is thin and soft; hence, incisions there heal very well. In other areas, such as the thick skin of the back and extremities, scars will be predictably wide and thick. Another factor is the direction of the scar. If a scar falls within a facial crease or in one of the body's "relaxed skin tension lines" it will be more favorable than if it crosses perpendicular to these lines. Genetics and age also are extremely important in scar formation and healing. Fair-complected individuals tend to have better scars than do those individuals with darker complexions, and older skin scars better than younger skin, probably owing to a decrease in collagen production.

Keloids

A keloid is a metabolic disorder affecting collagen deposition and maturation. People affected by this problem experience scars that blossom out beyond the area of injury. A good plastic surgeon is skilled in solving wound healing problems but cannot perform the miracle of scar erasure.

Cleft Lip and Palate

There is probably no joy greater than the birth of a child. When a child is born with a birth defect, apprehension and fear take over. Doctors, hospitals, and operations suddenly become part of the family life-style. Since obstetricians, family practitioners, and other primary care clinicians are the first to see the affected child, parents often will seek their advice. This section is designed to provide familiarity with the reconstructive surgery available to correct these defects.

Clefts of the upper lip and palate are common birth defects. They occur as a result of a failure of the middle third of the face to close during the fourth to seventh week of intrauterine life. Since the lip and palate close at different times during this period, it is possible to have only a cleft lip, only a cleft palate, or both. Also the severity can vary from small notches to complete splits, and can be unilateral or bilateral.

The timing of repair should be arranged to have minimal impact on future facial growth and yet carry the least risk from surgery and anesthesia. The lip usually is repaired at three months of age. At this time the child can easily withstand the 2- to 3-h procedure. The palate usually is closed shortly after the first birthday. This time is chosen because it is prior to the onset of sound formation and organized speech, for which an intact palate is needed. This procedure takes approximately 2 h. Both types of surgery require general anesthesia and a 2- to 3-day period of hospitalization.

References and Selected Readings

1. Smith JW, Aston SJ (eds): *Grabb and Smith's Plastic Surgery,* 4th ed. Boston: Little, Brown, 1991.
2. Regnault P, Daniel R (eds): *Aesthetic Plastic Surgery.* Boston: Little, Brown, 1984.
3. Serafin D, Georgiade NG (eds): *Pediatric Plastic Surgery.* St Louis: CV Mosby, 1984.
4. Goldwyn R (ed): *The Unfavorable Result in Plastic Surgery.* Boston: Little, Brown, 1972.
5. Peck G (ed): *Complications and Problems in Aesthetic Plastic Surgery.* New York: Gower, 1992.

61 Sports Medicine and Minor Orthopedic Problems

David B. Hale
Melody Toth
Ralph W. Hale

During any physical activity there is a risk of injury. This may vary from a minor abrasion or strain to a severe spinal injury or death. In contact sports such as football, basketball, and soccer, or sports utilizing apparatus such as gymnastics, the risk of serious injury is far greater than for the individual who jogs 2 to 3 miles or participates in an aerobic dance class. The purpose of this chapter is to concentrate on the more common and less severe problems of the type that would be likely to be seen in a primary care office practice.

Exercise injuries usually occur in bone, muscle, tendon, ligaments or skin, and often are the result of a misapplication of force or overuse. They also may occur from outside sources, e.g., being hit by a bicycle while jogging. Whatever the cause, one of the major impacts of such injuries is the interruption of the exercise program, leading to a loss of conditioning or a failure to resume exercising. Therefore, it is important to recognize early injury and its potential effect as soon as possible. Complaints of a physical nature that are found in a routine health screen should be investigated further. In most instances, this will require very little additional time; when identified early, most problems are easily managed.

History Taking

During an initial health screen, the physician should always inquire about whether the patient is pursuing an exercise program. If the answer is a negative, then one should be recommended. There are many pamphlets and local resources including the YWCA, local fitness centers, sporting goods stores, etc. The physician can easily identify several sources in the community that can be recommended.

If the patient does have an exercise program, she should be asked about any problems. These may be acute or chronic. Whichever, the physician should attempt to determine their extent and severity. The following questions have proved very helpful and can serve as a guide. However, as with any question format, individual physicians will need to develop their own routine. Following each question, an explanation of its purpose is included.

Do you participate in a regular exercise program? This establishes whether the patient is currently exercising or allows for recommendation of consideration of a program. If the answer is yes, the physician should continue with further questions.

What type of program do you use? This will help the physician understand the intensity level and make a judgment regarding its effectiveness (see Chap. 12).

How often do you exercise and for how long? This further defines the level of exercise.

Have you ever had any injuries as a result of your exercise program? This gives a past history and can alert the physician to areas of potential chronic injury.

Do you currently have any injuries or problems as a result of your exercise program? If the answer is no, please proceed to the last question. If the answer is yes, further questions about where, when, and other specifics are needed. Specific areas and the necessary investigations are covered later in the chapter.

Do you have any questions about your exercise program? If the answer is no, then no further questions are needed. If the answer is yes, then a specific discussion regarding the concern should ensue.

These six questions are enough to identify and investigate the vast majority of injuries related to exercise. They can be easily presented, either orally as part of the clinical history or in a questionnaire given to the patient when she registers. The questionnaire format should require yes-or-no answers, with space for any explanations. Since many physicians utilize the questionnaire approach, this is often the simplest method. For those who are still concerned about how these questions should be approached, substitute the word "contraception" for "exercise" and it will be noted immediately that the format is identical to a follow-up of contraception: Do you use contraception? What type? How often and for how long? Any history of problems? Any current problems? Any questions?

Physical Examination

Most physicians can readily examine any minor exercise injury without referral to an orthopedic surgeon. The principles are the same as with any other problem. However, when the basic examination fails to identify or diagnose the problem, a referral is warranted. As with all physical examinations, begin with observation. The following areas, which are not intended to be all-inclusive, need to be considered:

Color: Is there any discoloration?

Contour: Is there any obvious change in normal appearance? Any swelling?

Mobility: Is the patient having any difficulty moving the affected area? (This evaluation should include active and passive range of motion.)

Strength: Has there been a change, or is there a difference between the left and right side that indicates injury?

Following inspection, palpation is performed. Depending on the area of suspected injury, this may vary from simple palpation to establishing a range of motion.

Is there any palpable dislodgement or displacement?

Is there any pain on palpation?

If there is pain on palpation, is it point specific or diffuse?

Are there any limitations to the range of motion?

Is the area painful on motion?

Is the pain referred? If so, to where?

Are there any crepitations or effusions?

Is there any change in sensation? For example, is there numbness, a complaint of burning in the muscles or a joint, or any increase or decrease in sensation?

Obviously, when a specific site of injury is noted, a more direct examination of the site may be warranted.

Definitions

Before identifying specific complaints and their diagnosis and management, the physician needs to review several basic definitions.

Abrasion: A scraping of the epidermis that results in a mildly painful denuding of the skin.

Laceration: An incision into the skin that is usually described by length and depth. It is often contaminated if it occurs during exercise.

Strain: An injury to a muscle and/or tendon that usually occurs at the muscle tendon junction or at the tendinous insertion on the bone. Strains are classified into grades I, II, and III. Grade I: Mild with minimal disability; Grade II: Anything between grades I and III; Grade III: Complete disruption of the muscle or tendon unit.

Sprain: An injury to a ligament. Usually this results in an unstable joint. The degree of injury is divided into three grades. Grade I: Painful ligament but no instability; Grade II: Painful ligament with partial instability; Grade III: Painful ligament with complete instability including possible dislocation.

Contusion: A disruption of the blood vessels, usually veins, secondary to injury, resulting in extravasation of blood into the tissues. To the patient, a "bruise." This term is used by some to indicate the blow or injury that caused the disruption as well as its appearance.

Ecchymosis: A small nonelevated discoloration of the skin. It is indistinguishable from a contusion and may lead to confusion since both terms are used in medical and lay literature.

Dislocation: The dislodgment of the articular surfaces of a joint such that the proximal and distal articular surfaces are no longer in apposition.

Avulsion: The tearing away of a part of a structure; for the patient, it is usually the complete loss of a portion of the skin.

Injury Evaluation

Most injuries associated with exercise are found in the head/neck or in one of the four extremities and their attachments to the trunk. Injuries to the trunk may occur but these are less frequent. However, injuries to the ribs, breast, and back have been described and must not be overlooked. It is not the purpose of this chapter to review treatment or management of serious or severe injuries or fractures, some of which occur secondary to trauma, while others may occur during high-intensity exercise programs.

However, the diagnosis of a fracture or dislocation may be essential to minimize subsequent damage to surrounding tissues. Most fractures or dislocations will be associated with the acute, sudden onset of pain in the area of the injury. It is critical for the physician to assess how the injury occurred, since this can be a key to diagnosis. Some patients may even describe a sudden popping or snapping.

Immediate assessment by observation and palpation to determine any obvious deformity of a bone or joint should be performed. Gross instability or inability to use a joint may indicate serious injury. Since the major diagnostic tool is an x-ray, when in doubt, treat any injury as a fracture and either order radiographs or refer the patient.

The initial treatment is immobilization of the bone or joint and restriction of weight-bearing or use until the diagnosis is made. The general principles of first aid apply until definitive care is available.

One type of fracture to be aware of is the stress fracture. This is most common in the metatarsal, and is a result of extensive and prolonged intensive work-outs. X-rays rarely reveal the fracture, and bone scans are necessary. If pain in the foot persists after conservative therapy, a stress fracture should be considered.

Treatment of Acute Minor Injuries

In general, acute minor injuries occurring with exercise should all be treated by *R I C E,* either totally or partially. These initials refer to:

R = rest
I = ice
C = compression
E = elevation

Rest allows the affected part to recuperate on its own, employing the body's own recuperative powers. If the injury is mild, the rest can be limited to a short time span. Recurrence or absence of pain can be helpful in determining the length of time necessary for rest.

Ice is the modality of choice for treating acute injuries. It decreases inflammation and swelling while providing pain relief. In the past, heat was applied for pain relief; now we know that in reality it increases the swelling and delays healing. Ice is best applied by either an ice pack or ice massage. In the former, the ice is wrapped in a protective coating, usually a plastic bag or towel, to avoid direct skin contact, and then applied to the injury site. In massage, ice can be applied directly but is moved constantly around the area to prevent skin damage. A styrofoam cup is an excellent method. As the ice melts the styrofoam is gradually peeled away. Ice therapy usually is applied for 15 to 20 min, or to the point of skin anesthesia. The frequency will vary with the severity of the injury, but three to four times a day—until the pain and swelling have disappeared— usually is adequate. For chronic injuries, many athletes apply ice to the affected area before and after exercise on a daily basis. Although there is some debate about the effectiveness of this approach, it appears to work for some athletes. An important aspect of ice therapy is to begin treatment as soon as possible after the injury. For reasons still completely unknown, immediate treatment with ice has resulted in a much more rapid recovery.

Compression with or without a support helps to reduce the swelling associated with acute injuries. An Ace bandage applied to the area also can be an excellent way to hold an ice bag in place. Bracing or support is required only when immobilization or support of a joint is indicated. Compression is rarely used in chronic injury rehabilitation. Elevation is essential in the early phases of acute injury. By changing the level of the injury, a reduction in swelling is facilitated. The reduced swelling will then facilitate healing.

Although not part of the R I C E formula, the use of anti-inflammatory medications is an important aspect of treatment. For mild irritation or inflammation, aspirin is the drug of choice. For more severe irritation or inflammation, especially chronic cases, nonsteroidal anti-inflammatory drugs are indicated.

Rehabilitation is an essential component of any injury therapy program. This is best carried out by a certified athletic trainer or a physical therapist. Most minor injuries do not require this service. However, chronic injuries or repetitive injuries may benefit from this treatment.

Foot Problems

Most exercise programs involve use of the lower extremities. The frequency of walking, jogging, running, and aerobic dance make this area one of the most susceptible for injury. For convenience, the lower extremity is described anatomically, although it is important to remember that it is a unit; problems in one area may result in difficulties in another (e.g., a contusion on the heel may alter running mechanics, causing excessive strain on the knee, ankle, or hip). It is only by remembering the mechanics involved that the underlying cause of some problems can be identified.

Tendons

Inflammation of a tendon (tendonitis) is extremely common. This often results from excessive pressure on the tendon during active flexion/extension of the extremity. As the tendon moves back and forth in its fascial sheath or canal, it creates friction and irritation. The most serious of these in the foot/ankle occurs in the Achilles tendon. This injury is usually disabling and markedly reduces the ability to exercise. It results in acute pain in the Achilles tendon, usually at about the level of the malleoli. When palpated, it is point-tender; when the foot is dorsiflexed, the pain is intensified. Occasionally there is swelling in the posterior part of the ankle and slight crepitations may be felt. Other than the treatment described in the previous section, prolonged rest and anti-inflammatory drugs are indicated. Treatment is difficult, owing to the patient's inability to rest the tendon completely while participating in everyday activities. In the acute stages of Achilles tendonitis, a heel wedge may be added; this takes some of the stress from the tendon. Mild stretching exercises should be prescribed to keep full range of motion of the tendon. This can be accomplished by having the patient stand with her toes on a two-inch block, heels down, for one minute and repeating this three times a day. In the extreme case, referral for cast immobilization is indicated, as well as modification of shoes.

Rupture of the gastrocnemius or soleus muscles can occur with forceful dorsiflexion (i.e., after missing a step during aerobics or "stepping"). The patient will complain of pain. Physical exam will not always reveal a tendon defect or inability to plantar flex. Simply have the patient lie prone; then palpate the calf and the Achilles attachment on the foot. It is important to compare both sides in order to identify partial tears. Splinting often will be effective when there has not been complete disruption. Occasionally, the Achilles tendon will rupture. This is an acute event, and may occur without warning. Examination reveals a defect in the tendon and an inability to plantar flex the foot. Treatment usually is surgical.

Another tendon injury of the foot/ankle is rupture of the tibialis posterior tendon. The patient complains of pain on the medial aspect of the ankle with point tenderness. This may be misdiagnosed as a sprain, but any sprain in this area with point tenderness and limited swelling should cause suspicion of a tendon rupture.

Fascia

One of the more common complaints of the foot/ankle occurs in the fascial sheath that covers the plantar surface. A fasciitis results from excessive weight-bearing on the arch of the foot. The constant pressure stretches the fascia, causing inflammation and swelling. The patient complains of pain; when pressure is applied to the plantar surface, a diffuse pain is elicited. Treatment is symptomatic and occasionally requires arch support. If fasciitis is left untreated, bone spurs may develop along the calcaneus. If this does happen, a spur pad will provide some comfort. Exercises such as toe raises and towel curls will be beneficial; they will help redevelop the arch, thereby reducing the strain placed on the fascia by the falling arch.

Toe Raises: Stand with feet shoulder-width apart, rise up on toes, hold for three counts. Three sets of 10 should be performed daily.

Towel curls: Stand on the edge of a towel lengthwise, moving only your toes; curl the towel up under your arches; keep going to the end of the towel. When the exercise becomes easy, adding a weight will help. The exercise should be performed three to five times a day.

Rest for a short period is also helpful. The patient should be asked about her shoes and how long they have been used. Most running shoes should be changed every 500 miles or 6 months. One word of caution: mild plantar fasciitis may result in changes in running mechanics that result in excessive stress on the knee and lower extremities; this may be the patient's major complaint.

Others

Pain in and around the metatarsal area is not uncommon. It is usually due to excessive pressure on the toes, either by the type of exercise or the shape of the foot. It must be differentiated from plantar fasciitis, which is more diffuse. Metatarsalgia is point-specific. Treatment usually consists of changing the exercise pattern or padding the area with metatarsal pads. If the pain is localized to a specific metatarsal, Morton's neuroma or foot should be suspected. Initial treatment is with foot pads, followed by referral if no relief is obtained. Stress fractures always must be considered when foot pain is present. The diagnosis can be made only by x-ray or bone scan. When suspected, referral is indicated.

Ankle Injuries

The ankle is one of the most susceptible—and thus most often injured—anatomical areas. Since most exercise programs involve the lower extremity, this is not unexpected. The ankle itself contributes to the problem since it is composed of a series of nonarticulated bones held together by ligaments that sustain forces from all directions.

Strains and sprains are the usual injuries to the ankle. These injuries occur when the ankle bones are twisted or turned in such a fashion that abnormal stresses are placed on the ligaments and tendons. Frequently, this abnormal position occurs when the full weight of the body is placed on the ankle, thus creating tremendous forces. The resultant strain or sprain is graded as previously described. Treatment of the acute injury relies on the RICE principle. To facilitate the healing process, range-of-motion exercises should be started as soon as possible. These exercises are non-weight-bearing and can be done in the early stages of RICE. If swelling can be controlled and range-of-motion exercises started within 24 h, recovery time will be dramatically decreased.

Range-of-Motion Exercises

A.B.C.: With the big toe, write the alphabet. Be sure that the ankle is used, not the leg. This should be repeated at least three to four times a day.

Towel stretch: Roll a towel up and place it around the ball of the foot. Hold the towel in both hands and gently plantar flex the foot. Next relax the pressure and let the foot fall. When the foot is relaxed, turn the foot inside and then outward. Repeat this exercise 4 to 6 times, several times a day.

As the injury heals, external support such as taping may be necessary. Once a sprain has occurred, the ankle is more susceptible to repeat injury, and many coaches insist that all ankles be taped once an injury has occurred. In severe injuries, such as Grade III, casting and immobilization may be necessary.

It is important to remembr that children (before closure of the growth plate) usually do not get ankle sprains. Rather, if they complain of pain around the ankle joint and if x-rays are negative, the injury should be treated as a Salter *T* fracture (fracture through the growth plate) with immobilization for 2 weeks and orthopedic referral.

Lower Leg Problems

The anterior fascial compartment of the tibia may swell during exercise. This swelling produces acute pain and limits use. The common term is "shin splints." Treatment consists of rest and ice. For some people the swelling is frequent and limits exercise activity. One common problem that may increase shin splint pain in women is fallen arches. When shin splint pain is present, the physician should check first to see if the arch support is gone. If so, arch exercises should be initiated using toe raises and towel curls as noted previously. In addition, some type of arch support may be beneficial. For others, shin splints is only an occasional problem. Although the etiology is vague, an adequate warm-up prior to vigorous exercise is thought to be a beneficial preventive measure. If a young person continually develops lower calf pain with exercise, particularly running, this may indicate a more serious problem and an orthopedic referral should be made.

Cramping

The calf is a common site of cramps during exercise. Relief is obtained by gently stretching the calf muscle, by dorsiflexing the foot, and by massaging the calf. Relief will occur promptly. The etiology of the cramp is thought to be the result of lactic acid buildup. It usually occurs following prolonged exercise or with extreme heat. Recurrence is common if the exercise program is not interrupted. Mild stretching by flexing and extending the foot will also help relax and restore the leg to normal function. Usually after several minutes of light activity the muscle will be able to function normally with no recurrence. It is important to recommend to the woman that she should not bounce when stretching; also, she should not forcefully stretch nor have someone else forcefully stretch the muscles.

Knee Problems

Injuries to the knees are also common. The anatomy of the knee makes it extremely susceptible to injuries related to any application of external force. As a result, twisting or turning can be as responsible for problems as can blows to the knee. In addition, the knee, like the ankle, absorbs tremendous pressure when the weight of the upper body is transmitted through the distal femur to the proximal tibia. Since these two bones only rest on each other and do not form a true joint, the potential for injury is multiplied.

Ligament Injuries

Any history of injury during or as a result of twisting should suggest a ligamentous injury. In a typical history, the leg would have been planted down and the body turned with the foot in place. This would result in acute knee pain. Examination of the knee usually will reveal swelling as well as pain on motion. This pain is accentuated by placing tension on the suspected ligament. Treatment requires referral to an orthopedic surgeon.

Meniscus

The meniscus serves as internal support to the knee. It is susceptible to injury by twisting. However, as opposed to ligament injury, this pain is more internal and is increased by flexing or extending the knee. The patient occasionally will complain that the knee locks or collapses unexpectedly. This is most frequent in chronic injuries, and the patient will indicate that while doing a normal activity her knee locked and she stumbled or actually fell. Treatment is surgical.

Inflammation

Occasionally the patellar tendon will become irritated. When this occurs, the pain is in the ligament or under the patella. Motion of the patella is painful; occasionally there is crepitation on palpation. A similar problem occurs when the bursa becomes irritated. Often, careful palpation will provide the only differentiation between bursitis and tendonitis. In this instance, a careful history is most helpful. Prolonged kneeling is a frequent preceding event. Treatment is conservative, with anti-inflammatory agents and ice. Occasionally, the bursa will swell to such a degree that it requires drainage.

Chondromalacia

Anterior knee pain is often a symptom of chondromalacia. In the usual history, the patient has been participating in jumping sports or exercise. The cause is related to the patella's constant motion over the anterior tibial and femoral surfaces. The pain is directly over the patella and may be reproduced by compressing the patella against the femur. Radiographs will confirm the diagnosis. Initial therapy includes rest, ice, and anti-inflammatory drugs. If significant improvement does not occur in a short time, referral is necessary, because physical therapy, bracing, and occasionally surgery may be indicated. In mild cases, a patellar brace that stabilizes the kneecap will provide additional comfort and can be purchased at most sporting goods dealers. This will help in both tendonitis and chondromalacia.

The two most useful exercises to help strengthen and prevent tendonitis of the knee, chondromalacia, and even surgery, are quad sets and straight leg raises.

Quad sets: With the leg straight, tighten the thigh muscles. Hold for a count of three and relax. It is recommended that 200 be performed daily in sets of 10 done throughout the day.

Straight leg raises: While leaning against a table, place the leg straight out with the heel on the ground. Keeping the knee locked, raise the leg to waist level; then lower. Start at 3 sets of 25 daily, eventually increasing to 6 sets of 50 each day.

Hip and Thigh Injuries

Injuries to the thigh are almost always muscular. They result from excessive pressure on a major muscle or muscle group that results in tearing of either the tendon or muscle belly. These injuries occur most frequently in exercise or athletic events that require sudden explosive efforts, such as starts in a race. The most common area is the hamstring or quadriceps. Therapy is ice, compression, and rest. Stretching exercises and adequate pre-exercise warm-ups are helpful as preventive measures.

The hip joint is one of the most stable in the body. The ball and socket structure virtually guarantees limited injury. As a result, most injuries to the hip are either strains of the adjacent muscles or inflammations of the adjacent bursa. One of the most common hip injuries, caused by excessive running or by a direct blow, is greater trochanter bursitis. As the bursae become inflamed, the iliotibial band slips over it, instead of gliding smoothly, thus creating a snapping and giving-out sensation. It is easily cured. The therapy is rest, ice, and anti-inflammatory drugs. Occasionally, cortisone injections are indicated, but these are of limited value owing to their side effects.

Shoulder Injuries

The shoulder, like the knee, is composed of a large number of ligaments holding the bones in close approximation. As opposed to the hip, there is no deep ball and socket joint; thus, the ligaments must support the joint against external as well as internal forces. This results in a potential for exercise injuries similar to that found in the ankle and knee.

Dislocations are commonly seen with pick-up football or city basketball league games. It is important to know that these injuries can have significantly morbidity. The best treatment is to place the arm in a sling so the arm is in a position of comfort, and obtain immediate referral. Do not try to relocate the arm; this can result in serious nerve or artery injury.

Bursitis

This common problem results in shoulder pain, especially when lifting the humerus above shoulder level. It is also called ''impingement syndrome'' and is seen most frequently in patients who participate in sports that require the arm to be lifted above the head. The etiology is the rubbing of the humeral head against the undersurface of the acromion. The rotator cuff then becomes compressed in this area, and the resultant inflammation and erythema cause pain. Therapy includes rest, anti-inflammatory drugs, and ice. Frequently cortisone injections are required. In the milder form of bursitis, conservative therapy often is all that is needed. However, for moderate to severe forms, referral is indicated.

Clavicle

The clavicle is susceptible to fractures and separations. Fractures usually result from falls during an exercise program. When they occur, pain and deformity result. It is rare for complete separation to take place. Treatment consists of shoulder immobilization for six weeks via a specially designed appliance and pain relief. Occasionally, the junction of the clavicle and the acromion will separate as a result of a direct blow to the shoulder either from a collision or a fall, causing complete separation. Therapy is controversial, and referral is required. Minor separations can be treated conservatively with rest, immobilization, and analgesics.

Upper Extremities

The upper extremity, like the lower, is at risk for injury during exercise. This occurs primarily at the elbow and hand. Although injuries to the upper arm occur, they are unusual and most frequently are contusions or tendonitis.

Elbow

The most common cause of pain in the elbow is lateral epicondylitis. The etiology is the excessive torques produced at the elbow by the muscles of the forearm. Commonly called ''tennis elbow,'' the pain occurs when the wrist is dorsiflexed. Treatment consists of rest, ice, anti-inflammatory drugs, and a tennis elbow strap. As a precaution, lifting of bulky or heavy items is to be avoided. Should the pain be unresponsive, more aggressive therapy is indicated.

Bursitis

Swelling of the olecranon bursa may cause an apparent distortion of the elbow. This condition is rarely painful, but cosmetically it creates much concern. Drainage may or may not be effective. Therapy with compression and anti-inflammatory medication should be initiated and careful follow-up should be obtained because some cases of bursitis are septic.

Ulnar Nerve

Exercise that requires repeated throwing can result in irritation of the ulnar nerve. This causes a paresthesia of the hand where the ulnar nerve innervates. Like hitting the "crazy bone," the paresthesia soon resolves. Treatment is rest of the elbow and anti-inflammatory drugs. If symptoms persist, they may be due to a condition called ulnar nerve entrapment. In severe cases, surgical intervention is required.

Dislocation

After dislocations of the fingers, elbow dislocations are the most common. This injury occurs most often with falling on an extended forearm. It is important to assess peripheral nerve and artery function as these structures are often injured as well. Radiographs must be taken, and immediate referral for early reduction is essential to minimize long-term sequelae.

Wrist

Most discomforts of the wrist are the result of repeated wrist actions. Except for ball sports or grasping sports, such as gymnastics, the wrist is rarely a concern. Tendonitis may occur if repeated flexion-extension is performed. Ganglions are frequently seen, but rarely are exercise-related.

A specific entity of which the physician should be aware is *carpal tunnel syndrome.* The presenting complaint is a paresthesia of the palmar aspect of the hand and occasionally the wrist. It may also be associated with pain in the wrist or lower forearm, and occasionally with a sensory deficit or weakness in the fingers served by the median nerve. Although the pain may occur at any time, it is especially noticeable at night or in the late evening. The etiology is compression of the median nerve as it passes from the lower forearm and wrist into the hand. It is a relatively common occurrence, and has been reported more frequently in women. The antecedent events are those that require repeated wrist motion, especially if they are prolonged and require moderate to extensive force. This problem is common in office workers. A careful history is essential. Treatment consists of discontinuation of the task and occasionally use of splints to elevate the hand and relieve the compression. If this fails to relieve the symptoms, referral is indicated. Injection of corticosteroids or even decompression surgery may be required.

Hand

A common injury to the fingers is "mallet" or "baseball" fingers. This injury results when the distal interphalangeal joint is forced into flexion and the extensor tendon is avulsed with or without bone. The diagnosis is simple as the patient cannot dorsiflex the distal phalanx. Treatment, after radiographic confirmation of lack of a fracture, consists of 6 to 8 weeks of splinting.

Other hand injuries are sprains and strains. These respond to rest, immobilization, and anti-inflammatory drugs. Occasionally, the patient will dislocate one of the distal interphalangeal joints. Immediate treatment is to grasp the digit and reapproximate the joint by pulling while slightly twisting the digit. If immediate replacement fails or if there is any possibility of a fracture, a radiograph must be taken before any further attempt at replacement.

The thumb is also very mobile, and dislocations at the base of the metacarpalphalangeal joint are quite common. It is also important to assess the collateral ligaments of the metacarpalphalangeal joint after relocation because treatment varies considerably if they are injured. Splinting is required for minor lateral instability, but more than 40 degrees of lateral instability may require surgery. This injury, which leads to the development of severe disability, is frequently missed. Remember, if there is a possibility of a fracture, radiographs should be taken *prior* to realignment.

Back Pain

Back pain is one of the most common complaints in the exercising patient. Its location is usually in the lower back between L4 and S1. Diagnosis is helped by a careful history of the activity that immediately preceded the onset of pain. When examining a patient with back pain, it is important to test the flexibility of the hamstrings. Low back pain can be caused by hamstring tightness, especially in runners and very athletic persons. If the athlete is unable to touch her toes while in a sitting position or while standing with her leg straight, encourage a stretching program to increase flexibility in the hamstrings.

It is important to determine the site of the pain, whether it is constant or intermittent, and if there is radiation, especially in the sciatic area. Pain in the midline should make the physician suspicious of a disk problem. Examination should consist of testing for range of motion, straight leg raising, reflexes, motor and sensory effects. Most cases of midline pain or pain with sciatic radiation require referral. Often the first indication of scoliosis in a female will be found during evaluation of back pain that occurs during exercise. Treatment of backache includes rest, Williams flexion exercises, anti-inflammatory drugs, muscle relaxants, heat, and ice. If the back pain persists or increases, it is best to refer the patient. Most back injuries require at least 2 weeks to recover.[2] A lengthier discussion regarding back pain is found in Chap. 53.

Bone Tumors

No person's bone structure is identical to another's. As a result, bony prominences may appear throughout the body. They are most noticeable on the exposed long bones, but also may be noted with problems of fitting clothes or footwear. It is essential to determine whether these prominences are "normal" or the result of a bony tumor or exostosis. This is especially important if the prominence is increasing in size or causing pain. Causes vary from benign cysts or chondromas, to Paget's disease, to primary malignancy. Radiography is the primary diagnostic tool, and many of these "lumps" are found on radiographs obtained for other reasons. Referral is necessary unless the radiographic diagnosis is obvious.

Pregnancy

The same injuries that can occur to the nonpregnant woman can occur during pregnancy. However, there are a few special concerns about which the physician should be aware. During pregnancy the effect of progesterone causes a gradual relaxation of the ligaments. This occurs earlier with repeated pregnancies than with the first. The resulting relaxation increases the risk of damage to ligaments of the ankle and knee during exercise. With the added weight of pregnancy, the patient should be cautioned to avoid sudden turning and twisting. Appropriate ankle support is also indicated, especially if there is a previous history of ankle injury. Instability of the pelvis in late pregnancy as the pubic symphysis changes can change running and walking mechanics. As a result, the patient increases her injury susceptibility. Finally, the marked lordosis that occurs with later pregnancy alters the body mechanics by changing the center of gravity. It becomes more difficult to stop forward motion as well as change direction. Any of these may increase the injury potential for a pregnant patient who is actively exercising. These factors should also be considered when a pregnant patient comes into the office with a nonspecific musculoskeletal complaint.

Team Physician

With the increasing emphasis on sports programs for women, many physicians are asked to serve as team physicians. There are three essentials for the physician who elects to take this role. First, establish a referral relationship with a knowledgeable orthopedic surgeon who will be willing to take care of any patient whenever a problem arises that is beyond your expertise. Depending on the type of activity, this could be infrequent or usual. Second, become familiar with the common problems associated with the sport and develop an expertise in their diagnosis and treatment. If a certified athletic trainer is associated with the team, they will be an invaluable resource in this area and probably can describe 90 percent of the problems you will encounter. Finally, be available.

Summary

Most physicians can manage the common injuries and problems that occur during exercise. By taking a simple history and performing a brief examination, a diagnosis can be made. Treatment for almost all such injuries consists of rest, ice, and anti-inflammatory drugs. When the injury is beyond the scope of your expertise or when it requires a more specialized approach, a referral is appropriate and expected.

References and Selected Readings

1. American College of Obstetrics and Gynecology Patient Education Pamphlet, *Women and Exercise: A Guide for Women,* December 1992.
2. Richardson AB, Toth M: Orthopedic problems and office management of minor injuries of women who exercise, in Hale R (ed): *Caring for the Exercising Woman.* New York: Elsevier, pp 119–135, 1991.

62 The Care of Women with Physical Disabilities

Angeles Badell
Sandra Welner

According to the National Health Interview Survey (NHIS)[6] in 1990, there were 33.8 million persons, 13.7 percent of the total U.S. noninstitutionalized population, who were very limited in physical activity because of a chronic health condition. The prevalence of disability is fairly consistent between genders for persons under 65. Limitation in activity increases with age, and by the age range 65 to 69, 33.5 percent of females were limited in activity. The NHIS survey data document the extent of the need for primary health care for the physically challenged.

Disability is defined as any long- or short-term reduction of a person's activity as a result of an acute or chronic condition. Limitations in mobility are a common means by which a person's activity is reduced. Affected individuals are often in need of medical rehabilitation for aerobic conditioning.

The first part of this chapter will describe health problems related to the most frequent type of disabilities, i.e., disabilities caused by neurologic impairments and by musculoskeletal disorders. The second part of the chapter will address sexual and reproductive issues as they relate to women with physical disabilities.

Disabilities Caused by Neurologic Impairments and by Musculoskeletal Disorders

Individuals affected by traumatic brain injury (TBI), stroke, and any other static or progressive central nervous system disorder will have decreased or abnormal mobility of their body and limbs. Particularly pertinent for health care are the deficits affecting oral, pharyngeal, and esophageal motion as well as laryngeal and respiratory movements. These problems should alert the physician to the need for prevention and treatment of such disorders as chronic malnutrition, deficits in dental hygiene, gastroesophageal reflux, recurrent atelectasis, aspiration pneumonia, chronic constipation, and related disorders.

Spinal cord injuries (SCI) cause complete or incomplete sensory and motor deficits below the level of the injury, as well as neurogenic bowel and bladder incontinence. The high cord levels of quadriplegia affect respiratory function, and may require assisted ventilation. Persons with low cervical quadriplegia or paraplegia above T-6 share a high risk for episodes of autonomic dysreflexia (autonomic hyperreflexia). Autonomic dysreflexia is a serious and relatively common problem in individuals with spinal cord injuries above T-6. It is induced by noxious stimuli acting below the level of the lesion. The symptoms are uncontrolled sympathetic activity. The associated hypertension may become life-threatening. Management calls for the use of short- or long-acting sympathetic outflow blockers and a search for and removal of the noxious causative factors. One particular cause of autonomic dysreflexia may be acute abdominal disease. It is important to note that the diagnosis of acute abdomen may be masked in SCI patients by the neurological changes in abdominal muscle tone and the absence of pain.

Neurogenic bowel incontinence in SCI patients often results in constipation, and impaction can cause autonomic dysreflexia. The person with SCI needs to be trained in the management of constipation and the use of techniques to trigger evacuation at predetermined times to avoid socially unacceptable incontinence. The physiatrist who managed the training of the patient should be contacted for guidance in difficult cases.

Another serious potential problem in the SCI patient is renal disease. Chronic bladder, ureteral, and eventually renal damage may occur. This course of events can be prevented by attention to adequate hydration and periodic bladder emptying with clean intermittent catheterization. A low-grade bladder infection is not uncommon and may not always require chronic antibiotic treatment. Continued urologic follow-up is a must for all SCI patients.

A major health issue related to all SCI patients is skin care. The most serious skin problems are caused by decubitus ulcers due to prolonged pressure, usually on areas with underlying bony prominences. The rehabilitation management of the paraplegic includes education in avoiding traumatic and thermal injuries and the provision of equipment that can reduce the effect of pressure. However, all precautions may fail, and the examination of the skin is basic in all individuals with sensory deficits.

The pharmacologic management of spasticity is of particular concern. The most frequently used antispastic medications are baclofen, diazepam, and dantrolene sodium. Modifications of the dosage may be required if the severity of spasticity changes or if the side effects demand a change.

Pain is often the cardinal symptom associated with musculoskeletal impairments. Joint inflammation results in decreased mobility, causing secondary muscle atrophy and a progressive cycle of pain and disability. The appropriate pharmacologic management of rheumatic and other musculoskeletal disorders should be complemented with attention to the deleterious effects of prolonged rest, muscle atrophy, and aerobic deconditioning. Physically challenged persons who do not participate in regular aerobic conditioning activities are at risk for early onset of osteoporosis, obesity, hypertension, and atherosclerotic heart disease. The primary care physician should be alert to the early onset of these health problems as well as to the need for anticipatory preventive care.

Gynecologic Care and the Disabled Woman

Office Design and Equipment

A number of key points are important in designing an office to cater to women with physical limitations. The office should have accessible doorways, adequate spacing of furniture, and no projecting obstacles. An important feature of the gynecologic exam is an accessible table. This table should lower to 19 in in height to facilitate the transfer of patients from wheelchairs, and should have safety and security features to allow an adequate exam of a mobility-impaired individual. When low tables are not available and the patient needs to be lifted to a higher table, adequate personnel must be available to allow safe and dignified transfer.

Patients with extreme spasticity may be more easily examined in the knee-chest position, with an assistant holding the spastic legs away from the perineum to allow access for the speculum. When patients are examined in bed, a rolled blanket can be used to elevate the pelvis. Because of the different angle of the pelvis in relation to the speculum in this position, the speculum inserted handle downward may not expose a mid-position or anteverted cervix. It often is helpful to reverse the speculum so that the blade that ordinarily pushes down will now be pushing up, exposing the cervix.

In elderly or spinal cord-injured patients, xylocaine gel applied liberally to the perineal surface while talking to the patient before the exam may be of great benefit in decreasing perineal pain. In spinal cord-injured patients, application of xylocaine gel has been reported to decrease the incidence of spasticity.[13] As with all female patients, it is important to empty the bladder prior to the pelvic exam. However, this is particularly important for women with spinal cord injuries, since a full bladder and constipation can trigger spasticity.

If hip mobility is difficult, which is quite common in elderly women, patients may need to have one leg abducted and one knee flexed. If this maneuver is performed gently and slowly, adequate visualization usually can be achieved.

Sexuality

Some physiologic changes seen in women with disabilities include loss of innervation to the vagina; inadequate lubrication; decreased vaginal accommodation; and reduced, delayed, or absent orgasmic sensation.[26] For the woman who becomes disabled later in life, sexual identity adjustments can be extremely difficult. A newly disabled woman often feels that she has not changed and, on an emotional level, may not accept that her body has changed. The disabled woman may experience some anxiety about her ability to satisfy her partner. Her sexual partner, who may perceive her as fragile, may be afraid to touch her or to find ways to achieve their mutual satisfaction. If a disabled teenager or adult woman feels undesirable, she may become vulnerable to exploitation, particularly in sexual relations.[23] For example, before the woman became disabled, she may have refused to participate in unprotected sexual intercourse; now she may feel that if she does not consent, no one else will approach her. She may hesitate to discuss such fears with her physician, who should give her the opportunity to express her concerns.

Open communication is especially important when dealing with sexual difficulties, so that problems can be clearly identified and solutions explored. A careful history may differentiate between an impairment in genital functioning, and a situational dysfunction.

Contraception

Primary care physicians should explore contraceptive options when caring for the disabled woman. Choice should depend on the patient's mobility status as well as her dexterity and coordination. Patients with certain chronic diseases may have special considerations. Oral contraceptives used by spinal cord-injured women have been associated with a high incidence of thrombosis and should be avoided.[24] Patients with lupus also may have an increased risk of developing thrombosis when using oral contraceptives.[20] Packaging is important when selecting oral contraceptives for a patient because of potential problems with dexterity. The simplest package is the best.

Two kinds of IUDs are available in the United States: Progestasert and Paragard. These methods are useful for monogamous women with no history of pelvic infections in the past and whose pelvic sensation is intact. The use of condoms should be encouraged. Barrier methods such as sponges and diaphragms may be difficult for two reasons. Dexterity and range of motion can interfere with proper insertion, and sensory loss in the pelvis may preclude the patient's ability to detect proper positioning of the device: Medroxyprogesterone acetate in a Depo form is safe and effective if repeated administrations are given every three months. The Norplant system also appears to be safe, and is effective for five years in most women.

Pregnancy

Pregnancy in women with physical disabilities may range from routine to complex. Complications reported to be increased in disabled women include urinary tract infections, pyelonephritis, decubitus ulcers, and premature labor. Some disabilities result in pelvic deformities that may necessitate cesarean section.

Spinal cord injury is also associated with a life-threatening syndrome, autonomic hyperreflexia, which can masquerade as preeclampsia.[11,12] Patients with autonomic hyperreflexia have distention of the visceral organs, resulting in activation of the autonomic nervous system. A noxious stimulus dilates large blood vessels above the level of the lesion and constricts blood vessels below the level of the lesion. There is profuse sweating, headaches, and severe muscle spasms. These patients may have seizures and hemorrhagic stroke, and the mortality risk is substantial.[5,23,26]

Medical issues surrounding postpartum care in a woman with mobility impairments include thrombophlebitis, urinary tract infections, constipation, decubitus ulcers, and poor episiotomy healing.[5]

The pregnant woman who is disabled may encounter a significant amount of societal prejudice because her disability, in others' eyes, would make it impossible for her to be a competent mother. This is in fact not the case.

Sexually Transmitted Diseases (STDs)[22]

All sexually active women are at risk for contracting a sexually transmitted disease. In a woman with a disability this infection may go undetected for a number of different reasons. Sensory deficits in the pelvis may not specifically alert the patient to the usual symptoms of infection. She may have to learn to recognize such vague cues as an increase in spasticity and abdominal discomfort. A woman with mobility impairment may be reluctant to seek assistance, even if she suspects an infection, because of transportation difficulties or privacy concerns.

When prescribing antibiotics for women with physical limitations, consider her dexterity and coordination. Remember to designate easy-open packaging for patients whose finger dexterity is impaired. If a patient has a vision impairment, ask that a family member or friend assist her in monitoring her temperature. Some patients who have dysphagia may benefit from unit dose packaging of liquid medications.

Infertility

The infertility concerns of the woman with a physical disability are no different from those of any other woman. Fertility usually is not affected by physical disability. Tubal factors, ovulation dysfunction, sperm-mucus interaction, and male factors all require the same thorough evaluation performed for any other woman. If a couple has been attempting pregnancy for a year or more without success, an infertility work-up is appropriate.

Menopause, Osteoporosis, and Hormone Replacement

Women with disabilities are living longer. Therefore, the impact of aging in people with underlying disabilities requires significantly more consideration than in the past. Women with mobility impairment have a higher risk for osteoporosis. In some cases it is useful to evaluate this bone loss with quantitative digitized radiography measurements.[19] Long-term steroid use in patients with autoimmune disorders may compound osteopenia.[8] Calcium supplementation with vitamin D must be included in all regimens unless significant impairment in creatinine clearance or calcium excretion is present.

Women with physical disabilities are less likely to participate in exercise; they are thus at risk for cardiovascular deconditioning, excessive weight gain, and a higher risk for cardiovascular morbidity and mortality. Menopausal women lose the protective effects of estrogen on the cardiovascular, urologic, and skeletal systems, and on the skin. Estrogen replacement therapy is an important preventive intervention for these conditions. Unfortunately, this therapy has been inappropriately linked with thrombotic episodes in data derived from research on high-dose oral contraceptives.[1] Many studies of coagulation function in estrogen replacement therapies have found no significant alterations.[1,12] Even in patients with a history of thrombotic events in the distant past, a transdermal form of estrogen therapy can sometimes be used safely.[21]

Emotional Adjustment

A woman may have different emotional adjustment problems, depending on her age at the onset of the disability. The young girl who has had a congenital impairment or one that developed at a very early age may have incorporated her existing, accepted limitation into her identity. Though many women may accept such challenges with a positive outlook and strive for excellence within their capacities, others may feel they will never be able to aspire to the achievements of their unaffected counterparts.

A woman or teenager who becomes physically challenged experiences many losses that she is reminded of daily. These may be exacerbated by other adults and teenagers who frequently feel uncomfortable around the disabled individual. This may lead to blatant rejection by long-standing friends and coworkers, which in turn may result in severe isolation and depression. The role of the physician in trying to understand the patient's perception of these losses and how they affect her functioning is crucial in directing appropriate support and intervention if required. Key sensitive areas for focus include dissolution of long-standing friendships, leaving work with its activities and coworkers, and needs to adapt life-style to accommodate newly acquired and often frustrating physical limitations.

Grief and loss are natural and appropriate feelings. The clinician should not attempt to negate, discount, or ignore these emotions. Careful attention, however, is mandatory to prevent this normal frustration-depression from developing into a pathologic, paralyzing, isolating, possibly even suicidal depression. The health care provider must be empathetic and understanding to these women and must address their individual needs and concerns in a supportive manner. If the clinician senses that the patient's depression is becoming unstable or exacerbated and the primary care physician cannot manage the problem, the patient should be immediately referred to an appropriate specialist. However, the primary care physician must maintain a strong supportive relationship with the patient. This continuity is crucial in the emotional healing stage.

Social Issues

The physician's attention to the disability should not impair the value assessment of the person who is disabled. Handicaps are barriers that society and the environment place in the path of any person, preventing their participation in activities expected for their age and social condition. Individuals with disabilities are not intrinsically handicapped, and many are able to overcome societal and environmental obstacles.

Being sensitive to the person's needs and what can be done to reduce and eliminate handicaps that could affect the function of physically challenged individuals is what the 1990 Americans with Disabilities Act is all about.[2]

References and Selected Readings

1. Alkjaersig N, Fletcher A, DeZiegler D, et al: Comparison of transdermal and oral administration. *J Lab Clin Med* 3:224–228.
2. Batavia A, DeJong G, Eckenhoff EA, Haterson RS: After the Americans with Disabilities Act: The role of the rehabilitation community. *Arch Phys Med Rehabil* 71:114, 1990.
3. Burns T, Batavia A, Smith Q, DeJong G: Primary health care needs of persons with disabilities. What are the research and service priorities? *Arch Phys Med Rehabil* 71:138–142, 1990.
4. Collins P, Rosano GM, Jianh C, et al: Cardiovascular protection by oestrogen—A calcium antagonist effect? *Lancet* 341:1264–1265, 1993.
5. Cross LL, Meythaler JM, Tuel SM, Cross AL: Pregnancy following spinal cord injury. *West J Med* 154:607–611, 1991.
6. *Disability Statistics Abstract*—University of California, San Francisco. Published by U.S. Department of Education. National Institute of Disability and Rehabilitation Research (NIDRR), 1992.
7. Dunn SF, Gilchrist VJ: Sexual assault. *Primary Care* 20:359–373, 1993.
8. Hicks JE: Exercise in patients with inflammatory arthritis and connective tissue disease. *Rheum Dis Clin North Am* 16:845–870, 1990.
9. Julkunen HA, Kaaja R, Friman C: Contraceptive practice in women with systemic lupus erythematosus. *Br J Rheumatol* 32:227–230, 1993.

10. Kable WR, Gallagher JC, Nachtigall L, Goldgar D: Lipid changes after hormone replacement therapy for menopause. *J Reprod Med* 35:512–518, 1990.
11. Kotte FJ, Lehman JF: *Krusen's Handbook of Physical Medicine and Rehabilitation,* 4th ed. Philadelphia: WB Saunders, 1990.
12. Lobo RA: Estrogen and the risk of coagulopathy. *Am J Med* 92:283–285, 1992.
13. McGregor JA, Meeuwsen J: Autonomic hyperreflexia: A mortal danger for spinal cord-damaged women in labor. *Am J Obstet Gynecol* 151:330–333, 1985.
14. Notelovitz M: Estraderm for osteoporosis. *Geriatr Nurs* 13:337–338, 1992.
15. Pines A, Fisman EZ, Ayalon D, et al: Long-term effects of hormone replacement therapy on Doppler-derived parameters of aortic flow in postmenopausal women. *Chest* 102:1496–1498, 1992.
16. Pines A, Fisman EZ, Levo Y, et al: The effects of hormone replacement therapy in normal postmenopausal women: Measurements of Doppler-derived parameters of aortic flow. *Am J Obstet Gynecol* 164:8706–8712, 1991.
17. DeLisa JA: *Rehabilitation Medicine, Principles and Practice.* Philadelphia: JB Lippincott, 1993.
18. Rogers J, Matsumura M: *Mother to Be: A Guide to Pregnancy and Birth for Women with Disabilities.* New York: Demos Publications, 1991.
19. Scialli AR, Gestila KJ, Simon JA: Luprolide acetate in bone mineral density measured by quantitative digitized radiography. *Fertil Steril* 59:674–676, 1993.
20. Sipski ML, Alexander CJ: Sexual function and dysfunction after spinal cord injury. *Traum Spinal Cord Inj* 3:811–828, 1992.
21. Stampfer MJ, Colditz GA, Willett WC, et al: Postmenopausal estrogen therapy and cardiovascular disease. *N Engl J Med* 325:756–762, 1991.
22. Verduyn WH: Spinal cord injured woman: Pregnancy and delivery. *Paraplegia* 24:231–240, 1986.
23. Welner S: Gynecologic care of the disabled woman. *Contemp OB/GYN* 38:55–67, 1993.
24. Welner S: Treatment of sexually transmitted diseases in the physically disabled woman in, *Reproductive Issues for Persons with Physical Disabilities,* Baltimore: Brookes, 1993.
25. Wren BG: The effects of oestrogen on the female cardiovascular system. *Med J Australia* 157:204–208, 1992.
26. Yarkony GM: Spinal cord injured women: Sexuality, fertility and pregnancy, in Goldstein PJ, Stern BJ: *Neurological Disorders of Pregnancy.* Mount Kisco: Futura, pp 203–222, 1992.

63 Office Assessment and Management of Pain

Ronald Kanner

Scope of the Problem

Pain is one of the most common symptoms for which patients seek medical help. Intermittent headache is nearly ubiquitous, and over 75 percent of the general population has had at least one episode of back pain. Unfortunately, physicians frequently are poorly trained to manage patients in pain. While they usually have an adequate knowledge of pharmacology, they often prescribe analgesics inadequately and use a limited range of therapeutic modalities. The problem is compounded further by lack of clarity in terminology and in syndrome definitions.

Definitions

Pain is defined by the International Association for the Study of Pain as "an unpleasant sensory and emotional experience which we primarily associate with tissue damage or describe in terms of such damage, or both." The two most important considerations are that there is an emotional component to all pain and that actual tissue damage is not necessary for the experience of pain.

Nociception is the perception of a noxious stimulus. Pain, therefore, is the conscious experience of nociception.

Dysesthesia is the experience of an abnormal noxious sensation. It differs from nociception in that it does not feel like a normal pain response to a stimulus. Patients describe burning, tingling, or tight feelings.

Allodynia is the perception of a nonnoxious stimulus as painful. This commonly occurs in neuropathic pain syndromes, such as postherpetic neuralgia.

Hyperpathia is an exaggerated and abnormal pain response to a noxious stimulus. It is a type of dysesthesia in response to a noxious stimulus.

Hyperalgesia is similar to hyperpathia, but the

response is aberrant only in magnitude, not in type. That is, the patient recognizes more intense pain than would be expected from the stimulus.

Hypalgesia is diminished sensitivity to noxious stimuli.

Clinical Classification of Pain Syndromes

The most clinically relevant classifications of pain syndromes sort them according to location (topographic), time course (acute versus chronic), or presumed pathophysiology. Each has its advantages and disadvantages.

Topographic

Classification of pain syndromes by their location is useful in that it follows the manner in which patients present (e.g., with headache, backache, or abdominal pain). The drawback is lack of specificity.

Temporal

Acute and chronic pain differ in both quality and consequences. Acute pain usually is in proportion to tissue damage and is expected to resolve with healing of the underlying process.

Pathophysiologic

Certain pain characteristics allow the clinician to infer the underlying pathophysiology and to direct treatment accordingly.

In broadest terms, pain syndromes can be divided into nociceptive and nonnociceptive. Nociceptive pain syndromes are due to ongoing tissue damage that stimulates normal pain perception pathways. Pain tends to be localized and aching in quality. Bone and muscle pains are typical examples of somatic nociceptive pain, while bowel obstruction is an example of visceral nociceptive pain.

The two most common types of nonnociceptive pain are neuropathic pain and psychogenic pain. Neuropathic pain syndromes are those in which injury to the peripheral or central nervous system sets up an abnormal, self-perpetuating pain that may be independent of the original stimulus. Pain is felt as dysesthetic and is in the distribution of a nerve or nerves. Common examples are postherpetic neuralgia (shingles), diabetic peripheral neuropathy, and trigeminal neuralgia.

The term "psychogenic pain" is used to imply a pain syndrome in which there either is no underlying structural pathology or the response to the pathology is far beyond what would be expected.

Approach to the Patient in Pain

Appropriate pain management requires a guided history and physical examination, a clear syndrome diagnosis, and a therapeutic plan based on that diagnosis.

Guided History

A guided history must elicit pain location, character, temporal characteristics, intensity, exacerbating and relieving factors, and functional impairment.

The location of the pain is the easiest part of the history for the patient to supply. If there is difficulty with the verbal description, she can stand and outline the pain with one hand. This yields not only the location of the pain, but its radiation, if there is any. The patient should then be asked whether the pain is superficial or deep; comparing it to a muscle cramp or a sunburn can be helpful. The next step is to decide whether the pain is due to local pathology or referred. Local pain often is accompanied by focal tenderness; visceral, nociceptive pain often is referred to cutaneous sites. When patients are entirely unable to describe the location of their pain, or if the location is not in keeping with any anatomical possibility, the diagnosis of psychogenic pain should be entertained. The same is true when there seems to be "total body pain."

The character of the pain is the most difficult part for the patient to describe, but verbal descriptors of pain are among the most important points in making an accurate diagnosis. Certain pain qualities are so characteristic that they are sufficient to allow one to make the diagnosis. Burning, dysesthetic pain, superimposed on a numb or tight feeling is almost invariably neuropathic, as are sharp, lancinating jabs in a dermatomal distribution. Crampy, episodic pain is likely to be visceral, nociceptive pain. Localized, aching pain is likely to be somatic nociceptive. Pain that is described entirely in terms of emotional content (e.g., torturing, punishing) often has a large psychogenic component. If, despite lists and guided questioning, the patient is still unable to describe the character of her pain, she should be asked to liken it to some past pain experience that can provide a common language (e.g., toothache, stomach cramps).

The most significant temporal characteristics are onset, diurnal variation, and course. The onset of a change in character of pain is of equal importance. Posttraumatic pain is immediate. Weeks to months later, however, the pain may gradually change from an aching quality to a burning, dysesthetic one, heralding the start of reflex sympathetic dystrophy.

Most patients with chronic pain state that the pain is more severe at night than in the morning or during the day. Certain pain syndromes have specific diurnal variations. The pain of rheumatoid arthritis is almost invariably worse in the morning, easing as the day progresses; pain from osteoarthritis follows the opposite pattern. Cluster headaches may come on at a specific time each day, whereas brain tumor headaches classically are characterized by early morning awakening, and tension-type headaches may be present all day long.

Acute and chronic pain are separate entities, not only in their temporal patterns, but in their pathophysiology as well. No clear temporal cut-off determines when acute pain becomes chronic. It is more useful to decide when the concomitants of acute pain (response to a noxious stimulus, autonomic responses, anxiety, and appropriate pain behavior) give way to the concomitants of chronic pain (responses outlasting the stimulus, depression, and abnormal illness behavior).

Because pain is a subjective experience, efficacy of treatment often is judged by the patient's perception of changes in intensity. This can be achieved via such systems as numerical rating scales or verbal descriptors of visual analog scales, as long as the type of evaluation remains constant for a given patient.

Whether pain is constant, certain factors can make it more or less intense. A history of pain exacerbations with changes in the weather is common in patients with arthritic disorders. Any form of the Valsalva maneuver (straining against a closed glottis) exacerbates pain from a herniated intervertebral disc. Patients with sympathetic-dependent pain, as in reflex sympathetic dystrophy, causalgia, and some cases of postherpetic neuralgia, have marked exacerbations of pain with cold drafts. Other types of neuropathic pain are exacerbated by any light touch that normally would not be painful (allodynia).

There are a few other specific pain precipitants, such as alcohol in cluster headaches, tyramine-containing foods in patients taking monoamine oxidase inhibitors, and cutaneous triggers in patients with neuromata; but the majority of others (hot/cold, stress/relaxation, etc.) are nonspecific and idiosyncratic.

Functional impairment is not necessarily related to pain intensity, but recovery of function may be the prime goal of pain therapy. On the initial visit, one of the most important details to determine is what the patient cannot do now because of the pain that she could do before it started. A small disc bulge may be of no importance to a typist, but completely disabling for a construction worker. A mild carpal tunnel syndrome would be just the opposite.

The medical history should be focused on three major issues: (1) possible medical explanation for the current pain syndrome; (2) possible contraindications for certain analgesic therapies (e.g., peptic ulcer disease with nonsteroidal anti-inflammatory drugs or arrhythmias with tricyclic antidepressants); and (3) prior painful illnesses.

The psychosocial history has two goals: to determine the factors that influence treatment (prior pain history, coping skills, support structures, history of substance abuse, and psychological profile); and to establish a working psychological diagnosis. The goal of establishing a psychosocial profile is not simply to decide whether a pain complaint is "organic" or "functional," but to identify patterns that may impede recovery and to address them specifically.

Anxiety is the most common psychological concomitant of acute pain and of flare-ups of chronic pain. A patient who requires progressively higher doses of analgesics for what appears to be a stable process may be suffering from anxiety, and may be using the analgesics for their sedating effects.

Depression is the most common concomitant of chronic pain and may even have a similar neurophysiologic substrate. Patients may deny depression or indicate that it is purely a result of the chronic pain. A careful history of premorbid affect may be revealing.

Hypochondriasis is defined as the fear of having (or belief that one has) a serious disease. It is based on the person's interpretation of her physical signs or sensations as evidence of physical illness, despite medical reassurance to the contrary. It may also be considered more broadly in patients who over-react to minor illnesses. It is an emotional issue, not an attempt to deceive.

Somatization, or the somatoform pain disorder, is quite common. It is defined as the preoccupation with pain for at least 6 months when appropriate medical investigation rules out the presence of organic pathology, or when the disability is far out of proportion to any pathology. This is the most common type of "psychogenic" pain.

Malingering is the false claim of pain in hope of secondary gain (usually monetary). It is not a psychological syndrome, but a deliberate attempt to deceive.

Physical Examination

Examination of the patient with pain includes a guided medical examination, a neurologic exam, and a psychological evaluation. The two most crucial aspects of the examination are the inspection of the painful site and the demonstration of associated signs. Physical examination of the painful site serves three purposes: it reassures the patient that the complaint is being addressed directly, it provides information on immediate causative and associated lesions, and it helps the examiner to decide whether the pain is local or referred.

The site is examined for direct causative lesions. This is also part of the functional assessment. The affected part should be inspected at rest and then put through its full range of active and passive motion. In somatic nociceptive pain, the causative lesion usually is at the site of pain, whereas visceral nociceptive pain has cutaneous referral points that may be distant from the source. It may be necessary to reproduce the pain. Tenderness to percussion of the spine indicates a destructive lesion, while pain only on Valsalva is more compatible with disc protrusion. Tender points along the paraspinal muscles and trigger points in other muscles are characteristics of the myofascial pain/dysfunction syndrome, or fibromyalgia. Sympathetically mediated neuropathic pain is associated with trophic changes in the skin and, sometimes, in the underlying bone. Temperature changes are almost invariably present, with the affected extremity appearing cooler than the healthy one.

Physical signs can be misleading in patients with psychogenic pain syndromes. The most difficult patients are those who have some underlying organic lesion that is compounded by abnormal pain behavior.

Specific Pain Syndromes

Headache

Headaches are the most common recurrent pain problem and are more common in women than in men. The vast majority are benign, and structural intracranial pathology accounts for less than 1 percent of headache visits. The most important issues in headache management are to make an accurate syndrome diagnosis and to recognize rapidly the few cases that require emergency treatment.

Benign headache syndromes tend to have a chronic, recurrent temporal pattern, are devoid of neurologic findings, and have stereotyped symptoms. More dangerous headaches are acute and progressive, and may present with stiff neck, papilledema, or a focal neurologic deficit. These require emergency intervention.

Chronic/Recurrent Headache Syndromes These syndromes make up the vast majority of headache visits to physicians and, since they are rarely cured, require long-term management. If the correct diagnosis is made, most cases can be managed easily in the office. The strongest historical datum leading to diagnosis is the temporal pattern of the headache.

Tension-type headache (aka "muscle contraction") is the least defined of the headache syndromes. The temporal pattern is vague, and patients are unable to be precise about time of onset or duration. It may last as little as an hour or may be present nearly all the time. Pain is most often described as an aching or tight band around the head. Interestingly, small daily hassles seem to be more important than major life stressors in headache pathogenesis.

Physical examination is normal, except for the occasional appearance of tender points in the muscles of the neck or the muscles surrounding the temporomandibular joint. Self-medication is the rule, but may actually perpetuate the headaches. Cognitive/behavioral techniques, such as relaxation training and biofeedback, can decrease the frequency and intensity of headaches. Simple relaxation techniques can be taught in the office. Tricyclic antidepressants, such as amitriptyline, usually are considered the first-line drugs. They should be started in doses of 10 to 25 mg at bedtime and titrated up by similar increments every few days.

Migraine is an episodic headache syndrome characterized by throbbing or pounding pain that is usually unilateral and accompanied by photophobia, phonophobia, nausea, and anxiety. The headache may be preceded by focal neurologic symptoms (aura) that most commonly are visual (scotoma, fortification spectra, or photopsias), but may include numbness or weakness. Migraine with aura is what was called "classic migraine" in older classifications.

Migraine is significantly more common in women than in men. It often fluctuates with hormonal changes, often ceasing with menopause. Migraine may begin in childhood, but the majority of patients have the onset in adolescence or early adult life. In susceptible patients, some specific foods may precipitate headaches, and a careful history may be sufficient to identify and then eliminate the provoking factors.

Treatment of migraine can be divided into abortive and prophylactic measures. Ergot alkaloids were among the first specific abortive therapies for migraine. Ergotamine dosing usually begins with 2 mg orally at the onset of the attack, followed by 1 mg every half-hour until the headache ceases or the patient has taken a maximum of 6 mg in a day or 12 mg in a week. Higher dosing raises the risk of ergotism or other vascular complications. The drug also can be used sublingually or rectally. Long-term use should be avoided because it may lead to tolerance and physical dependence—as well as to chronic daily headache.

Naproxen (375 to 1100 mg, po) and ketorolac (60 mg, IM) are nonsteroidal anti-inflammatory drugs that can abort acute migraine episodes.

Sumatriptan, a 5-HT1 receptor agonist, is available as an autoinjector and, in doses of 6 mg, effectively aborts about 70 percent of attacks. It is contraindicated in patients with angina, uncontrolled hypertension, and peripheral vascular disease.

Prophylactic therapy usually is begun with beta-adrenergic blockers (e.g., propranolol, 10 mg qid) on the theory that eliminating the vasodilatory phase of the migraine eliminates the pain. They are contraindicated in patients with asthma and congestive heart failure.

Methysergide may be effective in patients refractory to other ergots. Dosing is with one pill (2 mg) three to four times a day. It should not be used for more than a few months at a time because of the risk of retroperitoneal fibrosis.

Tricyclic antidepressants can be used in the same way as in tension headaches. Calcium channel blockers, such as verapamil, also may be used.

Non-pharmacologic measures, such as relaxation techniques and the elimination of identified dietary precipitants, can be helpful. Patients should be instructed to eat regularly and to avoid sleep deprivation.

Cluster headaches are the only headache syndrome far more common in men than in women. Pain is piercing in nature, retroorbital, and invariably unilateral. It is accompanied by nasal congestion, tearing, ptosis, and miosis. Pain reaches maximum intensity within a few minutes and lasts 20 min to 1 h. Alcohol and high altitudes precipitate attacks. The clinical picture is so stereotyped that no further testing is needed.

Prophylactic therapy can be started with methysergide, as for migraine. Lithium is also quite effective, but the dose must be adjusted carefully and can range from 300 to 1500 mg/day.

Chronic daily headache usually evolves from tension or migraine as the result of frequent use of short-acting analgesics over a long period. The quality is similar to that of tension headache. Therapy is directed at withdrawing the offending agents and providing a regimen similar to that used for tension headache.

Temporomandibular Joint Disease (TMJ) Pain is described as aching and originating in the joint or ear. It is exacerbated by movement, and there may be evidence of jaw deviation or abnormal noises. It is probably best to consider it as a myofascial syndrome. Invasive therapies should be avoided and treatment should be based on conservative physical modalities, cognitive/behavioral techniques, and tricyclic antidepressants.

Acute or Progressive Headache Syndromes These syndromes are harbingers of serious neurologic impairment and are seen more commonly in the emergency room than in office practice. The historical data that should raise suspicion are sudden onset and rapid progression of a new headache or a change in pattern of an existing headache syndrome. These often are life-threatening problems, and it is essential that the diagnosis be considered when patients complain of headaches of these symptom patterns.

Subarachnoid hemorrhage should be considered in an otherwise healthy person who presents with sudden onset of a severe headache. The headache may have begun during a Valsalva maneuver, as with coitus or straining at stool. Computed tomography must be performed immediately; it demonstrates blood in the subarachnoid space in more than 90 percent of cases. Lumbar puncture is confirmatory in the remainder.

Metastatic brain tumors present with headaches that are not qualitatively different from tension headaches. The clinical differentiation is that the syndrome is progressive over weeks to months and is accompanied by an abnormal neurologic exam.

Pseudotumor cerebri (benign intracranial hypertension) is a disease most commonly seen in obese young women. The syndrome is characterized by headache and papilledema in a person with normal brain imaging. This problem requires urgent attention since it can result in loss of vision.

Temporal arteritis presents in elderly patients (it is very unusual before the age of 60) and is accompanied by jaw claudication and a general feeling of malaise. Polymyalgia rheumatica (aching around the shoulders and hips) is a common concomitant. The diagnosis should be suspected in any elderly patient with a new headache and systemic symptoms. Tenderness around the temporal artery is variable. The erythrocyte sedimentation rate (ESR) is markedly elevated in the majority of patients; if the clinical picture and elevated ESR appear together, treatment with prednisone 80 to 100 mg daily should be given emergently. Delay in treatment can lead to retinal artery occlusion and permanent blindness.

Low Back Pain

Accurate diagnosis depends on a directed history and physical examination, supplemented by the judicious selection of ancillary procedures. The approach to the patient with back pain is discussed in Chap. 53.

Neuropathic Pain Syndromes

These syndromes, caused by injury to the central or peripheral nervous system, have a stereotypical symptomatology. Patients complain of dysesthetic pains that are burning, tingling, or viselike, often unlike anything they have previously experienced. Occasionally, there is a lancinating (stabbing) or shooting, shocklike quality. Trigeminal neuralgia (tic douloureux) is usually purely lancinating, diabetic neuropathy purely dysesthetic, and postherpetic neuralgia a combination.

Neuropathic pain syndromes are best treated with adjuvant medications (described below). Anticonvulsants are most often used for the lancinating pains. In particularly refractory cases, opioids may be given a trial, but should be prescribed by physicians well versed in their use and possible side effects.

Psychogenic Pain Syndromes

Purely psychogenic pain (delusional pain) is uncommon. More commonly, there are psychological factors that influence the patient's perception and experience of pain. Therefore, little or nothing is to be gained by trying to decide whether or not pain is "real." With the exception of malingering, described earlier, all pain is real in that the patient is suffering.

If an accurate psychological diagnosis can be reached, specific therapies can be employed. Antidepressant medications for pain are more efficacious in depressed than in nondepressed patients, and the judicious use of anxiolytics may reduce dysfunction in distraught patients. Under no circumstances should the establishment of a psychiatric diagnosis be used as a confrontational tool; that will only reinforce abnormal illness behavior and destroy the physician-patient relationship. These are the cases in which a multidisciplinary pain center becomes useful.

Analgesic Interventions

Adequate pain management requires appropriate coordination of pharmacologic, psychological, and physical measures. The systemic pharmacologic agents used for the treatment of pain fall into three groups: the nonopioid analgesics (primarily the nonsteroidal anti-inflammatory drugs), opioid analgesics, and adjuvant drugs (primarily the antidepressants and anticonvulsants).

Nonsteroidal Anti-Inflammatory Drugs

The nonopioid analgesics are characterized by their peripheral site of action, ceiling effect, and side effect profiles affecting mainly the gastrointestinal tract (including bleeding). The ceiling effect implies that there is a level after which further dose escalation will produce intolerable side effects without increased analgesia.

Acetaminophen and the nonsteroidal anti-inflammatory drugs (NSAIDs) are the most commonly used agents. Acetaminophen has an analgesic potency similar to aspirin, but is only minimally anti-inflammatory. It has fewer gastrointestinal side effects than aspirin and does not affect platelet function. Total daily dosing should be kept below 4 g, to avoid the risk of analgesic nephropathy.

The nonsteroidal anti-inflammatory drugs (NSAIDs) are most effective in somatic nociceptive pain, presumably because of their antiprostaglandin activity and peripheral site of action. It is usually advisable to start with a loading dose to achieve therapeutic serum levels quickly. The drug dosage should then be titrated until there are effects or side effects. The ceiling dose varies from drug to drug and from patient to patient, and must be established individually. Furthermore, patients unresponsive to drugs in a given group may be responsive to drugs in a different group.

The most appropriate drug to use is usually the one with which the physician is most familiar. Occasionally, one particular drug has been studied better than others for a given syndrome (indomethacin for chronic paroxysmal hemicrania and naproxen for migraine), but the analgesic profiles appear similar.

The major side effects of the NSAIDs are gastrointestinal; these increase with the age of the patient and the duration of treatment. Misoprostol (Cytotec) can be used to avoid some of the gastric side effects, but may cause diarrhea. Renal impairment may occur with prolonged use at high levels. The main central nervous system side effects are dizziness and occasional confusion.

Opioid Analgesics

Fears of addiction and abuse make many physicians reluctant to use opioid analgesics for patients in chronic pain. However, in selected patients with refractory pain syndromes, opioids can provide relief with an acceptable and manageable risk of side effects.

Constipation is the most troublesome side effect of opioid therapy and requires prophylactic treatment. Stool-softeners are not sufficient by themselves, and all patients being treated with opioids should also be given a laxative, e.g., one of the senna compounds. Severe somnolence and respiratory depression are extremely uncommon at therapeutic opioid doses.

Some opioids have side effects peculiar to the drug. Meperidine (Demerol), the most-prescribed parenteral opioid analgesic, is metabolized to normeperidine, which can cause hyperreflexia, myoclonus, and seizures. The mixed agonist-antagonist narcotic analgesics, such as pentazocine (Talwin) and butorphanol (Stadol) can precipitate withdrawal in physically dependent patients and can have psychotomimetic effects in the elderly.

Opioids vary widely in their serum half-lives, from 2 to 3 h for hydromorphone (Dilaudid) to up to 54 h for methadone (Dolophine). Analgesic efficacy, however, does not directly parallel serum half-life. Even the long serum half-life drugs only provide 4 to 6 h of analgesia.

Controlled-release morphine preparations can provide gradual release of morphine over eight to 12 hours. Immediate-release morphine may be used prn for breakthrough pain.

All opioid analgesics are at least twice as potent when administered intramuscularly as when administered orally, owing to a first pass effect in the liver. Therefore, doses must be adjusted when the route is changed.

Adjuvant Medications

Adjuvant medications are those whose primary indication is for something other than pain but that have analgesic efficacy. Tricyclic antidepressants, anticonvulsants, anxiolytics, and lidocaine derivatives (mexiletine) have all been used in specific pain states, primarily in neuropathic pain.

The tricyclic antidepressants are the most widely used and most adequately studied of the adjuvant medications for pain. While the most recognized indication is for burning, neuropathic pain, they have also been used successfully in chronic low back pain, headache, and other pain syndromes. The analgesic effects are more evident in patients who have a concomitant depression, but nondepressed patients also respond. Dosing of the tricyclic antidepressants should be started at low levels (10 mg at bedtime in the elderly and 25 mg in the young) and titrated up every few days by similar increments. Analgesic effects appear earlier and at lower doses than do the antidepressant effects. Amitriptyline, a tertiary amine tricyclic, is the most widely used; but secondary amine tricyclics, such as nortriptyline and desipramine, are less anticholinergic and also have analgesic efficacy.

Anticonvulsant drugs such as carbamazepine (Tegretol) and phenytoin (Dilantin) are the drugs of choice for trigeminal neuralgia and, by extrapolation, are used for other lancinating pains. Carbamazepine should be started at 100 mg twice daily, and titrated up to effect, which usually is at 200 mg three to five times a day. Phenytoin, on the other hand, can be started at 300 mg daily.

Anxiolytics should be used for the control of anxiety in patients with pain, particularly when anxiety is leading to increased analgesic intake. The evidence for a primary analgesic effect is not as strong as with the antidepressants.

Mexiletine, an orally administered lidocaine derivative, is currently under study for painful diabetic neuropathy and other types of burning, neuropathic pain.

Anesthesiologic Procedures

Anesthesiologic procedures can be used to provide regional blockade in somatic nociceptive syndromes or for sympathetic blockade in certain neuropathic syndromes. They should be considered when the diagnosis is in question and should always be used before any ablative therapy is considered.

Physical Techniques

There are no adequately controlled and blinded studies to demonstrate the efficacy of physical techniques for the treatment of pain. The existing studies on therapies as diverse as transcutaneous nerve stimulation (TENS), massage, acupuncture, trigger point injections, and traction are all flawed. In anecdotal reports, all have been beneficial for a number of pain problems. Physical techniques should be adapted to the specific pain problem, such as trigger points techniques for myofascial pain, support for articular derangements, and exercises for weakened or immobilized areas.

Psychological Techniques

Anxiety, immobility, and protective postures are often appropriate for acute pain, but may represent abnormal illness behavior in chronic pain. After an adequate psychosocial assessment, one of the main goals in the psychological management of chronic pain is to provide the patient with tools to recognize and alter the behaviors that perpetuate her suffering. A pain diary is helpful to identify issues that may otherwise go unnoticed or unreported. Simple relaxation techniques can decrease the intensity and frequency of headaches and myofascial pain syndromes. Meetings with family members can identify interpersonal interactions that are perpetuating the pain. Patients who can recognize their role in pain treatment and feel that they are in control of their environment are more likely to benefit from pain rehabilitation.

Some patients simply cannot be managed by an individual practitioner and require referral to a specialized pain center. In general, these are patients with combined psychosocial, medical, and pharmacologic problems that need the multidisciplinary approach that is frequently ideally provided in a center.

References and Suggested Readings

1. Foley KM, Inturrisi CE: Analgesic drug therapy in cancer pain: Principles and practice. *Med Clin North Am* 71:207–232, 1987.
2. Getto CJ, Sorkness CA, Howell T: Issues in drug management. Part I. Antidepressants and chronic nonmalignant pain: A review. *J Pain Sympt Manag* 2:9–18, 1987.
3. Kanner RM: Evaluation and treatment of headache. *Primary Care Update for OB/GYNS* 1:33–38, 1994.
4. Portenoy RK: Mechanisms of clinical pain: Observations and speculations. *Neurol Clin* 7:205–230, 1989.
5. Portenoy RK: Chronic opioid therapy in nonmalignant pain. *J Pain Sympt Manag* 5:46S–62S, 1990.

64 Occupational and Environmental Medicine

Arthur L. Frank

THE OCCUPATIONAL AND ENVIRONMENTAL HISTORY
PRINCIPLES OF TOXICOLOGY
PREVENTION OF EXPOSURE
SOURCES OF INFORMATION

The role of women in the workplace is rapidly evolving. The majority of children now born in the United States are born to women who are employed outside of the home, and there is a rising recognition of reproductive hazards related to workplace exposures. In addition, the general public and women of reproductive age are much more aware than previously of potential risks to reproduction from environmental exposures. There are now concerns regarding exposure to electromagnetic fields, lead in drinking water, pesticides, and a wide range of other potentially noxious agents. In addition to concerns relating to the well-being of future offspring, the workplace and the environment may pose risks to the woman herself.

Unfortunately, most clinicians now practicing have had little training in obtaining information about occupational and environmental exposures. Ongoing uncertainty about many types of exposures complicates matters further. In the one-on-one setting of an office practice, it can be extremely difficult to provide useful information to patients regarding potential hazards to pregnancy and to their own well-being from occupational and environmental exposures.

The Occupational and Environmental History

Although traditionally poorly taught and reinforced, taking an occupational and environmental history is an important aspect of the overall assessment of a woman's well-being and that of any current or potential pregnancies. Physicians are routinely reminded that the medical history is perhaps the most significant part of the patient/physician encounter, but the area of exposure assessment often is neglected.

The patient/physician encounter often puts the patient in a dependent role; however, when it comes to knowledge and experience about her workplace and her environmental exposures, the patient is clearly on a more equal footing. When discussing workplace exposures the patient, who is also the worker, is often the best source of information about what is used at the workplace and what occupational health hazards may exist. The worker can give her physician information about specific materials to which she has been exposed by providing access to material safety data sheets (MSDS) required by law to be made available to workers for their information and to share with their physician. The clinician should also know that a variety of specialists are knowledgeable about workplace and environmental hazards, and that through such colleagues, e.g., occupational health physicians, occupational health nurses, and industrial hygienists, information can be obtained that may be of assistance in dealing with individual patients.

An Italian physician, Bernadino Ramazzini, in the early 1700s produced his great treatise on the diseases of workers, reminding physicians that it was incumbent upon them to ask what the patient did for a living.[7] In the modern world this can be expanded to include other exposures that may occur away from the worksite. There has been an ever-increasing blurring of distinctions between workplace and nonworkplace exposures; toxins leave the confines of a factory through the air, water, and finished products. Other significant exposures, such as second-hand smoke, can be found in settings as private as one's own home.

The physician should ask the patient what type of work she does, and then have the patient fully describe her work if the physician has any questions whatsoever about the exact nature of her job description or title. It is useful specifically to ask about any exposures to chemicals, dusts, fumes, vapors, radiation, etc. If the physician feels concern that the patient may, in fact, be harmed by such exposures, it is prudent to ask about fellow workers and any possible work-related health problems. Also, ask if the worker is required to wear any special protective equipment—especially a respirator—that might prevent inhalation or ingestion of substances that could be harmful.

It is important to know about all former jobs as well as the current job, and the next step is to undertake a comprehensive review of previous employment. In some cases, health problems may persist from prior exposures and are not attributable to the current one.

It is also important to ask about her spouse's employment and the possibility that hazardous materials are brought home on his work clothing or skin. If the spouse is in the military, dioxins may be relevant. Spousal exposure may pose a significant risk to reproduction.[8] This is an appropriate time to ask if the patient knows of any local environmental contamination or if she lives near a factory, hazardous waste site, or utilizes a known contaminated water supply.

Other questions have to do with home-related exposures. These include recent renovations or remodeling, the potential for exposure following installation of new home insulation with materials containing formaldehyde, and information regarding hobbies. It is also appropriate to ask about a spouse's hobbies, since these may be a source of exposure as well.

Figure 64-1 presents a framework for asking these questions. Questions of occupational and environmental exposure obviously need to be assessed along with other aspects of the patient's history, including her prior reproductive history, regular medical history, demographic history, and related environmental exposures (i.e., cigarette smoking and alcohol consumption).

Principles of Toxicology

The basic principles of toxicology govern reproductive outcomes, just as they affect other organ systems. Important issues include the chemical and physical properties of the possible toxin; exposure characteristics, such as dose, route of entry, and metabolic fate; and other related factors. Issues of individual susceptibility and synergism also may be operative.

Hazards to reproduction may come from both chemical and physical agents, and they affect both sexes. Among these materials are heavy metals, solvents, and pesticides. Table 64-1 lists some of the risk factors associated with adverse reproductive outcomes. For certain more narrowly focused groups, such as hospital personnel, there may be hazards from exposure to waste anesthetic gases and chemotherapeutic agents. The physical agent of primary concern for this group would be ionizing radiation, with concern developing over the past years for possible effects from nonionizing radiation as well. The last group of agents causing concern are biological agents, including viruses, parasites, and some bacteria. For a more detailed description of these

Current work: ____

How long at this job? ____

Description of work: ____

____

Any contact with dust, fumes, chemicals, radiation, noise, etc?

____ Yes ____ No If yes, describe: ____

____

Describe any adverse effects noted: ____

____

Are any fellow workers ill? ____ Yes ____ No If yes, describe: ____

____

Do you use any protective equipment at work? ____ Yes ____ No

Previous Job History	From	To	Exposures
1st regular job	______	______	
Next job	______	______	
Next job	______	______	
Vacation or temporary job	______	______	
Vacation or temporary job	______	______	

Military service or related exposures: ____

____

Have you lived near an industrial facility or has a family member worked in a setting where hazardous materials have been brought home? ____ Yes ____ No If yes, describe: ____

____

Hobby history:

Smoking history:

Alcohol and drug use history:

Comments:

Figure 64-1 Environmental and Occupational Exposure History

TABLE 64-1 Factors Associated with Adverse Female Reproductive Effects

Risk Factors Associated with Menstrual Disorders	
Antineoplastics	Tobacco
Fluorine	Formaldehyde
Carbon disulfide	Trinitrotoluene
Chloroprene	
Risk Factors Associated with Spontaneous Abortions	
Alcohol	Smoking
Medications	Infections
Risk Factors Associated with Low Birth Weight or Prematurity	
Alcohol	Smoking
Altitude	Infections
Exposures that May Be Associated with Adverse Outcomes	
Anesthetic gases	
Ionizing radiation	
Solvents (e.g., carbon disulfide)	
Heavy metals (e.g., lead, mercury)	
Pesticides (e.g., dibromochloropropane, dioxin)	

SOURCE: Adapted from Lemasters.[5]

exposures, see the work of Paul and Kurtz, which contains various specific "case studies."[6] Other case study materials are also available.[2]

A basic principle of toxicology is the classic dose-response relationship, which states simply that as the dose escalates, the likelihood of a biological response also rises. The concept of dose can be measured in different ways, including the doses found in the environment, the internalized dose following the route of entry, the dose of a specific toxic agent following metabolism of a xenobiotic, or some combination of these types of exposures. Potential complications are exposures to mixtures of materials—either complex mixtures found in the environment, such as gasoline, or synergism resulting from combinations of workplace toxins and risky personal habits, such as interaction with cigarette smoke or alcohol.

Individual susceptibilities are hard to define and often difficult to quantify. Susceptibility to toxins may vary by age, sex, nutritional status, genetics, concurrent disease, hormonal and immunologic status, and, as noted above, possible synergisms with personal habits and additional exposures.

Prevention of Exposure

Depending on the nature of the exposure to toxins, there may be a variety of basic approaches to eliminating or reducing exposures, whether before a woman becomes pregnant, during her pregnancy, or at all times. For such personal habits as smoking, alcohol use, and nutrition, each individual has considerable control over exposure. At the workplace, exposure control can take several forms. As a basic principle, it is not ideal to have a women who is pregnant, or who is trying to become pregnant, need to stop working. There may well be circumstances that require a woman to discontinue or curtail her normal activities, including work; but a ban on working is often the least acceptable alternative to the woman of many that exist. According to federal law, each worker is entitled to a safe and healthful workplace; given recent court decisions, this includes making the workplace safe for pregnant women and women who wish to become pregnant. This issue has gone to the Supreme Court, which found that a healthful and safe workplace is appropriate care.

There are times, however, when administrative controls are necessary. These may include job transfer, restriction of physical hazards during pregnancy, or modification of a job assignment. Compared with engineering controls, which are the ideal way of reducing exposure, the least comfortable alternative is to require personal protective equipment as the major means of controlling harmful exposures. Although potentially quite effective, in reality the use of a respirator over a typical 8-h shift is extremely difficult. The use of a lead apron to minimize radiation exposure is far less acceptable than engineering modifications that do not allow taking a radiograph unless the worker is in a sheltered or protected area that minimizes exposure.

Although the obstetrician/gynecologist may be the major source of medical information for pregnant women, such specialists may have been insufficiently trained to render judgments about specific exposures. Therefore, such physicians must have access to specialized information and personnel to assist with medical management of their patients. Documents available from the Agency for Toxic Substances and Disease Registry (ATSDR) list many such sources of information, including state health departments, university programs, and poison control centers.[1,2]

Sources of Information

As noted earlier, the worker is often the best source of information regarding specific exposures. Workers have access to material safety data sheets, which review issues such as routes of entry, reactivity, flammability, and recognized adverse biological effects. This is often a good place for the physician to start learning about specific toxins. Other more general references can help physicians develop an information base regarding reproductive hazards.[4–6,9] In addition to text resources, computer databases can be accessed for information. One such example is the Reprotoxline, which contains summaries and references on reproductive data for over 800 chemical and physical agents. The National Library of Medicine in Bethesda, Maryland, on the National Institutes of Health campus, also has several computer databases, including one on developmental reproductive toxicology, a hazardous substance databank, Medline and Toxline. There are other U.S. reproductive centers or pregnancy risk information services that can be accessed. Also, government agencies, such as the National Institute for Occupational Safety and Health, and the Occupational Safety and Health Administration, can be contacted for assistance about specific hazards. Although traditionally there have not been many resources of this type, significant numbers now exist to assist the practicing physician in dealing with pregnancy and reproductive issues as well as general health and safety.

However, even with all that is available one should also recognize that, for the vast majority of substances, little if anything is known about potential reproductive hazards. One is left with a need to make individualized judgments regarding a given case with a complex set of parameters; often there is a limited amount of information to help the patient. These same limitations apply to the area of regulatory toxicology and, when all issues are considered, there are relatively few compounds or potentially hazardous exposures for which there are significant databases. This lack of good scientific data, coupled with the potential anxiety of patients and the very real need to give good advice, is one of the great challenges to physicians—not only in reproductive toxicology, but also with many similar issues of toxic exposure where reproduction is not an immediate or even a future concern.

References and Selected Readings

1. Frank AL: ATSDR. Case studies in environmental medicine: Taking an exposure history. No 26. Frank AL, editor. U.S. Department of Health and Human Services. 1992, pp 1–56.
2. Welch LS: ATSDR. Case studies in environmental medicine: Reproductive and developmental hazards. No. 29. Welch LS, editor. U.S. Department of Health and Human Services. 1993, pp 1–41.
3. Frank AL: The occupational and environmental history, in Rom WN (ed): *Environmental and Occupational Medicine.* Boston: Little, Brown, 1992, pp 29–34.
4. Kurzel RB: Disorders of the female reproductive system and developmental disorders, in Tarcher AB (ed): *Principles and Practice of Environmental Medicine.* New York: Plenum, 1992, pp 413–435.
5. Lemasters GK: Occupational exposures and effects on male and female reproduction, in Rom WN (ed): *Environmental and Occupational Medicine.* Boston: Little, Brown, 1992, pp 147–170.
6. Paul M, Kurtz S: Reproductive hazards in the workplace. Occupational and environmental reproductive hazards center. Worcester: University of Massachusetts Medical Center, 1990.
7. Ramazzini B: Diseases of workers (*De morbis artificum diatriba, 1713*). Wright WC, translator. New York: Hafner, 1964.
8. Robaire B, Hales BF: Paternal exposure to chemicals before conception. *Br Med J:* pp 341–342, 1993.
9. Steinberger E: Disorders of the male reproductive system, in Tarcher AB: *Principles and Practice of Environmental Medicine.* New York: Plenum, 1992, pp 437–457.

65 Common Medical Emergencies

Thomas Kwiatkowski
William Rennie

This chapter describes the basic approach to the evaluation and treatment of a selected group of traumatic conditions and medical emergencies that may be encountered in the primary care setting.

Trauma is the most common cause of death and disability for all patients under age 40. Over 60 million injuries occur in the United States every year, with half of these requiring some kind of medical treatment. As patients grow older, other medical problems may account for the majority of physician visits, but dealing with trauma of all types still plays a major role in the health care of every sector of the population. Of the 30 million injuries each year that require medical treatment, only 12 percent need in-hospital care, leaving over 20 million patients cared for in some kind of ambulatory setting. The dramatic statistics of death and severe disability may not apply to these patients, yet real problems with temporary disability, loss of income, and occupational issues are often confronted in the primary care arena. In addition to treating trauma, primary care physicians can play a major role in reducing death and disability from trauma by making certain to emphasize preventive issues.

In addition to traumatic injuries, the primary care clinician also will encounter acute medical problems ranging from such environmental exposures as smoke inhalation and insect stings to adverse drug reactions and toxic ingestions. A thorough understanding of the approach to patients with these problems is important for establishing early treatment priorities and making appropriate referrals. Anaphylaxis and cardiac arrest can occur in the office setting. Understanding the general approach to these life-threatening conditions will give the primary care physician the necessary skills to treat an increasingly complex and chronically ill patient population.

Minor Head Trauma

Head trauma is extremely common, with a spectrum of injuries ranging from trivial to life-threatening. More severely injured patients will be transported to medical facilities or trauma centers, but patients with minor wounds or those seeking care at a time significantly delayed from the injury itself will present to the primary care physician. It is important to assess these patients completely and to recognize the signs of more severe or possibly occult injury.

Pathophysiology

The tightly closed bony calvarium provides good protection for the brain, but its rigidity also contributes to the injury patterns seen with head trauma. These injuries can be focal or diffuse. Focal lesions can occur within the brain itself or, more commonly, in the surrounding tissues. These lesions begin as bleeding in a specific area; then, as the hematoma expands, intracranial pressure rises. The brain tissue is compressed as a result of this increased pressure, giving rise to a continually worsening injury with focal neurologic findings. Subdural, epidural, and parenchymal hematomas as well as cerebral contusions fall into this category. Diffuse injury usually is the result of rapid acceleration/deceleration, with the resultant energy shock being absorbed by the brain. This causes a temporary widespread loss of neurologic function. Brief periods of unconsciousness are seen in the milder forms of diffuse injury, while more severe diffuse axonal injury can produce prolonged coma and eventual death. Concussion is the most common form of diffuse injury.

Clinical Evaluation

In the primary care setting, the head-injured patient should be screened for any potentially serious injuries and treated and followed for the more common minor injuries. Typical patients will present with recent minor injuries, often involving scalp lacerations or with previously sustained trauma that for one reason or another was not evaluated near the time of the injury. The clinician should always complete a thorough neurologic exam on all head-injured patients, which must include an assessment of the patient's mental status.

Scalp Injuries

The layers of the scalp can be described by the letters S.C.A.L.P. The *skin* is followed by a layer of *connective tissue* containing nerves and vessels. Beneath this is the *aponeurosis,* a tough layer made up of fascia from the frontal and occipital muscles. *Loose areolar tissue* is below this and separates it from the *periosteum* of the skull. It is important to ascertain the depth of scalp injuries before attempting repair, since lacerations through the aponeurosis will require an additional layer of closure. As with all wounds, thorough cleansing and debridement of foreign material is of primary importance. In addition, scalp wounds should be gently explored with a gloved finger to determine if any bony discontinuity is present. Skull films have been shown to be of little if any value in the evaluation of patients with head trauma. If mental status changes or focal findings are present, or if an examining finger detects depression, step-off, or crepitus of the underlying bone, the physician should immediately consider CT scanning and referral of the patient to a physician with special expertise in the management of head trauma patients.

In cases of uncomplicated lacerations, closure of the aponeurosis can be achieved with interrupted absorbable suture (3-0 or 4-0), and skin closure should be with 3-0 nylon or other similar material. Pressure dressings and head wraps generally should be avoided, allowing the patient to observe for any complications, which can then be reported quickly to the physician for management. A standard set of head-injury patient instructions should be given (Table 65-1) and should be discussed thoroughly with both the patient and a family member.

TABLE 65-1 **Head Injury Instructions**

You have sustained a head injury, but do not require hospital admission at this time. Following head injury or concussion, you may develop headache, dizziness or nausea, or vomit once or twice. If these symptoms continue over 48 h, you should return to the Emergency Department or your personal physician for reevaluation.

Contact your personal physician or return to the Emergency Department immediately for:

1. Confusion, difficulty waking up, restlessness, or trouble with speech
2. Persistent vomiting
3. Continuing or increasing headache
4. Weakness of arms or legs
5. Stiff neck, with or without a fever
6. Seizure
7. Clear or bloody fluid from ears or nose
8. Fever over 101°F
9. Pupils of unequal size

There *must* be a responsible person with you for the next 24 h. You should be awakened every 2 h to check for above symptoms.

For a headache you may use acetaminophen (Tylenol) 2 pills every 4–6 h or ibuprofen (Advil) 1–2 pills every 4–6 h with food. Do *not* drink any alcohol. Take only medication prescribed by the doctor. Take only a clear liquid diet for the next 12 h.

Loss of Consciousness

Most patients who have sustained a head injury significant enough to cause loss of consciousness will be evaluated initially in an emergency department. Patients who ask for telephone advice soon after sustaining such an injury should be encouraged to seek emergency evaluation. Many patients, for whatever reason, will seek medical attention hours to days later, and will report their previous loss of consciousness at this time. This can create a dilemma for the primary care physician, who must then assess the significance of the injury. Obviously, one would like to be able to rule out potentially dangerous lesions quickly and with some measure of assurance.

The most devastating of focal injuries that cause loss of consciousness are subdural hematomas. These result from the tearing of venous structures and are often associated with lacerations of the brain substance itself. For injuries this severe, a transient loss of consciousness is not unusual. The one exception to this rule is found in the elderly. These patients have longer and more vulnerable bridging veins, due to cerebral atrophy with age; damage to these vessels from a fall may result in subdural bleeding. Loss of consciousness may be only brief, with the slow bleeding giving rise to the so-called chronic subdural. Patients may experience a gradual deterioration of function, including mental status changes, over several days to weeks. It is of prime importance to consider this entity when evaluating any post-head trauma patient, particularly one who is elderly. Any changes in mood, clarity of thought, or motor function following such an injury should prompt the clinician to look for a subdural collection with CT scanning.

Epidural hematomas are characterized by rapid, arterial bleeding and do not present as chronic debilitation. They are usually associated with a fracture through the temporal bone, with subsequent disruption of the middle meningeal artery. Loss of consciousness is usual immediately after the blow to the head, but patients may regain consciousness for variable lengths of time before rapid deterioration takes place. This is the so-called lucid interval seen with epidural hematomas. Patients may present to the primary care physician during this interval, making recognition of this potentially fatal injury extremely important. The first thing for the clinician to realize is that the "lucid interval" is somewhat of a misnomer. Patients may be able to function, but their mental status is never completely normal. The interval also is short-lived, unlike the pattern seen with chronic subdural hematomas, lasting only minutes to hours. The clinician should keep consideration of this injury in the forefront when any head trauma appears to involve the temporal bone above the ear. Signs of increasing intracranial pressure and compression of brain tissue may occur quickly. Tip-offs are a dilated or sluggishly reactive pupil on the side of the head lesion and muscular weakness of the contralateral side. If the timing of the injury and the clinical findings, especially abnormal mental status, suggest this as a possible injury, immediate neurosurgical and/or CT evaluation are necessary.

The most common injury producing a loss of consciousness is a cerebral concussion. This diffuse injury is always transient, with return to normal mental status occurring within minutes. The patient who has had loss of consciousness for less than five minutes and returns to normal following this can be safely observed at home, provided neurologic and mental status examinations are totally normal and that the patient is in a home environment conducive to observation over the next 24 h. In the immediate post-injury period, a patient who has had more than 5 min loss of consciousness, has an altered mental status, or who has an abnormal neurologic exam requires more in-depth evaluation. Patients impaired by drugs or alcohol also fall into this category. Most of the time the additional evaluation will consist of CT scanning and/or inpatient observation for 24 h. When patients present more than 24 h after the initial loss of consciousness, there is less concern for significant occult injury. Usually such an injury will already have declared itself. The obvious exception is the elderly patient who may be harboring a chronic subdural hematoma, as described above. The evaluation for delayed presentation of loss of consciousness should consist of a thorough search for focal neurologic findings and a complete mental status exam. Individuals with normal exams may then be given standard head injury instructions and followed as outpatients (see Table 65-1).

Summary

Head trauma is very common, and those patients with minor injuries will most often be the ones who present for care to the primary care physician. With proper evaluation and knowledge of the natural history of potentially serious injuries, these patients can be managed appropriately in this setting. Primary care physicians can also play a key role in preventing head and other injuries by emphasizing the importance of bicycle helmets, seatbelt use, not driving while intoxicated nor being the passenger of an intoxicated driver, etc.

Neck and Spinal Injuries

Although it is unlikely that patients with spinal injuries will come to the primary care physician for evaluation and treatment, opportunities for preventing these injuries should not be overlooked. Injuries to the neck and spine occur most often from motor vehicle accidents and from falls. The elderly population is especially at risk for injury from falls, and "fall reduction" programs are now in place in many geriatric institutions. The primary care physician can help in the education of both patients and families by suggesting simple measures to be taken to guard against potentially debilitating falls. Inside the home, area rugs and small, low stools should be avoided as they may easily contribute to unsure footing or stumbling. Particular attention should be paid to familiar paths within the house so that they are kept clear of clutter. Any unsteady patient should have access to a walker or a tripod cane to increase their stability. Open stairways should be avoided, and inclined ramps installed whenever possible.

If a family member calls to report that a patient has fallen down, the physician should stress to that person the importance of not hastily moving the patient. Any patient not fully awake after a fall should be kept in position until trained professionals (EMS) can safely move them. Likewise, any impairment of normal movement in any extremity requires that the patient be moved only after adequate spine immobilization. Fully alert patients who can move all their extremities and have no complaint of neck pain are the only ones who can be moved by untrained personnel. Immobilizing the head and neck can be done in the home, provided it does not interfere with the patient's ability to maintain an open airway. Heavy bags of sugar or flour can be placed on either side of the head to limit lateral motion, and a thick towel roll can be placed under the chin to prevent neck flexion. Most cervical spine injuries are more stable in extension than in flexion, so the motion to warn against is movement of the chin toward the chest.

As with all traumatic injuries, prevention is the key to reduction of morbidity and mortality from spinal injuries. Primary care specialists should take advantage of their ongoing relationships with patients and families to provide education aimed at the reduction of these and other potentially serious injuries.

Fractures and Soft Tissue Injuries

Fractures and soft tissue injuries are encountered commonly in younger, athletic, more adventurous patients, and are seen as the result of motor vehicle accidents and falls in all age groups. Evaluation of patients with complaints related to musculoskeletal trauma can be guided by knowledge of injury patterns and by diligently searching for those suspected injuries. Many simple soft tissue injuries can be treated and followed by the primary care physician; most fractures will be best referred to an orthopedic specialist for management. Knowing how to sort out these problems from an unselected patient population is one of the challenges of primary care. There is an extensive discussion about this in Chap. 61. Therefore, the problem will be addressed in this chapter in a more abbreviated fashion, focusing on a few common injuries.

Pathophysiology

Fractures occur when a direct impact either applied externally or sustained from a fall exceeds the ability of the bone to resist deformation. The history of injury as well as the radiographic appearance of the fracture usually will give information about the mechanism of injury. A direct blow to the shaft of a bone likely will produce a transverse or oblique fracture. When associated with a twisting injury, a spiral fracture may be seen. Crush injuries or compression due to falls may produce fractures that are comminuted as the force of impact dissipates through the bony structure. Small avulsion fragments may be seen in fractures occurring from strain across a joint, with the often stronger ligamentous attachments remaining intact while the bone at the site of attachment gives way. The usual clinical triad seen in all types of fractures is pain, deformity, and disability.

Soft tissue injuries may also be characterized by the same clinical signs of pain and disability, but deformity usually is limited to generalized soft tissue swelling. These injuries most often involve joints, as with sprains and strains, and the mechanism of injury is more often related to an overstressing of the particular joint than to a direct impact to the area.

Clinical Evaluation

Of primary importance in the evaluation of patients with traumatic injuries is a clear, concise history of the injury. As referred to above, direct impact injuries may lead the physician to suspect a fracture more than injuries sustained from stress across a joint. Age is also an important factor. Older patients with osteopenic bones are less able to tolerate deforming forces than are younger patients with denser bone. In lower extremity injuries, the ability to bear weight on the affected limb militates against fracture, although isolated fibular fractures and some minor pelvic ramus fractures may still allow the patient to ambulate.

Several general findings on physical exam can help the clinician differentiate between soft tissue injuries and fractures. Localized point tenderness is a hallmark of a fracture, while soft tissue injuries may exhibit more diffuse pain. Likewise, crepitus in the area of injury suggests fracture. Ecchymosis of overlying tissue is common with fractures and more severe ligamentous injuries. Also, if both the patient and the examiner have difficulty in consistently localizing the pain, a fracture is less likely. For lower extremity injuries, as mentioned above, an ability to bear weight usually indicates soft tissue injury.

Two of the most frequently encountered clinical scenarios involving musculoskeletal injury are: 1. the patient who has fallen on an outstretched hand, 2. the patient who has a twisting injury of the lower extremity with an associated fall. The evaluation of these two types of patients will be illustrative of how the physician should approach patients with either upper or lower extremity injuries. With ambulatory patients who have sustained injuries from these two mechanisms, the clinician should suspect fractures in the upper extremity and sprains and strains in the lower extremity.

Upper Extremity Injuries

The classic "fall on the outstretched hand" should be thought of as an impact injury. This history alone should raise the clinician's suspicion of a fracture. As the patient lands on the outstretched hand, the force of impact is transmitted through all bony structures from carpus to clavicle. This mechanism can be responsible for the following fractures: scaphoid; distal radius; radial head (at the elbow); supracondylar humerus; surgical neck humerus; and clavicular. All these areas should be evaluated in a systematic way in a patient who has sustained such a fall. Soft tissue injuries associated with this mechanism of injury include lunate and perilunate dislocations, posterior elbow dislocation, dislocation of the shoulder, and tears of the rotator cuff.

When examining a patient who has fallen on her outstretched hand, the physician should first note how she is using or protecting the involved extremity. Most of the injuries above will cause the patient to present with the affected arm at her side, flexed at the elbow and being supported by the opposite arm. The only exception is a posterior elbow dislocation, which may be held away from her body. Keeping in mind all of the possible injuries, the physician should then ask the patient which area is most painful and begin the examination at a site removed from this area. This will allow other injuries to be quickly ruled out.

From distal to proximal the examination should include maneuvers to rule out the many possible fractures that can occur in a fall on the outstretched hand. The soft tissue injuries sustained from this mechanism of injury can be easily assessed at the same time.

Knowing the possible injuries from a classic "fall on the outstretched hand" will help in the quick office evaluation of patients injured by this mechanism. When asked for telephone advice from such patients, the possibility of fracture should be strongly considered. Patients should be instructed to apply ice packs to the affected area, to immobilize the arm in a sling if possible, and to come for examination as soon as possible. The clinician should anticipate the need for radiographic evaluation until a systematic exam reveals no areas of local pain or deformity and good range of motion of all joints involved.

Lower Extremity Injuries

A twisting of the lower extremity, usually accompanied by a fall, is a classic history. Injuries sustained as a result of the twisting force are usually ligamentous and occur across joints. In the ankle, sprains occur from twisting such that the sole of the foot is either directed inward (inversion injuries) or outward (eversion injuries). Distal fibular and tibial fractures also may be encountered as a result of this mechanism. The knee can sustain the bulk of a twisting force, with both medial and lateral ligaments as well as cartilage at risk for injury. Finally, from the ensuing fall, both hip and pelvic fractures must be considered.

When evaluating patients with a twisting/falling mechanism of injury, the clinician must first note the patient's willingness to bear weight on the affected extremity. Fracture is much less likely if the patient, although in pain, is still ambulatory. Most lower extremity injuries will be ligamentous, and evaluation should proceed in a systematic manner, both to confirm the suspected injury and to rule out possible associated skeletal injuries. In general, point tenderness over bony landmarks and crepitus in the involved area are indicative of fractures. Injuries to ligaments may cause point tenderness as well, but the painful area will be away from the nearby bony prominence. Ligamentous sprains are often classified as first-, second-, or third-degree sprains. First-degree injuries are characterized by stretching or microscopic tears to the ligament and exhibit minimal tenderness and swelling. Second-degree sprains have definite point tenderness over the ligament, and some instability of the joint is noted when stressed by the examiner. A partial tear of the ligament has occurred with this degree of injury. Third-degree sprains are severe injuries with marked swelling and tenderness, often of more than one ligament surrounding a joint. The joint is very unstable, and more aggressive immobilization measures and timely orthopedic involvement are necessary for complete treatment.

Hip and Pelvis Injuries

Younger patients tend to sustain ligamentous injuries from the twisting aspect of a "twisting and falling" injury, but older patients are at risk for fractures from the impact of the fall. This is especially true for fractures at the hip. Patients with this injury cannot ambulate or even get up from the site of the fall. For this reason, it is unlikely that the primary care physician will see this injury in the office or clinic. Telephone advice for family members who call to report the patient's condition should center around keeping the patient warm and relatively immobile until EMS workers can move her safely. Classically, the patient with a fracture of the hip will have a shortened and externally rotated appearance to the involved extremity and pain in the hip can easily be elicited by a simple heel strike.

A patient who gives a similar history of a fall yet eventually is able to get up and come to the office for evaluation should arouse suspicion of a pubic ramus fracture of the pelvis. She will be noted to have pain on compression of the pelvis and will exhibit no signs of hip involvement. Radiographs will confirm the diagnosis, and urinalysis should complete the evaluation to ensure that no associated bladder damage has occurred. These patients can be treated with analgesia and allowed to bear weight as tolerated. They can be managed by a primary care physician, who should be concerned with the complications of pain medications, prolonged bed rest, and, most importantly, how the home environment may have contributed to the original fall. Older patients should be given a walker. Area rugs and other potential obstacles should be removed from frequently traveled paths in the house (e.g., bedroom to bathroom). As always with older patients, a search for medical reasons for a fall also should be diligent.

Minor Burns

Of the more than 2 million burns that occur annually in the United States, approximately 95 percent are treated in the outpatient setting. Though most minor burns will heal uneventfully with minimal therapy, it is important for the primary care physician to recognize which burns can be treated in the office, which should be referred to a specialist in burn care, and which require hospitalization.

Classification

There are several ways to classify burn injuries. The most common form of burn injury is thermal injury, and these wounds are classified according to three major criteria: 1. extent of body surface area (BSA) involved, 2. depth of skin involvement, and 3. anatomical location.

The simplest method to estimate the extent of a burn injury is to use the Rule of Nines. This method divides the adult body surface into 11 areas, each equal to 9 percent or multiples thereof (Fig. 65-1) The genitalia are assigned a value of 1 percent. Burn wounds may involve only the epidermis or may tra-

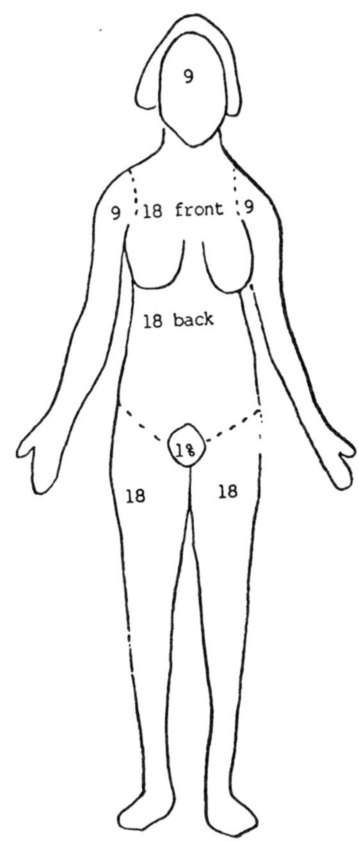

Figure 65-1 Rule of nines.

verse all layers of the skin and involve deeper structures as well. Accordingly, burns are classified as first-, second-, third-, or fourth-degree.

First-degree burns are the mildest and involve the epidermis only. Examples include most sunburns, brief exposures to hot liquids, or minor flash burns.

Second-degree burns are also referred to as partial-thickness burns and are subdivided into superficial and deep partial thickness injuries. They involve the epidermis and varying amounts of the dermis.

Superficial partial-thickness burns involve the upper portion of the dermis or papillary dermis. On examination, these burns are red, moist, and blanch with pressure. Frequently there is blister formation, and the wounds are very painful. Deep partial thickness burns involve the lower portion of the dermis or reticular dermis. On examination, the skin appears mottled or waxy-white. These burns are typically sensitive to pressure, but insensitive to pinprick. They may be very difficult to distinguish from full-thickness injuries.

Third-degree burns are also referred to as full-thickness injuries. They involve destruction of the epidermis, dermis, and a varying amount of the underlying subcutaneous tissues. The epithelial appendages (hair follicles, sweat glands, sebaceous glands) are destroyed, so that epithelial regeneration cannot occur from these sites as with partial-thickness injuries. The burns appear white, black, or cherry-red, and have a dry, leathery texture.

Fourth-degree burns extend deeply beneath the skin surface, involving fascia, muscle, or bone. On the surface they may be difficult to distinguish from third-degree burns.

Accurate assessment of burn depth may not be possible on initial evaluation. Repeated observations over the first 1 to 3 days often are necessary for an accurate assessment.

The American Burn Association divides burn injuries into the following categories: major—those requiring referral to a burn center; moderate—those that can be treated in a community hospital environment; minor—those that are amenable to outpatient treatment. Minor burns include: 1. Partial-thickness burns covering less than 15 percent BSA of an adult or 10 percent BSA of a child; 2. Small full-thickness burns less than 2 percent BSA of an adult.

Excluded from this definition are burns to critical areas (eyes, ears, face, hands, feet, perineum), inhalation injuries, electrical burns, and burns in patients who are at higher risk for complications (infants, elderly, patients with chronic diseases).

Treatment

The treatment of minor burn injuries has three primary objectives: relief of pain; prevention of infection and additional trauma; minimizing scarring and contracture.

Home Management/Phone Advice Patients who sustain minor burn wounds should be instructed to cover the involved area with cool compresses. This not only will provide pain relief but also will minimize edema. Any constricting jewelry, especially rings, must be removed to prevent vascular compromise. Home remedies such as butter, grease, or over-the-counter preparations should not be used; they will make physician evaluation more difficult, if not more painful. In addition, they may promote bacterial growth. Prompt physician evaluation should be encouraged, except for trivial injuries, so that an appropriate treatment plan can be developed and followed.

Office Management The initial evaluation and management of the minor burn injury should accomplish the following objectives: the safe and rapid removal of devitalized tissue through cleansing and debridement; the preservation of epithelial elements buried by the original injury; the provision of an optimal environment for epithelial regeneration; and the prevention of complications. After a complete history and physical exam, the burn wound should be approached in the following manner:

1. The extent and depth of the burn injury should be determined.
2. Tetanus prophylaxis should be provided for all minor burn wounds (Table 65-2). It is important to remember that patients without prior tetanus immunization require both tetanus immune globulin (TIG) and tetanus-diphtheria toxoid (Td) at the time of injury. They will also require Td booster injections at three weeks and three months post-injury to complete the immunization schedule.

TABLE 65-2 Tetanus Prophylaxis

History of Tetanus Immunization	Administer Td[a]	Administer TIG[b]
Unknown or less than 3 doses	Yes	Yes
3 or more doses		
> 5 years since last dose	Yes	No
< 5 years since last dose	No	No

[a]Td dose is 0.5cc IM

[b]TIG dose is 250 units IM

3. The wound should be covered with cool compresses for patient comfort.
4. In preparation for cleansing and debridement, the patient should be given appropriate analgesics.
5. In a sterile manner the burn should be gently cleansed with a wet gauze pad. A mild detergent (e.g., Ivory, Hibiclens) may be utilized. Following cleansing, the wound should be flushed with normal saline.
6. Debridement of remaining devitalized tissue should be performed with a forceps and scissors.
7. Treatment of blisters is controversial. The following is one recommended approach:
   a. debride all ruptured blisters initially;
   b. allow intact blisters to rupture spontaneously, at which point the dead skin should be debrided;
   c. after 5 to 7 days, debride all remaining blisters.

Burn Dressings With the open method, the burn wound is left exposed to air following initial cleansing and debridement. Wounds cared for in this manner should be washed 2 to 3 times daily. A topical antibacterial agent (e.g., bacitracin) usually is applied after each washing. This technique is especially useful for wounds of the face and neck, where the closed method would be cumbersome.

With the closed method, the burn wound is covered with one of several types of dressings. This is the most common method of treatment for minor burn injuries and is conducive to management in the ambulatory care setting. The application of dressings is also generally well accepted by the patient because it provides protection for the injured area and allows her to wear her usual clothing. The following method can be utilized for the application of burn dressings:

1. After cleansing and debridement, the burn wound should be covered with a topical antibacterial agent such as silver sulfadiazine, if indicated. It should be applied with a sterile tongue blade and spread to a thickness of 1/8 to 1/16 in.
2. The wound should then be covered with a nonadherent dressing; this will make subsequent dressing changes easier. If a topical antibacterial agent is used, a dry nonadherent absorbent dressing (e.g., Telfa) is very useful. If a topical antibacterial agent is not used, a petrolatum-based nonadherent dressing (e.g., Xeroform) can be utilized.
3. The wound is then covered with loose sterile gauze. For burns of the hands and feet, each digit should be separately padded to prevent maceration.
4. The entire dressing is then wrapped in a semielastic mesh bandage (such as Kerlix). It should be tight enough to hold the dressing in place but should not constrict the area.
5. Burn wounds treated with topical antimicrobial agents (e.g., silver sulfadiazine) should have their dressings changed twice daily. Care should be taken to wash off all of the topical agent prior to the application of the new dressing. We advise that wounds treated without topical antimicrobial agents have their dressings changed daily, though some physicians feel that these dressings may be left in place for 48 to 72 h. Burn dressings should be continued until signs of epithelialization are evident on exam.

Follow-up Outpatient burn management requires close patient follow-up. Since patients will need to observe their wounds at home as well as perform dressing changes, complete step-by-step instructions and patient education must be provided (Table 65-3). Instructions must describe wound cleansing techniques, wound dressing techniques, and signs and symptoms of wound infection.

The severity of the burn injury determines the frequency of patient follow-up. Most burns should be reevaluated within 24 to 48 h to assure that the pa-

TABLE 65-3 Follow-Up Care of Burn Wounds

1. Remove old dressing. If it adheres to your skin, soak it in room-temperature water and gently remove.
2. Wash the wound gently with a mild soap and water.
3. Pat the wound dry with sterile gauze.
4. Look for signs of infection, including swelling, cloudy or foul-smelling drainage, pain, or increasing redness around the burn injury. If any of these are present, notify your doctor immediately.
5. If antibiotic cream (Silvadene) is prescribed by your doctor, apply it approximately 1/8-in thick with a sterile tongue blade. If your injury does not require this treatment, proceed to Step 6.
6. Apply the nonadherent dressing in a single layer.
   __ Telfa __ Xeroform
7. Cover generously with sterile gauze pads.
8. Wrap with Kerlix just tight enough to hold the dressing in place.

tient is able to comply with outpatient management, to assess for signs of early infection, and to better appreciate the extent and depth of the burn injury. Most minor burn wounds should fully heal in 2 to 3 weeks.

Special Burns

Chemical and electrical burns are common, and patients may seek treatment for these injuries in the primary care setting. The clinician should be aware of the unique nature of these burns so as to provide appropriate initial management and subsequent referral.

Chemical Burns Substances causing injury can be most easily divided into acids and corrosive bases; identifying the nature of the substance is important for the prediction of its potential for serious injury. Regardless of the agent, first aid measures suggested to the patient by telephone or undertaken in the office or clinic should center on copious irrigation with water. A shower or garden hose is a much more effective decontamination device than is typical irrigation with normal saline. It is also of utmost importance to irrigate the injured area early, in the first few minutes following the burn. Telephone advice to chemically burned patients should direct them to accomplish at least 20 minutes of copious irrigation BEFORE going to the emergency department or traveling to the clinic or office for further evaluation.

Once adequate decontamination has been accomplished, the management of minor burns from chemical agents is not significantly different from that for thermal burns. Similar dressings and frequent wound checks are required. Indications for tetanus immunization and antibiotics are the same. However, because these can be devastating injuries and can be deceptive in their extent at first glance, we recommend that they be referred to a burn care specialist early in the course of treatment.

Electrical Burns Burns due to electricity may occur by three basic mechanisms: conduction injury, arcing, and flash burns. Secondary thermal burns also are seen when the victim's clothing is ignited as a result of the electrical exposure.

The most severe injuries result from the conduction of electricity through the body after contact with a high voltage source. Household current is normally considered low voltage, but common appliances and electronic equipment may include capacitors that store sufficient charge to cause extensive tissue damage. These patients are at risk for extensive tissue loss and complications involving virtually every organ system. Because of the risk of cardiac arrhythmias, they should be transported from the primary care setting by ambulance in spite of what may appear to be a trivial injury.

Arcing occurs when two objects of different potential, usually a primary source and a "ground," are brought into proximity and a spark occurs between them. The temperature of this electrical arc is approximately 2500° C, and may therefore cause deep partial-thickness or full-thickness thermal burns at the point where it contacts the skin. There is less propensity for deep tissue destruction with burns due to arcing alone than with conduction-type injuries.

Flash burns occur when current passes over the surface of the skin without any concentrated entrance point. These injuries usually result in only superficial partial-thickness burns. Normally one would consider treating this type of burn in a primary care setting; in practice, it often is impossible to determine the exact mechanism of injury causing a given patient's burn. It is therefore very difficult to predict which injuries are indeed minor and which will go on to produce more severe complications. Even with minimal skin involvement and with a low-voltage source causing the injury, evaluation with ECG and urinary hemoglobin/myoglobin is a minimum requirement before considering the patient a candidate for outpatient management.

Electrical burns provide treatment challenges to even the most seasoned burn care specialists, yet patients sustaining these injuries may first present for treatment in a primary care setting. Any electrical burn must be considered a potentially serious injury and arrangements made for early involvement of qualified specialists.

Prevention

The primary care physician should take advantage of the office or clinic setting to provide a range of preventive medicine services for patients. Simple safety measures can be suggested in patient handouts or waiting room videotapes. Many offices rotate preventive literature by season, with burn-related handouts stressing barbecue safety, sun protection, and avoidance of overheated car radiator caps in summer months and fireplace and space-heater safety in the winter. Also, specific patient groups can be targeted with educational information. New mothers, for instance, should be instructed to adjust the thermostat on home water-heaters to the lowest possible setting in order to avoid scalding injuries to infants. Parents with toddlers should turn stove-top pot handles away from the room, and be sure that hot beverages are well out of the reach of children. Electric cords should be kept out of easy access to toddlers, and unused outlets should be plugged. Patients should be reminded to wear gloves when handling corrosive household chemicals, and all such agents should be kept in a child-proof cabinet. Smoke detectors and fire extinguishers should be strongly advised by medical professionals to all patients. Their importance is obvious and cannot be overemphasized.

One final area of preventive medicine concerning burn injuries involves the recognition and prevention of abuse. Although children and female spouses are most often considered as victims of abuse, there is a growing amount of abuse of the elderly as well. Small, circular burns suggestive of cigarette butts, well-demarcated extremity burns suggestive of immersion scalding, and historical details incompatible with the observed injury are all tip-offs to abuse for all ages. Also suggestive are frequent and variable injuries, delay in seeking medical attention, and known family stress. The astute clinician may help to prevent severe morbidity and possible mortality by recognizing and intervening in these circumstances.

Summary

The majority of burn injuries can be treated in the outpatient setting by primary care physicians. Though most of these injuries will heal uneventfully, appropriate evaluation and management is necessary to minimize patient morbidity. Figure 65-2 outlines one approach to the management of these patients. Patient education efforts directed toward the prevention of all types of traumatic injury, including burns, is of major importance in the delivery of comprehensive medical care.

Smoke Inhalation/Carbon Monoxide Poisoning

Smoke inhalation—more specifically, carbon monoxide (CO) poisoning—is the most common cause of fire-related mortality. In addition, CO poisoning is seen in many other settings that have one thing in common: the improper combustion of carbon-containing materials confined in a closed space. Noteworthy examples include automobile exhaust in a closed garage, malfunctioning home space heaters (e.g., kerosene heaters) and the use of charcoal briquette barbecues or stoves in poorly ventilated areas. Because CO is a colorless, odorless, and nonirritating gas, accidental exposures are common. Patients often will not recognize the presence of the toxin, accounting for the fact that many exposure deaths

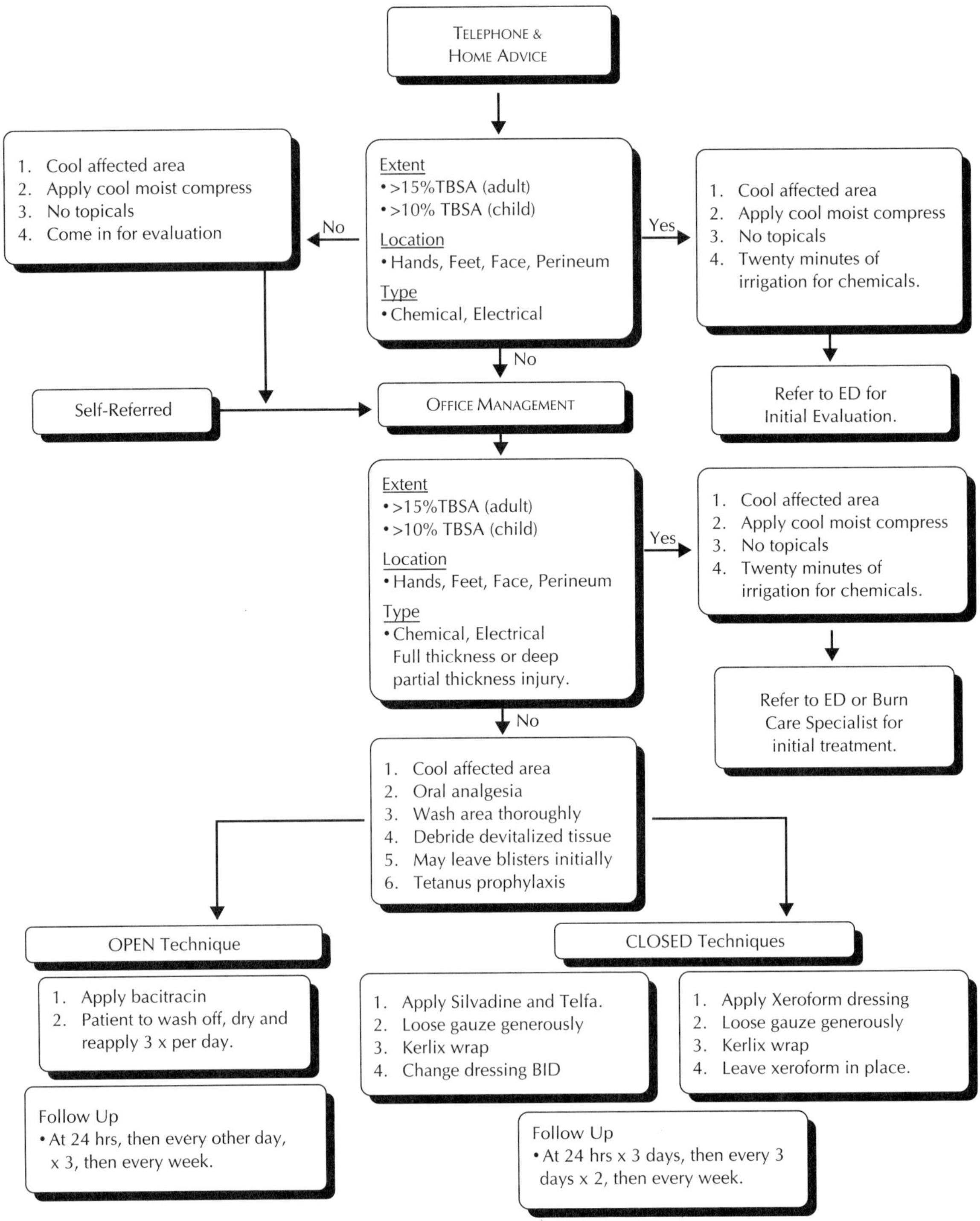

Figure 65-2 Management of minor burns.

occur during sleep. As will be discussed subsequently, the manifestations of CO poisoning are protean and can mimic many other common illnesses. However, owing to the frequency of this exposure, its potential severe morbidity and mortality, and the high likelihood that patients with less severe exposures will present in the outpatient setting, it is important for the primary care practitioner to understand the pathogenesis and management of this syndrome.

Pathophysiology

Carbon monoxide exerts its toxic effects primarily through its combination with hemoglobin, forming carboxyhemoglobin (COHB). The higher the level of COHB in the blood, the lower is the hemoglobin oxygen saturation, resulting in decreased oxygen transport and cellular hypoxia. The severity of the exposure depends on the concentration of inhaled CO, the duration of exposure, and various patient factors. Young children and household pets are more susceptible to severe toxicity because of their higher metabolic rates. Older patients with underlying vascular disease are more at risk because they are very sensitive to hypoxia.

Pregnant patients are also at increased risk because CO freely crosses the placenta and fetal hemoglobin has an even higher affinity for CO than maternal hemoglobin. Several fetal complications have been described following CO exposure, including various neurologic and somatic abnormalities, stillbirth, and spontaneous abortion.

The clinical effects of CO poisoning are related primarily to hypoxia. Organs with the greatest oxygen requirements, chiefly the heart and the brain, are most susceptible to toxicity. Cardiac ischemia and arrhythmias and various neurologic disturbances are common with significant CO exposures.

Patient Evaluation

All patients with smoke inhalation or CO exposure require a thorough evaluation. Patients in high-risk groups should always be referred to the local emergency department for evaluation owing to their higher risk of toxicity. Signs and symptoms of CO poisoning are related to the percentage of COHB in the blood (Table 65-4). However, blood levels do not always reflect maximal COHB levels; therefore, the patient's symptoms are a much better predictor of CO toxicity. Since the early symptoms of CO toxicity are nonspecific, many exposures are misdiagnosed as viral syndromes. Clinicians must have a high index of suspicion for this syndrome, especially in the winter months and when cases occur in clusters (e.g., an entire family awakes in the morning with various nonspecific complaints).

Management

The treatment of CO poisoning includes removal of the patient from the source of exposure and therapy directed at the rapid reduction of the patient's COHB level. The half-life of COHB at room air is approximately 4 to 6 h; on 100 percent oxygen, approximately 90 min; and with hyperbaric oxygen therapy, 15 to 20 min.

Patients with minor symptoms (e.g., mild headache that quickly resolves) require no therapy other than removal from the source of exposure. Patients with more severe symptoms should be placed on 100 percent oxygen and treated in the emergency department. A thorough evaluation including COHB level, arterial blood gas, electrocardiogram, and neurologic evaluation will be required. Depending on the

TABLE 65-4 Signs and Symptoms of Carbon Monoxide Poisoning

Carboxyhemoglobin Level (%)	Signs and Symptoms
0–10	Usually none
10–20	Mild headache
20–30	Throbbing headache, exertional dyspnea
30–40	Severe headache, impaired sensorium
40–50	Lethargy, confusion, syncope, tachycardia, tachypnea
50–60	Seizures, coma
> 60	Cardiorespiratory failure

patient's symptoms, COHB level, age, and pregnancy status, the need for hyperbaric oxygen therapy will be determined.

Prevention

Although CO poisoning in association with smoke inhalation is not always preventable, accidental exposures in the home can be minimized. Patients should be instructed regarding the proper use of space heaters that use fossil fuels. In addition, cooking with similar fuels or charcoal should be done only outside or in well-ventilated areas. And, most important, automobiles should never be allowed to run in a closed garage.

Drug Overdose/Toxic Ingestions

Drug overdose or poisoning by ingestion represent a leading cause of morbidity and mortality in the United States. For individuals under 45, it is second only to motor vehicle injuries as a cause of death secondary to accidents.[6] The epidemiology of toxic ingestion falls into two general categories: ingestions by children, which usually are accidental and typically have a good outcome; ingestions by middle-aged and older adults, where the ingestion usually is intentional and more likely to result in an adverse outcome. With the development of regional poison control centers beginning in the 1950s, poison information and advice are readily available to practitioners and the public. In addition, many public information campaigns have resulted in the introduction of child-proof containers and improved product labeling that have reduced accidental ingestions. Recent data, however, show that drug overdoses, both accidental and intentional, continue to be common and serious problems in all age groups.

Pathogenesis

Drug ingestions cause a multitude of clinical syndromes depending on the class and amount of drug ingested. The most frequently involved substances include analgesics, cleaning substances, cosmetics, plants, and cough and cold preparations. In contrast, the categories of drugs with the largest numbers of deaths include antidepressants, analgesics, stimulants and street drugs, sedative/hypnotics, and cardiovascular drugs.[11] Several poisoning syndromes or "toxidromes" are well described, and assist the clinician in determining the class or category of agent ingested. Many ingestions are nontoxic and require no specific therapy.

Patient Evaluation

Except for accidental nontoxic ingestions, all drug overdose patients require a thorough clinical evaluation. In addition, all intentional overdoses, regardless of clinical severity, require a complete psychiatric evaluation. Therefore, the vast majority of drug overdoses in adults require evaluation in an emergency department. In addition, it must be emphasized that many drugs have delayed clinical manifestations (e.g., acetaminophen, methanol) so that the absence of symptoms shortly after ingestion does not rule out a serious or life-threatening ingestion.

This is especially true for intentional overdoses in depressed middle-aged adults, who are less likely to give an accurate history regarding the agent ingested or the circumstances of the ingestion. Subtle nonspecific clinical signs and symptoms, including minor vital sign abnormalities, change in sensorium, pupillary abnormalities, or change in the temperature or moistness of the skin and mucous membranes may herald the early manifestations of a serious drug ingestion.

Management

Adult patients who have intentionally or accidentally ingested a potentially toxic substance must be brought to the nearest hospital emergency department. After serious or life-threatening ingestions, they should be taken to the hospital via ambulance. Many communities are served by advanced emergency medical service systems whose emergency medical technicians can deliver not only supportive care en route to the hospital but also specific therapeutic interventions including oxygen and airway maintenance, intravenous access, and the administration of specific medications including glucose and Narcan. In certain types of ingestions or exposures, specific therapy should be instituted prior to transport to the hospital. Included in this category are toxic exposures to the eyes or skin. Copious irrigation with tap water should be instituted immediately while awaiting ambulance transport. The routine use of syrup of ipecac to induce vomiting or the use of neutralizing substances (e.g., milk) is not recommended without professional advice. For potentially serious ingestions and in circumstances where transport to the nearest hospital is prolonged, patients should be instructed to contact their regional poison control center. If syrup of ipecac is recommended, the usual adult dose is 30 ml, followed by 16 to 32 oz of water. Ipecac can be purchased in most pharmacies and does not require a prescription.

Prevention

Most poison prevention activities have been directed at accidental poisonings in children. The prevention of intentional ingestions in adults is much more difficult. However, the primary care physician has an important role in poison prevention. This involves patient education efforts, drug prescribing practices, and identification of patients at risk.[2] Patients must be made aware of drug side effects and toxic symptoms.

As discussed in Chap. 39, it is important for the primary care physician to be alert for signs of depression and either treat or refer patients when appropriate. In addition, the physician should be prudent in prescribing practices for depressed patients. This is especially important when giving a patient a prescription for a lethal amount of a potentially toxic medication.

Animal and Human Bites

Dog bites account for the vast majority of bite injuries occurring in the United States, followed by cat bites and, less commonly, human and rodent bites. Most involve the extremities, though in children, because of their small size, facial injuries are not uncommon. The approach to most bite injuries is similar. However, certain types will require more intensive evaluation. For example, human bites—most importantly bites to the hand—often result in deep infections that require hospitalization. The risk of rabies transmission, especially from certain groups of wild animals, also must be determined, as will be discussed later in this section.

Pathogenesis

Unlike lacerations, bites tend to produce deeper injuries; as such, they are classified as either puncture wounds or crush injuries. The oral cavity of animals and humans also harbors a multitude of organisms, frequently resulting in polymicrobial infections. Certain organisms are more common in one species than another. For example, *Pasteurella multocida* is very common in cat bites and less common in dog bites. Human bites are usually polymicrobial, including *Staphylococcus aureus, Eikenella corrodens,* Streptococcus species, and several anaerobic organisms.

In addition to infection, more serious bite injuries can result in fractures, tendon damage, lymphangiitis, and osteomyelitis. Patient factors including older age, diabetes mellitus, and immunosuppression will also result in a greater likelihood of complications.

Patient Evaluation

All patients sustaining bite injuries require a thorough history. The age of the bite must be determined, as this will influence subsequent management. It is also important to identify the source of the bite. For dogs and cats, a history of current rabies vaccination must be determined. For other animals, the risk of rabies transmission must be assessed (Table 65-5). Consultation with local public health officials will assist the practitioner in determining the need for rabies vaccination.

The physical exam must be directed at determining the extent and depth of the bite injury. Particular attention must be paid to the detection of associated

TABLE 65-5 Risk of Rabies Transmission

High	Low
Skunks	Squirrels
Raccoons	Rats
Bats	Mice
Foxes	Rabbits
Woodchucks	Chipmunks
	Livestock

injuries, including fractures, tendon lacerations, and the involvement of joints, especially of the hand. These complicated injuries most likely will require referral to a specialist.

Management

Because of the high incidence of infection, all bite wounds require meticulous management. This includes copious irrigation and the removal of devitalized tissue. The decision to close a bite wound is determined by its age, location, and source. Superficial wounds to the face and extremities other than the hand that are evaluated within 8 to 12 h usually can be closed primarily and re-evaluated in 24 to 48 h. For facial wounds with potential cosmetic deformities, primary closure may be attempted up to 24 h after the injury, provided that close follow-up can be obtained. Deep puncture wounds and wounds to the hand should be left open because of the high incidence of infection and the inability to cleanse deeper wounds thoroughly. This is especially true for human bite wounds to the hand, where infection rates are very high. Many of these patients will require inpatient hospitalization for intravenous antibiotics, immobilization, elevation, and local wound care. All patients should receive tetanus prophylaxis if indicated (see Table 65-2), and all animal bites should be evaluated regarding the need for antirabies prophylaxis.

The use of prophylactic antibiotics is somewhat controversial, though in most circumstances they are given. The choice of antimicrobial agent(s) is determined by the source of the bite and the most likely pathogenic organism (Table 65-6). All patients treated in the outpatient setting should be reevaluated in 24 to 48 h.

TABLE 65-6 Antimicrobial Prophylaxis of Bite Wounds

Source	Likely Organisms	Antibiotic Choice
Cat	*Pasteurella multocida* *S. aureus*	Amoxicillin clavulanate Penicillin V or doxycycline
Dog	Viridans strep *Pasteurella multocida* Anaerobes	Penicillin V or ampicillin or doxycycline
Human	Viridans strep Staphylococci Corynebacterium Eikenella Anaerobes	Amoxicillin clavulanate or erythromycin

Prevention

Most preventive efforts directed at bite wounds involve control of rabies in domestic animals through vaccination programs. The control of rabies in wild animal populations usually is not possible. However, animals known to be common reservoirs of the rabies virus should be avoided and never kept as pets. In addition, houses and surrounding structures should be made "bat proof." If bats are found, they should be removed from the area.

Insect Bites

Insect bites are a common presenting complaint in the primary care physician's office. Most of these bites are mild and self-limited and require little treatment other than symptomatic medications and local wound care. Hymenoptera stings, in contrast, occasionally can cause serious systemic reactions, including anaphylaxis, and are the most common cause of fatalities in the U.S. secondary to venomous bites. Therefore, it is extremely important to differentiate local and systemic reactions to insect bites and to identify patients at risk for more serious or fatal systemic reactions in the future. Such patients require referral to a specialist for skin testing and possible immunotherapy and should be instructed in the use of other preventive measures, including the use of self-administered medications, e.g., EpiPen.

The evaluation and treatment of local and systemic reactions to Hymenoptera stings will be reviewed in this section, with special emphasis on the identification of patients at increased risk for the development of life-threatening systemic reactions.

Pathogenesis

The order Hymenoptera consists of three families of insects. Included are honeybees, hornets, yellow jackets, and wasps, found throughout the United States, and fire ants, which are primarily in the southeast. Reactions to a sting are secondary to various proteins in the venom. The severity of a reaction ranges from no signs or symptoms to life-threatening systemic reactions and anaphylaxis.

The immunologic reaction to the venom appears to occur in two stages. In the first stage, the patient is sensitized through the production of antibodies of the IgE class. This occurs with the first exposure to the venom, i.e., bite. On re-exposure, the second stage of the immunologic reaction may occur. In this stage, the preformed IgE antibodies are activated; through their interactions with basophils and mast cells, numerous mediators are released, including histamine and leukotrienes. Depending on host factors and the amount of venom absorbed, patients may develop only a local reaction (swelling and erythema) or full-blown anaphylaxis with pulmonary, cardiovascular, and gastrointestinal involvement.

Patient Evaluation

Hymenoptera stings may cause both local and systemic reactions.

Local Reactions Mild local reactions usually include a small area of redness, swelling, and pain. These symptoms are short-lived and resolve within 24 h. Severe local reactions involve a much larger area and more pronounced symptoms. Occasionally these patients also may complain of nausea and malaise, but there is no evidence of systemic involvement such as generalized urticaria or pruritus.

Systemic Reactions Systemic reactions also may be mild or severe. They usually occur within minutes of the sting. In their mildest form, the patient develops a generalized urticarial or erythematous rash that usually is pruritic. They may also develop gastrointestinal symptoms, including nausea, abdominal cramping, and diarrhea. Severe systemic reactions or anaphylaxis result in life-threatening pulmonary, cardiovascular, and other end-organ dysfunction (Table 65-7).

Patients also occasionally develop delayed reactions to Hymenoptera stings. These reactions occur from several hours to several days after the bite. Patients typically present with a serum sickness-like reaction, including urticaria or erythema, arthralgias, and joint effusions.

Management

Local Wound Care Patients with a recent sting should have the area of the bite inspected for any remnants of the stinger, which may contain unabsorbed venom. The stinger should be removed with a mild and repetitive scraping motion, best accomplished with a scalpel blade held parallel to the skin. With this method, the stinger can be lifted away from the skin without squeezing the venom sac. The stinger should never be grasped and squeezed with tweezers or a forceps as this could result in increased venom release. Following removal of the stinger, the area should be cleansed with a mild soap or antiseptic.

Local Reactions Local reactions that are mild require little therapy other than wound care. Ice may be applied to the area; if significant pruritus is present, an oral antihistamine, e.g., diphenhydramine or hydroxyzine, can be prescribed. Severe local reac-

TABLE 65-7 Anaphylaxis

End-Organ	Signs and Symptoms
Skin	Generalized urticaria, erythema, pruritus, swelling
Pulmonary	
Upper airway	Edema of tongue, larynx, upper airway with stridor, difficulty breathing
Lower airway	Bronchospasm, coughing, dyspnea
Cardiovascular	Hypotension, arrhythmias, chest pain, shock
Gastrointestinal	Nausea, vomiting, abdominal cramping, diarrhea
Central Nervous System	Confusion, altered mental status, occasionally seizures

tions with erythema and swelling greater than 5 cm may benefit from more aggressive therapy. Though still somewhat controversial, recent studies suggest a potential additional benefit with the use of an H2 blocker (e.g., cimetidine, 300 mg qid). With severe swelling and erythema, an oral steroid may be prescribed. A recommended regimen is prednisone, 1 mg/kg per day (maximum 60 mg/day) for five days.

Systemic Reactions Patients with moderate to severe systemic reactions should be brought to the emergency department. Initial management would include epinephrine, intravenous antihistamines, steroids, and aggressive fluid therapy. Patients with a very mild systemic reaction may be treated in the office. Most of these patients will respond to an initial 50 mg IM dose of diphenhydramine. If the patient is symptom-free after one hour, she can be sent home on an oral antihistamine for 1 to 3 days.

The patient with a more severe systemic reaction may be given subcutaneous epinephrine 0.3 to 0.5 ml (1:1000 solution) in addition to an antihistamine. This treatment should be used cautiously, if at all, in older patients or in those with underlying heart disease. If the patient responds to this initial dose and is symptom-free after one hour, she too can be discharged on an oral antihistamine. All patients discharged from the office after treatment for a systemic reaction should be given appropriate instructions to go to the nearest emergency department if their symptoms recur or worsen. In addition, they should be referred to an allergist for a more thorough evaluation.

Prevention

It is hard to predict which patients will develop severe systemic reactions or anaphylaxis to subsequent Hymenoptera stings. However, patients who have any type of systemic reaction are at greatest risk. Therefore, as previously mentioned, all patients who develop systemic reactions should be referred to an allergist for skin testing and possible immunotherapy (desensitization). In addition, an insect sting kit, e.g., EpiPen, should be prescribed and instructions given for its use. These patients should also avoid activities that place them at risk for subsequent stings.

Cardiopulmonary Arrest

Guidelines for Cardiopulmonary Resuscitation and Emergency Cardiac Care were most recently updated by the American Heart Association in 1992.[7] Included are recommendations for both basic and advanced cardiac life support.

For the practicing physician, the degree of familiarity with these guidelines will depend on the type and extent of one's practice. At the minimum, practicing physicians should be familiar with the technique of CPR and preferably be certified in Basic Life Support (BLS) by the American Heart Association or the American Red Cross. Communities with a high level of citizen CPR education have improved survival rates for cardiopulmonary arrest when linked with an appropriate Emergency Medical Service system. Physicians, as health care providers, should know the basics of CPR not only for the "health" of their communities but also as a resource for their high-risk patients.

Universal Algorithm for Adults (Table 65-8)

Table 65-8 summarizes the Universal Algorithm for Adults. An important point to be stressed is No. 2, Activation of the Local Emergency Medical Service (EMS) System. For patients in arrest, CPR has a very brief period of effectiveness. If advanced life support (ALS) is not available in 6 to 8 minutes, the chance of survival is near zero. Therefore, the institution of CPR without ready availability of ALS

TABLE 65-8 Summary of the Universal Algorithm for Adults

1. Assess responsiveness
2. If unresponsive, activate EMS
3. Call for a defibrillator, if available
4. Assess breathing
5. Open airway and give two slow breaths
6. Check for a pulse
7. If no pulse, begin CPR
8. Defibrillate if ventricular fibrillation or ventricular tachycardia is present

may not affect survival, although it certainly should be attempted if there is no alternative.

If a defibrillator is available, and the patient is in ventricular tachycardia or ventricular fibrillation, she should be defibrillated as soon as possible. This group of patients has the highest potential for survival following cardiac arrest, provided defibrillation is rapidly available. The initial defibrillator setting should be 200 joules. If she does not respond, the next defibrillation should be at 300 joules and, if unsuccessful, 360 joules. These three defibrillations should be given in rapid sequence. If the patient still does not respond, more aggressive intervention is required, including intubation and the administration of medications, including epinephrine, 1 mg, and lidocaine, 100 mg IV push.

For other types of cardiac arrest, e.g., asystole and pulseless electrical activity (formerly known as electrical-mechanical dissociation), the likelihood of success even with readily available ALS is much less than with ventricular fibrillation.

Recommendations for Primary Care Physicians

As previously stated, all practicing physicians should be certified in basic life support, especially those who treat high-risk patients. In addition, if a physician performs high-risk procedures in the office, including anesthesia or intravenous drug administration, adequate preparations for the possibility of cardiopulmonary arrest must be made. At the minimum, oxygen, intravenous access supplies, a defibrillator and basic cardiac arrest medications, e.g., epinephrine, lidocaine, and atropine, should be available. In addition, certification in advanced cardiac life support (ACLS) is desirable. Finally, the primary care physician must be fully familiar with the local EMS system and how to access it. Should an emergency occur in the office, the ready availability of ALS and transport to the hospital are the only means to maximize patient survival.

Prevention

Primary care physicians must ensure that their high-risk patients and their families are familiar with CPR. This often entails having family members certified in BLS or CPR. These courses are readily available in most communities and usually are sponsored by local hospitals or the American Red Cross. These families must also know how to access the local EMS system to ensure rapid availability of ALS.

Finally, patients must be instructed on how to respond appropriately to high-risk symptoms. If a patient develops chest pain or shortness of breath, she should be told to call 911 or her local EMS number and not go to the hospital via private transportation. Patients often do not appreciate the risk they are taking. As previously stated, ventricular fibrillation arrest may have a good outcome with ready availability of ALS. Primary care physicians also must not be reluctant to send a patient from the office to the hospital via ambulance who complains of chest pain or other high-risk symptoms. Even if she is stable, her course is unpredictable, and appropriate monitoring en route to the hospital is mandatory.

References and Selected Readings

1. Committee on Trauma: *Advanced Trauma Life Support, Instructor Manual.* Chicago: American College of Surgeons, 1993.
2. Braen R (ed): *Minor Burns, Evaluation and Treatment.* American College of Emergency Physicians. Place Marion Laboratories, 1979.
3. Centers for Disease Control: Compendium of animal rabies control, 1993. *MMWR* 42 (no. RR-3), 1993.
4. Crnkovich D, Carlson R. Anaphylaxis: an organized approach to management and prevention. *J Crit Illnes* 8:332–346, 1993.
5. Degowin EL, Degowin RL: *Beside Diagnostic Examination,* 4th ed. New York: Macmillan, 1981.
6. Eilers M, Garrison T: Toxicologic problems—general management principles, in Rosen P, Barkin R, et al: *Emergency Medicine—Concepts and Clinical Practice,* 3d ed. St Louis: Mosby-Year Book, 1992, pp 2470–2503.
7. Emergency Cardiac Care Committee and Subcommittees: Guidelines for cardiopulmonary resuscitation and emergency cardiac care. *JAMA* 268:2171–2302, 1992.
8. Goldfrank L, Flomenbaum N, Lewin N, et al: *Goldfrank's Toxicologic Emergencies,* 4th ed. Norwalk: Appleton & Lange, 1990.
9. Hoppensfeld S: *Physical Examination of the Spine and Extremities.* Norwalk: Appleton & Lange, 1976.

10. Kwiatkowski T, Rennie W: The outpatient management of minor burns. *Primary Care Update for OB/GYNS.* 1(4):173–181, 1994.
11. Litovitz TL, Schitz BF, Holm KC: 1988 annual report of the American Association of Poison Control Centers National Data Collection System. *J Emerg Med* 7(5):495–545, 1989.
12. Roberts J, Hedges J: *Clinical Procedures in Emergency Medicine,* 2d ed. Philadelphia: WB Saunders, 1991.
13. Rockwood CA, Green EP: *Fractures in Adults,* 2d ed. Philadelphia: JB Lippincott, 1984.
14. Rosen P, Barkin R, et al: *Emergency Medicine—Concepts and Clinical Practice.* 3d ed. St Louis: Mosby-Year Book, 1992.
15. Simon R, Koenigsknecht S: *Emergency Orthopedics: The Extremities,* 2d ed. Norwalk: Appleton & Lange, 1987.
16. Sinkinson C, French R, Graft D, McLean D: Individualizing therapy for Hymenoptera stings. *Emerg Med Rep* 11(14):134–142, 1990.

Part VII

Other Important Issues

66 Adverse Drug Reactions, Drug Interactions, and Cost-Effective Utilization of Drugs

Anne Y.F. Lin
Bruce G. Kay

Adverse Drug Reactions

Adverse drug reactions or side effects can occur despite the most careful use of drugs. Although some authors differentiate between the terms "adverse drug reactions" and "side effects," they will be used synonymously in this chapter. Many side effects are unavoidable, since they are an extension of the drug's pharmacologic effects and inseparable from its therapeutic actions. Such side effects are predictable on the basis of the drug's pharmacologic activity. Common examples of such reactions include chlorpropamide-induced hypoglycemia, captopril-induced hypotension, and diphenhydramine-induced urinary retention. There are, however, side effects which occur that are unpredictable since they are unrelated to the drug's pharmacologic activity. These effects can be subcategorized into allergic and idiosyncratic reactions.

Drug allergies account for approximately 20 percent of all adverse drug reactions. Although they are uncommon relative to predictable side effects, they are important since they may increase patient morbidity and mortality. Allergic reactions cannot be predicted, are not related to a drug's pharmacologic activity, and generally are not dose-related. For example, based on the ability of penicillin to inhibit bacterial cell wall synthesis, one cannot predict that anaphylaxis would occur. All clinicians recognize a rash as a potential allergic reaction to a drug. However, one should keep in mind that allergic reactions can affect many organ systems. Heparin-induced thrombocytopenia, nafcillin-induced interstitial nephritis, and phenytoin-induced hepatitis are all examples of allergic reactions. Allergic reactions (synonymous with hypersensitivity) are immune mediated; as such, an induction period is required for the production of antibodies or T cells that will recognize the specific drug. Therefore, reexposure or prolonged exposure is necessary for the development of allergic symptoms. Both humoral and cell-mediated immunity play a role in allergic reactions;

while humoral immunity does not carry life-long memory, cell-mediated immunity does. Therefore, a patient who reports having developed a rash 5 days into treatment with penicillin 20 years ago, may not develop a rash upon retreatment today. In contrast, reexposure to poison ivy after many years of exposure will still result in the development of contact dermatitis.

Upon obtaining patient medication histories, one question that always arises is whether patients with drug allergies will react to drugs that are within the same or similar pharmacologic class. Unfortunately, cross-reactivity among drugs is not always predictable, since for most drug allergies, we do not know what part of the chemical structure is responsible for the allergic reaction. This concept is best represented by patients with a sulfa allergy. The sulfur atom present in sulfa compounds is not the cause of the allergic reaction; if this were the case, such patients would have multiple allergies. It has been postulated that the para-amino group might be involved in this reaction. However, many compounds contain such a chemical group, and would present the potential for cross-reactivity with a large number of drugs. The small number of reported cases of cross-sensitivity among sulfonamides suggests that a unique metabolite or specific radical is the culprit. With the later mechanism, cross-sensitivity would be limited to only a few drugs that are very similar in structure. This may explain why some patients are allergic to hydrochlorothiazide but can tolerate furosemide. On the other hand, the first mechanism may explain why some patients with sulfonamide allergies are allergic to all PABA compounds (e.g., sunscreens). Overall, although cross-sensitivity among sulfonamides does occur, it is impossible to predict its frequency. History of a sulfonamide allergy is not an absolute contraindication to the use of potentially cross-reacting drugs. The clinical manifestation of the allergic reaction would determine whether a potential cross-reacting agent should be used. The use of other sulfonamide drugs would be contraindicated in patients with a prior history of Stevens-Johnson syndrome or any adverse effect associated with high morbidity and mortality. If a patient reports having had a rash after using a sulfonamide antibiotic, it would be prudent to use an alternative antibiotic. However, the use of thiazide diuretics or sulfonylureas may not be contraindicated.

Unfortunately, there are few confirmatory tests for drug allergy. Obtaining complete and accurate drug histories is critical to the diagnosis of drug-induced allergic reactions, or of any adverse effect. Whether cross-reacting drugs can be used or not will depend on the type of allergic reaction elicited. For example, patients who develop a maculopapular rash after several days of treatment with penicillin can complete the course of therapy. Symptomatic management of the rash may be all that is necessary. Therefore, in such patients, a penicillin may be used again if medically necessary. However, for a patient with a history of a reaction that is associated with a high mortality rate, such as anaphylaxis, penicillin would be contraindicated.

Idiosyncratic reactions typically do not involve the immune system. An anaphylactoid reaction is an example of such an adverse effect. Although the clinical presentation of an anaphylactoid reaction is the same as that of anaphylaxis, it is different in that it does not involve the immune system. Drugs (e.g., skeletal relaxants, contrast media, opiates) that cause anaphylactoid reactions have the ability to cause the release of histamine directly, without antibodies. Therefore, an induction period is not needed and patients can develop this reaction on first exposure. Additionally, patients can be pretreated with antihistamines and/or corticosteroids to prevent or minimize the reaction.

Often physicians need to determine whether a drug can cause a specific side effect. Upon reviewing the package insert or the *Physician's Desk Reference,* the side effect may not be listed. However, based on clinical judgment, it would appear that the drug, in fact, caused the problem. It is important to realize that, for several reasons, Phase II and III clinical trials cannot determine the complete safety profile of any drug. First, the number of patients enrolled in such trials is relatively small in comparison with the number of patients who will use the drug after marketing. Therefore, rare side effects may not be detected in these initial trials. Second, these trials are mostly short-term; side effects that occur only after long-term use will not be detected. Finally, for the most part, study patients are relatively healthy, except for the disease being treated. Thus, the influence of other disease states and organ dysfunction on the drug's safety profile is unknown at the time of initial marketing.

In order to determine if a patient is experiencing any adverse effect, five factors need to be taken into consideration: time sequence; serum drug concentration; known response pattern; dechallenge; and rechallenge. The first two factors are self-explanatory. The known response pattern is the typical clinical presentation of the adverse effect in question. This information can be obtained from case reports in the literature and from the manufacturer. The amount of information given will vary for each company. A manufacturer may have reports on file that have not been published. A drug information center, present in hospitals or colleges of pharmacy, can be contacted to determine what information is available in the literature. A comparison of the individual patient with this information will help the physician to determine causality. A positive dechallenge refers to resolution of the effect after the drug is discontinued, and a positive rechallenge refers to the reappearance of symptoms after the drug is restarted. In making this determination, one must keep in mind that patients may be taking more than one drug that could be associated with the side effect. One may not always be able to determine for certain which of those drugs caused the problem; in other cases, the known response pattern will identify the responsible drug.

Using drugs only when they are medically necessary is the key factor in minimizing the development of adverse drug reactions. When drugs are used, obtaining complete and accurate medication histories is critical to avoiding the development of or effectively managing a drug-induced adverse effect. The following pieces of data should be obtained: 1. names of all drugs (prescription and over-the-counter) and any "natural" remedies that the patient is taking; 2. dosage regimen and duration of treatment; 3. symptoms of adverse effects, including time of onset; 4. how the adverse effect was managed (if it occurred in the past); 5. history of previous drug reactions—with all the above information, if possible. Patients who have drug allergies should be treated with drugs that would not cross-react. However, the patient should be interviewed to determine if she did in fact have allergic symptoms. This would prevent the use of a less effective agent with a less desirable safety profile when it is not necessary.

Drug Interactions

The documentation of a drug interaction does not necessarily contraindicate the use of the two interacting agents. To avoid adverse reactions that are due to drug interactions, the clinician needs to be aware of the mechanism of the drug interaction, the time course of the interaction, and how the effects of the interaction can be monitored and minimized.

As with adverse effects, drug interactions can be divided into two types, pharmacodynamic and pharmacokinetic. Pharmacodynamic interactions occur when the administration of a second drug alters the patient's clinical response to the first drug. For example, the administration of a diuretic increases the potential for hypotension in a patient who is also taking captopril. Pharmacodynamic interactions have been studied to a much lesser extent than pharmacokinetic interactions because in many cases it is difficult to quantify a patient's response to a drug. Additionally, it is difficult to assess the clinical significance of such interactions in clinical studies.

More commonly, pharmacokinetic drug interactions are studied prior to drug marketing. These interactions will affect the absorption, distribution, metabolism, and elimination of a given drug. The resulting effects may or may not be clinically important. Usually, if a drug alters the rate of absorption of a medication given chronically, the interaction is clinically insignificant because the therapeutic serum concentration of the affected drug will not be altered. For example, concomitant administration of theophylline and magnesium-aluminum hydroxide antacids decreases the rate but not the extent of theophylline absorption. Clinically, this has no impact on patient management. In contrast, one would not want to delay the rate of absorption of morphine needed for immediate pain relief. Interactions that occur as a result of one drug's ability to decrease the percentage of absorption of another drug may be clinically significant. Coadministration of digoxin and cholestyramine results in decreased serum digoxin concentration. This interaction may be clinically significant because, in essence, this decreases the digoxin dose. However, these two drugs may still be used concomitantly if one separates their administration by at least 1.5 to 2.0 h. Drug bioavailability also can be affected by changes in enterohepatic circulation, as in the interaction between penicillin and oral contraceptives. Disruption of the gastrointestinal flora by penicillin decreases or eliminates the hydrolysis of estrogen conjugates; this impairs the enterohepatic circulation of the pharmacologically active drug. The clinical significance of this interaction has not been determined, although there have been reports of unintended pregnancies.

Most acidic drugs are reversibly bound, to a varying extent, to protein, primarily albumin. It is the free (unbound) drug that exerts the pharmacologic effects. Therefore, if a drug can be displaced from protein binding, there would not only be more free drug to exert its pharmacologic effect, but also more drug available for metabolism. However, the effects of drug displacement on drug metabolism are complex, and variable and depend on a number of factors.

Overall, changes in protein binding should result in a change in pharmacologic response. Generally, an interaction that occurs via this mechanism has potential clinical significance only for drugs that are highly protein-bound (>90 percent), such as warfarin. If a drug is bound to a lesser degree, any change in the percentage of free drug is not as great a relative change, and would not be clinically significant. For example, if a drug is 50 percent protein-bound, drug displacement of 5 percent results in only a 10 percent change of free drug. In contrast, if a drug is 95 percent protein-bound, an increase of 5 percent is a twofold increase in the amount of free drug.

Drugs also can alter the renal and hepatic elimination of other drugs. The offending drug must alter the major route of elimination of the affected drug in order for the interaction to be of potential clinical significance. In terms of metabolism, drugs may be either enzyme-inducers or enzyme-inhibitors. Generally, the effects of enzyme induction are slow and are dose-related. The clinical effect of this interaction is a decrease in efficacy of the affected drug. It may take up to 3 weeks before the maximal effects of the drug interaction are noted; corresponding to that, it would take some time for the effects of the drug interaction to dissipate. For example, the effects of enzyme induction by rifampin usually are seen within 2 to 4 days, with maximal effects occurring after approximately 6 to 10 days. Resolution of these effects occurs over two to three weeks. Therefore, a patient who is taking rifampin and oral contraceptives should continue to use additional contraceptive methods for several weeks after the discontinuation of rifampin. At the extreme, the effects of enzyme induction by phenobarbital occur gradually, with maximal effects being observed in two to three weeks. Phenobarbital's effects may take one month or more to dissipate. The onset and dissipation of the effects of other enzyme-inducers probably lie somewhere between rifampin and phenobarbital. Other examples of enzyme-inducers that cause clinically significant drug interactions include other barbiturates, carbamazepine, primidone, and phenytoin.

In contrast, enzyme inhibition, which is one of the most common mechanisms responsible for drug interactions, occurs as soon as the enzyme inhibitor reaches a critical serum concentration. Generally, the effects of enzyme inhibition can be seen, and dissipate, within 24 h of drug administration and discontinuation, respectively. The primary effect of this drug interaction results in increased serum drug concentrations and pharmacologic response. The most recent example of these interactions is the use of terfenadine and erythromycin. Erythromycin inhibits the metabolism of terfenadine and its carboxylic metabolite, resulting in cardiac arrhythmias. Concomitant administration of these two drugs obviously should be avoided.

As indicated, drugs also can affect the renal elimination of other drugs by altering the glomerular filtration, tubular secretion, or tubular reabsorption of a drug. The result of such an interaction can be used therapeutically. For example, probenecid competes for tubular secretion of penicillin and increases its therapeutic effect. On the other hand, probenecid can increase serum methotrexate concentration by two- to threefold, resulting in serious methotrexate toxicity.

In practice, one may not always be able to avoid the use of interacting drugs. However, several principles may be taken into consideration in order to minimize the potential for the development of subtherapeutic or toxic effects. First, the most critical time for monitoring the effects of any drug interaction is when the drug that causes the change is started or stopped. If the patient is already taking the drug that causes the change, the effects of an interaction may not be noticeable, because the physician will be titrating the dose of the affected drug according to patient response. The time of onset of the effects, as well as the time to maximal effects, of the interaction must be taken into account, since this can influence when and if steps need to be taken to manage the interaction. For example, nonsteroidal anti-inflammatory agents can decrease the response of antihypertensive agents over a period of one to two weeks. Therefore, the short-term use of ibuprofen or naproxen for dysmenorrhea or headache does not require any change in the patient's antihypertensive therapy.

Additionally, the time of onset also determines when laboratory monitoring is needed. For example, erythromycin increases serum theophylline concentrations generally over 3 to 5 days, and in many patients beyond 5 days. Therefore, it would not be cost-effective to draw a theophylline level on the same day or the day after erythromycin is started. If this information is not available for a given set of drugs, the physician may be able to predict the time course by the drugs' half-lives.

Third, the drug interactions most likely to result in an adverse effect are those that affect drugs with a narrow therapeutic range. In the case of drugs for which there is a correlation between serum drug concentrations and pharmacologic response, the patient who is at the extremes of the therapeutic range has a greater potential to be affected by the drug interaction.

Fourth, since some drug interactions are dose-related, unless an adequate dose is used the interaction may not occur. On the other hand, a large dose of a drug may result in a faster onset of the interaction. Fifth, a number of factors can affect a patient's response to the effects of the drug interaction. Factors such as age, genetics, and social habits (drinking, smoking) can increase the risk of drug interaction and can influence the extent of the effect.

Cost-Effective Utilization of Drugs

Physicians must consider drug costs in the management of patients. Several factors must be taken into account aside from the cost of the drug itself. When many "me too" drugs exist in a given pharmacologic category, such as the beta-blockers, it is important to determine if slight differences among the drugs are clinically significant in relation to patient management. If not, then the higher cost of the "new" and "better" drug will not be worth the additional investment. Second, if two drugs are equally effective, but one has a more risky side effect profile or requires additional laboratory monitoring, the additional cost of a drug without the latter two characteristics may be offset by the savings incurred from less laboratory monitoring and decreased potential for adverse drug reactions. Third, a dosage regimen that lends itself to improved patient compliance (once a day versus four times a day, or shorter treatment duration), potentially can decrease cost. Noncompliance can increase the risk for treatment failure, thereby increasing the cost of treatment. For example, 3-day antibiotic regimens are as effective as 7-day regimens in the management of uncomplicated cystitis in women, and are associated with fewer side effects and lower costs. In many cases, once the patient becomes asymptomatic there is an increased potential for the patient not to finish the course of therapy. Last, the availability of generic drugs should be taken into consideration. Manufacturers of generic drugs that have provided data to the FDA to be considered "therapeutically equivalent" are also bioequivalent to the proprietary product. Use of generic drugs can decrease the overall cost of therapy. A list of therapeutically equivalent agents can be found in the FDA's "Approved Drug Products with Therapeutic Equivalence Evaluations," which is updated annually.

Conclusion

The judicious use of drugs requires the physician not only to take the therapeutic effects of the drugs into consideration, but also to consider the potential for the development of adverse effects, to recognize and manage drug interactions and adverse effects, and to understand the costs of therapy. An understanding of some basic principles and the application of general guidelines as outlined above will aid the physician in the safe and effective use of medications.

References and Selected Readings

1. Assem E-SK: Drug allergy and tests for its detection, in Davies DM (ed): *Textbook of Adverse Drug Reactions.* New York: Oxford University Press, pp 689–732, 1991.
2. Boyd JR, Covington TR, Stanaszek et al: Drug defaulting. Part I. Determinants of compliance. *Am J Hosp Pharm* 31:362–367, 1974.
3. Hoigne R, Malinverni R, Sonntag R: Sulfonamides, other folic acid antagonists and miscellaneous antibacterial drugs, in Dukes MNG (ed): *Myler's Side Effects of Drugs.* New York: Elsevier, pp 715–725, 1992.
4. Hansten PD, Horn JR, Koda-Kimble MA, Young LY (eds): *Drug Interactions and Updates Quarterly,* vol 13. Vancouver: Applied Therapeutics, 1993.
5. Patterson R: Diagnosis and treatment of drug allergy. *J Allergy Clin Immunol* 81(2):380–384, 1988.
6. VanArsdel PP: Drug reactions: Allergy and near-allergy. *Ann Allergy* 57:305–311, 1986.
7. Witte KW, West DP: Immunology of adverse drug reactions. *Pharmacotherapy* 2:54–65, 1982.

67 Risk Management for Primary Care Physicians

Albert L. Strunk

Most physicians are well aware of the impact malpractice litigation has had on medicine.[1,2] Efforts at tort reform have been piecemeal on the state level and have not substantially alleviated the waste and cost of the present system. Several proposals have been made at the federal level, but none have been passed. A meaningful proposal to address issues of professional liability should be part of a comprehensive program of health care reform.

Larger issues of tort and product liability reform also cost U.S. taxpayers billions of dollars annually and have resulted, for example, in the unavailability of important pharmaceutical agents (e.g., vaccines), the curtailment of athletic programs (e.g., football, soccer), the closing of municipal facilities (e.g., swimming pools), and in some instances the bankruptcy of local government (e.g., multimillion dollar awards to public employees who successfully contended that their injuries were due to negligence by the governmental unit, as in the case of fire fighters, police officers, and sanitation workers).

Despite pressures to decrease the cost of health care, health care providers must find ways to maintain and improve the quality of care they provide while simultaneously improving their ability to defend successfully against the almost inevitable, although often non-meritorious lawsuit(s). Risk management is a tool to assist health care providers in their own defense and to assist patients as well. Risk management has been defined as "a style of practice wherein the physician minimizes the risk of lawsuits by practicing in a manner that reduces the possibility of actual error, ensures the best chance of obtaining desired results in patient care, and presents the most defensible treatment history."[3] While risk management has evolved in response to the malpractice litigation crisis, it is important to remember that the fundamental objective of risk management is quality assurance. The best and most defensible medicine is medical practice of the highest quality. If a patient chooses to assert a claim of negligent practice against her physician there is no mechanism to prevent the filing of the complaint. However, risk management tremendously improves the health care provider's chance of defending successfully against claims.

Risk management as part of the quality assurance process examines conformity to or deviation from accepted standards in the diagnosis and treatment of disease, whether medical or surgical. Physicians have believed historically that accepted medical standards are objectively ascertainable and are readily demonstrable to both professional colleagues and the lay public. Indeed, important aspects of risk management are directed specifically to the actual medical care received by the patient. On the other hand, a significant impetus today for litigation is a discrepancy between the patient's perception of her care and the actual care rendered. An equally important objective of risk management, therefore, is to increase the likelihood that the patient will *perceive* her care to have been good. In the best of all worlds both the actual care received and the patient's perception thereof will be good or excellent. Health care, formerly the practice of medicine, is now a consumer industry. How the health care consumer perceives her treatment is important. Moreover, such emotions as fear and anxiety may significantly color a patient's perception of her care and treatment—most often in a negative manner.

The Health Care Consumer

The patient is interested in several things in her encounter with her physician. First, she wants to have good professional rapport. She hopes her physician will be easy to talk to. She hopes and expects that her physician will be genuinely concerned about her health and welfare. When appropriate, she hopes her physician will be concerned about her family as well. The ability of the physician to engage the patient and project concern for her will likely improve the actual quality of care rendered and will certainly enhance the patient's perception of her care and treatment. Second, the patient wants to have ready access to medical care. Putting aside the issue of whether the individual patient is willing to pay for ready access, even for nonemergent problems, the patient increasingly has the expectation that she should be seen immediately upon calling or nearly so. In other words, the patient wants physicians to be available in sufficient numbers, in sufficient specialties, and in sufficient geographical distribution that she can and will be seen when she wants to be seen. (Notice that, from the patient's perspective, the issue is *not* whether she has a condition for which immediate medical care is required in the judgment of a physician.) Third, the patient is interested in cost of services. The advent of managed care has demonstrated to physicians that economic realities are more compelling than the notion of loyalty to a long-established physician-patient relationship. Fourth, the patient is interested in good care and, as previously noted, this has both a subjective and objective component. Board-certified obstetrician-gynecologists and other primary care physicians are generally well equipped to deal with the objective reality of the patient's medical condition; risk management enhances the physician's sensitivity to the patient's subjective perception of her health care experience as well.

The Physician-Patient Relationship

While it is essential to the physician-patient relationship that adequate time be available for each patient encounter, and while physician time with the patient has often been held out as a measurement of the quality of physician-patient interaction, it must be recognized that demands for greater efficiency in the delivery of health care may necessitate some curtailment of the physician component of the patient encounter. In other words, the patient will continue to seek a concerned physician who is easy to talk to, but it does not follow that the patient will be unwilling to accept the increasing involvement of certified nurse practitioners, midwives, physician's assistants, graduate nurses, and other paramedical personnel. If the use of such personnel enhances her access to the office, increases the quality of the history-taking and documentation of the office encounter, facilitates her diagnosis, speeds her treatment, meets or exceeds accepted standards of practice, and incurs less cost, the patient will in most cases feel that she has received excellent care and good value, even though her actual time with the physician may be less. The important thing is to avoid unnecessary delays in seeing the patient, to schedule in such a way as to minimize the impact of unexpected events on the physician's on-time availability in the office, and to be focused mentally and emotionally on the patient and her problems during the time available for direct physician-patient interaction.

Risk Management—A Team Effort

In order for such a schema to function effectively the physician, paramedical personnel, and office staff must function as an integrated team. All personnel must understand their respective roles and responsibilities if delivery of the highest quality care is to be achieved. To that end, duties and responsibilities must be delegated according to ability and must be well understood by all team members. Not infrequently, a lawsuit will arise because of an insensitive and uncaring act or remark by a staff member. Conversely, a well-trained team can handle unexpected events with care and concern, can detect complications, and can prevent injury.

Communication

The patient's initial encounter with the physician's office usually is by telephone. Effective risk management requires a review of procedures for handling telephone and written inquiries, the welcoming and integrating of new patients, and the scheduling of all patients whether established or new. Unfortunately, the telephone presents a significant liability risk because of the danger of misunderstanding and miscommunication. Telephone conversations should be clearly documented, and written notes and letters should be included in the patient's record, all in chronological order. Often telephone answering services maintain computerized logs of after-hour calls that can be used to ensure the completeness of records of patients who call during nonoffice hours.

Effective procedures for dealing with emergency situations must be in place. Patients should know what to do if telephone communications are temporarily interrupted. Likewise, coverage arrangements with other physicians must be clearly communicated to all patients.

Common sense dictates, when the physician is called away unexpectedly, that patients be told the reason for the delay beyond the blank statement that "the doctor has been called out." Some sense of the urgency or gravity of the situation must be conveyed if the patient is to understand and accept the notion that another patient's circumstance has a higher claim on the doctor's availability. Remember, the patient sees her time as no less valuable than your own.

Finally, though it may seem a small point, the office area where patients are received should be referred to as the "reception room," not the "waiting room." The latter connotes unnecessary delay and poor scheduling practices—factors that increase patient frustration, anxiety, and fear. Always ask yourself: Were I the patient, would I be pleased with the manner in which I was received in this office?

Medical Records

A good medical record will reflect not only the history of the present illness, but the medical, surgical, family, and social history as well. Checklists and patient-history forms are useful adjuncts and expedite the history-taking process. They may be utilized by a staff member, but at some point the physician must review the material and ask additional questions where indicated. The medical record is vital in documenting and defending the physician's diagnosis and treatment. Good records suggest good care; poor records suggest poor care and may necessitate the settlement of an otherwise defensible case.

Never alter the medical record. If an error is made, draw a single line through the entry, date and sign in the margin, and write the corrected entry after the last entry with an explanation of the error. An altered medical record will immediately convert a potentially defensible case into one which is difficult to defend. It is possible to defend a case with a less-than-optimal record; it usually is extremely difficult to defend even an otherwise nonmeritorious case once the record has been altered.

As to billing and financial records, keep these separate from the main chart. When patients or physicians request records, send only copies. Always retain originals. Obtain written authorizations for release of confidential information and, if there is uncertainty as to whether the patient understands the nature of the confidential information to be released, contact the patient before doing so, notwithstanding the previous written release.

Informed Consent

While informed consent has traditionally been more associated with hospital-based diagnostic and surgical procedures, primary care physicians are performing an increasing array of procedures in the office. Informed consent is often said to be a process rather than a form. In other words, the legal standard envisions that a patient will be educated about the specifics of her condition, the option(s) for treating the condition, risks and benefits of the various methods of treatment, and the reasons for her physician's recommendation of a specific medical or surgical approach. The law further requires that all this be done at a level the patients can understand. Moreover, an increasing number of jurisdictions are replacing the "reasonable physician standard" (what a reasonable physician would have told the patient) with the "materiality" or "patient viewpoint" standard (what a reasonable person in the patient's position would want to know under similar circumstances).

While it is true that failure to comply with the technicalities of an appropriate informed consent is not a frequent basis for recovery of an award in emergency circumstances, this is not true for elective procedures. In emergencies, juries simply do not believe a patient's contention that she would not have consented to emergency, often life-saving treatment. On the other hand, a large number of surgical procedures are elective. Diagnostic procedures are usually elective. Elective procedures require that the patient receive and understand the information necessary to make a fully informed decision about her treatment.

Unrealistic Expectations

Most patients have little understanding of the pathophysiology of the disease or condition that leads them to seek medical attention. Most healthy pregnant patients, for example, have a very limited concept of the risks of pregnancy. Physicians have an important task in educating patients about the realities of medical care and medical terminology. While physicians certainly should not exaggerate the risk of a particular disease or condition to the patient, neither should they minimize its seriousness or the risks and complications of treatments and surgical procedures. Physicians may contribute to a patient's unrealistic belief about her condition or about the result of medical or surgical intervention. Patients must understand that perfect outcomes cannot be guaranteed and that poor outcome despite good quality care is an inescapable reality for some conditions. Making the patient aware of the risks inherent in the presenting condition as well as the risks of treatment or nontreatment will minimize patient surprise and disappointment. Audiovisual aids, printed materials, and paramedical personnel may be employed to facilitate these educational goals and thereby to reduce the likelihood of litigation arising from failed expectations, surprise, and disappointment.

Conclusion

This chapter has discussed in a broad fashion some of the principal elements in an effective program of risk management. However, the implementation of such a program requires detailed examination of the specifics of a medical practice.[4] One must critically evaluate such things as telephone communications, appointments and scheduling, patient relations, billing and collections, equipment and drugs, personnel management, and medical records—to name just a few.

As emphasis on primary care increases and as managed care brings change to established physician-patient relationships, health care providers must remain alert to issues of professional liability. The concept that higher quality health care can be rendered to more citizens with increased efficiency at less cost remains untested in the marketplace of health care consumerism. No corresponding change is seen or anticipated in a tort system sorely in need of reform. Risk management reduces the possibility of actual error in medical diagnosis and treatment, optimizes desired results in patient care, and presents the most defensible treatment history in the unfortunate event of litigation. As such, risk management is a concept that commends itself to all physicians, but especially to those in the forefront of health care delivery, the primary care physicians.

References and Selected Readings

1. *Professional Liability and Its Effects:* Report of a 1992 Survey of ACOG's Membership, Washington, American College of Obstetricians and Gynecologists, 1992.
2. *Premium Ranges for Professional Liability Insurance for Ob-Gyns.* Telephone survey conducted by Department of Professional Liability Staff, Washington, American College of Obstetricians and Gynecologists, 1991.
3. The Assistant, Department of Professional Liability, American College of Obstetricians and Gynecologists. Washington: July, 1988.
4. Publications of The Department of Professional Liability, Washington, American College of Obstetricians and Gynecologists.

68 Ethics

Kenneth J. Ryan

The practice of medicine is a thoroughgoing ethical enterprise, with the physician having privileged access to intimate details of patients' lives and making judgments and taking actions that can significantly affect their present and future well-being. If anything, this is more true of primary care than of other branches of medicine, because primary care is concerned with all aspects of a patient's health in continuity over a lifetime. The primary care physician functions not only by the direct provision of medical care but also as a gatekeeper for referral to other medical or health services, as an educator, a confidante, and a facilitator in matters related to the patient's medical and health needs.

The purpose in the last quarter of the 20th century of a new emphasis on medical ethics in medical school education and in practice has been to make sure that physicians recognize the ethical problems that modern society poses for medicine and the problems that advances in medical science and technology pose for society. Once an aspect of medical care is recognized as an ethical problem, the challenge for the physician is to know how to reason about and deal with it so that ''right'' choices are made.

The Hippocratic Oath; Ethical Theories, Principles, and Reason

The Hippocratic oath and writings have been universal guides over the years for generally defining a physician's duties and the ethical practice of medicine. Such admonitions as to help one's patients if possible and at least not harm them, to maintain confidentiality, to treat first and worry about the fee later, and not to take advantage of patients are all timeless exhortations to the good doctor's conscience. Adherence to many but not all of the Hippocratic maxims remains necessary, but is not sufficient to practice medicine today. The modern world has a different view of the rights of individuals and of civil and women's rights, of physician's obligations, and of the limitations of the physician's authority than that reflected in the Hippocratic corpus.

Modern bioethics started in the 1960s in the United States, in the aftermath of the Holocaust and the Nuremberg code, and the failure of medical ethics to protect human subjects of medical research from harm or exploitation, even in the post-World War II era. Advances in medical technology, organ transplantation, and life-support systems and the public disputes over abortion all contributed to the interest in and expansion of medical ethics.

As a ''foundation'' for bioethics, several theories have been invoked, such as a Kantian respect for universal rules of conduct, or a John Millsian utilitarianism that bases ethics on the greatest good for the greatest number. These two theories contrast the outcome of any medical action versus the method used in achieving it. Ethical principles also have been promulgated that define ethical medicine in terms of respect for patients' rights and autonomy, or beneficent goals and outcomes for patients, and of seeking justice and fairness in the distribution of and access to medical benefits. The problem in the application of all these principles and theories in the real world is that they very often conflict. One has to make decisions when the choices cannot easily be pigeonholed into unambiguous "right" or "wrong." Decision-making then depends on experience and wisdom and sometimes compromise. In actual practice, we have to look at the ethical significance of both the outcomes and the means of our actions, and we need appropriate and convincing reasons for our choices. We all know that some reasons are better than others; to function well, we must justify our actions and decisions to our patients, to our colleagues, and to the larger community in which we live. There is also an inevitable ethical tension between the physician's obligation to the patient and the obligation with respect to resource allocation in society at large.

There are three general areas of medical practice where the new medical ethics has had a significant influence on the way physicians function: 1. The art of medicine has become more patient-oriented, and the physician-patient interaction has been redefined. 2. The goals of medicine have been recast in keeping with the changed social uses of medicine. 3. The science of medicine has set new standards by which to judge physician competence. Each of these will be considered in turn.

Ethics of the Art of Medicine

The relationship between physicians and patients used to depend largely on the good intentions of the physician and the willingness of the patient to listen to the doctor and do as he or she was told. This essentially parent-child balance of power favored the physician on the basis of his or her social privilege and superior knowledge. Patients, according to the prevailing social theory, were to play the "sick role." In the 1960s there was a change in the relationship of the public to such institutions as government and medicine. Discontent with the course of the Vietnam war and concern over minority and women's rights brought challenge to the old ways of doing business. For physicians, the challenge was to provide truthful and complete disclosure to their patients.

In the past physicians sometimes withheld information from their patients for the patients' "own good" and might not tell them if they had cancer or a fatal illness. Physicians might offer patients only one course of action to combat a disease and might not discuss other options and their consequences, including sometimes the value of no treatment at all. Patients might be used in research or for the education of medical or nursing students without their knowledge or consent. Physicians have at times had financial interests in laboratories or imaging centers and have referred patients preferentially and sometimes excessively to these medical businesses from which they directly profited. Most of these practices are now seen as unethical or at least ethically problematic.

Older physicians have had to change their ways, and younger physicians who came of age in the 1960s and later grew into an environment that naturally accepted the need to respect patients' rights and what that need entails. The Patient Bill of Rights of the American Hospital Association codified many of these changes in physician and hospital duties; while old ways die hard, patients are more apt today to insist on full disclosure and truth-telling. This is especially true in the case of women's health care, where, for example, women have insisted on more treatment options for breast cancer. Women now want more choice in medical care that affects their reproductive functions; they do not wish to be held captive to "male" perceptions of what is best, whether suggested by their physician, father, or spouse.

Research on women's medical problems has been systematically ignored or assumed to be the same as for men by the medical research community. Usually the possibility of pregnancy has excluded women from research studies because of fear of harm to the fetus or fear of litigation. For example, while men were studied for ways to avoid heart attacks and to deal with aging, women were simply ignored. This has made women medical orphans when it comes to dealing with illnesses during pregnancy, problems associated with the menstrual cycle, or where female physiology differs markedly from male. Fortunately, in the 1990s this pattern has been reversed. There is now a positive obligation by the Food and Drug Administration and federally funded medical research to involve reproductive-age and pregnant women in research on problems relevant to women's medical and health needs. From an ethical perspective, justice is now being served.

Ethics of the Goals and Social Role of Medicine

Of the innumerable ways society influences and uses medicine, several are worth consideration in a chapter on the ethics of primary care of women. These include those that are concerned with reproductive function, parenting, contraception, and abortion; rationing of and access to health care; dealing with terminal illness, euthanasia, and assisted suicide; and abuse and rape.

Reproductive Function

Over most of time, biology for women has been destiny, and social pressures have required them to do what nature supposedly "intended"—to reproduce and mother. Anything that medicine could do to further these goals was generally acceptable, and it was often considered wrong for medicine to frustrate them. Infertility services and midwifery or obstetrics were accepted; contraception and abortion generally were discouraged. As civilization advanced, a religious divide cast the issue in absolute terms. Starting with St. Augustine (for Catholics predominantly but not exclusively), the reproductive function was sanctified in marriage and natural coitus, and the fetus from conception came to have an inviolable right to life. This limits practicing Catholics to abstinence from sex and to the rhythm method for contraception; it simply prohibits abortion and the new assisted reproductive technologies such as in vitro fertilization. Others in society take a more naturalistic view of the reproductive process and have embraced the freedom from biological tyranny that contraception and abortion as well as assisted reproduction for the infertile have provided. Since abortion was legalized in the United States in 1973 by the Supreme Court *Roe* v. *Wade* decision, the ethical debate has been divisive and strident. On the other hand, most in our society accept contraception and some forms of assisted reproduction without much dissent. From an ethical perspective, it is my judgment that both sides to the abortion debate can adequately defend their positions depending on their religious beliefs in what God intended or requires. It is a true but rare instance of relativism in which both sides are correct for themselves—but they live in separate worlds. There may be excessive rhetoric on both sides, but it is not useful or correct to vilify either position.

The ethical responsibility of physicians is to be clear in their own minds how they view these issues and then to be straightforward and fair to their patients when they seek advice or services in this area. It would be a duty of physicians to explain to the patient the extent to which their own views on the matter influence the service or advice they provide. This is equally true with respect to questions about sexual orientation and life-style. No one expects physicians to perform abortions or give advice about sexual matters if they are morally opposed to them or are ignorant of such matters. Most would expect physicians to be consistent, to make their positions clear to the patient, and to refer as necessary.

With assisted reproduction, there are many social questions about who should parent; but, in reality, these cannot be much different from what pertains without medical assistance, except that by definition the assisted pregnancy usually is intended and wanted. Without going into all of the details of the issues raised by single parenting and same-sex rearing parents, gamete donation, and surrogacy, I have a simple test for the ethical acceptability of infertility services and reproductive assistance. If the child is wanted and can be adequately cared for, and if no one (including any party to the process and the expected child) is exploited in the process, there should be a general presumption of moral acceptability. It is sad but true that most naturally occurring pregnancies cannot meet this simple moral test.

Rationing

There will be an expectation by society that the primary care physician under health care reform and managed care will be the agent of conserving resources and limiting inappropriate use of medical services. There is a belief by many that this is possible without denying needed care or jeopardizing the quality of care. Many believe that there is even an ethical mandate to perform this husbanding of resources in order to provide adequate care for all. Nonetheless, there will be an ethical tension between the patient's needs and wants and the limits society chooses to place on physicians. Where this has been tried, contraception, abortion, and pregnancy services usually have been included as being cost-effective, while many forms of infertility services have been denied. It has even been claimed that infertility is not an illness—but nothing could be further from the truth. It is important that the physician not underestimate the incapacity, hurt, and need that infertility creates in patients and advocate for them where justified in order to obtain help for those who have no children.

There are of course many ethical questions about the process of rationing itself and whether those who can afford it should be allowed to purchase health services not available to others. The underlying assumption on the need for rationing is that in any society there are finite resources and that people will differ in how they might value and distribute them. It is expected, however, that a fair health care system will provide all citizens with a decent level of essential health services and that, in a free society, it should be possible and ethical to purchase additional health services as long as the basic needs of all are met.

Terminal Illness and Euthanasia

There may have been a time when one of the goals of medicine was to preserve life at all costs, but that position is no longer tenable. The goal society seems to have for medicine today is to provide relief from pain and suffering and not to prolong life by delaying death. The advent of the respirator and other life-support technologies has allowed preservation of vegetative life or the postponement of death, neither of which is highly prized by most patients. The change in public attitude evolved over time as various cases proceeded through the courts. In the case of Karen Ann Quinlan, the courts allowed the withdrawal of a respirator from a young woman who had been in a prolonged coma. Ironically, she continued to live for another 10 years. In the case of Brophy, it was a question of withdrawing food and fluid from a man in a persistent vegetative state. Finally, in the case of Cruzan, the United States Supreme Court ruled that an individual had the right to have their preferences with respect to life-support honored. Each of these cases was fought against by those who felt that life was sacred and should always be protected and maintained. Society, however, seems to accept the position that it is ethically permissible to give patients or their proxies a choice in the matter.

The advanced directive and living will are devices now being used to allow patients to indicate their preferences on how to be treated if faced with terminal illness. Patient preferences are generally accepted by the courts, and may be required by some courts before therapy is withdrawn. It is the responsibility of the physician—and especially the primary care physician—to determine the patient's preference and to honor them when she can no longer speak for herself. If physicians have a moral basis for disagreement, they should discuss this beforehand with the patient. When patients are referred to intensive care or coronary units, they very often lose all connections to their primary care doctor, and their preferences may be ignored unless forceful representation is made on their behalf. The same is true for cardiopulmonary resuscitation, which was designed to treat sudden *unexpected* cardiac arrest. It was not designed nor is it appropriate for everyone in the hospital whose heart stops beating.

The Netherlands has tolerated euthanasia by physicians for some time. From the ethical perspective, one is pitting an individual's need for relief of suffering against the abhorrence many feel toward kill-ing, and also to the fear that the process could easily be abused. It is further argued that generally one can provide relief of pain and suffering by adequate care and medication and that good hospice services obviate the need for euthanasia. It has been my judgment that our society and the medical profession will need a long time to discuss the need, objectives, and risks of euthanasia before considering its legalization. The same is true for assisted suicide, which accomplishes the same goal but makes the patient the active participant. This issue is particularly important to primary care physicians who take care of women. Women are susceptible to depression that might not be readily recognized and that could masquerade as a justifiable despondency. Such a patient might better be treated than done in. In cases where continued living is unbearably painful and can be relieved no other way, carefully controlled and documented euthanasia might be morally acceptable; but the case for legalizing should not be made without more study and societal review.

Abuse and Rape

Society has a sorry record in dealing with women's problems with rape and abuse. Male-dominated medicine may have been part of the problem. In the past, it was often assumed that women invited rape by their dress or behavior, which in turn was thought to justify the rape when it occurred. Often, complaining about a rape invited becoming even more of a victim, bringing loss of privacy and questioning about the victim's character and past sexual history by the police and courts. The idea that rape can occur in marriage has only recently been accepted, and "date" rape is an all too frequent occurrence. Rape seems to be part of an overall abuse problem, but physical abuse and murder of women by their husbands or boyfriends has become something of an epidemic in the United States. Just as society depends on pediatricians to alert authorities to child abuse, gynecologists and primary care physicians must fill that role for women. Physicians must be sensitive to the occurrence of abuse and must recognize how dependent the woman often is on her abuser. Seeing her physician may be an important mechanism in seeking help if the physician is prepared to deal with these issues.

Ethics of the Science of Medicine

Patients have a right to expect their physicians to be competent and up-to-date with the latest preventive, diagnostic, and treatment modalities; physicians have an obligation to meet those standards of competency. While much in medicine remains empirical, a good deal is now solidly grounded in carefully controlled randomized clinical trials, metaanalyses, and outcomes research. The challenge to the physician is to remain current with respect to medical knowledge and to integrate this knowledge into everyday practice. For example, the value of periodic health examinations has been reviewed by a Canadian Task Force; a United States Preventive Service task force has looked at the effectiveness of 169 interventions and diagnostic tests. There have been metaanalyses of studies of what constitutes effective care in pregnancy, childbirth, and newborn care. It is clear that the primary care physician should be most knowledgeable about the need for periodic examinations, tests, counseling, and immunizations. While many would recognize this as an essential component of practicing "good" medicine or being a "good" doctor, it should also be recognized as being an essential part of what medical ethics is all about.

References and Selected Readings

1. Evidence-Based Medicine Working Group: Evidence-based medicine. *JAMA* 268:2420, 1992.
2. Jonsen AR: The birth of bioethics. *Hastings Center Report* 23:S1, 1993.
3. Macklin R: Women's health: An ethical perspective. *J Law Med Ethics* 21:23, 1993.
4. Veatch RM (ed): *Medical Ethics*. Boston: Jones & Bartlett, 1989.
5. Wear S: *Informed Consent*. Dordrecht: Kluwer Academic Publishers, 1993.

69 Preventive Ethics

Frank A. Chervenak
Laurence B. McCullough

Preventive health care is an essential dimension of primary health care for women. Preventive ethics is an essential but sometimes overlooked component of preventive health care. Preventive ethics describes a set of clinical skills aimed at developing an excellent physician-patient relationship by emphasizing communication and the prevention of ethical conflicts.[2,5] This chapter describes the basic strategies of preventive ethics that should be mastered by all physicians who provide primary health care for women. These strategies are: 1. informed consent as an ongoing dialogue between the woman and her physician; 2. negotiation; and 3. respectful persuasion. Although the specific example used to illustrate the issues is an obstetric situation, the same basic principles of ethics apply to all patient-physician relationships.

Informed Consent as an Ongoing Dialogue

The informed consent process—undertaken over time and in anticipation of potential ethically conflicting decisions—is the basic strategy of preventive ethics. The goals of informed consent are for the patient to understand the physician's evaluation of her condition and the alternatives for managing her condition, to evaluate those alternatives on the basis of her values, to express her value-based preferences, and to have the benefit of the physician's recommendations.[1,3] These goals can be achieved in the following steps:

1. The physician initiates the process by eliciting from the patient what she believes about her condition, its diagnosis, alternatives available to manage it, and her prognosis under each alternative.
2. The physician corrects factual errors and incompleteness in the patient's fund of knowledge. This does not require that the patient receive a complete medical education.
3. The physician provides and explains his or her clinical judgment about the patient's condition and all available management strategies (including watchful waiting).
4. The physician works with the patient, as needed or requested, to help her to develop as complete as possible a picture of her condition and alternatives available (including watchful waiting).
5. The physician works with the patient, as needed or requested, to help her identify her relevant values.
6. The physician, as needed or requested, helps the patient, in a nondirective fashion, to evaluate her alternatives in terms of those values.

7. The patient undertakes to understand her condition, the available management strategies (including watchful waiting), and their prognoses; she expresses her value-based preferences.
8. The physician makes a recommendation, based on the clinical judgment already explained in Step 3.
9. A mutual decision is reached and implemented.[4,5]

At the present time, informed consent is at risk for becoming a meaningless bureaucratic ritual.[6] The nine steps of informed consent presented here should be seen as a powerful antidote to this disturbing tendency. It should be clear that informed consent is not to be equated with a signed consent form. Such an equation dehumanizes the patient and denigrates the physician-patient relationship.

To be sure, these nine steps sometimes can be time-consuming. However, building and sustaining a meaningful physician-patient relationship, which cannot occur in the absence of a genuine informed consent process, is worth the effort. Moreover, time spent on these nine steps will save time—and stress—involved in addressing ethical conflicts that occur when these nine steps are not followed.

Negotiation

Negotiation as a clinical strategy builds directly on informed consent.[2,5] Indeed, in the absence of ongoing informed consent, this strategy is likely to be much more difficult to implement.

Negotiation involves an ongoing dialogue in which a zero-sum game is not being played. A zero-sum game means that every advantage gained by one party occurs at the expense of or disadvantage to the other party.

Negotiation focuses primarily on the expression of values and then on their implications for shared clinical decision making. This simple step permits agreement on common values and mutual respect for different values. Common grounds between the pregnant woman and physician frequently can be found—something that may never be discovered if the two parties focus only on the conflict between differing decisions and on who will win the conflict. On the basis of this common ground, an atmosphere of good will and mutual respect can be fostered, thereby creating a context that encourages negotiation as a strategy for conflict resolution. An example would be a physician who recommends cesarean section for failure to progress in labor but agrees to extend a trial of continued labor for a specified period on the basis of the shared commitment to a healthy outcome of the pregnancy for both the pregnant woman and the fetus.

Respectful Persuasion

This kind of situation may become more difficult if the woman continues to refuse cesarean delivery after the specified period has elapsed. At this point, or shortly thereafter, obstetricians typically will become very uncomfortable about permitting labor to continue. In this situation, the probability for ethical conflict between the physician and the pregnant woman increases. Respectful persuasion is the appropriate response to such situations in preventive ethics.[2,5] Respectful persuasion involves the physician in the following steps:

1. Remind the woman about previous discussions about general issues that may be applied to the specific issue at hand. Ideally these should have occurred as a part of the ongoing informed consent process and prior negotiation.
2. Explain one's reasoning for taking the position.
3. Explain how other physicians may disagree.
4. Explain how one meets these objectives.
5. Show how the patient's values, including values she should reasonably adopt, support the recommendation.
6. Urge the patient to reconsider.

Identifying these elements of persuasion enables us to draw the ethically significant distinction between respectful persuasion and disrespectful persuasion. If any one or more of conditions 2 through

5 are not satisfied, the physician is engaging in disrespectful persuasion.

Advantages of Preventive Ethics

There are a number of important advantages to the preventive ethics approach to primary health care for women.

First, the primary focus of preventive ethics is on underlying values of both physician and patient, rather than specific decisions. There is a greater likelihood of discovering areas of commonality and negotiating disagreements if values are the starting point of the informed consent process rather than specific decisions.

Second, this approach reduces the emotional stress and ethical risks of decision-making in emergent situations wherein the woman is at risk for experiencing all at once the unexpected burdens of complicated clinical decisions. Complex matters require time and reflection if they are to be managed successfully and are therefore at high risk for being badly managed in a rush.

Third, preventive ethics focuses the patient-physician relationship on underlying matters of deep significance to both. It thus furthers the aim of humanizing the primary health care of women by avoiding the steering of women's choices under a false banner of respect for autonomy. This can occur, for example, when the physician offers cesarean delivery as a valid alternative when it is not indicated. Respect for autonomy does not create a positive obligation on the physician's part to perform risky medical and surgical procedures that are not indicated.

Fourth, like all primary care strategies, it is hoped that preventive ethics in the primary care of women will reduce the incidence of ethical conflicts and of unresolved ethical conflicts.

Finally, a preventive ethics approach will enhance the opportunity for the early detection of irreconcilable value-based differences between a particular woman and a particular physician. In these cases, the physician will have ample time and opportunity to help the woman find a physician whose values are more compatible with her own and to arrange for the transfer of her care with a minimum of bad feelings and a maximum of mutual respect if she decides to choose another physician.

References and Selected Readings

1. The American College of Obstetricians and Gynecologists: *Ethical Dimensions of Informed Consent (ACOG Committee Opinion 108)*. Washington, 1992.
2. Chervenak FA, McCullough LB: Clinical guides to preventing ethical conflicts between pregnant women and their physicians. *Am J Obstet Gynecol* 162:303–307, 1990.
3. Faden R, Beauchamp TL: *History and Theory of Informed Consent*. New York: Oxford University Press, 1986.
4. McCullough LB: An ethical model for improving the physician-patient relationship. *Inquiry* 25:454–465, 1988.
5. McCullough LB, Chervenak FA: *Ethics in Obstetrics and Gynecology*. New York: Oxford University Press, 1994.
6. Wear S: *Informed Consent: Patient Autonomy and Physician-Beneficence Within Clinical Medicine*. Dordrecht: Kluwer Academic Publishing, 1992.

Index

NOTE: Page numbers followed by a *t* indicate a reference to a table; those in italic indicate a reference to a figure.

ISBN 0-07-056225-3

90000>

9 780070 562257